EOC episode-of-care reimbursement
EPA Equal Pay Act of 1963
EPO exclusive provider organization
ERA electronic remittance advice
ERD entity relationship diagram
FASB Financial Accounting Standards Board
FDA Food and Drug Administration
FECA Federal Employees' Compensation Act
FEP Blue Cross and Blue Shield Federal Employee Program
FI fiscal intermediary
FLSA Fair Labor Standards Act of 1938
FOIA Freedom of Information Act
FPL federal poverty level
GAF geographic adjustment factor
GASB Government Accounting Standards Board
GIS geographic information system
GPCI geographic practice cost index
GPWW group practice without walls
GUI graphical user interface
HAVEN Home Assessment Validation and Entry
HCFA Health Care Financing Administration
HCPCS Healthcare Common Procedure Coding System
HCUP Healthcare Cost and Utilization Project
HEDIS® Health Plan Employer Data and Information Set
HH PPS home health prospective payment system
HHA home health agency
HHRG home health resource group
HHS Department of Health and Human Services
HI hospitalization insurance (Medicare Part A)
HIBCC Health Industry Business Communications Council
HIM health information management
HIMSS Health Information Management and Systems Society
HIPAA Health Insurance Portability and Accountability Act of 1996
HIPDB Healthcare Integrity and Protection Data Bank
HIS hospital information system

HISB Health Informatics Standards Board
HL7 Health Level Seven
HMIS health management information system
HMO health maintenance organization
HOLAP hybrid online analytical processing
HRSA Health Resources and Services Administration
ICD-9-CM International Classification of Diseases, Ninth Revision, Clinical Modification
ICR intelligent character recognition technology
IDS integrated delivery system
IEEE Institute of Electrical and Electronics Engineers
IHS Indian Health Service
IPA independent practice association
IPO integrated provider organization
IPS interim payment system
IRB Institutional review board
IRF inpatient rehabilitation facility
IRR internal rate of return
IRVEN Inpatient Rehabilitation Validation and Entry
IS information system
ISO United Nations International Standards Organization
ISS Injury Severity Score
IT information technology
JCAHO Joint Commission on Accreditation of Healthcare Organizations
K-NN k-nearest neighbor
LOS length of stay
LPC Least Preferred Coworker Scale
LUPA low-utilization payment adjustment
MBO management by objectives
MCO managed care organization
MDDBMS multidimensional database management system
MDS 2.0 Minimum Data Set for Long Term Care, Version 2.0
MDS-PAC Minimum Data Set for Post Acute Care
MEDIX Medical Data Interchange Standard

Health Information Management

Concepts, Principles, and Practice

Kathleen M. LaTour, MA, RHIA,
and Shirley Eichenwald, MBA, RHIA, CPHIMS
Editors

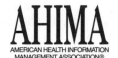

AHIMA

AMERICAN HEALTH INFORMATION
MANAGEMENT ASSOCIATION®

ISBN 1-58426-100-5
AHIMA Product Number AB103302

AHIMA Staff:
    Marcia Bottoms, Acquisitions Editor and Director of Publications
    Carol Brockman, Project Editor, Instructor's Guide
    Jill Burrington-Brown, MS, RHIA, Content Reviewer
    Michelle L. Dougherty, RHIA, Content Reviewer
    Sue Fiorio, Cover Designer
    Sandra Fuller, MA, RHIA, Content Reviewer
    Beth Hjort, RHIA, Content Reviewer
    Gwen Hughes, RHIA, Content Reviewer
    Katherine Kerpan, Project Editor, Textbook
    Linda L. Kloss, RHIA, CAE, Author of the Foreword
    Harry Rhodes, MBA, RHIA, Content Reviewer
    Dan Rode, MBA, FHFMA, Content Reviewer
    Rita A. Scichilone, MHSA, RHIA, CCS, CCS-P, CHC, Content Reviewer
    Jennifer Solheim, Assistant Editor
    Julia Wixtrom, Production Manager

American Health Information Management Association
233 North Michigan Avenue, Suite 2150
Chicago, Illinois 60601-5800

http://www.ahima.org

Contents

About the Editors and Authors

Kathleen M. LaTour, MA, RHIA, is an assistant professor and the chair of the department of health information management (HIM) at the College of St. Scholastica in Duluth, Minnesota. She is an active member of the Minnesota Health Information Management Association, where she was selected as the Distinguished Member in 1992. She has served as chair and member of many AHIMA councils and as a member of AHIMA's Board of Directors from 1993 to 1997. She participated in the development of the AHIMA Model Curricula for both bachelor's and master's level programs. She has authored several articles and recently contributed a chapter to *Health Information Management Technology: An Applied Approach,* a textbook published by AHIMA in 2001.

Shirley Eichenwald Maki, MBA, RHIA, CPHIMS, is an assistant professor and the coordinator of the healthcare informatics and information management graduate programs at the College of St. Scholastica in Duluth, Minnesota. Shirley has been an HIM professional and educator for over thirty years. She is the 2001 recipient of the College of St. Scholastica's Max H. Lavine Award for Teaching Excellence. She is a former president of AHIMA and the recipient of AHIMA's Distinguished Member Award in 1998. Shirley co-authored with Merida Johns, PhD, RHIA, AHIMA's White Paper on the Health and Well-being of HIM Education. She has held the position of director of education and accreditation at AHIMA and has served as an HIM consultant with Pyramid Health Solutions and Quadramed's HIM Division.

Margret Amatayakul, MBA, RHIA, FHIMSS, is the president of Margret\A Consulting, LLC, in Schaumburg, Illinois, a health information management and systems consulting firm specializing in computer-based patient records and associated standards and regulations, such as HIPAA. She has over thirty years of experience as an HIM professional, including having

formed and served as the executive director of the Computer-based Patient Record Institute (CPRI). Other positions held by Ms. Amatayakul include associate executive director of AHIMA, associate professor at the University of Illinois, and director of medical record services at the Illinois Eye and Ear Infirmary.

Elizabeth Bowman, MPA, RHIA, is a professor in the HIM program at the University of Tennessee Health Science Center in Memphis. Elizabeth has been an HIM educator for more than twenty-five years. She received her bachelor's degree from Millsaps College and her master's degree in public administration with a concentration in healthcare administration from the University of Memphis. She has served as the chair of the AHIMA Assembly on Education and received the AHIMA Educator Award in 1999. She was also awarded the Tennessee Health Information Management Association's Distinguished Member Award in 1998.

Bonnie S. Cassidy, MPA, FAHIMA, FHIMSS, is a principal consultant with the North Highland Company in Atlanta, Georgia. She received her bachelor of science degree in medical record administration from Daemen College in Amherst, New York, and her master's degree from Cleveland State University. Her achievements include the AHIMA 2000 Legacy Award, AHIMA's 1995 Professional Achievement Award, and the Distinguished Member Award from the Ohio Health Information Management Association (OHIMA). Bonnie is a former president of OHIMA. She has served AHIMA in numerous volunteer roles including chair of the Nominating and Professional Development committees, is currently a member of the E-Health Task Force, and is a frequent author in the *Journal of AHIMA* and popular presenter at AHIMA educational sessions and national conventions. Ms. Cassidy's career has included working as an educator for two major teaching hospitals and as a healthcare consultant for three professional services companies.

Nadinia Davis, MBA, CIA, CPA, RHIA, is an assistant professor of HIM at the College of Natural, Applied, and Health Sciences at Kean University in Union, New Jersey. She has worked as a coding consultant and auditor in acute settings and as a director of medical records at a rehabilitation institute. Prior to her HIM career, Nadinia worked in the financial services industry, most recently as an internal auditor. Nadinia is a former president and Distinguished Member of NJHIMA and a former member of the AHIMA Board of Directors. She is the co-author of *Introduction to Health Information Technology* and a contributor to *Effective Management of Coding Services.*

Mehnaz Farishta, MS, is the manager for marketing and communications at The Shams Group, Inc. (TSG), an award-winning knowledge management IT software and consulting company in the health information systems marketplace. Ms. Farishta has authored and co-authored several articles on the role of information technology in healthcare, especially in the areas of data warehousing, patient safety, and process automation. These articles have been published in noted healthcare publications, including *Journal of AHIMA* and *Topics in Health Information Management.* Prior to joining TSG, Ms. Farishta worked as an insurance analyst and consultant.

Susan H. Fenton, MBA, RHIA, is an adjunct instructor in the HIM graduate program at the College of St. Scholastica in Duluth, Minnesota. She is also a consultant to the medical informatics department at Scott and White Memorial Hospital in Temple, Texas. Prior to her current roles, Susan worked in medical information systems at the Mayo Clinic in Rochester, Minnesota, and was the national health information manager for the Veterans Health Administration in Washington, D.C. She has authored numerous articles and several book chapters.

Sandra R. Fuller, MA, RHIA, is the senior vice-president of professional development services and chief operating officer at AHIMA. Ms. Fuller's responsibilities include oversight of the *Journal of AHIMA* and the *In Confidence* newsletter, the development of HIM practice tools, the development and implementation of AHIMA House of Delegates resolutions and association position statements, the annual convention, continuing education and training, AHIMA's Web development, and online campus. She also serves as the association's point person on compliance issues related to the administrative simplification and information security provisions of the Health Insurance Accountability and Portability Act. Formerly director of patient data services at the University of Washington Medical Center in Seattle, Washington, Ms. Fuller completed her term as a member of AHIMA's Board of Directors at the end of 1996. She also served on AHIMA's Council on Education and its Alliance and Program committees. Ms. Fuller is a former president of the Washington State Health Information Management Association. She received both her master's degree in management and her bachelor's degree in HIM from the College of St. Scholastica in Duluth, Minnesota.

Michelle A. Green, MPS, RHIA, CMA, is a professor at Alfred State College in Alfred, New York. She received the State University of New York Chancellor's Award for Excellence in Teaching in 2000 and was included on the 1994, 1998, and 2000 lists of Who's Who among American Teachers. Mrs. Green thanks her husband and son "for understanding that being a teacher is what I am, not what I do."

J. Michael Hardin, PhD, is professor of statistics in the department of information systems, statistics, and management science at the University of Alabama in Tuscaloosa. He is also adjunct professor of health informatics in the Department of Health Services Administration at the University of Alabama at Birmingham (UAB). Prior to these positions, Dr. Hardin served for thirteen years as professor of health informatics, biostatistics, computer science, and preventive medicine at UAB and was selected as scholar in residence at Loyola University of Chicago. Additionally, he has been a visiting scholar at Trinity College, University of Dublin. He is a frequent speaker at AHIMA national meetings in the areas of database design, data modeling, and data mining. He has given over thirty presentations on various topics related to data mining and data warehousing and has taught decision support in health informatics for the past seven years. He has authored or co-authored over ninety publications and has served as a consultant to several major companies in the area of Medicare program integrity and utilization review.

Laurinda B. Harman, PhD, RHIA, is associate professor and chair of the department of health information management at the College of Allied Health Professions at Temple University in Philadelphia. She has been an HIM professional and educator for over thirty years and has directed HIM baccalaureate programs at George Washington University in Washington, D.C., and The Ohio State University in Columbus. She also served as director of education and human resource development at George Washington University and as a faculty member in the health information technology program at Northern Virginia Community College. Recently, she served as the editor of *Ethical Challenges in the Management of Health Information* and received the AHIMA 2001 Triumph Legacy Award for this important health information resource.

Linda L. Kloss, RHIA, CAE, is AHIMA's executive vice-president and chief executive officer, a position she has held since 1995. Before joining the AHIMA staff, Ms. Kloss served from 1976 to 1995 as a senior manager for Massachusetts-based MediQual Systems, Inc., and Chicago-based InterQual, Inc., where she participated in the design of computer-based tools for healthcare outcomes evaluation and consulted and lectured widely on quality improvement concepts and methods. Ms. Kloss has also held academic and HIM practice positions in Minneapolis and San Francisco. Ms. Kloss served on the AHIMA Board of Directors from 1980 to 1986 and was president in 1985. In addition to AHIMA, Ms. Kloss has served on the boards of directors for several not-for-profit organizations in healthcare and higher education. Her bachelor's degree in medical record science is from the College of St. Scholastica in Duluth, Minnesota. She obtained a master of arts in organizational development with a concentration in change leadership from DePaul University in Chicago.

Deborah Kohn, MPH, RHIA, CHE, CPHIMS, FHIMSS, is the principal consultant at Dak Systems Consulting in San Mateo, California, a national healthcare information technology advisory consultancy specializing in the analysis, planning, and design of electronic patient record component technologies and systems. Deborah has over twenty years of experience in healthcare management and information systems. She holds an undergraduate degree from The Ohio State University at Columbus and a graduate degree from UCLA in health services and hospital administration. She is certified in healthcare information and management systems and is a fellow of the Healthcare Information Management Systems Society. She is board certified in healthcare management and a diplomate of the American College of Healthcare Executives. She is an active member of AHIMA and the Association for Information and Image Management International (AIIM). In 1995, AHIMA awarded Ms. Kohn its prestigious Computer-based Patient Record Advancement Award for her efforts in promoting and implementing components of computer-based patient record systems. Ms. Kohn is also a recipient of AIIM's Master and Laureate of Information Technology designations, which recognize achievement in the area of document and Web content management.

Elizabeth Layman, PhD, RHIA, CCS, FAHIMA, is professor and chair of the department of health services and information management in the School of Allied Health Sciences at East Carolina University, Greenville, North Carolina. Between 1974 and 1990, she worked at Hennepin County Medical Center and the University of Minnesota Hospitals, Minneapolis, Minnesota, in such areas as third-party reimbursement, credit and collections, account auditing, outpatient registration, inpatient admissions, research studies, and quality management. Also during this time, she earned her associate's degree in medical record technology and her post-baccalaureate certificate in health information administration. In 1990, after obtaining a master's degree in organizational leadership, she joined the faculty of the Medical College of Georgia in Augusta, Georgia. In 1996, after earning her doctorate in higher education, she became the director of the HIM program at East Carolina University.

Madonna LeBlanc, MA, RHIA, is an assistant professor in the health informatics and information management program at the College of St. Scholastica in Duluth, Minnesota. Prior to her teaching role, Madonna managed health information services at St. Mary's/Duluth Clinic Health System in Superior, Wisconsin. Her responsibilities included a broad spectrum of acute care HIM functions, from physician education to JCAHO survey coordination. Her field experience also includes cancer registry and physician peer administration. Madonna is a graduate of the College of St. Scholastica's master of arts program in health information management.

Frances Wickham Lee, DBA, is an associate professor in the department of health information administration and policy at the Medical University of South Carolina. She received her master of business administration degree from Western Carolina University and her doctorate in business administration from the University of Sarasota. She is an active member of AHIMA and won a Distinguished Member Award from the Mental Health Section of AHIMA in 1995.

Mary Cole McCain, MPA, RHIA, is professor of health information management and chair of the health information management department at the University of Tennessee Health Science Center in Memphis. She has held this position since 1973. She also serves as assistant dean in the College of Allied Health Sciences. She served as chair of AHIMA's Assembly on Education and co-chaired the Model Curriculum Project for AHIMA. She is a recipient of the Tennessee Health Information Management Association's Distinguished Member Award.

Carol E. Osborn, PhD, RHIA, is the assistant director of coding and compliance at The Ohio State University Medical Center in Columbus. Ms. Osborn has been an HIM professional for over thirty years and is a former faculty member at both the University of Illinois at Chicago and The Ohio State University. Ms. Osborn has served AHIMA at both the state and national levels—she has participated as state president of AHIMA's Illinois education task force and as a member of both the AHIMA Council on Education and Item Writing Committee. She is the author of *Statistical Applications for Health Information Management,* as well as many articles that have appeared in the *Journal of AHIMA* and *Topics in Health Information Management.* She is a former president of the AHIMA Assembly on Education.

Karen R. Patena, MBA, RHIA, is a clinical assistant professor and undergraduate program coordinator in the HIM program, School of Biomedical and Health Information Sciences, at the University of Illinois at Chicago (UIC). Ms. Patena received her MBA degree with a concentration in management information systems from DePaul University and is currently pursuing a doctorate degree at UIC. She is an alumnus of the University of Illinois health information management program. Previously, Ms. Patena was director of the independent study division of AHIMA and was a faculty member at Indiana University and Prairie State College. She also has extensive experience in hospital medical record department management, including computer systems planning and implementation. Ms. Patena's areas of expertise include management, quality improvement and TQM, and the use of computers in healthcare and systems analysis. She has presented numerous tutorials at local, state, and national levels on the use of the Internet in HIM. She currently serves on the panel of surveyors for the AHIMA Council on Accreditation.

Lynda A. Russell, EdD, JD, RHIA, is the privacy manager at Cedars-Sinai Medical Center in Los Angeles, California. Lynda has been an HIM professional for over thirty years. Prior to her current position, she held positions as HIM department director, educator, risk manager, and practicing attorney. As an educator, she was director of the baccalaureate level health information administration program at the University of Central Florida in Orlando for nine of the eleven years she was on the faculty. Lynda has been active professionally on the national, state, and local levels in Florida and California. She serves as a frequent speaker and has numerous publications on a variety of health information and health information-related topics. Ms. Russell has served in numerous officer positions including president of the Florida Health Information Management Association and as a member of the Board of Directors of the California Health Information Association (CHIA). She has also held many committee appointments including chair of the CHIA Legislative Committee and CHIA Editorial Board and member of the AHIMA Editorial Board. Most recently, she has served on the AHIMA HIM Education Strategy Committee.

Patricia B. Seidl, RHIA, has more than seven years of project management experience and eighteen years of information technology experience. She has worked as a systems analyst for several healthcare institutions and as a consultant and project manager for a major healthcare software provider. Her project management consulting expertise also extends to disciplines outside healthcare settings. She was a contributing author to *Special Edition: Using Microsoft Project 2000* and has served as a visiting professor at the College of St. Scholastica. Ms. Seidl is currently working in clinical data management in the clinical research field.

Kam Shams, MA, is the chairman of The Shams Group, Inc. (TSG), an award-winning knowledge management IT software and consulting company in the health information systems marketplace. Kam has been a visionary and innovator in the IT industry for more than thirty years. He started his career in information technology in the early 1970s and has been in healthcare since 1981. Prior to establishing The Shams Group, Inc., Kam served as vice-president and chief information officer of noted healthcare integrated delivery networks. In the past, he has served on numerous IT user boards and coached CEOs on IT-related issues. He also is a visiting professor at the College of St. Scholastica in Duluth, Minnesota, for the department of healthcare informatics and information management, as well as at the University of Tennessee Health Sciences Center in Memphis, Tennessee. Mr. Shams has written extensively on how to leverage information technology to enhance healthcare processes for increased quality and best outcomes. He is a regular contributor to several healthcare periodicals and speaks frequently at conferences around the country.

David X. Swenson, PhD, is an associate professor in the management program at the College of St. Scholastica in Duluth, Minnesota, where he teaches strategic management, organizational development, leadership, and principles of management. He is also clinical associate professor of behavioral sciences at the University of Minnesota in Duluth and a forensic psychologist in private practice. Dr. Swenson has worked in the field of psychology for thirty years. He has served as director of student development at the College of St. Scholastica, director of clinical services at the Human Resource Center of Douglas County, Wisconsin, and co-director of the Institute for the Development of Human Resources, a training and consulting partnership. He is the author of over seventy publications, including the book *Stress Management for Law Enforcement.* A graduate of the University of Missouri at Columbia in counseling and personnel services, Swenson also has degrees in management and in educational media and technology and is a diplomate in forensic psychology.

Karen A. Wager, DBA, RHIA, is an associate professor in the department of health administration and policy at the Medical University of South Carolina in Charleston, where she received her master's degree in health information administration and finance. In 1998, she received a doctorate of business administration from the University of Sarasota. She is a member and has served on various committees of AHIMA. She was president of the South Carolina Health Information Management Association (SCHIMA) from 1991 to 1992.

Andrea Weatherby White, PhD, RHIA, is an associate professor and program director of the master's-level program in health administration in the department of health information administration and policy at the Medical University of South Carolina in Columbia. She was named Teacher of the Year by the university in 1995 and won the Excellence in Service Award in 2000. Ms. White has served for a number of years as an AHIMA accreditation site visitor for both the health information management and health information administration educational programs.

Vicki L. Zeman, MA, RHIA, is the academic coordinator of professional practice experience for the department of health information management at the College of St. Scholastica in Duluth, Minnesota. Ms. Zeman has been an HIM professional for thirty years and practiced in a variety of settings for thirteen years before becoming an educator. Her last six years in practice were focused on the area of hospitalwide quality improvement. While serving as an instructor in the HIM program for seventeen years, she has also provided administrative support as the coordinator of the RHIT progression program.

Preface

Health information management (HIM) professionals play a critical role in the delivery of healthcare in the United States. HIM professionals manage patient information systems in a variety of care settings including hospitals, ambulatory care, nursing homes, home care, hospice, behavioral health, correctional facilities, and so forth. In this role, HIM professionals collaborate with other members of the healthcare team to ensure that an individual's health information is accurate, accessible, confidential, and secure. In recent years, health information managers have been playing increasingly diverse roles in other health-related industries such as insurance companies, managed care, vendor settings, service organizations, and health-related consulting organizations. The dynamic nature of the HIM profession reflects the continuous change that characterizes the healthcare delivery system as a whole. The expansion of career opportunities has demanded new skill sets and competencies for HIM professionals.

While the expansion of the HIM profession has been a positive and rewarding trend, it poses unique challenges in preparing students in educational programs, especially at the baccalaureate level, to assume a variety of positions within the healthcare industry. Historically, the boundary between baccalaureate and associate degree programs in health information management has been ill defined. Course content and program outcomes have not been clearly differentiated, and the same textbooks have been used at both levels. This lack of distinction in educational preparation has led to a similar issue in the job market, as employers have not considered differences in credentials in the hiring process.

The need to respond to change has driven the efforts of the American Health Information Management Association (AHIMA) to develop model curricula for associate, baccalaureate, and master's level education. The model curricula create, for the first time, clear boundaries between the various levels of HIM education in terms of content, program outcomes, and professional competencies. Changes in both the accreditation process for HIM programs and the certification examinations for RHIAs and RHITs have served to support these deliberate differences between HIM credentials and educational programs. Over the past several years, HIM programs have been updating and developing their curricula to better reflect the AHIMA models.

This text is specifically directed toward baccalaureate degree programs in health information administration (HIA). Like the companion text for associate programs, *Health Information Management: An Applied Approach,* it is the result of AHIMA's ongoing efforts to provide rich resources for the education and training of students in HIA programs. It also offers a reference for current practitioners in the field. This textbook is designed to reflect HIM practice at the administrator level with emphasis on the core set of skills and knowledge set forth in the model curriculum. Its topics reflect the recommended content for HIA programs as defined in the Model Curriculum for Baccalaureate Degree Programs in Health Information Administration. The content and organization of the text allows for the effective integration of dynamic concepts into an existing HIA curriculum.

Central to the organization of this text is the information management model used by the Joint Commission on Accreditation of Healthcare Organizations (JCAHO), which presents health information management as an incremental process. This process begins with the collection of patient-specific data, is followed by the aggregation of data to generate information, the development of comparative data, and, finally, the utilization of such data and derived information to increase knowledge and support decision making. The use of the model curriculum and the information management model as the foundations of this textbook ensures that the content is covered in a logical and systematic way.

All of the content areas of the AHIMA Model Curriculum for Baccalaureate Programs are covered in this text with the exception of those related to the biomedical sciences (for example, anatomy, physiology, pathophysiology/disease processes, medical terminology, pharmacology, and so on), basic human resources management principles, and the skill-development aspects of classification systems. The editors recognize that in some content areas, specialized content-specific textbooks may be required as additional resources, especially for developing competence in coding, the use of basic computer systems, and human resources management.

A systems approach to the content is utilized in this text because the audience will be expected to develop skill in problem solving, decision making, systems thinking, and professional leadership. The structure used throughout this text is designed to help the student apply concepts and principles in practice in an organized and systematic way. The features used to accomplish this goal include the following:

- Examples and case studies used throughout the text reflect the contemporary spectrum of HIM practice environments.
- Each chapter begins with a section titled Theory into Practice, which includes a case study. The case study gives the learner an appreciation of how the major concepts and principles in the chapter are applied in a real practice-based situation.
- Each chapter contains sections called Check Your Understanding, which allow learners to verify their command of the information presented in the chapter. The sections also provide students with formative feedback as they proceed through the material.
- Each chapter contains either a Real-World Case developed from today's top stories in healthcare delivery or a profile of a health information administrator whose area of practice reflects the content area of the chapter, such as the profile of Matthew Greene in chapter 13.
- Each chapter provides Application Exercises that give learners an opportunity to put theory into practice themselves. The exercises also give instructors ideas for student activities and projects. These exercises are designed to help students develop critical thinking, problem solving, systems thinking, and leadership skills.
- Review Quizzes are included at the end of each chapter. They reflect the cognitive and competency levels identified in the model curriculum. The quizzes give students an opportunity to self-test their knowledge of the content area.

The text is presented in six parts. Part I introduces the concepts of informatics and information management as they apply to the healthcare industry. It also introduces the profession of health information management.

Chapter 1 introduces the concept of health information management, discusses the overall characteristics and challenges of today's modern healthcare environment, and provides a short history of AHIMA.

Chapter 2 provides an overview of the organizations that deliver, finance, and regulate healthcare services in the United States. It focuses on the impact of accreditation, licensure, regulation, reimbursement systems, and legal and ethical issues in creating the environment for managing and delivering healthcare services. This chapter provides a context for the concepts and applications presented in the remainder of the text.

Chapter 3 introduces the field of informatics as it is applied in healthcare. The chapter surveys the emerging technologies in the clinical environment, for example, imaging, natural language processing, artificial intelligence, and Web technologies. It explores the major issues associated with computerizing clinical data, and it presents an overview of the types of computer applications that are used to support clinical decision making. It also identifies the barriers and limitations associated with computerized clinical decision support.

Chapter 4 introduces the body of knowledge, competencies, and ethical principles that constitute the core of the HIM profession's contributions to the healthcare industry. The education, certifications, and associations that are identified with the health information management profession are discussed, as are the functions and roles of health information management professionals.

Chapter 5 introduces the concept of information as an organizational asset that must be managed effectively to provide and sustain its value. The chapter discusses principles and techniques for developing data, for creating a database infrastructure, and for establishing reporting capabilities that meet the needs of the various types and levels of information systems users within an organization. The essential characteristics of quality data as well as the principles, regulations, and techniques associated with ensuring data security are presented as the primary concerns of information managers.

The final chapter in this part, chapter 6, introduces the process of information systems development. It begins with a discussion of information systems planning as a component of an organization's strategic planning effort. This chapter focuses on the information systems life cycle: its phases, the activities within each phase, and the unique and complementary roles of information technology staff, information management professionals, and information users in the information systems development effort.

Part II of this text focuses on the development of health information systems from the perspective of individual patients. It addresses the development of personally identifiable health information and the basic concepts of managing health records in both a manual and computerized environment in today's healthcare facilities.

Chapter 7 addresses healthcare information standards including the concept of converting data into information in the healthcare environment. It also explores the development of uniform standards that guide data collection in healthcare. It discusses healthcare data sets, including the history, purpose, and use of each. It also introduces healthcare informatics standards that support the transition from paper-based to computer-based health records.

Chapter 8 focuses on the content and structure of patient-specific data and personally identifiable data and information, as collected in individual health records. It addresses data sources, capture of data in a health record, and documentation requirements. This chapter also addresses management issues related to paper-based record systems, including clinical documentation issues, medical word processing as a tool for documentation, forms design, storage and retrieval systems, and chart tracking.

Chapter 9 focuses on the development of health records in a computerized format, including issues related to the transition from paper-based records to electronic or computer-based records. Data capture, imaging, security, and user needs are among the topics addressed. Issues related to the creation and maintenance of computer-based patient records are also discussed.

Chapters 10 and 11 focus on the legal and ethical concepts and issues related to healthcare information systems and health information management practice. Current legal and regulatory issues are explored, including issues related to privacy, confidentiality, security, and access to healthcare data. Work processes related to release of information policies and procedures are addressed. Ethical issues such as those related to computerization of clinical information, the coding–reimbursement connection, and vendor–organization relationships are among those discussed in chapter 11.

Part III of the text focuses on the conversion of patient-specific data and information into aggregate data that are used for analysis, statistics, and research, as well as clinical and administrative decision making.

Chapter 12 focuses on impersonal uses of healthcare data, that is, data that have been abstracted from individual health records and captured in healthcare databases. Included in this chapter are secondary records such as indexes, registers, and registries, as well as exploration of data sources, data capture, and the healthcare information infrastructure. Information management concepts are applied to healthcare database development.

Chapter 13 provides an introduction to classification systems for healthcare data including ICD-9-CM, CPT, and SNOMED. Emerging clinical vocabularies are introduced, and the concept of data representation in computer-based systems is explored, as is medical linguistics as a basis for clinical classifications and vocabularies.

Chapter 14 provides an overview of the uses of coded data and health information in reimbursement systems. Included in this chapter are issues related to coding management, case-mix management, billing procedures, and severity-of-illness classifications. Methods for managing the quality of coded data are addressed.

Part IV of the text introduces the development and use of comparative data in healthcare and focuses on the development of statistical and research methodologies. It addresses professional competencies put forth in the AHIMA Model Curriculum for HIA Programs.

Chapter 15 emphasizes the collection, use, presentation, and verification of statistical healthcare data. Fundamentals of descriptive and inferential statistics are covered, as are standard formulae for facility-based statistics. This chapter focuses on the practical application of descriptive and inferential statistics in a healthcare environment and the application of information management concepts in developing comparative data.

Chapter 16 addresses basic research methods as they are applied to healthcare information. The chapter focuses on the steps in developing a research project, including defining a research problem, performing a literature review, determining research design and methodology, selecting measurement instruments, analyzing data, and presenting study results. Library research techniques and data search and access are also addressed.

Chapter 17 addresses the collection and use of aggregate data in the analysis and evaluation of healthcare services. Topics such as clinical quality assessment, clinical outcomes management, critical pathways and case management, utilization review, and risk management systems are explored. The chapter focuses on healthcare data as a resource in clinical decision making.

Part V explores knowledge-based healthcare data and information and applies the concepts of knowledge management to the use of healthcare information for biomedical and research support as well as for expert systems and decision support. The process of converting knowledge assets into wisdom to create a learning organization is explored.

Chapter 18 presents concepts associated with acquiring clinical knowledge-based data. This chapter addresses national research policy development, medical/health research and investigation, and research protocol data management. The role of health information management professionals in a research environment is explored.

Chapter 19 addresses the application of artificial intelligence concepts to support administrative, executive, and clinical decision making. Models for building such systems within healthcare organizations are reviewed. Current applications in each of these decision-making venues are presented along with a discussion of their strengths and limitations in practice.

Chapter 20 focuses on the transition of information into knowledge within an organization. It addresses the human factors that are key to using knowledge assets for the real benefit of an organization, and it explores the impact of corporate culture and values on the ability to translate knowledge assets into wise actions. The role of a knowledge manager in ensuring the availability of, as well as the wise and ethical use of, knowledge resources is explored. The role of the health information manager as both a broker of health information and a knowledge manager is also explored.

Part VI of the text addresses the tools, techniques, and strategies utilized in managing health information services. The chapter provides an overview of human resources management and focuses on applications of both operational and human resources management principles in the healthcare setting.

Chapter 21 introduces the management discipline, the evolution of management thought, and the functions of management. It focuses on the principles and basic tools associated with each management function as well as the theories and principles associated with leadership and decision making in organizations. Communications, problem solving, and change management models and techniques are explored.

Chapter 22 focuses on the systems nature of work processes in organizations. It introduces the concepts, tools, and techniques associated with designing (and redesigning) effective and efficient work processes, as well as those associated with implementing new or revised work processes. Performance measurement and performance improvement in terms of productivity, quality measurement, benchmarking, and work process redesign are presented as major topics.

Chapter 23 discusses the implementation of appropriate policies, procedures, and practices in each of the seven human resources (HR) activity areas: HR planning and analysis; equal employment opportunity; staffing; HR development; compensation and benefits; health, safety, and security; and employee and labor/management relations. Effective recruitment, selection, and hiring practices are also discussed, as well as orientation and ongoing training and the process of performance review.

Chapter 24 focuses on training and retaining a work force in a highly competitive environment. Topics include orientation programs, staff development, continuing education, and employee retention programs. Trends in staffing are also explored including outsourcing, home-based work processes, nontraditional scheduling, and contract workers.

Chapter 25 focuses on the concepts and tools associated with planning and controlling the financial resources required to operate a department or work unit within a healthcare organization. Operations, labor, and capital budgeting processes and techniques are presented. Organizational and departmental financial performance measures are reviewed. And, finally, techniques for improving financial performance at the department level are explored.

Chapter 26 addresses the topic of project management. The focus is on the various aspects of a project that must be integrated to effectively move it from an idea to a functioning reality. The processes that must be put in place to effectively manage a project are defined. The requisite skill set of project managers as well as the tools and techniques of project management are explored. The impact that project context, stakeholder needs and expectations, and competing demands have on the project manager's work is highlighted.

Chapter 27, the final chapter of the text, focuses on the role of the health information professional and manager as a visionary leader and strategist. The principles of strategic management are presented. Models for strategic planning and techniques for implementing a strategic management philosophy into a department or organization are explored.

Six appendices follow Part VI. Appendix A features sample health record documentation forms. Appendix B presents the sample position descriptions developed by AHIMA for HIM positions such as risk manager, quality improvement director, director of HIM academic program, coder, clinical data specialist, and several others. Appendix C presents the JCAHO and Medicare Conditions of Participation standards for the form and content of the health record. Appendix D provides a sample notice of health information practices. Appendix E lists all current AHIMA practice briefs, standards, and position statements. And finally, Appendix F provides an extensive list of online Web resources for HIM professionals.

A complete glossary of HIM terms is included at the end of the book. Throughout the text chapters, boldface type is used to indicate the first substantial reference to key terms included in the glossary. A detailed content index is also included at the conclusion of the text. Frequently used abbreviations, acronyms, and initialisms are spelled out on the inside covers of the book for easy reference.

Acknowledgments

Without the contributions of many individuals, this landmark textbook would not have been published.

The editors and publications staff would like to express appreciation to the many authors who contributed chapters to this textbook. They willingly shared their expertise, met tight deadlines, accepted feedback, and contributed to building the body of knowledge related to health information management. Writing a chapter is a time-consuming and demanding task, and we are grateful for the authors' contributions.

We would also like to thank the following reviewers who lent a critical eye to this endeavor:

Melanie S. Brodnik, PhD, RHIA
Jill Burrington-Brown, MS, RHIA
Jean S. Clark, RHIA
Claire R. Dixon-Lee, PhD, RHIA
Michelle L. Dougherty, RHIA
Kathleen A. Frawley, JD, MS, RHIA
Sandra R. Fuller, MA, RHIA
Robert Garrie, MS, RHIA
Debra Hamada, RHIA
Robert J. Hartl, MA

Anita Hazelwood, MLS, RHIA
Beth Hjort, RHIA
Gwen Hughes, RHIA
Elizabeth Layman, PhD, RHIA, CCS, FAHIMA
Mary Mike Pavoni, MS, RHIA, FAHIMA
Bonnie J. Petterson, MS, RHIA
Bryon Pickard, MBA, RHIA
Harry Rhodes, MBA, RHIA
Dan Rode, MBA, FHFMA
Rita A. Scichilone, MHSA, RHIA, CCS, CCS-P, CHC
Patricia L. Shaw, MEd, RHIA
Carol M. Spielman, MA, RHIA
Annette Valenta, PhD, RHIA
Carol A. Venable, MPH, RHIA
Valerie J. M. Watzlaf, PhD, RHIA
Karen Garrett Youmans, MPA, RHIA, CCS

Finally, the editors wish to acknowledge the guidance, patience, and expertise of Marcia Bottoms, director of publications for AHIMA. She is the glue that held the entire project together.

Foreword

To Tomorrow's Health Information Leaders

Communication and information management in healthcare are changing irrevocably. And it is about time. Before this decade is over, the electronic health record will be a reality for nearly all healthcare organizations, knowledge resources will be immediately accessible to caregivers, and citizens empowered by information will better understand their health and service options. Unencumbered by the physical limitations of a paper file, health information links departments, care levels, and entire healthcare organizations. It chronicles episodes and changes in the life of the individual and the health of families. It drives effective public health and public policy.

Health information management professionals will be on the front lines in shaping these revolutionary changes affecting healthcare, personal health, and the health of our society. *Health Information Management: Concepts, Principles, and Practice* is an urgently needed textbook for training the health information management revolutionaries who will herald in the information age of healthcare. Editors Shirley Eichenwald Maki, MBA, RHIA, CPHIMS, and Kathleen M. LaTour, MA, RHIA, designed a text that provides comprehensive coverage of the "science" of health information management and then added the "art" through a rich variety of case studies and exercises. They assembled twenty-five expert contributors representing the breadth of information management in healthcare as reflected in the AHIMA Model Curriculum for Baccalaureate HIA Programs.

The context within which information is managed—the healthcare system; concepts of informatics, information, and information systems management; and the profession of health information management—is expertly covered by contributors Bonnie S. Cassidy, MPA, FAHIMA, FHIMSS; Deborah Kohn, MPH, RHIA, CHE, CPHIMS, FHIMSS; Sandra R. Fuller, MA, RHIA; Frances Wickham Lee, DBA; and Karen A. Wager, DBA, RHIA. The content of health information and patient records, the laws, standards, and ethical values that affect how it is managed are presented by Kathleen M. LaTour, MA, RHIA; Mary Cole McCain, MPA, RHIA; Margret Amatayakul, MBA, RHIA, FHIMSS; Lynda A. Russell, EdD, JD, RHIA; and Laurinda B. Harman, PhD, RHIA. Contributors Elizabeth Bowman, MPA, RHIA; Susan H. Fenton, MBA,

RHIA; and Michelle A. Green, MPS, RHIA, CMA, address the development and use of coded and aggregate information for healthcare management and reimbursement. Authors Carol E. Osborn, PhD, RHIA; Elizabeth Layman, PhD, RHIA, CCS, FAHIMA; Vicki L. Zeman, MA, RHIA; J. Michael Hardin, PhD; Kam Shams, MA; and Mehnaz Farishta, MS, cover the development and use of statistical data to enable meaningful comparisons, support clinical and policy research, and improve the quality of healthcare. Finally, concepts and processes for managing health information services are explored by David X. Swenson, PhD; Madonna LeBlanc, MA, RHIA; Andrea Weatherby White, PhD, RHIA; Shirley Eichenwald Maki, MBA, RHIA, CPHIMS; Karen R. Patena, MBA, RHIA; Nadinia Davis, MBA, CIA, CPA, RHIA; Patricia B. Seidl, RHIA; and Linda L. Kloss, RHIA, CAE.

Publishing a text of this complexity is an unprecedented accomplishment for AHIMA. Special thanks to Marcia Bottoms, AHIMA's director of publications, for guiding this work and to Sandra R. Fuller, MA, RHIA, AHIMA's senior vice-president and chief operating officer, for the courage to launch this project.

Health information management professionals are highly specialized knowledge workers. The information revolution has expanded the breadth of the knowledge and skills required to be an effective HIM professional. It has also exploded the opportunities for further specialization into any number of information management subspecialty areas such as health statistics, leadership and management, compliance, and technology. This text is dedicated to you, the health information management student. You are tomorrow's professional leaders, and your efforts will ensure that information technology and informatics science are used fully and effectively to improve health and the quality of healthcare. This text is also dedicated to those who built and nurtured this profession and its legacy of service. As we complete the transition from a paper to a computer-based healthcare information systems, we will be fulfilling the dream of our profession's leaders—quality healthcare through quality information.

Linda L. Kloss, RHIA, CAE
Executive Vice-President, Chief Executive Officer,
AHIMA

Part I

Informatics and Health Information Management

Chapter 1
Introduction

*Shirley Eichenwald Maki, MBA, RHIA, CPHIMS,
and Kathleen M. LaTour, MA, RHIA*

The field of **health information management** (HIM) was originally called medical record science. Medical record science became a recognized field of study in healthcare only ten years after the hospital standardization movement began. Originally, members of the profession were called record librarians.

The **Association of Record Librarians of North America** was founded in 1928, and the association's first annual meeting was held in Chicago in 1929. The original objective of the association (and the profession) was to elevate the standards of clinical record keeping in hospitals, dispensaries, and other healthcare facilities. Since its founding, the association, now known as the **American Health Information Management Association** (AHIMA), and the professionals affiliated with it have been advocates for the effective management of clinical record content, structure, accuracy, integrity, and dissemination in every type of healthcare setting (Johns 2001).

As managed care became a driving force in American healthcare during the 1980s, effective information management began to emerge as a top priority for healthcare institutions. According to Blum (1986) and Protti (1984), 25 to 40 percent of an average hospital's operating costs were devoted to information handling at that time. Events affecting healthcare delivery and the management of healthcare delivery services in the 1990s have placed even greater pressure on healthcare organizations to improve their information-handling capacity and functionality. Johns (2002) emphasizes that the healthcare industry now fully recognizes the importance of information flow across departmental boundaries and the necessity of broad dissemination throughout the organization.

This chapter provides a brief introduction to the HIM profession and focuses on the changing nature of the profession's core domain of practice. It sets the stage for the remaining chapters in this textbook by providing a context for the broad range of topics that must be addressed in a textbook whose purpose is to describe the concepts, principles, and practices associated with the health information management profession in its current state of transformation. (A full discussion of the HIM profession and related professional associations is presented in chapter 4.)

The Modern Healthcare Environment

The 1990s brought several new forces to bear on the American healthcare industry, and each has had a transformational effect on the health information management profession. During that decade, competition among healthcare providers was stimulated by major changes in the reimbursement system used by **Medicare** and **Medicaid** (two federally mandated healthcare programs). **Integrated healthcare delivery systems** also began to emerge as a significant organizational model, and **managed care** delivery systems continued to expand. As a result of these developments, the availability of timely and accurate clinical information has become critical to the viability of healthcare organizations. Medical and administrative staffs now recognize that the information gathered from clinical records is an invaluable organizational asset. They also understand that it represents an important quality indicator and a vital tool for efficiently managing the business of healthcare in an increasingly tight financial environment.

During the 1990s, the wise application of increasingly sophisticated computer technology also received increased attention among healthcare professionals and organizations. Technology was the obvious solution to the need for greater efficiency in managing the ever-increasing volume of healthcare data. In addition, as diverse healthcare decision makers looked for flexibility in how they could access and analyze vast electronic repositories of clinical data, advanced **decision support technology** became available.

Today, these trends continue to affect the practice of health information management and healthcare in general as:

- New government regulations focus on administrative simplification strategies for healthcare
- New healthcare reimbursement systems are implemented
- The prevention of medical errors becomes even more important than in the past
- Work force shortages place an increasing emphasis on technological systems for improving productivity
- Integrated information system solutions as well as clinician-friendly hardware and applications are developed for healthcare applications
- The Internet and its derived technologies make connectivity across otherwise disparate information systems as well as access to application software and off-site maintenance even more affordable for healthcare organizations

Contemporary Health Information Management

The HIM profession is the only profession that has as its core professional concern the quality of the data collected and maintained in the course of delivering healthcare services. Although clinical and allied healthcare professionals depend on the availability of high-quality data to perform clinical decision making, their primary concern is providing diagnostic and therapeutic services, not managing clinical information per se. The administrators and managers of healthcare organizations also use collected clinical information to plan and manage healthcare services, but managing the quality of the data they use is not their major concern. Similarly, computer scientists and technicians are concerned primarily with the performance of software and hardware configurations; researchers are concerned primarily with the development of scientific solutions to important questions; third-party payers are concerned primarily with the control of financial resources; and policy makers are concerned primarily with incentives for cost-effectiveness, social justice, and ethical practice.

In an information-intensive, technology-driven environment, HIM professionals must concentrate on building their unique knowledge base and competencies in the following areas:

- Laws and regulations related to the accuracy, completeness, integrity, and security of healthcare information
- Healthcare data standards
- Healthcare statistical methods
- Clinical coding and classification systems
- Principles of health record and information systems
- Organizational and cross-disciplinary modes of functioning

Once applied in a world of paper-based records and manual systems for report generation, the HIM knowledge base

and competencies are now needed by healthcare organizations and computer application developers that seek to effectively transition vital clinical data resources into electronic clinical repositories and electronic health record systems. These modern technological systems support both the operational and strategic needs of the organization's work force and decision makers. (An expanded discussion of the emerging roles for HIM professionals is presented in chapter 4.)

The HIM profession today remains committed to its original goal of elevating health record standards and practices. It does so, however, in a healthcare environment that is becoming more and more technology driven in both its work processes and information flow, as well as more and more dependent on the quality and accessibility of the information contained within clinical records. HIM professionals work to ensure that their communities and customers are provided high-quality and cost-effective healthcare services.

Thus, to carry on the important legacy of their predecessors, today's HIM professionals must support an adapted vision of their unique contribution and build and maintain an accompanying set of strengthened competencies for the healthcare industry they serve. They must envision how the concepts, principles, and practices at the core of the HIM knowledge base and competencies continue to apply in their changing work environment and settings. In addition, they must assess their adaptive strength and weaknesses relative to that vision, and, most important, they must take action to position themselves appropriately to contribute their unique expertise to the organizations they serve.

Working in strong collaborative partnerships with specialists in information technologies and with specialized healthcare data and information users (nurses, physicians, pharmacists, therapists, administrators, researchers, policy makers, and others), health information managers have become key players within the emerging discipline of healthcare informatics. **Healthcare informatics** focuses on designing and implementing technology-based information systems to support the specialized activities associated with each type of healthcare worker. For example, nursing informatics focuses on systems that support the work of nurses, and medical informatics focuses on systems that support the work of physicians. Similarly, consumer informatics systems support the activities of patients, long-term-care residents, and healthcare clients (Shortliffe et al. 2000).

Summary

The health information management profession began with the founding of the Association of Record Librarians of North America in 1928. The association's original goal was to improve clinical record keeping in healthcare facilities. The association, now known as the American Health Information Management Association, and a new generation of health information management professionals has inherited a powerful legacy from those original medical records pioneers. They also have an extraordinary opportunity and obligation to build on that legacy by continuing to elevate the standards for clinical data and information systems in a healthcare environment that demands integrated, computer-based, user-focused data repositories and warehouses. The viability and vitality of the HIM profession in years to come will depend on the commitment of current professionals to think and act strategically in order to address the data and information needs of the evolving healthcare industry. HIM professionals must continually update their knowledge base and competencies through self-assessment and commitment to lifelong learning, and they must actively take part in their professional organizations' activities at the local, regional, state, and national levels.

References

Blum, B. I. 1986. *Clinical Information Systems.* New York City: Springer-Verlag.

Johns, M. L. 2002. *Health Information Management Technology: An Applied Approach,* chapter 1. Chicago: American Health Information Management Association.

Protti, D. J. 1984. Knowledge and skills expected of health information scientists: a sample survey of prospective employers. *Methods of Information in Medicine* 23:204–8.

Shortliffe, E. H., L. E. Perreault, G. Wiederhold, and L. M. Fagan. 2000. *Medical Informatics: Computer Applications in Health Care and Biomedicine.* New York City: Springer-Verlag.

Chapter 2
Healthcare Delivery Systems

Bonnie S. Cassidy, MPA, FAHIMA, FHIMSS

Learning Objectives

- To understand the history of the healthcare delivery system from ancient times until the present
- To understand the basic organization of the various types of hospitals and healthcare organizations
- To recognize the impact managed care has had on healthcare providers
- To recognize the impact that external forces have on the healthcare industry
- To identify the various functional components of an integrated delivery system
- To describe the systems used for reimbursement of healthcare services
- To recognize the role of government in healthcare services

Key Terms

Accreditation
Acute care
American Association of Medical Colleges (AAMC)
American College of Healthcare Executives (ACHE)
American Health Information Management Association (AHIMA)
American Hospital Association (AHA)
American Medical Association (AMA)
American Nurses Association (ANA)
Average length of stay (ALOS)
Blue Cross and Blue Shield Association
Case management
Chief executive officer (CEO)
Chief nursing officer (CNO)
Clinical privileges
Continuous quality improvement (CQI)
Continuum of care
Extended care facility
Hill-Burton Act
Home health care
Hospice care
Integrated delivery system (IDS)
Investor-owned hospital chain
Managed care
Managed care organization (MCO)
Medicaid
Medical staff bylaws
Medical staff classifications
Medicare
Mission (statement)
National Practitioner Data Bank (NPBD)
Prospective payment system (PPS)
Public health services
Reengineering
Rehabilitation services
Skilled nursing facility (SNF)
Subacute care
Tax Equity and Fiscal Responsibility Act (TEFRA)
Utilization Review Act
Workers' compensation

Introduction

A broad array of healthcare services is available in the United States today, from simple preventive measures such as vaccinations to complex lifesaving procedures such heart transplants. An individual's contact with the healthcare delivery system often begins before she or he is born with family planning and prenatal care and continues through end-of-life planning and hospice care.

Healthcare services are provided by physicians, nurses, and other clinical providers who work in ambulatory care, acute care, rehabilitative and psychiatric care, and long-term care facilities. Healthcare services are also provided in the homes of hospice and home care patients. Assisted living centers, industrial medical clinics, and public health department clinics also provide services to many Americans.

Integrated delivery systems (IDSs) provide a full range of healthcare services along a **continuum of care** to ensure that patients get the right care at the right time from the right provider. The continuum extends from primary care providers to specialist and ancillary providers. The goal of IDSs is to deliver high-quality and cost-effective care in the most appropriate setting (Sloane et al. 1999, p. 9).

Theory into Practice

In the 1990s, hospitals in the United States faced continued pressure to contain costs, improve quality, and demonstrate their contributions to the health of the communities they serve. Hospitals adapted to these pressures in various ways. Some hospitals merged with or bought out other hospitals and healthcare organizations. Others created integrated delivery networks to provide a full range of healthcare services along the continuum of care, from ambulatory care to inpatient care to long-term care. Still others concentrated on improving the care they provided by focusing on patients as customers. Many hospitals responded to local competition by quickly entering into affiliations and other risk-sharing agreements with acute and nonacute care providers, physicians' groups, and **managed care organizations.**

History of Western Medicine

Modern Western medicine is rooted in antiquity. The ancient Greeks developed surgical procedures, documented clinical cases, and created medical books. Before modern times, European, African, and native American cultures all had traditions of folk medicine based on spiritual healing and herbal cures. The first hospitals were created by religious orders in medieval Europe to provide care and respite to religious pilgrims traveling back and forth from the Holy Land. However, it was not until the late 1800s that medicine became a scientific discipline. More progress and change occurred during the twentieth century than over the preceding 2,000 years. The past few decades have seen dramatic developments in the way diseases are diagnosed and treated and in the way healthcare is delivered.

Before the advent of modern Western medicine, epidemics and plagues were common. Epidemics of smallpox, measles, yellow fever, influenza, scarlet fever, and diphtheria killed millions of people. Bubonic plague spread periodically through Europe and killed millions more. Disease was carried by rodents and insects as well as by the travelers who moved along intercontinental trade routes.

The medical knowledge that had been gained by ancient Greek scholars such as Hippocrates was lost during the Middle Ages. The European Renaissance, a historical period beginning in the fourteenth century, revived interest in the classical arts, literature, and philosophy as well as the scientific study of nature. This period also was characterized by economic growth and concern for the welfare of workers at all levels of society. With this concept came a growing awareness that a healthy population promoted economic growth.

North America's First Hospitals

Early settlers in the British colonies of North America appointed commissions to care for the sick, to provide for orphans, and to bury the dead. During the mid-1700s, the citizens of Philadelphia recognized the need for a place to provide relief to the sick and injured. They also recognized the need to isolate newly arrived immigrants who had caught communicable diseases on the long voyage from Europe.

In Philadelphia, Benjamin Franklin and other colonists persuaded the legislature to develop a hospital for the community. It was the first hospital in the British colonies of North America. The Pennsylvania Hospital was established in Philadelphia in 1752. (Almost 200 years earlier, Cortez established the first hospital in Mexico and it still serves patients today.)

Over its first 150 years, the Pennsylvania Hospital served as a model for the organization of hospitals in other communities. The New York Hospital opened in 1771 and started its first register of patients in 1791. Boston's Massachusetts General Hospital opened in 1821.

Standardization of Medical Practice

Human anatomy and physiology and the causes of disease were not well understood before the twentieth century. At one time, it was believed that four basic fluids, called humors, determined a person's temperament and health and that imbalances in the proportion of humors in the body caused disease. The therapeutic bleeding of patients was practiced until the early twentieth century. Early physicians also treated patients by administering a variety of substances with no scientific basis for their effectiveness.

An individual's early medical education consisted of serving as an apprentice to an established practitioner. Just about anyone could hang out a shingle and call himself a physician. The medical profession recognized that some of its members achieved better results than others, and leaders in the profession attempted to regulate the practice of medicine in the late 1700s. The first attempts at regulation took the form of licensure. The first licenses to practice medicine were issued in New York in 1760. By the mid-1800s, however, efforts to license physicians were denounced as being undemocratic, and penalties for practicing medicine without a license were removed in most states.

As the population of the United States grew and settlers moved westward, the demand for medical practitioners far exceeded the supply. To staff new hospitals and serve a growing population, many private medical schools appeared almost overnight. By 1869, there were seventy-two medical schools in the United States. However, these schools did not follow an established course of study and some graduated students with as little as six months of training. The result was an oversupply of poorly trained physicians.

The **American Medical Association** (AMA) was established in 1847 to represent the interests of physicians across the United States. However, the AMA was dominated by members who had strong ties to the medical schools and the status quo. Its ability to lead a reform of the profession was limited until it broke its ties with the medical schools in 1874. At that time, the association encouraged the creation of independent state licensing boards.

In 1876, the **American Association of Medical Colleges** (AAMC) was established. The AAMC was dedicated to standardizing the curriculum for U.S. medical schools and to developing the public's understanding of the need to license physicians.

Together, the AMA and the AAMC campaigned for medical licensing. By the 1890s, thirty-five states had established or reestablished a system of licensure for physicians. At that time, fourteen states decided to grant licenses only to graduates of reputable medical schools. The state licensing boards discouraged the worst medical schools, but the criteria for licensing continued to vary from state to state and were not fully enforced.

By the early twentieth century, it had become apparent that improving the quality of American medicine required regulation through curriculum reform as well as licensure. However, the members of the AMA were divided on this issue. Conservative members continued to believe that the association should stay out of the area of regulation. Progressive members supported the continued development of state licensure systems and the creation of a standardized model for medical education.

The situation attracted the attention of the Carnegie Foundation for the Advancement of Teaching. The president of the foundation offered to sponsor and fund an independent review of the medical colleges then operating in the United States. Abraham Flexner, an educator from Louisville, Kentucky, undertook the review in 1906.

Over the following four years, Flexner visited every medical college in the country and carefully documented his findings. In his 1910 report to the Carnegie Foundation, the AMA, and the AAMC, he described the poor quality of the training being provided in the colleges. He noted that medical school applicants often lacked knowledge of the basic sciences. Flexner also reported how the absence of hospital-based training limited the clinical skills of medical school graduates. Perhaps most important, he reported that huge numbers of graduates were being produced every year and that most of them had unacceptable levels of medical skill. He recommended closing most of the existing medical schools to address the problem of oversupply.

Several reform initiatives grew out of Flexner's report and from recommendations made by the AMA's Committee on Medical Education. One of the reforms required medical school applicants to hold a college degree. Another required that medical training be founded in the basic sciences. Reforms also required that medical students receive practical, hospital-based training in addition to classroom work. These reforms were carried out in the decade following Flexner's report, but only about half of the medical schools actually closed. By 1920, most of the medical colleges in the United States had met rigorous academic standards and were approved by the AAMC.

Today, medical school graduates must pass a test before they can obtain a license to practice medicine. The licensure tests are administered by state medical boards. Many states now use a standardized licensure test developed in 1968 by the Federation of State Medical Boards of the United States. However, passing scores for the test vary by state. Most physicians also complete several years of residency training in addition to medical school.

Specialty physicians also complete extensive postgraduate medical education. Board certification for the various specialties requires the completion of postgraduate training as well as a passing score on a standardized examination. The most common medical specialties include the following:

- Internal medicine
- Pediatrics
- Family practice
- Cardiology
- Psychiatry
- Neurology
- Oncology
- Radiology

The most common surgical specialties include these:

- Anesthesiology
- Cardiovascular surgery
- Obstetrics/gynecology
- Orthopedics
- Urology
- Ophthalmology

- Otorhinolaryngology
- Plastic and reconstructive surgery
- Neurosurgery

Some medical and surgical specialists undergo further graduate training to qualify to practice subspecialties. For example, the subspecialties of internal medicine include endocrinology, pulmonary medicine, rheumatology, geriatrics, and hematology. Physicians may also limit their practices to the treatment of specific illnesses. For example, an endocrinologist may limit his or her practice to the treatment of diabetes. Surgeons can work as general surgeons or as specialists or subspecialists. For example, an orthopedic surgeon may limit his practice to surgery of the hand, surgery of the knee, surgery of the ankle, or surgery of the spine.

Some physicians and healthcare organizations employ physician assistants (PAs) and/or surgeon assistants (SAs) to help them carry out their clinical responsibilities. Such assistants may perform routine clinical assessments, provide patient education and counseling, and perform simple therapeutic procedures. Most PAs work in primary care settings, and most SAs work in hospitals and ambulatory surgery clinics. PAs and SAs always work under the supervision of licensed physicians and surgeons.

Standardization of Nursing Practice

In the nineteenth century and the first part of the twentieth century, religious organizations sponsored more than half of the hospitals in the United States. Members of religious orders often provided nursing care in these organizations. As the U.S. population grew and more towns and cities were established, new hospitals were built. Older cities also grew, and city hospitals became more and more crowded.

In the late 1800s, nurses received no formal education and little training. Nursing staff for the hospitals was often recruited from the surrounding community, and many poor women who had no other skills became nurses. The nature of nursing care at that time was unsophisticated. Indeed, the lack of basic hygiene often promoted disease. Many patients died from infections contracted while hospitalized for surgery, maternity care, and other illnesses.

In 1868, the AMA called the medical profession's attention to the need for trained nurses. During the years that followed, the public also began to call for better nursing care in hospitals.

The first general training school for nurses was opened at the New England Hospital for Women and Children in 1872. It became a model for other institutions throughout the country. As hospital after hospital struggled to find competent nursing staff, many institutions and their medical staffs developed their own nurse training programs.

The responsibilities of nurses in the late nineteenth and early twentieth centuries included housekeeping duties. Nurses also cooked meals for patients in kitchens attached to each ward. Direct patient care duties included giving baths, changing dressings, monitoring vital signs, administering medications, and assisting physicians. During this time, nurses were not required to hold a license to practice.

In 1897, a group of nurses attending the annual meeting of the American Society of Superintendents of Training Schools for Nursing founded the Nurses Associated Alumnae of the United States and Canada. In 1911, the organization was renamed the American Nurses Association (ANA). During the early meetings of the association, members established a nursing code of ethics and discussed the need for nursing licensure and for publications devoted to the practice of nursing.

At the turn of the twentieth century, nurses also began to organize state nursing associations to advocate for the registration of nurses. Their goal was to increase the level of competence among nurses nationwide. Despite opposition from many physicians who believed that nurses did not need formal education or licensure, North Carolina passed legislation requiring the registration of nurses in 1903. Today, all fifty states have laws that spell out the requirements for the registration and licensure of nursing professionals.

Modern registered nurses must have either a two-year associate's degree or a four-year bachelor's degree from a state-approved nursing school. Nurse practitioners, researchers, educators, and administrators generally have a four-year degree in nursing and additional postgraduate education in nursing. The postgraduate degree may be a master's of science or a doctorate in nursing. Nurses who graduate from nonacademic training programs are called licensed practical nurses (LPNs) or licensed vocational nurses (LVNs). Nondegreed nursing personnel work under the direct supervision of registered nurses. Nurses in all fifty states must pass an exam to obtain a license to practice.

Today's registered nurses are highly trained clinical professionals. Many specialize in specific areas of practice such as surgery, psychiatry, and intensive care. Nurse-midwives complete advanced training and are certified by the American College of Nurse-Midwives. Similarly, nurse-anesthetists are certified by the Council on Certification/Council on Recertification of Nurse Anesthetists. Nurse practitioners also receive advanced training at the master's level that qualifies them to provide primary care services to patients. They are certified by several organizations to practice in the area of their specialty (for example, the National Board of Pediatric Nurse Practitioners).

Standardization of Hospital Care

In 1910, Dr. Franklin H. Martin suggested that the surgical area of medical practice needed to become more concerned with patient outcomes. He had been introduced to this concept in discussions with Dr. Ernest Codman. Codman was a British physician who believed that hospital practitioners should track their patients for a significant amount of time after treatment so that they could determine whether the end result had been positive or negative. Codman also supported the use of outcome information to identify the practices that led to the best results for patients.

At that time, Martin and other American physicians were concerned about the conditions in U.S. hospitals. Many observers felt that part of the problem was related to the lack of organization in medical staffs and to lax professional standards. In the early twentieth century, before the development of antibiotics and other pharmaceuticals, hospitals were used mainly by physicians who needed facilities in which to perform surgery. Most nonsurgical medical care was still provided in the home. It was natural, then, for the force behind improved hospital care to come from surgeons.

The push for hospital reforms eventually led to the formation of the American College of Surgeons in 1913. The organization faced a difficult task. In 1917, the leaders of the college asked the Carnegie Foundation for funding to plan and develop a hospital standardization program. The college then formed a committee to develop a set of minimum standards for hospital care. It published the formal standards under the title the *Minimum Standards.*

During 1918 and part of 1919, the college examined the hospitals in the United States and Canada just as Flexner had reviewed the medical colleges a decade earlier. The performance of 692 hospitals was compared to the college's *Minimum Standards.* Only eighty-nine of the hospitals fully met the college's standards, and some of the most well-known hospitals in the country failed to meet them.

The adoption of the *Minimum Standards* was the basis of the Hospital Standardization Program and marked the beginning of the modern **accreditation** process for healthcare organizations. Basically, accreditation standards are developed to reflect reasonable quality standards. The performance of each participating organization is evaluated annually against the standards. The accreditation process is voluntary. Healthcare organizations choose to participate in order to improve the care they provide to their patients.

The American College of Surgeons continued to sponsor the hospital accreditation program until the early 1950s. At that time, four professional associations from the United States and Canada decided to join forces with the college to create a new accreditation organization. This organization was called the Joint Commission on Accreditation of Hospitals. The associations were the American College of Physicians, the American Medical Association, the American Hospital Association, and the Canadian Medical Association. The new organization was formally incorporated in 1952 and began to perform accreditation surveys in 1953.

The Joint Commission, under the name Joint Commission on Accreditation of Healthcare Organizations, continues to survey several different types of healthcare organizations today, including the following:

- Acute care hospitals
- Long-term care facilities
- Ambulatory care facilities
- Psychiatric facilities
- Home health agencies

Several other organizations also perform accreditation of healthcare organizations. These include the American Osteopathic Association (AOA), the Commission on Accreditation of Rehabilitation Facilities (CARF), and the Accreditation Association for Ambulatory Health Care (AAAHC).

Professionalization of the Allied Health Professions

After the First World War, many of the roles previously played by nurses and nonclinical personnel began to change. With the advent of modern diagnostic and therapeutic technology in the middle of the twentieth century, the complex skills needed by ancillary medical personnel fostered the growth of specialized training programs and professional accreditation and licensure.

According to the AMA's definition of *allied health,* allied health incorporates the healthcare-related professions that function to assist, facilitate, and/or complement the work of physicians and other clinical specialists. The Health Professions Education Amendment of 1991 describes allied health professionals as health professionals (other than registered nurses, physicians, and physician's assistants) who have received either a certificate, an associate's degree, a bachelor's degree, a master's degree, a doctorate, or postdoctoral training in a healthcare-related science. Such individuals share responsibility for the delivery of healthcare services with clinicians (physicians, nurses, and physician's assistants).

Allied health occupations are among the fastest growing in healthcare. The number of allied health professionals is difficult to estimate and depends on the definition of allied health. Unlike medicine, women dominate most of the allied health professions, representing between 75 and 95 percent in most of the occupations. All fifty states require licensure for some allied health professions (physical therapy, for example). Practitioners in other allied health professions (occupational therapy, for example) may be licensed in some states, but not in others.

The following list briefly describes some of the major occupations usually considered to be allied health professions (Jonas and Kovner 1999, pp. 100–101):

- *Clinical laboratory science:* Originally referred to as medical laboratory technology, this field is now more appropriately referred to as clinical laboratory science. Clinical laboratory technicians perform a wide array of tests on body fluids, tissues, and cells to assist in the detection, diagnosis, and treatment of diseases and illnesses.
- *Diagnostic imaging technology:* Originally referred to as X-ray technology and then radiologic technology, this field is now more appropriately referred to as diagnostic imaging. The field continues to expand to include nuclear medicine technologists, radiation therapists,

sonographers (ultrasound technologists), and magnetic resonance technologists.

- *Dietetics:* Dietitians (sometimes called clinical nutritionists) are trained in nutrition. They are responsible for providing nutritional care to individuals and for overseeing nutrition and food services in a variety of settings, ranging from hospitals to schools.
- *Emergency medical technology:* Emergency medical technicians (EMTs) are responsible for providing a wide range of services on an emergency basis for cases of traumatic injury and other emergency situations and in the transport of emergency patients.
- *Health information management:* Health information management (HIM) professionals (formerly called medical record managers) oversee health record systems and manage health-related information to ensure that it meets relevant medical, administrative, and legal requirements. Health records are the responsibility of registered health information administrators (RHIAs) and registered health information technicians (RHITs).
- *Occupational therapy:* Occupational therapists (OTs) evaluate and treat patients whose illnesses or injuries have resulted in significant psychological, physical, or work-related impairment.
- *Physical therapy:* Physical therapists (PTs) evaluate and treat patients to improve functional mobility, reduce pain, maintain cardiopulmonary function, and limit disability. PTs treat movement dysfunction resulting from accidents, trauma, stroke, fractures, multiple sclerosis, cerebral palsy, arthritis, and heart and respiratory illness. Physical therapy assistants work under the direction of PTs and help carry out the treatment plans developed by PTs.
- *Respiratory therapy:* Respiratory therapists evaluate, treat, and care for patients with breathing disorders. They work under the direction of qualified physicians and provide services such as emergency care for stroke, heart failure, and shock, and treat patients with emphysema and asthma.
- *Speech-language pathology and audiology:* Speech-language pathologists and audiologists identify, assess, and provide treatment for individuals with speech, language, or hearing problems.

Check Your Understanding 2.1

Instructions: Choose the word or term that correctly completes each of the sentences below.

1. ____ The ancient ____ developed surgical procedures, documented clinical cases, and created medical books.
   a. Egyptians
   b. Greeks
   c. Phoenicians
   d. Chinese

2. ____ The ____ was established in 1847 to represent the interests of physicians across the United States.
   a. American Association of Medical Colleges
   b. American College of Surgeons
   c. Committee on Medical Education
   d. American Medical Association

3. ____ Today, medical school students must pass a test before they can obtain a ____ to practice medicine.
   a. Degree
   b. Residency
   c. Specialty
   d. License

4. ____ The first general training school for ____ was opened at the New England Hospital for Women and Children in 1872.
   a. Nurses
   b. Physician assistants
   c. Surgical specialists
   d. Surgeons

5. ____ Modern ____ must have either a two-year associate's degree or a four-year bachelor's degree from a state-approved nursing school.
   a. Nurse practitioners
   b. Licensed vocational nurses
   c. Registered nurses
   d. Licensed practical nurses

6. ____ In 1910, Dr. Franklin H. Martin suggested that the surgical area of medical practice needed to become more concerned with ____.
   a. Patient care
   b. Professional standards
   c. Patient outcomes
   d. Nonsurgical medical care

7. ____ The adoption of the *Minimum Standards* marked the beginning of the modern ____ process for healthcare organizations.
   a. Accreditation
   b. Licensing
   c. Reform
   d. Educational

8. ____ According to the AMA's definition, ____ incorporates the healthcare-related professions that function to assist, facilitate, and/or complement the work of physicians and other clinical specialists.
   a. Home health
   b. Nursing care
   c. Ambulatory care
   d. Allied health

Modern Healthcare Delivery in the United States

Until the Second World War, most healthcare was provided in the home. Quality in healthcare services was considered a product of appropriate medical practice and oversight by physicians and surgeons. Even the *Minimum Standards* used to evaluate the performance of hospitals were based on factors directly related to the composition and skills of the hospital medical staff.

The twentieth century was a period of tremendous change in American society. Advances in medical science promised better outcomes and increased the demand for healthcare services. But medical care has never been free. Even in the best economic times, many Americans have been unable to take full advantage of what medicine has to offer because they cannot pay for it.

Concern over access to healthcare was especially evident during the Great Depression of the 1930s. During the Depression, America's leaders were forced to consider how the poor and disadvantaged could receive the care they needed. Before the Depression, medical care for the poor and elderly had been handled as a function of social welfare agencies. During the 1930s, however, few people were able to pay for medical care. The problem of how to pay for the healthcare needs of millions of Americans became a public and governmental concern. Working Americans turned to prepaid health plans to help them pay for healthcare. However, the unemployed and the unemployable needed help from a different source.

Effects of the Great Depression

The concept of prepaid healthcare, or health insurance, began with the financial problems of one hospital, Baylor University Hospital in Dallas, Texas (AHA 1999, p. 14). In 1929, the administrator of the hospital had an idea. He arranged to provide hospital services to Dallas's schoolteachers for fifty cents per person per month. Before that time, a few large employers had set up company clinics and hired company physicians to care for their workers. But the idea of a prepaid health plan that could be purchased by individuals had never been tried before.

The idea caught on quickly, and new prepaid plans appeared across the country. Eventually, these plans became known as Blue Cross plans when the blue cross symbol used by some of the new plans was adopted officially as the trademark for all the plans in 1939.

Another type of prepaid plan, called the Blue Shield plan, was subsequently developed to cover the cost of physicians' services. The idea for the Blue Shield plans grew out of the medical service bureaus created by large lumber and mining companies in the Northwest. In 1939, the first formal Blue Shield plan was founded California.

Growth in the number of Blue Cross/Blue Shield plans continued through the Depression and boomed during the Second World War. During the war-related labor shortages, employers began to pay for their employees' memberships in the Blues as a way to attract and keep scarce workers.

The idea of public funding for healthcare services also goes back to the Great Depression. The decline in family income during the 1930s curtailed the use of medical services by the poor. In ten working-class communities studied between 1929 and 1933, the proportion of families with incomes under $150 per capita had increased from 10 to 43 percent. A 1938 Gallup poll asked people whether they had put off seeing a physician because of the cost. The results showed that 68 percent of lower-income respondents had put off medical care, compared with 24 percent of respondents in upper-income brackets (Starr 1982, p. 271).

The decreased use of medical services and the inability of many patients to pay meant lower incomes for physicians. Hospitals were in similar trouble. Beds were empty, bills went unpaid, and contributions to hospital fund-raising efforts tumbled. As a result, private physicians and charities could no longer meet the demand for free services. For the first time, physicians and hospitals asked state welfare departments to pay for the treatment of people on relief.

The Depression posed a severe test for the AMA. It was no easy matter to maintain a common front against government intervention when physicians themselves were facing economic difficulties. Many physicians became more willing to consider some form of government-sponsored health insurance. In 1935, the California Medical Association endorsed the concept of compulsory health insurance because health insurance promised to stimulate the use of physicians' services and help patients pay their bills.

The AMA's response to the economic crisis emphasized restricting the supply of physicians, rather than increasing the demand for their services, by instituting mandatory health insurance. The AMA reacted by pushing for the closure of medical schools and reductions in the number of new medical students.

By the mid-1930s, however, the AMA began to adjust its position on health insurance. Instead of opposing all insurance, voluntary or compulsory, it began to define the terms on which voluntary programs might be acceptable. Although accepting health insurance plans in principle, the AMA did nothing to support or encourage their development.

The push for government-sponsored health insurance continued in the late 1930s during the administration of President Franklin D. Roosevelt. However, compulsory health insurance stood on the margins of national politics throughout the New Deal era. It was not made part of the new Social Security program, and it was never fully supported by President Roosevelt.

Postwar Efforts toward Improving Healthcare Access

After the Second World War, the issue of healthcare access finally moved to the center of national politics. In the late 1940s, President Harry Truman expressed unreserved support for a national health insurance program. However, the issue of compulsory health insurance became entangled with America's fear of communism. Opponents of Truman's healthcare program labeled it "socialized medicine," and the program failed to win legislative support.

The idea of national health insurance did not resurface until the administration of Lyndon Johnson and the Great Society legislation of the 1960s. The Medicare and Medicaid programs were legislated in 1965 to pay the cost of providing healthcare services to the elderly and the poor. The issues of healthcare reform and national health insurance were again given priority during the first four years of President

Bill Clinton's administration in the 1990s. However, the complexity of American healthcare issues at the end of the twentieth century doomed reform efforts.

Influence of Federal Legislation

During the twentieth century, Congress passed many pieces of legislation that had a significant impact on the delivery of healthcare services in the United States.

Biologics Control Act of 1902

Direct federal sponsorship of medical research began with early research on methods for controlling epidemics of infectious disease. The Marine Hospital Service performed the first research. In 1887, a young physician, Joseph Kinyoun, set up a bacteriological laboratory in the Marine Hospital at Staten Island, New York. Four years later, the Hygienic Laboratory was moved to Washington, D.C. It was given authority to test and improve biological products in 1902 when Congress passed the Biologics Control Act. This act regulated the vaccines and sera sold via interstate commerce. That same year, the Hygienic Laboratory added divisions in chemistry, pharmacology, and zoology.

In 1912, the service, by then called the U.S. Public Health Service, was authorized to study chronic as well as infectious diseases. In 1930, reorganized under the Randsdell Act, the Hygienic Laboratory became the National Institutes of Health (NIH). In 1938, the NIH moved to a large, privately donated estate in Bethesda, Maryland (Starr 1982, p. 340).

Today, the mission of the NIH is to uncover new medical knowledge that can lead to health improvements for everyone. The NIH accomplishes its mission by conducting and supporting medical research, fostering communication of up-to-date medical information, and training research investigators. The organization has played a vital role in recent clinical research on the treatment of the following diseases:

- Heart disease and stroke
- Cancer
- Depression and schizophrenia
- Spinal cord injuries

Social Security Act of 1935

The Great Depression revived the dormant social reform movement in the United States as well as more radical currents in American politics. Unionization increased, and the American Federation of Labor (AF of L) abandoned its long-standing opposition to social insurance programs. The Depression also brought to power a Democratic administration. The administration of Franklin D. Roosevelt was more willing than any previous administration to involve the federal government in the management of economic and social welfare.

Even before Roosevelt took office in 1933, a steady movement toward some sort of social insurance program had been growing. By 1931, nine states had passed legislation creating old-age pension programs. As governor of New York State, Roosevelt endorsed unemployment insurance in 1930. Wis-

consin became the first state to adopt such a measure early in 1932.

Although old-age pension and unemployment insurance bills were introduced into Congress soon after his election, Roosevelt refused to give them his strong support. Instead, he created a program of his own. On June 8, 1934, he announced that he would appoint a committee on economic security to study the issue comprehensively and report to Congress in January 1935. The committee consisted of four members of the cabinet and the federal relief administrator. It was headed by the secretary of labor, Frances Perkins.

Although Roosevelt indicated in his June message that he was especially interested in old-age and unemployment programs, the committee included medical care and health insurance in its research. From the outset, the prevailing sentiment on the committee was that health insurance would have to wait. Abraham Epstein was the founder of the American Association for Social Security and a leading figure in the social insurance movement. In an article published in October 1934, he warned the administration that opposition to health insurance was strong. He advised the administration to be politically realistic and go slow on health insurance.

Sentiment in favor of health insurance was strong among members of the Committee on Economic Security. However, many members of the committee were convinced that adding a health insurance amendment would spell defeat for the entire Social Security legislation. Ultimately, the Social Security bill included only one reference to health insurance as a subject that the new Social Security Board might study. The Social Security Act was passed in 1935.

The omission of health insurance from the legislation was by no means the act's only conservative feature. It relied on a regressive tax and gave no coverage to some of the nation's poorest people such as farmers and domestic workers. However, the act did extend the federal government's role in public health through several provisions unrelated to social insurance. It gave the states funds on a matching basis for maternal and infant care, rehabilitation of crippled children, general public health work, and aid for dependent children under the age of sixteen.

Hospital Survey and Construction Act of 1946

Passage of the **Hill-Burton Act** was another important development in American healthcare delivery. Enacted in 1946 as the Hospital Survey and Construction Act, this legislation authorized grants for states to construct new hospitals and, later, to modernize old ones. The availability of federal financing created a boom in hospital construction during the 1950s.

Public Law 89-97 of 1965

In 1965, passage of a number of amendments to the Social Security Act brought Medicare and Medicaid into existence. The two programs have greatly changed how healthcare organizations are reimbursed. Recent attempts to curtail Medicare/ Medicaid spending continue to affect healthcare organizations.

Medicare is a federal program that provides healthcare benefits for people sixty-five years old and older who are covered by Social Security. The program was inaugurated on July 1, 1966. Over the years, amendments have extended coverage to individuals who are not covered by Social Security but are willing to pay a premium for coverage, to the disabled, and to those suffering from chronic kidney disease.

Medicaid is a federally mandated program that provides healthcare benefits to low-income people and their children. Medicaid programs are administered and partially paid for by individual states. Medicaid is an umbrella for fifty different state programs designed specifically to serve the poor. Beginning in January 1967, Medicaid provided federal funds to states on a cost-sharing basis to ensure that welfare recipients would be guaranteed medical services. Coverage of four types of care was required: inpatient and outpatient services, other laboratory and X-ray services, physician services, and nursing facility care for persons over the age of twenty-one.

Many enhancements have been made in the years since Medicaid was enacted. Services now include family planning and thirty-one other optional services such as prescription drugs and dental services. With few exceptions, recipients of cash assistance are automatically eligible for Medicaid. Medicaid also pays the Medicare premium, deductible, and co-insurance costs for some low-income Medicare beneficiaries.

An ongoing issue is the number of poor Americans who are not covered by Medicaid, Medicare, or private health insurance. Medicaid covers only about 40 percent of the poor (Jonas and Kovner 1999, p. 40). To address the healthcare needs of those who "fall through the cracks," at least twenty-five states have established bad-debt and charity care pools to pay for services to individuals not covered by any other program.

Public Law 92-603 of 1972

Utilization review was a mandatory component of the original Medicare legislation. Medicare required hospitals and **extended care facilities** to establish a plan for utilization review as well as a permanent utilization review committee. The goal of the utilization review process was to ensure that the services provided to Medicare beneficiaries were medically necessary.

In an effort to curtail Medicare and Medicaid spending, additional amendments to the Social Security Act were instituted in 1972. Public Law 92-603 required concurrent review for Medicare and Medicaid patients. It also established the professional standards review organization (PSRO) program to implement concurrent review. PSROs performed professional review and evaluated patient care services for necessity, quality, and cost-effectiveness.

Utilization Review Act of 1977

In 1977, the **Utilization Review Act** made it a requirement that hospitals conduct continued-stay reviews for Medicare and Medicaid patients. Continued-stay reviews determine whether it is medically necessary for a patient to remain hospitalized. This legislation also included fraud and abuse regulations.

Peer Review Improvement Act of 1982

In 1982, the Peer Review Improvement Act redesigned the PSRO program and renamed the agencies peer review organizations (PROs). At this time, hospitals began to review the medical necessity and appropriateness of certain admissions even before patients were admitted. Peer review organizations were given a new name in 2002 and are now called quality improvement organizations (QIOs). They currently emphasize quality improvement processes. Every state and territory, as well as the District of Columbia, now has its own QIO. The mission of the QIOs is to ensure the quality, efficiency, and cost-effectiveness of the healthcare services provided to Medicare beneficiaries in its locale.

Tax Equity and Fiscal Responsibility Act of 1982

In 1982, Congress passed the **Tax Equity and Fiscal Responsibility Act** (TEFRA). TEFRA required extensive changes in the Medicare program. Its purpose was to control the rising cost of providing healthcare services to Medicare beneficiaries. Before this legislation was passed, healthcare services provided to Medicare beneficiaries were reimbursed on a retrospective, or fee-based, payment system. TEFRA required the gradual implementation of a **prospective payment system** (PPS) for Medicare reimbursement.

In a retrospective payment system, a service is provided, a claim for payment for the service is made, and the healthcare provider is reimbursed for the cost of delivering the service. In a PPS, a predetermined level of reimbursement is established before the services are provided.

Public Law 98-21 of 1983

The PPS for acute hospital care (inpatient) services was implemented on October 1, 1983, according to Public Law 98-21. Under the inpatient PPS, reimbursement for hospital care provided to Medicare patients is based on diagnosis-related groups (DRGs). Each case is assigned to a DRG on the basis of the patient's diagnosis at the time of discharge. For example, under inpatient PPS, all of the cases of viral pneumonia would reimbursed at the same predetermined level of reimbursement no matter how long the patients stayed in the hospital or how many services they received.

Prospective payments systems for other healthcare services provided to Medicare beneficiaries have been gradually implemented in the years since 1983. Implementation of the ambulatory payment classification system for hospital outpatient services, for example, began in the year 2000.

Consolidated Omnibus Budget Reconciliation Act of 1985

The Consolidated Omnibus Budget Reconciliation Act made it possible for the Health Care Financing Administration (HCFA) to deny reimbursement for substandard healthcare services provided to Medicare and Medicaid beneficiaries. (HCFA's name was changed to the Centers for Medicare and Medicaid Services in June 2001.)

Omnibus Budget Reconciliation Act of 1986

The Omnibus Budget Reconciliation Act of 1986 requires peer review organizations to report instances of substandard care to relevant licensing and certification agencies.

Health Care Quality Improvement Act of 1986

The Health Care Quality Improvement Act established the **National Practitioner Data Bank** (NPDB). The purpose of the NPDB is to provide a clearinghouse for information about medical practitioners who have a history of malpractice suits and other quality problems. Hospitals are required to consult the NPDB before granting medical staff privileges to healthcare practitioners. The legislation also established immunity from legal actions for practitioners involved in some peer review activities.

Omnibus Budget Reconciliation Act of 1989

The Omnibus Budget Reconciliation Act of 1989 instituted the Agency for Health Care Policy and Research. The mission of this agency is to develop outcome measures to evaluate the quality of healthcare services.

Omnibus Budget Reconciliation Act of 1990

The Omnibus Budget Reconciliation Act of 1990 requires PROs to report actions taken against physicians to state medical boards and licensing agencies.

Health Insurance Portability and Accountability Act of 1996

The Health Insurance Portability and Accountability Act of 1996 (HIPAA) addresses issues related to the portability of health insurance after leaving employment, as well as administrative simplification. One of the provisions of the Health Insurance Portability and Accountability Act (HIPAA) was the creation of the Healthcare Integrity and Protection Data Bank (HIPDB). The mission of the data bank is to inform federal and state agencies about potential quality problems with clinicians and with suppliers and providers of healthcare services.

Biomedical and Technological Advances in Medicine

Rapid progress in medical science and technology during the late nineteenth and twentieth centuries revolutionized the way healthcare was provided. The most important scientific advancement was the discovery of bacteria as the cause of infectious disease. The most important technological development was the use of anesthesia for surgical procedures. These nineteenth-century advances laid the basis for the development of antibiotics and other pharmaceuticals and the application of sophisticated surgical procedures in the twentieth century. (Figure 2.1 offers a time line of key biological and technological advances at a glance.)

Although surgical procedures were performed before the development of anesthesia, surgeons had to work quickly on conscious patients to minimize risk and pain. The availability of anesthesia made it possible for surgeons to develop

Figure 2.1.   Key Biological and Technological Advances in Medicine

Time	Event
1842	First recorded use of ether as an anesthetic
1860s	Louis Pasteur laid the foundation for modern bacteriology
1865	Joseph Lister was the first to apply Pasteur's research to the treatment of infected wounds
1880s–1890s	Steam first used in physical sterilization
1898	Introduction of rubber surgical gloves, sterilization, and antisepsis
1895	Wilhelm Roentgen made observations that led to the development of X-ray technology
1940	Studies of prothrombin time first made available
1941–1946	Studies of electrolytes; development of major pharmaceuticals
1957	Studies of blood gas
1961	Studies of creatine phosphokinase
1970s	Surgical advances in cardiac bypass surgery, surgery for joint replacements, and organ transplantation
1971	Computed tomography first used in England
1974	Introduction of whole-body scanners
1980s	Introduction of magnetic resonance imaging
1990s	Further technological advances in pharmaceuticals and genetics; Human Genome Project

more advanced surgical techniques. The use of ether as an anesthetic was first recorded in 1842. At about the same time, nitrous oxide was introduced for use during dental procedures, and chloroform was used to reduce the pain of labor. By the 1860s, the physicians who treated the casualties of the American Civil War on both sides had access to anesthetic and pain-killing drugs.

In the 1860s, Louis Pasteur began studying a condition in wine that made it sour and unpalatable. He discovered that the wine was being spoiled by parasitic growths. His research proved that tiny, living organisms (called bacteria) increase through reproduction and cause infectious disease. Pasteur also demonstrated that bacteria can be destroyed by the application of heat and certain chemicals, for example, alcohol. In doing so, he laid the foundation for modern bacteriology. After twenty years of research into the biology of microorganisms, Pasteur began studying human diseases. In 1885, he developed a vaccine that prevented rabies.

Although the importance of cleanliness had been known since early times, the role that microorganisms played in disease was not understood until Pasteur conducted his research. In 1865, Joseph Lister was the first to apply Pasteur's research to the treatment of infected wounds. Lister began by protecting open fractures from infection by treating the wounds with carbolic acid (a disinfectant). His discovery was called the antiseptic principle. Antisepsis reduced the mortality rate in Lister's hospital after 1865 from 45 to 12 percent. He published his results in 1868, and soon carbolic acid was being used to prevent bacterial contamination during surgery.

During the 1880s and 1890s, physical sterilization through the use of steam was developed. This technological advance had a major impact on surgery and in other areas throughout the hospital. The sterile operative technique was further advanced through the introduction of rubber surgical gloves in 1898. Other advances included the use of sterile gowns, masks, and antibiotics and other drugs.

In 1895, the well-known physicist Wilhelm Roentgen made observations that led to the development of X-ray technology. He found that he could create images of the bones in his hand by passing X rays through his hand and onto a photographic plate. Radiographic technology is used extensively to diagnose illnesses and injuries today.

Many advances in laboratory testing occurred during the twentieth century. Equipment that allows the rapid laboratory processing of diagnostic and prognostic examinations was developed, and the number of diagnostic laboratory procedures increased dramatically. For example, studies of prothrombin time were first made available in 1940, electrolytes in 1941 through 1946, blood gas in 1957, creatine phosphokinase in 1961, serum hepatitis in 1970, and carcinoembryonic antigen (the first cancer-screening test) in 1974.

Diagnostic radiology and radiation therapy have undergone huge advances in the past fifty years. An enormous advance first used in 1971 in England is an imaging modality called computed tomography (CT). The first CT scanners were used to create images of the skull. Whole-body scanners were introduced in 1974. In the 1980s, another powerful diagnostic tool was added, magnetic resonance imaging (MRI). Magnetic resonance imaging is a noninvasive technique that uses magnetic and radio-frequency fields to record images of soft tissues.

Surgical advances have been remarkable as well. Cardiac bypass surgery was developed in the 1970s, as were the techniques for joint replacement. Organs are now successfully transplanted, and artificial organs are being tested. New surgical techniques have included the use of lasers in ophthalmology, gynecology, and urology. Microsurgery is now a common tool in the reconstruction of damaged nerves and blood vessels. The use of robotics in surgery holds great promise for the future (Sloane et al. 1999, pp. 6–7).

Check Your Understanding 2.2

Instructions: Match the descriptions with the appropriate legislation.

1. ___ Hill-Burton Act
2. ___ Tax Equity and Fiscal Responsibility Act
3. ___ Public Law 89-79 of 1965
4. ___ Utilization Review Act
5. ___ Omnibus Budget Reconciliation Act of 1989
6. ___ Public Law 92-603 of 1972
7. ___ Health Care Quality Improvement Act of 1986
8. ___ Omnibus Budget Reconciliation Act of 1990

a. Amendments to the Social Security Act that brought Medicare and Medicaid into existence

b. Authorized grants for states to construct new hospitals

c. Required concurrent review for Medicare and Medicaid patients

d. Required hospitals to conduct continued stay reviews for Medicare and Medicaid patients

e. Established the National Practitioner Data Bank

f. Required peer review organizations to report actions taken against physicians to state medical boards and licensing agencies

g. Required extensive changes in the Medicare program to control the rising cost of providing healthcare services to Medicare beneficiaries (PPS general implementation)

h. Instituted the Agency for Health Care Policy

Professional and Trade Associations Related to Healthcare

A number of trade and professional associations currently influence the practice of medicine and the delivery of healthcare services in the United States. Descriptions of a few of the numerous healthcare-related professional and trade associations that currently influence healthcare issues are provided below.

American Medical Association

The American Medical Association (AMA) was founded in 1847 as a national voluntary service organization. Today, its membership totals approximately 300,000 physicians from every area of medicine. The organization is headquartered in Chicago. Its mission is to promote the science and art of medicine and to improve public health. Its key objectives are these:

- To become the world leader in obtaining, synthesizing, integrating, and disseminating information on health and medical practice
- To remain the acknowledged leader in promoting professionalism in medicine and setting standards for medical ethics, practice, and education
- To continue to be an authoritative voice and influential advocate for patients and physicians
- To continue to be a sound organization that provides value to members, related organizations, and employees

In addition, the AMA acts as an accreditation body for medical schools and residency programs. It also maintains and publishes the *Current Procedural Terminology* (CPT) coding system. CPT codes are used as the basis of reimbursement systems for physician's services and other types of healthcare services provided on an ambulatory basis.

American Hospital Association

The **American Hospital Association** (AHA) was founded in 1899. At its first meeting, eight hospital superintendents gathered in Cleveland, Ohio, to exchange ideas, compare methods of hospital management, discuss economics, and explore common interests and new trends. The original group was called the Association of Hospital Superintendents. Its mission was "to facilitate the interchange of ideas, comparing and contrasting methods of management, the discussion of hospital economics, the inspection of hospitals, suggestions of better plans for operating them, and such other matters as may affect the general interest of the membership" (AHA 1999, p. 110).

The association adopted a new constitution in 1906 and a new name, the American Hospital Association. At that time, it had 234 members. Its major concerns were developing hospital standards and building the management skills of it members.

Today, the mission of the AHA is to advance the health of individuals and communities. The association has a current membership of approximately 5,000 hospitals and healthcare institutions, 600 associate member organizations, and 40,000 individual executives active in the healthcare field. The association's headquarters are located in Chicago.

The AHA publishes *Coding Clinic,* which provides official ICD-9-CM coding advice.

Joint Commission on Accreditation of Healthcare Organizations

Since its beginning in 1952, the Joint Commission has continually evolved to meet the changing needs of healthcare organizations. The organization changed its name from the Joint Commission on Accreditation of Hospitals (JCAH) to the Joint Commission on Accreditation of Healthcare Organizations (JCAHO) in the late 1980s in recognition of changes in the U.S. health delivery system. Today, the JCAHO is the largest healthcare standards-setting body in the world. It conducts accreditation surveys in more than 19,500 facilities, including ambulatory care facilities, long-term care facilities, behavioral health facilities, healthcare networks, and managed care organizations as well as acute care hospitals (JCAHO 2000).

In the late 1990s, the JCAHO moved away from traditional quality assessment processes and began emphasizing performance and quality improvement. The ORYX initiative reflected the new approach. The goal of the ORYX initiative was to incorporate the ongoing collection of quality and performance data into the accreditation process.

Today, the JCAHO's standards give organizations substantial leeway in selecting performance measures and improvement projects. Outcome measures document the results of care for individual patients as well as for specific types of patients grouped by diagnostic category. For example, an acute care hospital's overall rate of postsurgical infection would be considered an outcome measure. The outcome measures must be reported to the JCAHO via software from vendors that have been approved by the JCAHO for this purpose.

Blue Cross and Blue Shield Association

The forerunner of the **Blue Cross and Blue Shield Association** was a commission instituted by the AHA in 1939. In 1960, the commission was replaced by the Blue Cross Association and ties to the AHA were broken. In 1982, the Blue Cross Association merged with the National Association of Blue Shield Plans to become the Blue Cross and Blue Shield Association, often referred to as "the Blues."

The organization is the trade association for forty-seven locally operated Blue Cross and Blue Shield plans in the United States and Puerto Rico. The association's purpose is to coordinate the activities of the local plans. The association is headquartered in Chicago. Today, approximately 25 percent of the American population is enrolled in Blue Cross and Blue Shield health insurance plans.

American College of Healthcare Executives

The **American College of Healthcare Executives** (ACHE) is an organization for healthcare administrators. Like most of the organizations already discussed, it is headquartered in Chicago. Its mission is to serve as "the professional membership society for healthcare executives; to meet members' professional, educational, and leadership needs; to promote high ethical standards and conduct; and to enhance healthcare leadership and management excellence."

ACHE has nearly 30,000 members internationally. It also publishes books and textbooks on healthcare services management.

American Nurses Association

The **American Nurses Association** (ANA) was founded in 1897. It is headquartered in Washington, D.C. The ANA is a professional association as well as the strongest labor union active in the nursing profession. It represents the interests of the nation's 2.6 million registered nurses. The ANA's mission is to work for the improvement of health standards and the availability of healthcare services, to foster high professional standards for nurses, to stimulate and promote the professional development of nurses, and to advance the economic and general welfare of its members.

American Health Information Management Association

The **American Health Information Management Association** (AHIMA) is the professional membership organization for managers of health record services and healthcare information. It was founded in 1928 under the name of the Association of Record Librarians of North America. In 1929, the association adopted a constitution and bylaws. The name of the association was changed to the American Medical Record Association in 1970 and then to the American Health Information Management Association in 1991.

Today, with headquarters in Chicago, the association has more than 40,000 members. Its mission is to be a "community of professionals engaged in health information management, providing support to members and strengthening the industry and profession." The association's vision is of "a world in which the public values the contribution of health information management professionals and the American Health Information Management Association, in the advancement of health through quality information."

The association accredits two-year, four-year, and master's-level programs in health information management. It also certifies health information professionals as registered health information technologists (RHITs) for graduates of two-year programs and registered health information administrators (RHIAs) for graduates of baccalaureate programs. In addition, the AHIMA offers credentialing examinations for coding professionals as certified coding specialists (CCSs) and certified coding specialists for physicians' services (CCS-Ps).

Other Healthcare-Related Associations

Many other healthcare-related associations in the United States serve their professional members by providing educational, certification, and accreditation services. The best known include the following:

- The American Osteopathic Association
- The American Dental Association
- The American College of Surgeons
- The American League for Nursing
- The American Society of Clinical Pathologists
- The American Dietetic Association
- The Commission on Accreditation of Rehabilitation Facilities
- The American Association of Nurse Anesthetists

Check Your Understanding 2.3

Instructions: Match each organization with the description that best describes it.

1. ___ American College of Healthcare Executives
2. ___ American Hospital Association
3. ___ American Medical Association
4. ___ American Nurses Association
5. ___ American Health Information Management Association
6. ___ Blue Cross and Blue Shield Association

a. Part of this organization's mission is to "enhance healthcare leadership and management excellence."

b. This organization was originally called the Association of Hospital Superintendents.

c. This organization was originally a commission instituted by the AHA in 1939.

d. This association was founded in 1928 under the name of the Association of Record Librarians of North America.

e. Part of this organization's mission is to work for the improvement of health standards and the availability of healthcare services.

f. This organization's mission is to promote the art and science of medicine and to improve public health.

Organization and Operation of Modern Hospitals

The term *hospital* can be applied to any healthcare facility that has the following four characteristics:

- An organized medical staff
- Permanent inpatient beds
- Around-the-clock nursing services
- Diagnostic and therapeutic services

Most hospitals provide acute care services to inpatients. **Acute care** is the short-term care provided to diagnose and/or treat an illness or injury. The individuals who receive acute care services in hospitals are considered inpatients. Inpatients receive room-and-board services in addition to continuous nursing services. Generally, patients who spend more than twenty-four hours in a hospital are considered inpatients.

The **average length of stay** (ALOS) in an acute care hospital is thirty days or less. (Hospitals that have ALOSs longer than thirty days are considered long-term care facilities. Long-term care is discussed in detail later in this chapter.) With recent advances in surgical technology, anesthesia, and pharmacology, the ALOS in an acute care hospital is much shorter today than it was only a few years ago. In addition, many diagnostic and therapeutic procedures that once required inpatient care can now be performed on an outpatient basis.

For example, before the development of laparoscopic surgical techniques, a patient might be hospitalized for ten days after a routine appendectomy (surgical removal of the appendix). Today, a patient undergoing a laparoscopic appendectomy might spend only a few hours in the hospital's outpatient surgery department and go home the same day. The influence of managed care and the emphasis on cost control in the Medicare/Medicaid programs also have resulted in shorter hospital stays.

In large acute care hospitals, hundreds of clinicians, administrators, managers, and support staff must work closely together to provide effective and efficient diagnostic and therapeutic services. Most hospitals provide services to both inpatients and outpatients. A hospital outpatient is a patient who receives hospital services without being admitted for inpatient (overnight) clinical care. Outpatient care is considered a kind of ambulatory care. (Ambulatory care is discussed later in this chapter.)

Modern hospitals are extremely complex organizations. Much of the clinical training for physicians, nurses, and allied health professionals is conducted in hospitals. Medical research is another activity carried out in hospitals.

Types of Hospitals

Hospitals can be classified in many different ways, including the following:

- Number of beds
- Type of services provided
- Type of patients served

- For-profit or not-for-profit status
- Type of ownership

Number of Beds

A hospital's number of beds is based on the number of beds that it has equipped and staffed for patient care. The term *bed capacity* is sometimes used to reflect the maximum number of inpatients the hospital can care for. Hospitals with fewer than a hundred beds are usually considered small. Most of the hospitals in the United States fall into this category. Some large, urban hospitals may have more than five hundred beds. The number of beds is usually broken down by adult beds and pediatric beds. The number of maternity beds and other special categories may be listed separately. Hospitals also can be categorized on the basis of the number of outpatient visits per year.

Type of Services Provided

Some hospitals specialize in certain types of service and treat specific illnesses. For example:

- Rehabilitation hospitals generally provide long-term care services to patients recuperating from debilitating or chronic illnesses and injuries such as strokes, head and spine injuries, and gunshot wounds. Patients often stay in rehabilitation hospitals for several months.
- Psychiatric hospitals provide inpatient care for patients with mental and developmental disorders. In the past, the ALOS for psychiatric inpatients was longer than it is today. Rather than months or years, most patients now spend only a few days or weeks per stay. However, many patients require repeated hospitalization for chronic psychiatric illnesses. (Behavioral healthcare is discussed in more detail later in this chapter.)
- General hospitals provide a wide range of medical and surgical services to diagnose and treat most illnesses and injuries.
- Specialty hospitals provide diagnostic and therapeutic services for a limited range of conditions, for example, burns, cancer, tuberculosis, or obstetrics/gynecology.

Type of Patients Served

Some hospitals specialize in serving specific types of patients. For example, children's hospitals provide specialized pediatric services in a number of medical specialties.

For-Profit or Not-for-Profit Status

Hospitals also can be classified on the basis of their ownership and profitability status. Not-for profit healthcare organizations use excess funds to improve their services and to finance educational programs and community services. For-profit healthcare organizations are privately owned. Excess funds are paid back to the managers, owners, and investors in the form of bonuses and dividends.

Type of Ownership

The most common ownership types for hospitals and other kinds of healthcare organizations in the United States include the following:

- Government-owned hospitals are operated by a specific branch of federal, state, or local government as not-for-profit organizations. (Government-owned hospitals are sometimes called public hospitals.) They are supported, at least in part, by tax dollars. Examples of federally owned and operated hospitals include those operated by the Department of Veterans Affairs to serve retired military personnel. The Department of Defense operates facilities for active military personnel and their dependents. Many states own and operate psychiatric hospitals. County and city governments often operate public hospitals to serve the healthcare needs of their communities, especially those residents who are unable to pay for their care.
- Proprietary hospitals may be owned by private foundations, partnerships, or investor-owned corporations. Large corporations may own a number of for-profit hospitals, and the stock of several large U.S. hospital chains is publicly traded.
- Voluntary hospitals are not-for-profit hospitals owned by universities, churches, charities, religious orders, unions, and other not-for-profit entities. They often provide free care to patients who otherwise would not have access to healthcare services.

Organization of Hospital Services

The organizational structure of every hospital is designed to meet its specific needs. For example, most acute care hospitals are made up of a board of directors, a professional medical staff, an executive administrative staff, medical and surgical services, patient care (nursing) services, diagnostic and laboratory services, and support services (for example, nutritional services, environmental safety, and health information management services).

Board of Directors

The board of directors has primary responsibility for setting the overall direction of the hospital. (In some hospitals, the board of directors is called the governing board or board of trustees.) The board works with the chief executive officer (CEO) and the leaders of the organization's medical staff to develop the hospital's strategic direction as well as its **mission,** vision, and values:

- *Mission:* A statement of the organization's purpose and the customers it serves
- *Vision:* A description of the organization's ideal future
- *Values:* A descriptive list of the organization's fundamental principles or beliefs

Other specific responsibilities of the board of directors include the following:

- Establishing bylaws in accordance with the organization's legal and licensing requirements
- Selecting qualified administrators
- Approving the organization and makeup of the clinical staff
- Monitoring the quality of care

The board's members are elected for specific terms of service (for example, five years). Most boards also elect officers, commonly a chairman, vice-chairman, president, secretary, and treasurer. The size of the board varies considerably. Individual board members are called directors, board members, or trustees. Individuals serve on one or more standing committees such as the executive committee, joint conference committee, finance committee, strategic planning committee, and building committee.

The makeup of the board depends on the type of hospital and the form of ownership. For example, the board of a community hospital is likely to include local business leaders, representatives of community organizations, and other people interested in the welfare of the community. The board of a teaching hospital, on the other hand, is likely to include medical school alumni and university administrators, among others.

Increased competition among healthcare providers and limits on managed care and Medicare/Medicaid reimbursement have made the governing of hospitals especially difficult during the past two decades. In the future, boards of directors will continue to face strict accountability in terms of cost containment, performance management, and integration of services to maintain fiscal stability and to ensure the delivery of high-quality patient care.

Medical Staff

The medical staff consists of physicians who have received extensive training in various medical disciplines (for example, internal medicine, pediatrics, cardiology, gynecology/obstetrics, orthopedics, and surgery). The medical staff's primary objective is to provide high-quality patient care to the patients who come to the hospital. The physicians on the hospital's medical staff diagnose illnesses and develop patient-centered treatment regimens. Moreover, physicians on the medical staff may serve on the hospital's governing board, where they provide critical insight relevant to strategic and operational planning and policy making.

The medical staff is the aggregate of physicians who have been granted permission to provide clinical services in the hospital. This permission is called **clinical privileges.** An individual physician's privileges are limited to a specific scope of practice. For example, an internal medicine physician would be permitted to diagnose and treat a patient with pneumonia but not to perform a surgical procedure. Most members of the medical staff are not actually employees of the hospital. However, many hospitals do directly employ radiologists, anesthesiologists, and critical care specialists.

Medical staff classification refers to the organization of physicians according to clinical assignment. Depending on the size of the hospital and on the credentials and clinical privileges of its physicians, the medical staff may be separated into departments such as medicine, surgery, obstetrics, pediatrics, and other specialty services. Typical medical staff classifications include active, provisional, honorary, consulting, courtesy, and medical resident assignments.

Officers of the medical staff usually include a president or chief of staff, a vice-president or chief of staff-elect, and a secretary. These offices are authorized by vote of the entire active medical staff. The president presides at all regular meetings of the medical staff and is an ex officio member of all medical staff committees. The secretary ensures that accurate and complete minutes of medical staff meetings are maintained and that correspondence is handled appropriately.

The medical staff operates according to a predetermined set of policies. These policies are called the **medical staff bylaws.** The bylaws spell out the specific qualifications that physicians must demonstrate before they can practice medicine in the hospital. The bylaws are considered legally binding. Any changes to the bylaws must be approved by a vote of the medical staff and the hospital's governing body.

Administrative Staff

The leader of the administrative staff is the **chief executive officer** (CEO) or chief administrator. The CEO is responsible for implementing the policies and strategic direction set by the hospital's board of directors. He or she also is responsible for building an effective executive management team and coordinating the hospital's services. Today's healthcare organizations commonly designate a chief financial officer (CFO), a chief operating officer (COO), and a chief information officer (CIO) as members of the executive management team.

The executive management team is responsible for managing the hospital's finances and ensuring that the hospital complies with the federal, state, and local rules, standards, and laws that govern the delivery of healthcare services. Depending on the size of the hospital, the CEO's staff may include healthcare administrators with job titles such as vice-president, associate administrator, department director or manager, or administrative assistant. Department-level administrators manage and coordinate the activities of the highly specialized and multidisciplinary units that perform clinical, administrative, and support services in the hospital.

Healthcare administrators may hold advanced degrees in healthcare administration, nursing, public health, or business management. A growing number of hospitals are hiring physician executives to lead their executive management teams. Many healthcare administrators are fellows of the American College of Health Care Executives (ACHE).

Patient Care Services

Most of the direct patient care delivered in hospitals is provided by professional nurses. Modern nursing requires a diverse skill set, advanced clinical competencies, and postgraduate education. In almost every hospital, patient care services constitutes the largest clinical department in terms of staffing, budget, specialized services offered, and clinical expertise required.

Nurses are responsible for providing continuous, around-the-clock treatment and support for hospital inpatients. The quantity and quality of nursing care available to patients are influenced by a number of factors, including the nursing staff's educational preparation and specialization, experience, and skill level. The level of patient care staffing is also a critical component of quality.

Traditionally, physicians alone determined the type of treatment each patient would receive. However, today's nurses are playing a wider role in treatment planning and **case management.** They identify timely and effective interventions in response to a wide range of problems related to the patients' treatment, comfort, and safety. Their responsibilities include performing patient assessments, creating care plans, evaluating the appropriateness of treatment, and evaluating the effectiveness of care. At the same time that they provide technical care, effective nursing professionals also offer personal caring that recognizes the patients' concerns and the emotional needs of patients and their families.

A registered nurse qualified by advanced education and clinical and management experience usually administers patient care services. Although the title may vary, this role is usually referred to as the **chief nursing officer** (CNO) or vice-president of nursing or patient care. The CNO is a member of the hospital's executive management team and usually reports directly to the CEO.

In any nursing organizational structure, several types of relationships can be identified, including the following:

- Line relationships identify the positions of superiors and subordinates and indicate the levels of authority and responsibility vested with each position. For example, a supervisor in a postop surgical unit would have authority to direct the work of several nurses.
- Lateral relationships define the connections among various positions in which a hierarchy of authority is not involved. For example, the supervisors of preop and postop surgical units would have parallel positions in the structure and would need to coordinate the work they perform.
- Functional relationships refer to duties that are divided according to function. In such arrangements, individuals exercise authority in one particular area by virtue of their special knowledge and expertise.

Diagnostic and Therapeutic Services

The services provided to patients in hospitals go beyond the clinical services provided directly by the medical and nursing staff. Many diagnostic and therapeutic services involve the work of allied health professionals. Allied health professionals receive specialized education and training, and their qualifications are registered or certified by a number of specialty organizations.

Diagnostic and therapeutic services are critical to the success of every patient care delivery system. Diagnostic services include clinical laboratory, radiology, and nuclear medicine. Therapeutic services include radiation therapy, occupational therapy, and physical therapy.

Clinical Laboratory Services

The clinical laboratory is divided into two sections: anatomic pathology and clinical pathology. *Anatomic pathology* deals with human tissues and provides surgical pathology, autopsy, and cytology services. *Clinical pathology* deals mainly with the analysis of body fluids, principally blood, but also urine, gastric contents, and cerebrospinal fluid.

Physicians who specialize in performing and interpreting the results of pathology tests are called pathologists. Laboratory technicians are allied health professionals trained to operate laboratory equipment and perform laboratory tests under the supervision of a pathologist.

Radiology

Radiology involves the use of radioactive isotopes, fluoroscopic and radiographic equipment, and CT and MRI equipment to diagnose disease. Physicians who specialize in radiology are called radiologists. They are experts in the medical use of radiant energy, radioactive isotopes, radium, cesium, and cobalt as well as X rays, radium, and radioactive materials. They also are expert in interpreting X-ray, MRI, and CT diagnostic images.

Radiology technicians are allied health professionals trained to operate radiological equipment and perform radiological tests under the supervision of a radiologist.

Nuclear Medicine and Radiation Therapy

Radiologists also may specialize in nuclear medicine and radiation therapy. Nuclear medicine involves the use of ionizing radiation and small amounts of short-lived radioactive tracers to treat disease, specifically neoplastic disease (that is, nonmalignant tumors and malignant cancers). Based on the mathematics and physics of tracer methodology, nuclear medicine is widely applied in clinical medicine. However, most authorities agree that medical science has only scratched the surface in terms of nuclear medicine's potential capabilities.

Radiation therapy uses high-energy X rays, cobalt, electrons, and other sources of radiation to treat human disease. In current practice, radiation therapy is used alone or in combination with surgery or chemotherapy (drugs) to treat many types of cancer. In addition to external beam therapy, radioactive implants, as well as therapy performed with heat (hyperthermia), are available.

Occupational Therapy

Occupational therapy is the medically directed use of work and play activities to improve patients' independent functioning, enhance their development, and prevent or decrease their level of disability. The individuals who perform occupational therapy are credentialed allied health professionals called occupational therapists. They work under the direction of physicians. Occupational therapy is made available in acute care hospitals, clinics, and rehabilitation centers.

Providing occupational therapy services begins with an evaluation of the patient and the selection of therapeutic goals. Occupational therapy activities may involve the adaptation of tasks or the environment to achieve maximum independence and to enhance the patient's quality of life. An occupational therapist may treat developmental deficits, birth defects, learning disabilities, traumatic injuries, burns, neurological conditions, orthopedic conditions, mental deficiencies, and psychiatric disorders. Within the healthcare system, occupational therapy plays various roles. These roles include promoting health, preventing disability, developing or restoring functional capacity, guiding adaptation within physical and mental parameters, and teaching creative problem solving to increase independent function.

Physical Therapy and Rehabilitation
Physical therapy and rehabilitation have expanded into many medical specialties. Physical therapy can be applied in most disciplines of medicine, especially in neurology, neurosurgery, orthopedics, geriatrics, rheumatology, internal medicine, cardiovascular medicine, cardiopulmonary medicine, psychiatry, sports medicine, burn and wound care, and chronic pain management. It also plays a role in community health education. Credentialed allied health professionals administer physical therapy under the direction of physicians.

Medical **rehabilitation services** involve the entire healthcare team: physicians, nurses, social workers, occupational therapists, physical therapists, and other healthcare personnel. The objective is to either eliminate the patients' disability or alleviate it as fully as possible. Physical therapy can be used to improve the cognitive, social, and physical abilities of patients impaired by chronic disease or injury.

The primary purpose of physical therapy in rehabilitation is to promote optimal health and function by applying scientific principles. Treatment modalities include therapeutic exercise, therapeutic massage, biofeedback, and applications of heat, low-energy lasers, cold, water, electricity, and ultrasound.

Respiratory Therapy
Respiratory therapy involves the diagnosis and treatment of patients who have acute and/or chronic lung disorders. Respiratory therapists work under the direction of qualified physicians and surgeons. The therapists provide such services as emergency care for stroke, heart failure, and shock patients. They also treat patients with chronic respiratory diseases such as emphysema and asthma.

Respiratory treatments include the administration of oxygen and inhalants such as bronchodialators. They set up and monitor ventilatory equipment and provide physiotherapy to improve breathing.

Ancillary Support Services
The ancillary units of the hospital provide vital clinical and administrative support services to patients, medical staff, visitors, and employees.

Clinical Support Services
The clinical support units provide the following services:

- Pharmaceutical services
- Food and nutrition services
- Health information management (health record) services
- Social work and social services
- Patient advocacy services

- Environmental (housekeeping) services
- Purchasing, central supply, and materials management services
- Engineering and plant operations

Health information management services are managed by registered health information administrators (RHIA) and registered health information technicians (RHIT). The pharmacy is staffed by registered pharmacists and pharmacy technologists. Food and nutrition services are managed by registered dieticians, who develop general menus, special diet menus, and nutritional plans for individual patients. Social work services are provided by licensed social workers and licensed clinical social workers. Patient advocacy services may be provided by several types of healthcare professionals, most commonly, registered nurses and licensed social workers.

Administrative Support Services
In addition to clinical support services, hospitals need administrative support services to operate effectively. Administrative support services provide business management and clerical services in several key areas, including:

- Admissions and central registration
- Claims and billing (business office)
- Accounting
- Information services
- Human resources
- Public relations
- Fund development
- Marketing

Check Your Understanding 2.4

Instructions: Indicate whether the statements below are true or false (T or F).

1. ___ Ambulatory care is the short-term care provided to diagnose and/or treat an illness or injury.

2. ___ The influence of managed care and the emphasis on cost control in the Medicare/Medicaid programs have resulted in shorter hospital stays.

3. ___ Hospitals can be classified on the basis of their ownership and profitability status.

4. ___ Government hospitals are operated by a specific branch of federal, state, or local government as for-profit organizations.

5. ___ The board of directors has primary responsibility for setting the overall direction of the hospital.

6. ___ Medical staff classification refers to the organization of physicians according to clinical assignment.

7. ___ A registered nurse qualified by advanced education and clinical and management experience usually administers diagnostic services.

8. ___ Physicians who specialize in radiology are called radiology technicians.

9. ___ Occupational therapy is made available in acute care hospitals, clinics, and rehab centers.

10. ___ The ancillary units of the hospital provide vital clinical and administrative support services to patients, medical staff, visitors, and employees.

Forces Affecting Hospitals

A number of recent developments in healthcare delivery have had far-reaching effects on the operation of hospitals in the United States.

Growth of Subacute Care

Subacute care has come to represent a new movement in healthcare. In the past, the term was used in reference to the services provided to hospitalized patients who did not meet the medical criteria for needing acute care. Today, it refers to the level of skilled care needed by patients with complex medical conditions, typically Medicare patients who have multiple medical problems.

Traditionally, nursing homes, home care providers, and rehabilitation facilities have provided subacute care. Now some hospitals are developing subacute units in response to changing demographics that make it a cost-effective alternative to inpatient acute care.

Development of Peer Review and Quality Improvement Programs

The goal of high-quality patient care is to promote, preserve, and restore health. High-quality care is delivered in an appropriate setting in a manner that is satisfying to patients. It is achieved when the patient's health status is improved as much as possible. Quality has several components, including the following:

- Appropriateness (the right care is provided at the right time)
- Technical excellence (the right care is provided in the right manner)
- Accessibility (the right care can be obtained when it is needed)
- Acceptability (the patients are satisfied)

Peer Review

In peer review, a member of a profession assesses the work of colleagues within that same profession. Peer review has traditionally been at the center of quality assessment and assurance efforts. The medical profession's peer review efforts have emphasized the scientific aspects of quality. Appropriate use of pharmaceuticals, postoperative infection rates, and accuracy of diagnosis are among the measures of quality that have been used.

Peer review is a requirement of the Centers for Medicare and Medicaid Services (CMS), as well as of the Joint Commission on Accreditation of Healthcare Organizations (JCAHO).

Quality Improvement

Quality improvement (QI) programs have been in place in hospitals for years and have been required by the Medicare/Medicaid programs and accreditation standards. QI programs have covered medical staff as well as nursing and other departments or processes.

Efforts to encourage the delivery of high-quality care take place at the local and national levels. Such efforts are geared toward assessing the efforts of both individuals and institutions. Currently, professional associations, healthcare organizations, government agencies, private external quality review associations, consumer groups, managed care organizations, and group purchasers of care all play a role in trying to promote high-quality care.

Growth of Managed Care

Managed care is a generic term for a healthcare reimbursement system that manages cost, quality, and access to services. Most managed care plans do not provide healthcare directly. Instead, they enter into service contracts with the physicians, hospitals, and other healthcare providers who provide medical services to enrollees in the plans.

Managed care systems control costs primarily by presetting payment amounts and restricting patient access to healthcare services through precertification and utilization review processes. (Managed care is discussed in more detail in chapter 14.) Managed care delivery systems also attempt to manage cost and quality by:

- Implementing various forms of financial incentives for providers
- Promoting healthy lifestyles
- Identifying risk factors and illnesses early in the disease process
- Providing patient education

Although the most recent studies suggest that managed care results in lower costs with equal or better quality, most are limited because they have focused on short-term health outcomes (Weinerman et al. 1996, p. 1037). Very little is known about the long-term effects of specific reimbursement or organizational arrangements on quality of care. Further, recent evidence indicates that the quality of care provided under managed care systems may differ across population groups.

Efforts at Healthcare Reengineering

During the 1980s, healthcare organizations adopted **continuous quality improvement** (CQI) processes. Lessons learned from other areas of business were applied to healthcare settings. **Reengineering** came in many varieties, such as focused process improvement, major business process improvement and business process innovation, total quality management, and CQI. Regardless of its approach, every healthcare organization attempted to look inside and think "process" as opposed to traditional "department" thinking. Healthcare organizations formed cross-functional teams that collaborated to solve organizational problems. At the same time, JCAHO reengineered the accreditation process to increase its focus on process and systems analysis. Gone were the days of thinking in a "silo." All of those silos were turned over, and healthcare teams learned from each other. The drivers of reengineering included cost reduction, staff shortages, and automation.

Emphasis on Patient-Focused Care

Patient-focused care is a concept developed to contain hospital inpatient costs and improve quality by restructuring services so that more of them take place in the nursing units (patient floors) and not in specialized units in dispersed hospital locations. The emphasis is on cross-training staff in the nursing units to perform a variety of functions for a small group of patients rather than one set of functions for a large number of patients. Some organizations have achieved patient-focused care by assigning multiskilled workers to serve food, clean patients' rooms, and assist in nursing care. However, some organizations have experienced low patient satisfaction with this type of worker because the patients are confused and do not know who to ask to do what.

Hospital staff spend most of their time performing activities in the following nine categories:

- Medical, technical, and clinical procedures
- Hotel and patient services
- Medical documentation
- Institutional documentation
- Scheduling and coordination
- Patient transportation
- Staff transportation
- Management and supervision
- Ready-for-action activities

A study at Lakeland Regional Medical Center, a 750-bed hospital in central Florida, found that medical, technical, and clinical activity consumed one-sixth of the center's personnel-related costs. The study also showed that almost twice that amount of time was spent on writing things down. Scheduling and coordination took as much time as medical activity, and ready-for-action activities consumed even more.

The study suggested that restructuring services at Lakeland would reduce the number of staff required for patient care activities from 2,200 to 1,200 and improve care. The amount of physical space allotted to each unit would be sufficient to contain a minilab, diagnostic radiology rooms, linen and general supply, stockrooms, and so on. If such changes were carried out, medical documentation could be reduced by almost two-thirds, scheduling and coordination service by more than two-thirds, and ready-for-action time by two-thirds.

Hospitals have had difficulty in fully and rapidly implementing patient-focused care for the following reasons: the high cost of conversion; the extensive physical renovations required; resistance from functional departments; and other priorities for management, such as mergers and considering potential mergers.

Development of Integrated Healthcare Delivery Systems

Managed care and healthcare organization integration have placed enormous pressure on information systems. The need for cost data, as well as the integration of data from the various components of integrated systems, have placed many demands on systems technology and personnel. A healthcare provider that cannot completely analyze the cost of delivery when dealing with an insurer is at a distinct disadvantage. Similarly, an inability to integrate patient data across a system can produce increased costs and inefficiencies.

The role of computers has changed rapidly in healthcare organizations, just as it has in many service organizations. The more advanced systems, once called data-processing centers, became management information systems. As computer operations became more powerful and complex, it became possible to think about creating new services or greatly improving existing ones. Innovations were considered strategic uses of information systems because they helped an organization to compete or achieve its goals. Hospitals and integrated health systems have begun to use computers to serve in new functions. For example, a hospital can offer physicians the opportunity to connect to its computer system. Thanks to virtual private networks, a physician can connect to an integrated health system's intranet and work within the system in a private and secure environment without worrying about the downtime often experienced on the Internet.

Check Your Understanding 2.5

Instructions: Choose the best terms to complete the following sentences.

1. ___ Today, ___ refers to the level of skilled care needed by patients with complex medical conditions, typically Medicare patients who have multiple medical problems.
   a. Acute care
   b. Ambulatory care
   c. Subacute care
   d. High-quality care

2. ___ Quality has several components, including appropriateness, technical excellence, ___, and acceptability.
   a. Accuracy of diagnosis
   b. Continuous improvement
   c. Connectivity
   d. Accessibility

3. ___ ___ is at the center of quality improvement efforts.
   a. Quality assurance
   b. Peer review
   c. Managed care
   d. Continuous quality improvement

4. ___ ___ is a generic term for a healthcare reimbursement system that manages cost, quality, and access to services.
   a. Quality improvement
   b. Subacute care
   c. Managed care
   d. Patient-focused care

5. ___ Recent evidence indicates that the quality of care provided under managed care systems may differ across ___.
   a. Population groups
   b. Healthcare settings
   c. Medical facilities
   d. Integrated delivery systems

6. ___ ___ attempts to contain hospital inpatient costs and improve
quality by restructuring services.
   a. Continuous quality improvement
   b. Patient-focused care
   c. Managed care
   d. Acute care

7. ___ Managed care and healthcare organization integration have placed
enormous pressure on ___.
   a. Integrated delivery systems
   b. Acute care facilities
   c. Rehabilitation facilities
   d. Information systems

8. ___ The role of ___ has changed rapidly in healthcare organizations,
just as it has in many service organizations.
   a. Reengineering
   b. Computers
   c. Quality improvement programs
   d. Peer review efforts

Other Types of Healthcare Services

Thus far, this chapter has focused primarily on acute care
services delivered for the most part in the hospital setting.
However, healthcare delivery is more than hospital-related
care. It can be viewed as a continuum of services that cuts
across services delivered in ambulatory, acute, subacute,
long-term, residential, and other care environments. This section describes several of the alternatives for healthcare delivery along this continuum.

Ambulatory Care

Ambulatory care can be defined as:

> The preventive and/or corrective healthcare provided in a practi-
> tioner's office, a clinic, or a hospital on a nonresident (outpatient)
> basis. The term usually implies that patients go to locations outside
> their homes to obtain healthcare services and return the same day.

It encompasses all of the health services provided to individual patients who are not residents in a healthcare facility.
Such services include the educational services provided by
community health clinics and public health departments. Primary care, emergency care, and ambulatory specialty care
(which includes ambulatory surgery) can all be considered
ambulatory care. Ambulatory care services are provided in a
variety of settings, including urgent care centers, school-
based clinics, public health clinics, and neighborhood and
community health centers.

Current medical practice emphasizes performing healthcare services in the least costly setting possible. This change
in thinking has led to decreased utilization of emergency
services, increased utilization of nonemergency ambulatory
facilities, decreased hospital admissions, and shorter hospital
stays. The need to reduce the cost of healthcare also has led
primary care physicians to treat conditions they once would
have referred to specialists.

Physicians who provide ambulatory care services fall into
two major categories: physicians working in private practice

and physicians working for ambulatory care organizations.
Physicians in private practice are self-employed. They work
in solo, partnership, and group practices set up as for-profit
organizations.

Alternatively, physicians who work for ambulatory care
organizations are employees of those organizations. Ambulatory care organizations include health maintenance organizations, hospital-based ambulatory clinics, walk-in and
emergency clinics, hospital-owned group practices and health
promotion centers, freestanding surgery centers, freestanding
urgent care centers, freestanding emergency care centers,
health department clinics, neighborhood clinics, home care
agencies, community mental health centers, school and workplace health services, and prison health services.

Ambulatory care organizations also employ other healthcare providers, including nurses, laboratory technicians,
podiatrists, chiropractors, physical therapists, radiology technicians, psychologists, and social workers.

Private Medical Practice
Private medical practices are physician-owned entities that
provide primary care or medical/surgical specialty care services in a freestanding office setting. The physicians have
medical privileges at local hospitals and surgical centers but
are not employees of the other healthcare entities.

Hospital-Based Ambulatory Care Services
In addition to providing inpatient services, many acute care
hospitals also provide various ambulatory care services.

Emergency Services and Trauma Care
More than 90 percent of community hospitals in the United
States provide emergency services. Hospital-based emergency departments provide specialized care for victims of
traumatic accidents and life-threatening illnesses. In urban
areas, many also provide walk-in services for patients with
minor illnesses and injuries who do not have access to regular primary care physicians.

Many physicians on the hospital staff also use the emergency care department as a setting to assess patients with
problems that may either lead to an inpatient admission or
require equipment or diagnostic imaging facilities not available in a private office or nursing home. Emergency services
function as a major source of unscheduled admissions to the
hospital.

Outpatient Surgical Services
Generally, ambulatory surgery refers to any surgical procedure that does not require an overnight stay in a hospital. It
can be performed in the outpatient surgery department of a
hospital and in a freestanding ambulatory surgery center.
During the 1980s and 1990s, the percentage of surgeries
done on an outpatient basis rose dramatically. The increased
number of procedures performed in an ambulatory setting
can be attributed to improvements in surgical technology and
anesthesia and the utilization management demands of third-
party payers.

Outpatient Diagnostic and Therapeutic Services

Outpatient diagnostic and therapeutic services are provided in a hospital or one of its satellite facilities. Diagnostic services are those services performed by a physician to identify the disease or condition from which the patient is suffering. Therapeutic services are those services performed by a physician to treat the disease or condition that has been identified.

Hospital outpatients fall into different classifications according to the type of service they receive and the location of the service. For example, emergency outpatients are treated in the hospital's emergency or trauma care department for conditions that require immediate care. Clinic outpatients are treated in one of the hospital's clinical departments on an ambulatory basis. And referral outpatients receive special diagnostic or therapeutic services in the hospital on an ambulatory basis, but responsibility for their care remains with the referring physician.

Community-Based Ambulatory Care Services

Community-based ambulatory care services refer to those services provided in freestanding facilities that are not owned by or affiliated with a hospital. Such facilities can range in size from a small medical practice with a single physician to a large clinic with an organized medical staff.

Among the organizations that provide ambulatory care services are specialized treatment facilities. Examples of these facilities include birthing centers, cancer treatment centers, renal dialysis centers, rehabilitation centers, and so on.

Freestanding Ambulatory Care Centers

Freestanding ambulatory care facilities provide emergency services and urgent care for walk-in patients. Urgent care centers (sometimes called emergicenters) provide diagnostic and therapeutic care for patients with minor illnesses and injuries. They do not serve seriously ill patients, and most do not accept ambulance cases.

Two groups of patients find these centers attractive. The first group consists of patients seeking the convenience and access of emergency services without the delays and other forms of negative feedback associated with using hospital services for nonurgent problems. The second group consists of patients whose insurance treats urgent care centers preferentially compared with physicians' offices.

As they have increased in number and become familiar to more patients, many of these centers now offer a combination of walk-in and appointment services.

Freestanding Ambulatory Surgery Centers

Generally, freestanding ambulatory surgery centers provide surgical procedures that take anywhere from five to ninety minutes to perform and that require less than a four-hour recovery period. Patients must schedule their surgeries in advance and be prepared to return home on the same day. Patients who experience surgical complications are sent to an inpatient facility for care.

Most ambulatory surgery centers are for-profit entities. They may be owned by individual physicians, managed care organizations, or entrepreneurs. Generally, ambulatory care centers can provide surgical services at lower cost than hospitals can because their overhead expenses are lower.

Public Health Services

Public health services employ a variety of health professionals. Public health workers are concerned primarily with the health of entire communities and population groups. Most public health workers are educated in specific clinical disciplines, such as nursing and medicine. Some public health professionals are graduates of the nation's twenty-four accredited schools of public health (Jonas and Kovner 1999, p. 102).

Home Care Services

Home health care is the fastest-growing sector to offer services for Medicare recipients. The primary reason for this is increased economic pressure from third-party payers. In other words, third-party payers want patients released from the hospital more quickly than they were in the past. Moreover, patients generally prefer to be cared for in their own homes. In fact, most patients prefer home care, no matter how complex their medical problems. Research indicates that the medical outcomes of home care patients are similar to those of patients treated in skilled nursing facilities for similar conditions.

In 1989, Medicare rules for home care services were clarified to make it easier for Medicare beneficiaries to receive such services. Patients are eligible to receive home health services from a qualified Medicare provider when they are homebound, when they are under the care of a specified physician who will establish a home health plan, and when they need physical or occupational therapy, speech therapy, or intermittent skilled nursing care.

Skilled nursing care is defined as both technical procedures, such as tube feedings and catheter care, and skilled nursing observations. Intermittent is defined as up to twenty-eight hours per week for nursing care and thirty-five hours per week for home health aide care. Many hospitals have formed their own home health care agencies to increase revenues and at the same time allow them to discharge patients from the hospital earlier.

Voluntary Agencies

Voluntary agencies provide healthcare and healthcare planning services, usually at the local level and to low-income patients. Their services range from giving free immunizations to offering family planning counseling. Funds to operate such agencies come from a variety of sources, including local or state health departments, private grants, and funds from different federal bureaus.

One common example of a voluntary agency is the community health center. Sometimes called neighborhood health centers, community health centers offer comprehensive, primary healthcare services to patients who otherwise would not have access to them. Often patients pay for these services on a sliding scale based on income or according to a flat rate, discounted fee schedule supplemented by public funding.

Some voluntary agencies offer specialized services such as counseling for battered and abused women. Typically, these are set up within local communities. An example of a voluntary agency that offers services on a much larger scale would be the Red Cross.

Long-Term Care

Generally speaking, long-term care is the healthcare rendered in a nonacute care facility to patients who require inpatient nursing and related services for more than thirty consecutive days. Skilled nursing facilities, nursing homes, and rehabilitation hospitals are the principal facilities that provide long-term care. Rehabilitation hospitals provide recuperative services for patients who have suffered strokes and traumatic injuries as well as other serious illnesses. Specialized long-term care facilities serve patients with chronic respiratory disease, permanent cognitive impairment, and other incapacitating conditions.

Long-term care encompasses a range of health, personal care, social, and housing services provided to people of all ages with health conditions that limit their ability to carry out normal daily activities without assistance. People who need long-term care have many different types of physical and mental disabilities. Moreover, their need for the mix and intensity of long-term care services can change over time.

Long-term care is mainly rehabilitative and supportive rather than curative. Moreover, healthcare workers other than physicians can provide long-term care in the home or in residential or institutional settings. For the most part, long-term care requires little or no technology.

Long-Term Care and the Continuum of Care

The availability of long-term care is one of the most important health issues in the United States today. There are two principal reasons for this. First, thanks to advances in medicine and healthcare practices, people are living longer today than they did in the past. The number of people who survive previously fatal conditions has been growing, and more and more people with chronic medical problems are able to live reasonably normal lives. Second, there was an explosion in birth rate following World War II. Children born during that period, the so-called baby-boomer generation, are today in or entering their fifties. These factors combined mean that the need for long-term care can only increase in the years to come.

As discussed earlier, healthcare is now viewed as a continuum of care. That is, patients are provided care by different caregivers at several different levels of the healthcare system. In the case of long-term care, the patient's continuum of care may have begun with a primary provider in a hospital and then continued with home care and eventually care in a skilled nursing facility. That patient's care is coordinated from one care setting to the next.

Moreover, the roles of the different care providers along the patient's continuum of care are continuing to evolve.

Health information managers play a key part in providing consultation services to long-term care facilities with regard to developing systems to manage information from a diverse number of healthcare providers.

Delivery of Long-Term Care Services

Long-term care services are delivered in a variety of settings. Among these settings are skilled nursing facilities/nursing homes, residential care facilities, hospice programs, and adult day-care programs.

Skilled Nursing Facilities/Nursing Homes

The most important providers of formal, long-term care services are nursing homes. **Skilled nursing facilities** (SNFs), or nursing homes, provide medical, nursing, and/or rehabilitative care, in some cases, around the clock. The majority of SNF residents are over age 65 and quite often are classified as the frail elderly.

Many nursing homes are owned by for-profit organizations. However, SNFs also may be owned by not-for-profit groups as well as local, state, and federal governments. In recent years, there has been a decline in the total number of nursing homes in the United States, but an increase in the number of nursing home beds.

Nursing homes are no longer the only option for patients needing long-term care. Various factors play a role in determining which type of long-term care facility is best for a particular patient, including cost, access to services, and individual needs.

Residential Care Facilities

New living environments that are more homelike and less institutional are the focus of much attention in the current long-term care market. Residential care facilities now play a growing role in the continuum of long-term care services. Having affordable and appropriate housing available for elderly and disabled people can reduce the level of need for institutional long-term care services in the community. Institutionalization can be postponed or prevented when the elderly and disabled live in safe and accessible settings where assistance with daily activities is available.

Hospice Programs

Hospice care is provided mainly in the home to the terminally ill and their families. Hospice is based on a philosophy of care imported from England and Canada that holds that during the course of terminal illness, the patient should be able to live life as fully and as comfortably as possible, but without artificial or mechanical efforts to prolong life.

In the hospice approach, the family is the unit of treatment. An interdisciplinary team provides medical, nursing, psychological, therapeutic, pharmacological, and spiritual support during the final stages of illness, at the time of death, and during bereavement. The main goals are to control pain, maintain independence, and minimize the stress and trauma of death.

Hospice services have gained acceptance as an alternative to hospital care for the terminally ill. The number of hospices is likely to continue to grow because this philosophy of care for people at the end of life has become a model for the nation.

Adult Day-Care Programs

Adult day-care programs offer a wide range of health and social services to elderly persons during the daytime hours. Adult day-care services are usually targeted to elderly members of families in which the regular caregivers work during the day. Many elderly people who live alone also benefit from leaving their homes every day to participate in programs designed to keep them active. The goals of adult day-care programs are to delay the need for institutionalization and to provide respite for the caregivers.

Data on adult day-care programs are still limited, but there were about 3,000 programs in 2000. Most adult day-care programs offer social services, crafts, current events discussions, family counseling, reminiscence therapy, nursing assessment, physical exercise, activities of daily living, rehabilitation, psychiatric assessment, and medical care.

Behavioral Health Services

From the mid-nineteenth century to the mid-twentieth century, psychiatric services in the United States were based primarily in long-stay institutions supported by state governments, and patterns of practice were relatively stable. Over the past forty-five years, however, remarkable changes have occurred. These changes include a reversal of the balance between institutional and community care, inpatient and outpatient services, and individual and group practice.

Today, the number of long-stay residents in state mental hospitals is estimated to be well below 80,000. In 1955, it was more than 500,000. The shift to community-based settings began in the public sector and community settings remain dominant. The private sector's bed capacity increased in the 1970s and 1980s, including psychiatric units in non-federal general hospitals, private psychiatric hospitals, and residential treatment centers for children. Substance abuse centers and child and adolescent inpatient psychiatric units grew particularly quickly in the 1980s, as investors recognized their profitability. In the 1990s, the growth of inpatient private mental health facilities leveled off, and the number of outpatient and partial treatment settings increased sharply.

Some patients with treatment-resistant schizophrenia, severe mood disorders, or chronic cognitive impairment may be dangerous to themselves or others. State and county hospitals may be returning to their traditional role by providing asylum to disabled patients who are unable function in their communities.

Residential treatment centers for emotionally or behaviorally disturbed children provide inpatient services to children under eighteen years of age. The programs and physical facilities of residential treatment centers are designed to meet patients' daily living, schooling, recreational, socialization, and routine medical care needs.

Day-hospital or day-treatment programs occupy one niche in the spectrum of behavioral health care settings. Although some provide services seven days per week, many programs provide services only during business hours, Monday through Friday. Day-treatment patients spend most of the day at the treatment facility in a program of structured therapeutic activities and then return to their homes until the next day. Day-treatment services include psychotherapy, pharmacology, occupational therapy, and other types of rehabilitation services. These programs provide alternatives to inpatient care or serve as transitions from inpatient to outpatient care or discharge. They also may provide respite for family caregivers and a place for rehabilitating or maintaining chronically ill patients. The number of day-treatment programs has increased in response to pressures to decrease the length of hospital stays.

Insurance coverage for behavioral healthcare has always lagged behind coverage for other medical care. Although treatments and treatment settings have changed, rising healthcare costs, the absence of strong consumer demand for behavioral health coverage, and insurers' continuing fear of the potential cost of this coverage have maintained the differences between medical and behavioral healthcare benefits. Only 13 percent of the cost for treating behavioral health disorders is covered by private insurance dollars, compared with 28 percent for general medical care. States continue to play their traditional role by providing a safety net for uninsured and underinsured psychiatric patients. As a result, states and local governments pay 28 percent of the cost for behavioral mental health services but only 14 percent of the cost for other healthcare services (Jonas and Kovner 1999, p. 265).

Although the majority of individuals who are covered by health insurance have some outpatient psychiatric coverage, the coverage is often quite restricted. Typical restrictions include limits on the number of outpatient visits, higher copayment charges, and higher deductibles.

Behavioral health care has grown and diversified, particularly over the past forty years, as psychopharmacologic treatment has made possible the shift away from long-term custodial treatment. Psychosocial treatments continue the process of care and rehabilitation in community settings. Large state hospitals have been supplemented, and in many cases replaced, by psychiatric units in general hospitals, new outpatient clinics, community mental health centers, day-treatment centers, and halfway houses. Treatment has become more effective and specific, based on our growing understanding of the brain and behavior. Recent advances in the biological and behavioral sciences continue to improve opportunities for diagnosing, treating, and preventing psychiatric disorders (Jonas and Kovner 1999, pp. 243–73).

Instructions: Match the descriptions provided with the terms to which they apply.

1. ___   Behavioral health service
2. ___   Public health service
3. ___   Home care service
4. ___   Hospice program
5. ___   Skilled nursing facility
6. ___   Voluntary agency
7. ___   Residential care facility
8. ___   Day-treatment program
9. ___   Continuum of care
10. ___   Freestanding ambulatory care center

a. Fastest-growing sector of Medicare

b. Provides emergency services and urgent care for walk-in patients

c. Represents a reversal in the balance between institutional and community care

d. Environment that is more homelike and less institutional

e. Concerned primarily with the health of entire communities and population groups

f. Provides healthcare and healthcare planning services usually at the local level and to low-income patients

g. Provides alternatives to inpatient care or serves as transition from inpatient to outpatient care or discharge

h. Care provided mainly in the home to the terminally ill and their families

i   Care provided by different caregivers at several different levels of the healthcare system

j. Healthcare rendered in a nonacute care facility to patients who require inpatient nursing and related services for more than thirty consecutive days

Reimbursement of Healthcare Expenditures

Together, the Medicare and Medicaid programs and the managed care insurance industry have virtually eliminated fee-for-service reimbursement arrangements.

Evolution of Third-Party Reimbursement

Commercial health insurance companies (for example, Aetna) offer medical plans similar to Blue Cross/Blue Shield plans. Traditionally, Blue Cross organizations covered hospital services and Blue Shield covered inpatient physician services and a limited amount of office-based care. Today, Blue Cross plans and commercial insurance providers cover a full range of healthcare services, including ambulatory care services and drug benefits. (Healthcare reimbursement systems are discussed in more detail in chapter 14.)

Most commercial health insurance is provided in the form of group policies offered by employers as part of their fringe benefit packages for employees. Unions also negotiate health insurance coverage during contract negotiations. In most cases, employees pay a share of the cost and employers pay a share.

Individual health insurance plans can be purchased but usually are expensive or have limited coverage and high deductibles. Individuals with preexisting medical conditions often find it almost impossible to get individual coverage.

Commercial insurers also sell major medical and cash payment policies. Major medical plans are directed primarily at catastrophic illness and cover all or part of treatment costs beyond those covered by basic plans. Major medical plans are sold as both group and individual policies. Cash payment plans provide monetary benefits and are not based on actual charges from healthcare providers. For example, a cash payment plan might pay the beneficiary $150 for every day he or she is hospitalized or $500 for every ambulatory surgical procedure. Cash payment plans are often offered as a benefit of membership in large associations, for example, the American Association of Retired Persons (AARP).

Like the Blues, the commercial insurance companies are subject to supervision by state insurance commissioners. However, such supervision does not include rate regulation. One general requirement is that commercial plans establish premium rates high enough to cover all potential claims made under the insurance they provide.

Government-Sponsored Reimbursement Systems

Until 1965, most of the poor and many of the elderly in the United States could not afford private healthcare services. As a result of public pressure calling for attention to this growing problem, Congress passed Public Law 89-97 as an Amendment to the Social Security Act. The amendments created Medicare (Title XVIII) and Medicaid (Title XIX).

Medicare

Federal health insurance for the aged, called **Medicare,** was first offered to retired Americans in July 1966. Today, retired and disabled Americans who are eligible for Social Security benefits automatically qualify for Medicare coverage, without regard to income. Coverage is offered under two coordinated programs: hospital insurance (Medicare Part A) and medical insurance (Medicare Part B).

Medicare Part A is financed through payroll taxes. Initially, coverage applied only to hospitalization and home health care. Subsequently, coverage for extended care in nursing homes was added. Coverage for individuals eligible for Social Security disability payments for over two years and those who need kidney transplantation or dialysis for end-stage renal disease also was added.

Medical insurance under Medicare Part B is optional. It is financed through monthly premiums paid by eligible beneficiaries to supplement federal funding. Part B helps pay for physician's services, outpatient hospital care, medical services and supplies, and certain other medical costs not covered by Part A. At the present time, Medicare Part B does not provide coverage of prescription drugs. (Medicare Parts A and B are discussed in greater detail in chapter 14.)

Medicaid

Medicaid is a medical assistance program for low-income Americans. The program is funded partially by the federal government and partially by state and local governments. The federal government requires that certain services be provided and sets specific eligibility requirements.

Medicaid covers the following benefits:

- Inpatient hospital care
- Outpatient hospital care
- Laboratory and X-ray services
- Skilled nursing facility and home health services for persons over twenty-one years old
- Physician's services
- Family planning services
- Rural health clinic services
- Early and periodic screening, diagnosis, and treatment services

Individual states sometimes cover services in addition to those required by the federal government.

Services Provided by Government Agencies

Federal health insurance programs cover health services for several additional specified populations.

TRICARE, which was originally referred to as the Civilian Health and Medical Program for the Uniformed Services (CHAMPUS), pays for care delivered by civilian health providers to retired members of the military and the dependents of active and retired members of the seven uniformed services. The Department of Defense administers the TRICARE program. It also provides medical services to active members of the military.

The Department of Veterans Affairs (VA) provides healthcare services to eligible veterans of military service. The VA hospital system was established in 1930 to provide hospital, nursing home, residential, and outpatient medical and dental care to veterans of the First World War. Today, the VA operates more than 950 medical centers throughout the United States. The medical centers are currently being organized into twenty-two Veterans Integrated Service Networks (VISNs) to increase the efficiency of their services.

Through the Indian Health Service, the Department of Health and Human Services also finances the healthcare services provided to native Americans living on reservations across the country.

State governments often operate healthcare facilities to serve citizens with special needs, such as the developmentally disabled and mentally ill. Some states also offer health insurance programs to those who cannot qualify for private healthcare insurance. Many county and local governments also operate public hospitals to fulfill the medical needs of their communities. Public hospitals provide services without regard to the patient's ability to pay.

Workers' Compensation

Workers' compensation is an insurance system operated by the individual states. Each state has its own law and program to provide covered workers with some protection against the costs of medical care and the loss of income resulting from work-related injuries and, in some cases, illnesses. The first workers' compensation law was enacted in New York in 1910. By 1948, every state had enacted such laws. The theory underlying workers' compensation is that all accidents that occur at work, regardless of fault, must be regarded as risks of industry and that employer and employee should share the burden of loss (Jonas and Kovner 1999, p. 41).

Managed Care

The growth of managed care in the United States has had a tremendous impact on healthcare organizations and healthcare professionals. **Managed care** is a broad term used to describe several types of prepaid healthcare plans. Common types of managed care plans include health maintenance organizations (HMOs), preferred provider organizations (PPOs), and point-of-service (POS) plans.

Members of HMOs pay a set premium and are entitled to receive a specific range of healthcare services. In most cases, employers and employees share the cost of the plan. Coverage can be provided for an individual employee or his or her whole family. HMOs control costs by requiring members of the plan to seek services only from a preapproved list of providers, who are reimbursed at discounted rates. The plans also control access to medical specialists, expensive diagnostic and treatment procedures, and high-cost pharmaceuticals. They generally require preapproval for specialty consultations, inpatient care, and surgical procedures.

The development of managed care was an indirect result of the federal government's enactment of the Medicare and Medicaid laws in 1965. Medicare and Medicaid legislation prompted the development of **investor-owned hospital chains** and stimulated the growth of university medical centers. Both of these furthered the corporate practice of medicine by increasing the number of management personnel and physicians employed by hospitals and medical schools (Kongstevdt 1993, pp. 3–5).

The new healthcare programs for the elderly and poor laid the groundwork for increased corporate control of medical care delivery by third-party payers. This was done through the government-mandated regulation of fee-for-service and indemnity payments for healthcare services. After years of unchecked healthcare inflation, the government authorized corporate cost controls on hospitals, physicians, and patients, such as diagnosis-related groups (DRGs), prospective payment systems, and the resource-based relative value scale.

Further federal support for the corporate practice of medicine resulted from passage of the HMO Act of 1973. Amendments to the act enabled managed care plans to increase in numbers and expand enrollments through healthcare programs financed by grants, contracts, and loans. After passage of the HMO Act, strong support for the HMO concept came from business; the executive, legislative, and judicial branches of government; and several states where managed care proliferated, such as California, some northeast states, and particularly Minneapolis-St. Paul, Minnesota.

Bipartisan support for managed care was based on the concept that HMOs can decrease costs and encourage free-market competition in the medical care arena with only limited government intervention. One measure of success of this policy can be found in the virtual disappearance of some seventeen national health insurance bills introduced into Congress in the early 1970s (Kongstevdt 1993, pp. 3–5).

Cost and Quality Controls

The federal government became involved in the quality-of-care/malpractice issue through the establishment of the National Practitioner Data Bank under the Health Care Quality Improvement Act of 1986. Congress enacted this legislation to:

- Moderate the incidence of malpractice
- Allow the medical community to demonstrate new willingness to weed out incompetents
- Improve the base of timely and accurate information on medical malpractice

The act required hospitals to request information from the data bank whenever they are hiring, granting privileges, or conducting periodic reviews of a practitioner.

Check Your Understanding 2.7

Instructions: Indicate whether the statements below are true or false (T or F).

1. ____ Blue Cross plans and commercial insurance providers cover a limited range of healthcare services.

2. ____ Most commercial health insurance is provided in the form of group policies offered by employers as part of their fringe benefit packages for employees.

3. ____ Today, retired and disabled Americans who are eligible for Social Security benefits automatically qualify for Medicare coverage.

4. ____ Medicaid is a medical assistance program for upper-income Americans.

5. ____ The Department of Veterans Affairs administers the CHAMPUS program.

6. ____ State governments often operate healthcare facilities to serve citizens with special needs, such as the developmentally disabled and mentally ill.

7. ____ The development of managed care was a direct result of the federal government's enactment of the Medicare and Medicaid laws in 1965.

8. ____ The federal government became involved in the quality-of-care/malpractice issue through the establishment of the National Practitioner Data Bank.

Real-World Case

Executive leaders of healthcare organizations focused on growth during the 1990s, the period during which a number of new integrated healthcare networks emerged. Today, most of the physician practices, skilled nursing facilities, and home health agencies owned by integrated networks are suffering significant financial losses.

The University of Pennsylvania Health System in Philadelphia is an example of a system that achieved a financial turnaround. The system suffered a $187 million operating loss in 1999, but a $5.9 million operating profit during the first quarter of 2000. Similarly, Centura Health (in Englewood, Colorado) went from a $53 million operating loss in 1999 to a $47.2 million operating profit in 2000.

Discussion Questions

Read the special report on these turnarounds in the February 5, 2001, issue of *Modern Healthcare*. Then answer the following questions.

1. How did these two integrated delivery systems achieve such rapid financial turnarounds?

2. What changes did they make in their core operations?

3. How would your organization's mission, vision, and values affect your criteria?

Summary

Throughout history, humans have attempted to diagnose and treat illness and disease. As populations settled into towns and cities, early folk medicine traditions eventually led to the establishment of formalized entities specifically designed to care for the sick.

In the American colonies, enlightened thinkers such as Benjamin Franklin soon saw the need to establish hospitals and to regulate the practice of medicine. The nineteenth century saw the growth of organizations dedicated to standardizing medical practice and ensuring consistency in the quality of healthcare delivery. Organizations such as the American Medical Association and the American Nurses Association were created to represent the interests of their members and to further ensure the quality of their services.

The twentieth century ushered in a completely new concept in the provision of healthcare: prepaid health plans. For the first time, Americans could buy health insurance. However, during the Great Depression of the 1930s and the Second World War, it became obvious that millions of Americans could not afford to pay for healthcare. After the war, the federal government began to study the problem of healthcare access for all Americans. Finally, during the Johnson administration in the 1960s, Congress passed amendments to the Social Security Act of 1935 that created the Medicare and Medicaid programs. These programs were designed to pay for the cost of healthcare services to the elderly and the poor.

As the healthcare industry has grown, so have efforts to regulate it. Some regulation has come from professional and trade associations that are associated with the industry. However, much regulation has come from the federal government, particularly with regard to the Medicaid and Medicare programs. Moreover, the types and variety of healthcare services that are available today have increased dramatically. Every new type of service, and every new way to provide it, brings complex issues that must be addressed in order to ensure that Americans receive the highest-quality healthcare possible at the most affordable price.

Passage of the Medicare and Medicaid programs and establishment of the managed care industry have had a tremendous impact on the way that healthcare in the United States is delivered and paid for. The ramifications of these changes on the American healthcare industry have yet to be fully appreciated. The only thing that is certain is that the American healthcare system continues to be a work in progress.

References

American Hospital Association. 1999. *100 Faces of Health Care.* Chicago: Health Forum.

Cofer, Jennifer, editor. 1994. *Health Information Management,* tenth edition. Berwyn, Ill.: Physicians' Record Company.

Elliott, Chris, et al. 2000. *Performance Improvement in Healthcare: A Tool for Programmed Learning.* Chicago: American Health Information Management Association.

Joint Commission on Accreditation of Healthcare Organizations. 2000. *2001 Comprehensive Accreditation Manual for Hospitals.* Oakbrook Terrace, Ill.: JCAHO.

Jonas, Steven, and Anthony R. Kovner. 1999. *Health Care Delivery in the United States,* sixth edition. New York City: Springer Publishing.

Kongstevdt, Peter. 1993. *The Managed Care Handbook.* Gaithersburg, Md.: Aspen.

Leavitt, Judith Walzer, and Ronald L. Numbers, editors. 1997. *Sickness and Health in America: Readings in the History of Medicine and Public Health,* third edition. Madison, Wis.: University of Wisconsin Press.

Quality of health care, part 3: improving the quality of care. 1996. *New England Journal of Medicine* 335:1062.

Shryock, R. H. 1947. The beginnings: from colonial days to the foundation of the American Psychiatric Association. In *One Hundred Years of American Psychiatry,* J. K. Hall, G. Zilboorg, and H. A. Bunker, editors. New York City: Columbia University Press.

Sloane, Robert M., Beverly LeBov Sloane, and Richard Harder. 1999. *Introduction to Healthcare Delivery Organization: Functions and Management,* fourth edition. Chicago: Health Administration Press.

Starr, Paul. 1982. *The Social Transformation of American Medicine.* New York City: Basic Books.

Stevens, Rosemary. 1999. *In Sickness and in Wealth.* Baltimore, Md.: Johns Hopkins University Press.

Weinerman, E. R., R. S. Ratner, A. Robbins, and M. A. Lavenbar. 1996. Yale studies in ambulatory medical care: five determinants of use of hospital emergency services. *American Journal of Public Health* 56:1037.

Application Exercises

1. Based on what you learned in this chapter, what role do you think the government should play in financing healthcare services?

2. If you had been a hospital CEO in the mid-1990s, what key components would you have included in your strategic plan?

Review Quiz

Instructions: Choose the most appropriate answer for the following questions.

1. ____ Which of the following statements best describes an integrated delivery system?
   a. A system of healthcare delivery that ensures that patients obtain appropriate, cost-effective services
   b. A group of healthcare organizations that collectively provides a full range of coordinated health-related services
   c. A healthcare system that contracts directly with physicians in an independent practice or with one or more multispeciality group practices
   d. A healthcare system made up of two or more hospitals that are owned by the same organization

2. ____ Where was the first hospital organized in the British colonies of North America?
   a. Baltimore
   b. New York City
   c. Philadelphia
   d. Boston

3. ____ What was the primary objective of the original Social Security Act, which became law in 1935?
   a. To provide healthcare insurance for the elderly
   b. To finance the construction of new hospitals and the modernization of existing facilities
   c. To provide retirement income to the elderly
   d. To provide supplementary income to the disabled

4. ____ Why was the American Medical Association established?
   a. To represent the interests of physicians across the country
   b. To standardize the curriculum for U.S. medical schools
   c. To develop state licensure systems
   d. To close most of the existing medical schools to address the problem of oversupply

5. ____ Which of the following occupations is not usually considered to be an allied health profession?
   a. Dietitian
   b. Physical therapist
   c. Emergency medical technician
   d. Surgeon

6. ____ Under which president was legislation on national health insurance passed?
   a. Harry Truman
   b. Bill Clinton
   c. Franklin Roosevelt
   d. Lyndon Johnson

7. ____ Which of the following descriptions best describes the Medicaid program?
   a. Provides healthcare benefits for people aged sixty-five and older
   b. Provides healthcare benefits to low-income persons and their children
   c. Authorizes states to construct new hospitals
   d. Requires extensive changes in the Medicare program

8. ____ Individuals who receive acute care services in a hospital are considered what?
   a. Ambulatory care patients
   b. Outpatients
   c. Inpatients
   d. Long-term care patients

9. ____ Hospitals can be classified by which of the following?
   a. Type of services provided
   b. Type of ownership
   c. Number of beds
   d. All of the above

10. ____ Which of the following defines a hospital's mission statement?
    a. Describes the organization's purpose and the customers it serves
    b. Describes the organization's ideal future
    c. Describes the organization's fundamental principles
    d. Describes the organization's legal and licensing requirements

11. ____ In almost every hospital, the largest clinical department in terms of staffing, budget, specialized services offered, and clinical expertise required is which of the following?
    a. Diagnostic services
    b. Patient care services
    c. Occupational therapy services
    d. Rehabilitation services

12. ____ What was the intention of managed care?
    a. To manage cost, quality, and access to care
    b. To manage peer review efforts
    c. To manage Medicare and Medicaid programs
    d. To manage the accreditation process

13. ____ Which is the best definition of ambulatory surgery?
    a. Any surgical procedure that is done in an emergency department
    b. Any surgical procedure that does not require an overnight stay in a hospital
    c. Any surgical procedure that is done on a patient who is brought to the hospital in an ambulance
    d. Any surgical procedure that is performed in a surgicenter

14. ____ Why are home health care services the fastest-growing sector of Medicare?
    a. Because patients prefer to receive care at home
    b. Because of the impact of recent Medicare legislation
    c. Because of increased economic pressure from third-party payers
    d. Because hospitals prefer to send patients home early

15. ____ The VA hospital system was established to provide hospital, nursing home, residential, and outpatient medical and dental care to the veterans of which war?
    a. Second World War
    b. Korean War
    c. Vietnam War
    d. First World War

Chapter 3
Informatics in Healthcare

Deborah Kohn, MPH, RHIA, CHE, CPHIMS, FHIMSS

Learning Objectives

- To understand the field of informatics as it is being applied in healthcare
- To identify the major issues associated with computerizing health data and information
- To learn the types of computer applications and technologies being used to support the delivery of healthcare and the management of health data and information
- To identify the barriers/limitations associated with computerized health data and information

- To develop a working knowledge of the emerging technologies that support the creation and maintenance of computer-based patient record (CPR) systems
- To prepare for assuming a leadership role in the development of improved healthcare information systems, integrated patient information systems, and decision support tools

Key Terms

Analog
Application service provider (ASP)
Artificial intelligence (AI)
Autocoding
Bar coding technology
Bit-mapped data
Care Maps®
Clinical care plans
Clinical informatics
Clinical/medical decision support system
Clinical or critical pathways
Clinical practice guidelines
Clinical workstation
Clinician/physician portals
Consumer informatics
Continuous speech/voice recognition technology
Data
Data marts
Data mining
Data repositories
Data types
Data warehouses

Decision support systems
Dental informatics
Diagnostic image data
Digital
Discrete data
Document image data
E-commerce
E-health
Electronic data interchange (EDI)
Encryption
Enterprise master patient index (EMPI)
Evidence-based medicine
Executive information system (EIS)
Expert decision support system
Free-text data
Geographic information system (GIS)
Health information management (HIM)
Healthcare informatics
Informatics
Information
Information management
Information science

Information systems
Intelligent character recognition (ICR) (or gesture recognition) technology
Intranets
Logical
Management information system (MIS)
Master patient index (MPI)
Medical informatics
Metadata
Motion (or streaming) video/frame data
Multimedia
Natural language processing technology
Neural networks
Nursing informatics
Object-oriented databases
Online/real-time analytical processing (OLAP)
Online/real-time transaction processing (OLTP)
Optical character recognition (OCR) technology
Outcomes management

Personal digital assistants (PDAs)
Personal health record (PHR)
Pixel
Physical
Physiological signal-processing systems
Point-of-care information systems
Protocol
Public key infrastructure (PKI)
Raster image
Real audio (or sound) data
Relational databases
Structured data
Taxonomy
Text mining
Unstructured data
Vector graphic (or signal-tracing) data
Web browser–based systems
Web content management systems
Web-enabled systems
Wireless technology

Introduction

The relatively recent introduction and rapid evolution of the use of computer technology to manage data and information is spearheading healthcare delivery systems and services in the new millennium. This means that well-trained and skilled individuals with knowledge about both healthcare and computerized information technologies will be needed to design, develop, select, and maintain tomorrow's healthcare information management systems.

This chapter introduces the field of informatics as it is currently being applied in the healthcare industry. It also describes the current and emerging technologies used to support the delivery of healthcare and the management and communication of patient information. Finally, the chapter discusses health information management as a component of the health informatics infrastructure and the partnerships that HIM professionals will forge with information technology and health informatics professionals in the future.

Theory into Practice

A large, nonprofit, acute care organization in New Jersey currently employs Daryl, a health information manager, as a clinical systems analyst in its information systems (IS) department. Daryl supports all the health information management (HIM) department's applications from an IS perspective. This includes the organization's patient billing/accounts receivable (PB/AR) system's HIM applications, such as the master patient index (MPI). Additionally, this includes the department's encoder, dictation/transcription, and electronic document management systems (EDMS).

As such, Daryl plays a key liaison role between IS and HIM. She represents the HIM department's systems at all IS department meetings and chairs the organization's PB/AR and EDMS technical users groups.

In general, Daryl identifies HIMD's current and future information system needs, recommends and facilitates all system changes, implements and customizes new applications, and troubleshoots/resolves application system issues in both installation and production environments. She defines project plans and coordinates the resources to accomplish project plan objectives. Also, she improves and enhances HIMD's application software by participating in the direction, selection, conversion, and routine management of these applications.

To accomplish this, Daryl's typical day includes researching answers to problems, setting up meetings and appointments with HIM department users, coordinating demonstrations and training sessions, following up on tasks assigned at meetings, testing applications and interfaces, and working with vendors to make enhancements to existing products. She uses the following, important skills:

- Attention to detail
- Knowledge of HIM department fundamentals to understand how technology can be used and modified
- Knowledge of the department's business rules
- Knowledge of the flow of information throughout the organization
- Knowledge of the department's work flow
- Organizational skills
- Project management skills

Recently, Daryl took the lead in identifying HIM requirements for the organization's new clinical IS. Such requirements included providing interface specifications to and from the HIM department's transcription system and setting up the HIM department's security profiles.

Having implemented a transcription system at a former place of employment, Daryl learned how to work with people and analyze both manual and automated systems. The prior experience also gave Daryl more exposure to the fundamentals of project management and taught her how to develop a request for proposal (RFP), complete the steps required to evaluate software, and perform system administration functions.

Therefore, Daryl began the project by assembling an ad hoc committee of transcription users throughout the organization, whether or not these users would be required to interface to the clinical IS. After the first meeting, the committee determined that not only would all these users be required to interface with the clinical IS, but also there were other transcription users "hiding" in the organization who needed to be a part of the committee!

After performing a thorough inventory of every transcription system, the committee accounted for eight disparate word-processing systems that were used for organizational transcription. The HIM department's word-processing system was used to transcribe the majority of the organization's medical report dictation. However, the other systems were used to transcribe at least 30 percent of the organization's dictation. These systems ranged from one, old, non-Microsoft Windows operating system–based version of Corel's WordPerfect to two proprietary systems to three systems, each with different versions of Microsoft Word™.

Therefore, the analysis persuaded the committee to recommend to the organization's IS steering committee that, at this time, standardizing on one transcription system—the system used by the HIM department—would be the most appropriate, strategic solution for the organization, its clinical IS, and its clinical IS transcription interface requirements.

This recommendation was made after a lot of discussion and dissention. For example, all the committee members realized that the recommendation would be difficult to implement because the users of the remaining transcription systems involved care providers who were unaccustomed to change. Further, it would be expensive in the short term because it would require a significant amount of retraining, additional hardware and server capacity, and the potential consolidation of all transcription positions under the HIM department.

However, in the long term, the benefits of standardizing on one system would allow IS to develop one set of interface instructions as opposed to seven. The remaining systems needed to be upgraded anyway because some of the interfaces could not proceed unless more current operating systems and software versions were installed. In addition, because interfaces are extremely costly to develop and maintain, the long-term advantages of standardizing on one transcription system throughout the organization outweighed the short-term disadvantages of interfacing and maintaining seven, disparate systems.

As lead, Daryl realized that the short-term challenges had to be addressed immediately. These included changing provider behavior, retraining various transcriptionists and dictators, and reorganizing HIM department positions with job descriptions and salaries. In other words, solutions to these challenges needed to be designed—and even implemented—before the committee could begin to determine the systems' interface rules and HIM department security profiles for the clinical IS.

Based on her previous management and healthcare informatics experiences, Daryl knew that responsibilities for several tasks had to be delegated, including the required retraining, marketing of the recommendation, and working with HIM's director and transcription system vendor to expand the department's existing transcription area. Also, the tasks included amending the existing transcription system contract to add software licenses. The delegation took place primarily using existing ad hoc committee members. In addition, Daryl incorporated "outside" champions as well as "troublemakers" so that the tasks could be accomplished in tandem and any roadblocks could be dismantled along the way.

The Field of Informatics

Informatics is the science of information management. It uses a variety of techniques to automate—or, in other words, use—computers for the management of **data** and **information** to support decision-making activities. The management of data and information includes the generation, collection, organization, validation, analysis, storage, and integration of data, as well as the dissemination, communication, presentation, utilization, transmission, and safeguarding of information.

Healthcare informatics is the field of **information science** concerned with the management of all aspects of health data and information through the application of computers and computer technologies. The "science" of managing healthcare data and information is based on the fact that the healthcare industry is information intensive. One needs to spend only a day with a healthcare provider to realize that the largest percentage of healthcare professional activities relates to managing massive amounts of data and information. This includes obtaining and documenting information about patients, consulting with colleagues, staying abreast of the current literature, determining strategies for patient care, interpreting laboratory data and test results, and conducting research.

The influence of healthcare informatics is broad. Healthcare information technology (IT) is having a huge impact not only on the complex financial and administrative aspects of healthcare, but also on its unique clinical applications. For example, clinical **information systems,** which provide computerized communication and **information management** for such functions as order entry, results retrieval, care planning, and charting, are installed in every kind of healthcare organization—from major academic teaching hospitals and integrated delivery networks/systems to post–acute care facilities, physician practices, and managed care organizations. In addition, healthcare informatics is changing at the speed of thought. Current or existing computerized healthcare information systems become obsolete as they are installed.

However, the healthcare industry does not appear to value healthcare informatics to the same degree that other vertical market industries do. The healthcare industry is perceived as being slow to understand computerized information management and to incorporate it effectively into the work environment. Perhaps this is because the requirements of the healthcare industry are more demanding than those of other industries in a number of areas. These areas include implications of violations of privacy, support for personal values, responsibility for public health, complexity of the knowledge base and terminology, perception of high risk and pressure to make critical decisions rapidly, poorly defined outcomes, and support for the diffusion of power (Stead and Lorenzi 1999, p. 343).

Moreover, it is possible that the healthcare industry's stakeholders do not clearly understand healthcare informatics. Some observers charge that the people who manage the industry's information services are unable to put in place systems that meet its needs in a timely and cost-effective fashion. These observers claim that the ties between information and improved financial and healthcare outcomes are not being established. For example, they cite technology projects that stumble because of unreliable, fragmented, and nonstandardized medical, financial, and administrative data.

Health information managers are well positioned to play a key role in ensuring acceptance of healthcare informatics within the healthcare industry. They have the skills needed to exploit the computerized systems and technologies for their unique practical and strategic functionalities. Therefore, they can leverage chief information officers, the health information technology industry, and the field of healthcare informatics as partners to enable people to use information to improve health. In addition, they can provide the leadership needed to develop a better model for the healthcare delivery system.

The Informatics Revolution in Healthcare

Revolution is an overused word, but when applied to the effect of all that is digital, automated, or electronic in the healthcare industry, it is entirely accurate. Over the past several decades, established relationships, value chains, and strategies have been radically altered or swept away by computer technology.

Evolution of Healthcare Informatics

The term *informatics* was adopted in the early 1970s when European universities and research institutions offered programs to keep up with the introduction and application of computers and computer systems. Likewise, the term *healthcare informatics* as we know it today was based on an idea born in Europe. However, since the mid-1980s, some of the most original and creative minds in the healthcare professions in the United States have engaged healthcare informatics, giving rise to a discipline in its own right.

Today, the goal of the discipline is to understand the structure, dynamics, and design of information systems that are composed of people, technology, and organizational factors. This allows the flow and use of information to be individually optimized for every task in every context for every user (Turley et al. 2001, p. 48). Thus, the focus of the discipline is on the development of computer-based applications that are specifically designed to support specific types of users in performing their work or meeting their needs.

For example, some users of the discipline (for example, physicians) work in clinical medicine or medical research, where the term *medical informatics* is used. Other users work in nursing, where *nursing informatics* is becoming a more commonly recognized term. Some users work in dentistry, where the profession is taking new steps toward *dental informatics*. And still other users, including pharmacists and therapists, work in the allied healthcare professions, where the term *clinical informatics* has recently gained acceptance. Even *consumer informatics* is beginning to be represented as new relationships emerge between people and the health system. Consequently, the generic term *healthcare informatics* is seen as the broad domain, stressing the interdisciplinary nature of the field and underscoring the need to involve all healthcare professionals and patients.

The value proposition of healthcare informatics can be explained as the study, creation, and implementation of structures and algorithms designed to improve the communication and understanding of healthcare data and information, as well as to improve the management of the data and information. Thus, the value proposition covers the clinical, technical, public, and commercial aspects of healthcare.

As such, healthcare informatics can make it possible to achieve better outcomes for the healthcare delivery and IT industries. Its structures and communication methods allow information to be linked to healthcare work processes and managed as an asset outside the systems that automate those processes. Its data-mining techniques and filters locate information and limit reports to the immediate context. Its presentation metaphors can enhance healthcare users' exploration techniques and adapt to individual learning styles. Its education and training programs are beginning to produce people who know how to develop effective information-enabled work processes.

Examples of Calls to Action and Informatics Successes

Calls to action for the use of information technologies to improve the healthcare delivery system are not new. The 1990s began with the Institute of Medicine's (IOM) report, which was based on the findings of its Committee on Improving the Patient Record, which championed the computer-based patient record (CPR) (Dick and Steen 1991). (CPRs are discussed in detail in chapter 9.) The second portion (Title II) of Public Law 104-191, the Health Insurance Portability and Accountability Act of 1996 (HIPAA), addressed the requirements to support electronic information exchange with goals of administrative efficiency and process improvement. It also mandated the protection of health information. The millennium began with two additional IOM reports based on the findings of its Committee on Quality of Health Care in America. The first report shocked the nation with its estimated number of deaths each year resulting from preventable medical errors (Kohn, Corrigan, and Donaldson 1999). The second, follow-up report called for transforming America's "failing" healthcare industry (Committee on Quality of Health Care in America 2001). Each of these calls to action has identified IT needs and the potential for IT benefits.

Additionally, examples of healthcare informatics successes are steadily growing. Charge collection and billing, automated laboratory testing and reporting, clinical documentation, patient and provider scheduling, diagnostic imaging, and secondary data use make up a distinguished healthcare informatics "success" list, proving what is doable and supporting further investment.

Still, many of the healthcare informatics calls to action and successes have not produced compelling outcomes, especially those outcomes that communicate the feasibility of a better health system for more individuals at an affordable cost. Therefore, today's task for informatics is to design the information resources and systems that enable healthcare organizations to accomplish visions for providing the highest-quality care in the most effective way. To do so, the visions must make the benefits of the proposed systems more clear. In addition, they must establish explicit links between the promised benefits and the key enablers of the benefits—the information technologies.

Current and Emerging Information Technologies in Healthcare

To examine the information resources and systems that enable healthcare organizations to accomplish their visions in the most effective way, health information management (HIM) students must possess fundamental knowledge of computer-based information systems' components, regardless of industry. This includes knowledge of system hardware, software, and service components; communication and networking components; the Internet and its derived technologies; and system architectures. For the purposes of this book, it is assumed that students have acquired this knowledge through other, generic computer system courses and related textbooks.

Next, it is appropriate that students review some of the current and emerging information technologies used to support the delivery of healthcare as well as the management and communication of health data and information within the healthcare setting. To do this, five categories of current and emerging technologies in healthcare have been defined. These categories support:

- Different types of data and formats
- Efficient access to, and flow of, data and information
- Managerial and clinical decision making
- The diagnosis, treatment, and care of patients
- The security of data and information

Supporting Different Types of Data and Formats

The information technologies currently in use for healthcare applications as well as the new technologies being developed consist of different data types and formats, all used to support the creation, storage, dissemination, and analysis of information in every healthcare setting. Specific examples include emerging voice recognition and natural language processing technologies.

Different Data Types and Formats

Healthcare informaticists have agreed that a CPR system, as defined by the Institute of Medicine (IOM) in 1991 and redefined in 1997, is not one, or even two or more, "products." Rather, the CPR system is a concept that consists of a plethora of integrated, component information systems and technologies. The automated files that make up the CPR system's component information systems and technologies consist of different **data types,** and the data in the files consist of different data formats.

Some data formats are **structured** and some are **unstructured.** For example, the data elements in a patient's automated laboratory order, result, or demographic/financial information system are coded and alphanumeric. Their fields are predefined and limited. In other words, the type of data is **discrete,** and the format of these data is structured. Therefore, when a healthcare professional searches a database for one or more coded, discrete data elements based on the search parameters, the engine can easily find, retrieve, and manipulate the element.

However, the format of the data contained in a patient's transcribed radiology or pathology result, history and physical (H&P), or clinical note system using word-processing technology is unstructured. **Free-text data,** as opposed to discrete, structured data, are generated by word processors, and their fields are not predefined and limited. When a healthcare professional searches unstructured text, the search engine cannot easily find, retrieve, and manipulate one or more data elements embedded in the text.

Likewise, the format of the data contained in a patient's dictated radiology or pathology result, H&P, or clinical note system using continuous speech (also known as voice) recognition technology (real-time voice in–text out) is unstructured. However, the continuous speech/voice recognition technology's engine takes the unstructured, free-text-based voice data and codifies them, often with the help of templates. Hence, the format of the outputted text data becomes structured, with predefined and limited fields. Search engines can then easily find, retrieve, and manipulate one or more data elements embedded in the text.

Diagnostic image data, such as a digitized chest X ray or a computed tomography (CT) scan stored in a diagnostic image management system, represent a different type of data: **bit-mapped data.** Saving each bit of the original image creates the image file. In other words, the image is a **raster image,** the smallest unit of which is a picture element or **pixel.** Together, hundreds of pixels simulate the image. The format of these data is unstructured.

Some diagnostic image data are based on **analog,** photographic films, such as an analog chest X ray. These analog films must be digitally scanned, using film digitizers, to digitize the data. Other diagnostic image data are based on **digital** modalities, such as computed radiography (CR), computed tomography (CT), magnetic resonance (MR), or nuclear medicine.

Document image data are also bit mapped. These data are based on analog paper documents or on analog photographic film documents. Most often, analog paper-based documents contain handwritten notes, marks, or signatures. However, such documents can be preprinted (such as forms), photocopies of original documents, or computer generated, but available only in hard copy. Analog photographic film-based documents (that is, photographs) are processed using an analog camera and film, similar to analog chest X rays. Therefore, both the analog paper-based and the photographic film-based documents must be digitally scanned, using scanning devices that are similar to facsimile machines.

The CPR system's component information systems and technologies consist of additional data types. When this occurs, the data and the systems they represent are referred to as **multimedia. Real audio data** consist of sound bytes, such as digital heart sounds. **Motion or streaming video/frame data,** such as cardiac catheterizations, consist of digitized film attributes, such as fast forwarding. The files that consist of **vector graphic** (or **signal-tracing**) **data,** are created by saving lines plotted between a series of points, accounting for the familiar ECGs, EEGs, and fetal traces.

Figure 3.1 shows the different types of data and their sources found in CPR system component information systems and technologies.

Continuous Speech/Voice Recognition Technology

The concept of generating an immediately available, legible, final, signed note or report based on computer voice input has been the catalyst for the development and application of different forms of speech/voice recognition technology in healthcare for at least twenty years. Unfortunately, the technology remains inaccurate. Systems offering greater than 95 percent accuracy are not acceptable for efficient and often lengthy clinical dictation purposes. Consequently, many still consider speech/voice recognition an emerging technology.

Today, the most common form of speech/voice recognition technology is speaker independent with continuous speech input. Speaker-independent technology does not require extensive training. The software is already trained to recognize generic speech and speech patterns.

Continuous speech input does not require the user to pause between words to let the computer distinguish between the beginning and ending of words. However, the user still is required to be careful in the enunciation of words. Although continuous speech input vocabularies are expanding due to faster and more powerful computer hardware, only limited vocabularies have been developed. Limited vocabulary-based continuous speech input systems require the user to say words that are known or taught to the system. In healthcare, limited vocabulary-based specialties such as radiology, emergency medicine, and psychiatry have realized benefits for dictation from this technology.

Recent data indicate that **continuous speech/voice recognition technology** may be an acceptable alternative for producing outpatient notes. Although it takes longer to dictate and edit the outpatient notes on the computer compared with dictating and editing the notes for human transcription, decreased delays and costs associated with producing transcribed documents have been realized (Borowitz 2001, p. 102).

Other areas in healthcare have realized significant benefits from this input technology for specific programs. These programs include data-entry systems, navigating through pathways, pulling down menus, editing text, autodialing phone numbers, and completing multiple-choice-based forms. This usually requires exchanging data with the other applications through seamless, but complex, interfaces.

The ultimate goal in speech/voice recognition technology is to be able to talk to a computer's central processor and rapidly create vocabularies for applications without collecting

Figure 3.1.   CPR Data Types and Their Sources

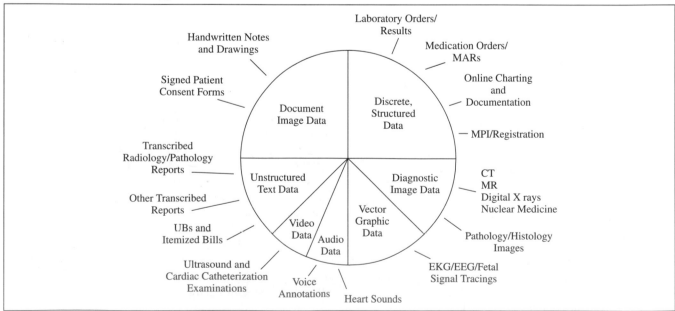

any speech samples (in other words, without training). It includes being able to talk at natural speed and intonation and in no specific manner. Additionally, it includes having the computer understand what the user wants to say (the context of the word or words) and then apply the correct commands or words as coded data, in a structured format. Finally, it includes identifying a user's voice and encrypting the voiceprint. Over the next years and decades, clinical vocabularies and algorithms will continue to improve, true speaker independence will be achieved, and natural language understanding will ultimately make structured dictation a reality.

Natural Language Processing Technology

One could argue that **natural language processing technology** is another name for continuous speech/voice recognition technology. When one talks at natural speed without pausing between words, the *natural language* voice bytes are, indeed, *processed* by this technology.

However, **autocoding** is the term commonly used to describe natural language processing technology's method of extracting and translating dictated and then transcribed free-text data, or dictated and then computer-generated discrete data, into ICD and CPT (E&M) codes for clinical and administrative applications such as patient billing and health record coding. **Text mining** and **data mining** are the terms commonly used to describe the process of extracting and then quantifying and filtering free-text data and discrete data, respectively.

Natural language processing technology differs from simple Boolean word search programs in that it considers sentence structure (syntax), meaning (semantics), and context to accurately extract the data. For example, the narratives "no shortness of breath, chest pain aggravated by exercise" and "no chest pain, shortness of breath aggravated by exercise" look the same to a Boolean word search engine when looking for occurrences of "chest" and "pain" in the same sentence. This approach retrieves approximately 20 percent of the answer 20 percent of the time. It is rife with false positives and false negatives.

On the other hand, natural language processing technology knows the difference in the narratives' meanings. For the health record coding application, it teaches computers to understand English well enough to "read" transcribed reports/notes and then find certain key concepts (not merely words) by identifying the many different phrasings of the concept. By "normalizing" these concepts, different phrases of the same content can all be compared with one another for statistical purposes. By employing statistical algorithms, natural language processing technology can then compare and code these similar expressions accurately and quickly, without the involvement of coding professionals. For example, "the patient thinks s/he has angina" and "the doctor thinks the patient has angina" have different meanings from a coding perspective (Schnitzer 2000, p. 96).

Early results of several formative studies suggest that natural language processing technology improves health record coding productivity and consistency without sacrificing quality (Warner 2000, p. 78). As such, vendors are frantically working to integrate natural language processing technology within health record coding reference tools, coding clinic guidelines, drug databases, and legacy information systems to provide complete and accurate patient billing or health record coding with little or no human intervention.

Check Your Understanding 3.2

Instructions: Answer the following questions on a separate piece of paper.

1. Give an example of each of the following data formats: structured, unstructured.

2. Give an example of each of the following data types: discrete, free text.

3. Explain the difference between a diagnostic image and a document image.

4. Give a healthcare example for each of the following data types: real audio data, motion or streaming data, signal or vector graphic data.

5. Explain the difference between (a) voice recognition technology and natural language processing technology and (b) natural language processing technology and Boolean text searching.

Supporting Efficient Access to, and Flow of, Data and Information

A plethora of current and emerging information technologies are used to support the efficient access to, and flow of, healthcare data and information. For purposes of this book, the following technologies are highlighted:

- Character/symbol recognition technologies
- Electronic data interchange and e-commerce
- Enterprise master patient indexes
- Data repositories
- Clinical workstations or clinician/physician portals
- Web-based systems and applications
- Intranets and Web content management
- Application service providers

Character/Symbol Recognition Technologies

Several "automatic identification" technologies recognize electronically scanned characters or symbols from analog items such as tangible materials or documents. Such technologies enable the identified data to be quickly, accurately, and automatically entered into digital systems. These automatic identification technologies include **bar coding, optical character recognition** (OCR), and **intelligent character recognition** (ICR) technologies.

Bar Coding Technology

Two decades ago, the bar code symbol was standardized for the healthcare industry, making it easier for the industry to adopt bar coding technology and to realize its potential. Since then, bar coding applications have been adopted for patient wristbands, specimen containers, business/employee/patient records, library reference materials, medication packages, dietary items, and more. Benefits have been realized by the uniform consistency in the development of commercially available software systems, fewer procedural variations in healthcare organizations using the technology, and the flexibility to adopt standard specifications for functions while retaining current systems. Because virtually every tangible item in the clinical setting, including the patient, can be assigned a bar code with an associated meaning, it is not surprising to find bar coding as the primary tracking, identification, or inventory data-capture medium in healthcare organizations.

With bar coding technology, an individual's computer data-entry rate can be increased by eight- to twelvefold in applications such as patient tracking, supply requisitioning, or chart/film tracking. For example, a function such as hand-keying chart/film locations into a computer that once took a healthcare professional eight hours to perform now can be done in thirty to forty-five minutes with bar coding technology.

In addition to eliminating time, bar coding technology eliminates most of the mounds of paperwork (worksheets, count sheets, identification sheets, and the like) that are still associated with traditional computer keyboard entry. When bar coding systems are interfaced to these types of healthcare information systems, the bar code can be used to enter the data, especially repetitive data, saving additional processing time and paper generation.

More important, the data input error rates with bar coding are as close to zero as most IT professionals think is possible. For all intents and purposes, bar-coded data, with an error rate of approximately three transactions in one million, can be considered error free. Thus, it is a most effective remedy for medication errors when used to make sure that the right medication dose is administered to the right patient.

Optical Character Recognition Technology

Like bar coding, optical character recognition (OCR) was invented to reduce hand-keying. It was initially used to automatically identify financial accounts consisting of Arabic numbers and Roman letters using the E13B font on thousands of paper-based documents, such as checks. OCR interprets the bit-mapped shapes of the numbers and letters captured by a scanner into their coded equivalents.

OCR has since been perfected to recognize the full set of preprinted/typeset fonts as well as point sizes. Moreover, it performs well with different Germanic and Romance languages. The best OCR systems compensate for imperfectly formed characters and scanned pages by employing characteristics such as deskewing, broken character repair, and redaction. Deskewing "straightens" oblique characters; broken character repair "fixes" incomplete characters; and redaction "hides" superfluous characters. OCR is used to perform everything from indexing scanned documents to digitizing full text. Its ability to dramatically reduce manual data input, or hand-keying, and at the same time increase input speed represents the best aspect of this technology.

Unfortunately, like other technologies, OCR has been perfected but is not perfect. The 90 to 95 percent recognition rate realized by most OCR systems may not be sufficient for the kind of text recognition applications OCR software is designed to perform. In addition, after an analog document is scanned by OCR technology, the data become unstructured, free-text data. As with all unstructured text data, when a healthcare professional needs to search the text, the search engine cannot easily find, retrieve, and manipulate one or more data elements embedded in text.

Intelligent Character Recognition Technology

The recognition of unconstrained, handwritten, English-language free text (print and/or cursive, upper and/or lower case, characters and/or symbols), known as intelligent character recognition (ICR) or gesture recognition technology and primarily stored on paper-based, analog documents, is quite an elaborate information-processing performance. An operation such as the detection of lines or the beginnings of words in sections of written text can be accomplished with relative ease in the normal case. However, subsequent tasks turn out to be extraordinarily complicated. These include the segmentation of the words into individual characters and the assignment of the individual characters to a definite class of characters, such as words. Consequently, error rates remain high. As such, ICR technology is being adopted slowly, primarily into the data-entry activities of certain types of pen-based computer devices, such as handheld devices.

Neural networks remain the leading ICR technology. These networks are modeled on the way synapses work in the brain: processing information by recognizing patterns of signals. As such, they adapt themselves into shifting configurations based on what they encounter. In other words, they change as they grow and learn.

Consequently, for each handwritten character or symbol recognized by ICR technology, a confidence level is internally expressed as a percentage. And a user picks the threshold below which he or she wants to flag uncertain characters or symbols. Like speech/voice recognition technology, a training or setup period is required for this emerging technology.

Electronic Data Interchange and E-Commerce

Electronic data interchange (EDI) allows the transfer (incoming/outgoing) of information directly from one computer to another by using flexible, standard formats. These formats function as a common language among many different healthcare "trading" or "business" partners (payers, government agencies, financial institutions, employer groups, healthcare providers, suppliers, and claims processors) who have agreed to exchange the information electronically but use a wide variety of application software with incompatible native formats. In the healthcare industry, with its traditionally strong reliance on paper-intensive processes, the goal of EDI is to eliminate the administrative nightmares of transferring paper documents back and forth between these partners and then hand-keying the information into the partners' disparate computer systems.

No EDI story has been told more often than that of the former American Hospital Supply Corporation (AHSC) in the late 1970s. AHSC pioneered an electronic connection with its customer hospitals that reinforced its position as the country's largest distributor of hospital supplies. Beginning as a "dumb terminal"–based utility for transmitting electronic purchase orders, over time this proprietary system evolved into a PC-based information system that served as the gateway for what became Baxter Healthcare's purchase orders and confirmations.

By the late 1980s, the healthcare industry's business partners expanded their EDI linkages beyond purchase orders to electronic invoices and payments. At the same time, the American National Standards Institute (ANSI) chartered the Accredited Standards Committee (ASC) X12 to create standard, electronic formats for all business transactions. ASC X12's Insurance Subcommittee (X12 N) Healthcare Task Group developed many standard healthcare transactions. These included healthcare claims (837), healthcare payments and remittance advices (835), and healthcare claim status requests (276).

However, acceptance by the healthcare industry to use these standards as the tools for conducting business electronically was atrociously slow. The unfortunate outcome of the industry's self-imposed obstacles to the adoption of standards-based EDI increased the need for paper-based and telephone callback business processes, resulting in even higher costs and less efficiencies than the older, manual systems.

In 1991, the Workgroup for Electronic Data Interchange (WEDI), a public/private task force, was established by the United States Department of Health and Human Services (HHS) to develop an action plan for healthcare standards-based EDI: standardizing and implementing electronic data exchange to reduce the healthcare industry's inefficient administrative processes and increasing costs. WEDI's 1993 report underscored the need to establish uniform content and coding so that healthcare data could be exchanged quickly, easily, and inexpensively via interconnecting networks. Also, the report recommended industrywide, standards-based EDI implementation guidelines. Such guidelines included establishing unique identification numbers for patients, providers, and payers; ensuring security to protect confidential medical and financial information; and enabling eligibility checking, verification of claim status and copayments, and referral information. The HHS secretary Louis Sullivan proposed that standards-based EDI would decrease paperwork and result in savings of $4 to $10 billion annually (Department of Health and Human Services 1993). These WEDI/HHS recommendations and proposals became the drivers that forced the enactment of Title II, Administrative Simplification, of the Health Insurance Portability and Accountability Act of 1996 (HIPAA).

HIPAA's proposed rule on the EDI/coding standard transaction set was published in August 2000. As of this writing, its original, third quarter, 2002 compliance date was extended to the third quarter of 2003. The rule mandates that healthcare "covered entities"/"business partners" implement a common standard (ASC X12 N) for the transfer of information and accept the standard-based electronic transaction. This regulation does not apply to the transfer of data and information within a healthcare organization, but it does apply to the transfer of data and information external to and between healthcare organizations.

By the new millennium, the term *EDI* (but not the concept) had become somewhat dated. With the mid- to late 1990s lightning-effect introduction and widespread acceptance of the Internet and its derived technologies, such as the web, the term **e-commerce** began to replace the term *EDI*. Today, e-commerce is used to describe the integration of all aspects of business-to-business (B2B) and business-to-consumer (B2C) activities, processes, and communications, *including* EDI.

In addition, the term **e-health** is now used to describe the application of e-commerce in the healthcare industry. Several principles and concepts of e-health directly relate to EDI principles and concepts. These include the links among the healthcare trading/business partners; the links to healthcare equipment and supply vendors, providers, and health plans; and the transactions for exchanging data on healthcare eligibility, referrals, claims, and so forth.

Enterprise Master Patient Indexes

Too often, breakdowns in patient identification cause patient record errors that threaten data integrity. The most common error occurs when healthcare provider organization registration personnel fail to locate existing patient information in the organization's **master patient index** (MPI), including the patient's unique identification number. The patient is then assigned another record (in other words, a duplicate record) and a new file is created in the database. When this error occurs, it is unclear into which database file the patient's data should be entered. This often results in unnecessary, duplicate tests, billing problems, and increased legal exposure in the case of adverse treatment outcomes.

Another common error occurs when registration personnel incorrectly register a patient under another person's existing, unique identification number. This error of overlay results in the merging of two different patients' data into one file. The clinical risks are obvious.

As healthcare organizations come together into integrated delivery networks (IDNs), the probability increases that information about a patient is spread across multiple databases, in multiple formats, and updated and accessed by multiple transaction processing systems and personnel. This distribution causes problems when the IDN begins to assemble information about a patient in order to deliver care across diverse systems and encounters. Longitudinal applications, such as the CPR system, cannot be successful.

Consequently, healthcare provider organizations are developing strategic initiatives for **enterprise master patient indexes** (EMPIs). EMPIs provide access to multiple repositories of information from overlapping patient populations that are maintained in separate systems and databases. The approach is through an indexing scheme to all the organizations' databases' unique patient identification numbers and information. As such, EMPIs become the cornerstones of healthcare system integration projects.

EMPIs work in two ways. In the back end, EMPIs coordinate record keeping. The indexes receive information from multiple systems that need no modification. The receiving is often performed through an integration gateway or engine. The enterprise index tests to see whether the patient is identified in all of the systems; if not, it may assign a unique identification number or other, related identifier as well as correlating records throughout the enterprise.

In the front end, EMPIs receive requests from existing registration systems to send data to these systems. Usually these existing registration systems need some reprogramming to enable them to request and receive data from the EMPI. Currently, there is no consistent, accepted trigger event and standard data format to do this.

EMPI building is complex. Variations in information systems, data capture, and organizational goals and objectives present multiple challenges to integrating patient data. For example, EMPI building involves a multitude of decision points. These include deciding whether to employ centralized or distributed data storage; whether to maintain limited, additional information such as allergies and encounter histories or robust information such as problem lists; and whether to establish batch processing or real-time communication between the registration system and the EMPI. EMPIs require many complex capabilities. These capabilities include merging records pertaining to the same person, maintaining source systems' pointers, removing duplicate records, and providing a common user interface. Finally, after technical and organizational issues are overcome, the purely operational task of linking patients across multiple entities and episodes of care and maintaining these linkages is difficult and can be costly.

Data Repositories

Data repositories are powerful databases that exist in every industry and are designed to store large amounts of data. Typically, these databases are organized into data fields, data records, and data files.

Typically, the model of these databases is relational. In other words, the data are stored physically in the database using two-dimensional tables that create a relation. Typically, the format of the data is structured and the type of data is discrete. Therefore, this model forces the database architect to predict how many data fields, records, and files will be stored about a particular event.

Some **relational databases** contain binary large objects (BLOBs) in their tables that consist of unstructured data, such as free-text data, bit-mapped data, real audio data, streaming video data, or vector graphic data. More commonly, relational databases contain pointers in their tables that indicate other, physical data repositories containing the unstructured data.

Typically, the other physical data repositories are **object-oriented databases.** An object can contain several types of unstructured data. Typically, these data types are stored in the database tables with specific behavior rules or procedures. For example, streaming video data are stored in the database tables with "fast-forward" or "rewind" behavior rules. This model cannot force the database architect to predict how many data fields, records, and files will be stored about a particular event.

Typically, in healthcare provider organizations, the term *data repository* is used to refer to databases that are relational and store structured, discrete, patient clinical, administrative, and financial data. As such, the repositories storing patient clinical data are often called clinical data repositories (CDRs), the repositories storing patient financial data are often called financial data repositories (FDRs), and so on. Sometimes one data repository physically stores all the organization's structured and discrete clinical, administrative, and financial data related to patients.

To provide continuous, high-quality care for patients, all the physical data repositories in healthcare provider organizations must be linked logically. These repositories include the relational databases that store structured, discrete, patient clinical, administrative, and financial data as well as the object-oriented databases that store unstructured, patient free-text, bit-mapped, real audio, streaming video, or vector graphic data. The EMPI primary index keys, the patients' unique identification numbers, are these links.

In addition, the organizations' logically linked, physical data repositories must be designed to allow **online/real-time transactions processing** (OLTP) of the data stored in the repositories. In other words, the data are entered into the repositories by the organizations' various "feeder" applications, and the users must be able to manipulate, update, retrieve, and otherwise act on the data in real time while the data are stored in the repositories. This requires data repositories to include tools designed to perform intricate data searches and retrievals.

For example, typically, a healthcare provider organization's CDR incorporates powerful, centralized, relational database management technology. In an online/real-time mode, the CDR allows providers of care to access and manipulate patient structured and discrete, administrative and clinical data, such as patient demographic data, physician orders, nursing care plans, and laboratory/radiology/pathology results. It also allows providers to access and manipulate patient unstructured, free-text data, such as transcribed clinical report data.

Clinical Workstations or Clinician/Physician Portals

No one information system or vendor can provide all the applications, data types, and data formats needed by all of the healthcare industry's diverse healthcare organizations and users. Consequently, healthcare provider organizations maintain multiple, disparate "feeder" applications for their repositories. Depending on their sizes and systems acquisition philosophies, some healthcare provider organizations maintain and often integrate large numbers of disparate feeder applications and others maintain and integrate at least two or three.

Each disparate feeder application for the repository has a unique user interface, uses different data nomenclature, and takes limited advantage of data standards. Therefore, it is not only difficult to integrate the information from the disparate systems into the repositories, but it is also difficult for the organizations' users to learn and interact with the different systems.

The concept of the **clinical workstation** evolved during the early 1990s so that one single point of access to the data in the repositories and to the applications "feeding" the data into the repositories would be deployed at the clinician's workstation or desktop. This single point of access would include a common user interface to view the information from the disparate applications as well as to launch the applications.

During this time, Microsoft's Windows® operating system products became ubiquitous for PC client workstations. Consequently, the Windows-based graphical user interface (GUI) was originally deployed at the clinical workstation. With the mid- to late-1990s introduction and widespread acceptance of the Internet and its derived technologies, the Web browser began to be deployed as the user interface of choice.

Today, clinical workstation is still used to describe the presentation of healthcare data and the launching of applications in the most effective way for healthcare providers. However, the concept of Web-based, clinician/physician portals is beginning to replace the concept of the clinical workstation.

Like clinical workstations, **clinician/physician portals** were first seen as a way for clinicians to easily access (via a Web browser) the healthcare provider organizations' multiple sources of structured and unstructured data from any network-connected device. Like clinical workstations, clinician/physician portals evolved into an effective medium for providing access to multiple applications as well as the data. But because clinician/physician portals are based on intranet and Internet technologies, they also became the access points to sources of data and applications both internal and external to the organization, respectively.

In short, clinician/physician portals have become, and can be considered analogous to, internal, private Webs. As such, the portals provide centralized security both internal and external to the organization. This is accomplished by restricting access to data and applications contained within the portal to authorized users. Examples of authorized users for healthcare provider organizations include a role (for example, physician), an individual (for example, Chris Jones, MD), a group of individuals (for example, all the physicians in the organization), a department (for example, internal medicine), or a group of departments.

In addition, clinician/physician portals provide simplified, automated methods of creating **taxonomy,** or classifying data. Consumer portals, such as Yahoo.com, provide good examples of this, whereby files and data corresponding to food, fashion, and travel are organized for easy access. Finally, true portals have at least one search engine and allow customization at the role and individual level. As such, search engines must be able to search e-mails, file servers, Web servers, and databases; and customization must allow users to create individual, relevant views. The clinical benefits of these portal features and functions are obvious.

Web-Based Systems and Applications

In the past decade, healthcare information system vendors were forced to migrate their existing systems and products from proprietary, centralized processing-based architectures running on mainframe computers, minicomputers, and microcomputers to open, client/server–based architectures. This required a lot of time and money in terms of company research and development (R&D). In many cases, it involved a total rewrite of the systems' code. For those healthcare information system (HIS) companies that designed their systems based on client/server architectures, they, too, were required to expend a lot of R&D time and money. This was because, typically, such firms had to transition from 16-bit to 32-bit hardware and software components, which also involved a total rewrite of the systems' code.

Ironically, at the same time that thousands of computer components were being "thickened" to 32 bits, maintaining thick client workstations and their multitude of corresponding servers became an IS department's worst nightmare. Also, during this time, the Internet and its derived technologies began to be introduced, offering a simpler and more cost-effective alternative to computer system development and maintenance.

However, the mass introduction and acceptance of the Internet and its derived technologies once again forced HIS companies to make another transition: to Web browser-based architectures. This, again, required a lot of R&D. In all cases, it involved a total rewrite of the systems' code.

Unfortunately, many HIS companies with legacy and/or client/server–based systems no longer could afford to make the next transition to Web-based architectures. Consequently, many of these companies began to "transition" their existing systems and products to Web browser–based architectures by **Web-enabling** the systems.

With Web enabling, the HIS companies do not rewrite their systems' code in the newer, Web-based programming languages, such as HTML, SGML, XML, or Java and its derivatives. Instead, when an authorized user logs onto the system, he or she is presented with a Web page. From the Web page, the companies' systems applications (for example, applications written in Microsoft's 32-bit Visual Basic) are launched.

Web browser–based systems are more complex. These are systems where companies have either written or rewritten their systems' code using one or more of the above-mentioned, Web-based programming languages. In Web browser–based systems, the Web browser acts as the primary desktop interface for access to a healthcare organization's repositories. The Web browser is used to display and query (for example, to drill-down via hypertext) information stored in databases as quickly as client/server–based systems. (For comparison purposes, in Web browser–based systems, the retrieval application typically resides on the server. In client/server–based systems, the retrieval application typically is loaded on standard, thick client workstations.)

Web browser-based systems accept data inputs from other systems and send them to other databases over the network using plug-ins or display controls, such as Active X or CORBA. Web browser–based systems are OLTP systems and have been proven to reduce network administration and workstation maintenance costs.

Intranets and Web Content Management

Web-based information systems and applications cannot continue to proliferate without creating **intranets** designed to enhance communication among an organization's employees and facilities. This is because intranets link every employee within an organization via an easy-to-navigate, comprehensive network devoted to internal business operations.

Just as portals are analogous to internal, private Webs, intranets are analogous to internal, private Internets. Access to data and applications contained within the intranet is restricted to authorized users. This is so that the general Internet public cannot access this private, secure network. However, through its intranet, a healthcare organization can access the Internet's servers for general Internet mail and messaging.

Intranets are growing at an astounding rate. They offer better security than use of the "public" Internet. Moreover, they are less expensive to implement and easier to use than most private networks of proprietary mail and messaging software products. In fact, today, intranets have become so important that almost every healthcare provider organization uses them as some form of development platform.

For example, these private, secure networks provide every healthcare organization employee basic information, such as message boards, employee handbooks, manuals, mail, cafeteria menus, newsletters, directories, and contact lists. Also, they are used for the development of the organization's computerized patient record. Here, the challenge is to evolve from the intranet's "static," informational, and brochureware-based Web pages to "dynamic" Web pages where authorized intranet users can access the private network's Web-based applications from anywhere and at anytime. This requires a powerful, stable infrastructure that can handle the transmission of larger amounts of data and support dynamic applications during times of peak use. It also requires continuous management of all the information and content on the intranet so that its users can find what they need to do their jobs better and so that the intranet information is kept current.

Publishing a few static or dynamic pages on an organization's intranet-based Web site is relatively easy. However, getting a group of people to do this effectively is challenging. Getting many groups of people to create the pages, track the revisions, set up the work flow, and scale and secure the intranet's framework is quite difficult from an organizational perspective.

Web content management systems label and track the exponential increase in and variety of information that is placed on a Web site so that the information can be easily located, modified, and reused. These systems are a critical component in personalizing an organization's intranet-based Web portals and page content for site users and visitors. They also provide crucial versioning and globalization capabilities. *Versioning* enables each of the Web site's content components to be tracked individually. Then, as the content changes, each iteration of the content can be identified, and the overall Web site can be recreated as it existed at any specific point in time. *Globalization* enables the look and feel of an organization's Web site to be managed centrally, while specific content is managed for local requirements, such as regional healthcare language or procedure differences.

Like other, traditional technologies and systems, intranets and Web content management systems have inherent benefits. Similarly, the issues surrounding the successful deployment of the technologies and systems in healthcare provider organizations are complex. For example, technical hurdles that must be overcome in using intranets and Web content management are found at every point of the compass; some are obvious, and some are hidden. More important, the implementation of the business processes that breathe new life into healthcare organizations via these technologies and systems is difficult. Developing intranets and using Web content management take time and commitment, usually without obvious, upfront, hard-dollar benefits.

Application Service Providers

Application service providers (ASPs) are service firms that deliver, manage, and remotely host standardized (prepackaged) applications software through centralized servers via a network, not exclusively but more commonly, the Internet. The software is provided through an outsourcing contract. As such, the ASP is viewed as a type of outsourcing. The contract is based on fixed, monthly usage, "rental-like" fees (for example, flat rate and per registered user fees) or transaction-based fees (for example, per transaction or percentage of revenue). The emphasis of this arrangement is on the functional use, rather than on the ownership, of a system (Nussbaum 2001, p. 3).

ASPs share many characteristics with the other types of outsourcing. The former service bureaus, which provided remote time-sharing services, existed during a time when hardware costs and knowledge to operate the hardware were expensive and not widely available. Service bureaus were a type of outsourcing that allowed healthcare provider organizations to concentrate management attention on its core business of patient care and not become distracted or diverted into IT challenges.

Times changed, and the high connectivity costs plus substantial monthly fees associated with service bureaus became less attractive than smaller, more robust and flexible systems that could be operated locally. But the concept of outsourcing did not dissipate. The remote computing option became an extension of the service bureau concept. Currently, this type of outsourcing is offered by many of the major HIS vendors. The difference is that remote computing outsourcing requires a substantial cadre of healthcare organization–employed and local IT professionals to operate the organization's software while the system's hardware and software reside in the vendor's data center.

The appeal of the ASP to both IT buyers and sellers is based on its position as a type of outsourcing somewhere between remote computing and full-asset outsourcing, which involves the transfer of all staff, long-term relationships, and accountability from internal IT management to a contracted third party. For example, major, capital, IT expenditures are the responsibility of the ASP. Consequently, healthcare organizations no longer need to fund large, upfront IT expenditures. Traditionally, chief financial officers crafted leases or similar arrangements to help mitigate some of the cash-flow impact of IT purchases. However, the ASP is also responsible for all the systems' maintenance and upgrades, which, under a leasing arrangement, are the responsibility of the healthcare organization. In addition, the ASP offers various payment methods, such as fixed monthly fees or transaction-based fees. Consequently, the ASP outsourcing model permits a more predictable monthly cost, potentially over a shorter duration.

Although the ASP model offers many benefits, a number of issues must be understood as detracting from its appeal. Perhaps the least favorable aspect of the ASP outsourcing model is the likelihood that the healthcare organization must accept a standard, off-the-shelf product. For the ASP to maintain its system efficiently and effectively for all its customers, often users are not allowed the level of customization or tailoring to which they are accustomed. Often healthcare organizations lose control on the time of system upgrades as well as the response time for changes to the software. The ASP may be faced with conflicting priorities among its customers in terms of demand for specific features and functions.

Given the need for integration and interfacing between and among a healthcare organization's disparate information systems, it is not a trivial exercise to consider how to integrate and interface ASP offerings into healthcare organizations' existing or future IT environments. Virtually all ASPs in healthcare limit their deliveries to their owned applications. Where multiple source applications are delivered and customer owned, virtually none is provided with a common user interface.

It is also not trivial to change an ASP in the event it files for bankruptcy or no longer participates with its customers in a partner-based relationship. Last but not least, security is a major concern, with the healthcare organization still maintaining full responsibility for firewalls and HIPAA compliance.

Many ASP delivery models reflect the application breadth, source, level of integration, interfaces, customer risks, and associated services. Thus, the delivery of the ASP model varies based on the organization's current environment and the value. Currently, the most significant targets for ASP consideration appear to be healthcare provider organizations with smaller investments in IT and/or that have difficulty retaining technical expertise and resources. This includes physician practices, small acute or specialty care facilities, and stand-alone clinics.

Check Your Understanding 3.3

Instructions: Answer the following questions on a separate piece of paper.

1. Give a healthcare example for each of the following automatic identification technologies: bar coding, OCR, and ICR.
2. How are the concepts of EDI, e-commerce, and e-health interrelated?
3. What is driving the heightened interest in EMPI technology within the healthcare industry?
4. What types of data are commonly maintained in an object-oriented database associated with a clinical data repository?
5. What is the primary purpose of the clinical workstation and the clinician/physician portal?
6. How are Web browser-based systems different from Web-enabled systems?
7. Why are intranets becoming so popular in healthcare organizations?
8. What are the benefits and drawbacks of choosing to use the application service provider (ASP) model for providing IT applications to a healthcare organization?

Supporting Managerial and Clinical Decision Making

Many current and emerging information technologies are used to support managerial and clinical decision making. For the purposes of this book, the following technologies and systems are highlighted:

- Data warehouses and data marts
- Decision support systems
- Artificial intelligence

Data Warehouses and Data Marts

Data warehouses are large, centralized, enterprisewide collections of all the historical, demographic, and transactional data and information about businesses that are used to support managerial or, in the case of healthcare provider organizations, clinical decision-making processes. Data warehousing is the acquisition of all the business data and information from potentially multiple, cross-platform sources such as legacy databases, departmental databases, and online transaction-based databases and then the warehouse storage of all the data in one consistent format. Data mining is the probing and extracting of all the business data and information from the warehouse and then the quantifying and filtering of the data for analysis purposes.

Like data repositories, data warehouses are powerful databases. And, like data repositories, typically the format of the data in the warehouse is structured and the type of data is discrete.

However, typically, the model of the data warehouse database is subject oriented. In other words, the data within the data warehouse are organized along subject lines (customer, product, patient, clinician) rather than along operational lines (accounting, management, medicine, surgery) in order to be accessible and useful across the enterprise. For example, healthcare provider organizations use data warehouses to centrally organize patient information to establish wellness plans supporting community medicine to reduce costs.

In addition, the data are stored in the warehouse database using multidimensional tables rather than two-dimensional tables that create a relation as in relational databases. For example, if a surgeon performs a certain procedure several times during a period of time, the data query also may need to include the average length of stay (ALOS) for the procedure. Therefore, the warehouse data must be structured so that the identifying data (such as a procedure or time period or ALOS) resides in the database dimension headers (which are comparable to the row and column headers of a spreadsheet) rather than being repeated for each record as in relational databases. This multidimensional model, sometimes referred to as a physical cube, lends itself to trend analysis and forecasting.

Generally, for day-to-day operations, a healthcare organization needs relatively current data, and each operational unit needs only its own data. That is why relational and object-oriented database models for data repositories are well suited for OLTP. But for large-scale, retrospective data analysis, for which **online/real-time analytical processing** (OLAP) is designed, a healthcare organization generally needs not just its current status but also a historical record over time or time variance, encompassing all the organizational operating units by subject for comparison purposes.

In addition, for large-scale data analysis, a healthcare organization generally requires summary data, not detail data. Using the above surgeon and procedure example, the data query may need to know only the summary figure for the ALOS.

Finally, warehouse data, when correctly recorded, cannot be updated like repository data. Generally, only two kinds of operations occur in a data warehouse: data warehousing and data mining. This is referred to as the nonvolatility of warehouse data.

In healthcare, data warehouses have been used primarily for the following applications (Henchey 1998, p. 68):

- *Clinical management:* For example, every day, patient clinical data are fed into the warehouse from multiple sources to contribute to enterprisewide best practices and to identify areas of excessive variation from best practices.
- *Operations management:* For example, sophisticated analytical tools, such as cost accounting, case-based budgeting, and variance analysis tools, are included with the warehouse to determine new healthcare market opportunities.
- *Outcomes management:* For example, data mining is conducted to study patient health status or other factors, such as satisfaction, that contribute to clinical outcomes.
- *Population management:* For example, to proactively manage the health of plan members, data mining helps the organization to predict utilization or identify at-risk members requiring case management.
- *Revenue management:* For example, the data warehouse assists healthcare financial analysts in addressing all the different contractual and regulatory reimbursement formulas. With revenue based on a mix of several dimensions, such as fee-for-service, capitation, and risk pooling, only the data warehouse can provide a complete picture of the enterprise's revenue stream and the factors controlling it.

A data warehouse cannot simply be bought and installed. Its implementation requires the integration of many products within its architecture. For example, data warehouses often require advanced data warehousing and mining techniques and tools. The software must be able to locate data that are often stored on multiple servers that may include any type of machine or operating system. The software must be able to maintain **metadata** (indexed data about the data), such as what indexes the acquired data uses. Further, the software must be able to recognize data duplication and exceptions as well as issue alerts when data are not present or have been corrupted.

Data marts can be thought of as miniaturized data warehouses. Data marts are usually geared to the needs of a specific department, group, or business operational unit. Because data marts are considerably smaller in both size and complexity than data warehouses, some healthcare organizations build data marts as a way of testing data warehouses on smaller, more focused scales. What many are finding, though, is that data marts can easily proliferate into a collection of incompatible data stores with accessibility or utility limited to the department or operational unit that designed the mart.

Decision Support Systems

Decision support systems (DSSs) are interactive computer systems that intend to help decision makers use data and models to identify and solve problems and make decisions. A great deal of innovation is occurring related to DSSs, and the technologies that make them up are changing rapidly.

Generally, DSSs are based on either a data repository model or a data warehouse model. Both transfer data from an operational environment (either in real time or retrospectively, in batches at fixed intervals) to a decision-making environment, and both organize the data in a form suitable to decision support applications.

Power (1997) suggests that DSSs can be classified based on one or more of the following five categories:

- *Communications-driven DSSs* emphasize communications, collaboration, and shared decision-making support. A simple Internet bulletin board or threaded e-mail is the most elementary level of functionality in this type of DSS.
- *Data-driven DSSs* emphasize access to and manipulation of internal, and sometimes external, structured business data. Simple file systems accessed by query and retrieval tools provide the most elementary level of functionality in this type of DSS.
- *Document- or graphics-driven DSSs* focus on the retrieval and management of unstructured business data. Basic document- or graphics-driven DSSs exist in the form of Web-based search engines.
- *Knowledge-driven DSSs* can suggest or recommend actions to decision makers. These DSSs are person-to-computer systems with specialized problem-solving expertise. The expertise consists of knowledge about a particular domain, understanding of problems within that domain, and skill at solving some of these problems.
- *Model-driven DSSs* emphasize access to and manipulation of a model, for example, statistical, financial, optimization, and/or simulation models. Simple statistical and analytical tools provide the most elementary level of functionality in this type of DSS.

A wide variety of DSSs and related tools and technologies exist in healthcare, most of which can be classified as hybrids of the above categories. These systems include, but are not limited to, clinical/medical decision support systems, management information systems (MIS), executive information systems (EIS), geographic information systems (GIS), and expert decision support systems.

Clinical/Medical Decision Support Systems

Typically, **clinical/medical decision support systems** are data driven. They assist clinicians in applying new information to patient care through the analysis of patient-specific clinical/medical variables. Clinical/medical decision support systems can be characterized simply by providing reminders and alerts, clinical guideline advice, or benchmarking tools. However, many of these systems are used to enhance diagnostic efforts and include computer programs that provide extensive differential diagnoses based on the clinical/medical data and information entered by the clinician (Barnett et al. 1987). Other forms of clinical/medical decision support systems seek to prevent medical errors and improve patient safety. These DSSs include tools such as antibiotic management programs and anticoagulation dosing calculators (Hunt et al. 1998).

Management Information Systems

Typically, **management information systems** (MISs) refer to the broad range of data-, document-, or knowledge-driven DSSs that provide information concerned with an organization's administrative functions (in other words, those functions that are associated with the provision and utilization of services). In addition, DSS-based MISs enable management to interrogate the computer on an ad hoc basis for various kinds of information within the organization so as to predict the effect of potential decisions. As such, DSS-based MISs provide information to people who must query these systems to make disposition decisions about valuable resources in a timely, accurate, and complete manner. Such systems are crucial for the effective administration of any organization and include, but are not limited to, general accounting and financial systems, customer relationship management (CRM) systems, enterprise resource planning (ERP) systems, and operations/plant management systems.

Executive Information Systems

Executive information systems (EISs) are DSSs that support the decision making of senior managers. As such, EISs provide direct online access to timely, accurate, and actionable information about aspects of a business that are of particular interest to a senior healthcare manager. Typically, this information is provided in a useful and navigable format so that managers can identify broad strategic issues and then explore the information to find the root causes of those issues. According to Kelly (2001), the following EIS features and functions are essential:

- The system must be specifically tailored to executives' information needs.
- The system must be able to access data about specific issues and problems.
- The system must be able to aggregate data into meaningful reports.
- The system must provide extensive online analysis tools including trend analysis, exception reporting, and drill-down or data-mining capabilities.
- The system must be able to access a broad range of internal and external data.
- The system must be easy to use (typically mouse or touchscreen driven).
- The system must be able to be used directly by executives without assistance.
- The system must be able to present information in a graphical form.

Geographic Information Systems

In the strictest sense, **geographic information systems** (GISs) are DSSs capable of assembling, storing, manipulating, and displaying geographically referenced data and information. In other words, GISs identify data according to their locations. The applications of GIS in healthcare extend from practical community-based services to sophisticated studies on a global scale. For example, pediatricians consult community-based GISs to observe neighborhoods with high concentrations of lead and decide whether lead screenings would be appropriate for certain patients.

Expert Decision Support Systems

Expert decision support systems (also referred to as systems that use principles of artificial intelligence) use a set of rules or encoded concepts to construct a reasoning process. Such rules or concepts are based on knowledge developed from consultation with experts on a problem and the processing and/or formalizing of this knowledge in such a manner that the problem can be solved. In other words, expert DSSs provide the kind of problem analysis and advice that an expert might provide if he or she were present as a consultant.

Some of the various rules-based processing techniques used by expert DSSs are neural networks and data mining, defined earlier in this chapter. Other techniques include (Siwicki 1996, p. 47):

- *Fuzzy logic:* A rules-based system that mimics human thought and enables a computer to "think" in inexact terms rather than in a definitive, either-or manner
- *Genetic algorithms:* Tools that examine data and determine by programmed stipulations which data best match a stated goal and which data do not
- *Symbolic reasoning:* A method of deduction that follows an explicit line of inferences

Expert systems "learn" based on the continual addition of data to the system. Therefore, in its simplest model, the technologies of continuous speech/voice recognition or ICR can be considered expert. These technologies adapt themselves into shifting configurations based on what they encounter, and they change as they grow and learn.

Throughout the past decade, federal grants have been awarded to healthcare organizations to develop clinical/medical, managerial, executive, geographical, and expert DSSs. For example, in 1997, the Seattle-based Fred Hutchinson Cancer Research Center received more than $1.5 million to develop a clinical/medical DSS that can be accessed by care providers over the Internet. The University of North Carolina Medical Center received almost $900,000 to expand and evaluate an existing guideline-based DSS for childhood preventive services. Duke University Medical Center received almost $800,000 to rewrite an existing DSS-based EIS using Internet technologies (Chin 1997, p. 24).

Artificial Intelligence

In other disciplines and industries, the term *artificial intelligence* is often used synonymously with the term *expert decision support systems.* Because expert decision support systems, especially those using neural network techniques, "learn" as humans do by processing information through recognizing patterns of signals, there are only a few differentiators.

The field of **artificial intelligence** (AI) is the branch of computer science concerned with endowing computers with the ability to simulate human intelligence and behavior. As such, AI attempts to understand intelligence and intelligent entities and then design computer systems to perform functions normally associated with language, learning, reasoning, and problem solving.

This involves developing systems that think and act like humans. This human-centered approach to AI involves empirical science, which, in turn, involves hypothesis creation and experimental confirmation. This also involves developing systems that think and act rationally. A rationalist approach to artificial intelligence involves a combination of mathematics and engineering.

Exploring and furthering the application of AI to clinical situations is lofty because of the vital and crucial nature of medical science as well as the need for accurate and timely data and information to support clinical decisions. Consequently, AI to support clinical decision making focuses on the gathering, availability, security, and use of medical information throughout the human life cycle and beyond.

Check Your Understanding 3.4

Instructions: Answer the following questions on a separate piece of paper.

1. What features differentiate a data warehouse from a data repository?
2. What is the primary difference between expert decision support systems and the more common clinical decision support systems?
3. What functional capabilities are associated with applications that use artificial intelligence technology?

Supporting the Diagnosis, Treatment, and Care of Patients

Many current and emerging information technologies are used to support the diagnosis, treatment, and care of patients. For the purposes of this book, the following technologies are highlighted:

- Physiological signal processing systems
- Point-of-care information systems and wireless technology
- Automated care plans, clinical practice guidelines, clinical pathways, and protocols
- Telemedicine/telehealth
- Computer-based patient record systems
- Computer-based patient information and education

Physiological Signal Processing Systems

The human body is a rich source of signals that carry vital information about underlying physiological processes. Traditionally, such signals have been used in clinical diagnosis as well as in the study of the functional behavior of internal organs.

Earlier in this chapter, **physiological signal processing systems,** such as ECG, EEG, EMG, and fetal trace systems, were mentioned because these systems store data based on the body's signals and create output based on the lines plotted between the signals' points. The data type used by these systems is referred to as signal tracing or vector graphic data.

Physiological signal processing systems measure biological signals. Also, they help to integrate the medical science of analyzing the signals with such disciplines as biomedical engineering, computer graphics, mathematics, diagnostic image processing, computer vision, and pattern recognition. The integration of these disciplines allows these systems to electronically compile measurement equations, estimate the signals' parameters, and characterize the feedback elements. For example, the computer-based analysis of the neuromuscular system, the definition of cardiovascular system models, the control of cardiac pacemakers, the regulation of blood sugar levels, and the development of artificial organs not only serve patient diagnostic and care purposes, but they also support the development and simulation of instrumentation for physiological research and clinical investigation.

Point-of-Care Information Systems and Wireless Technology

Computer systems that allow healthcare providers to capture and retrieve data and information at the location where the healthcare service is performed have come a long way since hard-wired computer terminals with green screens were first placed at the patient's bedside more than twenty years ago. Functionally, almost every type of patient clinical and administrative application has been introduced to provide care services at the bedside, in the exam room, at the home, or even on the patient, as in medical monitoring. Technologically, massive changes have occurred in these systems' platforms, footprints, and networking capabilities.

For example, many acute care facilities have installed clinical **point-of-care information systems** that, among other services, provide online medication order entry, profiles, administration schedules, and records. The records include information about medications not given (with reasons) as well as related information such as fluid balances, physical assessments, laboratory test results, and vital signs. All medications, including unit doses, are bar coded and scanned at or near the patient's bedside along with the patient's wristband and caregiver's identification badge. This prompts a safety edit, documents administration of the medication, and generates the charge.

Other acute care facilities have installed administrative point-of-care (or service) systems that have eliminated admitting areas. Inpatients are greeted at the door with their room assignments, and roving admissions representatives visit patients in the assigned rooms to complete all the admission procedures.

Typically, point-of-care information systems use portable, handheld, wireless devices to enable entry of the data by a bar code scanner, keypad, or touch screen. Also, the devices are used to upload and download information to and from hard-wired workstations. Retrieval of the data occurs at the wireless device or on wall-mounted or portable monitors. The data also can be entered and retrieved on hard-wired workstations located in areas outside the point of care, such as central areas at patient care units, back offices, central or satellite pharmacies, and physician lounges/homes/offices.

Most care providers maintain that it takes more time to enter data into point-of-care information systems than into manual systems. However, recently, providers have accepted the increased data-entry times because they realize impressive benefits from quicker data retrieval times. They also realize, for example, improved safety benefits from screening medications before administration, such as lowered medication error rates, improved and more legible records, improved scheduling of medications, improved communication between staff members, and more accurate and timely billing. In addition, other organization and team partners, such as quality assessment personnel, case managers, and third-party payers, are able to access these systems simultaneously for authorized data retrieval purposes.

Perhaps the biggest change influence on, as well as challenge for, point-of-care information systems and their use comes from recent, significant advances in wireless technology and smaller, mobile devices. For the healthcare industry, the successful integration of wireless technology and smaller, mobile devices with point-of-care software supports and enhances the clinician's decision-making processes.

True wireless systems use wireless networks and wireless devices to access and transmit data in real time. At the basic level, **wireless technology** is based on the use of radio waves. For the purposes of this chapter, the technology is divided into two categories: (1) regulated and unregulated, and (2) wide area and in-building.

For the general benefit of the country, Congress has charged the Federal Communications Commission (FCC) with regulation of the radio spectrum. This regulation encompasses licenses for the use of the radio frequencies for commercial radio, television, walkie-talkies, and mobile telephones. Specific portions of the radio spectrum may be assigned to specific users, such as individual radio stations, or set aside for general and usually low power use, such as Citizens Band (CB) radio.

For years, healthcare organizations have used in-building wireless point-of-care information systems, such as telemetry systems. These systems were based on existing technologies and use a portion of the radio spectrum reserved for industrial, scientific, and medical purposes (ISM band). Individual licenses are not required for these types of systems.

Also, provider organizations have long used wide-area wireless technology to support information systems, such as point-of-care systems. This technology involves microwave systems that are based on fixed, point-to-point wireless technology used to connect buildings in a campus network.

Microwave systems are regulated and require licenses and compliance with FCC procedures.

Until recently, most in-building wireless systems were proprietary. However, adoption of the IEEE 802.11 wireless technology standard has begun to provide a reasonable level of standardization. The IEEE 802.11 standard allows data transmission speeds up to 11 megabits per second; it is relatively low power; and it does not require licenses for installation and use. The IEEE 802.11b is an international standard that provides a method for wireless connectivity to fixed and portable devices within a local area. As such, this standard allows interoperability among multiple vendor products.

But it is the widespread adoption of cellular telephone technology that has significantly advanced the development of wireless technology and, consequently, its support for point-of-care systems. A brief look at most healthcare organizations today turns up mobile phones, two-way pagers, Internet-enabled telephones, and **personal digital assistants** (PDAs).

Currently, the majority of these devices are used to meet personal, individual needs. For wireless technology and the smaller mobile devices to be integrated into larger corporate projects such as point-of-care information systems, they must significantly enhance the function and use of existing information systems. Therefore, to date, only a few healthcare organizations have successfully taken advantage of the technology and devices for point-of-care projects. Impediments that have prevented a more widespread use of the technology and devices for point-of-care systems include:

- Impediments preventing widespread use of wireless technology
  —Vendor difficulty in packaging wireless technology with specific clinical software applications that demonstrate a significant return on investment and added value to the clinician
  —The use of proprietary wireless technology
  —Inconsistent technology deployment
  —The need to make a large investment for the deployment of wireless on a wide scale
  —The need to make a large investment for the underlying network infrastructure to support wireless
- Impediments preventing widespread use of smaller, portable, point-of-care devices
  —Battery life, weight, and screen real estate
  —How and when the batteries will be recharged, where the devices will be stored when not in use, and how updated data will be accessed
  —Application functionality, for example, how the data are delivered in bits and are not presented in a page-oriented fashion, how the processing of the data must be transactional, and how an abundance of frivolous graphics or poor-quality content cannot be tolerated

Automated Clinical Care Plans, Practice Guidelines, Pathways, and Protocols

The terms used to describe practice mandates, care process guides and documents, disease management decision algo-rithms, and quality improvement tools are not well standardized. They tend to be used informally and interchangeably, resulting in miscommunication among healthcare professionals. Consequently, when clinical care plans, practice guidelines, pathways, and protocols are automated and used by multidisciplinary teams, the effects on patient care can be detrimental unless the definitions are uniformly applied. For example:

- Healthcare providers create **clinical care plans** for individual patients for a specific time period. Typically, clinical care plans are based on provider training.
- **Clinical practice guidelines** are recommendations based on systematic statements or clinical algorithms of proven care options. Often professional organizations and associations, health plans, and government agencies such as the Agency for Health Care Policy and Research develop these guidelines.
- For a specific time period, **clinical or critical pathways** or **Care Maps** delineate standardized, day-to-day courses of care for a group of patients with the same diagnosis or procedure to achieve consistent outcomes. Typically, pathways or Care Maps are developed by the local healthcare organization or health plan.
- Clinicians often use the term **protocol** to refer to the written documents that guide or specify a practice, including clinical practice guidelines and pathways. Strictly speaking, however, protocols are more detailed care plans for individual patients based on investigations performed by professional societies, drug companies, or individual researchers (Bufton 1999, p. 258).

Providers are now recognizing the enormous variation in how they diagnose, treat, and care for patients. Consequently, there is a trend to adopt **evidence-based medicine** and **outcomes management** based on more use of guidelines, formalized pathways, and protocols. Automating these guidelines, pathways, and protocols for easier access and use is the first step. Also, there is a trend to incorporate care plans into providers' notes. This is being recognized as automated clinical documentation systems are being introduced into and used by more healthcare organizations.

In short, care plans, guidelines, pathways, and protocols, as well as formularies and other knowledge bases, are becoming automated for easier access and use and for easier maintenance. In particular, practice guidelines and knowledge bases that are available through subscriptions from agencies, societies, and research companies can be kept more current because users can incorporate periodic downloads into their transaction-based or analytic systems.

The challenge for automated care plans, practice guidelines, pathways, and protocols is that, like clinical workstations and portals, no one form of clinical documentation or one view of the information suits everyone or all situations. For example, the wide variability of clinical documentation is obvious in H&Ps versus consultations. Such documentation suits some providers, but not others, or some situations, but not all. Similarly, views of data are requested in page, narrative, table, flowchart, or graphic formats. Therefore, automated plans, guidelines, pathways, and protocols require customization capabilities to help individuals and groups better share knowledge to reach similar decisions about patient care. Automated drawing tools and anatomical diagrams are other documentation options.

Another challenge is that it is difficult to convert intricate clinical care processes and guideline, pathway, and protocol content into computer architecture. An even higher level of complexity occurs when the content is merged with reengineered processes, instead of just automating the existing or status quo processes. This is because these actions represent a translation of specific and conceptual clinical information and interpretations into data fields. Therefore, it is recommended that clinicians work with information systems analysts, such as health information managers, to ensure that the integrity of the clinical content is preserved during the conversion.

In addition, the task of seamlessly embedding reminders or alerts or defaulted, guideline-based clinical orders into information systems as well as the care processes is challenging. According to Bufton (1999, p. 266), this requires in-depth knowledge of the following:

- The computer system's capabilities and limitations, such as data dictionaries, field lengths, screen builders, data retrieval/analysis/reporting capabilities
- The processes of care, local caseloads, and local practice environments
- The many diverse guidelines, pathways, and protocols

Telemedicine/Telehealth

Interactive, patient–provider consultations across gulfs of time and space represent what is often referred to as classic telemedicine or telehealth. However, the field has always encompassed a plethora of strategies for moving clinical knowledge and expertise instead of moving people. As such, telemedicine/telehealth systems, like CPR systems, are concepts made up of several cost-effective technologies used to bridge geographic gaps between patients and providers.

In other words, telemedicine/telehealth is not video-conferencing technology. Rather, it is clinically adequate, interactive, media conferencing (for example, video conferencing) integrated with other technologies. It can be dynamic and include interactive (or real-time processing) technology, or it can be static and include store-and-forward (or batch-processing) technology. It includes telecommunications and remote control-based biomedical technologies. It utilizes in-room systems, rollouts, desktop systems, and/or handheld units. Often it is integrated with component technologies of the CPR system and/or derived technologies of the Internet. The access and ability to transmit patient records and the integration with reference databases on the Internet all play into the telemedicine/telehealth model.

Telemedicine/telehealth is not a new way to deliver healthcare. It is the taking of existing ways of delivering healthcare and enhancing them, such as enhancing patient–provider consultations via "electronic house calls." It is the extending of care to underserved populations, whether they are located in rural or urban areas, and the redefining of the healthcare organization's community. It is the transferring of clinical information between places of lesser and greater medical capability and expertise.

Like medicine in general, telemedicine/telehealth technology is made up of a number of specialties and subspecialties. Some examples include:

- Telecardiology
- Teledermatology
- Telehome healthcare
- Teleneurology
- Telenursing healthcare
- Teleophthalmology
- Telepathology
- Telepsychiatry
- Teleradiology
- Telesurgery

The telemedicine/telehealth specialty that has been around for the longest time and, perhaps, is the most notable is teleradiology. However, since the early 1990s, the University of Pittsburgh Medical Center, the Mayo Clinic, and other prestigious provider organizations have employed dynamic telepathology interactions. Teleradiology and telepathology specialties are considered first-generation telemedicine/telehealth systems and services because they do not rely on patient interaction.

The second-generation telemedicine/telehealth systems and services involve those specialties relying on patient interaction and consultations. These include teleophthalmology, telepsychiatry, telehome healthcare, and so on.

The latest generation of telemedicine/telehealth systems and services involves patient interaction beyond the consultation. For example, in October 2001, telesurgeons in New York City performed the world's first complete (that is, from start to finish) telesurgery by successfully operating on the gallbladder of a patient in France. This was accomplished by sending high-speed signals through fiber-optic cables across the Atlantic Ocean to robots in a Strasbourg clinic.

As both a clinical and technological endeavor, telemedicine/telehealth plays a key role in the integration of managing patient care and in the more efficient management of the information systems that support it. However, overcoming multiple technical challenges remains a concern. These challenges include the lack of systems interoperability and network integration as well as metropolitan broad bandwidth limitations. Physician resistance, proven cost-effectiveness, proven medical effectiveness, and safety are other challenges that require overcoming complex behavioral, economic, and ethical constraints.

Computer-Based Patient Record Systems

In 1991, the Institute of Medicine (IOM) defined the CPR as "an electronic patient record that resides in a system specifically designed to support users by providing accessibility to complete and accurate data, alerts, reminders, clinical decision support systems, links to medical knowledge, and other aids" (Dick and Steen 1991, p. 11). Although a common definition of the CPR was under way by various groups by the end of the decade, no universal term for it has emerged.

Following are some of the terms currently used synonymously (and sometimes incorrectly) with the term CPR:

- Automated medical record (AMR)
- Electronic medical record (EMR)
- Electronic patient record (EPR)
- Electronic health record (EHR)

Despite the fractionalization of the vocabulary leadership, the idea is the same. The CPR is "electronically stored information about an individual's lifetime health status and health care. It replaces the paper medical record as the primary record of care, meeting all clinical, legal and administrative requirements. . . . [It] provides reminders and alerts, linkages with knowledge sources for decision support, and data for outcomes research and improved management of health care delivery" (Dick, Steen, and Detmer 1997, p. 11).

Fortunately, there is agreement that the CPR system is not one or even two or more products. According to Dick and Steen (1991, p. 12), the CPR system is a "set of components that form the mechanism by which patient records are created, used, stored and retrieved. . . . It includes people, data, rules and procedures, processing and storage devices, and communication and support facilities." According to Dick, Steen, and Detmer (1997, p. 11), the CPR system is "an evolving concept that responds to the dynamic nature of the healthcare environment and takes advantages of technological advances." In other words, the CPR system is a concept consisting of an array of integrated, component information systems and technologies.

Unfortunately, no universal understanding of the CPR system's components exists. Information technology professionals understand the system's components as elements of an information technology infrastructure by which the patient's CPR is created and managed. The infrastructure represents an aggregation of information from multiple, often disparate, databases and systems within and across the healthcare enterprise. It incorporates a messaging standard for common representation of all pertinent patient data. Stored data are indexed with sufficient detail to support retrieval for patient care delivery, management, and analysis. It includes hardware, application software, system software, user interfaces, networks, communications protocols, and so on.

CPR System Infrastructure

Technically, the CPR system infrastructure consists of multiple **physical** data repositories. Typically, these repositories are organized into data fields, data records, and data files. They store structured, discrete, clinical, administrative, and financial data as well as unstructured, patient free-text, bit-mapped, real audio, streaming video, or vector graphic data. They must be linked to form one, **logical** (or conceptual) repository. Typically, the EMPI primary index keys constitute these links. (See figure 3.2.)

Technically, the CPR system infrastructure also consists of multiple data types, information systems, software applications, and technologies. Examples of multiple data types were explained earlier in this chapter. Examples of multiple information systems include most of those discussed in this chapter, such as medical information systems, hospital information systems, ambulatory care information systems, practice management systems, electronic document management systems, picture archive and communication systems, telemedicine systems, patient appointment and resource scheduling systems, physiological signal processing systems, registration/eligibility/enrollment systems, decision support systems, and clinical information systems. Examples of multiple software applications and technologies also include

Figure 3.2.   Physical and Logical Data Repositories for CPR Systems

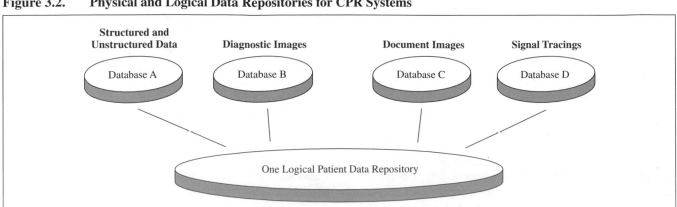

most of those discussed in this chapter, such as work-flow and messaging software, security/access to information technologies, single log-on software, Internet-derived technologies, and electronic signature software.

Currently, one or more CPR system infrastructure component technologies or systems have been installed in healthcare organizations. However, the existing components may not be integrated.

Typically, several components are implemented in parallel. Solely technical attributes of CPR system infrastructure component systems and technologies must not be considered to determine whether and when to implement various components. Instead, the value of the component to improve the quality of patient care, the fiscal priorities of the organization, the available technical and organizational resources, and the unique business motives and strategies of the organization must be considered.

CPR System Attributes

The 1991 IOM report identified twelve attributes for the CPR system. These attributes represent the elements essential to provide the required functionality that supports healthcare providers with a robust CPR system. Since then, the attributes have been revised and expanded. This is to ensure their completeness as tools with enhanced utility for providing high-quality patient care in light of the ever-changing healthcare environment and technological advances.

Following are the 1991 IOM report's twelve attributes for the CPR system (Dick and Steen 1991):

1. The CPR system offers a problem list.
2. The CPR system measures health status and functional levels (in other words, it measures clinical outcomes).
3. The CPR system documents clinical reasoning and the rationale for patient care decisions.
4. The CPR system provides longitudinal and timely linkages with other patient records.
5. The CPR system protects the privacy of the individual by guaranteeing that the information is confidential (in other words, indicating that the information is sensitive) and the confidential information is secure (for example, by providing audit trail capabilities).
6. The CPR system provides continuous, authorized user access.
7. The CPR system supports simultaneous, multiple user views into the CPR.
8. The CPR system supports timely access to local and remote information resources.
9. The CPR system facilitates clinical problem solving, using specific rule sets or decision support systems.
10. The CPR system supports direct data entry by providers of care, especially physicians.
11. The CPR system supports practitioners in measuring or managing costs and improving quality.

12. The CPR system is flexible to support existing and evolving clinical specialty needs.

According to Dick and Andrews (1995, pp. 66, 78), revised and expanded CPR system attributes also are considered crucial to the establishment of robust CPR systems. If any one of them were ignored or inadequately addressed in the design and development of the CPR system, the CPR might be jeopardized. Some of these subattributes include:

- The CPR system includes a substantial, flexible, and extensible clinical data dictionary.
- The CPR system supports a well-designed CDR so that the CDR is capable of supporting the extensive and diverse needs of all healthcare practitioners.
- The CPR system includes an array of powerful input capabilities to allow for the direct data entry of caregivers at the point of care.
- The CPR system supports a user-friendly, ergonomically designed presentation of the information for all intended users, including a presentation tailored to the type of individual and to personal preferences.
- The CPR system includes automated, intelligent support that anticipates and facilitates all clinical processes and thinking.

Current Status of Computer-Based Patient Record Systems

No one disputes the fact that CPR systems have the potential to improve the quality of care at lower costs. Furthermore, technologically, the chances of realizing the CPR vision are better today than ever before, primarily thanks to the advent of the Internet and its derived technologies model. As such, much can be done today to prepare and continue to implement the CPR system's component systems and technologies. For example, implementing clinical decision support systems, medication administration systems, and patient registries can provide huge advantages in patient care and safety.

However, today, ten years after the original IOM report, CPR systems are far from the standard for patient medical records. In addition, it is anticipated that still more years will pass before healthcare organizations realize the potential of CPR systems.

Perhaps the biggest challenge is that the return on investment has not yet been demonstrated. Others argue that, as originally defined, a CPR system is not what is needed and the objective of the CPR system should not be a theoretical ideal or concept but, rather, a focus on patient care processes and related systems and technologies that produce immediate, clear benefits and value (Drazen 2001).

Consequently, there remains a bewildering array of CPR initiatives, activities, and debates with no good assessment vehicles. For example, provider organizations continue to buy huge, difficult-to-implement systems from one large vendor for millions of dollars, which does little to restore the confidence that there will be a future market for other, more focused products. As long as the healthcare industry continues to do this, the CPR system will not advance quickly.

Computer-Based Patient Information and Education

Over the past decade, the use of e-commerce (in other words, the use of the Internet and its derived technologies to integrate all aspects of business-to-business and business-to-consumer activities, processes, and communications) has transformed every vertical market industry. In the healthcare industry, the following examples illustrate this transformation:

- Increasing numbers of patients access the Internet for information about healthcare providers, treatment options, and personal health information.
- Health Web sites provide patients with tools to develop and maintain personal, online health records independent of providers.
- Healthcare providers and patients correspond via e-mail, with each viewing and contributing information to the health record.
- Health plans, disease-specific groups, and professional associations use Web sites to provide education and interact with patients.

As a result, plausible scenarios regarding a patient's health information include the following:

- Personal, patient information might be obtained and used inappropriately by unauthorized individuals or organizations. Examples of targeted marketing based on unauthorized use of individually identifiable health information have already been cited.
- A patient's information might be accessed fraudulently and altered without detection. Also, the accessed information might be incomplete, incorrect, out-of-date, or misinterpreted, potentially resulting in financial or health-related harm to the patient.
- A patient might inadvertently enter the wrong medication in an allergy portion of a personal health record. In a subsequent episode of care, this information might be accessed and used to make prescribing decisions. The patient might have an allergic reaction and file suit.
- A hacker might break into the records of a provider and make entries in numerous records indicating a serious, chronic disease. The patient's credit rating, employment, or ability to get health insurance might be affected.

Contrary to popular belief, the information patients share with their care providers has never been completely private and protected. A national survey released in January 1999 found that one in five people believes that his or her personal health information has been used inappropriately, without his or her knowledge or consent. More striking, one in six Americans engages in some form of privacy-protective behavior to shield themselves from what they consider to be harmful and intrusive uses of their health information (California Health-Care Foundation 1999).

But because of the Internet and its e-commerce transformation, the situation has become more acute. For example, traditional, organizational health information management (HIM) processes have become inadequate. Centrally controlled processes such as release of information in accordance with a valid authorization are not easily administered in cyberspace. Authentication of health record entries to verify responsibility and accuracy is more complex when managing an Internet-connected longitudinal, rather than episodic, health record. Safeguarding against misinterpretation of treatment findings is more difficult when patients have online access to information, potentially even seeing test results before the provider.

Computer technology can offer suitable solutions to traditional HIM problems. However, technology without effective policy will neither meet patients' requirements nor be adequate for providers who remain legally responsible for much of the information. According to Goldman and Hudson, without ubiquitous and strong privacy rules and their enforcement, the promise of the Internet and e-commerce to transform the quality of healthcare people receive might become just another failed venture that further disempowers people (2000, pp. 140–48).

Consequently, the quality of care that people receive as well as the integrity of information needed to improve the health of the larger community are at stake. Therefore, more than ever, promoting health through education and protecting patient information are values that must go hand in hand.

E-Health

Simply stated, e-health is the application of e-commerce to the healthcare industry. E-health offers businesses and consumers the opportunity to provide or engage in a number of services, including:

- Personal health records
- Patient appointment scheduling
- Patient registration
- Previsit health screening, evaluations, and assessments
- Postvisit patient education
- Information on health conditions, diseases, wellness, or new healthcare developments
- Support for handheld, point-of-care devices

E-health offers businesses and consumers clear, potential benefits, including:

- Enabling patients and staff to do more with less support
- Streamlining managed care contract administration, EDI, and claims processing
- Building relationships and brand equity with patients, physicians, and affiliated providers
- Improving access to vital patient information
- Reducing care costs
- Improving care delivery
- Building market image and position
- Improving employee productivity and morale

- Facilitating pharmaceutical research, clinical trials, and regulatory submission
- Promoting direct contact with patients

Healthcare organizations must be able to provide high-quality services through e-health to realize the above benefits. Although most organizations have the necessary technology to provide these services, e-health initiatives are often hindered by an organization's culture to accept the profound changes that e-health can bring about.

Following are key qualities required of an e-health culture:

- *Quick:* The growth of e-health requires that organizations respond more quickly to communications from patients and customers. Because of e-health technologies' speed and ease of use, the people served by healthcare organizations have come to expect equally fast replies. To promote this level of speed within the organization's culture, healthcare professionals must support and encourage quick decision making, helping the organization to become accustomed to a faster pace of operation.
- *Patient focused and service oriented:* Although all healthcare organizations are in the business of serving people, many information systems still are not truly patient focused and thus not e-compatible. As e-health technologies continue to allow patients to seek help through a wider variety of sources, organizations that, in the past, did not provide high-quality service through patient-centered systems are going to fall behind. To promote greater patient focus and service orientation in the organization's culture, healthcare professionals must determine where the service shortcomings lie and then make the necessary improvements. For example, a new e-health-based patient appointment and resource scheduling system will not enhance patient service if patients still have to wait an hour to be seen by a provider after they arrive at the point of service.
- *Partnership-friendly:* To implement many of the e-health technologies and systems to support the delivery of healthcare and the management and communication of health data within the healthcare organization, many partnerships and outsourcing relationships with vendors have developed. To promote better relationships with these partners, healthcare organizations must develop other partnerships for purposes other than technology. As such, an organization that is comfortable working with all kinds of partners has a much broader range of tools available because it employs high-tech means to improve service to patients.

As the wave of e-health continues, the challenge to HIM professionals is clear. They can understand the potential of e-health in the industry and can control and direct its power to the benefit of their customers, health plan members, and patients. Or they can allow the technologies to roll uncontrolled through and around their organizations. If they choose the latter, they will effectively hand over their rich knowledge base and expert skills to faster-moving, better-focused professionals, some of whom may not even exist yet.

Personal Health Records

Personal health records (PHRs) electronically populate elements or subsets of personal health information from provider organization databases into the electronic records of authorized patients, their families, other providers, and sometimes health payers and employers. A range of people and groups maintain the records, including the patients, their families, and other providers. The development of PHRs parallels the consumer-centrism long evident in other vertical market industries, such as banking, where consumers maintain and examine their activities twenty-four hours a day in a secure electronic environment.

PHRs come in a variety of forms and formats, with no single design or sponsorship model yet to emerge. Currently, the most common PHR variations and models include:

- *Shared data record:* The shared data record model consumes the largest number of PHRs and is the most effective. Here, both provider (or employer or health plan) and patient maintain the record. In addition, the provider (or employer or health plan) supports the record. As such, the patient receives and adds information over time. The focus of this model is to keep track of health events, medications, or specific physiological indicators, such as exercise and nutrition.
- *CPR extensions:* The CPR extensions model extends the CPR into cyberspace so that an authorized patient can access the provider's record and check on the record's content. Often this model also allows an authorized patient to extract data from the healthcare provider's record. The record is still maintained by the provider but is available to the patient in an online format.
- *Provider-sponsored information management:* The provider-sponsored information management model represents provider-sponsored information management by creating communication vehicles between patient and provider. Such vehicles can include reminders for immunizations or flu shots, appointment scheduling or prescription refill capabilities, and monitoring tools for disease management in which regular collection of data from the patient is required.

Several issues are at stake. The first is whether a provider organization will be willing to work with a PHR. For example, increasing consumer demand for useful PHRs will make it mandatory that a CPR is capable of sending and receiving data from a PHR. Another issue is whether a patient can trust the network that is transmitting his or her information. Certainly, large-scale deployment of Internet-based PHRs will be slow because of ongoing privacy and security challenges.

(As of this writing, the American Society for Testing and Materials [ASTM] Committee E31 [Healthcare Informatics],

Subcommittee 26 is close to establishing a standard for PHRs on the Internet. Content for the standard was based on the e-health tenets developed by the American Health Information Management Association in 2000.)

PHRs have tremendous implications for the future of HIM professionals. HIM professionals will become the custodians of the online dimension of PHRs and their information on top of the organization's CPR and the organization's paper records. Consequently, HIM professionals must answer a number of questions as they begin to create PHRs for consumers/patients, link PHRs to education and the healthcare community, and integrate the PHRs with other patient or health plan member information. For example (Hagland 2001):

- Who will be the stakeholders who will be developing and implementing PHRs?
- How will the PHRs fit into the organization's existing culture and processes for patient information access?
- If the organization has installed component technologies of the CPR system, how will PHRs integrate with those existing components?
- How will PHRs fit into the organization's strategic IT plan?
- What will be the privacy, security, and confidentiality dimensions of the PHRs?
- What will be the budgetary implications?
- What will be the organization's marketing and public relations implications?
- What will be the medicolegal implications?
- If an outsourcing partner maintains the PHRs at least partly or fully, what will be the practical and strategic implications of that decision?

Check Your Understanding 3.5

Instructions: Answer the following questions on a separate piece of paper.

1. Give at least five distinct examples of diagnostic tests that involve physiological signal processing?

2. What patient data are typically collected and viewed (accessed) by care providers using point-of-care systems?

3. What is driving the increased use of computerized care protocols in healthcare?

4. Describe how second- and third-generation tele-health applications differ in functionality from first-generation applications such as teleradiology.

5. Why doesn't an electronic medical record created by scanning/faxing analog paper documents into digitized, bit-mapped images fit the description of a computer-based patient record as defined in the 1991 and 1997 IOM reports?

6. Give at least five examples of services healthcare organizations are offering their customers utilizing e-health technology?

7. What are the characteristics of an e-health culture in a healthcare organization?

8. Describe the differences among the following three common models for the PHR: shared data record, CPR extensions, and provider-sponsored information management.

Supporting the Security of Data and Information

Many current and emerging information technologies are used to support the security of healthcare data and information. They are the same technologies used to support the security of data and information in most vertical market industries. What sets the healthcare vertical market industry apart is the application of the technologies according to the second portion (Title II) of HIPAA, which mandates the protection of health information.

For the purposes of this book, the following technologies are highlighted:

- Encryption/cryptography
- Biometrics technology
- Firewall systems
- Audit trails

Encryption/Cryptography

Computer technology's greatest strengths also are its greatest weaknesses. For example, computer technology, especially the Internet and its derived technologies, easily allows anyone to send and receive information. However, it also easily allows anyone to intercept a transmission.

Cryptography is an applied science in which mathematics transforms intelligible data and information into unintelligible strings of characters and back again. **Encryption** technology uses cryptography to code digital data and information. This is so that the information can be transmitted over communications media and the sender of the information can be sure that only a recipient who has an authorized decoding "key" can make sense of the information.

There are two broad categories of encryption. The first category is symmetric or single-key encryption. Here, each computer uses software that assigns a secret key or code. One computer uses the key to code the message, and the other computer uses the same key to decode the message before the recipient can read it. This form of encryption requires both computers to have the same key.

The second category is asymmetric or **public key infrastructure** (PKI) encryption. PKI does not require that both computers have the same key to decode messages. A private key is known to one computer, which gives a public key to the other computer with which it wants to exchange encrypted data. The public key can be stored anywhere it is convenient, such as on a Web site or with an e-mail. The second computer decodes the encrypted message by using the public key and its own private key.

To prevent abuse, some type of authority is needed to serve as a trusted third party. A certification authority (CA) is an independent licensing agency that vouches for the individual's identity and relationship to the individual's public key. Acting as a type of electronic notary public, a CA verifies and stores a sender's public and private encryption keys and issues a digital certificate or "seal of authenticity" to the recipient.

These keys come in various strengths or levels of security. The strengths vary not only according to the algorithm that codes the data, but also on how well the encoding and decoding keys are maintained. The more bits a key has, the harder it is to break the code without massive computer assistance.

For Internet sites, the use of private and public keys is handled behind the scenes by users' computer browsers and the Web servers for the sites. For example, when a healthcare Internet user performs an online, interactive business transaction, a secure socket layer (SSL) PKI is used to exchange sensitive healthcare data and information.

PKI is becoming the de facto encryption technology for secure data transfers and online authentication. As such, its use will enable healthcare organizations to meet HIPAA's regulations concerning the security of data and electronic signatures.

Biometrics Technology

Biometrics technology verifies a person's identity by measuring (comparing different mathematical representations of) biological and physical features or traits unique to the individual. For example, in signature verification technology, the biometrics of a handwritten signature are measured to confirm the identity of an individual. In data access technology, the biometrics of a hand (hand geometry), fingerprint (fingerprint matching), eye (iris or retinal scanning), voice (voice verification), or facial feature (facial image recognition) are measured to confirm the individual's identity.

Unique, positive identification or verification without the fear of replication or duplication for access to confidential health information is critical. As such, HIPAA requires a mechanism to ensure the authentication of the user and to restrict the user only to those systems that he or she is authorized to access. But because positive identification is so reliable as a personal identifier, individuals might feel that their privacy is threatened or compromised.

Fingerprint matching is the oldest and most popular type of biometrics technology. Everyone has unique, immutable fingerprints made of a series of ridges, furrows, and minute points or contours on the surface of the finger that form a pattern. Retinal scanning is quite accurate because it involves analyzing the layer of blood vessels at the back of the eye. But it is not as popular an identification technology because of the close contact users must make with a scanning device and thus is unfriendly for users wearing eyeglasses or contact lenses. Iris scanning is less intrusive than retinal scanning but is considered clumsy to use.

Facial image recognition requires an unobtrusive, digital camera to develop a dynamic, facial image of the user. Unfortunately, matching dynamic images is not as easy as matching static images, such as two or more fingerprints or iris scans. Therefore, currently, positive identification based on multiple biometrics technologies has the most promising potential for authentication purposes.

Firewall Systems

Firewalls are hardware and software security devices situated between the routers of a private and public network. They are designed to protect computer networks from unauthorized outsiders. However, they also can be used to protect entities within a single network, for example, to block laboratory technicians from getting into payroll records. Without firewalls, IT departments would have to deploy multiple-enterprise security programs that would soon become difficult to manage and maintain.

Firewalls originated during the 1980s and were used to screen a network's incoming data from unwanted, outside addresses. At that time, networks were not large and complicated. Consequently, firewalls were not foolproof and were easy to circumvent.

By contrast, today's massive and complex networks demand firewall systems fortified with software applications that, for example, authenticate users, encrypt messages, scan for viruses, and produce audit trails. Technically, most firewalls are made up of proxy and filtering services. Proxy services are special-purpose programs allowing network administrators to permit or deny specific applications or features of applications. They screen user names and all information that attempts to enter or leave the private network. Filtering allows the routers to make permit/deny decisions for each piece of information that attempts to enter or leave the private network.

Firewalls are based on preestablished rules that allow or deny access to the network or exchange of information between the networks. As such, firewalls enforce security policies so that everything not explicitly permitted is denied. For example, firewall systems determine which inside services may be accessed from the outside, which outsiders are permitted access to the permitted inside services, and which outside services may be accessed by insiders. For a firewall to be effective, all traffic to and from the networks must pass through the firewall, where it can be inspected.

The firewall itself must be immune to penetration. Unfortunately, a firewall cannot offer protection after an attacker has gotten through or around it.

Audit Trails

Audit trails are chronological sets of records that provide evidence of computer system utilization. Data are collected about every system event, such as log-ins, log-outs, file accesses, and data extractions. As such, audit trails are used to facilitate the determination of security violations and to identify areas for improvement. Their usefulness is enhanced when they include trigger flags for automatic, intensified review.

Today, audit trails serve as strong impediments to computer data abuse. For example, the presence of these tools promotes awareness that people who access confidential information can be tracked and held accountable.

Care must be taken to determine which audited data elements are required by law or which ones are exceptions. Following are some suggested data elements to track activity in healthcare information system audit trails:

- Date and time of event
- Patient identification
- User identification
- Access device used
- Type of action (view/read, print, update/add)
- Identification of patient data access by a category of content
- Source of access and software application used
- Reason for access by category (patient care, research, billing)

Practical issues concerning the use of audit trails involve trust. For example, healthcare organizations must be able to distinguish between users who access patient records for patient care and those who access them for unauthorized purposes. Frequent sampling by organizational managers or "tiger teams" is one way to determine system usage within an environment of trust. Delegating to users the responsibility to examine their own audit histories is another way to determine this. It is recommended that the results of audit trails be published and included in employee performance reviews.

Healthcare Informatics and Health Information Management

Health information management is the healthcare industry's professional field that ensures that high-quality data and information are available to every type of authorized user who depends on the data/information to deliver high-quality healthcare services and to make high-quality healthcare-related decisions. HIM professionals serve not only the healthcare industry, but also the public. By managing, compiling, analyzing, and utilizing data from many sources, HIM professionals identify ways to better utilize healthcare resources, more accurately provide patient billing and reimbursement services, reveal public health patterns, and establish new medical treatments vital for improved patient care and administrative purposes.

Trained HIM professionals manage the quality of the data/information content, including its timeliness, appropriateness, accuracy, relevance, and integrity. In addition, HIM professionals develop policies to meet information management standards as mandated by the government and other regulatory and accrediting organizations. Most important, HIM professionals work diligently to protect the privacy of the individual and the confidentiality of the data/information they make available to legitimate users.

Historically, healthcare and healthcare-related data and information have been collected, stored, and transmitted using paper technologies. Currently, paper technology is still used as the primary source for data/information management purposes. Consequently, having to maintain dual technologies and related systems—part manual, part electronic—is providing the most angst for HIM professionals who are fighting hard to maintain their existing territories. However, as more and more healthcare and healthcare-related data/information are being collected, stored, and transmitted using computer technologies, the HIM discipline is increasingly becoming a professional field within the domain of healthcare informatics.

Because healthcare informatics is the healthcare industry's professional field that is concerned with the management of all aspects of health data and information, it includes and, in fact, cannot ignore HIM as one of its components. However, healthcare informatics is focused solely on the application of computers and computer technologies to support authorized users in their healthcare and related practices, research, and education. Consequently, HIM is the component of the healthcare informatics infrastructure by which authorized users' information needs are electronically created and managed.

As such, HIM professionals must be viewed as intimate partners with IT professionals, who, together, form strong alliances with each type of authorized user (physicians, nurses, clinicians, dentists, consumers, and administrators) to develop the required hardware/software and to manage the data/information content. Also, HIM professionals must be viewed as intimate partners with healthcare informatics professionals, who, together, support each type of authorized user's unique information needs and, concurrently, support the overall information needs of the healthcare organizations in which they work. Only in this context will HIM professionals continue to assume a leadership role in the development of improved healthcare information systems, integrated patient information systems, accurate decision support tools, or any or all of the current and emerging information technologies and systems highlighted in this chapter.

Check Your Understanding 3.6

Instructions: Answer the following questions on a separate piece of paper.

1. What is public key infrastructure (PKI), and why is it receiving so much attention within the healthcare industry?

2. What are the benefits and drawbacks of using each of the following human features for authentication purposes: fingerprints, iris images, and facial images?

3. Firewalls protect network access by employing proxy and filtering services. What are proxy services and filtering services?

4. What are two practical ways to instill user trust in healthcare organizations when deploying information system audit trails?

5. The HIM discipline is becoming a professional field within the domain of healthcare informatics. What is driving this transition?

Real-World Case

The following case study is based on an article by E. Simendinger, J. C. Ruckdeschel, and D. Vizzi (2000).

The future of e-health has become a major area of speculation for Frank Day, the CEO at the Diablo Medical Foundation Clinic (DMFC) in California. His interest has become magnified as the technology continues to change. For example:

- Initially, video conferencing between fixed projection rooms allowed long-distance consultations between physicians or between physicians and patients at DMFC. However, the Internet, with its total democratization of the communication process, is supplanting video conferencing.
- Beginning around 1998, DMFC's patients began to present printouts to their physicians of information from the Internet's health-related Web sites. Today, patients are wondering why they cannot communicate electronically with their physicians as they do with their accountants, attorneys, and others.
- The number of incoming requests over the Internet for clinical information on individual patients, specific diseases, clinical studies, and so on is expected to grow, and DMFC must be ready to respond to the challenges of patient privacy that this will generate.

Frank caught up with DMFC's health information manager, Terry Green. Terry explained that the product for the provision of healthcare is information, similar in the e-business context to Amazon.com. But Frank was not convinced. Healthcare information, he said, is graphic, textual, and/or structured. It was not something one could neatly bundle to send to people via UPS.

On the other hand, Frank's business acumen told him that DMFC had to better define its product. He asked Terry how DMFC could get paid for its healthcare information product.

According to Terry, DMFC had to provide information to its patients about general health, prevention, early detection, and treatment. Therefore, DMFC had to continue to offer complimentary, traditional products to patients, such as pamphlets and brochures, medical supplies, and sample pharmaceuticals. However, physician consults for reviewing pathology, radiology exams, and individual records could be reimbursable. Also, the supervision of DMFC's chat rooms for patients' responses to specific diseases on DMFC's Web site might generate compensation.

With this information, Frank gathered his management team, and he and the team identified the following physician-related services that could be fairly and appropriately billed and reimbursed:

- Accounting for the time physicians spend on the telephone: A large amount of time is spent in this activity, and, currently, physicians are not being reimbursed for

it. Traditionally, patients consider billing for telephone time insulting; physicians do not.
- Accounting for the time physicians spend on billing for new patients or for services for a person who is unlikely to become a patient: Although a nominal amount of time is usually spent in these activities, currently, physicians are not being reimbursed for it.
- Accounting for the time physicians spend reviewing records: Again, a large amount of time is spent in this activity and, currently, physicians are not reimbursed for it.
- Accounting for the time physicians would spend commenting via e-mail: Electronic correspondence could consume a significant amount of physician time.

Also, team members realized they had to research the implications of the following physician-related services:

- Physicians providing diagnoses across state lines, where the physicians are not licensed to practice
- Physicians providing information across international borders, which foreign governments might view as an intrusion

Finally, the team decided to investigate uses for e-health outside the clinical realm. At the meeting, Terry provided additional information to help weigh the benefits of e-health, including:

- To maintain a modest inventory, DMFC could purchase services via the Web and reduce the costs associated with current purchasing groups for such items as pharmaceuticals, bandages, topical medications, and linens.
- Computer systems and technologies to perform standard office functions such as billing could be available using Web services, and the software could be supported online as part of the administrative processes.
- Wider recognition of DMFC on the Web could introduce newer and broader marketing opportunities.

However, Frank was still not convinced that e-health could work to DMFC's benefit. In addition, he was sure that the technology would be so short-lived that it would not be a useful investment. The following questions from the team added to Frank's hesitancy:

- Could purchasing be handled entirely over the Web, thus allowing a reduction or elimination of the current purchasing department?
- If Web-based computer programs replaced DMFC's billing and informational areas, how would they be used?
- Even though DMFC's Information Services Department (ISD) is technically competent, the implementation of DMFC's existing computer systems was clearly expanding beyond ISD's ability to manage well an e-health project for the organization. Consequently, how could ISD maintain a new Web-based administrative and/or clinical product on a day-to-day basis?

Discussion Questions

1. As DMFC's health information manager, how would you have answered each of the above questions?

2. What other options, if any, does Frank have?

3. As DMFC's health information manager, what would you recommend to Frank?

4. What risks does DMFC face by moving into this new area of business?

5. What are the critical success factors if e-health is pursued?

Summary

Making the benefits of the current and emerging information technologies and systems and their application in the healthcare industry more clear requires significant changes. Such changes are technological, organizational, social, and attitudinal.

Demonstrating the return on investment in computer technologies requires methodical planning. This comes in light of their staggering capital and operating costs as well as the expense of human resources in installing, integrating, managing, and maintaining increasingly complex systems.

Accepting the trade-offs associated with computer technologies requires massive education and training. For example, CPR systems will never exactly replicate the flexibility of paper technology. However, increased legibility, increased access to the information, and the ability to use the information simultaneously for other purposes will be provided in return. All the confidential information cannot be locked in drawers and file cabinets. However, the growing volume of information stored electronically and accessed remotely results in the need for ongoing attention to privacy and security concerns.

Accomplishing the organization's visions for providing the highest-quality care in the most effective way requires providing healthcare professionals the authority to establish the links between the promised benefits and the key enablers of the benefits, the information technologies.

Depicting the art of the possible requires patience.

These requirements are how well-trained and highly skilled individuals with knowledge about both healthcare and computerized information technologies will design, develop, select, and maintain tomorrow's healthcare information management systems and apply technology to the management of healthcare information. This is how HIM professionals will contribute to the important field of informatics in healthcare.

References

American Health Information Management Association. 2000. AHIMA's basic operational tenets for protecting the privacy of personal health information on the Internet. Available at http://www.ahima.org/infocenter/guidelines/tenets.html.

Barnett, G. O., J. Cimino, J. Hupp, and E. Hoffer. 1987. DXplain: An evolving diagnostic decision-support system. *Journal of the American Medical Association* 258(1):67–74.

Borowitz, S. 2001. Computer-based speech recognition as an alternative to medical transcription. *Journal of the American Medical Informatics Association* 8(1):101–2.

Bufton, M. 1999. Electronic health records and implementation of clinical practice guidelines. In *Electronic Health Records: Changing the Vision,* Gretchen F. Murphy, Mary Alice Hanken, and Kathleen A. Waters, editors. Philadelphia: W. B. Saunders Company.

California HealthCare Foundation. 1999. *National Survey: Confidentiality of Medical Records.* Available from www.ehealth.chcf.org. Accessed December 2001.

Chin, T. 1997. Federal grants to aid work on decision support systems. *Health Data Management* 5(2):24.

Committee on Quality of Health Care in America, Institute of Medicine. 2001. *Crossing the Quality Chasm: A New Health System for the 21st Century.* Washington, D.C.: National Academy Press.

Department of Health and Human Services. 1993. A push toward paperless processing in healthcare. *HHS News* press release, November 23, 1993.

Dick, R., and W. Andrews. 1995. Point of care: An essential technology for the CPR. *Healthcare Informatics* 12(5):64–66, 78.

Dick, Richard S., and Elaine B. Steen, editors. 1991. *The Computer-Based Patient Record: An Essential Technology for Health Care,* 1st ed. Washington, D.C.: National Academy Press.

Dick, Richard S., Elaine B. Steen, and Don E. Detmer, editors. 1997. *The Computer-Based Patient Record: An Essential Technology for Health Care,* rev. ed. Washington, D.C.: National Academy Press.

Drazen, E. 2001. Is this the year of the computer-based patient record? *Healthcare Informatics* 18(2):94–98.

Goldman, J., and Z. Hudson. 2000. Virtually exposed: Privacy and e-health. *Health Affairs* 19(6):140–48.

Hagland, M. 2001. Getting more personal. *Journal of the American Health Information Management Association* 72(8):35.

Health Insurance Portability and Accountability Act of 1996. Public Law 104-191. Available at www.access.gpo.gov/nara/cfr/index.html.

Henchey, P. 1998. Maximizing ROI in data warehouses. *Advance for Health Information Executives* 2(1):60–70.

Hunt, D., R. Haynes, S. Hanna, and K. Smith. 1998. Effects of computer-based clinical decision support systems on physician performance and patient outcomes: A systematic review. *Journal of the American Medical Association* 280(15):1339–46.

Kelly, F. 2001. Implementing an EIS. Available from www.ceoreview.com. Accessed September 2001.

Kohn, Linda T., Janet M. Corrigan, and Molla S. Donaldson, editors. 1999. *To Err Is Human: Building a Safer Health System.* Washington, D.C.: National Academy Press.

Nussbaum, G. 2001. Bitten by the ASP: Application service providers. *Proceedings of the Healthcare Information and Management Systems Society,* Vol. 1 (Session 7), pp. 1–9. Chicago: HIMSS.

Power, D. J. 1997. What is a DSS? *DSstar, The On-Line Executive Journal for Data-Intensive Decision Support* 1(3). Available from www.dssresources.com. Accessed September 2001.

Schnitzer, G. 2000. Natural language processing: A coding professional's perspective. *Journal of the American Health Information Management Association* 71(9):95–98.

Simendinger, E., J. C. Ruckdeschel, and D. Vizzi. 2000. Does e-commerce belong in a cancer and research institution? *The Journal of Healthcare Management* 45(3).

Siwicki, B. 1996. Artificial intelligence: A new generation of health care applications. *Health Data Management* 4(4):47–52.

Stead, W., and M. Lorenzi. 1999. Health informatics: Linking investment to value. *Journal of the American Medical Informatics Association* 6(5):341–48.

Turley, J., C. Johnson, T. Johnson, and J. Zhang. 2001. A clean slate: Initiating a graduate program in health informatics. *MD Computing* 18(1):47–48.

Warner, H. 2000. Can natural language processing aid outpatient coders? *Journal of the American Health Information Management Association* 71(8):78–81.

Application Exercises

1. Using the CPR data types and their sources model (figure 3.1) as a guide, interview an HIM director and/or an IT director at a local healthcare organization to determine the extent to which that organization has computerized the various components of the CPR.

2. Visit the Web sites of at least three healthcare organizations in your area to identify and compare (a) the various types of data presented on the site and (b) the extent to which each organization uses its Web site to transact business activities.

3. Search the Internet for personal health record sites; select at least two sites to visit and review these sites to (a) experience their functionality, (b) assess their user-friendliness, and (c) assess their privacy policies and practices.

Review Quiz

Instructions: Choose the best answer for the following questions.

1. ___ The use of computers to manage data and information that supports healthcare practices is called ___.
   a. Medical informatics
   b. Dental informatics
   c. Healthcare informatics
   d. Nursing informatics

2. ___ The data elements in a patient's automated laboratory result are examples of ___.
   a. Unstructured data
   b. Free-text data
   c. Financial data
   d. Structured data

3. ___ ___ is an example of analog data.
   a. CT scan
   b. Photographic, chest x-ray film
   c. MRI exam
   d. EKG tracing

4. ___ The computer-based process of extracting, quantifying, and filtering discrete data that reside in a relational database is called ___.
   a. Text mining
   b. Data mining
   c. Autocoding
   d. Bar coding

5. ___ Computer-based recognition of handwritten, free-text characters is known as ___.
   a. Optical character recognition
   b. Intelligent character recognition
   c. Voice recognition
   d. Natural language processing

6. ___ Online/real-time transaction processing (OLTP) is a functional requirement for a ___.
   a. Data repository
   b. Data mart
   c. Data warehouse
   d. Data dictionary

7. ___ HTML, SGML, and XML are programming languages used to create ___.
   a. Web-enabled applications
   b. Expert decision support systems
   c. Web browser-based applications
   d. Artifical intelligence systems

8. ___ In healthcare, one of the primary uses for data warehouses is ___.
   a. Utilization review
   b. Accounts receivable management
   c. Outcomes management
   d. Materials/inventory management

9. ___ The field of artificial intelligence is most closely related to ___.
   a. Expert decision support systems
   b. Geographic information systems
   c. Executive information systems
   d. Medical decision support systems

10. ___ The computerized analysis of heart functioning, blood sugar levels, and brain wave activity is an example of ___.
    a. Point-of-care documentation
    b. Artificial intelligence
    c. Online analytical processing
    d. Physiological signal processing

11. ___ The technology that allows a healthcare organization to logically (or conceptually) link multiple physical data repositories is ___.
    a. MPI
    b. OLAP
    c. OLTP
    d. EMPI

12. ___ All of the following are examples of potential e-health applications, except ___.
    a. Bedside nursing care
    b. Appointment scheduling
    c. Patient education
    d. Personal health record

13. ___ The personal health record model that maintains provider control on content while allowing online access to the authorized patient is the ___.
    a. Shared data record model
    b. CPR extension model
    c. Provider-sponsored information management model
    d. Smart card model

14. ___ Of the following human features, the one that is most unobtrusive to obtain but most difficult to match for authentication purposes is ___.
    a. Retinal image
    b. Fingerprints
    c. Facial image
    d. Iris scan

15. ___ The security devices situated between the routers of a private network and a public network to protect the private network from unauthorized users are called ___.
    a. Audit trails
    b. Passwords
    c. Firewalls
    d. Encryptors

Chapter 4
The Health Information Management Profession

Sandra R. Fuller, MA, RHIA

Learning Objectives

- To understand the professional definition of health information management (HIM)
- To recognize the components of HIM
- To differentiate HIM from information technology and health science
- To identify the types of data relevant to the HIM profession
- To understand the functions within the HIM professional domain
- To understand the media and forms in which health information is found
- To recognize the components of the HIM body of knowledge
- To identify the characteristics of a profession that apply to HIM
- To identify the key HIM professional associations
- To understand the importance of a professional code of ethics and what the HIM Code of Ethics means
- To recognize the importance of lifelong learning in the HIM profession
- To understand the process and benefits of certification and the requirements for maintaining certification
- To recognize the importance of continuing education and the options available to HIM professionals

Key Terms

Access control
American Health Information Management Association (AHIMA)
American Medical Information Association (AMIA)
Certification
Certified coding specialist (CCS)
Certified coding specialist—physician based (CCS-P)
Clinical data
Coded data
College of Healthcare Information Management Executives (CHIME)
Data capture
Data dictionary
Data display
Data modeling
Data quality management
Demographic data
Epidemiological data
Financial data
Health Information Management and Systems Society (HIMSS)
Health science librarians
Informatics
Information technology professionals
Medical informaticians
Nosology
Process and work-flow modeling
Registered health information administrator (RHIA)
Registered health information technician (RHIT)
Research data
Reference data

Introduction

In 1928, the Association of Record Librarians of North America was organized under the sponsorship of the American College of Surgeons. The objective of the new organization was "to elevate the standards of clinical records in hospitals, dispensaries, and other distinctly medical institutions" (Huffman 1941, p. 18). This precursor to the **American Health Information Management Association** (AHIMA) began to define the qualifications, duties, and training for individuals working in medical records. In 1941, Huffman (pp. 185–87) categorized the responsibilities of the medical record librarian as:

- Organization and management
- Numbering, filing, and cross-indexing
- Ethics and medicolegal
- Statistics, comparative studies, and research
- Secretarial duties
- Correlation of the medical records library and the medical reference library

Many of these elements are still included in today's professional definition of health information management (HIM). Other elements of the 1941 definition are irrelevant or of limited importance. The longevity of this professional definition documents the unique role of the health information manager and the resilience of the profession through time.

This chapter focuses on the professional definition and scope of health information management. It also discusses the characteristics of a profession, such as belonging to professional organizations, and provides specific examples that apply to health information management.

Theory into Practice

Joe was faced with a dilemma. For the past fifteen years, he had been director of medical records in the largest community hospital in the small city where he lived. During that time, he had completed his master's degree in health information management and was now looking for a new challenge. However, Joe already had the most senior–level HIM job in his organization. Moreover, moving to another city was out of the question because his wife had a great job and they did not want to relocate their family.

Then Joe learned that a new position was being created in the information systems (IS) department. The hospital was planning to acquire a new clinical IS and the chief information officer (CIO) was looking for someone to lead the project. Joe had worked with the IS department on a number of projects in the past and had always liked project management, application specification, and ensuring that new systems met the organization's needs. He felt that the IS position was just what he was looking for, but there were a few obstacles. First, the CIO was looking for a nurse to fill the position. Second, Joe did not want to leave HIM. And third, he was uncertain how the IS role would prepare him for the future.

Joe decided to gather some information. He spoke with someone from his master's program who had a made a similar move, talked with a friend at the annual convention about nontraditional roles, met with a recruiter to discuss career paths, and did some reading on evolving HIM careers.

Finally, Joe applied for the job. Despite his skepticism, the CIO agreed to interview Joe because of his strong performance with the organization. However, Joe explained how his education had prepared him for both the technical and project management elements of the job. Also, he pointed out that he already had established relationships with a number of the clinical staff with whom he would be working. Moreover, he had excelled at putting together a team with diverse skills and getting the job done. Joe was offered the job and began two months later.

Because of the job's critical nature, the system's high profile, and Joe's qualifications, he was able to make the move without a salary cut. Further, he negotiated an increase in six months if the implementation was on schedule and within budget. His talks with friends and colleagues had persuaded him that he would not be leaving HIM but, rather, would be moving into a different phase of his career and the profession. A growing number of HIM professionals are working outside their departments within hospitals and outside hospitals altogether.

What's more, Joe now sees new possibilities for his future. Working with the IS department continues to develop his technical expertise. He is fine-tuning his project management skills, and the new position has already provided opportunities to practice his presentation skills. He is planning ahead and considering how he might leverage these new talents to apply for the CIO role at another healthcare organization in town or perhaps go into consulting to help other organizations with their system implementations.

Professional Definition

In the past fifty years, numerous changes have affected the responsibilities of the health information manager. The advent of computers, government sponsorship and regulation of healthcare, advances in medical practice, and socioeconomic changes and progress in higher education have all affected the health information management (HIM) profession. In 2000, AHIMA's Committee on Professional Development completed the most recent update of the professional definition for HIM. (See figure 4.1.) Changes in the healthcare environment, information technology, and information management continue to have an impact on the practice of health information management. The new definition reads:

> Health information management improves the quality of healthcare by ensuring that the best information is available to make any healthcare decision. Health information management professionals manage healthcare data and information resources. The profession encompasses services in planning, collecting, aggregating, analyzing, and disseminating individual patient and aggregate clinical data. It serves the healthcare industry including: patient care organizations, payers, research and policy agencies, and other healthcare-related industries (Russell 2001, 48B).

Figure 4.1.   **Update of the Professional Definition of Health Information Management**

Health Information Management: Professional Definition
Developed by the 1999 and 2000 Committees on Professional Development

Effective January 2001

Health information management improves the quality of healthcare by ensuring that the best information is available to make any healthcare decision. Health information management professionals manage healthcare data and information resources. The profession encompasses services in planning, collecting, aggregating, analyzing, and disseminating individual patient and aggregate clinical data. It serves the following healthcare stakeholders: patient care organizations, payers, research and policy agencies, and other healthcare-related industries.

HEALTH	Domain Description	Unique Impact
The field of health is broad, including everything from birth to death and wellness to illness. Health information management deals largely with patient data.	Health information includes: • **Clinical data** captured during the process of diagnosis and treatment. • **Epidemiological databases** that aggregate data about a population. • **Demographic data** used to identify and communicate with and about an individual. • **Financial data** derived from the care process or aggregated for an organization or population. • **Research data** gathered as a part of care and used for research or gathered for specific research purposes in clinical trials. • **Reference data** that interacts with the care of the individual or with the healthcare delivery systems, like a formulary, protocol, care plan, clinical alerts or reminders, etc. • **Coded data** that is translated into a standard nomenclature or classification so that it may be aggregated, analyzed, and compared.	Health information professionals manage a variety of types of information across the healthcare industry. Their expertise uniquely impacts the value of this data as evidenced in the examples below: • **Clinical Data**—Organization of information supports direct patient care and serves a variety of industry needs like reimbursement, planning, and research. • **Epidemiological Databases**—Aggregate statistics reveal disease trends. • **Demographic Data**—Attention to data quality provides unique identification of patients in a healthcare enterprise and accurate information available to run the business of healthcare. • **Financial Data**—Understanding the clinical context of costs and the rules for reimbursement improves organizational decision making. • **Research Data**—Planning for future use of data improves the quality and reduces the cost of data capture and analysis. • **Reference Data**—Providing current literature and research outcomes enhances clinical knowledge at the point of care and in operational decision making. • **Coded Data**—Aggregate statistics enhance analysis for epidemiological patterning. Combining knowledge of the clinical content, documentation principles, coding systems, and data use provide accurate information for the industry.
INFORMATION	Domain Description	Unique Impact
Health information is captured and stored in a variety of media and forms.	The management of information relates to all of these forms: • **Data**—Individual and aggregate • **Reports** • **Medical records**—An aggregation of reports and data that describe an individual patient usually within one delivery site or system • **Data dictionaries** • **Vocabularies** Information may be stored using a variety of media: • **Paper** • **Databases** • **Microfilm/microfiche** • **Computer stored**	**FORMS** **Data** • Healthcare generates enormous amounts of data that are only useful if well managed. **Reports** • Summarization of data into relevant reports quickly communicates vital information. **Medical Records** • Developing uniform definitions of the most critical information gathered about a patient to create a legal document. **Data Dictionary** • Creating standards to define critical content. **Vocabularies** • Defining the language of healthcare. **MEDIA** **Paper** • Managing the historic and pervasive method of healthcare communication. **Databases** • Constructing relevant collections of data. **Microfilm/Microfiche** • Reduction of storage space required for maintaining legal documents. **Computer Stored** • Assuring preservation of a legal standard when applying new technologies.

(Continued on next page)

Figure 4.1.   (Continued)

MANAGEMENT	Domain Description	Unique Impact
Management of health information uniquely stems from a knowledge of clinical, management, and informatics principles and is performed by individuals focused at the strategic, management, and technical levels.	**PLANNING** **Administration** • Managing data collection and storage • Managing information retrieval and release **Policy Development** • Establishing security, confidentiality, retention, integrity, and access standards • Developing training programs that empower others to carry out the information policies • Advocating for privacy, confidentiality, and access **Strategic Planning** • Identifying the organization or projects that need information support for current and future strategic operations and initiatives • Planning capture, storage, and display of data to ensure operational effectiveness, including use of technology **INFORMATICS** **Data Modeling** • Determining data needs and identifying the relationships among these data **Process and Work-Flow Modeling** • Identifying the flow of work and information required to perform a function including: decomposition diagrams, dependency diagrams, and data flow **Data Capture and Display Design** • Focusing on system design, screen design, report design, and forms design **Data Dictionary Maintenance** • Maintaining dictionary design, standardization, update, and dissemination **Access Control** • Designing, implementing, and monitoring the map between information and user access **Data Quality Management** • Effecting the collection, application, warehousing, and analysis of data to improve information quality **Nosology** • Analyzing and interpreting disease and procedure classifications and terminologies for accuracy of translation of healthcare data **TECHNICAL** **Classification and Coding** • Assigning the appropriate code or nomenclature term for categorization **Abstracting** • Compiling the pertinent information from the medical record based on predetermined data sets **Registry Development** • Assembling a chronological set of data for an express purpose **Storage** • Implementing and providing oversight of electronic and paper-based filing systems **Retrieval** • Making accessible information that is stored in various media and sites **Release** • Appropriately responding to requests for information based on laws and policy **Analysis** • Performing qualitative and quantitative analysis of documentation against standards and policy	**PLANNING** **Administration** • Reducing the cost of health information • Successfully implementing an enterprisewide master person index **Policy Development** • Participating in national policy discussions on health information privacy • Drafting organizational policies that conform with state and federal regulations **Strategic Planning** • Initiating market position strategies influenced by sound outcomes data • Ensuring easy access to health information by care providers across an enterprise **INFORMATICS** **Data Modeling** • Improving access to healthcare data • Improving the quality of information **Process and Work-Flow Modeling** • Ensuring faster access to cash through improved revenue cycles • Providing for less time spent by clinicians in charting, more time for patient care **Data Capture and Display Design** • Improving patient safety through reduced documentation error • Reducing training time for clinicians in how to chart **Data Dictionary Maintenance** • Making accurate and timely data available for clinical and business decisions • Increasing access to data **Access Control** • Protecting patients' right to privacy • Complying with state and federal laws and regulations • Improving access when appropriate **Data Quality Management** • Consistently and methodically improving the quality of data • Improving decision making influenced by reliable information **Nosology** • Providing access to clinically relevant aggregate data **TECHNICAL** **Classification and Coding** • Reducing the threat of fraud and abuse litigation • Improving data accuracy • Establishing processes for accurate reimbursement **Abstracting** • Providing access to key data at the patient and aggregate levels **Registry Development** • Providing information to support long-term care of chronic disease • Providing research information for the value of treatment of chronic disease **Storage** • Reducing costs of storing records • Complying with state and federal laws **Retrieval** • Making information available for healthcare emergencies • Providing the most cost-effective access to information **Release** • Protecting patients' rights to privacy of health information • Reducing risk of litigation from inappropriate release **Analysis** • Allowing for meaningful interpretation of statistical data • Presenting both business and clinical information with appropriate content and context review **EXTENDED ROLES** *As with any robust profession, individuals evolve into divergent roles to develop, support, and nurture aspects of the profession. Although related to the profession, additional skills are developed to contribute to health information management without directly managing health information. For example, they support the core definition by:* • *Teaching others to manage health information* • *Developing and marketing products and services that help to manage health information* • *Developing software that manages health information* • *Consulting with others in the management of health information*

HIM deals primarily with information that is created during the diagnosis and treatment of individual patients. Closely related, but different, fields include information technology, health science libraries, and medical informatics.

The *information technology* field provides computing hardware, software, and data transmission technology for all industries, including healthcare. Although HIM professionals routinely work with **information technology professionals** and study some computer science courses, HIM does not require the same depth of computer skill that information technology does. However, HIM's unique focus on healthcare requires clinical information and healthcare industry training, along with the core HIM curriculum, described later.

Health science is a specialized area of library science that evolved from the enormous volume of reference materials published in medical and health literature. **Health science librarians** provide access to library resources and teach people how to use them (Chronicle Guidance Publications 1999, p. 8). The provision of reference material to aid in health decision making is an increasingly important function of computer-based patient records (Institute of Medicine 1997, p. 88). As the demand for faster access to health literature increases, HIM professionals will continue to work closely with health science librarians to integrate these information resources with information on a specific patient or patient population.

Medical informatics is the "field that concerns itself with the cognitive, information processing and communication tools of medical practice, education and research including the information science and technology to support these tasks" (Greenes and Shortliffe 1990). **Medical informaticians** are physicians who specialize in medical information processing. Other postgraduate specialties include nursing and pharmacy informatics.

Scope of Health Information

Health information includes information from birth to death and from the individual patient record to aggregate data on a patient population that can span the globe. Health information managers play a unique role that involves a wide variety of data types. Within the professional definition of HIM, health information includes the following types of data:

- **Clinical data,** the most common type of health information, document the signs, symptoms, diagnoses, impressions, treatments, and outcomes of the care process. They are captured during diagnosis and treatment and are stored in the medical record. Clinical data serve a variety of industry needs beyond direct patient care, including reimbursement, planning, and research. They may be collected and stored in paper or computer formats. Although the health information manager rarely collects or uses clinical data directly in the delivery of care, one of his or her principal roles is that of developing systems that collect accurate and timely information and make it available to decision makers.

- **Epidemiological data** are used to describe health-related issues or events, such as disease trends, found in specific populations. The information then may be used to inform the public or to generate actions that could affect a trend. For example, data on the incidence of sexually transmitted diseases might be used to measure the impact of a teen education program. HIM professionals could establish systems to transmit such information accurately and appropriately while maintaining patient confidentiality. They also could be involved in data analysis and display.

- **Demographic data** provide statistical information about a population, such as age, place of residence, gender, and so on. Accurate and complete demographic data perform two important information functions in healthcare. First, data such as age and gender have their own value when combined with clinical information. For instance, a gender designation can make a diagnosis commonplace, rare, or impossible. Breast cancer, a common diagnosis in a certain age of female, is rare, albeit possible, in males. However, pregnancy is only possible in females. Second, demographic data may be used to uniquely identify individuals so that all of the other health information attributed to them can be collected and accessed accurately.

- **Financial data** are either derived from the care process or aggregated for an organization or population. Healthcare is a business. It is, in fact, a business that consumed 10.1 percent of the gross domestic product in 2000 (Bureau of Economic Analysis 2001). Although accounting and financial management are not within the HIM domain, understanding the rules for reimbursement and the relationship between clinical services and costs is important to the health information manager role.

- **Research data** may be collected as a part of care and then used in research or collected for specific research purposes in clinical trials. HIM professionals play a role in the collection and use of research data from existing records. In addition, they consider research needs when planning for future types and uses of data as a research tool. In this way, HIM professionals improve access to data while reducing the costs of research at the same time.

- **Reference data** are commonly created and maintained by someone outside health information management. They interact with the care of the individual or with the healthcare delivery system in the form of a formulary, protocol, care plan, clinical alert, or reminder. The nursing staff or the medical staff generally create care plans; the pharmacy normally administers the formulary, although ensuring that reference data are available for the care provider is a critical HIM role. Health information managers also are responsible for incorporating elements of this static information into the patient's medical record to support clinical documentation and to create a complete record.

- **Coded data** are data that have been translated into a standard nomenclature of classification so that they can be aggregated, analyzed, and compared. To facilitate the analysis of large amounts of information, coded data frequently are grouped into meaningful categories. The categories may be as simple as M for male and F for female or as extensive as those used to code diagnoses and procedures. The grouping may be age range or the complex methodology used for prospective payment systems.

All of these data result from, or interact with, clinical data captured about an individual patient. HIM professionals may specialize in working with one data type, or their responsibilities may affect all of the various data types. Whatever the type of health information, HIM professionals are likely to perform a variety of tasks.

Check Your Understanding 4.1

Instructions: Answer the following questions on a separate piece of paper.

1. What factors have influenced the change in the professional definition of health information management?
2. What are the differences between HIM professionals and information technology professionals?
3. What role does the HIM professional play in working with clinical data? How does the HIM professional's role differ from roles assumed by other healthcare professionals?
4. How are reference data different from other types of healthcare data?

Domains of Health Information Management Practice

The management of health information is based on a knowledge of clinical management and informatics principles. HIM can be practiced at the planning level, addressing the administrative elements of health information as well as policy development. When focused on informatics, HIM includes several functions that administer information systems. When practiced at a technical level, HIM manipulates data to be used by others for a variety of decision-making purposes. (See figure 4.1.)

Planning

The practice of health information management at the planning level involves the administration of information systems and the development of policies to ensure that those systems are administered effectively and confidentially today and in the future.

Administration

Planning in HIM covers the administration of systems that collect and store data and the management of information

retrieval and release. Effective administration of these systems makes information available and ensures appropriate access, security, and confidentiality. Effective planning also makes healthcare delivery more efficient because of reduced waste in clinical time and administrative processes. Administration may involve staff, space, equipment, and procedures for a large integrated delivery system or may be focused on ensuring the effective utilization of a single information resource.

Policy Development

Along with the administration of systems and people, the development of policies specific to health information is among the HIM professional's job functions. Policy development includes:

- Establishing data security, confidentiality, retention, integrity, and access standards
- Developing training programs that empower others to carry out the information policies
- Advocating for data privacy, confidentiality, and access

Strategic Planning

Finally, strategic planning for future information needs is a role for the HIM professional involved in the planning function. This role involves identifying information needs for an organization or a project to support current and future strategic operations or in support of compliance with regulations or laws. It also involves planning the capture, storage, and display of data to ensure operational effectiveness, including the use of technology.

Informatics

Informatics is the science of information management. It uses computers to automate the collection, storage, utilization, and transmission of information.

The information management tasks that actually involve handling data and information fall into the arena of informatics. These tasks include:

- *Data modeling:* Process of determining data needs and identifying the relationships among the data
- *Process and work-flow modeling:* Method for identifying the flow of work and information required to perform a function, including decomposition diagrams, dependency diagrams, and data flow
- *Data capture and display:* Function that includes system design, screen design, report design, and form design
- *Data dictionary maintenance:* Task that encompasses dictionary design, standardization, update, and dissemination
- *Access control:* Process for designing, implementing, and monitoring the map between information and user access
- *Data quality management:* Function that encompasses the collection, application, warehousing, and analysis of data to improve information quality

- *Nosology:* Function of analyzing and interpreting disease and procedure classifications and terminologies for accurate translation of healthcare data

These informatics functions can be illustrated using a simple information system (IS) example. A patient presents to the emergency department and needs to be registered. **Data modeling** would indicate what information is needed to identify the patient, to collect insurance information for payment, to provide demographic information needed for patient care, and to identify the person the patient would want contacted in the event his or her condition worsened. An example of the relationship among the data might be that the patient's address is the same for identification, billing, and contact purposes. Thus, this information would need to be collected only once.

Continuing with the example, **process and work-flow modeling** would involve identifying how this information is collected. In the emergency department, a critical patient may have a different process model than a patient with a less serious condition. Certain information, such as name, date of birth, and Social Security number, might need to be collected before any clinical treatment could begin, whereas insurance information could be collected prior to disposition.

Data capture and **data display** for collecting the registration information might involve a form the patient fills in and returns to the registration clerk. It is easy to see how such a form should be designed to easily transform written patient information to the data fields on a computer screen. Also, information should be collected in the most convenient manner for the patient. For example, all of the insurance information should be collected at one time, rather than making the patient repeatedly refer to his or her insurance card throughout the interview.

A **data dictionary** defines all of the unique data elements in the data set. For instance, the data field for Social Security number would indicate that it is nine characters long, numeric, and the unique identifier assigned by the Social Security Administration. Having a complete and specific data dictionary allows for data field design and editing. An edit for the Social Security number would be to ensure that all of the characters are numbers. A data dictionary also may record other types of data attributes (for example, weight recorded in pounds rather than grams) or stipulate that an entry must be authenticated or signed by the person collecting the information.

Access control is a critical function within HIM relative to information security. This function maps the relationship between information and the individuals authorized to use it. It may be established at a variety of levels. For instance, an attending physician may have access to a patient's entire medical record, but a lab technician may have access to lab data only. Understanding the information contained in the medical record and the roles of the different individuals authorized to use it allows the health information manager to design mechanisms that enable users to access the information they need and also safeguard patient confidentiality.

In the emergency department example, it is clear how data quality management plays a key role in high-quality care and the effective delivery of medicine. **Data quality management** considers each of the steps of the data cycle: collection, application, warehousing, and analysis. HIM professionals first look at how the data are used and then design the required data set, through data modeling, to ensure that they are collected at the most logical point. Application (use) of the data is considered to ensure that the information is available when and where it is needed. Warehousing (storage) of the data ensures that the information from this emergency visit is available for a follow-up visit to either the patient's primary care provider or the hospital inpatient unit should the patient require hospitalization. Making the data available for analysis may be required to determine staffing levels in the emergency department, to address quality of care concerns, or to improve patient satisfaction questionnaires.

Nosology, the final informatics function in the HIM professional definition, does not deal directly with the information collected in the emergency department encounter. As a nosologist, the HIM professional puts in place a standard terminology or description of the diagnoses and procedures used so that information can be stored and analyzed. Suppose the HIM professional wanted to find all of the patients who came to the emergency department for a myocardial infarction. Care providers use a number of different terms to refer to a myocardial infarction, including an MI, a heart attack, a coronary, and so on. By developing and using a standard terminology to describe this condition, the nosologist can ensure that every case of myocardial infarction will be found.

Health Information Technology

Health information professionals also work in technical roles that process health data and records. Much of this technical work is the focus of the associate-level education in health information technology. For example, health information technology includes the following functions:

- *Classification and coding:* Process of assigning the appropriate code or nomenclature term for categorization
- *Abstracting:* Function of compiling the pertinent information from the medical record based on predetermined data sets
- *Registry development:* Process of assembling a chronological set of data for an express purpose
- *Storage:* Implementation and oversight of computer-based and paper-based filing systems
- *Retrieval:* Process of making information stored in various media and sites accessible
- *Release:* Function of appropriately responding to requests for information based on laws and policy
- *Analysis:* Process of conducting qualitative and quantitative analysis of documentation against standards and policy

Health Information Media and Forms

The final domain of HIM professional practice concerns the forms in which health data are captured and stored. The management of information relates to all of these forms:

- Data (individual and aggregate)
- Reports
- Health records
- Data dictionaries
- Clinical vocabularies

Information may be stored using a variety of media, including paper, database, microfilm/microfiche, and electronic (computer systems).

Check Your Understanding 4.2

Instructions: Answer the following questions on a separate piece of paper.

1. What benefits are gained from HIM planning?
2. How are data modeling and process or work-flow modeling related?
3. What are some of the elements of a data dictionary?
4. What are some examples of how understanding the content of health information relates to the informatics functions?

Health Information Management Body of Knowledge

To carry out the professional definition, HIM professionals study a defined curriculum or body of knowledge. There are distinct curriculum models of each educational level within the field: associate, baccalaureate, and master's. The health information administration (HIA) model (baccalaureate level) is presented here and can be categorized into eleven topics (figure 4.2):

- Biomedical sciences
- Information technology
- Healthcare delivery systems
- Organization and management
- Quantitative methods and research
- Healthcare information requirements and standards
- Healthcare information systems
- Health data content and structures
- Clinical quality assessment and performance improvement
- Biomedical research support
- Health information services management

Like the professional definition of HIM, the HIM curriculum is examined and updated periodically to ensure its relevance to the demands of the field. The AHIMA accredits educational institutions that offer associate and baccalaureate degrees in health information administration and health information technology. This accreditation process ensures that the appropriate curriculum is being taught,

along with other essential elements of a high-quality educational experience.

Two elements make this curriculum unique: (1) the specialization to healthcare throughout the curriculum and (2) the combination of studies in the biomedical sciences, management, and information fields. In addition to this specific HIM curriculum, HIM students are required to have an understanding of additional general education topics to prepare them for the workplace, including:

- Oral and written communications
- Social and behavioral sciences
- Humanities
- Microcomputer literacy, including word processing, spreadsheets, database management, and graphic presentation
- General sciences
- Mathematics

These content areas do not represent individual courses but, rather, define the scope of instruction required of all accredited HIA programs.

Check Your Understanding 4.3

Instructions: Answer the following questions on a separate piece of paper.

1. What is the purpose of quantitative methods and research in the HIA curriculum?
2. Data information and file structures are included in what topic of the curriculum?
3. What are the elements within health data content and structures?
4. List all of the curriculum topics that would be important to performing research?

Characteristics of a Profession

The term *profession* may be defined in a number of ways. *Merriam-Webster's Collegiate Dictionary* (1995) defines it as "a calling requiring specialized knowledge and often long and intensive academic preparation." In *The Qualifying Association,* Millerson describes a profession as "a type of higher grade, non-manual occupation, with both subjectively and objectively recognized occupational status, possessing a well-defined area of study or concern and providing a definite service, after advanced training and education" (1964, p. 10). There are certainly characteristics of a profession that apply to health information management:

- Professional associations
- A code of ethics
- A unique body of knowledge that must be learned through formal education
- A system of training with entry by examination or other formal prerequisites (certification)
- Professional cohesion
- Professional literature

Figure 4.2   Curriculum Content for Health Information Administration

Biomedical Sciences
Intent: To develop understanding of the clinical knowledge base through study of the structure and function of the healthy human body, pathophysiology, diagnostic and treatment modalities, and pharmacy therapy available for clinical management of patient care and to enhance professional communication in healthcare environments.

- Anatomy
- Physiology
- Language of medicine
- Medical sciences
- Pharmacology

Information Technology
Intent: To introduce the major concepts of computer programming, computer architectures, operating systems, and application software. The core emphasizes the use of tools and techniques for the development of higher-level content in database processing, data communication technologies, and systems analysis.

- Computer concepts—hardware
- Processors
- Primary and secondary stage peripherals
- Architectures (e.g., client-server)
- Computer concepts—software
- Operating systems and utilities
- Application development systems (e.g., procedural and nonprocedural languages, SQL programming)
- Networks and data communications
- Local-area networks (LANs) and wide-area networks (WANs)
- Data, information, file structures
  —Data administration
  —Database structures
  —Data definitions
  —Data dictionary
  —Data modeling
  —Database management systems concepts
- Data security
  —Information privacy
  —Prevention and control methods
  —Risk assessment
  —Business contingency planning
- Data retrieval
  —Data access (e.g., query languages and security)
  —Report design
- Mainframe operating systems

Healthcare Delivery Systems
Intent: To describe the organization, financing, and delivery of healthcare services.

- Organization of healthcare delivery
- Healthcare organizations
- Accreditation standards
- Licensure/regulatory requirements
- Payment and reimbursement systems
- Legal aspects and issues
- Professional ethics

Organization and Management
Intent: To develop understanding of the business aspects of the healthcare organization, studying principles of human resources, management theory, and concepts relating to organizational behavior and culture, financial management, and accounting. Business techniques introduced are cost-benefit analysis, quality improvement, strategic planning and forecasting, and organizational assessment and benchmarking.

- Principles of management
- Strategic planning and forecasting
- Marketing
- Human resources management
- Education and training
- Organizational behavior
  —Entrepreneurialism
  —Leadership

  —Motivation
  —Team/consensus-building
  —Change management
  —Negotiation techniques
- Interpersonal skills techniques
- Quality/performance improvement methods/TQM
- Financial management
- Cost-benefit analysis
- Organizational assessment and benchmarking
- Cost accounting
- Work redesign/reengineering

Quantitative Methods and Research
Intent: To provide a foundation in concepts and techniques related to statistical analysis of data and basic research methods used for health services and clinical research. Includes practical application of descriptive and inferential statistics using computerized statistical packages.

- Vital statistics
- Descriptive statistics
- Inferential statistics
- Epidemiology
- Data presentation techniques
- Statistical reliability and validity
- Computerized statistical packages
- Research methodologies
- Knowledge base/library research techniques

Healthcare Information Requirements and Standards
Intent: To study regulations and standards associated with health information management that are promulgated by private and government entities.

- Standards for accreditation and licensure
- Government regulations in healthcare

Healthcare Information Systems
Intent: To study the clinical and business information applications in healthcare. Concepts, techniques, and tools associated with the systems development life cycle are included.

- Clinical and business applications of computing in healthcare
- Systems theory and development
- Systems planning
- Systems analysis
- Systems design
- Systems implementation and testing
- Systems selection processes
- Human factors and user–interface design

Health Data Content and Structures
Intent: To develop skills in identifying information needs and uses through techniques of data flow analysis and data mapping and assessment of the continuum of data integrity. Techniques and tools for the conceptual configuration and modeling of health information are studied, and concepts and methods for data administration and interfacing are developed. The technical standards for data structures and knowledge representation and content of the computer-based patient record systems are emphasized. Classifications, nomenclatures, and medical vocabularies are studied.

- Content of the health record
- Aspects of the computer-based patient record
- Decision-making processes
- Vocabulary standards
- Medical linguistics
- Healthcare information models
- Extra-enterprise healthcare information infrastructures
- Data validity and integrity
- Healthcare data sets
- Case mix
- Severity-of-illness systems
- Classification systems and nomenclatures
- Primary versus secondary records
- Registries and indexes

(Continued on next page)

Figure 4.2   (Continued)

Clinical Quality Assessment and Performance Improvement	Health Information Services Management

Intent: To present the principles of quality management and to develop knowledge, skills, attitudes, and values needed to coordinate quality and resource management programs.
 	
• Quality assessment and performance improvement (collection tools, data analysis, reporting techniques)
• Utilization and resource management
• Risk management
• Clinical outcomes management and research
• Critical path concepts/case management
• Accreditation and licensing quality/performance improvement standards
 	
Biomedical Research Support
Intent: To study design concepts and information systems to support biomedical and health services research and investigation (e.g., drug companies, genetic engineering firms, academic institutions, and individual researchers). Major national research policy-making bodies, their research protocols, and their management of information are included.
 	
• Data search and access techniques
• National research policy making
• Biomedical/health research and investigation
• Research protocol data management
	Intent: To develop the "intrapreneurial" role and customer service orientation for support of the management of health information resources and brokering of health information services.
	
	• "Intrapreneurial" role
	• Leading development of health information resources and systems
	• Strategic planning for information systems
	• Security management
	• Education and training of staff
	• Brokering of information services
	   —Assessment of information needs
	   —Identification of information sources
	   —Integration of multiple information sources
	   —Retrieval of information
	   —Interpretation of data appropriate to user needs
	   —Statistical interpretation
	   —Presentation of information
	   —Decision support system use
	• Managing and communicating with professionals
	• Resolving organizational information issues
	   —Problem solving and decision making

Adapted from Assembly on Education. 1995. *Entry-Level Baccalaureate Degree Education in Health Information Management: Reform for the 21st Century.* Chicago: American Health Information Management Association.

Professional Associations

Accepting the rewards of a profession means accepting its responsibilities. One of the ways to ensure professional success is through membership in a professional association. The following professional associations are particularly important to individuals working in the field of health information management.

American Health Information Management Association

The **American Health Information Management Association** (AHIMA) represents more than 40,000 HIM professionals who work throughout the healthcare industry. HIM professionals serve the healthcare industry and the public by managing, analyzing, and utilizing data vital for patient care and making them accessible to healthcare providers when they are needed most.

AHIMA members play many diverse roles, yet share a common purpose: to provide reliable and valid information that drives the healthcare industry. They are specialists in administering information systems, managing medical records, and coding information for reimbursement and research. As leaders in the field of health information management, AHIMA members work to ensure that healthcare is based on accurate and timely information. Building on the profession's strong tradition, they also are prepared to be a driving force in a changing healthcare industry.

The AHIMA works not only to strengthen the profession, but also to improve healthcare by:

• Supporting members with practice guidance and lifelong learning opportunities

• Providing a professional network through Communities of Practice for members to reach out to their colleagues
• Guaranteeing excellence to the healthcare industry through certification and relevant resources
• Disseminating best practices and innovations
• Promoting education and research in the field
• Providing public policy leadership
• Advocating for the profession and for HIM issues

The AHIMA supports a system of component organizations in every state plus Washington, D.C., and Puerto Rico. Component state associations (CSAs) provide their members with local access to professional education, networking, and representation. They also serve as an important forum for communicating national issues and keeping members informed of regional affairs that affect health information management. For more information, visit the AHIMA Web site at www.ahima.org.

American Medical Information Association

The **American Medical Information Association** (AMIA) is a membership organization composed of individuals, institutions, and corporations that develop and use information technologies in healthcare. Founded in 1990, AMIA was created when the American College of Medical Information and the Symposium on Computer Applications in Medical Care merged. Its members include physicians, nurses, computer and information scientists, biomedical engineers, medical librarians and academic researchers, and educators. AMIA represents the United States to the International Medical Informatics Association. Further, AMIA sponsors educational sessions and publishes *JAMIA*, the *Journal of the American*

Medical Informatics Association. For more information, visit the AMIA Web site at www.amia.org.

College of Healthcare Information Management Executives

The **College of Healthcare Information Management Executives** (CHIME) was formed in 1992 through a collaborative effort by the Healthcare Information and Management Systems Society (HIMSS) and the Center for Health Information Management (CHIM). CHIME serves two purposes: (1) to serve the professional development needs of healthcare chief information officers (CIOs) and (2) to advocate more effective use of information management within healthcare.

CHIME offers its members professional development opportunities through its biannual CIO Forums and through courses in information technology strategies, architecture, and best practices. Other resources include member-to-member surveys, online reference documents, and various presentations made available online. CHIME also participates in the Joint Healthcare Information Technology Alliance. For more information, contact www.cio-chime.org.

Healthcare Information and Management Systems Society

The **Healthcare Information and Management Systems Society** (HIMSS) provides leadership in healthcare for the management of technology, information, and change. Members include healthcare professionals in a variety of healthcare settings, including hospitals, corporate healthcare systems, clinical practice groups, vendor organizations, and consulting firms. Although HIMSS offers a variety of benefits, it is best known for its annual conference and exhibition, which is the largest in the industry. HIMSS has forty-three chapters organized on geographical areas. HIMSS also offers certification as a Certified Professional in Health Information Management Systems (CPHIMS).

The Center for Health Information Management (CHIM), which has been an independent association composed of health information technology vendors and businesses, has begun the transition to become a section of the HIMSS. For more information, visit the HIMSS Web site at www.himss.org.

Joint Health Information Technology Alliance

The Joint Health Information Technology Alliance (JHITA) is composed of the American Health Information Management Association (AHIMA), the American Medical Informatics Association (AMIA), the College of Healthcare Information Management Executives (CHIME), and the Healthcare Information and Management Systems Society (HIMSS). Two areas of focus for JHITA are (1) "to provide appropriate advocacy for legislation/regulation promoting the effective use of technology and its management, telecommunications, and business process re-engineering" and (2) "to be a dynamic force in our industry by developing jointly sponsored offerings including educational programs, market focus groups, research, services and activities relating to infor-

mation technology and management, telecommunications, and business process re-engineering" (www.JHITA.org).

JHITA monitors national legislative and regulatory activities and reports on them to its membership through routine summaries, advocacy papers on topics of particular interest to the membership, and presentations at selected member organization events. An additional JHITA focus is professional development and education on topics that span the industry.

Code of Ethics

An important element of any profession is its commitment to a code of ethics. Today's HIM professionals can face a variety of ethical dilemmas regarding payment and reimbursement systems, confidentiality and privacy, facility accreditation and licensure, and fair employment practices. A formal code of ethics ensures that professionals understand and agree to uphold an ethical standard that puts the best interests of the profession before their personal best interests.

The AHIMA has developed a code of ethics for certified HIM professionals. (See figure 4.3.) A violation of the code of ethics is grounds for disciplinary action, including revocation of credentials. AHIMA's professional conduct committee evaluates and responds to reports of ethical violations through a formal hearing process.

Figure 4.3.   AHIMA Code of Ethics

Preamble: This Code of Ethics sets forth ethical principles for the health information management profession. Members of this profession are responsible for maintaining and promoting ethical practices. This Code of Ethics, adopted by the American Health Information Management Association, shall be binding on health information management professionals who are members of the Association and all individuals who hold an AHIMA credential.

 I. Health information management professionals respect the rights and dignity of all individuals.
 II. Health information management professionals comply with all laws, regulations, and standards governing the practice of health information management.
 III. Health information management professionals strive for professional excellence through self-assessment and continuing education.
 IV. Health information management professionals truthfully and accurately represent their professional credentials, education, and experience.
 V. Health information management professionals adhere to the vision, mission, and values of the Association.
 VI. Health information management professionals promote and protect the confidentiality and security of health records and health information.
 VII. Health information management professionals strive to provide accurate and timely information.
 VIII. Health information management professionals promote high standards for health information management practice, education, and research.
 IX. Health information management professionals act with integrity and avoid conflicts of interest in the performance of their professional and AHIMA responsibilities.

Revised and adopted by AHIMA House of Delegates—October 4, 1998.

Education

An educational requirement is part of the definition of a profession. Indeed, it is the entry into any profession. Additionally, ongoing education is a responsibility of any professional. This is especially true of HIM professionals challenged by new regulations, revolutionary technologies, and an industry in transition. In October 1997, the AHIMA House of Delegates passed a resolution calling for its members to embrace lifelong learning:

> That AHIMA members make the commitment to lifelong learning and professional development so that HIM professionals continue to be vital players in ensuring quality healthcare through quality information.

This learning may be formal education through the pursuit of a master's or doctoral degree. There are a few master's programs in health information management. Continuing professional development also can be gained through continuing education gained from conferences, workshops, reading, or new distance training opportunities. Seeking challenging work assignments and making professional development a goal in career choices all add to professional development.

Certification

Certification is a process by which a nongovernment agency or association recognizes the competence of individuals who have met certain qualifications as determined by the agency or association. In health information management, AHIMA certification provides both personal validation and validation to employers and consumers of professional competence. Specifically, certification:

- Demonstrates to colleagues and superiors a dedication to high-quality healthcare and to the highest standards of health information management.
- Presents solid evidence to employers that an employee has trained and been tested to implement best practices and apply current technology solutions, abilities that in turn advance the organization.
- Sets a person apart from uncredentialed job candidates. In recent AHIMA-sponsored research groups, healthcare executives and recruiters cited these reasons for preferring credentialed personnel: (1) assurance of current knowledge through continued education, (2) possession of field-tested experience, and (3) verification of base-level competency.
- Has value for employers because it supports a worker's ability to uphold industry standards and regulations, thereby potentially saving organizations from fines and penalties due to errors or noncompliance.
- Catalyzes career development by augmenting resumes and adding recognition to candidates' capability. Because credentials appear after a person's name, they announce expertise with every signature.

To achieve certification from the AHIMA, individuals must meet certain eligibility requirements and successfully complete an examination. Until 2002, the AHIMA awarded four credentials:

- Registered health information administrator (RHIA)
- Registered health information technician (RHIT)
- Certified coding specialist (CCS)
- Certified coding specialist—physician based (CCS-P)

In fall 2002, the AHIMA added a new entry-level coding credential, the certified coding associate (CCA). This credential was developed to address the shortage of qualified coders. It creates the first step on a coding career ladder that could lead to a CCS or a CCS-P with more training and experience. Moreover, CCAs may choose to diversify their interests in health information management beyond coding and continue their education and apply for the RHIT or RHIA credentials.

Also in the fall of 2002, the AHIMA began offering an advanced specialty credential in information privacy and security. In a joint effort with HIMSS, the AHIMA will offer the following privacy certifications: Certified in Healthcare Privacy (CHP) and Certified in Healthcare Privacy and Security (CHPS). HIMSS offers a certification in healthcare security called Certified in Healthcare Security (CHS). These new certifications address the industry demand created by the Health Insurance Portability and Accountability Act (HIPAA) and increasing public demand for a comprehensive approach to protecting patient confidentiality.

Registered Health Information Administrator

Registered health information administrators (RHIAs) are skilled in the collection, interpretation, and analysis of patient data. Additionally, they receive the training necessary to assume managerial positions related to these functions. RHIAs interact with all levels of an organization—clinical, financial, administrative—that use patient data in decision making and everyday operations.

In a recent membership survey, the AHIMA found that more than half of the RHIA respondents were directors, managers, or consultants, with nearly 31 percent serving as HIM directors. Historically, most RHIAs have held the title of director of the HIM department of an acute care facility, but today other career opportunities abound. As patient records evolve toward computerization and as more entities such as third-party payers require health data, RHIAs benefit from a wide selection of roles in the industry. Information security and storage, data quality assurance, and advanced assistance to consumers with their health information are among the new domains. The AHIMA's Vision 2006 identifies and describes emerging HIM roles that parallel changes in the healthcare industry.

RHIAs enjoy job placements in a broad range of settings that span the continuum of healthcare, including office-based physician practices, nursing homes, home health agencies, mental health facilities, and public health agencies. The growth of managed care has created additional job opportunities in health maintenance organizations (HMOs), preferred provider organizations (PPOs), and insurance companies. Prospects are especially strong in these settings for RHIAs who possess advanced degrees in business or health administration.

To become eligible to take the RHIA examination, applicants must meet one of the following educational requirements:

- Baccalaureate degree from an AHIMA/CAAHEP-accredited health information administration (HIA) program
- Baccalaureate degree from an accredited college or university and a certificate in HIA from an accredited program
- Degree from a foreign HIA baccalaureate program with which the AHIMA has a reciprocal agreement (The AHIMA currently has an agreement with the Health Information Management Association of Australia at the baccalaureate level.)
- Baccalaureate degree in any field with current RHIT certification (This special window of opportunity is available from 1999 to 2004.)

The RHIA exam is offered continually through computer testing sites throughout the country. An application must be filed with the AHIMA, and then an identification number and password are assigned.

Registered Health Information Technician

Registered health information technicians (RHITs) are health information technicians who ensure the quality of medical records by verifying their completeness, accuracy, and proper entry into computer systems. RHITs also may use computer applications to assemble and analyze patient data for the purpose of improving patient care or controlling costs. These technicians often specialize in coding diagnoses and procedures in patient records for reimbursement and research. Moreover, they may serve as cancer registrars, compiling and maintaining data on cancer patients. In a recent AHIMA membership survey, the majority of RHIT respondents held job titles in one of the following categories: coding/technician or manager/supervisor. With experience, the RHIT credential holds solid potential for advancement to management positions, especially if it is combined with a bachelor's degree.

Although most RHITs work in hospitals, they also work in a variety of other healthcare settings, including office-based physician practices, nursing homes, home health agencies, mental health facilities, and public health agencies. In fact, employment opportunities exist for RHITs in any organization that uses patient data or health information, including pharmaceutical companies, law and insurance firms, and health product vendors.

RHITs can look forward to expanding career opportunities in health information technology. According to the Bureau of Labor Statistics, health information technicians occupy one of the top ten health occupations, with the fastest potential growth between now and year 2010 (Wing 2002, p. 40).

Certified Coding Specialist

Certified coding specialists (CCSs) are professionals skilled in classifying medical data from patient records, generally in the hospital setting. CCSs review patient records and assign numeric codes for each diagnosis and procedure. To perform this task, they must possess expertise in the ICD-9-CM coding system and the surgery section within the CPT coding system. In addition, the CCS must be knowledgeable in medical terminology, disease processes, and pharmacology.

Hospitals or medical providers report coded data to insurance companies or the government (in the case of Medicare and Medicaid recipients) for reimbursement of their expenses. Researchers and public health officials also use coded medical data to monitor patterns and explore new interventions. Thus, coding accuracy is highly important to healthcare organizations because of its impact on revenues and describing health outcomes. Accordingly, the CCS credential demonstrates tested data quality and integrity skills in a coding practitioner. The CCS certification exam assesses mastery or proficiency in coding rather than entry-level skills.

Certified Coding Specialist—Physician-Based

The **certified coding specialist—physician based** (CCS-P) has expertise in physician-based settings such as physician offices, group practices, multispecialty clinics, or specialty centers. The CCS-P reviews patient records and assigns numeric codes for each diagnosis and procedure. To perform this task, he or she must possess in-depth knowledge of the CPT coding system and familiarity with the ICD-9-CM and HCPCS Level II coding systems. The CCS-P is also expert in health information documentation, data integrity, and quality. Because patients' coded data are submitted to insurance companies or the government for expense reimbursement, the CCS-P plays a critical role in the health provider's business operation. Moreover, the employment outlook for this coding specialty looks highly favorable with the growth of managed care and the movement of health services delivery beyond the hospital.

The AHIMA will continue to develop relevant certification programs in response to market demand. Future initiatives will likely lead to other advanced specialty certification in focused HIM topics.

Certification Maintenance

The purpose of a continuing education (CE) program is to offer the public a form of assurance that individuals practicing a profession maintain competence following certification in that profession. In the health professions, maintaining competence is especially critical because of the rapid growth in technology, changes in social policies, and the expanding roles of health professionals in all areas of healthcare.

Participants are responsible for self-assessment of their personal strengths and weaknesses and for developing individual CE programs designed to ensure their own professional competence. The number of CE hours that can be obtained in any particular activity is unlimited. It is recommended that participants attempt to increase their knowledge and skills through a balanced variety of educational methods.

Continuing Education Requirements

All credentialed health information professionals (RHIAs and RHITs), including active, inactive, and student members of the AHIMA, as well as nonmembers, maintain their credentials by:

1. *Completion of acceptable CE credits during a two-year period (cycle):* RHIAs must earn 30 CE clock hours/credits; RHITs must complete 20 CE clock hours/credits. To receive credit, activities must be completed within the assigned cycle period. All cycles begin on January 1 and end on December 31 the following year.
2. *Payment of CE assessment fees:* AHIMA members are charged a CE assessment with annual membership dues. Nonmembers pay a CE fee, set by the AHIMA Board of Directors, at the end of each CE cycle.
3. *Validation of CE report:* Participants must submit their CE Report Forms to the AHIMA by January 31, following the end of the CE cycle. (It is suggested that participants keep a photocopy of the form.) Participants who are not audited will receive a CE Validation Certificate to retain as evidence of meeting CE requirements. Participants selected for audit do not meet requirements until they have complied with the audit procedures. A CE Validation Certificate will be forwarded to audited participants after documentation has been received and approved.

Reporting Requirements and Cost

Four to six weeks prior to the end of the CE cycle, participants will receive a Continuing Education Report Form from the AHIMA. Participants must record the number of clock hour credits received in each of the core content areas, the number of hours received in other HIM areas, and the total hours earned during the reporting period.

Although only the number of hours earned needs to be reported, it is important that participants maintain complete personal files of CE activities in case they are audited. The AHIMA provides a Continuing Education Tracking Form that members may use to track their hours throughout the reporting period.

Currently, non-AHIMA members pay a $100 CE assessment per cycle. AHIMA members currently pay an annual $10 assessment with their membership dues.

Revocation and Restoration of Certification

The RHIA or RHIT credential will be revoked for failure to comply with CE requirements. Revocation is effective the year following the end of the applicable CE cycle. Before revocation, a Notice of Intent to Revoke is sent to the participant. If there is no response to the notice of intent, credentials are revoked.

Any individual whose credential is revoked may request an Application for Restoration of Credential from the AHIMA. To restore a credential, applicants must either document earning the applicable number of CE credits for the credential (discussed above) within the restoration period or apply to rewrite the next RHIA/RHIT examination.

No one may use the RHIT or RHIA credential after it has been revoked. During restoration, the individual is listed as an RHIT or RHIA restoration candidate for a maximum period of one year.

Continuing Education Audits

As CE hours are entered into the membership files, approximately two percent of the candidates are randomly selected for audit. An individual selected for audit is required to submit verifiable documentation for each activity listed on the CE Report Form. Auditors will seek verification of attendance or participation, content description, and CE credits earned. Thus, CE participants are advised to retain all records in their files for at least one year following the cycle end date.

Prior Approval of Activities

Unless otherwise indicated, programs or activities do not need prior approval from the AHIMA. If the program or activity has not received AHIMA prior approval, candidates can judge for themselves whether it meets AHIMA requirements.

Professional Cohesion

Another aspect of a profession is professional cohesion, which is characterized by the members of a profession acting in a unified way. The existence of a professional association is one expression of professional cohesion as it embodies the members of the profession who act as a profession rather than as individuals. Professional cohesion can be witnessed in AHIMA's position statements or in advocacy positions that are taken with regulators or legislators. The recognition and adoption of best practices is another example of professional cohesion.

Professional Literature

The final element of a profession is the existence of professional literature. This textbook is one example of professional literature. The *Journal of AHIMA* is the most well known source of health information management knowledge. Published since the 1930s, the *Journal* is distributed to all AHIMA members and is available as a subscription to nonmembers. In addition to AHIMA there are several other publishers of books and periodicals dealing with health information management. However, research and publication of health information management topics is in short supply when compared to other professions. This is an area of concern and opportunity for health information management professionals.

Instructions: Answer the following questions on a separate piece of paper.

1. Which professional HIM association offers professional certification to its members?

2. Why might someone belong to more than one professional association?

3. What are some of the key services provided by professional associations?

4. Why would professional associations gain from forming an alliance?

5. Why is it important to understand the HIM Code of Ethics?

6. How is the importance of continuing education addressed in the AHIMA's Code of Ethics?

7. What elements of the Code of Ethics relate to the individual's participation with the AHIMA?

8. What are the benefits of certification, and how does one maintain it?

9. Who is eligible for RHIA certification?

10. How frequently are certification records audited?

11. How does someone report continuing education activities?

Current and Evolving Professional Roles

In 1996, AHIMA's Board of Directors took on an ambitious project: looking into the future and envisioning HIM practice and roles in the next millennium. Logically, the board's first step was to ask, "Exactly what does a health information manager do?" To answer that question and to continue to build a definition of the profession, the association began an initiative called Vision 2006. Vision 2006 is built on the work of a prior initiative, Vision 2000, which in 1991 sought to describe how HIM practice would evolve in the 1990s. Vision 2006 takes over for Vision 2000 and looks even further into the future.

Traditional HIM practice has been based on physical records, files filled with paper forms and documents. Although some information based on current health records may be electronically stored and manipulated, most HIM functions today are still built around the existence of a physical record. New practice will be based on data management. As HIM practice evolves from its traditional base and aligns itself with changes in the healthcare delivery system and information technology, exciting career opportunities will emerge. Vision 2006 defined seven roles for the future:

- A *health information manager in an integrated delivery system* is responsible for the organizationwide direction of HIM functions. The role may be a line or staff management position. It includes working with the chief information executive and information system users to advance systems, methods, and applications support and to improve data quality, access, confidentiality, security, and usability.

- A *clinical data specialist* concentrates on data management functions in a variety of applications including

clinical coding, outcomes management, specialty registries, and research databases.

- A *patient information coordinator* helps consumers manage their personal health information, including personal health histories and release of information; this individual also helps customers understand managed care services and access to health information resources.

- A *data quality manager* is responsible for data management functions that involve formalized continuous quality improvement activities for data integrity throughout the organization, beginning with the data dictionary and policy development, as well as data quality monitoring and audits.

- A *data resource administrator* represents the next generation of records and data management and uses technological tools such as the computer-based patient record, data repositories, and data warehouses to meet current and future care needs across the continuum, provide access to the needed information, and ensure long-term data integrity and access.

- A *research and decision support analyst* ensures the quality of data and information generated through clinical investigations and other research projects. The decision support specialist provides clinicians and senior managers with information for decision making and strategy development. Both specialists use a variety of analytical tools.

- A *security officer* is responsible for managing the security of electronically maintained information, including promulgation of security requirements, policies and privilege systems, and performance auditing.

Since the launch of Vision 2006 in 1996, new roles have emerged: *compliance officer* and *privacy officer.* Roles for HIM professionals are developing in e-health companies and the pharmaceuticals industry. The key is that the profession continues to respond to the needs of the healthcare industry and continually advances the quality of health information.

Real-World Case

Jane Rogers, age 31, is supervisor for clinical coding in the health information service at Memorial Medical Center in Chicago. She left her job as a clinical coder at Community General Hospital six months ago to take this newly created position. Jane graduated from the Health Information Administration program at Chicago University ten years ago and is credentialed as a registered health information administrator (RHIA) and clinical coding specialist (CCS) by the AHIMA. She is an active member in good standing of the association and serves on the Coding Roundtable for the Chicago Area Health Information Management Association. The position at Memorial was a significant promotion, increasing her salary by $11,000 a year and offering her a chance to be a supervisor. The new level of earnings allowed Jane to live on her own and to purchase her own car, a four-year-old bright-red Saturn.

Jane reports to Steve Murray, manager of patient accounts and the health information service. Steve is the nephew of Memorial's chief financial officer, John Murray III, who was brought in to turn around the medical center, which was in significant financial trouble in the mid-1990s. Steve has an MBA from the University of Chicago but, unlike most managers at Memorial, including his uncle, no formal training in healthcare administration, health information, or financial management. However, he is young and ambitious and has shown himself to be an effective manager. He has streamlined operations in patient accounts and health information services, increasing revenues by 20 percent, increasing collections and cash flow, automating many functions, and reducing clerical staff.

Jane is responsible for the staff that review medical records of patients treated at Memorial to identify the diagnoses and procedures involved in inpatient, outpatient, and emergency treatment. Staff assign codes that are the basis for the bills submitted for reimbursement to the federal and state government and to private insurance companies.

Steve told Jane that her first priority was to make coding functions more current. Further, he wanted to cut in half the twenty or more days that it currently took to complete coding and billing functions. To that end, Jane reorganized processing procedures, taught staff new techniques for speeding up record review, and within three months had achieved her goal. In a meeting with Steve at the end of her three-month probationary period, Jane was awarded a $1,000 spot bonus for her achievement. Even John Murray stopped by to congratulate her. Jane was so proud of her achievement that she presented her approaches at the monthly meeting of the Coding Roundtable and received words of encouragement from many of her colleagues.

With processing now running smoothly, Jane turned to coding accuracy. She undertook a study in which she randomly sampled the coded records of all six of her coding staff and recoded them herself without looking at the original codes. She found that accuracy rates ranged from 78 to 92 percent. Although benchmark standards are difficult to come by, Jane knew that the coders at Community General met a standard of 90+ percent and that their evaluations and merit increases depended on maintaining it. Despite standard guidelines for correct code assignment, payer requirements do not always conform to them. Payers are constantly issuing instructions about what codes they will and will not accept, and coders sometimes do not have the latest instructions. Further, medical record documentation is not always clear or complete, and accurate code assignment requires some individual judgment. Because the codes assigned to a case determine reimbursement, it is possible to increase the organization's revenue by using codes representing more complex diagnoses or procedures. These must be supported by documentation in the medical record. However, code assignment is seldom a black-and-white decision and thus it is possible to assign unsupported codes, thereby increasing reimbursement, and to fail to assign an appropriate code, thereby decreasing reimbursement.

In her weekly meeting with Steve, Jane reviewed the findings and proposed a plan for retraining and ongoing data quality control, including an adjusted compensation plan that would reward accurate work by her staff members. Her plan also called for developing a set of written guidelines that would reinforce Memorial's official guidelines and be presented to administration and the medical staff for approval. In this way, the coders would know the ground rules and the basis on which their performance was to be measured. Steve indicated that he would support the plan provided it did not result in slower processing time or reduced levels of reimbursement. Jane agreed to make certain that training did not slow down processing. She also suggested that improving accuracy would likely have a neutral effect on reimbursement because coders were undoubtedly missing reimbursable diagnoses and procedures.

With her plan in hand, Jane thought that it would be wise to focus on the clinical areas most vulnerable to inaccurate coding. She began by conducting another interrater reliability study of cardiac surgery cases because these cases always present a challenge to coders. Again, she found wide variability in coder performance, this time ranging from 68 to 89 percent. She developed guidelines and obtained approval for them from the cardiac surgery clinical staff and administration. Then, she conducted a training program for her staff, who were paid overtime to attend so they did not fall behind in their work.

With another success under her belt, Jane next tackled the area of respiratory disease, another area of coding complexity and a major clinical service at Memorial, representing nearly 10 percent of its discharges. Further, Jane knew from reading her *Journal of the AHIMA* that bacterial pneumonia was the focus of investigations of Medicare fraud and abuse being conducted by the Department of Justice (DOJ). In fact, a number of healthcare organizations had paid substantial fines for having coded pneumonia cases with codes not supported by documentation in the medical records. Jane pulled a sample of records coded as "bacterial pneumonia," "other bacterial pneumonia," and "viral pneumonia." She worked late into the night for a week coding, recoding, checking, and double-checking her findings, which showed that cases were being consistently coded with the "bacterial" and "other bacterial" codes even though very few of the records had culture reports verifying bacterial infection. She calculated that with 150 cases a year and $5,000 in additional billings per case, this pattern of inaccurate coding was resulting in $750,000 in unsubstantiated revenue. The sheer volume of such cases made it unlikely that Memorial could claim random error if the DOJ chose to investigate.

Jane spent the weekend rechecking her findings and preparing a report with guidelines for accurate coding. She decided she had better talk to the coding staff before her regular weekly meeting with Steve on Monday afternoon. So first thing Monday morning, she met with her staff and reviewed her findings. Jane was shocked when Sally, the most tenured coder nodded and said, "We're just doing what we're told." When pressed, Sally acknowledged that the chief of respiratory medicine, Dr. Barrows, and Steve Murray had met with the coding staff the year before to discuss the coding of pneumonia cases. Jane asked, "Do you have anything in writing from the meeting?" "No," Sally replied, "they just told us that there were other ways to determine bacterial pneumonia than by culture and that Memorial was the major referral center for treating bacterial pneumonia." Needing time to digest what she had learned, Jane rescheduled her meeting with Steve, claiming a headache and upset stomach. She went home early to consider what to do next.

Concluding that the best approach would be to let the facts speak for themselves, Jane presented her report to Steve the next day along with her pneumonia coding guidelines. Steve was quiet and did not interrupt her, taking notes as she went through her findings. She concluded by saying, "Steve, we must implement the new guidelines at once, and we must also submit corrected bills for the cases we inaccurately submitted over the past year. This is the only way we can be sure that a fraud and abuse investigation will not be brought against Memorial." Steve replied, "Thank you, Jane. I'd like a copy of the report, and I'll discuss it with Dr. Barrows and John Murray. We'll get back to you. In the meantime, don't say anything about this to anyone."

Three weeks have passed, and Steve has canceled three weekly meetings in a row and barely spoken to Jane when they meet informally in the hallway or cafeteria. He has asked no further questions and has given no indication of his intention to act on Jane's findings or proposals for action.

Discussion Questions

1. What codes of ethical conduct apply to Jane's behavior in this situation?
2. What are Jane's duties to the public? The organization she works for? Her employees? Herself?
3. What are Jane's possible courses of action?
4. What course of action should she pursue?

Summary

Health information managers work with clinical, epidemiologic, demographic, financial, research, reference, and coded healthcare data. Health information administrators plan information systems, develop policy, and identify current and future information needs. In addition, they apply the science of informatics to the collection, storage, use, and transmission of information.

HIM professionals prepare for their careers through mastering a well-defined body of knowledge expressed in a formal curriculum. This curriculum covers, though is not limited to, content which addresses biomedical sciences, informatics, management, and research principles. Once finished with their formal education, most HIM professionals achieve certification by passing a certification examination offered by AHIMA. Maintenance of certification demonstrates a lifelong commitment to continuing education and adherence to the HIM Code of Ethics.

As the professional association that represents most health information managers, AHIMA provides numerous services to its members and to the healthcare industry. Through accreditation of academic programs and certification of individual members, AHIMA ensures a qualified workforce. AHIMA works to improve healthcare by disseminating best practices, promoting research, and providing public policy leadership.

The HIM profession continues to evolve and change in response to healthcare trends, information technology, and government regulation. In the 1980s, most HIM professionals worked in hospitals; today, almost half of the AHIMA's members work outside hospitals in a growing variety of health information practice sites. Health information management is a dynamic profession facing many current and future challenges, transitions, opportunities. The ongoing conversion from paper files to computer-based records has brought with it a shift in roles (from managers and supervisors to more high-level technical specialists) for HIM leaders.

References

American Health Information Management Association. www.ahima.org.

American Medical Informatics Association. www.amia.org.

Assembly on Education. 1995. *Entry–Level Baccalaureate Degree Education in Health Information Management: Reform for the 21st Century.* Chicago: American Health Information Management Association.

College of Healthcare Information Management Executives. www.chime.org.

Chronicle Guidance Publications. 1999. *Health Sciences Librarians Brief 516,* pp. 8–11. Moravia, N.Y.: Chronicle Guidance Publications, Inc.

Degoulet, P., and M. Fieschi. 1997. *Introduction to Clinical Informatics.* New York City: Springer.

Greenes, R. A., and E. H. Shortliffe. 1990. Medical informatics: an emerging academic discipline and institutional priority. *JAMA* 263:1114.

Health Information Management and Systems Society. www.himss.org.

Huffman, Edna K. 1941. *Manual for Medical Records Librarians.* Chicago: Physicians' Record Company.

Institute of Medicine, Committee on Improving the Patient Record in Response to Increasing Functional Requirements and Technological Advances. 1997. *The Computer-Based Patient Record: An Essential Technology for Health Care.* Washington, D.C.: U.S. National Academy of Sciences.

Joint Healthcare Industry Technology Alliance. www.jhita.org.

Kloss, L. 2000. Ethics in the age of compliance. *AHIMA Program in a Box.* Chicago: American Health Information Management Association.

Merriam-Webster's Collegiate Dictionary. 1995. Springfield, Mass.: Merriam-Webster.

Millerson, G. 1964. *The Qualifying Association: A Study in Professionalization.* London: Routledge & Paul.

National Income and Product Accounts: Second quarter 2001 Gross Domestic Product: Revised Estimates: 1998 through first quarter 2001. Bureau of Economic Analysis News Release, July 27, 2001. Available from www. bea.doc.gov.

Russell, L. A. 2001. Not what we were in 1928: a new professional definition. *Journal of the American Health Information Management Association* 72(4):48A–48D.

Webster, Berenika. 1999. Records management: from profession to scholarly discipline. *Association of Records Managers and Administrators Information Management Journal* 4(33):20.

Wing, P., and E. Salsberg. 2002. How trends shape the work force today and tomorrow. *Journal of the American Health Information Management Association* 73(4):38.

Application Exercises

1. Search the Internet or use the library to find other examples of professional definitions or descriptions from other healthcare disciplines. Write a summary of how these other definitions compare with the HIM professional definition.

2. Review the elements of the HIA curriculum and identify those elements that would have been added since the introduction of computers. Summarize the differences in a one-page review.

3. Search the Internet for HIM job ads. Complete a grid that lists, by job, the type of HIM function that would be prominent and the types of health information that would be primarily used.

4. Review the curriculum models for the HIT, HIA, and master's-level programs. Write a brief paper that compares and contrasts the curriculums.

5. Interview an HIM professional regarding the professional development activities that he or she pursues.

6. Conduct a survey of HIM professionals to determine whether educational preparation and credentials affect salary.

Review Quiz

Instructions: Choose the best answer for the following questions.

1. ___ Which field concerns itself with the cognitive information process and communication tools of medical practice, education, and research, including the information science and technology to support these tasks?
   a. Medical information management
   b. Health informatics
   c. Health science librarians
   d. Information technology

2. ___ Data used to describe a specific population are called what?
   a. Reference data
   b. Financial data
   c. Clinical data
   d. Epidemiological data

3. ___ Establishing security, confidentiality, retention, integrity, and access standards are examples of which HIM function?
   a. Policy development
   b. Data modeling
   c. Strategic planning
   d. Classification and coding

4. ___ Which of the following statements is true of data quality management?
   a. It affects the collection, application, warehousing, and analysis of data to improve information quality.
   b. It analyzes and interprets disease and procedure classifications and terminologies.
   c. It includes system design, screen design, and report and forms design.
   d. Involves appropriately responding to requests for information based on laws and policy.

5. ___ Which curriculum topic involves the study of clinical and business information applications in healthcare?
   a. Biomedical research support
   b. Health information services management
   c. Healthcare information systems
   d. Health data content and structures

6. ___ Guaranteeing excellence in the healthcare industry through certification and relevant resources is one of the functions of which professional association?
   a. HIMSS
   b. AHIMA
   c. CHIME
   d. JHITA

7. ___ The College of Healthcare Information Management Executives was formed in 1992 through a collaborative effort between the Center for Health Information Management and which organization?
   a. AHIMA
   b. JHITA
   c. CHIM
   d. AMIA

8. ___ Historically, the position of HIM director has been held by individuals with which AHIMA credential?
   a. RHIA
   b. CCS
   c. RHIT
   d. CCS-P

9. ___ In recent AHIMA-sponsored research groups, healthcare executives and recruiters cited which of the following reasons for preferring credentialed personnel?
   a. Association membership
   b. Assurance of current knowledge through continued education
   c. Required they pay a higher salary
   d. Credentials required by law

10. ___ Under which conditions does a profession continue to grow and develop?
    a. When it maintains a static curriculum model
    b. When it remains constant and resists change
    c. When it focuses on increasing the number of people in the profession
    d. When it responds to the needs of the industry

Chapter 5
Data and Information Management

Frances Wickham Lee, DBA

Learning Objectives

- To understand the differences among data, information, and knowledge
- To discuss the basic principles of information management
- To list and give examples of seven characteristics of quality data
- To discuss how the design of a database can affect data quality
- To compare a relational database and its characteristics with other database models
- To discuss how data modeling, particularly using an entity relationship diagram (ERD), can help ensure high-quality data
- To discuss the role of a data dictionary in ensuring both the quality of enterprisewide data and data within a specific database application
- To describe and compare the roles of database administrator, data administrator, and data resource manager
- To discuss how to ensure the integrity and security of data within a database

Key Terms

Attributes
Authorization management
Conceptual data model
Data
Data administrator
Data definition language (DDL)
Data dictionary
Data integrity
Data manipulation language (DML)
Data models
Data resource manager
Database
Database administrator
Database life cycle (DBLC)
Database management system (DBMS)
Derived attribute
Entity
Entity relationship diagram (ERD)
Foreign key
Information
Information management
Integrity constraints

Key attributes
Knowledge
Logical data model
Many-to-many relationship
Normalization
Object
Object-oriented database (OODB)
Object-oriented database management system (OODBMS)
One-to-many relationship
One-to-one relationship
Physical data model
Primary key
Relational database
Relational database management system (RDBMS)
Seven dimensions of data quality
Structured query language
System catalog
Unified modeling language (UML)

Introduction

Health information managers have numerous roles within the healthcare industry. Most, if not all, of these roles involve managing information that is shared by a diverse and sometimes widely dispersed group of end users. Meeting the challenge of managing the data and information needed to deliver or support high-quality healthcare is not a simple task. Frequently, end users have different views, not only of the various uses of data and information, but also of the basic definitions of the data elements. These different views must be reconciled in order to develop high-quality healthcare information systems.

This chapter introduces data and information as organizational assets that must be managed effectively to provide and sustain their value. It looks at the relationship between data and information, the basic principles of information management, managing data quality through database design techniques and data dictionaries, the role of the data manager, and the importance of securing healthcare data stored in a database system.

Theory into Practice

The following true story appeared in "Tools for Defining Data," an article by Abdul-Malik Shakir and published in the *Journal of the American Health Information Management Association* in September 1999. It clearly illustrates the need for end users to agree on data definitions and some of the problems that can be created when such definitions are not in place.

In 1991, a large national health maintenance organization (HMO) was planning to create a disease management program for pediatric care. As part of the planning effort, the HMO decided to conduct a survey of its regional sites to determine the utilization pattern for pediatric care. It sent a questionnaire to each of the 12 regional offices asking these two questions:

1. How many pediatric members were enrolled as of year-end 1990?
2. How many pediatric visits took place in 1990?

On the surface, the questions seemed quite simple and appropriate. The HMO would determine the number of pediatric members and the number of pediatric visits by region. It could then compute pediatric utilization by region—and across the program as a whole. This data would then be used to determine a baseline for development of utilization management programs and would assist in comparative analysis of pediatric utilization across regions.

There was only one problem—the absence of common data definitions. Each of the regions operated somewhat autonomously and interpreted the request for information differently. As a result, the regional offices raised a number of questions and revealed numerous discrepancies in their interpretations of data definitions:

1. What is a pediatric member?
   —a dependent member under the age of 18
   —a dependent member under the age of 21
   —a dependent child member, regardless of age
   —a patient under the age of 18

2. What is a pediatric visit?
   —a visit by a pediatric member
   —a visit by a patient under the age of 18
   —any visit to the pediatric department
   —a visit with a pediatrician

Attempts to answer these questions only raised more questions. What is a member? What does it mean to be enrolled? What is a dependent? How is patient/member age calculated? What is a visit? What is a patient and how does one differ from a member? What is a department? What are the department types? What is a pediatrician?

This story shows us how important it is that suppliers and consumers of data agree on data definitions before exchanging information. Had the regions not revealed their assumptions, the discrepancies in their interpretations of the data definitions might never have been recognized, and the organization would have unknowingly compared apples to oranges. In the long term, a business strategy with significant implications would have been based upon invalid information.

From Data to Information

Where does information come from? The simple answer is that **information** is processed **data.** Data are the raw facts, generally stored as characters, words, symbols, measurements, or statistics. Unprocessed data are not very useful for decision making. Take, for example, the numerals 6, 5, and 0. What do they mean? If seen together as "650," the data might be processed into the number six hundred and fifty. When processing this number further by looking it up in the ICD-9-CM codebook or entering it into an encoder software program, it takes on even more meaning. It is now known that 650 is the code that represents a completely normal delivery. Is this information? That depends. When looking for a particular patient's diagnosis to process a claim, 650 may, in fact, be providing the information an insurance clerk would need. However, for the medical researcher looking for patient characteristics that contribute to completely normal deliveries, 650 on one patient's chart is not yet "processed" enough to provide useful information. (See figure 5.1.)

Figure 5.1.   From Data to Knowledge

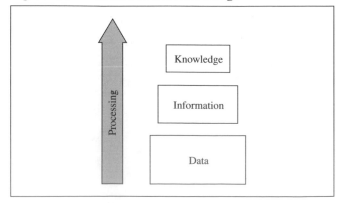

Some texts include a third, higher level in the data-to-information hierarchy: knowledge. Johns (1997, p. 53) defines **knowledge** as "a combination of rules, relationships, ideas, and experience." People use knowledge to make decisions. In the 650 example above, the medical researcher might use his or her experience, diagnostic rules (written or not), and statistical rules to determine the relationships between patient characteristics and the 650 diagnosis. Computer systems that combine an expert knowledge base and some type of rule-based decision analysis component are sometimes referred to as "knowledge systems" to differentiate them from more traditional transaction-based or analytical information systems. Although computerized decision support systems (DSS) in healthcare are not always knowledge systems, knowledge systems are almost always used for decision support. (See chapter 19 for more information on decision support systems.)

Where does "data" end and "information" begin? How are the two concepts related? Do the data collected and stored affect the information available within the organization? To answer these questions, one must first know who needs the data/information to perform what job function or functions. What people and what decisions are involved?

Information is a valuable asset at all levels of the healthcare organization. Personnel, both clinical and support staff, who perform the day-to-day operations related to patient care or administrative functions rely on information to do their jobs. This is truly the information age, and nowhere is this more apparent than in healthcare. Healthcare managers at both the middle management level and the executive level make extensive use of information, both to carry out day-to-day operations and in strategic planning for the organization. An interesting point to think about is that the same data may actually provide different information to different users. In other words, one person's data may be another person's information.

To illustrate this point, consider a small data set that represents some patient demographic data. It might be a subset of data from a hospital master patient index (MPI) system. (See table 5.1.)

This single set of data could be used at all levels of the hospital, beginning with the admissions process, a day-to-day operation of the facility. Admission personnel would use the data set to verify previous admissions or the spelling of a name. They also would be responsible for data entry and updating the MPI to ensure that it contains accurate, timely data. The MPI data set, as is, would provide useful information to the admissions personnel.

At the middle management level, the director of outpatient services might want information about where recent patients live and how far they travel to use this hospital. He or she might further process or query the data set to classify patients by zip code. After the query is completed, the director of outpatient services has useful information to help identify where patients live.

The CEO is interested in patient mix as well but wants to see trend data over time showing the percentage of Medicare patients versus the percentage of private-pay and nonpaying patients. Once again, the same data set is used, but the query process is more complex and the data set must be linked to another data set that contains payment information. The data in the MPI data set must be processed more extensively before any truly useful information is available to meet the CEO's needs.

Moreover, the data from the MPI might be used in strategic planning for the hospital. Any number of complex queries about the patient population could contribute to strategic marketing or development decisions. The organization might even combine the MPI data set with external data sets using sophisticated decision support systems that compare its performance with the performance of other facilities in the region or state.

Check Your Understanding 5.1

Instructions: Answer the following questions on a separate piece of paper.

1. Give an example of data that are found in a patient medical record. How could these data become information?

2. Explain the statement that "one person's information can be another person's data."

Basic Principles of Information Management

With so many different uses of the same data and information, it is critical that healthcare organizations manage their information resources wisely. Today, they recognize that

Table 5.1.   Subset of a Master Patient Index Table

MRN	SSN	Last Name	First Name	Middle Name	DOB	Payment Type	Zip Code
096543	123-23-2345	Jones	Georgia	Louise	11/21/1957	Self	29425
065432	789-99-3456	Lexington	Milton	Robert	08/12/2000	Private	29425
467345	022-45-5378	Lovingood	Jill	Karen	10/14/1992	Medicaid	29401
678543	222-56-7777	Martin	Chloe	Mary	05/30/1978	Private	29465
234719	654-33-2222	Martin	John	Adams	06/22/1961	Private	29401
786543	435-89-0034	Nance	Natalie	JoAnn	11/27/1902	Medicare	29464

information is a valuable resource that must be managed carefully and deliberately, just as other categories of resources, such as financial and human resources, are. Before the design and development on any information system (IS), it is important to understand and embrace some basic principles of **information management.**

Austin and Boxerman (1998) cite three "overarching" principles for managing information resources:

1. Treat information as an essential organizational resource, on a par with human resources, financial resources, and capital facilities and equipment.
2. Obtain top executive support for IS planning and management.
3. Develop an IS strategic vision and plan.

These three principles may be considered steps in setting the stage for effective information management within the healthcare organization. However, planning for information systems involves other important considerations, including:

- The value of information lies in its application to decision making within the organization.
- Quality data is the foundation of quality information.
- Integration of systems enhances IS quality and efficiency.
- Information users must be involved in defining needs and designing information systems.

All of these principles are highly intertwined. Strategic IS planning is key to managing information resources wisely and ensuring that systems are compatible with one another and can be integrated. Moreover, planning ensures that the information systems the organization is developing are in line with its overall mission, goals, and strategic plan. The entire strategic IS planning process is only effective if the organization's top-level executives are supportive and actively involved.

It is the enterprisewide nature of information that dictates the importance of systems integration and of involving users in defining and designing information systems. Too often, information systems are built for one particular unit within the organization, which can lead to inefficient management of information or even inaccurate information. If the users are not involved in all aspects of systems design and development, the resulting IS may function very well technically, but be of no use to anyone. Which is worse, a technically weak and cumbersome computer system that provides the information needed or a technically savvy system that does not? Invariably, end users choose the cumbersome system that provides the "right" information. (For a more complete discussion of strategic information systems planning, read chapter 6.)

The concept of data quality is closely tied to the ability of an IS to support decision making at all levels of the organization. The adage "Garbage in, garbage out" is very true. The next sections of this chapter discuss the characteristics of data quality and controlling it through database design, data modeling, and data dictionaries.

Check Your Understanding 5.2

Instructions: Answer the following questions on a separate piece of paper.

1. What are the basic principles of information management?
2. Why is it particularly important for healthcare organizations to understand the basic principles of information management?

Data Quality Management

How can one know when data quality has been achieved? The quality of the data is tied to the use, or application, of the data. Again, quality data is the foundation of quality information and the value of information lies in its *application* to decision making within the organization.

Recognizing the Characteristics of Data Quality

Data quality is evaluated using a set of characteristics called the **seven dimensions of data quality.** These seven dimensions, or characteristics, are as follows:

- *Relevancy:* Data must be relevant to the purpose for which they are collected. Very accurate, timely data may be collected about a patient's color preferences or choice of hairdresser, but are they relevant to the patient's care?
- *Granularity:* Data granularity is sometimes referred to as data "atomicity," which means that the individual data elements cannot be further subdivided; they are "atomic." For example, a typical patient's name should generally be stored as three data elements—last name, first name, middle name ("Smith" and "John" and "Allen"), not as a single data element ("John Allen Smith"). Again, granularity can be related to the purpose for which the data are collected. Although it is possible to subdivide a person's birth date into separate fields for the month, the date, and the year, this is usually not desirable. The birth date is at the lowest level of granularity when used as a patient identifier.
- *Precision:* Precision often relates to numerical data. It denotes how close to an actual size, weight, or other standard a particular measurement is. Some healthcare data must be very precise. For example, in figuring drug dosage, it would not be acceptable to round up to the nearest gram if the drug were to be dosed in milligrams.
- *Timeliness:* Timeliness is a critical dimension in the quality of many types of healthcare data. Take, for example, a patient's discharge diagnoses recorded as ICD-9-CM codes. These codes must be recorded in a timely manner in order to facilitate reimbursement for the healthcare facility.
- *Currency:* Many types of healthcare data become obsolete after a period of time. A patient's admitting diagno-

sis is often changed by the time he or she is discharged. If a clinician needed a current diagnosis, which one would he or she choose?

- *Consistency:* Data quality needs to be consistent. A difference in the use of abbreviations provides a good example of how the lack of consistency can lead to problems. For example, a nurse may use CPR to mean cardiopulmonary resuscitation one time and computer-based patient record another time, leading to confusion if the chart were audited.
- *Accuracy:* Data that are free of errors are accurate. Typographical errors in discharge summaries or misspellings of names are examples of inaccurate data.

Establishing Data Quality Requirements for Information Systems

It has already been noted that users must be involved in defining their information needs and designing information systems. One of the first steps in systems analysis is to identify the users' specific data needs. As a part of this process, it is important to identify the level of quality the user requires for each data element. Another way to view this is to evaluate the use of the data along the seven dimensions of quality. This evaluation eventually will be translated into technical performance requirements for the information system.

Consider a billing information system. A patient's principal diagnosis is a critical piece of data that must be contained within the billing system. Which of the seven dimensions of quality must this principal diagnosis meet when it is recorded on the patient's bill? A principal diagnosis code is relevant to the bill and is, by nature, a granular, or atomic, data element. It is precise because it has only one meaning. However, the remaining dimensions of timeliness, currency, consistency, and accuracy also must be achieved. A billing system would be considered functioning well only if these quality dimensions for the principal diagnosis could be demonstrated.

Controlling Data Quality through Effective Database Design

Today's healthcare information systems are generally built on an underlying database structure. A **database** is a collection of data that is organized so that its contents can be easily accessed, managed, and updated (Whatis.com 2001). This type of IS structure can be found in computer applications ranging from a large enterprisewide clinical data repository to a small desktop application designed to track delinquent signatures on patient records. Regardless of the scope or size of the database used in an application, the theoretical constructs are the same and a good database design is equally important.

"A good database does not just happen"(Rob and Coronel 2002). The structure of the database must be designed carefully. A poorly designed database can lead to redundant data and information errors, which in turn can lead to poor man-

agement or patient care decisions. Redundant data within a database result from storing unnecessarily duplicated data.

Revisit the master patient index (MPI) subset described earlier. Think of it as representing a portion of a table within a database that provides the data for an integrated hospital-wide IS. Assume that this table stores all of the patients' demographic information. This should be the only place where the patient's name, date of birth, and address are stored. If this information is needed in other applications, such as billing, the unique identifier (in this case, the medical record number [MRN]) should be used to link the table to other tables with the accounting and billing information. Storing a data element in one location within the database enables accurate data updates and deletions.

Suppose there was a separate storage table for patient demographic information for each department-level application. The patient's demographic information would be stored in a billing database and in the MPI database. What if a patient's name was misspelled or a birth date was incorrect? Someone would have to go to each table separately and update the information. If the MPI was updated without also updating the billing database, this would lead to reports yielding inconsistent, if not inaccurate, results. How would anyone know which table had the correct information?

It is no exaggeration to say that a poorly designed database can lead to poor decision making. The database is the source from which information is created. To repeat, one of the basic principles of information management is that the value of information lies in its application to decision making within the organization.

Database Life Cycle

Chapter 6 introduces the concept of a systems development life cycle (SDLC), which is used in systems analysis to illustrate the stages of development for an information system. The general SDLC provides a framework for developing any type of IS project. When dealing with a database project, the SDLC is often referred to as the **database life cycle** (DBLC) (Rob and Coronel 2002). The phases of the DBLC correspond to those of the general SDLC but include the specific tasks needed to develop an effective database.

Figure 5.2 (p. 88) illustrates a six-phase DBLC. The phases of this life cycle are as follows:

1. *Database initial study:* In the initial study phase, the database developer meets with key users and develops a list of user requirements. Technical requirements are discussed and an analysis of how this database fits with existing systems is conducted.
2. *Database design:* In the design phase, the type of database is determined (relational or object oriented, for example). Conceptual-level and logical-level data models are developed during this phase. User interface also is designed. User–developer interaction is critical during this phase. Depending on the scope of the project, a prototype database may be developed and tested.

3. *Database implementation:* The database is actually loaded onto the network or workstation where it will reside. Test users are assigned user and access rights at the time of implementation.

4. *Testing and evaluation:* The importance of testing the database and evaluating the results of the testing cannot be overemphasized. Many times, even after careful design, problems are not discovered until the database is being used in a "live" environment.

5. *Database operation:* After the database is implemented, tested, and evaluated, it can be put into full operation.

6. *Database maintenance and evaluation:* The final phase of the life cycle is maintenance and evaluation. The database must be continually maintained, evaluated for its usefulness and efficiency, and updated as enhancements or changes are required.

It is important to recognize that this life cycle is an iterative, rather than a sequential, process. Each phase can lead to modifications in other phases. This chapter focuses on activities related primarily to the second phase in the DBLC, the design phase. However, the design phase is closely related to the other phases. For example, the importance of user involvement in defining the objectives and constraints of the database cannot be overemphasized. Moreover, users are critical to development of a complete and accurate data dictionary. (Data dictionaries are defined and discussed later in this chapter.)

Data models, which are "pictures" or abstractions of real conditions, are used extensively during database design. A good analogy for a data model is a blueprint of a new building. No reputable builder would construct a building without a detailed blueprint. Of course, some changes may occur along the way, but the basic foundation and ways in which the building units will be put together are worked out in the blueprint. The use of data models facilitates communication between the technically oriented database designer and the end users. Data models also enable the individuals involved in database design to explore the features and characteristics of the database before actual implementation occurs.

Types of Databases

Before beginning a more detailed discussion of using and developing data models, the common types of databases and their associated **database management systems** (DBMS) should be defined. This section defines and describes two database structures: relational and object oriented. Two other structures, hierarchical and network, are older types that no longer have a significant presence in the database market. They may be found as legacy systems within healthcare organizations but not in newer systems.

Relational Database Structure

The **relational database** model was developed in 1970 (Rob and Coronel 2002). It was not considered a practical design at the time because it required significant processing power. As computers became more powerful in the late 1980s and 1990s, the relational database became the predominant type used in healthcare and in other industries. A relational database is implemented through a **relational database management system** (RDBMS). The major advantage of the RDBMS is that it allows a database designer to operate at a logical, rather than a physical, level. (See section on levels of data models.) Microsoft Access® is an example of an RDBMS for developing desktop applications. Oracle®, DB2™, and Sybase™ are examples of more robust systems for developing larger applications.

The RDBMS consists of three distinct components: the interface, the data manipulation "engine," and the tables. (See figure 5.3.) The interface component of the RDBMS is developed using a wide variety of software. In Microsoft Access, for example, Visual Basic for Applications (VBA) is built into the RDBMS and used to create the forms and reports that comprise the majority of the user interface. The tables within a relational database are created using a special type of software, a **data definition language** (DDL). In between the user interface and the data tables is the database

Figure 5.2.   Database Life Cycle

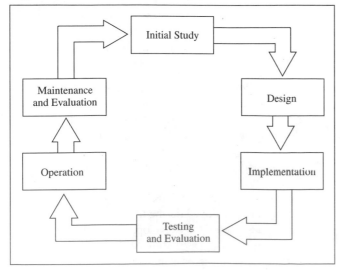

Figure 5.3.   RDSMS Components

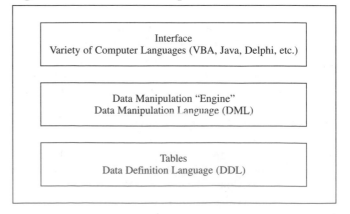

"engine," the component that retrieves, edits, and updates the data from its underlying tables. The type of software used for these functions is called a **data manipulation language** (DML).

The most common language used for both DDL and DML for relational databases today is **structured query language** (SQL). All RDBMSs support SQL, and many RDBMS vendors have created extensions to the language that are specific to their product. The SQL used in Access looks slightly different from the SQL used in Oracle. SQL is a nonprocedural, or fourth-generation, language. The user specifies what must be done, but not how it is to be done. In other words, the SQL user does not have to know about the complex actions that actually are occurring when an SQL command is executed by the computer (Rob and Coronel 2002).

Tables (sometimes called relations) provide the foundation of a relational database. Each table consists of rows and columns. Rows represent each record within the table; columns represent the data fields or attributes of each table.

Tables in a relational database are related to one another by sharing a common field, or **key attribute.** In the earlier example involving the MPI and the billing system, these two tables could be linked by the key attribute, MRN.

The relational database has several advantages over its predecessors, the network and hierarchical databases. The most important advantages include:

- *Structural independence:* It is possible to make changes to the database structure without affecting how the RDBMS accesses the data. In other words, data elements can be changed in the tables without affecting the data manipulation features or interface with the user.
- *Improved conceptual simplicity:* Through its use of logical tables, the relational database makes it easier for the developer and the user to understand the data.
- *Easier database design, implementation, management, and use:* Relational databases are much easier to design and manage than their predecessors were.
- *Ad hoc query capability:* The common data manipulation language, SQL, is simple to use and understand because it so closely resembles the English language.
- *A powerful database management system:* A good RDBMS makes it possible to hide a system's physical complexity from the developer and the user (Rob and Coronel 2002).

Object-Oriented Database Structure

The newest type of database structure is the **object-oriented database** (OODB). The basic component in the OODB is an object, not a table. An **object** includes both data and their relationships within a single structure; it is conceptually more difficult to understand than a table. **Object-oriented database management systems** (OODBMS) utilize classes and subclasses that "inherit" characteristics from the parent class. The goal of using objects in programs and database management systems is to promote reuse of program codes

and to store the data with the methods (procedures) that use the data. Object-oriented database concepts are beyond the scope of this chapter, but experts believe that they will have a definitive impact on healthcare applications in the near future (Duffy 1997). The OODB has not replaced the relational database in the healthcare market, but many products are incorporating elements of the OODB with their relational databases.

Data Models

Data modeling serves as a link between "real" things about which the organization wants to collect and maintain data and the actual database structure. One of the problems with database design is that designers, programmers, and users do not necessarily see data the same way. Different users have different views of the organization's data, depending on their particular needs. Different views of data can lead to poorly constructed information systems that fail to meet the needs of many users. Ensuring that communication among the designers, programmers, and users is as unambiguous as possible can prevent this. Data modeling is an excellent communication tool for reducing complex data structures to easy-to-understand "pictures" or abstractions.

Levels of Data Models

There are three levels of data models: conceptual, logical, and physical. The levels are based on the degree of abstraction represented by the data model. The **conceptual data model** is the one with the highest level of abstraction. In other words, it is neither hardware nor software dependent. In theory, the same conceptual model can be developed whether the organization develops its database as a relational database or an object-oriented database. The conceptual model also implies that it defines requirements for the entire enterprise or organizational unit under consideration. End users should be intimately involved in the development of conceptual data models. The level of abstraction should be high enough that end users with little or no computer programming experience can visualize the data requirements.

The next level of data model is the **logical data model.** The logical data model is still hardware independent but will be drawn to match the type of database management system (DBMS) that will be used. There are differences in the way logical models are depicted, depending on whether the DBMS is relational or object oriented. For example, the **entity relationship diagram** (ERD), described in detail in later sections of this chapter, was developed to depict relational database structures. It can be used to depict conceptual-level models for any type of database but would only be used to model a relational database at the logical level. A common notation used for modeling object-oriented databases is **unified modeling language** (UML). UML can be used for depicting a conceptual data model and a logical OODB model.

Another characteristic of the logical data model is that it is drawn to represent a view of the data by a specific group within the enterprise. The group might be a department or a unit within a department. Of course, the logical data model should be based on the conceptual model for the enterprise. Another way to think about logical data models is that they are components of the conceptual model with more DBMS-related detail.

The **physical data model** is concerned with the lowest level of abstraction, including how data are physically stored on storage media such as disks or tapes (Rob and Coronel 2002). This level of modeling is generally done by programmers or database developers with little interaction with users (Johns 1997). As relational and object-oriented databases have become more widely used, the physical data model has decreased in importance. One of the strengths of the relational and object-oriented databases is that they do not require the physical modeling details required by the older hierarchical and network database structures.

Data Modeling Process

The importance of data modeling cannot be overstated. Not only does the data model serve as a communication tool among IS developers and users, but it also provides the developer an opportunity to work out conceptual and design issues and problems *prior to beginning the actual design process.* This is an important step in ensuring the quality of the data and, subsequently, the information that can be gathered from the information system. The data themselves constitute the most basic units within an IS.

As stated earlier, one of most common data models, the ERD, is associated with relational database design. The ERD modeling technique is used to develop both conceptual and logical data models for relational databases. Several different sets of notations are used for drawing an ERD. Two of the most common methods are the Chen model and the Crow's foot model. Peter Chen developed his notation for ERDs in the 1970s (Rob and Coronel 2002). The Crow's foot model was developed by C. W. Bachman and is based on the same modeling concepts as the original Chen model; the Crow's foot model depicts the data relationships at a slightly higher level of abstraction than the Chen does, making it a very effective communication tool for users and developers (Rob and Coronel 2002). The models used for illustration throughout this chapter are drawn using the Crow's foot symbols.

Figure 5.4 illustrates a simple ERD drawn using the conventions associated with the Chen model and with the Crow's feet symbols. These models show that the relationship between the data table (or entity) HOSPITAL and the data table (or entity) DIVISION is one to many. This relationship means that for every instance of HOSPITAL stored in the database, there can be many related instances of DIVISION stored. Reading the diagram in the other direction, each instance of DIVISION stored in the database is related to only one instance of HOSPITAL. Think about a multihospital system that has three hospitals—A, B, and C. Each hospital has multiple divisions within it, and each specific division (for example, the finance division in A) is related to only one hospital.

Although a detailed discussion of the conventions and steps associated with developing an ERD are beyond the scope of this chapter, the basic steps for developing an ERD for a simple end-user database is outlined. Readers desiring a more complete discussion should refer to a database development textbook, such as *Database Systems: Design, Implementation, and Management* (Rob and Coronel 2002).

An ERD is a graphical representation of the entities, attributes, and relationships that comprise a database. It is used as a planning and communication tool throughout the database development process. As stated earlier, an ERD can be used as a conceptual-level data model for any type of database and as a logical-level data model for a relational database. This discussion examines a simple ERD being developed for a patient-tracking system in a rural healthcare system that operates three clinics. The proposed tracking system will be developed as a relational database. Its purpose will be to track patient visits within the three clinics.

Entities

Entities in the ERD are represented by a rectangle. An **entity** is a person, place, or thing about which data are to be collected in the database being designed. What would the entities for the patient-tracking database be?

Another way to think about entities is that they eventually will be transformed into the tables within the database. The entities for the visit-tracking database would be PATIENT, CLINIC, and VISIT. There could be more entities, depending on the data to be stored. For example, if one wanted to collect information about the provider of care for the visit, one would

Figure 5.4.   ERD Notations

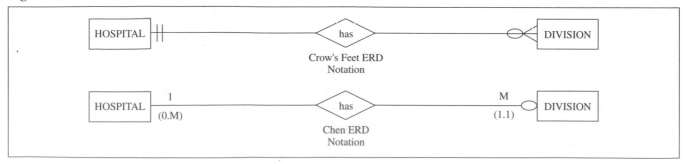

likely have an entity, PROVIDER, or even two entities, PHYSICIAN and NURSE. Selecting the entities for an ERD depends on the purpose of the proposed database. This example limits data collection to VISIT, PATIENT, and CLINIC.

Attributes

Attributes are the characteristic or data elements to be collected about each entity. They can be depicted in an ERD as oval shapes coming off an entity. This method is not practical when there are many attributes per table; therefore, many designers use a separate list to document attributes. In the Crow's foot notation, attributes are sometimes listed within the entity rectangle.

In this example, what would be some likely attributes? For the PATIENT table, one would want to store a unique identifier for the patient, such as a Social Security number or a medical record number. This unique identifier is called a **primary key.** A primary key cannot be duplicated within the table and cannot contain a null value. Each table row or record within the database must have a unique primary key.

Continuing with the example, one also would want to store at least basic demographic information such as address, phone number, and date of birth. Figure 5.5 shows simplified, partial lists of attributes for the three tables. Attributes become the fields or column headings within the data tables of a relational database. Notice that the names of the attributes in figure 5.5 adhere to a common naming convention for database fields. The name of the table makes up the first part of the name followed by an underscore. This way, it is easy to identify where a particular data element is stored by looking at its names. Also note that these attributes are all "atomic," meaning they cannot be further subdivided.

Another type of attribute is a **derived attribute.** Derived attributes are not stored in the database table but, instead, are calculated when the database is accessed. An example of a derived attribute is age. A patient's age at the time of a visit could be calculated using the date of birth attribute, the admission date, and the visit date. A patient's current age could be calculated using date of birth and today's date.

In this example, the primary key (PK) for PATIENT, PATIENT_MRN, is repeated in VISIT, as is the PK for CLINIC, CLINIC_ID. These keys are called **foreign keys** (FK) in the VISIT table. By having the foreign keys in VISIT, the information in PATIENT and CLINIC is linked through the VISIT table. Figure 5.6 illustrates the ERD for this example.

Relationships

Relationships are represented in an ERD by a diamond shape or as text across the relationship line. The name of the relationship is usually a verb that describes the relationship between two or more of the entities in the diagram. A conceptual ERD contains three types of relationships:

- One to one
- One to many
- Many to many

A **one-to-one relationship** exists when an instance of an entity (a row or record) is associated with one instance of another entity, and vice versa. This type of relationship is illustrated in figure 5.7. The relationships shown in figure 5.7 are taken from a current bed assignment database. There is only one bed per patient and one patient per bed. One-to-one relationships are rare in logical-level data models because they often indicate that a separate entity is unnecessary. Often a one-to-one relationship can be implemented as an attribute or field within a single table. In other words, a field, PATIENT_BED, could be added in the PATIENT table in this example to collect this information.

Figure 5.5.   Partial Attribute Lists for PATIENT, VISIT, and CLINIC

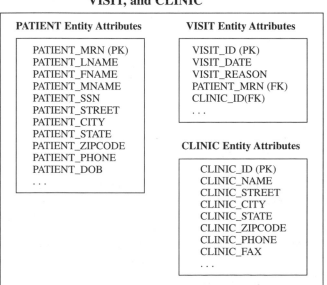

PATIENT Entity Attributes
PATIENT_MRN (PK)
PATIENT_LNAME
PATIENT_FNAME
PATIENT_MNAME
PATIENT_SSN
PATIENT_STREET
PATIENT_CITY
PATIENT_STATE
PATIENT_ZIPCODE
PATIENT_PHONE
PATIENT_DOB
. . .

VISIT Entity Attributes
VISIT_ID (PK)
VISIT_DATE
VISIT_REASON
PATIENT_MRN (FK)
CLINIC_ID(FK)
. . .

CLINIC Entity Attributes
CLINIC_ID (PK)
CLINIC_NAME
CLINIC_STREET
CLINIC_CITY
CLINIC_STATE
CLINIC_ZIPCODE
CLINIC_PHONE
CLINIC_FAX
. . .

Figure 5.6.   Sample ERD

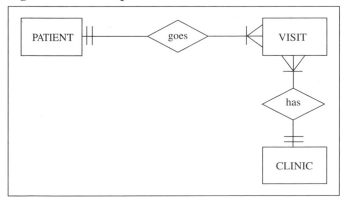

Figure 5.7.   One-to-One Relationship

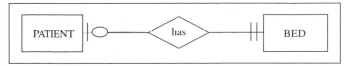

The **one-to-many relationship** exists when one instance of an entity is associated with many instances of another entity. In the example shown in figure 5.6, the relationship between PATIENT and VISIT is one to many. For each instance of PATIENT in the database, there could be many instances of VISIT. In other words, each patient may have many visits, but each visit is associated with only one patient. The relationship between CLINIC and VISIT is also one to many. For each instance of CLINIC, there can be many VISITS, but each visit only occurs in one clinic. One-to-many relationships also can be optional. In this example, however, they are not because each patient must have a visit before he or she is entered into the database and each clinic must have visits before it is entered into the database.

Whether a relationship is optional is determined by the "business rules" of an organization. If one said that patients were entered into the database before they had any visits, this relationship would change to optional. This might occur in a family-oriented clinic where children or spouses of patients were registered, but never seen.

A **many-to-many relationship** only occurs in a data model developed at the conceptual level. In the example shown in figure 5.6, suppose the need for a separate VISIT entity was not recognized. The relationship between PATIENT and CLINIC is many to many. For each instance of PATIENT, there could be many instances of CLINIC because patients can be seen in more than one clinic. For each instance of CLINIC, there could be many PATIENTS because the clinic sees many patients. Figure 5.8 shows the many-to-many relationship between PATIENT and CLINIC.

Well-structured databases consist primarily of one-to-many relationships. Many-to-many relationships cannot be implemented in a relational database and, as discussed, one-to-one relationships are rare. The process of ensuring that the data model can be implemented as relational tables in a database is called **normalization.** By normalizing the data tables to ensure that data are stored in only one location, except for the planned redundancy inherent in key attributes, database developers decrease the possibility of data anomalies resulting from additions and deletions.

Check Your Understanding 5.3

Instructions: Answer the following questions on a separate piece of paper.

1. List the seven dimensions of data quality.
2. Give one example of the importance of each dimension in ensuring the quality of patient information.
3. Which type of database is the most common today?
4. How does database design affect the quality of the data stored in the database?
5. What is a data model?
6. Discuss the differences among a conceptual-level, logical-level, and physical-level data model.
7. What are some common uses of an ERD? What is UML?
8. Define the basic components of an ERD.
9. How are the entities and relationships depicted in an ERD?
10. Using the Crow's feet notation, draw an ERD to depict the following relationship: Each patient has one physician, but each physician has many patients.

Figure 5.8.   Many-to-Many Relationship

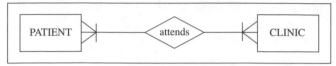

Controlling Data Quality through the Use of a Data Dictionary

An important tool in controlling the quality of data in healthcare is the data dictionary. Whenever a set of data is created, it should have an accompanying data dictionary. Revisit the brief scenario described at the beginning of this chapter. The problems encountered because of a lack of data definitions could have been avoided had the organization invested time and resources into developing a data dictionary.

Types of Data Dictionaries

There are two general types of data dictionaries: the DBMS data dictionary and the organizationwide data dictionary.

DBMS Data Dictionary

The DBMS data dictionary is developed in conjunction with the development of the database. Modern DBMSs have built-in data dictionaries that go beyond data definitions and store information about tables and data relationships. These integrated data dictionaries are sometimes referred to as **system catalogs,** reflecting their technical nature.

Figure 5.9 is an example of a portion of a designer-defined data dictionary developed in Microsoft Access for the simplified PATIENT table discussed earlier. The database developer would use this portion of the software to define the data to be stored in the database's system catalog.

A typical data dictionary associated with a DBMS allows for at least documentation of the following:

- Table names
- All attribute or field names
- A description of each attribute
- The data type of the attribute (text, number, date, and so on)
- The format of each attribute, such as DD_MM_YYYY for the date
- The size of each attribute, such as 11 characters in a Social Security number with dashes
- An appropriate range of values, such as integers 100000–999999 for the health record number
- Whether the attribute is required
- Relationships among attributes

Other descriptions that might be stored in the data dictionary associated with a database include:

- Who created the database
- When the database was created

Figure 5.9.   Partial Data Dictionary for PATIENT Table

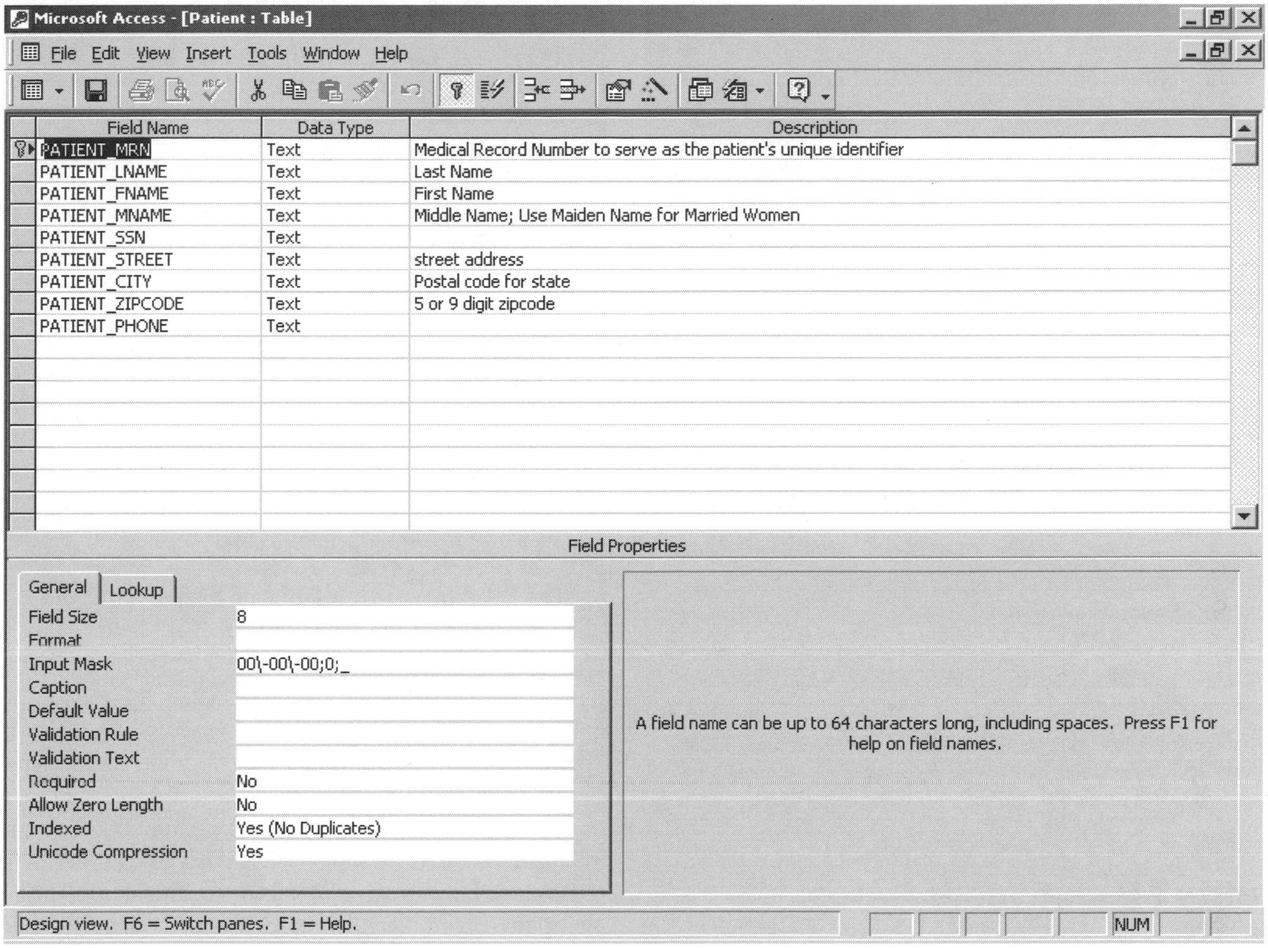

- Where the database is located
- Which programs can access the database
- Who the end users and administrators of the database are
- How access authorization is provided to all users

Organizationwide Data Dictionary

The second type of data dictionary is developed outside the framework of a specific database design process. This data dictionary serves to promote data quality through data consistency across the organization. Individual data element definitions are agreed upon and defined. It leads to better-quality data and facilitates the detailed, technical data dictionaries that are integrated with the databases themselves. Ideally, every healthcare organization will develop a data dictionary to define common data and their formats. This organizationwide document becomes a valuable resource for IS development.

Looking at the MPI example discussed earlier, what would need to be defined for each field? Although everyone may think they know the definition of a Last Name, can they all agree that it will be stored as no more than twenty-five characters? How should the Middle Name be handled? Will it be the maiden name for married women? Is the med-

ical record number to be stored with leading zeros or not? Is the Social Security number required? If so, what will be used when it is not available? These are all issues that can be settled with the development of an organizationwide data dictionary.

Another challenge for healthcare managers results from interorganizational projects or the merger of healthcare organizations. Suppose a multifacility organization wanted to merge its MPI systems. Imagine the challenges involved in not only defining data elements, but also uncovering existing definitions. What if the organizations in question had built other systems based on internal MPI definitions?

The true story of the HMO quoted at the beginning of this chapter could have been prevented if the HMO had developed an organizationwide data dictionary. Each regional office then would have been using the same definitions.

Development of Data Dictionaries

The health information manager would be a key member of any data dictionary project team. Developing a data dictionary can be an overwhelming task when considering the diversity of data users and the size and scope of some healthcare organizations. However, a few simple steps can be taken at the beginning of the data dictionary development project to get it under way:

1. *Define the scope of the project.* Is the project related to one application, one facility, or the entire organization?
2. *Determine the members of the project team.* The scope of the project will dictate who needs to be involved. If multiple facilities are involved, each one will need adequate representation on the team. The team should have representatives from all user groups, including clinicians and administrative personnel.
3. *Set priorities.* Which group of data elements is most critical to the project? Making this determination will clarify where to begin.
4. *Learn from the experience of others.* Investigate how other organizations have developed data dictionaries (Duffy 1997). The Internet and published journal articles, as well as personal contacts, can be helpful for this step.

Check Your Understanding 5.4

Instructions: Answer the following questions on a separate piece of paper.

1. What is a data dictionary? What is its importance in ensuring data quality?
2. What type of information would be listed in an organizationwide or enterprisewide data dictionary? What other types of information would be stored in a system catalog?

Quality Management Roles

This chapter focuses on the importance of maintaining high-quality data that will lead to high-quality information and decisions. High-quality data do not just happen. Healthcare organizations must establish mechanisms and policies for managing their data resources. Such mechanisms and policies must encompass not only the technical aspects of implementing and maintaining the databases within the organization, but also ensure that the data conform to established standards of quality. Several roles within the healthcare information systems team can be used to manage the quality of healthcare data. These include database administrator, data administrator, and an emerging role for HIM professionals, as defined by the AHIMA (1999), data resource manager.

Database Administrator

The technical aspects of managing a database are usually assigned to a **database administrator** (DBA). Typical DBA functions include defining and developing the database, implementing the technical aspects of the DBMS, monitoring the performance of the database, creating and enforcing the security measures associated with the DBMS, and managing the system catalogs or data dictionaries that are internal to the DBMS (Johns 1997).

DBAs typically have information technology backgrounds and may not be equipped to deal with managing the less technical side of data quality, particularly healthcare data. This has led some healthcare organizations to create a new position—the data administrator (DA).

Data Administrator

According to Johns (1997), the functions of the **data administrator** include:

- Planning for the database, including identifying the major entities, attributes, and relationships among entities, and developing the conceptual data models for the organization
- Evaluating and selecting an appropriate DBMS
- Managing an enterprisewide data dictionary
- Training database users
- Developing and implementing database security policies and procedures

The DA must work closely with the DBA, but the focus of the DA role is on managing the data and the database rather than on the technical implementation and maintenance issues that are the DBA's responsibility.

Data Resource Manager

In 1998, the AHIMA described an emerging data management role for HIM managers in its Vision 2006 document—the **data resource manager** (DRM). The AHIMA defines a DRM as the person who "uses technical tools, such as computer-based health record systems, data repositories, and data warehouses . . . (to) ensure that the organization's information systems meet the needs of those who provide and manage patient services along the continuum of care and that the organization's data resources are secure, accessible, accurate, and reliable"(AHIMA 1999).

The role of the DRM is specifically defined as having two primary goals: (1) to provide leadership for the data resource management functions and (2) to ensure that the data are secure, accessible, accurate, and reliable.

The DRM role is very similar to the DA role described by Johns (1997), with a few differences in focus. As defined by the AHIMA, the DRM is not only concerned with managing the quality and security of the healthcare data in an organization, but also very involved in retrieving data from the systems within the organization. The skill set required to perform the data resource management function in a healthcare organization includes a thorough understanding of health information administration and a working knowledge of the technical aspects of health information systems, particularly databases and DBMSs. The DRM should be comfortable as a participant in healthcare database management and design. Further, he or she should have a thorough understanding of HIM issues such as confidentiality, access, release of information, and security.

Safeguards for Ensuring the Integrity and Security of Data

Nowhere is ensuring the integrity and security of data more important than in healthcare. Healthcare organizations have an obligation to protect patient privacy and to maintain the confidential nature of the physician–patient relationship. Healthcare privacy and confidentiality are regulated by state and national laws and standards, as well as by standards of care. Other chapters in this text discuss confidentiality and privacy from a legislative and regulatory perspective. This section focuses on the safeguards that should be implemented in a healthcare database system.

Data Integrity

Data integrity is the assurance that data have only been accessed or modified by those authorized to do so (Whatis.com 2001). Databases contain conditions known as **integrity constraints** that must be satisfied by the data stored there. Database integrity constraints include:

- *Data type:* The data entered into a field should be consistent with the data type for that field. For example, if a field is a numeric field, it should only accept numbers. If the field is a date field, it should only accept a legitimate date.
- *Legal values:* For many fields there is a limited number of "legal" values. For example, a health record number may only be entered as 000001 through 999999.
- *Format:* Certain fields, such as Social Security numbers, must be entered in a certain format, such as 999-99-9999.
- *Key constraints:* Key constraints are the constraints placed on the primary and foreign keys within the database. A foreign key, for example, cannot be entered into the database unless a corresponding primary key already exists (Pratt and Adamski 2000).

These constraints help ensure that the originally entered data and changes to these data follow certain rules. DBMSs today include the functionality to enforce integrity constraints (Pratt and Adamski 2000). After the parameters for the types of integrity have been set within the database, users cannot violate them. For example, they cannot enter nonnumeric data into a number field. An error message will result. Likewise, a user cannot add a VISIT entry to the database described earlier unless a corresponding PATIENT has already been entered.

Data Security

Modern DBMSs also have built-in mechanisms to enforce security rules. Within healthcare organizations, most of the database systems are shared systems with multiple users. This makes implementing the security features of the DBMS critical.

Protecting the security and privacy of data in the database is called **authorization management.** Two of the important aspects of authorization management are user access control and usage monitoring (Rob and Coronel 2002).

User access control features within the database are designed to limit access to the database or some portion of it. They generally provide the DBA or DA responsible for security with the tools to:

- Define each user of the database. The DBA can create log-in information for each user.
- Assign passwords to users.
- Define user groups. By defining user groups, the DBA can limit access to certain groups. For example, some users may have read-only privileges. These users can see the data in the database but cannot enter or change them. Other users may be granted read–write privileges, so they can enter and change data.
- Assign access privileges. This can be done according to user groups as described above or on an individual basis. The highest level of privilege is the administrative level, which should be reserved for the DBA. Persons with administrative permissions can change the underlying structure of the database (Rob and Coronel 2002).

This list represents the security features that are part of the DBMS. The database also can be secured at the network operating system level. In many cases, a database user will first log in to the network system with one log-in and password and then log in to the database with a second log-in and password. The database also can be secured through physical security protections, such as locked rooms and password-protected workstations. The level of sensitivity of the data within the database should determine the level of security.

Usage monitoring is another aspect of authorization management. One of the most commons ways that database administrators monitor the use of the database is to use audit trails to determine whether there have been any actual or attempted access violations. These audit trails should be able to tell the DBA when and where the attempted breech occurred.

Real-World Case

Medical Associates (MA) is a physician group for a large academic medical center located in the southeastern United States. MA provides services ranging from prevention and wellness to highly specialized care at outpatient clinics and facilities both on the medical center campus and in the surrounding community. Several years ago, after a major lawsuit involving the possibility of coding and billing inconsistencies, the MA executive committee voted to adopt a formal organizational compliance plan, with the goal of ensuring that their physicians, providers, and billing staff understood their legal responsibilities with regard to professional billing. One of the key features of the plan was to provide "coordinated training of clinical staff and billing personnel concerning applicable billing requirements and MA policies."

As outlined in the MA compliance plan, approximately 3,000 clinical and nonclinical employees need compliance education and training. Each of approximately twenty departments has a compliance coordinator responsible for tracking its employees' compliance education to ensure that all preestablished yearly requirements are met. Employees with patient care responsibilities must accrue four hours of training per year—one hour of general training and three hours of training related specifically to billing compliance. However, different categories of employees may have different training requirements. For example, some nonclinical employees only need one hour of general training. Any of this training can be obtained in a number of different settings: sessions offered by the employee's own department, departmental meetings with a compliance topic discussed, sessions offered by another department, sessions offered by the Compliance Office, videotape sessions, Internet sessions, or reading articles and other documents. Every employee must have documented evidence, including a signed attendance sheet, that he or she actually attended approved educational sessions to accrue the hours. Another complicating factor in maintaining quality-tracking records is the fact that each training session may count for more than one type of training. Some sessions may last for only fifteen minutes, others for three hours.

Originally, each department developed its own system for tracking employees. Recognizing that the education tracking and documentation would be an arduous task, several MA departments developed Excel applications for tracking and reporting; others developed small Access databases for this purpose.

Several significant issues emerged as compliance coordinators gained experience in tracking and reporting compliance education for their departments. They began to recognize a need to share their data across departments. As they began to share their spreadsheets and small databases, they soon realized that there were no standard definitions for the fields within the disparate tracking systems and no means for easily uploading one department's data into another's system. Multiple problems related to redundant data were identified. Any one employee might have education documented in more than one department's education tracking system. The MA Compliance Office had to spend a great deal of time trying to clean and merge the data that came in from the various departments. The central Compliance Office could not easily identify who actually needed what type of education. These issues and others led the MA Compliance Office to consider the development of a central, shared database for all coordinators to use.

After several months of planning, a centralized, shared compliance education database was developed. Figure 5.10 shows the underlying table structure of its final version. In addition, a user-friendly interface was developed for data entry and information retrieval. The database was designed as a relational database, and the relationships are included in the schema. The infinity symbol shows the "many" sides of each one-to-many relationship. Because of the relational nature of the database, redundancy was reduced and the chance for data-entry update and deletion errors was all but eliminated.

The centralized education database has worked well for the MA compliance coordinators since its implementation a year ago. Multiple standard reports have been developed. These can be customized to show data by department, by cost center, or by divisions within departments. The MA compliance coordinators meet periodically to discuss multiple issues, including database issues. The database developer has continued to work under contract for MA compliance and has made various enhancements to the interface and standard reports. However, the underlying data structure has remained the same. The MA Compliance Office has expressed its confidence in the quality of the data and, consequently, in their reports since the database was implemented. The departmental coordinators also are happy in knowing that each employee for whom they are responsible is only in the database one time and that regardless of which department provided the education they can track the total required hours accrued.

Discussion Questions

1. List the types of data quality errors the compliance coordinators and the Compliance Office were experiencing prior to implementation of the shared relational database.

2. How did implementation of the relational database help improve the quality of the compliance data?

3. No mention is made of the development of a data dictionary for the MA compliance group. Do you think the group should consider developing one? Why or why not? Although the entire development process is not outlined in this scenario, list some of the activities you would have expected the database developer and compliance team members to participate in as the database was developed. How might these activities affect data quality?

4. How does the relational schema shown in this scenario compare to an ERD? Draw an ERD to represent this database.

Figure 5.10.   Relational Schema for Compliance Education Database

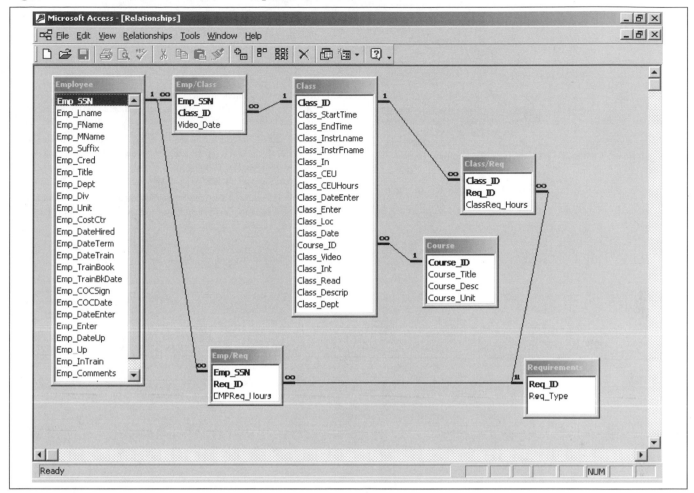

Summary

Health information managers must manage information that is shared by diverse and widely dispersed groups of end users. The different uses and views of these various end users must be reconciled in order to develop high-quality healthcare information systems.

Information is derived from data, or raw facts, and then used by any number of individuals within healthcare organizations in making decisions about patient care. Thus, information is a valuable resource that must be managed carefully following certain basic principles. Essential to the management of information is the organization's ability to ensure the quality of the data it maintains. Data quality is evaluated, in part, by meeting the seven dimensions of quality: relevancy, granularity, precision, timeliness, currency, consistency, and accuracy. Eventually, the evaluation of the data is translated into technical performance requirements for the information system.

Data quality can be controlled through effective database design found in computer applications. The design organizes the data in a way that facilitates their use. Two common types of database structures are the relational database and the object-oriented database. Each database structure is implemented through a specific management system. Key to database design is the process of data modeling, which links the "real" things about which the organization wants to collect and maintain data and the database structure.

An important tool in controlling data quality is the data dictionary. There are two general types: the DBMS (database management system) data dictionary, which is developed at the same time the database is developed, and the organizationwide data dictionary, which promotes data consistency throughout the organization.

To manage their data resources, healthcare organizations must set up mechanisms and policies that address not only database implementation and maintenance, but also standards of data quality. Three roles involved in data and information management are the database administrator, the data administrator, and the data resource manager. In 1998, the American Health Information Management Association identified the latter as an emerging role for health information managers.

References

American Health Information Management Association. 1999. *Evolving HIM Careers.* Chicago: AHIMA.

Austin, C. J., and S. B. Boxerman. 1998. *Information Systems for Health Services Administration,* fifth Edition. Chicago: Health Administration Press.

Duffy, P. G. 1997. Data dictionaries: an overview. *Journal of the American Health Information Management Association* 68(2):30–32, 34.

Johns, M. L. 1997. *Information Management for Health Professions.* Albany, N.Y.: Delmar.

Pratt, P. J., and J. Adamski. 2000. *Concepts of Database Management,* third edition. Cambridge, Mass.: Course Technology, Thomson Learning.

Rob, P., and C. Coronel. 2002. *Database Systems: Design, Implementation, and Management.* Cambridge, Mass.: Course Technology, Thomson Learning.

Shakir, A. M. 1999. Tools for defining data. *Journal of the American Health Information Management Association* 70(8):48–53.

Whatis.com. 2001.

Application Exercises

1. Interview a database administrator at a local healthcare facility. Discuss the major functions of this individual's job and the types of databases used in the facility.

2. Search the Internet under the key words "entity relationship diagrams." What types of sites discuss these data models?

3. Review several patient medical records (paper-based or electronic). Discuss whether you believe the patient medical record represents data or information. Defend your answer.

4. Select one electronic medical record report that was created from a database. Evaluate the report using the seven dimensions of data quality. Do you think the fact that the report was created from a database improved the data quality? Why or why not?

5. Use the Internet or a literature search to find an example of a relational database that is in used in healthcare and an example of an object-oriented database used in healthcare.

Review Quiz

Instructions: Choose the best answer for the following questions.

1. ___ Which of the following examples illustrates data that have been transformed into meaningful information?
   a. 45%
   b. .3567 units of penicillin
   c. $5 million
   d. The average length of stay at Holt Hospital is 5.6 days

2. ___ Which of the following is not one of the three basic principles for managing information as a resource, according to Austin and Boxerman (1998)?
   a. Treat information as an essential organizational resource, on par with human resources, financial resources, and capital facilities and equipment
   b. Obtain top executive support for information systems planning and management
   c. Develop an information systems strategic vision and plan
   d. Hire a CIO to manage information as a resource

3. ___ Which of the following lists represents the dimensions of data quality?
   a. Relevancy, granularity, timeliness, currency, accuracy, precision, and consistency
   b. Relevancy, granularity, timeliness, currency, atomic, precision, and consistency
   c. Relevancy, granularity, timeliness, concurrent, atomic, precision, and consistency
   d. Relcvancy, granularity, equality, currency, precision, accuracy, and consistency

4. ___ Which dimension of data quality is defined as "data that is free of errors?"
   a. Accuracy
   b. Granularity
   c. Precision
   d. Currency

5. ___ A ___ is a collection of data that is organized so that its contents can easily be accessed, managed, and updated.
   a. Spreadsheet
   b. Database
   c. File
   d. Data table

6. ___ Which of the following is not one of the six phases of the database development life cycle?
   a. Database initial study
   b. Database design
   c. Data modeling
   d. Operation

7. ___ Which of the following is considered to be a major advantage of relational databases?
   a. Structural independence
   b. Conceptual simplicity
   c. Easier database design
   d. All of the above

8. ___ Which of the following statements is not true of structured query language (SQL)?
   a. It is both a data manipulation and data definition language
   b. It is a fifth-generation computer language
   c. It is the computer language associated with relational databases
   d. It allows a user to query a relational database

9. ___ The basic component of a (an) ___ is an object, which contains both data and their relationships in a single structure.
   a. Object-oriented database
   b. Relational database
   c. Access database
   d.. None of the above

10. ___ The data model that is most widely used to illustrate a relational database structure is an ___.
    a. UML
    b. ERD
    c. Object model
    d. All of the above

11. ___ Within an entity relationship diagram, an entity is drawn as a ___.
    a. Rectangle
    b. Triangle
    c. Diamond
    d. Line

12. ___ When an ERD is implemented as a relational database, an entity will become a (an) ___.
    a. Query
    b. Form
    c. Object
    d. Table

13. ___ When an ERD is implemented as a relational database, an attribute will become a (an) ___.
    a. Column heading
    b. Field
    c. Object
    d. Both a and b

14. ___ At the conceptual level, relationships between database tables can be expressed as 1:M, 1:1, or M:M. Which of the following is an example of a M:M relationship?
    a. Patients to hospital admissions
    b. Patients to consulting physicians
    c. Patients to hospital medical records
    d. Primary care physicians to patients

15. ___ Which of the examples listed in 13 represents a 1:1 relationship?

16. ___ Which of the examples listed in 13 represents a 1:M relationship?

17. ___ A (An) ___ is developed outside the framework of a specific database and is used to define individual data elements used throughout a healthcare facility.
    a. System catalog
    b. Organizationwide data dictionary
    c. DBMS data dictionary
    d. All of the above

18. ___ Which of the following individuals would be most likely to be responsible for the technical aspects of the DBMS?
    a. Database administrator
    b. Data administrator
    c. Data resource manager
    d. Network administrator

19. ___ Authorization management ___.
    a. Is the process used to protect the privacy and security of a database
    b. Involves limiting user access to a database
    c. Involves monitoring the use of the database
    d. All of the above

20. ___ Which of the following statements is true?
    a. Because of the existence of user-friendly software packages, such as Microsoft Access, the importance of data modeling has diminished
    b. Data modeling is an essential step in database design
    c. ERD and data modeling are identical
    d. Conceptual data modeling requires an extensive technical background

Chapter 6
Information Systems Development

Karen A. Wager, DBA, RHIA

Learning Objectives

- To understand the importance of strategic information systems planning to healthcare organizations
- To describe the purpose and major activities within each phase of the systems development life cycle: analysis, design, implementation, and maintenance and evaluation
- To identify the resources needed to effectively manage information systems within healthcare organizations
- To discuss the roles and responsibilities of information system professionals, including chief information officers, analysts, programmers, and network and database administrators
- To identify the health information manager's role in planning, selecting, and implementing healthcare information systems

Key Terms

Analysis phase
Chief information officer (CIO)
Component alignment model (CAM)
Database administrators
Design phase
Electronic medical record (EMR)
Healthcare information systems steering committee
Implementation phase
Information system (IS)
Information systems (or services) department
Information technology (IT)
Information technology strategy
Maintenance and evaluation phase
Network administrators
Organizational pull model
Programmers
Request for information (RFI)
Request for proposal (RFP)
Strategic IS planning
Systems analysts
Systems development life cycle (SDLC)
Technology push model
Webmasters

Introduction

Healthcare organizations are beginning to embrace information systems (IS) technology for a host of different reasons. Besides the increased pressure to control costs and improve efficiency, healthcare organizations are looking for ways to ensure patient safety, reduce medical errors, improve the quality of care, and demonstrate compliance with new privacy and security regulations.

Given the diverse and competing IS priorities within a healthcare organization and the fact that implementing an IS is a substantial investment, how should decisions be made regarding which IS initiatives to support? How can healthcare administrators be reasonably assured that the information systems selected will meet their organization's current and future needs and be accepted by end users? After the decision is made to implement an IS, what resources are needed to adequately support it?

This chapter introduces a framework for addressing these important questions, including a description of the process that should be used to select a new IS, large or small. It also describes the people, policies, and organizational structure needed to maintain information systems and to manage information resources effectively. Finally, it discusses strategic planning for information systems, the systems development life cycle, information resource management, and the role of the health information manager in planning, selecting, and implementing healthcare information systems.

Theory into Practice

This case is based on a comprehensive study of five primary care physician practices that implemented the same **electronic medical record** (EMR) product (Wager, Lee, and White 2001). Family Medicine Center (FMC) was the one practice out of the five studied that was dissatisfied with its choice of EMR. This brief synopsis provides a good illustration of the notion that factors beyond the functionality of the healthcare information system may cause system failure or success.

FMC implemented its EMR system in 1994. The center purchased the system from a reputable vendor and expected that it would reduce personnel costs and enable FMC to realize numerous other efficiencies. Instead, FMC invested more than $400,000 in the system and spent several frustrating years trying to get it to work right. Now key personnel within the clinic want to pull the plug on the system and start over with a brand-new one (Wager, Lee, and White 2001).

What went wrong? As with most system failures, the authors of this case discovered that multiple factors, organizational and other, contributed to the frustrations and dissatisfactions with the use of the EMR at FMC. One factor may have been the disastrous implementation phase. FMC's lead physician, Dr. Barron, selected the system based on the advice of a colleague in the field. The other physicians working in the practice knew very little about computers and trusted Dr. Barron's judgment. No planning group was identified and no real strategic decision process was used to make the EMR choice.

To complicate matters further, Dr. Barron agreed with the EMR distributor that it would be best to implement the scheduling and billing components of the system concurrently with the EMR components. It was the distributor's first sale and much of his time was spent handling conversion problems from the old billing system to the new one, with little time left to train nurses, physicians, and support staff on proper use of the EMR.

Years later, common complaints among the nurses and physicians include:

- The initial training was grossly inadequate.
- The system is too cumbersome to use.
- Our patients do not like us typing in the exam room.
- Half the record is electronic and half is on paper.
- Rather than save time, the system has actually created more work.
- No one is available to help when we have problems with the system.

It would be easy to assume that FMC's EMR failed because the product was not appropriate for the facility. When examined within the context of the larger study in which the majority of practices were pleased or very pleased with the same EMR product that was installed at FMC, this conclusion seems too simplistic. What could FMC have done to improve its chances for a successful implementation of the EMR? Subsequent sections of this chapter outline some of the ways healthcare organizations can improve their chances of system success.

Overview of Today's Environment and Challenges

In 1993, the healthcare industry spent $7.5 billion on IS technology; by 2003, spending is projected to be $23 billion. A recent national survey found that 22 percent of IS managers believe that their budgets will continue to grow because of an increased emphasis on IS technology in their organizations' strategic plan (HIMSS 2001). However, the increase in budgets does not mean that healthcare organizations or IS departments are in a freewheeling spending environment. In fact, the pressure to demonstrate the cost–benefit or return on investment of IS technology has never been greater (Baldwin 2000; Kastens and Gray 1998).

With healthcare managers at all levels looking to IS technology as the means to providing services more efficiently and effectively, it is not uncommon for multiple competing priorities to exist within a single institution. For example, the director of the pharmacy wants to replace the pharmacy information system with one that will alert providers to possible drug interactions; the administrator in the patient accounting office wants to upgrade the patient billing system so that patients can access their accounts online; the director of nursing wants handheld electronic notepads to aid nurses in documentation; the director of health information services wants to implement a new document imaging system; and the chief executive officer is eager to use decision support systems that will help prevent and track medical errors. These same managers often work in facilities that are part of a larger integrated delivery network and find themselves competing with each other for limited IS resources. To complicate matters, senior executives are urging managers to adopt a systemwide perspective on information management issues with the expectation that the organization should be able to integrate clinical and financial information across the continuum of services at both the individual (patient) level and the population level.

Healthcare information systems can be costly to implement and resource intensive to support. Therefore, it is unrealistic to expect a healthcare organization to fund all identified IS efforts. In addition to the up-front costs associated with acquiring the systems, there are substantial costs associated with maintaining and supporting them. As studies have shown (Anderson 1997; Anderson and Aydin 1997; Wager et al. 2000), choosing the right healthcare IS is not enough to ensure its success. Adequate technical support services also must be available to maintain the system. Moreover, numerous costs are associated with integrating new information systems with other computerized systems already in place. Many clinical information systems were developed separately from existing financial and administrative systems, and merging data from these different systems can be extremely difficult, time-consuming, and expensive. Yet, in today's competitive environment, healthcare organizations that are unable to integrate clinical and financial information for decision-making purposes are at a tremendous disadvantage. In fact, some experts argue that the true benefits of integrated delivery systems may not be fully realized until integrated information systems are built to support them (Shortell, Gillies, and Anderson 1994; Shortell, Gillies, and Devers 1995).

Healthcare information systems are not only costly to implement and support, but nearly half of them fail because of user resistance and other, nontechnical issues, despite the fact that the systems are technologically sound (Anderson 1997; Anderson, Aydin, and Jay 1994). Some healthcare information systems have actually been removed from organizations because they were too costly to maintain or because the costs far exceeded the perceived benefits (Lawler et al. 1996; Williams 1992). Forsythe and Buchanan (1992, p. 10) contend that "automated systems rarely stand alone—they need to work with people. This means that people have the

power to make a system work or to sabotage it; systems are only successful if people are willing to work with them." Clearly, experience has shown that the success of a new IS and its acceptance among clinicians and other users depends heavily on a variety of social and organizational factors, not just technological ones (Anderson 1997; Kaplan 1997; Wager et al. 2000).

Strategic Planning for Information Systems

No board of directors would ever recommend building a new healthcare facility without an architect's blueprint and an extensive assessment of community/market needs and resources. The architect's blueprint helps ensure that the new facility has a strong foundation, a well-planned organizational basis, and the potential for growth and expansion. The external assessment helps ensure that there is a need for the new facility and that adequate resources are available to support it.

Similarly, it is critical that healthcare organizations establish a vision of how the system will support their mission and goals before developing or purchasing a new **information system** (IS). Organizations also should allocate sufficient organizational and **information technology** (IT) resources to support the new system.

To develop a blueprint for IS technology, the healthcare organization should engage in strategic planning for information systems. **Strategic IS planning** is the process of identifying and prioritizing the organization's IS needs as based on its strategic goals. The intent of strategic planning for information systems is to ensure that all IS technology initiatives are well integrated and aligned with the organization's overall strategic plan.

In years past, relatively few healthcare organizations engaged in strategic planning for information systems. If an IS plan existed at all, it probably had been developed by the staff in the **information systems department,** people who had not participated in the organization's overall strategic planning process. Having two separate plans often led to redundant systems, duplication of effort, and the acquisition of information systems that could not interact with each other.

Most healthcare leaders today realize the contribution of information management to the achievement of their strategic plans and business goals. No longer is it acceptable to develop an IS plan independent of the strategic plan for the organization. IS plans must be an integral part of the organization's overall strategic plan and must specify not only where the organization should go, but also how it should make the transition from the systems of today to the systems of tomorrow (Martin, Wilkins, and Stawski 1998).

Role of the Healthcare Information Systems Steering Committee

Strategic planning for information systems should involve a range of individuals across the organization, including senior administrators, physicians, nurses, and key people from the ancillary services departments (for example, radiology, laboratory medicine, and pharmacy) as well as IS and health information management (HIM) professionals. Generally, these individuals are organized as a team or a committee known as the **healthcare information systems** (HIS) **steering committee.** The HIS steering committee's primary role is to identify and prioritize IS needs, ensure that all new IS initiatives support the organization's strategic goals, and monitor the progress of new system implementations and upgrades to existing systems.

Opinions vary as to who should lead the planning effort. Some authors believe that the **chief information officer** (CIO) or another designated senior-level administrator should assume this role (Austin and Boxerman 1998). Others believe that it is better to have a clinician or medical staff leader who is "further removed" from the IS department (Martin 1998) or to contract with an outside consultant organization to oversee the process. Whoever is chosen to organize or lead the planning effort should be someone who has strong communication and organizational skills, is well respected by clinicians and the administrative team, and is viewed as a leader within the organization. Ideally, the person chosen should have enough power or clout to make things happen.

Strategic Planning Process

The HIS steering committee should begin strategic planning with a discussion of the organization's view of the role that IS technology will play in the organization's future. Leaders generally view IS technology in either of two primary ways: as a tool that helps them work more efficiently and effectively or as a tool that enables them to expand their business plans.

The first viewpoint, often referred to as the **organizational pull model,** allows the organization to "do what it does better" (Martin, Wilkins, and Stawski 1998). In other words, the healthcare institution sets its business objectives and then looks to the IS department to develop an IT plan that meets the information system requirements implied in the business plan. Information technology in this model is used to support and improve the operation of the organization.

Other organizations may view information technology more strategically; that is, they may look at how information technology could be used to "to change what they do." This view is known as the **technology push model** (Martin 1998). In this model, IT technology is viewed as being able to "push" an organization into new business areas, perhaps areas never before thought possible. For example, a healthcare organization might explore how telemedicine or remote access to an electronic medical record (EMR) system could be used to expand its service area.

One view is not necessarily better than the other. What is important is that the view be aligned with the organization's strategic plan. The view should reflect the organization's vision and goals as identified by the senior leadership team and the board of directors. Having an understanding of the organization's view of IS technology can help guide the HIS steering committee in the strategic IS planning process.

Component Alignment Approach

There are several different models or approaches to strategic planning for information systems (Glaser and Hsu 1999). One model is the **component alignment model** (CAM) developed by Martin (1998). The CAM is based on the premise that it is critical that the healthcare organization adopt a systems perspective to implementing IS technology. That is, the organization should see itself as a part of a whole entity rather than as a conglomeration of independent departments or units.

Historically, this has not been the approach to systems development within healthcare. Many information systems were developed or acquired by healthcare organizations in a rather piecemeal fashion. Early systems were primarily administrative or financial in nature and often developed in-house by what was then the data processing department. With the advent of microcomputers in the mid-1980s, healthcare organizations began to invest more extensively in clinical information systems. However, these systems were often purchased by outside vendors based on individual department needs and not on the needs of the organization as a whole or on its strategic plans. For example, the radiology department might have purchased the best radiology information system on the market and the laboratory department, the best laboratory IS, with little, if any, consideration of whether the organization had an appropriate IT infrastructure to adequately support the two systems. The systems were thought of quite independently.

Today, it is vital that the leadership team adopt a system-wide perspective on information management and view each major IS acquisition within the context of the larger picture, that is, how the system supports the organization's overall mission and strategic goals. The goal is to build systems, not disparate applications. In fact, one of the major challenges facing IS staff is that of integrating data from disparate systems and getting the systems to "talk to each other." Clinicians are often frustrated at being unable to pull together clinical and financial data from among the various systems used within the healthcare enterprise.

To help ensure that information systems support the organization's strategic plan and not be acquired in isolation, Martin (1998) suggests in his CAM model that healthcare leaders examine both the external and internal environment and business plans before establishing IS priorities or making IS investments. He argues that seven major components must be aligned with each other. These include:

- *External environment:* External forces affecting healthcare organizations (for example, government regulations, changes in payment mechanisms, competitive forces)
- *Emerging information technologies:* IT with the potential to influence the way a healthcare organization delivers its services (for example, speech recognition, handheld computing devices, telemedicine)
- *Mission:* The underlying goals the healthcare organization is committed to achieve
- *Organizational infrastructure and processes:* How the healthcare organization is organized to deliver its services
- *IT infrastructure and processes:* The healthcare organization's IT resources and how they are organized
- *Business strategy:* The rationale the healthcare organization uses to define its business activities
- *Information technology strategy:* The rationale the healthcare organization uses in its procurement and propagation of IT

Two of these components—the external environment and emerging information technologies—are external factors and beyond the organization's control; therefore, they are considered uncontrollable components. These elements may have a direct impact on the other controllable CAM components within the organization. For example, increased government regulation, demand for accountability, advances in information technology, the changing demographics of the country, and the emergence of managed care are all factors external to the organization and beyond its control. However, facility leaders, including members of the HIS steering committee, should consider the effects of these environmental changes on the organization's infrastructure and processes, mission, business strategy, IT infrastructure and processes, and IT strategy.

All of the components in the CAM model are interdependent and should be responsive to changes in the external environment and the organization's mission and direction. (See figure 6.1.)

CAM is only one approach. The steering committee might take many other approaches to develop the actual strategic IS plan. The approach chosen depends on the time, financial resources, and personnel the organization wants to invest in the planning process, as well as other constraints. Whatever approach is taken should involve senior-level leadership within the organization.

Generic Approach

The following steps represent a generic approach to developing a strategic IS plan. (See figure 6.2, p. 106.) This approach can be modified or adapted to meet the healthcare organization's individual needs. The steps include the following:

1. Review the organization's strategic plan and assess the organization's current external environment.

Figure 6.1.   Component Alignment Model

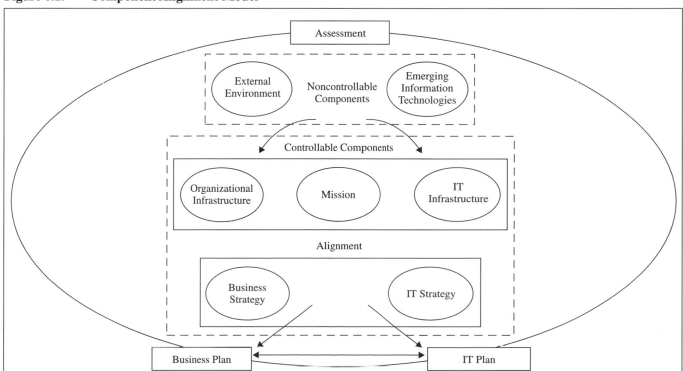

Source: Martin et al. (1998)

2. Evaluate the organization's existing information systems and current internal environment.
3. Identify the organization's IS needs and prioritize current and future IS projects.
4. Gain approval from the organization's leaders (executive management and board of directors) of the prioritized plan for completing IS projects.

Reviewing the Strategic Plan and Assessing the External Environment

To begin the planning process, the HIS steering committee should review the organization's current strategic plans, goals, and objectives and evaluate its current external environment. The overall strategic plan should include an environmental assessment that analyzes the external forces that may affect the organization. External forces include changes in reimbursement methodologies, new government regulations, and changes in the demographics or healthcare needs of the community.

In addition, an environmental assessment should be performed to explore emerging information technologies and their potential impact on the ways the healthcare organization delivers its services. In conducting this assessment, a subgroup of the committee may wish to review the literature, visit trade shows, network with colleagues in the field, or meet with leading vendors in the marketplace. A number of consultant groups also can provide vendor/product information to the organization.

Evaluating Existing Information Systems and Assessing the Internal Environment

In addition to the external environmental assessment, it is equally important for the HIS steering committee to conduct an internal environmental assessment of the organization's current IS environment. The committee should consider questions such as:

- Which information systems are currently used within the organization?

Figure 6.2.   Strategic Information Systems Planning Process

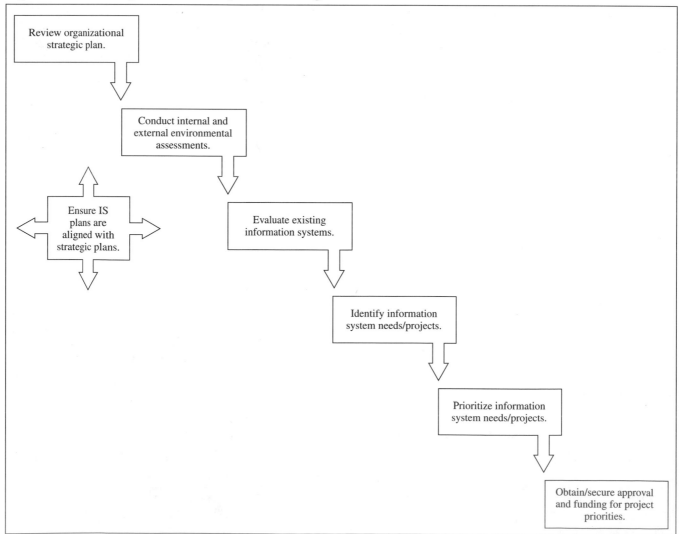

- To what extent do these systems meet the needs of end users?
- Which systems are likely to need replacement or upgrades? Which ones are likely to become obsolete within the next few years?
- To what extent is the organization able to support and maintain its current systems? Does it have the people, equipment, and network infrastructure needed to support its current systems?
- To what degree are the current systems cost-effective and efficient?
- How well do the existing information systems support the organization's strategic goals?

As part of the analysis of the current internal environment, the committee also may want to compare the organization's IT functionality and performance against external benchmarks. For example, the committee might compare the organization's ratio of end users to technical support personnel with industry averages. It also might compare the organization's performance in key areas with the performance of other, similar organizations. The committee might wish to consider the following questions:

- How secure are patient information systems?
- How much downtime does the facility experience?
- How much IT staff time is spent troubleshooting system problems?
- In what ways, if any, have the major systems adversely affected patient care?
- To what degree are existing systems in compliance with the new Health Insurance Portability and Accountability Act (HIPAA) privacy and security regulations?

It is essential that the organization evaluate existing systems to accurately identify its needs, problems, and opportunities for improvement. Otherwise, it runs the risk of installing a new IS to fix a perceived problem only to discover that the new system never addressed the actual problem and, instead, created a host of new problems.

Identifying IS Needs and Prioritizing IS Projects

After the committee has developed a good understanding of the organization's strategic goals, emerging information technologies, and existing information systems, it should begin to identify IS needs throughout the organization. This internal needs assessment can be formal or informal. For example, if the committee wants to conduct a formal assessment, it might conduct structured interviews with key users or administer surveys in key areas throughout the organization. A less formal approach would be to ask all HIS steering committee members to list the information needs within their respective areas. The outcome of this assessment is a fairly comprehensive list of the organization's information management needs. Eventually, the list can be used to identify projects and establish IT priorities.

The next step in the planning process is to establish priorities. Again, the committee might take different approaches to accomplish this very important task. One approach is to identify all proposed IS projects and hold an intensive retreat where all interested stakeholders (HIS steering committee members and other interested clinicians and staff) score and rank each project. Sufficient information concerning each project should be given to the stakeholders ahead of time to help them make informed choices. This particular approach was used successfully by an enterprisewide steering committee in establishing IS priorities at a large academic medical center and is discussed further in the case study at that end of this chapter.

Gaining Approval for the Plan

Whether the approach described above or another approach to priority setting is used, the strategic IS planning process should result in a list of identified project priorities. These priorities then should be developed further and forwarded to the senior administration and/or the board of directors for approval and funding. It is important to note that the priority list is not static. It should be reviewed periodically and modified accordingly based on changes in the environment and the growing needs of the organization.

Check Your Understanding 6.1

Instructions: Answer the following questions on a separate piece of paper.

1. Why is strategic planning for information systems important to organizations in today's healthcare environment? What risks are associated with not having an IS plan?
2. Who should be involved in the strategic planning process? Who should lead the effort?
3. Why is it important for the IS plan to be integrated with the healthcare organization's overall strategic plan?
4. Explain the difference between the organizational pull model and the technology push model.
5. Briefly describe the seven major components of the component alignment model.
6. Why is it important for healthcare organizations to examine their existing information systems? What aspects of the existing system(s) should be examined during the planning process?
7. How might a healthcare organization go about prioritizing its IS projects or needs?

Information Systems Development

After information system priorities have been established as part of the strategic plan, the healthcare organization should follow a structured project management process for selecting and implementing new systems. The structured approach enables the organization to identify viable alternatives, gain user buy-in, select a system that meets the needs of the users, and implement the system in a well-organized, systematic way.

Because several new system projects may be going on at the same time and people may be involved in more than one project, it is important that the projects be organized and managed consistently. Ideally, the IT staff or the project leader should maintain a project repository for every IS initiative. Included in the project repository would be all minutes, notes, survey results, and other relevant information used in managing the project. The project repository is particularly important in healthcare organizations that experience high turnover among IT staff.

Systems Development Life Cycle

One process for IS development is the **systems development life cycle** (SDLC). Although there are many different models of the SDLC, all generally include a variation of the following four phases: analysis, design, implementation, and maintenance and evaluation. As the activities that occur in each phase are discussed, it should become apparent that the process does not end when the new IS is implemented. Rather, the SDLC is an ongoing process that requires ongoing assessment and planning. Figure 6.3 illustrates the cyclical nature of the SDLC.

Like the strategic IS planning process, the SDLC involves the participation of myriad people with different backgrounds and areas of expertise. Depending on the nature and scope of the project, representatives from the key clinical and administrative areas should be involved. For example, if the organization plans to replace its pharmacy IS, in addition to key people from the pharmacy department, the process might include individuals from the medical staff, nursing, and other ancillary areas that depend on or use pharmacy information. Representatives from IT and HIM services also should be involved.

Analysis Phase

After senior administration or the board gives the go-ahead for the project, the **analysis phase** begins. During the analysis phase, the need for a new IS is explored further, problems with the existing system are solidified, and user needs are identified. The primary focus in this beginning phase of the SDLC is on the business problem, independent of any technology that can or will be used to implement a solution to that problem.

In this phase, it is important to examine the current system and to identify opportunities for improvement or enhancement. Even though an initial assessment was completed as part of the strategic information planning process, the analysis phase of the SDLC involves a more extensive evaluation. Typically, the existing system is evaluated by asking people who routinely use it to identify its strengths and limitations. Completion of this task can help to ensure that the organization does not make a significant investment in a new system only to later discover that what was needed was better communication, additional training, and more extensive technical support, not a new information system.

When it is clear that a new IS is needed, the next step is to assess the information needs of users and to define functional requirements. It is best to have a structured method for accomplishing this task. For example, the project team might administer a questionnaire, conduct focus groups, or hold joint-requirements planning sessions. A joint-requirement planning session is a highly structured group meeting that is conducted to analyze problems and define functional requirements. Whatever method or combination of methods is used to solicit user input, the process should result in a detailed list of user specifications.

Design Phase

After the users' needs have been identified, the process generally moves into the **design phase.** During this phase, consideration is given to how the new system will be designed or selected. Questions to ask include:

- Will the new system be built in-house?
- Will the organization contract with an outside developer to build the system?
- Will the facility purchase an information system from a vendor?

Because of time, cost, and personnel restraints, most healthcare organizations first look at what IS products are available in the vendor community. For this reason, this discussion focuses on selecting an IS from a vendor rather than building one in-house. (Should a facility decide to build a system in-house, it is generally because the facility's needs are unique and it has the technical expertise to design and support the system.)

A facility that wishes to explore the systems available in the vendor community might begin by obtaining information from exhibits at professional conferences, directories or publications, the Internet, vendor user groups, consulting firms, and contacts with colleagues in the health information systems field. A **request for information** (RFI) is generally sent to a fairly extensive list of vendors that are known to offer products or systems that meet the organization's needs. The RFI is used to obtain general product information and to prescreen vendors. Responses to the RFI are used to narrow the

Figure 6.3.   Systems Development Life Cycle

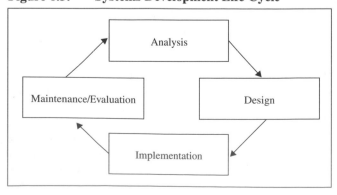

list to a smaller number of vendors who will be invited to respond to the **request for proposal** (RFP).

The RFP generally includes much more detail on the requirements of the system and provides guidelines for vendors to follow in bidding. For a major system acquisition, Austin and Boxerman (1998, p. 223) recommend that the RFP include the following elements:

- An introduction to the organization in which the system will be used, including organizational charts, operating statistics, number of personnel, and financial information
- A statement of functional requirements, categorized as mandatory or desirable, and listed in priority order
- Specification of the content and format to be followed in proposals, including vendor profile, software and hardware descriptions, training plans, documentation to be provided, maintenance coverage, a list of other clients who have used similar products or services, a cost schedule, and performance guarantees
- A statement describing the criteria to be used in evaluating proposals
- The requirements for on-site demonstrations and system testing
- The requirements for the vendor's role in system implementation
- General contractual requirements, including warranties, performance bonds, payment, schedule, and penalties for failure to meet schedules specified in the contract

After the RFP has been distributed to the vendors, the organization may wish to hold a bidders' conference to answer the vendors' questions about the RFP and to give all vendors the opportunity to receive the same information.

Concurrent with the development of the RFP, the project team should establish the criteria with which to evaluate the vendors' responses to the RFP. For example, the team may wish to evaluate the extent to which each vendor's product meets the functional requirements of the new system, the vendor's track record of performance, and the extent to which the vendor's philosophy of systems development is congruent with the organization's IT strategy. In addition, the team may wish to evaluate system reliability, costs, and projected benefits. However, the evaluation of the vendor and its products should not depend solely on its response to the RFP. Other formal and informal mechanisms should be used to evaluate each vendor and its products. For example, the project team may hold vendor presentations, check references, attend user group meetings, and make site visits to other facilities that use the product. The purpose of these activities is to gather as much relevant information as possible to make an informed decision. Interested clinicians, administrators, and other end users, as well as members of the project team, should have the opportunity to participate in as many of these activities as possible.

As part of the system selection process, the project team should conduct a cost–benefit analysis for each viable alternative. Costs should include acquisition costs, such as hardware, software, network, training, in addition to operating or maintenance costs, such as system upgrades, technical support, supplies, and equipment. Most costs can be identified and measured reasonably accurately. However, the benefits to implementing an IS can be much more difficult to identify. Some benefits, such as increased productivity or improved access to information, are tangible and can be measured (albeit not easily); others are intangible and very difficult to quantify. For example, a new EMR system might lead to improved employee morale or increased patient satisfaction, but these potential benefits might be more difficult to isolate and quantify. Consequently, when comparing different vendor systems or alternatives, it is important to evaluate and measure costs and benefits to the extent possible. A variety of standard cost–benefit analysis methods may be used to evaluate different IT options that are beyond the scope of this book. A fairly complete explanation of different cost–benefit analysis methods is provided in *Systems Analysis and Design* (Whitten, Bentley, and Dittman 2001).

When the top two or three vendors have been identified, leadership within the healthcare organization generally initiates the contract negotiation process. It is generally a good idea for the organization to begin contract negotiations with more than one vendor. This provides leverage during the negotiation process and affords the organization an alternative should it and the vendor not agree on the terms of the contract. A host of very detailed and technical issues are generally addressed in the contract—everything from when the system is to be delivered and installed, to warranties and guarantees, to who is responsible for ensuring that the product interfaces with other institutional systems. Internal legal counsel generally reviews the contract carefully before it is signed and commitments are made.

Implementation Phase

After contract negotiations have been finalized, the **implementation phase** begins. In this phase, a comprehensive plan for implementing the new system is developed. An interdisciplinary implementation team is generally established and led by a project manager. The implementation team will likely include some of the same individuals who were involved in selecting the new system, but other key people should be involved in the process as well. Ideally, the project manager should be someone who is well respected and knowledgeable, has experience with implementing new systems, and has the political influence and power to make things happen. He or she also should have strong organizational and communication skills and be able to work effectively with the vendor. The importance of selecting the right person to lead the effort cannot be overemphasized. Even though a good implementation does not guarantee user acceptance of the new system, as illustrated in the FMC case study described earlier, a poor implementation can lead to frustration, dissatisfaction, and disillusionment. Some organizations never recover fully from a disastrous system implementation.

One of the implementation team's priorities is to identify all of the tasks that must be completed before the go-live date. Depending on the type of system, the number of users, and the complexity of the conversion process, the tasks may vary in scope and complexity. However, many system implementation projects require at least the following tasks:

- Preparing the site (for example, work-flow patterns, noise, space, telephone lines, and electrical power)
- Installing the necessary hardware and software
- Preparing data tables
- Building interfaces
- Establishing an IT infrastructure (for example, stable network, secure database) to support the system
- Ensuring that adequate security and confidentiality practices are in place
- Training managers, technical staff, and other end users
- Testing the new system
- Identifying and correcting errors
- Preparing documentation to support system use (for example, procedure manuals)
- Implementing conversion plans
- Developing and testing backup and disaster recovery procedures

Although each of these major tasks is very important, a few should be highlighted to stress their importance during the implementation phase. First, it is critical to thoroughly test any new system before the go-live date. This means testing, testing, and retesting the new system with real patient data, not sample data that the vendor may have provided or that your institution may have created. Even though it is nearly impossible to identify and correct all of the errors before a system goes live, it is essential to identify and correct as many of them as possible. It is often much easier to correct a problem in the test mode than after the system is fully operational.

Second, adequate training is essential. As seen in the FMC case, a healthcare organization may be implementing a solid, highly reputable new system, but if the staff who will be using it are not thoroughly trained, it can result in dissatisfaction with the system and low staff morale. For any new system to be successful, it must be accepted and used by the staff. Different organizations and vendors might use different approaches to training, but one common approach is to train the trainer. This approach involves identifying key people in the various functional areas (for example, nursing units, laboratory, billing), training them on the system, and then having them train others in their area (with guidance from the vendor or a "superuser").

The train the trainer method can be effective because after the vendor is gone, staff must be available who are comfortable with the system and can assist others. It is equally important to allow adequate time for training. Staff should not have to squeeze in training on their lunch break, with little or no time to practice using the new system. Just as it is important to use real data in testing the system, it is critical to give staff practice using the new system with real patients or real data.

In addition to providing training, the organization must have the IT infrastructure and processes in place to support the system. The infrastructure should include a stable network, a sufficient number of workstations appropriately located throughout the organization, adequate security measures, up-to-date procedural manuals, and a process for reporting problems with the system.

Finally, it is important to develop plans for converting the old system to the new one. Conversion to a new system often requires major changes in the work flow and organizational structure and places increased demands on staff during this period. Therefore, it is essential to plan appropriately for the conversion and to ensure that adequate technical and support staff members are available to assist managers and end users, as needed.

Throughout the implementation process, many tasks or activities may occur simultaneously; others will need to be completed before other activities can begin. Because of the number of different tasks occurring, it is generally a good idea for the project manager to use a Gantt chart or project management tool that identifies the major tasks, their estimated start and completion dates, the individuals responsible for performing them, and the resources needed to complete them. Again, activities or tasks that depend on the completion of other tasks should be readily identified. Project management software such as Microsoft Project® is useful for creating Gantt charts, is easy to use, and enables the manager to track project resources (for example, staff, equipment) and expenditures.

Maintenance and Evaluation Phase

The final phase of the SDLC is the **maintenance and evaluation phase.** Regardless of how well designed and tested a new system may be, errors or bugs will inevitably occur after it goes into operation. IT support staff must be available to find potential problems and take steps to correct them. Whether the technical staff are in-house or employed through a contract service, well-trained staff must be available to maintain or support the new system. For critical systems such as patient care or clinical information systems, technical support should be available twenty-four hours a day, seven days a week. Sufficient technical staff also should be available to oversee system backups and upgrades, replace outdated equipment, respond to new regulatory requirements, and provide ongoing training and assistance. Some experts estimate that at least 25 percent of the total technical staff time may be devoted to maintenance activities when several information systems are in place (Austin and Boxerman 1998).

As the organization hires new people, its technical or support staff must be available to train them on the system. Likewise, all staff will need additional training on a regular basis to ensure that they are current with system upgrades, enhancements, and new features or procedures. Ideally, the organization should have a plan in place outlining how staff will receive initial and ongoing training on any new or existing IS. Many healthcare organizations now appoint an individual within key clinical and administrative departments whose primary role is to ensure that the department staff have adequate training and technical support available to them. For example, the radiology department might have a radiological technician with strong computer skills who serves as the information technician and assists and trains other staff in the department. Such an approach can be effective in increasing response time to user requests and alleviating user frustration.

In addition to providing adequate training and support, the healthcare organization should monitor data quality and integrity and ensure that the system is secure and safe. Specifically, emergency backup procedures should be in place in the event the system fails or goes down for any reason. All staff should know what to do in such circumstances. The backup procedures should be well documented and readily available to staff.

However, maintaining and supporting the new systems is not enough. Information systems should be evaluated on an ongoing basis to determine whether they are contributing to the institution's overall goals and meeting user needs. Healthcare administrators today are demanding to know whether the return on investment (ROI) to the organization has been realized since the systems were implemented. Being able to measure ROI is becoming increasingly important as healthcare institutions struggle to manage limited resources more effectively. Consequently, as a part of the system evaluation process, institutions are looking at the organizational, technological, and economic impact of information systems on the enterprise as a whole (Anderson, Aydin, and Jay 1994; Friedman and Wyatt, 1997; Kaplan, 1997).

HIM Contributions to Information Systems Development

Health information managers can make unique contributions to the SDLC process. Because HIM professionals understand the origins and content of patient data contained in health records as well as the financial impact of coding, they are in an ideal position to speak to the need to integrate clinical and financial information. HIM professionals also have a broad understanding of healthcare organizations and their major components and frequently interact with the clinicians and administrators who need access to relevant information for decision-making purposes.

Perhaps the best way to describe the different contributions HIM professionals could make to the SDLC is to walk through a simple example. Let's say that the healthcare organization has decided to select and implement an enterprisewide EMR system within the next two years. During the analysis phase, the HIM professional could assist in identifying problems with the current health record system and in assessing the needs of various user groups. Because this individual understands the major components of an EMR system and many of the problems associated with paper-based health record systems, she or he could assist the project team in identifying user specifications for the RFP.

During the design phase, the HIM professional could share knowledge and insight into the EMR selection process. Most likely, he or she would attend several professional conferences each year to visit vendor exhibits, network with colleagues throughout the nation, and attend educational sessions on various aspects of EMR development and implementation. The HIM professional could bring back to the institution the insight and lessons learned from others in the field. Throughout the EMR selection process, the HIM professional could attend vendor demonstrations, conduct site visits, and evaluate vendor responses to the RFP. In addition, he or she could provide valuable input when security and confidentiality issues are addressed.

During the implementation phase of the EMR project, the HIM professional should become part of the implementation team or could participate in system testing, train staff, identify errors, develop backup and disaster recovery plans, and, again, ensure that all staff members are aware of patient confidentiality and system security. Finally, in the maintenance and support phase of the project, the HIM professional could evaluate the system's impact on the department on an ongoing basis, identify and communicate problems to the appropriate individuals, and develop an ongoing training program for staff. These are just a few of the many ways in which a HIM professional could make significant contributions to the SDLC of a new system.

Check Your Understanding 6.2

Instructions: Answer the following questions on a separate piece of paper.

1. What is the relationship between strategic information systems planning and the systems development life cycle?

2. Identify the four main phases of the SDLC and describe the purpose or intent of each.

3. What is the difference between an RFI and an RFP?

4. Briefly describe the HIM professional's contributions to the SDLC.

Management of Healthcare Information System Resources

Managing information resources is a vital function of any healthcare organization. Within hospitals or health systems, an in-house information services or information systems department often coordinates this function, although a growing number of healthcare organizations outsource IT functions to outside vendors. In fact, a recent survey of health information leaders revealed that two-thirds of healthcare organizations currently outsource at least some of their IT functions (HIMSS 2001). Web site development and management is the most frequently outsourced function, followed by applications development and workstation support. Advantages to outsourcing often include cost reductions and accessability to highly competent IT staff.

Organizational Structure

Despite the trend to outsource some IT functions, many healthcare organizations have an IS department that provides a wide range of technical support functions to users throughout the organization. These functions include systems development and implementation, systems support/maintenance, user support, database administration, communications and network administration, and Web support. (See figure 6.4.)

Chief Information Officer

Generally, the IS department is managed by the chief information officer (CIO) or director of IS, who in turn reports to the chief executive officer (CEO) or some other senior-level individual. The CIO is responsible for helping to lead the strategic IS planning process, managing the major functional units within the IS department, and overseeing the management of information resources throughout the enterprise.

IS Department Staff

In years past, most of the staff working in the IS department typically had backgrounds in programming and computer science. Today, the department is likely to include individuals with unique sets of skills and specialized areas of interest. These positions include:

- *Systems analysts:* Systems analysts investigate, analyze, design, develop, install, evaluate, and maintain the

organization's healthcare information systems. They typically are involved in all aspects of the SDLC and serve in a liaison role between end users and programmers, database administrators, and other technical personnel. Systems analysts with a clinical background in nursing, medicine, or other health professions are often called clinical systems analysts. They understand the language of clinicians and typically have an in-depth understanding of the patient care process.
- *Programmers:* Programmers are responsible primarily for writing program codes and developing applications. They typically perform the function of systems development and work closely with system analysts.
- *Network administrators:* Network administrators are involved in installing, configuring, managing, monitoring, and maintaining network applications. They are responsible for supporting the network infrastructure and controlling user access.
- *Database administrators:* Database administrators are involved in database design, management, security, backup, and user access. They are responsible for the technical aspects of managing a database
- *Webmasters:* Webmasters are the most recent additions to the IS department. They provide support to Web applications and to the healthcare organization's intranet and Internet operations. Some of their responsibilities include designing and constructing Web pages, managing hardware and software, and linking Web-based applications to the organization's existing information systems.

All IS staff must have an opportunity to keep current in the IS field by attending conferences, gaining certification in specialized areas, and enrolling in formal academic or continuing education courses. IT applications serving the healthcare industry are emerging at a phenomenal rate, so the professional development of IS staff is critical.

Figure 6.4.   Typical Organizational Structure for IS Department

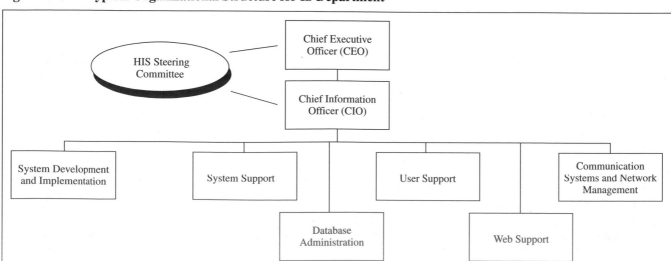

Real-World Case

The Medical University of South Carolina (MUSC) is a large academic medical center composed of a tertiary care hospital, a children's hospital, a psychiatric hospital, a cancer center, multiple outpatient clinics, and six academic colleges: Medicine, Nursing, Pharmacy, Dentistry, Health Professions, and Graduate Studies. It is a public institution whose primary mission is to educate future healthcare professionals, provide comprehensive healthcare services to the citizens of South Carolina, and conduct health science research. Specific units at MUSC, such as the Department of Family Medicine, have a long history of using electronic medical record (EMR) systems or clinical information systems to support patient care and facilitate research. Most of the units with the most advanced information systems have a physician or clinician champion who was instrumental in the adoption of the tech-

nology. As a side note, MUSC contracts with an outside facilities management firm to oversee nearly all of its computing and information technology needs and has done so since the mid-1980s. This group is known as the Center for Computing and Information Technology (CCIT).

In 1994, MUSC developed its first comprehensive strategic IS plan for the clinical enterprise. (See figure 6.5 for the time line.) The clinical enterprise included all key inpatient and outpatient areas. At the time, more than 110 interviews were conducted with key clinicians and administrators throughout the enterprise. The purpose of the interviews was to identify the needs of the users. Twenty-three clinical enterprise projects emerged from these interviews, including the need to implement order entry, document imaging, an ambulatory EMR system, radiology imaging, and a referral communication system for physicians. The IT strategy that MUSC adopted was based on the concept of open-systems

Figure 6.5.   MUSC Information Systems Planning Timeline

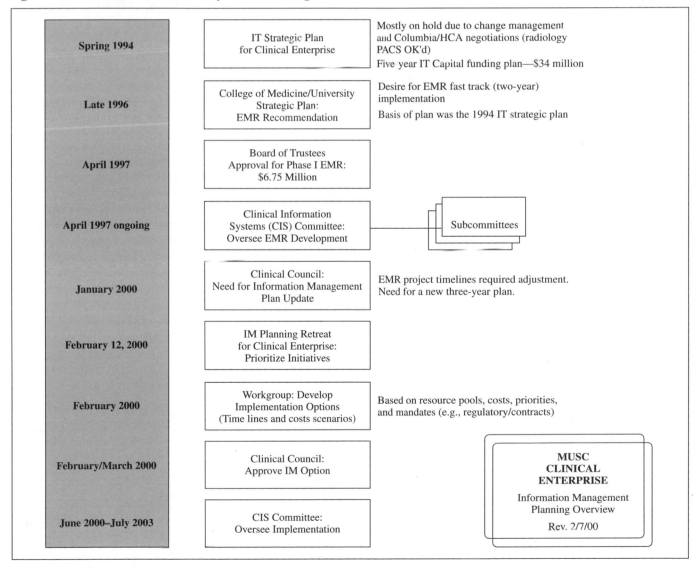

architecture. That is, MUSC permitted ancillary departments to specify, select, and implement information systems that best suited their needs. However, the systems had to be able to interface with the existing MUSC hospital IS for the purposes of admission, discharge and transfer (ADT), and patient billing.

By 1996, the College of Medicine had expanded the IS plan and had recommended that MUSC implement an EMR system throughout the clinical enterprise. The dean of the College of Medicine at the time was the driving force behind the recommendation. Soon afterward, the board approved $6.75 million to support the first phase of the EMR system project (also known as EMERALD). MUSC's approach to implementing an enterprisewide EMR was (and continues to be) through the development of a clinical data repository (CDR). The CDR software collects a copy of clinical results and stores the data in a permanent patient database or repository. The CDR has actually been accumulating data since early 1993. It began with laboratory, microbiology, pathology, radiology, and discharge summaries and operative reports. More recently, several clinical areas have integrated their clinic notes and letters into the CDR.

To oversee and manage implementation of the EMR, an enterprisewide clinical information systems (CIS) steering committee was established in 1997. A well-respected physician and associate dean in the College of Medicine initially chaired the committee. This physician was not a "computer person" but recognized the value of information technology in managing information more effectively. He insisted that the IT staff speak in nontechnical or lay terms at the CIS steering committee meetings. When this physician stepped down as chair, another physician member of the CIS steering committee assumed the role as chair. The new physician chair is a computer guru. He has a background in computer science and wrote much of the program code for the first computerized medical record used on campus.

Over the years, the strategic IS plan has been reviewed and updated, with the most recent revision occurring in February 2000. Initiated by the chair of the CIS steering committee in collaboration with the director of healthcare computing services at CCIT, a half-day retreat was held on a Saturday. The primary goal of the retreat was to identify the information management (IM) priorities for the next three years. These are referred to as IM priorities because the MUSC president felt strongly that the organization should think in terms of IM priorities rather than IS or IT priorities.

More than 150 key stakeholders throughout MUSC were invited to participate in the retreat, including physicians, nurses, and clinicians from other ancillary departments, as well as IT staff, administrators, health information managers, and educators/researchers. Those unable to attend also were given the opportunity to rank the projects and cast their votes.

Prior to the retreat, each stakeholder was given a packet of materials that described each project. The packet included the following elements:

- A project description and one-time costs (capital costs, not operating costs)
- The goal/scope of the project
- Prerequisites (a description of what activities must be done for the system to be installed)
- Considerations (additional relevant information concerning the proposed project)
- Key benefits (a description of the anticipated benefits)
- Facilities affected (a list of the facilities at the medical center that would be affected by the proposed system, for example, inpatient, outpatient/ambulatory care, entire enterprise)
- Constituencies affected (major stakeholders who would be affected, including clinicians, clinical students and trainees, patients, managers and administrators, health services researchers, other researchers, referring physicians)
- Percentage complete (when project is currently under way, percentage of project that has been completed to date)
- IT level of effort (used five-point range of very low [less than one man-week] to very high [less than three man-years] to define the level of effort)
- Non-IT level of effort (used the same scale the IT level of effort)
- Score (stakeholders asked to score each project on scale of one [lowest priority] to five [highest priority])

Prior to and again during the retreat, each stakeholder was asked to prioritize each project on the basis of three established criteria: (1) potential impact on patient care and safety, (2) potential impact on cost reduction and improved efficiency, and (3) compliance with regulations.

Stakeholders were instructed to score and rank each project on the basis of its overall impact on the organization, not the system's impact on individual departments or units. The projects were grouped into five categories: (1) core EMR initiatives, (2) interfaces with the clinical data repository, (3) administrative reporting systems, (4) infrastructure, and (5) related IM initiatives.

More than a hundred stakeholders from across the academic medical center participated in the half-day retreat. Each stakeholder was assigned to a small interdisciplinary team that included a physician, a nurse, an IT representative, an administrator, an educator/researcher, an ancillary department representative, and an HIM professional. With the help of a facilitator to keep the group on task and to ensure that adequate time was allocated to discuss each project and of a resource person to provide additional background information, each group reviewed thirty-seven different projects. Seven of the thirty-seven projects were actually removed from the voting process because they were considered mission critical and had to proceed regardless of other projects. Picking the top eight from the remaining thirty projects was not an easy task. The small groups met for nearly two hours to discuss each project.

After the small group discussion, each stakeholder then voted for his or her top project priorities using a nominal group technique. That is, each stakeholder was given eight colored stickers and asked to place one next to each of his or her top eight priorities. The outcome of the retreat was a list of the top eight IS priorities for the institution, which the CIS steering committee then reviewed and forwarded to the board of trustees for consideration and funding.

Eighteen months later, according to CCIT's healthcare computer services director, the top eight priorities established at the retreat will not be implemented in the three-year time frame because of insufficient funds. However, some of the lower-cost initiatives have progressed (albeit at a lower priority) and the top-priority initiatives have moved ahead one at a time as they have become critical. For example, a lab system server that was getting too old/slow was replaced, and radiology imaging equipment was upgraded. Some of the lower-priority projects will be completed ahead of the higher-priority projects because they cost less. The cost of the project became the determining factor with only critical/high-priority needs receiving funding. In the midst of it all, the vendor that historically supported the CDR decided to stop supporting this product. Therefore, MUSC must decide what to do to replace the CDR interface engines and results-review browser. The CIS steering committee continues to oversee the progress of all projects in its monthly meetings.

Discussion Questions

1. What is the primary role of the CIS steering committee at MUSC? How does this role compare with that of the HIS steering committee described in this chapter?

2. What are the advantages to the way MUSC identified its IS priorities? The disadvantages? How else might an organization as complex as MUSC prioritize IS projects?

3. What was MUSC's IT strategy? What are the benefits and challenges to its approach?

4. Would you consider MUSC's planning effort to be a success or a failure? Please explain.

5. Do you think the approach MUSC took to strategic IS planning and IS priority setting would work in other healthcare institutions? Explain.

6. How should the results of the February 2000 retreat be communicated to stakeholders? To others in the organization?

7. What are the advantages and disadvantages of having a physician as chair of the CIS or HIS steering committee? Is it important for the chair to have a strong background or knowledge of computers? What knowledge and skills are important for the chair to possess? Please explain.

Summary

In today's environment, healthcare organizations look to information systems technology as a way to help them provide high-quality care in a cost-effective manner. However, healthcare managers at all levels often find that they are competing with their colleagues for limited IS resources. Senior administrators are encouraging healthcare managers to work together to build integrated information systems that will support patient care and enable them to control costs across the enterprise. Clearly, in today's environment, information systems should not be developed or selected in isolation. Healthcare organizations should engage in strategic IS planning to ensure that systems are available to support their goals and plans and to prioritize IS needs. The IS plans should be well aligned and integrated with the organization's overall strategic plans. This process should involve key stakeholders throughout the organization, including clinicians/administrators, as well as HIM and information technology leaders.

After the decision has been made to develop or select a new information system, a project manager should be appointed to oversee and manage the SDLC process. Again, key stakeholders throughout the organization should be involved in the analysis, design, implementation, and maintenance/support phases of the SDLC. Adequate technical and organizational resources should be in place to ensure that the new systems are sufficiently maintained and supported. Systems should be reviewed and evaluated on an ongoing basis to determine their technological, organizational, and economic impact on the enterprise. Project management is discussed in detail in chapter 26.

References

Anderson, J. G. 1997. Clearing the way for physicians' use of clinical information systems. *Communications of the ACM* 40(8):83–90.

Anderson, J. G., and C. E. Aydin. 1997. Evaluating the impact of health care information systems. *International Journal of Technology Assessment in Health Care* 13(2):380–93.

Anderson, J. G., C. E. Aydin, and S. J. Jay, editors. 1994. *Evaluating Health Care Information Systems: Methods and Applications.* Thousand Oaks, Calif.: Sage Publications.

Austin, C. J., and S. B. Boxerman. 1998. *Information Systems for Health Services Administration,* fifth edition. Chicago: Health Administration Press.

Baldwin, G. 2000. CIOs' secrets to calculating return on investment. *Health Data Management* 8(7):54–59, 62–54, 66–57.

Forsythe, D. E., and B. G. Buchanan. 1992. Broadening our approach to evaluating medical information systems. *Symposium on Computer Applications in Medical Care* 15:8–12.

Friedman, C. P., and J. C. Wyatt. 1997. *Evaluation Methods in Medical Informatics.* New York City: Springer.

Glaser, J. P., and L. Hsu. 1999. *The Strategic Application of Information Technology in Healthcare Organizations: A Guide to Implementing Integrated Systems.* Boston: McGraw-Hill.

Health Information Management Systems Society. 2001. Twelfth Annual HIMSS Leadership Survey Sponsored by Superior Consultant Company and Dell Computer Corporation. Available from www.himss.org.

Kaplan, B. 1997. Addressing organizational issues into the evaluation of medical systems. *Journal of the American Medical Informatics Association* 4(2):94–101.

Kastens, J. M., and S. P. Gray. 1998. Juggling act: six IT strategies for managing IDS into the next century. *Healthcare Informatics* 15(2):123–24, 126–27.

Lawler, F., J. Cacy, N. Viviani, R. Hamm, and S. Cobb. 1996. Implementation and termination of a computerized medical information system. *Journal of Family Practice* 42(3):233–36.

Martin, J. B. 1998. Creating a strategic plan. In *Guide to Effective Healthcare Information and Management Systems and the Role of the Chief Information Officer,* third edition, J. Shapiro, editor. Chicago: Health Information Management Systems Society.

Martin, J. B., A. S. Wilkins, and S. K. Stawski. 1998. The component alignment model: a new approach to health care information technology strategic planning. *Topics in Health Information Management* 19(1):1–10.

Shortell, S. M., R. R. Gillies, and D. A. Anderson. 1994. The new world of managed care: creating organized delivery systems. *Health Affairs* 13(5): 46–64.

Shortell, S. M., R. R. Gillies, and K. J. Devers. 1995. Reinventing the American hospital. *Milbank Quarterly* 73(2):131–60.

Waegemann, C. P. 1996. The five levels of electronic health records. *M.D. Computing* 13(3):199–203.

Wager, K. A., F. W. Lee, and A. W. White. 2001. Life after a disastrous electronic medical record implementation: one clinic's experience. *Annals of Cases on Information Technology* 3:153–68.

Wager, K. A., F. W. Lee, A. W. White, D. M. Ward, and S. M. Ornstein. 2000. Impact of an electronic medical record system on community-based primary care practices. *Journal of the American Board of Family Practice* 13(5):338–48.

Whitten, J. L., L. D. Bentley, and K. C. Dittman. 2001. *Systems Analysis and Design Methods,* fifth edition. Chicago: McGraw-Hill.

Williams, L. S. 1992. Microchips versus stethoscopes: Calgary Hospital MDs face off over controversial computer system. *Canadian Medical Association* 147(10):1534–47.

Application Exercises

1. Interview a local CIO at a healthcare facility. Find out whether the organization has a strategic information systems plan, how the plan was developed, and the process used to establish IS priorities. Discuss the role of senior leadership and the medical staff in this process.

2. Interview a local health information manager in a healthcare facility. Discuss his or her role in the strategic information planning process and selection/implementation processes.

3. Review the literature on strategic information systems planning in healthcare. Compare and contrast at least two approaches to strategic IS planning other than the approaches discussed in this chapter.

4. Find and critique an example of an RFP for a healthcare information system. You may wish to visit local healthcare facilities, search the Internet, and/or review the literature.

5. Investigate different methods or tools that may be used to (1) analyze current information systems, (2) identify user needs, (3) compare and evaluate vendor products, and (4) conduct cost-benefit analyses of different options/information systems.

Review Quiz

Instructions: Select the correct answer to each of the following questions.

1. ___ Which of the following best describes the intent of strategic information systems planning?
   a. To provide the potential for growth and expansion
   b. To ensure that all IS technology initiatives are integrated and aligned with the organization's overall strategy
   c. To assess community/market needs and resources
   d. All of the above

2. ___ On what premise is Martin's component alignment model based?
   a. That the organization acquire information systems in a piecemeal fashion
   b. That the organization adopt a systems perspective to implementing IS technology
   c. That the organization purchase systems based on individual department needs
   d. That the organization focus primarily on systems that are financial in nature

3. ___ Which components in Martin's CAM model are considered uncontrollable?
   a. Emerging information technologies and external environment
   b. Business strategy and external environment
   c. Mission and information technology strategy
   d. IT infrastructure and processes and emerging information technologies

4. ___ What is the primary role of the healthcare information systems steering committee?
   a. To identify and prioritize the organization's IS needs
   b. To ensure that all new IS initiatives support the organization's strategic goals
   c. To monitor the progress of new system implementations and upgrades to existing systems
   d. All of the above

5. ___ Which of the following is *not* a phase of the systems development life cycle?
   a. Design
   b. Maintenance and evaluation
   c. Alignment
   d. Analysis

6. ___ What does the view that healthcare organizations might use information technology to "change what they do" refer to?
   a. The technology push model
   b. The organizational pull model
   c. Either of the above
   d. Neither of the above

7. ___ Which of the following is not included in an RFP?
   a. Requirements for on-site demonstrations and systems testing
   b. General product information
   c. General contractual requirements
   d. Statement describing the criteria to be used in evaluating proposals

8. ___ Which of the following is the first step in a generic approach to developing a strategic IS plan?
   a. Identify the organization's IS needs and prioritize current and future IS projects
   b. Gain approval from the organization's leaders for the prioritized plan for completing IS projects
   c. Review the organization's strategic plan and assess the organization's current external environment
   d. Evaluate the organization's existing information systems and assess its current internal environment

9. ___ Which of the following positions is *not* a role within today's IS department?
   a. A programmer
   b. A database administrator
   c. A project leader
   d. A network administrator

10. ___ What are the functions of the chief information officer in a healthcare organization?
    a. Oversees management of the organization's information resources
    b. Helps lead the strategic IS planning process
    c. Manages the major functional units within the IS department
    d. All of the above

Part II

Development of Healthcare Information

Chapter 7
Healthcare Information Standards

Kathleen M. LaTour, MA, RHIA

Learning Objectives

- To explain healthcare data sets and to describe their purpose
- To recognize the basic data sets used in acute care, ambulatory care, and long-term care settings
- To understand the unique use of the Minimum Data Set for Long-Term Care and Resident Assessment Protocols in defining and addressing the care of residents in long-term care facilities
- To understand the differences between the data sets— Data Elements for Emergency Department Systems and the Essential Medical Data Set—and how they are used in hospital-based emergency departments
- To understand the purpose and use of the Health Plan Employer Data and Information Set (HEDIS)
- To understand the intent of the ORYX initiative and to give examples of the core measures identified through ORYX

- To understand the role that HEDIS and ORYX play in healthcare quality and performance improvement
- To recognize the key players in current efforts to develop standards for computer-based health records
- To define the term healthcare informatics standards and to explain vocabulary standards, content and structure standards, transaction (communication) standards, and security standards
- To identify data sets and/or standards appropriate for specific care settings for use in developing health records and health information systems
- To understand the relationship of code sets to healthcare informatics standards in computer-based environments
- To recognize the impact of the Health Insurance Portability and Accountability Act of 1996 (HIPAA) on the development of health informatics standards

Key Terms

Accreditation
Accreditation Standards Committee X12
Aggregate data
Ambulatory care
American College of Radiology—National Electrical Manufacturers Association (ACR-NEMA)
American National Standards Institute (ANSI)
American Society for Testing and Materials (ASTM)
ASTM Standard E1384
Bills of Mortality
Centers for Medicare and Medicaid Services (CMS)
Computer-based Patient Record Institute (CPRI)
Core measure/core measure set
Data elements
Data Elements for Emergency Department Systems (DEEDS)
Data set
Department of Health and Human Services (HHS)
Digital Imaging and Communication in Medicine (DICOM)

Electronic data interchange (EDI)
Essential Medical Data Set (EMDS)
Extensible markup language (XML)
Health Care Financing Administration (HCFA)
Health Industry Business Communications Council (HIBCC)
Health Information Standards Board (HISB)
Health Insurance Portability and Accountability Act of 1996 (HIPAA)
Health Level Seven (HL7)
Health Plan Employer Data and Information Set (HEDIS)
Healthcare informatics standards
Hospital discharge abstract system
Identifier standards
Inpatient
Institute of Electrical and Electronics Engineers (IEEE)

Joint Commission on Accreditation of Healthcare Organizations (JCAHO)
Long-term care
Medical Data Interchange Standard (MEDIX)
Medicare prospective payment system
Messaging standards
Minimum Data Set for Long Term Care—Version 2.0 (MDS 2.0)
National Center for Health Statistics (NCHS)
National Committee for Quality Assurance (NCQA)
National Committee on Vital and Health Statistics (NCVHS)
National Council on Prescription Drug Programs (NCPDP)
National Information Infrastructure—Health Information Network Program (NII-HIN)
National provider file (NPF)
National provider identifier (NPI)

ORYX initiative
Outcomes and Assessment Information Set (OASIS)
Outpatient
Performance improvement
Resident Assessment Protocols (RAPs)
Security standards
Social Security number (SSN)
Standards development organizations (SDOs)
Structure and content standards
Transaction standards
Uniform Ambulatory Care Data Set (UACDS)
Uniform Hospital Discharge Data Set (UHDDS)
United Nations International Standards Organization (ISO)
Unique physician identification number (UPIN)
Unique identification number
Vocabulary standards
Workgroup on Electronic Data Interchange (WEDI)

Introduction

Data and information pertaining to individuals who use healthcare services are collected in virtually every setting where healthcare is delivered. Data represent basic facts and measurements. In healthcare, these facts usually describe specific characteristics of individual patients. The term *data* is plural. Although the singular form is *datum,* the term that is frequently used to describe a single fact or measurement is **data element.** For example, age, gender, insurance coverage, and blood pressure are all data elements concerning a patient. The term *information* refers to data that have been collected, combined, analyzed, interpreted, and/or converted into a form that can be used for specific purposes. In other words, data represent facts; information represents meaning.

In healthcare settings, data are stored in the individual's health record. The numerous data elements in the health record are then compared, combined, and interpreted by the patient's physician and other healthcare providers. For example, test results are combined with the physician's observations and the patient's description of his or her symptoms to form information about the disease or condition that is affecting the patient. Clinicians use both data and information to diagnose diseases, develop treatment plans, assess the effectiveness of care, and determine the patient's prognosis.

Data about more than one patient can be extracted from health records and combined as **aggregate data,** which then are stored in a database. Aggregate data are used to develop information about groups of patients. For example, data about all of the patients who had suffered an acute myocardial infarction during a specific time period could be collected in a database. From the aggregate data, it would be possible to identify common characteristics that might predict the course of the disease or provide information about the best way to treat it. For example, researchers identified the link between smoking and lung cancer by analyzing aggregate data about patients with a diagnosis of lung cancer.

The first known efforts to collect and use healthcare data to produce meaningful statistical profiles date back to the seventeenth century. In the early 1600s, Captain John Graunt gathered data on the common causes of death in London. He called his study the **Bills of Mortality.** However, few systematic efforts were undertaken to collect statistical data about the incidence of disease until the twentieth century, when technological developments made it possible to collect and analyze large amounts of healthcare data.

Modern efforts at standardizing healthcare data began in the 1960s. At that time, healthcare facilities began to use computers to process larger amounts of data than could be handled manually. The goal was to make comparisons among data from multiple facilities. It soon became evident that healthcare organizations needed to use standardized, uniform data definitions in order to arrive at meaningful data comparisons.

The first data standardization efforts focused generally on hospitals and specifically on hospital discharge data. Discharge data were collected in **hospital discharge abstract systems.** These systems used databases compiled from aggregate data about all of the patients discharged from a particular facility. The need to compare uniform discharge data from one hospital to the next led to the development of **data sets,** or lists of recommended data elements with uniform definitions.

Today, hospitals and other healthcare organizations collect more data and develop more information than ever before. Moreover, data and information from the health records of individual patients are used for more purposes than ever before. The demand for information is coming from users within the organizations as well as from external users such as third-party payers, government agencies, accreditation organizations, and others.

This chapter describes the principal standardized data sets that have been developed for use in different types of healthcare settings, including acute care, long-term care, and ambulatory care. It then discusses standards developed to meet the data collection needs of today's computer-based environment. Finally, the chapter looks at data collection standards that are still evolving.

Theory into Practice

In a large Midwestern health system, the director of health information services chaired the system's clinical data standards committee. The committee had recently decided to develop a data dictionary as a first step toward implementing a computer-based patient record (CPR) system.

Data dictionaries include the following components:

- A list of data elements collected in individual health records
- Definitions of the data elements
- Descriptions of the attributes of each data element
- Specifications for the size of the data field in the information system
- Descriptions of the data views to be accessed by various users

The committee began the process with what it considered to be a simple data element—patient gender. The committee members looked at the two standard references for patient data sets in acute care settings: the Uniform Hospital Discharge Data Set (UHDDS) and the Uniform Ambulatory Care Data Set (UACDS). Both data sets indicated that gender should be recorded as either "male" or "female." However, this either–or choice presented a problem.

The healthcare system included a number of hospitals and clinics. One of the hospitals offered a gender reidentification program that treated patients who were in the process of transitioning from one gender to the other. Another hospital provided neonatal intensive care services for a large geographical region. Some of the infants treated in the neonatal intensive care unit had been born with congenital defects that made it difficult to determine their gender.

During discussions of the problem, the clinical laboratory representative on the committee stressed the importance of documenting the gender of every patient. She explained that the normal range for most laboratory tests varies by gender. This information was a surprise to many committee members.

After the committee's initial discussion, the health information management professional agreed to research other data sets and standards. He found that recent healthcare informatics standards for electronic and computer-based patient records recommended using four gender descriptors: male, female, undetermined, and unknown.

The committee decided to adopt the four descriptors for gender. In the data collection process, if the term *undetermined* or *unknown* were selected, the individual doing data entry would be referred to another screen that would explain the data choice in more detail and include another data element to describe the patient's genitalia.

The challenges the committee faced in defining this relatively simple data element raised its awareness of how difficult it would be to adequately define every data element to be included in the new CPR system. The committee members gathered information on every available standardized healthcare data set and healthcare informatics standard and carefully compared the data definitions recommended. They discovered that implementation of the CPR system would be a huge project. However, they were committed to the process because it would improve the quality of the data collected in the system. The collection of consistent, reliable, and valid data would improve administrative and clinical decision making and make it possible to perform meaningful **performance improvement** comparisons.

Standardized Data Sets

The concept of data standardization became widely accepted during the 1960s, and data sets were developed for a variety of healthcare settings. Data sets for acute care, long-term care, and ambulatory care were the first to be created. In healthcare, data sets have two purposes: (1) to identify the data elements that should be collected for each patient and (2) to provide uniform definitions for common terms. The use of uniform definitions ensures that data collected from a variety of healthcare settings will share a standard definition.

The standardization of data elements and definitions makes it possible to compare the data collected at different facilities. Comparison data are used for a variety of purposes, including external accreditation, internal performance improvement, and statistical and research studies. However, data sets are not meant to limit the number of data elements that can be collected. Most healthcare organizations collect additional data elements that have meaning for their specific administrative and clinical operations.

Uniform Hospital Discharge Data Set

In 1969, a conference on hospital discharge abstract systems was sponsored jointly by the **National Center for Health Statistics** (NCHS), the National Center for Health Services Research and Development, and the Johns Hopkins University. Conference participants recommended that all short-term general hospitals in the United States collect a minimum set of patient-specific data elements. They also recommended that these data elements be reflected in all databases formulated from hospital discharge abstract systems. They called the list of patient-specific data items the **Uniform Hospital Discharge Data Set** (UHDDS).

In 1974, the federal government adopted the UHDDS as the standard for collecting data for the Medicare and Medicaid programs. When the Prospective Payment Act was enacted in 1983, UHDDS definitions were incorporated into the rules and regulations for implementing diagnosis-related groups (DRGs). The **National Committee on Vital and Health Statistics** (NCVHS) revised the UHDDS in 1984. The new UHDDS was adopted for all federal health programs in 1986.

The intent of the UHDDS is to list and define a set of common, uniform data elements. The data elements are to be collected in the health records of every hospital inpatient. They are subsequently abstracted from the health record and included in databases that describe aggregate patient characteristics. Most short-term, general hospitals in the United States collect patient-specific data in the format recommended by the UHDDS.

The UHDDS has been revised several times since 1986. The current version includes the recommended data elements shown in figure 7.1, p. 124.

Uniform Ambulatory Care Data Set

Ambulatory care includes medical and surgical care provided to patients who return to their homes on the same day they receive the care. It is provided in physicians' offices, medical clinics, same-day surgery centers, outpatient hospital clinics and diagnostic departments, emergency treatment centers, and hospital emergency departments. Patients who receive ambulatory care services in hospital-based clinics and departments are referred to as **outpatients.** (Patients who are admitted to hospitals for overnight stays are referred to as **inpatients.**)

Since the 1980s, the number and the length of inpatient hospitalizations have declined dramatically. At the same time, the number of healthcare procedures performed in ambulatory settings has increased. There are several reasons for this trend, including:

- Technological improvements in diagnostic and therapeutic procedures and the development of short-acting anesthetics have made it possible to perform many medical and surgical procedures in ambulatory facilities. Surgical procedures that once required inpatient

Figure 7.1.   UHDDS Data Elements

Data Element	Definition/Descriptor
01. Personal identifier	The unique number assigned to each patient within a hospital that distinguishes the patient and his or her hospital record from all others in that institution.
02. Date of birth	Month, day, and year of birth. Capture of the full four-digit year of birth is recommended.
03. Sex	Male or female
04. Race and ethnicity	04a. Race American Indian/Eskimo/Aleut Asian or Pacific Islander Black White Other race Unknown 04b. Ethnicity Spanish origin/Hispanic Non-Spanish origin/Non-Hispanic Unknown
05. Residence	Full address of usual residence Zip code (nine digits, if available) Code for foreign residence
06. Hospital identification	A unique institutional number used across data collection systems. The Medicare provider number is the preferred hospital identifier.
07. Admission date	Month, day, and year of admission.
08. Type of admission	Scheduled: Arranged with admissions office at least 24 hours prior to admission Unscheduled: All other admissions
09. Discharge date	Month, day, and year of discharge
10 & 11. Physician identification • Attending physician • Operating physician	The Medicare unique physician identification number (UPIN) is the preferred method of identifying the attending physician and operating physician(s) because it is uniform across all data systems.
12. Principal diagnosis	The condition established, after study, to be chiefly responsible for occasioning the admission of the patient to the hospital for care.
13. Other diagnoses	All conditions that coexist at the time of admission or that develop subsequently or that affect the treatment received and/or the length of stay. Diagnoses that relate to an earlier episode and have no bearing on the current hospital stay are to be excluded.
14. Qualifier for other diagnoses	A qualifier is given for each diagnosis coded under "other diagnoses" to indicate whether the onset of the diagnosis preceded or followed admission to the hospital. The option "uncertain" is permitted.
15. External cause-of-injury code	The ICD-9-CM code for the external cause of an injury, poisoning, or adverse effect (commonly referred to as an E code). Hospitals should complete this item whenever there is a diagnosis of an injury, poisoning, or adverse effect.
16. Birth weight of neonate	The specific birth weight of a newborn, preferably recorded in grams.
17. Procedures and dates	All significant procedures are to be reported. A significant procedure is one that is: • Surgical in nature, or • Carries an anesthetic risk, or • Carries a procedural risk, or • Requires specialized training. The date of each significant procedure must be reported. When more than one procedure is reported, the principal procedure must be designated. The principal procedure is one that is performed for definitive treatment rather than one performed for diagnostic or exploratory purposes or was necessary to take care of a complication. If two procedures appear to be principal, the one most closely related to the principal diagnosis should be selected as the principal procedure. The UPIN must be reported for the person performing the principal procedure.
18. Disposition of the patient	• Discharged to home (excludes those patients referred to home health service) • Discharged to other healthcare facility • Discharged to acute care hospital • Left against medical advice • Discharged to nursing facility • Alive, other; or alive, not stated • Discharged home to be under the care of a home health service (including a hospice) • Died All categories for primary and other sources are: • Blue Cross/Blue Shield • Health maintenance organization (HMO) • Other health insurance companies • CHAMPUS • Other liability insurance • CHAMPVA • Medicare • Other government payers • Medicaid • Self-pay • Worker's Compensation • No charge (free, charity, special research, teaching) • Self-insured employer plan • Other
19. Patient's expected source of payment	Primary source Other sources
20. Total charges	All charges billed by the hospital for this hospitalization. Professional charges for individual patient care by physicians are excluded.

hospitalization and long recovery periods are now being performed in same-day surgery centers.

- Third-party payers have extended coverage to include most procedures performed on an outpatient basis.
- The **Medicare prospective payment system** limits reimbursement for inpatient care and, in effect, encourages the use of ambulatory and/or outpatient care as an alternative to more costly inpatient services.

Like hospitals, ambulatory care organizations depend on the availability of accurate data and information. A standardized data set to guide the content and structure of ambulatory health records and data collection systems in ambulatory care was needed.

In 1989, the National Committee on Vital and Health Statistics approved the **Uniform Ambulatory Care Data Set** (UACDS). The committee recommended its use in every facility where ambulatory care is delivered. Several of the data elements that make up the UACDS are similar to those used in the UHDDS. However, the UACDS also includes data elements specific to ambulatory care, such as the reason for the encounter with the healthcare provider. For example, the UACDS data elements that describe the personal identifier, residence, date of birth, gender, and race/ethnicity of the patient are the same as the definitions in the UHDDS. The purpose of keeping the same demographic data elements is to make it easier to compare data for inpatients and ambulatory patients in the same facility.

The UACDS also includes optional data elements to describe the patient's living arrangements and marital status. These data elements (shown in figure 7.2) are unique to the UACDS. Ambulatory care practitioners need information about the living conditions of their patients because patients and their families often need to manage at-home nursing care, for example, activity restrictions after a surgical procedure. Hospital staff provide such nursing services in acute care settings.

The goal of the UACDS is to improve data comparison in ambulatory and outpatient care settings. It provides uniform definitions that help providers to analyze patterns of care. The data elements in the UACDS are those most likely to be needed by a variety of users. Unlike the UHDDS, the UACDS has not been incorporated into federal regulations. Therefore, it is a recommended, rather than a required, data set.

Minimum Data Set for Long-Term Care and Resident Assessment Protocols

Uniform data collection is also important in the long-term care setting. **Long-term care** incorporates the healthcare services provided in residential facilities for individuals who are unable to live independently owing to chronic illness or disability. Long-term care facilities also provide dietary and social services as well as housing and nursing care.

For a long-term care facility to participate in the Medicare and Medicaid programs, the **Centers for Medicare and Medicaid Services** (CMS) (formerly, the Health Care Financing

Figure 7.2.   UACDS Data Elements

Data Element	Definition/Descriptor
Provider identification, address, type of practice	Provider identification: Include the full name of the provider as well as the unique physician identification number (UPIN). Address: The complete address of the provider's office. In cases where the provider has multiple offices, the location of the usual or principal place of practice should be given. Profession: • Physician, including specialty or field of practice • Other (specify)
Place of encounter	Specify the location of the encounter: • Private office • Clinic or health center • Hospital outpatient department • Hospital emergency department • Other (specify)
Reason for encounter	Includes, but is not limited to, the patient's complaints and symptoms reflecting his or her own perception of needs, provided verbally or in writing by the patient at the point of entry into the healthcare system or in the patient's own words recorded by an intermediary or provider at that time.
Diagnostic services	All diagnostic services of any type.
Problem, diagnosis, or assessment	Describes the provider's level of understanding and the interpretation of the patient's reasons for the encounter and all conditions requiring treatment or management at the time of the encounter.
Therapeutic services	List, by name, all services done or ordered: • Medical (including drug therapy) • Surgical • Patient education
Preventive services	List, by name, all preventive services and procedures performed at the time of encounter.

Disposition	The provider's statement of the next step(s) in the care of the patient. At a minimum, the following classification is suggested:
	
	1. No follow-up planned
	2. Follow-up planned
	  • Return when necessary
	  • Return to the current provider at a specified time
	  • Telephone follow-up
	  • Return to referring provider
	  • Refer to other provider
	  • Admit to hospital
	  • Other

Administration [HCFA]) require the development of a comprehensive functional assessment for every resident. From this assessment, a nursing home resident's plan of care is developed.

The **Minimum Data Set for Long-Term Care—Version 2.0** (MDS 2.0) is a federally mandated standard assessment form used to collect demographic and clinical data on nursing home residents. It consists of a core set of screening and assessment elements based on common definitions. To meet federal requirements, long-term care facilities must complete an MDS for every resident at the time of admission and at designated reassessment points throughout the resident's stay.

The MDS uses some of the same data elements and definitions used in other data sets. However, it is far more extensive and includes more clinical data than either the UHDDS or the UACDS. The data collected via the MDS are used to develop care plans for residents and to document placement at the appropriate level of care.

The MDS organizes data according to twenty main categories. Each category includes a structured list of choices and/or responses. The use of structured lists automatically standardizes the data that are collected. The major categories of data collected in the MDS include:

- Demographic information
- Identification and background information
- Cognitive patterns
- Communication/hearing patterns
- Vision patterns
- Mood and behavior patterns
- Psychosocial well-being
- Physical functioning and structural problems
- Continence in past fourteen days
- Disease diagnoses
- Health conditions
- Oral/nutritional status
- Oral/dental status
- Skin condition
- Activity pursuit patterns
- Medications
- Special treatments and procedures
- Discharge potential and overall status
- Assessment information
- Therapy supplement for Medicare PPS

The data collected via the MDS are used to develop a **Resident Assessment Protocol** (RAP) summary for each resident. The MDS provides a structured way to organize resident information and develop a resident care plan. Problems identified through the assessment process are documented, and a RAP is triggered. For each triggered RAP, the facility must describe the following factors:

- Nature of the condition (may include presence or lack of objective data and subjective complaints)

- Complications and risk factors that affect the decision to proceed to care planning
- Factors that must be considered in developing individualized care plan interventions
- Need for referrals/further evaluation by appropriate healthcare professionals

Nursing home personnel use the data from the MDS and RAP to plan, carry out, and assess the care given to individual residents.

Other practice settings, such as rehabilitation and post-acute care, are considering versions of the MDS for use in patient assessment, but none has been implemented to date. Modifications to the MDS are expected with implementation of MDS Version 3.0, anticipated in 2003.

Data Elements for Emergency Department Systems

Emergency and trauma care in the United States has become very sophisticated over the past few decades. Emergency services represent a significant part of the healthcare delivery system. As emergency and trauma care services have been developed, it has become increasingly important to collect relevant aggregate data. Many states require the reporting of trauma cases to state agencies.

In 1997, the Centers for Disease Control and Prevention (CDC) published a data set called **Data Elements for Emergency Department Systems** (DEEDS). This data set was developed with input from the American College of Emergency Physicians, the Emergency Nurses Association, and the American Health Information Management Association. Its stated purpose is to support the uniform collection of data in hospital-based emergency departments.

DEEDS recommends the collection of 156 data elements in hospitals that offer emergency care services. As with the UHDDS and UACDS, this data set contains recommendations on both the content and the structure of the data elements to be collected. The data are organized into the following eight sections:

- Patient identification data
- Facility and practitioner identification data
- Emergency department payment data
- Emergency department arrival and first-assessment data
- Emergency department history and physical examination data
- Emergency department procedure and result data
- Emergency department medication data
- Emergency department disposition and diagnosis data

Essential Medical Data Set

The **Essential Medical Data Set** (EMDS) was created as a complement to DEEDS. It was developed as part of the **National Information Infrastructure—Health Information**

Network Program (NII-HIN) in 1997. The EMDS gives healthcare providers a concise medical history data set for each individual patient. The goal is to enhance the effectiveness of emergency care. The EMDS is different from DEEDS. DEEDS is designed to collect data about a specific emergency encounter; EMDS is designed to create a health history for an individual patient.

The EMDS is intended for use in electronic and computer-based health record systems. During the course of an emergency, the emergency department's information system queries a data repository for the patient's past medical history. The documentation for the visit is recorded according to the DEEDS format, and the data are sent to a regional data repository when the emergency care episode is complete.

Emergency care often has a critical impact on patient survival. Therefore, it is important to collect standardized, comparable data. These data then can be used to assess the effectiveness of treatment modalities, response time, and patient survival rates.

Trauma registries and statewide trauma database systems have grown incrementally over the past several years. State departments of public health as well as the federal agencies involved in oversight of emergency care are interested in statistical data about the efficacy of emergency treatment.

Health Plan Employer Data and Information Set

The **Health Plan Employer Data and Information Set** (HEDIS) is sponsored by the **National Committee for Quality Assurance** (NCQA). HEDIS is a set of standard performance measures designed to provide purchasers and consumers of healthcare with the information they need for comparing the performance of managed healthcare plans. The most recent version, called HEDIS 2000, was released in 1999.

HEDIS is designed to collect administrative and claims data as well as health record review data. The data are used to analyze and assess the outcomes of treatment. HEDIS focuses specifically on how effectively health plans improve the functional status of patients.

HEDIS contains more than fifty measures related to conditions such as heart disease, cancer, diabetes, asthma, chlamydia infection, smoking cessation, and menopause counseling. It includes data related to patient outcomes in addition to data about the treatment process used by the clinician in treating the patient.

Standardized HEDIS data elements are abstracted from health records in clinics and hospitals. The health record data are combined with enrollment and claims data and analyzed according to HEDIS specifications.

The purpose of HEDIS is to collect standardized data about specific health-related conditions or issues so that the success of various treatment plans can be assessed and compared. HEDIS data form the basis of performance improve-

ment efforts for health plans. HEDIS data also are used to develop physician profiles. The goal of physician profiling is to positively influence physician practice patterns.

Examples of HEDIS clinical measures include:

- Adolescent immunizations
- Smoking cessation programs
- Antidepressant medication management
- Breast cancer screening
- Cholesterol screening after a heart attack
- Prenatal care during the first trimester

Data from HEDIS studies are often released publicly by health plans to document substantial positive effects on the health of their clients. Results are compared over time and with data from other sources. From the data, health plans determine opportunities for performance improvement and develop potential interventions.

HEDIS is an example of a population-based data collection tool. It illustrates the need for developing standardized data definitions and uniform collection methods. It also emphasizes the importance of data quality management.

Core Measures for ORYX

The **Joint Commission on Accreditation of Healthcare Organizations** (JCAHO) is one of the largest users of healthcare data and information. Its primary function is the **accreditation** of hospitals and other healthcare organizations. In 1997, the JCAHO introduced the **ORYX initiative** to integrate outcomes data and other performance measurement data into its accreditation processes. (The initiative was named ORYX after an African animal that can be thought of as a different kind of zebra.) The goal of the initiative is to foster a comprehensive, continuous, data-driven accreditation process for healthcare facilities.

The ORYX initiative uses nationally standardized performance measures to improve the safety and quality of healthcare. The program's objectives include:

- Establishing a national comparative database to support benchmarking, health services research, and internal performance improvement activities
- Fostering standardization of performance measures
- Encouraging the use of evidence-based treatment protocols

The five **core measures** to be implemented by the JCAHO as part of the ORYX initiative include:

- Acute myocardial infarction (including coronary artery disease)
- Heart failure
- Pneumonia (community acquired)
- Surgical procedures and complications
- Pregnancy and related conditions (including newborn and maternal care)

The goal of the ORYX initiative is to develop data sets for each core measure so that data collection can be standardized among all healthcare facilities.

The core measurement set will include the minimum number of data elements needed to provide an accurate and reliable measure of performance. Core measures will rely on data elements that are readily available or already collected. Data elements, core measurement sets, and measures will be clearly defined in understandable terms.

An example of data collected for the ORYX initiative is the core measurement set for acute myocardial infarction. Data elements for the following areas will be collected:

- Smoking cessation advice/counseling
- Intrahospital mortality
- Mortality within thirty days after an acute myocardial infarction
- Time from arrival to initiation of reperfusion therapy
- Administration of beta blocker at arrival
- Prescription for beta blocker at discharge
- Lipid profile
- Prescription for aspirin at discharge
- Administration of aspirin at arrival
- Patients with a left ventricular ejection fraction lower than 40 percent prescribed ace inhibitor at discharge
- Cholesterol management

Outcomes and Assessment Information Set

In 1999, the Health Care Financing Administration (HCFA) (renamed the Centers for Medicare and Medicaid Services [CMS]) implemented a standardized data set for use in the home health industry. The **Outcomes and Assessment Information Set** (OASIS) is designed to gather data about Medicare beneficiaries who are receiving services from a home health agency. OASIS includes a set of core data items that are collected on all adult home health patients. The data are used in measuring patient outcomes in order to assess the quality of home healthcare services. Under the prospective payment program for home health, which was implemented in 2000, data from OASIS also form the basis of reimbursement for provided services.

OASIS data are grouped into the following categories:

- Demographics and Patient History
- Living Arrangements
- Supportive Assistance
- Respiratory
- Neurological
- Psychological
- Integument
- Pain
- Activities of Daily Living (ADLs)/Instrumental Activities of Daily Living (IADLs)
- Medications
- Elimination Status
- General Information
- Emergent Care

Data collected through OASIS are used to assess the patient's ability to be discharged or transferred from home care services and to evaluate the quality and outcome of services given to the patient.

The standardized collection of common data elements can provide valuable information about the effectiveness of interventions and treatments for specific diseases. Healthcare facilities can compare their success rates with those of other facilities to determine areas for performance improvement. This type of analysis can provide critical information that may eventually have a positive impact on clinical outcomes.

Check Your Understanding 7.1

Instructions: Answer the following questions on a separate piece of paper.

1. What is the difference between patient-specific data and aggregate data?

2. Why is it important for data from various sources to be defined in a standardized or uniform way?

3. How does a data set make it possible to standardize data in healthcare organizations?

4. What organization took the lead in developing a minimum data set for hospitals?

5. What factors led to the movement to develop uniform data sets in healthcare?

6. What role has the growth of technology played in the development of data sets?

7. Why was it necessary to develop a new data set for ambulatory care facilities? Why was the UHDDS inadequate in the ambulatory care setting?

8. What data elements are different in the UACDS compared to the UHDDS?

9. What organization sponsored the development of the UACDS?

10. In what way is the use of the MDS for Long-Term Care different from the use of either the UHDDS or the UACDS?

11. How does the MDS indicate potential problems that must be addressed by the nursing home patient's caregivers?

12. What organization mandates the use of the MDS for Long-Term Care?

13. Why is it important to have a specific data set for use in emergency departments? Why is the UHDDS inadequate in this type of setting?

14. What is the primary difference between DEEDS and the EMDS?

15. How are aggregate data about emergency and trauma care used?

16. What is the common purpose for the use of data generated through HEDIS, ORYX, and OASIS?

17. Which organizations sponsor HEDIS, ORYX, and OASIS?

18. Why does each of these outcomes measurement systems focus on the collection of clinical data elements in their databases?

Standards for Electronic Data and Electronic Data Interchange

The National Center for Vital and Health Statistics (NCVHS) has led the development of standardized data sets since the early 1960s. The data sets developed by the NCVHS have become standards for data collection in specific sites of care such as hospitals, ambulatory care clinics, and long-term care facilities.

Although the NCVHS uniform data sets have been the industry standard for data collection, they were created for use in paper-based (manual) health record systems. They were not designed to accommodate the data needs of the current healthcare delivery system or the demands of CPR systems. To fulfill current demands for information, universal standards are needed in the areas of health record content and structure; uniform vocabulary; electronic data interchange (EDI); and data confidentiality, privacy, and security.

Data Needs in a Computer-Based Environment

Healthcare organizations often have several different data-processing and computer systems operating at the same time. For example, a hospital's laboratory system might be entirely separate from its billing system. In fact, the various departments of large healthcare organizations often use different operating systems and are serviced by different vendors.

Healthcare organizations must integrate data that originate in various databases within facilities as well as in databases outside the facility. They also must be able to respond to requests to transfer data to other facilities via EDI. These goals can only be accomplished when every database system is operating on the same platform or using common standards. It is impractical to require all systems to use a common operating platform; thus, the adoption of information/data standards is the method of choice for facilitating communication across information systems.

Healthcare Informatics Standards

Healthcare informatics standards describe accepted methods for collecting, maintaining, and/or transferring healthcare data between computer systems. Standards use common definitions for data elements so that data can be linked from one system to another. For example, a **unique physician identification number** (UPIN) used to identify a specific physician makes it possible to transmit data about that physician from one system to another. Standards are the key to exchanging data throughout the healthcare delivery system.

Health informatics standards fall into four categories: vocabulary standards, structure and content standards, transaction/messaging standards, and security standards.

Vocabulary Standards

Vocabulary standards establish common definitions for medical terms to encourage consistent descriptions of an individual's condition in the health record. Medical terminology is extremely complex, and establishing medical vocabulary standards is a challenging task. Various synonymous medical terms are often used in different areas of the country. In fact, medical terminology can vary among physicians working in the same organization, depending on where and when each physician was trained and which medical specialty he or she practices. For example, one physician might describe a patient's diagnosis as Parkinson's disease, another might describe it as Parkinsonism, and a third might use the term *paralysis agitans*. All three terms are correct, but using the terms interchangeably would adversely affect data quality. In addition, data comparison among the physicians' patients would be very difficult, if not impossible.

The use of clinical classification codes (for example, CPT and ICD-9-CM codes) to represent health-related conditions and procedures is common in healthcare. The use of standardized, uniform terminology is critical to accurate coding. Vocabulary standards not only provide guidance in code selection, but they also set the stage for future automated coding systems.

Structure and Content Standards

Structure and content standards establish the data elements to be collected and provide clear descriptions of the data elements to be included in CPR systems. Moreover, they specify the type of data to be collected in each data field, the width of each data field, and the content of each data field.

For example, **Standard E1384** from the **American Society for Testing and Materials** (ASTM) defines the content and structure for computer-based health records. This standard was developed to fulfill five goals:

- To identify the content and structure of computer-based patient records
- To define the relationships of data coming from diverse source data systems
- To provide a common vocabulary, perspective, and references for those developing or using CPRs
- To describe examples of a variety of data views by which the logical data structure might be accessed or displayed
- To relate the logical structure of the CPR to the documentation currently used in health records

ASTM Standard E1384 identifies basic information categories for health records and organizes the categories into segments. Specific data content is then identified for each segment. Part of the E1384 data administration category is illustrated in figure 7.3, p. 130.

Transaction Standards

Transaction standards facilitate **electronic data interchange** (EDI). EDI is the exchange of data between two or more independent computer systems. Transaction standards, sometimes referred to as message format standards, transmission standards, or communication standards, establish a format and sequence of data during electronic transmission.

One of the purposes of the HIPAA Administrative Simplification rules is to standardize information exchange and in August of the year 2000, the Department of Health and Human Services (HHS) published regulations for electronic transactions. These regulations apply to transactions that occur between healthcare providers and healthcare plans and payers (Rode 2001). The long-term goal of the transaction standards is to allow providers and plans or payers to seamlessly transfer data back and forth with little intervention. To do this, HHS has adopted the electronic transactions standards

Figure 7.3.   Example of E1384 Content and Structure Standard

Category: Administrative Data

Segment 1: Demographics

These are personal data elements, sufficient to identify the patient, collected from the patient or patient representative and not related to health status of services provided. Some elements may require updating at each encounter or episode and must satisfy various national standards and regulations such as JCAHO standards, Conditions of Participation for Medicare, UHDDS, UACDS, and LTCDS.

Sample Data Elements:

1.01   Name of patient
1.02   Multiple birth marker
1.030   Unique identification number
.
.
.
1.06   Date of birth
1.07   Place of birth

Segment 3: Financial Elements

These are identifying data elements on all parties responsible for payment of patient healthcare services.

3.01   Primary payment source (may include address)
3.02   Insurance group number
3.03   Insurance identification number

ASC X12 (Accredited Standards Committee X12) and NCPDP (National Council for Prescription Drug Programs).

Electronic data interchange (EDI) is the electronic transfer of information, such as health claims transmitted electronically, in a standard format between trading partners. EDI originated when a number of industries identified cost savings through the electronic transmission of business information. They were convinced that the standardization of formatted information was the most effective means of communicating with multiple trading partners. EDI allows entities within the healthcare system to exchange medical, billing, and other information and to process transactions in a manner that is fast and cost-effective. With EDI there is a substantial reduction in handling and processing time compared to paper, and the risk of lost paper documents is eliminated. EDI also can eliminate the inefficiencies of handling paper documents, which would significantly reduce administrative burden, lower operating costs, and improve overall data quality.

The **American National Standards Institute** (ANSI) coordinates voluntary standards in the United States. Many standards developers and participants support ANSI as the central body responsible for the identification of a single consistent set of voluntary standards called American National Standards. ANSI provides an open forum for all concerned interests to identify specific business needs, plan to meet those needs, and agree on standards. Although ANSI itself does not develop standards, its approval of standards does indicate that the principles of openness and due process have been followed in the approval process and that a con-

sensus of those participating in the approval process has been achieved.

In 1979, ANSI chartered a new committee, known as the **Accredited Standards Committee (ASC) X12, Electronic Data Interchange** (referred to as ASC X12). The charge of the committee is to develop uniform standards for the electronic interchange of business transactions. The work of ASC X12 is conducted primarily by a series of subcommittees and task groups whose major function is the development of new, and the maintenance of existing, EDI standards. The standards adopted for EDI are called ANSI ASC X12N and include:

• Professional/institutional X12N 837 Healthcare Claim Transactions, version 4010
• X12N 837 Coordination of Benefits (COB) transactions
• X12N 835 Health Care Claim (HCC) Payment/Advice (or remittance advice, RA) transactions

To implement the HIPAA administrative simplification provisions, the above transaction standards are included under part 162 of title 45 of the **Code of Federal Regulations** (CFR) as the standard for processing electronic healthcare claims, coordination of benefits, and **remittance advice** (RA) transmissions. All other formats for electronic healthcare claims, **coordination of benefits** (COB) **transactions,** and remittance advice (RA) transmissions will become obsolete for submission of claims data, exchange of COB data, and submission of remittance data within two years after the effective date of the publication of part 162 in the *Federal Register.* Under federal law, most providers have two years to comply with each set of HIPAA standards after the final rule is published (small health plans have an additional year to comply). For most providers, compliance is required by October 2003 for the electronic transaction rule.

The NCPDP standards govern transmission of prescription information from pharmacies to payers for prescription management and for receiving approval and payment information in return.

The Administrative Simplification rule of the 1996 HIPAA legislation mandated compliance with transaction standards by all healthcare entities. In December 2001, the Administrative Simplification Compliance Act provided the opportunity for delaying compliance with HIPAA transaction requirements until October 2003 (Amatayakul 2002). The purpose of the extension is to allow healthcare facilities to have a compliance plan in place by April 2003 to fully comply with the HIPAA standards.

Security Standards

Security standards ensure that patient-identifiable health information remains confidential and protected from unauthorized disclosure, alteration, or destruction. Effective security standards are especially important in computer-based environments because patient information is accessible to many users in many locations.

The **Health Insurance Portability and Accountability Act of 1996** (HIPAA) mandated the adoption of security standards, including administrative procedures, physical safeguards, and technical security mechanisms. Many standards organizations—most notably, the ASTM and **Health Level Seven** (HL7)—have developed security standards, but no single standard currently addresses all of the HIPAA provisions. The **Department of Health and Human Services** (HHS) developed a comprehensive security standard for electronic health data, but it has not yet been adopted. (The security and privacy provisions of HIPAA are discussed in detail in chapters 10 and 11.)

Standards Development

Many organizations are involved in the development of healthcare informatics standards. These organizations are referred to as **standards development organizations** (SDOs). Both private organizations and government agencies are involved in the process of developing standards. Many standards are created through a voluntary consensus process that involves identifying the need for a standard, negotiating the content of the standard, and drafting a proposed standard. The final standard is published after undergoing a comment and revision period.

A number of organizations play key roles in coordinating standards development. They do not develop standards but, rather, coordinate the efforts of other SDOs. The **American National Standards Institute** (ANSI) coordinates the development of voluntary standards in a variety of industries, including healthcare. Most SDOs in the United States are members of the ANSI. The **Health Information Standards Board** (HISB) is a subgroup of the ANSI that acts as an umbrella organization for groups interested in developing healthcare computer messaging standards.

The **United Nations International Standards Organization** (ISO) coordinates international standards development. The ANSI represents the United States at the ISO.

Many organizations are involved in the process of setting standards within specific industries and areas of expertise. The U.S. healthcare industry is no exception. Table 7.1 (p. 132) provides a list of the organizations that are actively involved in developing standards for health-related information management. The ISO has several healthcare-related committees working on standards development for the healthcare industry.

Many private and government organizations influence the development of standards by taking positions on proposed standards and setting policies that lend credibility to standards. The government agencies that influence standards development include the Centers for Medicare and Medicaid Services (formerly, the Health Care Financing Administration), which is the overseer of the Medicare/Medicaid programs; the Food and Drug Administration (FDA); the Agency for Health Care Policy and Research (AHCPR); and the National Center for Health Statistics (NCHS).

Check Your Understanding 7.2

Instructions: Answer the following questions on a separate piece of paper.

1. What is the difference between a data set and a healthcare informatics standard?

2. What changes in the healthcare industry have prompted the focus on developing healthcare informatics standards?

3. How would ASTM Standard E1384 be helpful during the development of a computer-based patient record system?

4. What SDOs have been most active in developing structure and content standards for computer-based patient records?

5. What is the role of the ANSI, HISB, and ISO in developing healthcare informatics standards?

New and Evolving Standards

The development of healthcare informatics standards is far from complete. The Health Insurance Portability and Accountability Act of 1996 mandated adoption of privacy and security standards for health information. Leading standards groups are continuously working to reach consensus on a variety of standards, but many issues are still to be resolved.

Identifier Standards

Identifier standards recommend methods for assigning unique identification numbers to individuals, including patients, healthcare providers (for example, physicians and dentists), corporate providers (healthcare organizations), and healthcare vendors and suppliers. Identifiers usually use a combination of numeric or alphanumeric characters such as a hospital number or a billing number. At present, most identifiers are used only within one facility or within a single healthcare system. HIPAA regulations will require the development of unique identification numbers that can be used across information systems.

It is generally agreed that unique identification numbers are needed for patients, but there is no consensus on the method of identification. Much of the controversy relates to the use of the **Social Security number** (SSN) as the identifier for patients. Many groups favor use of the SSN because it is an existing number and most U.S. citizens either have or can easily obtain one.

Opponents object to using the SSN as a unique identification number because of privacy concerns. Social Security numbers are widely used for purposes unrelated to healthcare, and it is relatively easy to discover an individual's SSN in public documents such as motor vehicle records. Many experts believe that unauthorized users would use SSNs to find and access the health records of specific individuals. Another problem with use of the SSN is the simple fact that the Social Security Administration has not approved its use as a unique identification number, and this use does not fit the categories of usage it has already approved.

Table 7.1.   Standards Development Organizations

Organization	Types of Standards	Description
Accredited Standards Committee X12 Data Interchange Standards Association (DISA) 333 John Carlyle Street, Suite 600 Alexandria, VA 22314 Telephone: (703) 548-7005 www.disa.org	Electronic data interchange for billing transactions The committee's particular area of focus has been computer-to-computer communications between healthcare providers and third-party payers	Chartered in 1979 by ANSI, the X12N subcommittee develops and maintains X12 standards, interpretations, and guidelines. X12N is one of the standards for EDI that is specified in the regulations of the Health Insurance Portability and Accountability Act of 1996. Subgroups of X12N include: *WEDI: Workgroup on Electronic Data Exchange* WEDI has been the prime mover in the development of insurance industry standards. In 1995, WEDI became a private standards advocacy group. *HIBCC: Health Industry Business Communications Council*
American College of Radiology—National Electrical Manufacturers Association (ACR-NEMA) American College of Radiology 1891 Preston White Drive Reston, VA 20191 Telephone: (703) 648-8900 www.acr.org National Electrical Manufacturers Association 1300 N. Seventeenth Street, Suite 1847 Rosslyn, VA 22209 Telephone: (703) 841-3200 www.nema.org	Exchange of digitized images	ACR is a professional association, and NEMA is a trade association. They have worked collaboratively to develop the Digital Imaging and Communications in Medicine (DICOM) standard, which promotes a digital image communications format and facilitates development by the American College of Radiology of picture archive and communications systems. DICOM may be used for electronic exchange of X rays, computed tomography (CT), magnetic resonance imaging (MRI), ultrasound, nuclear medicine, and other radiology images. Work is under way to support other diagnostic images.
American Society for Testing and Materials (ASTM) 100 Barr Harbor Drive West Conshohocken, PA 19428 Telephone: (610) 832-9585 www.astm.org	Multiple health informatics standards, including clinical content of patient records, exchange of messages about clinical observations, data security and integrity, healthcare identifiers, data modeling, clinical laboratory systems, Arden syntax (a coding system), and system functionality	Organized in 1898, the ASTM is one of the largest SDOs in the world. It provides a forum for vendors, users, consumers, and others to develop standards for a wide range of materials, products, systems, and services. It is composed of more than 140 subcommittees or working groups identified as E31 and E32. Since 1990, Committee E31 on Healthcare Informatics has developed standards for health information and health information systems. Standard E1384, discussed earlier, is a product of the E31 subcommittee of ASTM.
Health Level Seven (HL7) 3300 Washtenaw Avenue, Suite 227 Ann Arbor, MI 48104 Telephone: (734) 677-7777 www.hl7.org	Electronic interchange of clinical, financial, and administrative information among disparate health information systems	HL7 is an ANSI-accredited SDO. Level 7 refers to the highest level of the Open System Interconnection (OSI) model of the International Standards Organization. The HL7 standard addresses issues that occur within the seventh, or application, layer.
Institute of Electrical and Electronics Engineers (IEEE) 445 Hoes Lane P.O. Box 1331 Piscataway, NJ 08855-1331 Telephone: (732) 981-0060 www.ieee.org	Medical device information and general informatics format	The IEEE's Medical Data Interchange Standard (MEDIX) is a standard set of hospital system interface transactions based on the ISO standards for all seven layers of the OSI model. Another IEEE standard for a medical information bus (MIB) links bedside instruments in critical care with health information systems.
National Council on Prescription Drug Programs (NCPDP) 4201 N. Twenty-fourth Street, Suite 365 Phoenix, AZ 85016 Telephone: (602) 957-9105 www.ncpdp.org	Data interchange and processing standards for pharmacy transactions	The NCPDP has defined standards for transmitting prescription information from pharmacies to payers for prescription management services and for receiving approval and payment information back in near-real time. Other standards address adverse drug reactions and utilization review.

Adapted from Brandt 2000, p. 39.

The most commonly used provider identifier is the **unique physician identification number** (UPIN). The UPIN was originally created by HCFA for use by physicians who bill for services provided to Medicare patients. The Centers for Medicare and Medicaid Services (CMS) (formerly HCFA) is currently developing a **national provider file** (NPF) that will include all healthcare providers (including nonphysicians) and sites of care.

In 1993, HCFA initiated the National Provider Identification Initiative to develop a provider identification system to meet Medicare and Medicaid needs and, ultimately, the needs of all users. The workgroup investigated all existing identifiers and designed a new **national provider identifier** (NPI). The NPI uses an eight-character alphanumeric identifier. The CMS is working on implementing the NPI for the Medicare program.

Messaging, Transaction, and Communication Standards

The ability to transmit data from one computer system to another continues to be one of the greatest challenges in implementing CPR systems. Messaging, transaction, and communication standards are in various stages of development but have not been generally accepted by users.

The following communications and **transaction standards** are the most advanced and have formed the basis of the electronic transaction standards mandated by HIPAA:

- Accreditation Standards Committee X12 message format standards for transactions between providers and payers
- ASTM message format standards
- HL7 transaction standards

Many other transaction and communication standards are being developed to address billing and claims submission processes.

Vocabulary Standards and Clinical Data Representation (Codes)

The classification systems used to code medical diagnoses and procedures must be considered in the development of healthcare informatics standards. ICD-9-CM and CPT/HCPCS codes represent clinical information and are used to communicate patient-identifiable information between healthcare organizations and payers. Coded aggregate data also are communicated among healthcare organizations, researchers, policy makers, and government agencies. The ICD-9-CM and CPT/HCPCS systems are used most widely, but many other healthcare classifications systems have been developed.

The Codes and Structures Work Group of the **Computer-based Patient Record Institute** (CPRI) did an evaluation of clinical coding systems. This project evaluated eight major clinical classifications. None of the systems currently available appeared to fulfill every user's needs. The Systematized Nomenclature of Human and Veterinary Medicine International (SNOMED), however, demonstrated the highest score in all categories of the evaluation.

HIPAA requires implementation of standardized code sets as part of its mandate.

Privacy and Security Standards

Recent technological advances have made it possible to collect, store, and transmit enormous amounts of healthcare data. Healthcare organizations of all kinds must implement effective systems to protect the confidentiality, privacy, and security of their information systems. Privacy and security issues have been addressed at the national level by a variety of organizations. For example, the ASTM developed privacy and security standards through its Subcommittee E31.17.

The Health Insurance Portability and Accountability Act (HIPAA) contains provisions that address EDI and data security. The act specifically directs the HHS to protect the confidentiality and security of transmitted health information. The proposed HIPAA data security standards consider the following factors:

- Technical capabilities of record systems
- Costs of security measures
- Training people with access to health information about data confidentiality and security
- Value of audit trails

The intent of HIPAA is to improve the efficiency and effectiveness of the U.S. healthcare system by standardizing the electronic exchange of health information and at the same time maintaining its confidentiality and security. HIPAA regulations apply to every individual and facility involved in maintaining and transmitting patient-identifiable healthcare data and information. The full implementation of HIPAA will take several years. A full discussion of the HIPAA privacy rule is included in chapter 10.

Development of Extensible Markup Language (XML)

Recent advances in standards development have occurred in the area of extensible markup language (XML). XML was developed as a universal language to facilitate the storage and transmission of data published on the Internet. Markup languages communicate electronic representations of paper documents to computers by inserting additional information into text (Sokolowski 1999). The best known markup language is hypertext markup language (HTML), which is used to convert text documents into Internet-compatible format.

Pothen and Parmanto (2002) describe XML as "an easy-to-learn, standardized mark-up language with customizable tags that describe data within documents." In other words, XML provides a context for data through the use of a tag. In the context of health data, XML tags each item of data with a descriptor that differentiates, for example, between a number that is a Social Security number from a number that represents the medical record number. XML allows data to be communicated from one computerized system to another without losing the integrity of the data. In addition, according to Sokolowski, XML provides structure and rules that are "important for healthcare informatics because they will provide context for narrative text, a document information model, agreement on high level structures, and a facility for standardizing formats" (Sokolowski 1999, p. 22).

As computer-based patient records continue to evolve in somewhat disjointed manner (as described by Amatayakul in chapter 9), XML has the potential to solve some of the difficulties posed by the lack of standardized vocabulary and the need to transmit data among disparate computer systems. Some of the characteristics that make XML relevant to the development of a CPR were described by Pothen and Parmanto (2000):

- XML combined with existing classification systems such as ICD-9-CM can improve the completeness of health records by providing a clear description of the content of data in the record
- XML allows data in the health record to be organized in a meaningful and searchable form

XML also can serve as a standard for exchange of health information over the web because it is not impeded by disparate computer systems. A test project conducted in Canada utilized XML for data exchange among three remote health-related organizations that each used a different set of applications, databases, and technology. The organizations mapped each system to standard templates in XML and were able to seamlessly transfer data from one location to the other (Smith 2001). The implementation of XML within the healthcare industry has the potential to address many of the issues of both vocabulary and transmission.

Check Your Understanding 7.3

Instructions: Answer the following questions on a separate piece of paper.

1. What is the relationship between data standards and the coding of healthcare data?

2. What is the reason for creating a unique identification number for every healthcare consumer?

3. Why is use of the Social Security number as a unique identification number controversial?

4. What characteristics of XML make it a potential solution for many of the problems of storing and transmitting health information?

Real-World Case

According to a recent article published in *Modern Healthcare,* a Winona, Minnesota, healthcare system and a healthcare information company have developed a health information network that improves communication between patients and local physicians and other healthcare providers. The system relies on an already-existing high-speed network to provide interactive health records that can be used by local facilities,

physicians, pharmacies, and patients. Patients are able to make appointments, check their health records for test results, and communicate with their physicians via the Internet. Physicians also will be able to communicate with one another and with local hospitals, nursing homes, and clinics. The system was designed to ensure the security and confidentiality of data.

Because over 60 percent of Winona residents use the Internet, the population is well prepared to use this health network to improve healthcare. Residents who do not own computers will have access to computer labs in schools, libraries, and other public locations.

Baseline data for the project will be gathered through health risk assessments, and patients will gain access to the health information network via a sign-in process. The results of the health risk assessments will provide a baseline of data about the community and also allow the community to assess the impact of this project on its health status.

Discussion Questions

1. The Winona project is an example of the use of technology to link healthcare consumers with their care providers. What role do healthcare informatics standards play in this type of project?

2. As the Winona project links prescription data into the database, what standards development organization would be the best resource for guiding these pharmacy-based data?

3. Discuss the specific need for each of the following types of standards in this project: vocabulary standards, content and structure standards, messaging standards, and security standards.

4. Confidentiality, privacy, and security are of special concern when a large number of individuals access a database containing personally identifiable data. What sources would provide information that would be helpful in designing a data security program?

5. What role could a health information management professional play in the development of the Winona project?

6. Because this database links data from a variety of sites of care such as hospitals, nursing homes, and physicians' offices, what data sets should be used to define data elements? If data elements were defined differently in various data sets and/or healthcare informatics standards, which resource should take precedence in designing the system?

Summary

According to Brandt (2000), "the vision is clear: a longitudinal, or lifetime, health record for each person that is computer-based, secure, readily accessible when needed, and linked across the continuum of care [is needed]. In reality, we are a long way from that model." It is impossible to develop a longitudinal CPR that meets Brandt's specifications without standards that guide the development. The complexity of technology, the variations in computer platforms from one system to the next, and the differing (and sometimes conflicting) data needs of users demand flexible health data/information systems. The systems must be able to store volumes of data in a standardized format, communicate across vendor-specific systems, and keep data in a secure manner that protects individual privacy and information confidentiality.

The need for standardized data definitions was recognized in the 1960s, and the National Committee on Vital and Health Statistics took the lead in developing uniform minimum data sets for various sites of care. As technology has driven the development of the data/information systems, the early data sets have been supplemented with healthcare informatics standards that focus on computer-based data systems. A number of standards-setting organizations have been involved in developing uniform definitions, data fields, and views for health record content and structure. Standards for developing medical vocabularies, messaging/communications systems, and data/information security, privacy, and confidentiality are being created and implemented. These standards are dynamic and in constant development by various groups. Standards development generally takes place as a consensus-driven process among various interested parties. In most cases, implementation is voluntary.

Some data sets and standards have been incorporated into federal law and are thus required for use by affected healthcare organizations. For example, in 1983, the standardized definitions of the Uniform Hospital Discharge Data Set were incorporated into the Prospective Payment Act (PL98-603) and are still required for reporting inpatient data for reimbursement under the Medicare program.

The Health Insurance Portability and Accountability Act of 1996 mandated the incorporation of healthcare informatics standards into all electronic or computer-based health information systems. Of particular importance under HIPAA are transaction/messaging standards for communication of data across systems and security standards that protect individual privacy and confidentiality. The rules and regulations for HIPAA are still in development, and, to date, only the transaction and privacy standards have been finalized.

Work will continue on the development of healthcare informatics standards well into the twenty-first century. It is a complex task. The rapid growth of technology and the increasing need for healthcare data/information makes the task a daunting one.

References

Amatayakul, M. 2002. Practice brief: The transactions extension: no reason to procrastinate. *Journal of the American Health Information Management Association* 73(3):16A–C.

Brandt, M. D. 1999. Standards for EHR content, systems, and data exchange. In *Electronic Health Records: Changing the Vision,* G. F. Murphy et al., editors. Philadelphia: W. B. Saunders Company.

Brandt, M. D. 2000. Health informatics standards: a user's guide. *Journal of the American Health Information Management Association* 71(4):39–43.

Dougherty, M. 1999. Reimbursement. In *Long-Term Care Handbook: Resources for the Health Information Manager,* Teresa Ganser, editor. Chicago: American Health Information Management Association.

Linck, J. C. 1996. Patient and health care data. In *Health Information: Management of a Strategic Resource,* M. Abdelhak et al., editors. Philadelphia: W. B. Saunders Company.

Morissey, J. 2000. Minnesota town to get health data online. *Modern Healthcare,* June 12, 2000.

Murphy, G., and M. Brandt. 2001. Practice brief: Health informatics standards and information transfer: exploring the HIM role. *Journal of the American Health Information Management Association* 72(1):68A–D.

Peters, R. M. 2000. XML: defining the transition from paper to digital records. *Journal of the American Health Information Management Association* 71(1):34–38.

Pothen, D. J., and B. Parmanto. 2000. XML furthers CPR goals. *Journal of the American Health Information Management Association* 71(9):24–29.

Rulon, V., and J. Sica. 1997. The evolution of HEDIS: 3.0 and beyond. *Journal of the American Health Information Management Association* 68(6):32–39.

Rode, D. 2001. Understanding HIPAA transactions and code sets. *Journal of the American Health Information Management Association* 72(1):26–32.

Smith, D. A. 2001. Data transmission: a world of possibilities. *Journal of the American Health Information Management Association* 72(5):26–27.

Sokolowski, R. 1999. XML makes its mark. *Journal of the American Health Information Management Association* 70(10):21–24.

Application Exercises

1. Identify four data elements about yourself and/or another individual and convert them into information as shown in the following example:

   Data elements: Age: 32
   Gender: Female
   Height: 5 feet, 3 inches
   Weight: 152 pounds

   Information: The individual is overweight according to standardized height/weight charts.

2. Using four sample health records from an acute care facility, determine whether the facility is collecting data according to the Uniform Hospital Discharge Data Set.

3. Have a classmate play the role of a nursing home resident at the time of admission and conduct an interview on the basis of the Minimum Data Set for Long-Term Care. Use the data collected in the MDS to complete a Resident Assessment Protocol summary, and identify at least two RAP triggers. The current version of the MDS may be found at www.hcfa.gov/medicaid/mds/default.htm.

4. Use the library to access one article about an HEDIS outcomes study and one article about a core measure study using ORYX indicators. Summarize each of the articles in a one-page review.

5. Develop a table or grid that identifies relevant healthcare informatics standards that should be used to design a computer-based patient record (CPR) in an acute care setting. The CPR should include data from the following systems, and the data will be used for claims processing/billing as well as for patient care:

   - Clinical data from caregivers (for example, history and physical exam, nurse's notes, physician's progress notes, physician's orders, consultations, final diagnosis)
   - Pharmacy
   - Laboratory
   - Radiology
   - Emergency/trauma center (for patients admitted through the emergency department)
   - Coded data for statistics, research, and billing

6. Write a memo to the chief executive officer of a data committee to oversee implementation of healthcare informatics standards. In a maximum of one and one-half pages, persuade the CEO that the committee is needed.

Review Quiz

Instructions: Choose the answer that best completes the following statements.

1. ____ The name of the government agency that has led the development of basic data sets for health records and computer databases is the ____.
   a. Centers for Medicare and Medicaid Services
   b. Johns Hopkins University
   c. American National Standards Institute
   d. National Committee on Vital and Health Statistics

2. ____ The primary purpose of a minimum data set in healthcare is to ____.
   a. Recommend common data elements to be collected in health records
   b. Mandate all data that must be contained in a health record
   c. Define reportable data for federally funded programs
   d. Standardize medical vocabulary

3. ____ Data that are collected on large populations of individuals and stored in databases are referred to as ____.
   a. Statistics
   b. Information
   c. Aggregate data
   d. Standards

4. ____ The data set that has been incorporated into federal law and is required for Medicare reporting is the ____.
   a. Ambulatory Care Data Set
   b. Uniform Hospital Discharge Data Set
   c. Minimum Data Set for Long-Term Care
   d. Health Plan Employer Data and Information Set

5. ____ Both HEDIS and the JCAHO's ORYX program are designed to collect data to be used for ____.
   a. Performance improvement programs
   b. Billing and claims data processing
   c. Developing hospital discharge abstracting systems
   d. Developing individual care plans for residents

6. ____ ASTM Standard E1384 provides guidance to healthcare organizations in developing ____.
   a. Data security
   b. Medical vocabulary
   c. Transaction standards
   d. Content and structure of health records

7. ____ Standardizing medical terminology to avoid differences in naming various medical conditions and procedures (such as the synonyms *bunionectomy, McBride procedure,* and *repair of hallus valgus*) is one purpose of ____.
   a. Transaction standards
   b. Content and structure standards
   c. Vocabulary standards
   d. Security standards

8. ____ The federal law that directed the Secretary of Health and Human Services to develop healthcare standards governing electronic data interchange and data security is the ____.
   a. Medicare Act
   b. Prospective Payment Act
   c. Health Insurance Portability and Accountability Act
   d. Social Security Act

9. ____ The number that has been proposed for use as a unique patient identification number but is controversial because of confidentiality and privacy concerns is the ____.
   a. Social Security number
   b. Unique physician identification number
   c. Health record number
   d. National provider identifier

10. ____ Most healthcare informatics standards have been implemented by ____.
    a. Federal mandate
    b. Consensus
    c. State regulation
    d. Trade association requirement

Chapter 8
Paper-Based Health Records

Mary Cole McCain, MPA, RHIA

Learning Objectives

- To describe the traditional (paper-based) health record and to identify its primary uses and users
- To identify the organizations that publish standards on the content of the health record
- To describe the major content areas of the health record, including administrative and demographic data, clinical data, and specialized content
- To outline the flow of health record information from initial encounter to final format
- To contrast methods that providers use to contribute information to the health record
- To give examples of general requirements for the primary documentation required in most health records, including the history and physical, progress notes, orders, and discharge summary
- To define quantitative and qualitative record analysis
- To compare the purposes and advantages of the following processes: concurrent analysis and discharge analysis, open-record review, and closed-record review
- To compare an incomplete health record and a delinquent health record
- To identify forms and documentation requirements specific to facilities other than acute care hospitals, including ambulatory care, home care, hospice care, rehabilitation care, and long-term care facilities
- To explain the role of the health information management professional in the forms control program
- To compare internal and contract word-processing services
- To summarize how new developments in medical word processing, such as telecommuting and voice recognition technology, will change the role of the medical transcriptionist
- To define the unit, serial, and serial-unit systems of record numbering and filing and the appropriate use of each, including methods of number assignment
- To explain the basic rules of terminal digit filing and the reasons why it is used
- To describe policies and procedures on health record storage, retention, and destruction
- To define the functions of the master patient index

Key Terms

Administrative information
Advance directives
American Association for Medical Transcription (AAMT)
American College of Surgeons (ACS)
Authentication
Authorization
Autoauthentication
Bar coding
Bylaws
Care path
Case manager
Certified medical transcriptionist (CMT)
Chart tracking
Closed-record review
Closed records
Compliance
Concurrent analysis
Conditions of Participation
Consent
Consultation
Contract service
Delinquent health record
Demographic information
Digital dictation
Discharge analysis
Discharge summary
Disposition
Do not resuscitate (DNR) order
Electronic signature
Family numbering
Health Insurance Portability and Accountability Act of 1996 (HIPAA)
History

Incentive pay
Informed consent
Integrated health record
Licensure
Longitudinal record
Master patient index
Master population index
Medical transcriptionist
Medicare
Microfilming
Open-record review
Optical imaging
Outsourcing
Principal diagnosis
Problem-oriented health record (POMR)
Progress notes
Qualitative analysis
Quantitative analysis
Retention schedules
Scanning
Serial filing system
Serial numbering system
Serial-unit numbering system
Source-oriented health record
Telestaffing
Terminal-digit filing system
Transcription
Unique identifier
Unit filing system
Unit numbering system
Universal chart order
Universal patient identifier
Voice recognition technology
Word-processing services

Introduction

The patient health record is in the process of transition from a paper-based to a computer-based format. Indeed, most health-care facilities currently maintain their health records using a combination of the two formats in order to accommodate the many different ways in which patient information is provided. Today's health records include computer printouts as well as handwritten notes. Data now arrive via electronic transfer from computerized laboratory or radiological testing or examination, through direct voice entry into a word-processing system, and from provider wireless devices and/or handheld personal computers. But as this chapter describes, the paper-based health record is a long way from being obsolete.

This chapter traces the evolution of the health record and describes the different kinds of information it contains and the different formats in which it is kept. The chapter also focuses on the health information management professional's role in managing patient information, from the creation and storage of information to its long-term retention and eventual destruction, and in ensuring its accuracy, completeness, and security. Finally, the chapter describes the functions of the master patient index.

Theory into Practice

The director of health information management (HIM) at one hospital was promoted to the newly created position of HIM director for the corporate system, which involved oversight responsibility for HIM services at five facilities located within a single metropolitan area. The purpose of the new position was to standardize patient health record procedures and formats and to create the foundation for the transition to a paperless record system.

The system's leadership recognized that computerization would not solve all of its HIM problems. There first had to be an excellent manual system to computerize. At the largest facility, optical imaging technology had been purchased along with word-processing software to enable reports to upload directly into the imaging system. The laboratory and radiology results were entered into the system automatically.

The new director had to use her basic knowledge of HIM principles to assess the current systems in all five facilities. She found that although the facilities were a part of one system administratively, the individual HIM departments operated in different ways. The first phase of the process was to inventory forms and then standardize and index them so that records could be scanned into the imaging system immediately following patient discharge. This involved all of the HIM professionals at all five facilities working together as a team to review the forms. Imaging procedures then were implemented in all five facilities. The word-processing systems were standardized and upgraded, with experienced transcriptionists given the option of working from home. Further, all departmental policies and procedures were standardized for all five facilities. These myriad activities took three years to complete. When the Health Insurance Portability and Accountability Act (HIPAA) regulations were published, the focus of the job shifted from operational decisions for health information managers to the training of personnel in all five hospitals on the confidentiality and security of health information.

The HIM director's new job reflects the constant changes and opportunities for growth presented to many HIM professionals. Health information managers must be flexible and willing to grow professionally as technology changes the field and new challenges arise. The HIM professional's foundation knowledge is important to ensure that excellent documentation and records management processes are instituted and continued in the transition steps to a computer-based patient record.

Evolution of the Health Record

The paper-based patient health record has evolved as medicine and medical technology have evolved. Once simply the notation of the patient's name and a brief description of his or her illness or injury, the health record today is a detailed collection of handwritten entries, typed reports, and computer printouts reflecting the contributions of numerous healthcare providers.

Historical Overview

Health records have existed as long as there has been a need to communicate information about patient treatment. Archeological evidence indicates that maintaining information on patient care and treatment techniques is an ancient art.

Health records are maintained by all organizations that deliver health care including physician and provider offices, long-term care facilities, emergency clinics, rehabilitation facilities, home health, correctional institutions, and numerous types of delivery systems and organizations. Records vary depending on the type of facility. Healthcare records in acute care hospitals, for example, require rapid documentation by many providers. Patients are often in the hospital for life-threatening injuries or conditions, and many different providers access and record information in the patients' health records, on average, within a five-day time span. Although format and content of the health record may differ, all providers of care must maintain information to meet patient care needs and comply with relevant laws, standards, and regulations.

Today's HIM professional is responsible for records that contain more paper than ever before and are maintained in a variety of formats other than paper.

Documentation and Maintenance Standards for the Health Record

Health records provide proof of what has been done for the patient. As the complexity of care has evolved, so has the need for improved documentation. Standards for record documentation and maintenance have been established and are refined and revised constantly.

The American College of Surgeons and the Joint Commission on Accreditation of Healthcare Organizations

The **American College of Surgeons** (ACS) provided the impetus for standardizing health records when it developed minimum standards for hospitals early in the twentieth century. It was evident to the ACS that standards were needed because candidates for membership were unable to produce proof of their experience with various types of surgical cases. Records were either nonexistent or of poor quality. The ACS Minimum Standard of 1917 included specific requirements for maintaining patient health records. The Joint Commission on Accreditation of Healthcare Organizations (JCAHO) standards for documentation evolved from this original standard.

The JCAHO (formerly called the Joint Commission on Accreditation of Hospitals) is the successor organization to the ACS. It assumed responsibility for the accreditation process in 1952 as a joint effort of the ACS, the American College of Physicians, the American Medical Association, and the American Hospital Association. Initially responsible for the accreditation of hospitals, the JCAHO has since expanded its accreditation process to home health, long-term care, and other types of healthcare facilities.

The major source of information on the work of the hospital or any healthcare facility is the health record. JCAHO surveyors routinely review the health records of current patients to obtain knowledge about the facility's performance and process of care.

Medicare Conditions of Participation

The federal government passed **Medicare** legislation in 1965 to provide healthcare insurance coverage to Americans over sixty-five years of age. Since then, the legislation has been expanded to cover persons disabled for two years as well as persons with chronic kidney disease. The Centers for Medicare and Medicaid Services (CMS), until 2001 known as the Health Care Financing Administration (HCFA), is the division of the federal Department of Health and Human Services responsible for developing and enforcing regulations regarding the participation of healthcare providers in the Medicare program.

The Medicare regulations for health record content and documentation were originally established in the **Conditions of Participation.** As health record documentation became increasingly important, the CMS began to focus on reviewing it for medical necessity and **compliance** with the decision-making rules established by the federal government. In addition, the CMS published guidelines for documenting histories and physical examinations and medical decision making that affect physician reimbursement.

State Licensure

Every state has certain **licensure** regulations that healthcare facilities must meet in order to remain in operation. Licensure regulations may include very specific requirements for the content, format, retention, and use of patient records. These regulations are established by state governments, usually under the direction of state departments of health.

Internal Standards

Bylaws, rules, and regulations are developed by the medical staff and approved by the board of trustees or governing body in every type of healthcare facility. In addition to describing the organization's manner of operation, bylaws delineate the content of patient health records, the exact personnel who can write or enter information in health records, and restate applicable JCAHO and Medicare requirements. In addition, bylaws describe the time limits for completing patient health records. Surveyors review the bylaws to ensure that healthcare facilities abide by their own established rules and regulations and that the bylaws are in agreement with current JCAHO standards.

The Modern Health Record

The modern health record includes the contributions of numerous healthcare providers. In addition, it includes information provided by the patient or a person acting on his or her behalf describing the reasons for the patient's visit to the healthcare provider and other pertinent background facts. The modern health record is patient centered, meaning that the patient is the focus of all documentation on the activities that revolve around him or her while under the provider's care.

Definition of the Health Record

The information in the health record must outline and justify the patient's treatment, support diagnosis of the patient's condition, describe the patient's progress and response to medications and services, and explain the outcomes of the care provided. As documentation of all of the activities that revolve around the patient, the health record promotes continuity of care among all the providers who treat the patient.

The health record itself is the property of the healthcare facility. However, the patient has the right to be informed about the use of his or her personal health information.

Functions of Health Records and Health Information

To providers, the health record is valuable as the principal source of information in determining care for the patient. To the healthcare facility, it is valuable as a key source of information in determining the reimbursement for care.

The primary functions of the health record are:

- To facilitate the ongoing care and treatment of individual patients
- To support clinical decision making and communication among clinicians
- To document the services provided to patients in support of reimbursement
- To provide information for the evaluation of the quality and efficacy of the care provided
- To provide information in support of medical research and education

- To help facilitate the operational management of the facility
- To provide information as required by local and national laws and regulations

Ongoing Care and Treatment of Individual Patients

The most important use of the health record is patient care and the person to whom the record is of most value is the patient. The care and treatment of individual patients reflected in the record is of paramount importance.

When physicians were the only caregivers, they knew the patient and family and decided how detailed the patient's records needed to be. Often a small card or a ledger listing the patient's problem at a particular time was all the record keeping physicians needed. As healthcare has come to depend on technology and the skilled personnel to use it, health records have become more complex. Providers cannot remember all the information provided by the available technology, and fast access to past information about the patient's care is vital to the continuity of care.

Clinical Decision Making and Communication

Health information serves the vital function of allowing all the patient's providers to enter and analyze information and to make decisions. Each member of the healthcare team has equal access to the information and can review what others are doing and communicate with them through the record. Thus, the health record is the healthcare team's primary reference and communication tool.

Reimbursement

Information in the health record is used to document the services provided to the patient so that payment for the care provided can be made by those responsible for the bill. Insurance companies, managed care organizations, and Medicare require that specific information be submitted to support the bill and to prove that the care provided was medically necessary.

Evaluation of the Quality and Efficacy of Care

The health record is used as a legal document to prove the quality of care rendered by the healthcare provider. The documentation in the record provides information for accrediting and licensing activities.

Medical Research and Education

Data from many health records can be aggregated and analyzed for research studies and to provide statistical information on medical conditions and treatment modalities. As an example, public health agencies need health information. Certain diseases and conditions must be reported to the department of health in order to develop prevention and control procedures and to monitor disease trends. Moreover, the information in health records serves to provide continuing education for students in a variety of health professions.

Operational Management

Information gathered from health records helps facilities plan for the future based on the types of patients and diagnoses treated. Aggregate statistical information provides data on the use of services, provider patterns, and other important issues. Management often uses the information to make comparisons with other facilities. Finally, the quality of information in the health record aids managerial decision making in terms of improving the quality of patient care.

Legal Purposes

The health record serves the legal interests of the patient, the provider, and the facility. It serves as evidence in legal cases addressing the treatment received by the patient. It serves to prove the patient's allegations in a malpractice case and also is used by the clinical provider and the facility to defend the care they provided the patient. The record is admissible as evidence because it is considered a business record in that documentation occurs routinely as part of the healthcare facility's daily operation.

The Longitudinal Health Record

The term **longitudinal health record** refers to as a record that is compiled about an individual from birth to death. It is valuable because all the information about a patient is maintained and accessible. It serves as a reference of past history and avoids repetition of details and duplication of testing for the same conditions. Moreover, the longitudinal health record helps to prevent medical errors because information on allergies, drug interactions, surgeries, and past medical problems can be made available before treatment decisions are made. The physician can review the details of a patient's care and retrieve information needed at a later date.

A longitudinal health record is difficult to achieve in a paper-based record system because the patient typically has records at a variety of provider locations, such as physicians' offices, clinics, and hospitals, each of which often has a totally separate paper system. The different records are not linked, making it difficult to access all needed patient information. A longitudinal electronic health record would be especially valuable because it would allow information to be accessed from different locations.

Responsibility for Quality Documentation

The provider of care is responsible for ensuring that entries made in the record are of high quality. Although the facility's medical staff bylaws establish the rules and regulations for record content, the individual care providers are ultimately responsible for the quality of entries they make and authenticate. Figure 8.1 presents general documentation guidelines that every provider who writes or enters information in the patient health record should follow.

The quality of provider entries includes legibility. If an entry cannot be read, it must be assumed that it cannot or was not used in the patient care process.

The HIM professional is responsible for ensuring that providers understand the regulations and standards for proper documentation and for educating providers as changes occur. He or she should be involved in training residents and others who enter information so that standards are maintained and the record remains in its proper format.

The facility's administration is responsible for providing the equipment and support personnel to assist physicians in proper documentation. This includes computers and dictating and transcription equipment services, as well as HIM staff and other staff members who assist in creating a high-quality record and the proper coding and billing for reimbursement.

Except in facilities owned by individuals or the government, a board of trustees has ultimate legal responsibility for the quality of care rendered in the facility. However, responsibility for patient care decisions and documentation of these decisions is delegated to the physician responsible for the patient.

Check Your Understanding 8.1

Instructions: Answer the following questions on a separate sheet of paper.

1. What is the primary purpose of patient health information?
2. What are six other purposes or uses of patient health information?
3. What is the role of each of the following in the development of standards for health information: American College of Surgeons, Joint Commission on Accreditation of Healthcare Organizations, Centers for Medicare and Medicaid Services, state licensure, and medical staff bylaws?
4. Why is a longitudinal health record valuable?
5. Who is responsible for ensuring the quality of health record documentation?

Figure 8.1.   Guidelines for Documenting and Maintaining the Patient Health Record

These guidelines are considered standard or typical health information practices. Individual facilities develop their own policies based on institutional needs and laws and regulations.

1. All entries in the health record must be authenticated to identify the author (name and professional status) and dated.
2. No erasures or deletions should be made in the health record.
3. All entries in the paper health record should be in ink. Photocopying or scanning should be considered when colored ink or colored forms are used because some colors do not reproduce well.
4. Blank spaces should not be left in progress/nursing notes. If blanks are left, they should be marked out with an X so that additional information cannot be inserted on the paper out of proper date sequence.
5. If a correction must be made in a paper health record, one line should be neatly drawn through the error, leaving the incorrect material legible. The error then should be initialed and dated so that it is be obvious that it is a corrected mistake.
6. The original report should always be maintained in the health record. Cumulative laboratory reports or computerized nursing notes may be replaced with the latest cumulative report. Faxed copies of admission orders and histories and physicals may be used as originals in the record. The usual signature requirements should be followed.
7. All blanks on forms should be completed, especially on consent forms.
8. When health records are filed incomplete (as directed by medical staff/health record committee policy), a statement should be attached to indicate that this is the case. The statement should be signed by the chief of staff/chair of the health record committee as specified in the policy.
9. Chart folder labeling, dotting, or other methods of identifying at a glance a particular type of patient, such as one with a drug or alcohol diagnosis or HIV-positive status, should be discouraged to prevent inadvertent breaches of patient confidentiality.

Content of the Health Record

All health records contain information that can be classified into two broad categories: administrative/demographic data and clinical data. All health record entries must be legible, complete, dated, and authenticated according to the healthcare organization's policies.

Administrative and Demographic Information

Administrative and demographic information is generally found on the front page of the patient health record. The information entered provides facts that identify the patient and data related to payment and reimbursement and other operational needs of the healthcare facility.

Registration Data

Registration data represent one type of **administrative information.** They are collected prior to, or at the time of, hospital admission and/or treatment in an emergency department or a physician's or clinician's office. This is the first information the facility collects. Payment information is part of the administrative information. Administrative information also includes the various consents for treatment and the use of patient information, notification of patient rights, and other nonclinical information.

Demographic information is a type of administrative information. Demographic information includes facts such as:

- The patient's name
- The patient's address
- The patient's telephone number
- The patient's date of birth
- The patient's next of kin
- Other identifying information specific to the patient

A **unique identifier** number is assigned to the health record that allows all information about the patient to be inserted in the correct record or to be accessed when a query is entered into the computer system. Demographic information helps to specifically identify the patient and provides statistical information that is vital for planning, research, statistics, and other needs.

Demographic information may be entered directly into the computer by admission or registration personnel. In cases where the patient is coming to the facility for elective, or voluntary, treatment and/or an operative procedure, he or she can provide this information prior to arrival at the facility. The patient usually provides the information directly, but in cases where the patient is a minor or is incapacitated or in an emergency situation, another individual may provide the information. In such cases, the record must state the name and relationship of the person providing the information in case the information has to be verified or amended.

The demographic information in a totally paper-based health record environment is usually on the first page, which is called the face sheet or front sheet. This term also is used to refer to the computer view containing the information in facilities that have a computer-based admissions and discharge system in which a printout of the computer screen becomes the face sheet of a paper record. Figure 8.2 shows the face sheet of a paper-based record.

Consent to Treatment

Through the **consent** process, the patient agrees to undergo the treatments and procedures to be performed by clinical caregivers. This general consent is often part of the admission or entry process into the healthcare facility. However, the consent does not replace the individual consent forms the patient must complete and sign for each operation or special procedure to indicate that he or she is fully informed about the care to be provided. Written consents signed by the patient for experimental drugs and treatment and for participation in research must be included in the health record. Refusal of treatment or procedures likewise must be written to ensure that the consequences of the decision have been explained and the patient is aware of them.

Consent to Use or Disclose Protected Health Record Information

With regulatory changes put into place under the **Health Insurance Portability and Accountability Act** (HIPAA) of 1996, upon admission to the facility or prior to treatment by the provider, patients must be informed about the use of personally identifiable health information. This notice of privacy practices must explain and give examples of the uses of the patient's health information for treatment, payment, and healthcare operations, as well as other disclosures for purposes established in the regulations (see appendix D). If a particular use of information is not covered in the notice of privacy practices, the patient must sign an **authorization** form specific to the additional disclosure before his or her information can be released.

Consent to Special Procedures

In cases where the patient is coming to the facility for a specific procedure, an **informed consent** spelling out the exact details of the treatment must be signed by the patient or his or her legally authorized representative. This consent must show that the patient or the person authorized to act for the patient understands exactly what the procedure, test, or operation is going to be, including any possible risks, alternative methods, and outcomes.

Advance Directives

An **advance directive** is a written document, such as a living will, that states the patient's preferences for care. It also can be in the form of a durable power of attorney for healthcare in which the patient names another person to make medical decisions on his or her behalf in the event he or she is incapacitated. When the patient has a written advance directive, its existence must be noted in the health record. Patients or family members may bring the document to the facility to show the patient's wishes in case of terminal disease, trau-

matic injury, or cardiac arrest. The advance directive can be included as a part of the health record, although its inclusion may not be required. There may be documentation by the physician of a discussion with the patient or the family about the patient's wishes, rather than a formal written document.

Patients must be informed that they have the right to have an advance directive. Further, they must be notified of the provider's policies regarding its refusal to comply with advance directives.

Acknowledgment of Receipt of Patient's Rights Statement

Medicare requires that patients be informed of their rights, including the right to know who is treating them, the right to confidentiality, and the right to be informed about treatment. The patient's rights statement also must explain the patient's right to refuse treatment, to participate in care planning, and to be safe from abuse. The patient must sign a statement that these rights have been explained, and the signed statement must be made part of the health record. States often have laws and regulations regarding the rights that must be explained to patients, such as the right to privacy in treatment, to refuse treatment, and to refuse experimental treatments and drugs.

Property and Valuable List

Although facilities encourage patients to leave jewelry and other valuables at home, patients will have with them needed property such as clothing, teeth, eyeglasses, hearing aids, and other personal articles. Patients may be asked to sign a release of responsibility form to absolve the facility of responsibility for loss or damage to their personal property. This form then becomes part of the patient health record.

Birth and Death Certificates

The collection of birth information is often the responsibility of admitting personnel, nursing, or HIM personnel who prepare the certificate for submission to the state department of health. Many states use birth certificate software that has the fields required for the collection of such information. Birth certificates do not necessarily require a physician's signature; some states allow each facility to select a designated person, such as an HIM professional, to certify births. In most states, official birth certificates are maintained permanently by the department of health.

The funeral home director or the coroner is responsible for completing the death certificate in many states. The funeral director must obtain the signature of the attending physician or the physician who declared the patient dead for the death certificate. Death certificates are usually maintained permanently by the department of health.

Clinical Data

Clinical data include information related to the patient's condition, course of treatment, and progress. The patient health record includes mainly clinical data.

Figure 8.2.   Face Sheet of a Paper-Based Record

ADMISSION/DISCHARGE RECORD

Medical Record No.

| Last Name | First Name | Middle Name | Maiden Name | Soc. Sec. No. | Room No. | Admitting no. |

| Address | City | State | ZIP Code | Home Phone | Sex: ☐ M ☐ F |

| Age-Yrs | Birth Date Mo. Day Year | Birthplace | Marital Status: ☐ Married ☐ Div ☐ Single ☐ Sep ☐ Widowed ☐ Unknown | Religion |

Race: ☐ American Indian or Alaskan Native ☐ Asian or Pacific Islander ☐ Black ☐ White ☐ Other

Ethnicity: ☐ Spanish Origin/Hispanic   ☐ Non-Spanish Origin/Non-Hispanic

| Occupation | Employer or Employer of Spouse | Address of Employer - Phone |

| Name of Spouse | Address if Other Than Above | Birthplace |

| Notify in Case of Emergency | Relationship | Address | Phone |

| Name of Father | Birthplace | Maiden Name of Mother | Birthplace |

| Name of Blue Cross and/or Blue Shield Plan | Group No. | Contract No. | Effective Date | Subscriber ☐ Dependent ☐ | Family Member ☐ Comprehensive Coverage ☐ |

| Other Hospitalization Insurance | Cert. or Policy No. | Group No. | Effective Date | Medicare No. |

| Referring Physician's Name and Address | Attending Physician | AH. Phys. Code | Date of Last Admission |

| Smoker: ☐ Yes ☐ No | Nature of Admission: ☐ Emergency ☐ Urgent ☐ Elective ☐ Newborn | Service | Admission Date | Hour ☐ AM ☐ PM | Discharge Date | Hour ☐ AM ☐ PM |

Admitting Diagnosis   Completed by

Principal Diagnosis: The condition established after study to be responsible for occasioning the admission of the patient to the hospital for care.

Code Name

Other Diagnoses:

Principal Procedure: The procedure performed for definitive treatment rather than for diagnostic or exploratory purposes, or to treat a complication; the procedure most related to the principal diagnosis.

Date

Other Procedures:
   Date(s)

Coded By

Disposition:

Discharged
☐ To Home or Self Care
☐ Against Advice
Transferred:
☐ To Short Term Hosp.
☐ To Skilled Nurs. Fac.

Transferred (cont.)
☐ To. Int. Care/Nurs. Home
☐ To Home Health Ser.
☐ To Other Fac. (specify)

☐ Died ☐ Autopsy
☐ No Autopsy

Medical History

The **history** is a summary of the patient's illness from his or her point of view. Its purpose is to allow the patient or his or her authorized representative to give the physician as much background information about the patient's illness as possible. The physician usually tailors the physical examination to symptoms described in the patient's history and begins an assessment. Thus, the history provides a base on which the physician can develop a plan.

Documentation guidelines for histories and physical examinations and medical decision making published by the Centers for Medicare and Medicaid Services (CMS) affect physician reimbursement and are discussed further in chapter 14.

Components of the Medical History

The medical history has several components, including:

- *Chief complaint:* Told in the patient's own words (or those of the patient's representative), the chief complaint is the principal reason the patient is seeking care.
- *Present illness:* This component addresses what the patient feels the problem is and includes a brief description of the duration, location, and circumstances of the complaint.
- *Past medical history:* This consists of questions designed to gather information about past surgeries and other illnesses that might have a bearing on the patient's current illness. The physician asks about childhood and adult illnesses, operations, injuries, drug sensitivities, allergies, and other health problems.
- *Social and personal history:* The social history uncovers information about habits and living conditions that might have a bearing on the patient's illness, such as marital status, occupation, environment, and so on. Consumption of alcohol or tobacco products also may affect a patient's health. This section also should address the patient's psychosocial needs.
- *Family medical history:* The questions in this component allow the physician to learn whether other family members have conditions that might be considered genetic. Common questions concern cardiovascular diseases or conditions, renal diseases, history of cancer or diabetes, allergies, health of immediate relatives, and ages of relatives at death and causes of their deaths.
- *Review of systems:* This component consists of questions designed to cue the patient to reveal symptoms he or she may have forgotten, did not think were important, or neglected to mention when providing the historical information.

It is important that the person recording the history document whether the information was given by the patient or by another person in cases where the patient is unable to communicate.

Physical Examination

The physical examination is the actual comprehensive assessment of the patient by the physician. Its purpose is to obtain initial signs and symptoms so that appropriate treatment can begin. The end of the physical examination should indicate the impression based on the information obtained and the initial plan for the patient's care while in the hospital.

Components of the Physical Examination

The physical examination is conducted by observing the patient, palpating or touching the patient, tapping the thoracic and abdominal cavities, listening to breath and heart sounds, and taking the blood pressure. The patient is examined thoroughly. If the patient is admitted for a particular procedure, a more focused physical examination will take place.

Time Frame of the History and Physical Examination

The facility must have a policy that establishes a time frame for completing the history and physical. Most facilities set the time frame as the first twenty-four to forty-eight hours following admission and require that the history and physical be completed by the provider who is admitting the patient. It is acceptable to the JCAHO when the history and physical examination are completed within thirty days before the patient is admitted. Medicare regulations require that the history and physical examination be performed no more than seven days prior to admission or within forty-eight hours after admission of the patient. Any new information or changed information should be addressed.

The JCAHO requires the history and physical examination to be recorded and made part of the patient health record prior to any operative procedure. When the physician chooses to dictate the history and physical, the dictated report must be transcribed and attached to the chart before the procedure. When the report is dictated, but not transcribed, a written preoperative note covering the history and physical is acceptable only in an emergency. The attending physician must write an explanation of the emergency circumstances.

The HIM professional is responsible for ensuring that the most stringent time requirements are followed so that the facility is in compliance with state and federal laws and regulations, licensure standards, Medicare Conditions of Participation, and accreditation requirements for the specific type of facility. When the patient is readmitted within thirty days after discharge for the same condition, some hospitals allow the previous history and physical examination to be updated and signed and dated by the physician. This is called an *interval history* and is acceptable to the JCAHO. However, using a history and physical more than seven days old will not meet the more stringent regulation established by Medicare.

Table 8.1 lists the information usually included in a complete medical history, and table 8.2 (p. 146) shows the information usually documented in the report of a physical examination.

Diagnostic and Therapeutic Orders

Physicians' orders drive the healthcare team. Orders may be for treatments, ancillary medical services, laboratory tests, radiological procedures, drugs, devices, related materials, restraint, or seclusion. Orders change according to the patient's needs and responses to previous treatment. In the case of drugs, the physician orders a specific drug in a particular dosage stating how often the drug is to be given, by what means (orally, intravenously, or by other method), and for how long. Certain categories of drugs, such as narcotics and sedatives, have an automatic time limit or stop order. This means that these medications must be discontinued unless the physician gives a specific order. This prevents patients from receiving drugs for a longer period of time than is necessary.

Orders for tests and services must demonstrate the medical necessity and explain the reason for the order. The legibility of orders is important to ensure that they are clearly understood by the personnel who must carry them out. Some facilities use a computerized order-entry system. Verbal orders entered into the record or computer system by non-physician personnel must be signed or authenticated by the provider authorized to give orders. If providers have not signed in a timely manner, the computer will not let them access the system until the orders are signed.

Clinicians Authorized to Give and Receive Orders

Orders must be written by the physician or verbally communicated to persons authorized to receive verbal orders either in person or by telephone. The person accepting the order should sign and give his or her title, such as RN, PT, LPN, as appropriate. In some states, certified registered nurse practitioners and physician assistants are allowed to write or give verbal orders.

Table 8.1.   Information Usually Included in a Complete Medical History

Components of the History	Complaints and Symptoms
Chief complaint	Nature and duration of the symptoms that caused the patient to seek medical attention as stated in his or her own words
Present illness	Detailed chronological description of the development of the patient's illness, from the appearance of the first symptom to the present situation
Past medical history	Summary of childhood and adult illnesses and conditions, such as infectious diseases, pregnancies, allergies and drug sensitivities, accidents, operations, hospitalizations, and current medications
Social and personal history	Marital status; dietary, sleep, and exercise patterns; use of coffee, tobacco, alcohol, and other drugs; occupation; home environment; daily routine; and so on
Family medical history	Diseases among relatives in which heredity or contact might play a role, such as allergies, cancer, and infectious, psychiatric, metabolic, endocrine, cardiovascular, and renal diseases; health status or cause and age at death for immediate relatives
Review of systems	Systemic inventory designed to uncover current or past subjective symptoms that includes the following types of data: • *General:* Usual weight, recent weight changes, fever, weakness, fatigue • *Skin:* Rashes, eruptions, dryness, cyanosis, jaundice; changes in skin, hair, or nails • *Head:* Headache (duration, severity, character, location) • *Eyes:* Glasses or contact lenses, last eye examination, glaucoma, cataracts, eyestrain, pain, diplopia, redness, lacrimation, inflammation, blurring • *Ears:* Hearing, discharge, tinnitus, dizziness, pain • *Nose:* Head colds, epistaxis, discharges, obstruction, postnasal drip, sinus pain • *Mouth and throat:* Condition of teeth and gums, last dental examination, soreness, redness, hoarseness, difficulty in swallowing • *Respiratory system:* Chest pain, wheezing, cough, dyspnea, sputum (color and quantity), hemoptysis, asthma, bronchitis, emphysema, pneumonia, tuberculosis, pleurisy, last chest X ray • *Neurological system:* Fainting, blackouts, seizures, paralysis, tingling, tremors, memory loss • *Musculoskeletal system:* Joint pain or stiffness, arthritis, gout, backache, muscle pain, cramps, swelling, redness, limitation in motor activity • *Cardiovascular system:* Chest pain, rheumatic fever, tachycardia, palpitation, high blood pressure, edema, vertigo, faintness, varicose veins, thrombophlebitis • *Gastrointestinal system:* Appetite, thirst, nausea, vomiting, hematemesis, rectal bleeding, change in bowel habits, diarrhea, constipation, indigestion, food intolerance, flatus, hemorrhoids, jaundice • *Urinary system:* Frequent or painful urination, nocturia, pyuria, hematuria, incontinence, urinary infections • *Genitoreproductive system:* Male—venereal disease, sores, discharge from penis, hernias, testicular pain, or masses; female—age at menarche, frequency and duration of menstruation, dysmenorrhea, menorrhagia, symptoms of menopause, contraception, pregnancies, deliveries, abortions, last Pap smear • *Endocrine system:* Thyroid disease; heat or cold intolerance; excessive sweating, thirst, hunger, or urination • *Hematologic system:* Anemia, easy bruising or bleeding, past transfusions • *Psychiatric disorders:* Insomnia, headache, nightmares, personality disorders, anxiety disorders, mood disorders

Table 8.2.   Information Usually Documented in the Report of a Physical Examination

Report Components	Content
General condition	Apparent state of health, signs of distress, posture, weight, height, skin color, dress and personal hygiene, facial expression, manner, mood, state of awareness, speech
Vital signs	Pulse, respiration, blood pressure, temperature
Skin	Color, vascularity, lesions, edema, moisture, temperature, texture, thickness, mobility and turgor, nails
Head	Hair, scalp, skull, face
Eyes	Visual acuity and fields; position and alignment of the eyes, eyebrows, eyelids; lacrimal apparatus; conjunctivae; sclerae; corneas; irises; size, shape, equality, reaction to light, and accommodation of pupils; extraocular movements; ophthalmoscopic exam
Ears	Auricles, canals, tympanic membranes, hearing, discharge
Nose and sinuses	Airways, mucosa, septum, sinus tenderness, discharge, bleeding, smell
Mouth	Breath, lips, teeth, gums, tongue, salivary ducts
Throat	Tonsils, pharynx, palate, uvula, postnasal drip
Neck	Stiffness, thyroid, trachea, vessels, lymph nodes, salivary glands
Thorax, anterior and posterior	Shape, symmetry, respiration
Breasts	Masses, tenderness, discharge from nipples
Lungs	Fremitus, breath sounds, adventitious sounds, friction, spoken voice, whispered voice
Heart	Location and quality of apical impulse, trill, pulsation, rhythm, sounds, murmurs, friction rub, jugular venous pressure and pulse, carotid artery pulse
Abdomen	Contour, peristalsis, scars, rigidity, tenderness, spasm, masses, fluid, hernia, bowel sounds and bruits, palpable organs
Male genitourinary organs	Scars, lesions, discharge, penis, scrotum, epididymis, varicocele, hydrocele
Female reproductive organs	External genitalia, Skene's glands and Bartholin's glands, vagina, cervix, uterus, adnexa
Rectum	Fissure, fistula, hemorrhoids, sphincter tone, masses, prostate, seminal vesicles, feces
Musculoskeletal system	Spine and extremities, deformities, swelling, redness, tenderness, range of motion
Lymphatics	Palpable cervical, axillary, inguinal nodes; location; size; consistency; mobility and tenderness
Blood vessels	Pulses, color, temperature, vessel walls, veins
Neurological system	Cranial nerves, coordination, reflexes, biceps, triceps, patellar, Achilles, abdominal, cremasteric, Babinski, Romberg, gait, sensory, vibratory
Diagnosis(es)	

Medical staff policies and procedures must specifically state the categories of personnel authorized to accept orders. Verbal orders for medication are usually required to be given to, and to be accepted only by, nursing or pharmacy personnel. Some categories of personnel that may accept verbal or oral orders for services within the specific area of practice include physical therapists, registered nurse anesthetists, dietitians, and medical technologists.

Moreover, orders for tests and treatments must justify the condition of medical necessity because payers may not reimburse the facility if the reason for the test or treatment is not properly documented.

The time the order was given should be in writing. Some facilities do not allow verbal orders for treatments or procedures that might put the patient at risk. Other facilities require verbal orders to be repeated by the person accepting them to verify that they are clearly understood.

Signatures on Orders

Generally, orders must be dated and signed—or authenticated—by the provider or providers responsible for the patient's care and who either wrote or gave the orders. In the case of verbal or telephone orders, the provider should sign them as soon as possible after giving them. Many facilities require the ordering provider to indicate that the telephone orders are accurate, complete, and final by signing them within twenty-four hours. The timing requirements for signatures on orders are governed by state law, facility policy, accreditation standards, and government regulations and may vary from facility to facility.

For years, HIM department personnel carefully reviewed each order and marked those with missing signatures so that each could be individually signed by the responsible provider after discharge. However, signing orders after discharge does not affect the patient's care process, so many facilities no longer routinely review orders for signature following patient discharge. A review of orders is part of the concurrent or **open-record review** process; thus, orders can be signed in a timely manner and providers with patterns of unsigned orders can be detected. A comparison of orders to laboratory and other ancillary reports and to nursing documentation is another way to ensure that all orders are carried out.

Some facilities are developing standing, or standard, orders for certain procedures that all physicians can use when performing the particular procedure. Other facilities require an additional order to implement the standing orders, and still others allow a registered nurse to initiate the standing orders because the medical staff has previously approved them.

Special Orders

Do not resuscitate (DNR) orders must contain documentation that the decision to withhold cardiopulmonary resuscitation (CPR) was discussed, when the decision was made, and who participated in the decision. This discussion is often documented in the progress notes. Generally, patients are presumed to have consented to CPR unless a DNR order is present in the record. This may be part of the advance directives in the record.

Orders for seclusion and restraint, including drugs used for restraint, must comply with facility policies and Medicare regulations, state laws, and JCAHO requirements. These should never be standing or as-needed orders but, instead, must be ordered only when necessary to protect the patient or others from injury or harm. Specific time limits for these orders must be followed, and there must be continuous oversight of the patient under restraint or seclusion.

Discharge Orders

Discharge orders for hospital patients must be in writing and can only be issued by a physician. When a patient leaves against medical advice, this fact should be noted in lieu of a discharge order because the patient was not actually discharged. In the case of death, some facilities require that a discharge to the morgue order be written.

Clinical Observations

Clinical observations of the patient are documented in the health record in several formats, including progress notes, consultation reports, and ancillary notes, as described below.

Medical Services

Progress notes are chronological statements about the patient's response to treatment during his or her stay in the facility. Facility procedures and policies must state exactly what categories of personnel are allowed to write or enter information into progress notes. Generally, these personnel include physicians, nurses, physical therapists, occupational therapists, respiratory therapists, social workers, case managers, dietitians, nurse anesthetists, pharmacists, radiologic technologists, speech therapists, and others providing direct treatment or consultation to the patient. Each person authorized to enter documentation into the progress notes must write or enter his or her own note, authenticate and date it, and indicate authorship by signing his or her full name and title.

Each progress note reviews changes in the patient's condition, findings based on the facts of the case, test results, and response to treatment, as well as an analysis of the findings. The final part of the note contains the decisions or actions planned for future care. When writing in a paper patient record, providers must avoid leaving blank spaces between progress notes to prevent information from being added out of sequence.

Flowcharts are an effective way to illustrate the patient's progress and can be computerized to demonstrate progress or to keep track of certain data. Many physicians and other providers use handheld personal computers to maintain ongoing flowchart information about patients, such as blood glucose levels over time.

How often progress notes are written depends on the patient's condition, and the frequency is generally established by the healthcare facility or payers of care. In a hospi-
tal, the physician primarily responsible for the patient's care is often required to write a progress note daily. Doing so shows the physician's involvement and that he or she is aware of changes in the patient's condition.

Consultations are additional opinions of specialists. The attending physician may request that the specialist see the patient and prepare a consultation report. Each consultant is responsible for writing, dictating, or entering his or her own report. The report should show evidence of the consultant's review of the record and the patient and any pertinent findings, opinions, and recommendations. Moreover, the documentation should show that the physician requesting the consultation reviewed the report.

Nursing Services

Nursing personnel have the most frequent contact with patients, and their notes provide the complete record of the patients' progress and condition and demonstrate the continuity of care. Licensed registered nurses, licensed practical nurses, and nursing assistants record the facts of the physician's orders being carried out, observe the patient's response to treatment interventions, and describe the patient's condition and complaints as well as the outcome of care as reflected in the patient's status at discharge or termination of treatment. The method most commonly used by nurses to enter notes is narrative detailed documentation.

Nursing personnel begin recording information in the health record when the patient is admitted to the facility. They coordinate the patient's care to ensure that orders are carried out. The initial nursing assessment must summarize the date, time, and method of admission; the patient's condition, symptoms, and vital signs; and other information. Many nurses use a variation of the problem-oriented health record format (discussed later in this chapter) when recording notes. All nursing notes must be signed by the individuals who provided the service or observed the patient's condition. Full names and titles are required.

Charting by exception, or focus charting, is a method of charting only abnormal or unusual findings or deviations from the prescribed plan of care. A complete assessment is performed every shift or every eight hours. When events differ from the assessment or the expected norm for a particular patient, the notes should focus on that particular event and include the data, intervention, and response. Flow sheets and care plans may be used to illustrate changes in the patient's condition. The purpose of charting by exception is to reduce repetitive record keeping and documentation of normal events. Bedside terminals and direct input of monitoring information and other computerization of nursing observations and medication distribution save nurses a great deal of time because information does not have to be rewritten numerous times.

Medication records are maintained for all patients and include medications given, time, form of administration, and dosage and strength. The records are updated when the patient is given his or her medication. The health record must reflect when a medication is given in error, indicating what was done about it and the patient's response. Adverse drug reactions must be fully documented and reported to the provider and to the performance improvement/risk management program according to guidelines established by the facility.

Flow sheets are often used in addition to narrative notes for intake and output records showing how much fluid the patient consumed and how much was eliminated. In addition, blood glucose records are often flowcharted for ease of comparison. Degree of pain is another aspect of the patient's condition that is commonly flowcharted.

Nurses are responsible for maintaining records of patient transfers (to surgery, to another room, or level of care) as well as visits to physician or treatment offices and other locations outside the facility.

Case managers are nurses, social workers, or other personnel who are responsible for assisting the patient through the care process. The case management process improves quality of care because care is scheduled in an orderly way and fragmentation is reduced. Hospitals, managed care organizations, and other facilities use case managers to improve coordination of care, scheduling, and discharge planning. Many facilities use predetermined **care paths,** that are specific to diagnoses or conditions; case managers ensure that patients receive care according to the care path. Care paths are also called clinical pathways, critical paths, and clinical algorithms.

Ancillary Services

Laboratory and radiology reports and reports from other ancillary services, such as EKGs (electrocardiographs) and EEGs (electroencephalographs), must be signed by the physician responsible for the interpretations. A pathologist is responsible for the work of the clinical laboratory; a radiologist is responsible for the work of the radiology department. Many states have separate **retention schedules** for the actual X rays that differ from the retention time frames for other health records. The typed interpretations of the radiology or other reports become part of the health record and are kept as long as the health records are kept.

Laboratory results in a computerized environment are available to the provider as soon as they are entered into the computer. In most facilities, a laboratory summary is generated consistently throughout the patient's stay, with a final summary completed within twenty-four hours after discharge. These multipage summaries are printed and made part of the patient health record. Some facilities use manually completed laboratory forms divided into several sections. The original report is the one that should be included in the record. The laboratory conducts tests on blood, urine, sputum, and other body fluids. Many specialized tests are performed in the laboratory to provide information the physician can use to make a diagnosis, including analyses of specimens removed during surgery. Most facilities require the original

laboratory report to be placed in the health record within twenty-four hours.

Healthcare facility policies and procedures must state that the practitioner approved by the medical staff to interpret diagnostic procedures, such as nuclear medicine procedures, MRIs, EEGs, and EKGs, should sign and date his or her interpretations. The interpretations then become part of the health record. Scans and videotapes, tracings, or other actual recordings are often fed directly into the computer system. Providers may view such recordings, but the recordings do not become part of the permanent record. It is important that all tests or procedures ordered have corresponding reports in the health record.

Orders and records of services rendered to patients from rehabilitation, physical therapy, occupational therapy, audiology, or speech pathology should be included in the record as appropriate to the patient. These reports must contain evaluations, recommendations, goals, course of treatment, and response to treatment. Nutritional care plans need to be developed in compliance with a physician order, and information on nutrition and diet should be included in the discharge plan and transfer orders.

Surgical Services

The operative section of the health record includes the anesthesia record, the intraoperative record, and the recovery record. The history and physical examination, informed consents signed by the patient or his or her authorized representative, and the postoperative progress note also are part of the documentation about the operative procedure. Every patient's chart must include a complete history and physical examination prior to surgery or invasive procedure unless there is an emergency. When the history and physical report was dictated, it must be included in the record in a typed version. Advance directives and organ donation forms also must be included in the chart before surgery.

Moreover, the anesthesiologist or the certified registered nurse anesthetist must write a preanesthesia evaluation or an updated evaluation prior to surgery. This evaluation must cover information on the anesthesia to be used, risk factors, allergy and drug history, potential problems, and a general assessment of the patient's condition. An intraoperative anesthesia record must be maintained of all events during surgery, including complete information on the anesthesia administration, blood pressure, pulse, respiration, and other monitors of the patient's condition. Finally, after surgery, the appropriate anesthesia personnel must write a postoperative anesthesia follow-up report. Outpatient surgical cases also must include postanesthesia evaluations. Records of postanesthesia visits should indicate any unusual events or complications.

The operative report itself must be written or dictated by the surgeon immediately after surgery and must include the names of the surgeon and assistants, technical procedures, findings, specimens removed, estimated blood loss, and postoperative diagnosis. The surgeon must write a brief postoperative progress note in the record immediately after surgery before the patient leaves the operating suite. Most facilities have dictation areas set up near the operative suite or cardiac catheterization laboratories to allow surgeons to dictate the operative reports immediately. However, the written postoperative progress note must be completed to provide information for patient care until the typed report is placed in the patient record, usually twelve to twenty-four hours after surgery. Some facilities use a preprinted postoperative progress note form with the required elements listed to remind the surgeon of the items that must be included. The postoperative progress notes and the dictation and transcription of operative reports must be carefully monitored to ensure that they are placed in the health record in a timely manner.

Pathology reports are required for every case in which a surgical specimen is removed or expelled during a procedure and must include a microscopic and gross evaluation of the tissue. These reports are part of the operative section of the health record and must be signed by the pathologist. The preoperative diagnosis and pathological diagnosis can then be compared.

Information on the patient's discharge from the postoperative or postanesthesia care unit must be documented and signed by the licensed independent practitioner responsible for the discharge or by the provider verifying that the patient is ready for discharge according to specific discharge criteria. The operative section also will contain data on implants, including product numbers, and additional information for follow-up.

Organ Transplantation

Medicare requires hospitals to inform families of the opportunity to donate organs, tissues, or eyes. Documentation showing that the organ procurement organization has been notified regarding a patient near death must be included in the health record so that anatomical gifts can be preserved and used. In the case of living donor transplants of kidneys or other organs, an operative report must be written for both donor and recipient following all the standards for operative records.

Conclusions at Termination of Care

The health record must summarize the patient's condition at the beginning of treatment and basic information about tests, examinations, procedures, and results occurring as a result of treatment. The conclusion at termination of care is called the discharge summary.

Discharge Summary

The **discharge summary,** also called the clinical resume, provides details about the patient's stay in the facility and is the foundation for future treatment. It is prepared when the patient is discharged or transferred to another facility or when the patient expires. The summary states the patient's reason for admission and gives a brief history explaining why he or she needed to be hospitalized. Pertinent laboratory, X-ray, consultation, and other significant findings, as well as the patient's response to treatment or procedures, are included. In addition to a description of the patient's condition at discharge, the discharge summary delineates specific instructions given to the family for future care, including information on medications, referrals to other providers, diet, activities, follow-up visits to the physician, and the patient's final diagnoses. The discharge summary must be signed and dated by the physician.

Some facilities require the final diagnoses to be recorded and the discharge summary to be dictated or written at discharge or they immediately consider the chart delinquent. The information in the discharge summary is extremely important to meet the facility's coding, billing, and reimbursement needs. In some facilities, a paper discharge summary form with an outline of contents is used to ensure that all items are included. The form has three parts so that the part with follow-up instructions can be given to the patient.

When a patient dies in the hospital, hospitals often require the physician who pronounced death to write a note that gives the time and date of death. The death note is in addition to the discharge summary required in all death cases no matter how long the patient was in the facility. Most facilities do not require a discharge summary for normal newborns and obstetrical cases without complications, as long as there is a final progress note.

A discharge summary is not required for patients who are in the hospital for forty-eight hours or less. Such patients usually have a short-stay or short-service record or a final discharge progress note. This one-page form can be used to record the history and physical examination, the operative report, the discharge summary, and discharge instructions. When the patient is admitted to the facility, the reason for admission must be recorded. When the patient dies forty-eight hours or less after admission, the short-stay record is insufficient and a complete discharge summary must be prepared.

The discharge summary must be completed within thirty days after the date of discharge. When a patient is transferred, the physician should complete the discharge summary within twenty-four hours.

The principal diagnosis and other diagnoses should be recorded completely without symbols or abbreviations on the health record summary sheet (the face sheet) or discharge summary or on another form prescribed by the facility. The **principal diagnosis** is defined as the condition determined, after study, to be chiefly responsible for occasioning the patient's admission to the hospital.

Healthcare facilities must determine what information goes with the patient when he or she is transferred to another level of care. When the transfer is to an affiliated institution that is part of the same healthcare system, the original patient record is transferred with the patient and new orders are written at the receiving institution to initiate care. A discharge summary is generally required.

Discharge Plan
Discharge planning information regarding further treatment of the patient should be part of the acute care health record. The discharge planning process begins at admission and must include information on the patient's ability to perform self-care as well as other services needed by the patient. The case manager, the social worker, utilization review personnel, or nursing personnel may write this plan.

Records Filed with the Health Record
Debate is ongoing about whether patient records received from other facilities should be made part of the receiving facility's health record. Some facilities release all the information because all of it was used in treatment decisions. Other facilities maintain that they are responsible only for the information originating in their own facilities and have requestors obtain original records from the originating facility. New federal regulations under HIPAA require that all information, including information from other facilities, is part of the health record.

Facilities maintain information on the release of information from the patient record explaining what was released, to whom the information was released, and the date. This required information is often filed with the health record but should not be released when the patient record is released.

Specialized Health Record Content

The format of the patient health record varies according to the type of care provided. Many facilities offer specialized services requiring special documentation that is not found in every patient's record. JCAHO standards and regulations often specify particular content to include in the record. The following sections describe various specialized services and their records.

Obstetrical Care
The prenatal and labor record, which is kept in the physician's office, serves as the history and physical for an obstetrical patient. When the patient requires a Cesarean section, the record must include a full history and physical or a detailed admission progress note explaining the need for a C-section.

A delivery record indicates the name of the patient, maiden name, date of delivery, sex of infant, name of physician, name of persons assisting, any complications, type of anesthesia used, name of person administering anesthesia, and names of others present at delivery. In the case of a stillborn infant, a separate patient record is not created; rather, information is recorded in the mother's delivery record. A fetal death certificate is completed on the appropriate form.

Neonatal Care
Newborns are considered separate patients with separate health records. The newborn patient record must include an admission examination and a discharge examination. Usually, special chart forms for progress notes, orders, and nursing notes are included. When the patient has been in the newborn intensive care unit, a complete discharge summary is required.

Emergency Care
Emergency health records may be filed separately or incorporated into the health record when the patient is admitted to the same facility. When the records are filed separately, the emergency record must be available when the patient is readmitted or appears for care in the future. Most of the emergency information is recorded on one sheet in a paper health record format. Additional sheets include laboratory, radiology, and other tests; consent forms; and follow-up instructions.

The content of the emergency health record should include:

- Identification data
- Time of arrival
- Means of arrival (by ambulance, private automobile, or police vehicle)
- Name of person or organization transporting patient to the emergency department
- Pertinent history, including chief complaint and onset of injury or illness
- Significant physical findings
- Laboratory, X-ray, and EKG findings
- Treatment rendered
- Conclusions at termination of treatment
- Disposition of patient, including whether sent home, transferred, or admitted
- Condition of the patient upon discharge or transfer
- Diagnosis upon discharge
- Instructions given to the patient or the family regarding further care and follow-up
- Signatures and titles of the patient's caregivers

When the patient leaves before being seen or against medical advice, this fact should be noted on the emergency department form. Consent forms for treatment must be included. In cases where there is an emergency or the patient is in critical condition or otherwise unable to sign the consent, an explanation should be documented. A copy of the emergency record should be made available to the provider of follow-up care.

Most states require facilities to maintain an additional chronological record or to register all patients visiting the emergency department with name, date, time of arrival, and record number. This registration also includes the names of patients who were dead on arrival.

Emergency patients must be made aware of their rights. Transfer and acceptance policies and procedures must be delineated to ensure that facilities comply with the Emergency Medical Treatment and Active Labor Act (EMTALA) and state regulations regarding transfers. Patients cannot be transferred or refused treatment for reasons related to ability to pay or source of payment nor can hospitals determine that space is unavailable based on ability to pay or source of payment. Anyone who requests or requires an examination must be provided an appropriate medical screening examination by hospital staff to determine whether a medical emergency exists. Further, the hospital must stabilize the medical emergency by ensuring an airway and ventilation, by controlling hemorrhage, and by stabilizing and/or splinting fractures before a patient can be transferred. The hospital must maintain screening examinations for a period of five years.

Appropriate transfer means that the receiving hospital agrees to receive the patient and provide appropriate medical treatment. Records must be provided to the receiving hospital, and the patient or responsible person must understand the medical necessity of the transfer.

Ambulatory or Outpatient Care

Ambulatory or outpatient care means that patients move from location to location. Patients arrive for treatment and leave after treatment has been administered; they do not stay overnight. Ambulatory or outpatient care may be given in a freestanding clinic, a clinic that is part of a larger hospital system, or a physician's or other provider's office. When patients are in a clinic affiliated with a hospital, the entire health record should be available. The JCAHO requires ambulatory patients to have a summary list by the third visit that includes known diagnoses, conditions, procedures, drug allergies, and medications. It also requires each ambulatory care record to contain a history and physical examination, operative reports, diagnostic and therapeutic procedures, consultations, follow-up notes, observations of patients, and discharge notes at the conclusion or termination of treatment. Contents vary depending on the treatment received.

Ambulatory facilities that only perform surgery are called ambulatory surgery clinics (ASCs). Patients having surgery at any type of ambulatory facility must have a history and physical examination prior to surgery, consents, an operative note, a postoperative progress note, and the same anesthesia information as an operative patient in the hospital. In addition, the record must document instructions for postoperative care and postoperative follow-up. Clinics often call patients after surgery, and these calls should be documented in the record. The Accreditation Association for Ambulatory Health Care requires that the history and physical examination, laboratory reports, radiology reports, operative reports, and consultations be signed in a timely manner. Laboratory and other reports must be included in the patient record as soon as possible.

Traditionally, physician office records have been less comprehensive than hospital medical records. Physicians must develop standardized formats and comprehensive documentation practices.

The focus of ambulatory care is to see or treat patients quickly and then move them efficiently out of the facility. Because of the brief nature of ambulatory care, rapid access to information is vital.

Behavioral Health Care

Behavioral health records, also known as mental health records or psychiatric records, must include diagnostic and assessment information. Medicare requires that the records contain a provisional or admitting diagnosis and the reason for admission, as well as the names of the persons involved in making the admission decision. In addition, a goal-oriented treatment plan must be in place.

Medicare further requires that social service records assess family and home information and community resources available to the patient. Special requirements for a psychiatric evaluation include history, mental status, information on the present illness, and intellectual and memory function. Progress notes must be recorded at least weekly for the first two months and at least once monthly thereafter. Finally, a discharge summary should be written. Special attention must be paid to orders for restraint and seclusion as noted in the discussion on orders.

Home Health Services

According to the National Association for Home Care, the term home care covers many types of services "delivered at home to recovering, disabled, chronically or terminally ill persons in need of medical, nursing, social, or therapeutic treatment and/or assistance with the essential activities of daily living" (NAHC 2001). Physicians order home care services that may include visits from many types of healthcare providers, including physicians and nurses. Patient health records must contain a legible record of each visit describing what was done to or for the patient during the visit.

The providers working with patients must develop and document periodic plans of care. Specific forms developed by the CMS (formerly, the HCFA) are used in home care to document and update the plan of care. Verbal orders must be signed before the home health agency submits a bill for payment.

Hospice Care Services

The National Hospice and Palliative Care Organization (NHPO) defines hospice care as a "team-oriented approach to expert medical care, pain management, and emotional and spiritual support expressly tailored to the patient's needs and wishes." Because hospice care is delivered to patients with all types of terminal illnesses, the family is involved in the care and support is given by the hospice organization. Hospice services are provided in numerous types of settings, including homes, hospitals, and long-term care facilities (NHPO 2001). Special documentation for the election of hospice care is required for Medicare to pay for hospice care.

Rehabilitation Services

Rehabilitation covers a wide range of services provided to build or rebuild the patient's abilities to perform the usual activities of daily life. Among these services are physical therapy, occupational therapy, and speech therapy.

Physical therapists work in numerous types of facilities, ranging from acute care to long-term care and patient homes, setting goals for patients and helping them reach their goals by building muscle strength and respiratory and circulatory efficiency. Their patients include those who have been disabled for a number of reasons, including birth defect, trauma, and illness. Treatments include exercise, manipulation, heat therapy, light therapy, the use of electricity, and therapeutic massage. In addition to setting treatment goals, physical therapists have to document patient progress.

Occupational therapists are part of the rehabilitation team and work with patients to restore their ability to perform the usual functions of daily life, such as eating, dressing, preparing food, working, and handling other activities specific to the patient. Speech therapists and other specialized therapists are important members of the rehabilitation team and work together to achieve a variety of patient goals.

Long-Term Care

Long-term care describes the care provided for extended periods of time to patients recovering from illness or injury. Long-term care facilities offer a combination of services, ranging from independent living to assisted living to skilled nursing care. Rehabilitation services are often part of the long-term care plan. The long-term care record must document a comprehensive assessment that includes items in the minimum data set (MDS) to meet Medicare requirements stated in 42 CFR 483.20. Chapter 7 addresses MDS standards for data collection.

In addition, long-term facilities must meet state requirements. Individualized patient care plans must be developed and included in the health record. These plans must cover the potential for rehabilitation, the ability to perform activities of daily living, medications prescribed, and other aspects of care.

As with acute care facilities, the frequency of notes depends on the patient's condition. The focus in long-term care is on the achievement of goals. The HIM functions are similar to those in other types of facilities, but a great deal of concurrent review is required. Paper records of patients who have been in the facility for an extended period of time must be divided with the most current information maintained on the nursing unit, with the rest filed elsewhere to save space at the nursing station.

Check Your Understanding 8.2

Instructions: Match the contents with the appropriate part of the record by placing the letter for the form in the blank preceding the description of the form's content.

a. Care path
b. History
c. Physical examination
d. Orders
e. Consultations
f. Nursing notes
g. Advance directives
h. Emergency record
i. Discharge summary
j. Ancillary notes

1. ___ Directions given for drugs, devices, and healthcare treatments
2. ___ Comprehensive assessment of patient to determine signs and symptoms

3. ___ Records maintained by physical therapists, speech therapists, respiratory therapists, and other providers of special services
4. ___ Protocol for the process of care
5. ___ Summary of background information about the patient's illness
6. ___ Statement of patient's wishes and/or instructions for care
7. ___ Conclusions at the termination of care
8. ___ Observations of the patient's response to treatment
9. ___ Record that must contain the time and means of arrival and the name of the person transporting the patient to the facility
10. ___ Opinions of specialists

Format of the Paper-Based Health Record

The term *format* refers to the organization of information in the health record. There are many possible formats, and most facilities use a combination of arrangements.

Source-Oriented Health Records

The **source-oriented health record** is the conventional or traditional method of maintaining paper-based health records. In this method, health records are organized according to the source, or originating, department that rendered the service (for example, all lab reports are filed together, all radiological reports are filed together, and so on).

When the patient is in active treatment in the hospital, for example, the record is often maintained in reverse chronological order, with the most recent information on top. Tabs allow easy reference to the grouped reports, enabling staff to quickly find the patient's response to treatment.

After the patient is discharged, many facilities rearrange the record in chronological order. However, the arrangement is still source oriented with all labs together, all progress notes together, and all other related reports filed together in date order. Figure 8.3 shows the arrangement of forms for records maintained in a large acute care hospital.

Problem-Oriented Health Records

Lawrence Weed developed the **problem-oriented medical record** (POMR) in the 1970s. The POMR comprises the problem list, the database (the history and physical examination and initial lab findings), the initial plan (tests, procedures, and other treatments), and progress notes organized so that every member of the healthcare team can easily follow the course of patient treatment.

A distinctive feature of the problem-oriented health record is the problem list, which serves as the record's table of contents. All relevant problems—medical, social, or other—that may have an impact on the patient are listed with a number. As problems are resolved, the resolution is noted; new problems are added as they occur. The problem list serves as a permanent index that providers can quickly check to review the status of past and current problems. The JCAHO requires ambulatory records to have a problem list.

The most recognizable component of the POMR is the SOAP format, which is a method for recording progress notes. SOAP is an easy acronym that helps providers remember the specific and systematic decision-making process. **S** stands for *subjective findings* and includes statements about the patient and symptoms. The subjective findings are followed by *objective findings* (the **O** in the acronym) such as laboratory and test results and observations and findings from the physical examination. **A** stands for *analysis,* which consists of appraisals and judgments based on the findings and observations. The **P** stands for *plan,* which states the need for continuing care or revision of care. Although the full problem-oriented medical record as championed by Weed has not been adopted universally, many physicians and providers routinely use the SOAP method or an adaptation of it to document progress notes and include a problem list in the record.

Integrated Health Records

The content of the **integrated health record** is arranged in strict chronological order. Different types of information and sources of information are mixed together according to the dates on the entries. The order of the record is determined by the date the information was entered, the date of the service, or the date the report was received, not by the source department; and the record gives the sequence of the patient's care as delivered. Although this system makes it difficult to find a particular document unless one knows the date, it does provide a better picture of the story of the patient's care. Physicians' offices often use this format.

Figure 8.3.   Patient Record Content

This is not a complete list but does show the types of forms found in most acute care hospitals.

Admission record
Discharge diagnosis information
Identification data
General conditions of admission form
Medicare statements
History
    Chief complaint
    Present illness
    Review of systems
    Past history
    Family history
    Social history
Physical examination
Impression or working diagnosis (part of history and physical or
      admission note)
Plan of care (part of history and physical or admission notes)
Prenatal and labor record
    Labor and delivery summary
    Admission assessment
    Labor progress record
    Infant identification sheet
Reports of tests and results
    Laboratory
      Transfusions
      Bone marrow
      Toxicology
      Other special reports
    Radiology includes scans, ultrasounds, arteriograms, MRI, and so on
      EEG
      EKG
      Echocardiograms
      Treadmill
      Holter monitor
      Doppler
Therapy reports
    Physical therapy
    Occupational therapy
    Cardiac rehabilitation
    Respiratory therapy
Progress notes, clinical observations, and patient's response to care
Consultation reports
Informed consent
Anesthesia record
Operative room clinical record
Intraoperative report
Postoperative or recovery record

Pathology report
Discharge summary
Final diagnosis
Death
    Consent for autopsy
    Autopsy report, if done
    Release of body
Discharge instructions
Nursing notes and observations
    Medication administration records
    Graphic charts
    Intake-output, temperature, pulse, respirations
Nursing assessments
    Admission assessments
    Care plans
    Critical pathways
Records of donation or receipt of transplants or implants
Advance directives (if brought to the facility by the patient)
Living will (if brought to the facility by the patient)
Power of attorney
Special consents
    Anatomical gifts
    AMA release
    Leave of absence
    Consent to photograph
Emergency record
    Treatment record
Newborn records
    Admission record
    Discharge summary
    Consultation
    Consents
    Physician orders/progress notes
    Lab
    Radiology
    Newborn record
    Estimated gestational age
    Medication record
    Initial assessment
    Labor and delivery record
    Infant identification—footprints and photographs
    Newborn ICU delivery room
    Flow sheet
      Observation, neonatal, ICU
    Nursery progress record
    Pediatrician selection form

Courtesy Methodist Health Systems, Memphis, Tenn.

Strengths and Weaknesses of Paper-Based Health Records

The main benefit of paper-based health records is that they are the usual way that records are maintained. Professionals do not need technological training to begin documenting in the record.

However, paper-based records have numerous disadvantages. The main disadvantage is that only one person at a time can access information. In addition, there are problems with tracking and monitoring locations of the paper record when it is checked out of the HIM department. The filing of loose reports also presents a problem. Attaching loose reports is not always a priority in a busy patient care area, and this can result in numerous loose pieces of paper arriving in the HIM department. HIM personnel must route or deliver the forms to the patient care treatment area if the patient is still present or must sort and file stacks of loose paper forms. Organizing loose reports and attaching them to many individual records can be a formidable job. Finally, an entire record or a volume of a paper record can be lost or misfiled, making important patient information unavailable to providers when they need it.

Figure 8.4 lists the steps in the usual flow of the paper-based health record in a traditional acute care facility.

Check Your Understanding 8.3

Instructions: Fill in the blanks with the appropriate terms.

1. ____ This is the conventional or traditional method of maintaining paper-based health records.

2. ____ This record is maintained in the same format while the patient is hospitalized and after discharge.

3. ____ This record is maintained in strict chronological order.

4. ____ This record begins with a problem list that serves as the table of contents for the record.

5. ____ This organization provides care to patients who are terminally ill.

6. ____ These services include physical therapy, occupational therapy, and speech therapy.

7. ____ These services range from independent living to assisted living and skilled nursing care.

Staffing of the Health Information Department

The HIM department's organization varies according to the type of organization. Long-term care facilities may have a very small HIM department with one person in charge or with responsibility for records that are assigned as part of an administrative position. Some long-term care facilities use outside consultants to handle the functions of record keeping.

In contrast, large acute care facilities often employ many HIM professionals, including a department director. Other HIM professionals manage specific areas or functions such as coding, analysis, assembly, transcription, release of information,

Figure 8.4.   Steps in the Flow of the Paper-Based Patient Health Record Following Discharge

1. Records of discharged patients arrive or are delivered to HIM department.

2. Receipt of records is verified by comparing discharge lists to actual charts received.

3. Folder corresponding to records is pulled.

4. Record is assembled according to prescribed format ensuring that all pages belong to the correct patient and that forms are in correct date order.

5. Deficiencies such as signatures, reports needing completion, and so on are assigned to the responsible provider.

6. Diagnoses and procedures are coded.

7. Record is held for final completion by providers either in incomplete chart area or some other filing area.

8. Charts are rechecked after the providers have done their work to ensure that all have been completed.

9. The complete record is filed in the permanent filing area.

imaging, storage, filing, and retrieval. In addition, large facilities sometimes use contract personnel to perform transcription, coding, release of information, and other activities.

In facilities with large ambulatory patient populations and paper-based record systems, health records frequently move in and out of the HIM department. Records must be pulled from the file for clinic appointments and for walk-in patients without appointments; the records need to be delivered and picked up, and then refiled. Any reports of tests or treatments that arrive separately from the record must be attached to the record quickly. Patients may have several appointments in several different clinics, resulting in many transfers of patient records to various providers. Tracking chart location is critical because so many providers, including resident physicians, use the record.

Management of Health Record Content

The HIM professional manages health record content through oversight responsibilities of medical word processing, in which dictated information is converted into usable output that becomes part of the record. The responsibilities for incomplete records include analyzing and monitoring incomplete records to ensure that they are properly completed to meet facility standards and patient healthcare needs and controlling the design and production of forms to ensure that all records are in a standardized format.

Medical Word Processing

Completion of the health record is greatly enhanced by the sophisticated word-processing equipment in use today. Physicians and other providers first dictate the necessary reports, including history and physical examinations, operative reports, discharge summaries, consultations, progress notes, clinic notes, pathology reports, and radiology reports. The dictation then is converted to final printed output to become a part of the original health record. In the healthcare field, word processing is often called **transcription** and the personnel who type the dictation are called **medical transcriptionists.** Facilities should encourage providers to dictate so that reports can be accessed electronically.

Components of a Medical Word-Processing System

The word-processing system encompasses both the dictation and transcription process. The physician or provider dictates into a telephone by calling a special number connected to the facility's dictation system or by using a special phone dedicated only to dictation. The dictation also may be recorded using a separate handheld recorder onto a tape that is delivered to the department. Input from personal computers (PCs) or handheld computer devices is becoming more prevalent. Whatever the means of input, a transcriptionist retrieves the dictated voice and converts it into words. The transcription may be performed on-site at the facility or off-site at a remote location. The final product is sent for review to the physician or provider, who signs the report authenticating it as the final approved original for inclusion in the health record. Authentication may be done on the printed report or electronically in the computer system. The facility's policies must specify that the signature indicates that the provider who dictated the report has reviewed and edited it (if necessary) and approves its content.

The latest development in medical word-processing systems is **digital dictation.** In this system, vocal sounds are recorded and converted to digital form. The physician or provider begins the dictation process using a telephone, a microphone attached to a PC, or a hands-free microphone. He or she enters digits to indicate certain basic information, such as identification of the author, identification of the patient, and the type of report to be dictated (a history and physical examination, a discharge summary, an operative report, and so on).

The dictation then is transmitted to a computer that digitizes the voice. After the voice sounds have been digitized, the dictation is accessed by the transcriptionist who listens to the voice and converts it to typed output. Special software features allow the transcriptionist to produce output with as few keystrokes as possible, using techniques such as word expanders. Word expanders are shortened versions of phrases. For example, the keystrokes WDWN are changed to produce typed output as "well-developed, well-nourished." Some facilities use normal reports or macros that the physician can direct the transcriptionist to edit and tailor to the individual patient. This improves the quality of the final output and ensures that all necessary documentation is included.

Digital systems allow the dictated information to be managed so that emergency work or reports that have to be completed quickly are produced first. The dictation can be easily located in any random order. Digital systems automatically time-stamp the time the work was dictated and the time the transcription was started and completed. Random access by the transcriptionist allows the workload to be shared and distributed among several transcriptionists. Physicians can dial in and listen to the recorded information, rather than waiting until the typing is done. Coders can listen to the dictated recorded information and code from the discharge summary and other dictated reports, rather than waiting for the actual transcribed reports. The possibility of work being lost is reduced because of the time-stamping features. The typed output can be faxed automatically to the physician's office, printed out in the transcription area, printed out to clinics or patient floors, uploaded into the electronic medical record (EMR), and tied into the chart completion system.

Physicians can review transcribed documents online and may have editing capabilities. In some systems, both the original and the final edited versions become part of the health record.

There is movement toward using PCs as recording devices rather than using a dedicated dictation station. A radiologist can view an image on the PC screen and dictate into either a headset or a handheld mike plugged into the PC, rather than using a separate station for dictation. The advantage is that the equipment can be used for purposes other than dictation.

Speech recognition, or voice recognition technology, is used increasingly as the accuracy of input improves. In **voice recognition technology,** the spoken word is transmitted immediately to a database and converted to typed output, which eliminates the need for the transcriptionist to listen to and type the information. The quality of the output is very dependent on the quality of the dictation. The speaker must speak clearly and distinctly. The role of the transcriptionist will change as this new technology increases in accuracy. In time, the transcriptionist will become primarily an editor and proofreader.

The HIM department establishes turnaround times for transcribing dictated reports for different types of work. For example, history and physical examination reports must be completed quickly because they have to be attached to the record prior to surgery. Consultation reports also often have a very short turnaround time. Operative reports, on the other hand, may be assigned a turnaround time of twelve hours or less. And discharge summaries may have a lower priority for transcription if the digital system allows coders and other personnel to access and listen to them. Whatever turnaround times are set, meeting the time frames is an important measure in assessing the quality and productivity of the transcription area.

Planning for and Selecting Medical Word-Processing Equipment

When faced with the prospect of purchasing or upgrading a word-processing system, the HIM professional must be aware of the long-range consequences of this important decision.

Equipment vendors can provide a wealth of information based on their experience and work in various facilities. They can help the HIM department determine the number of ports, or entry points, that need to be available based on the number of dictators and transcriptionists requiring simultaneous access. The system needs to have sufficient accessibility to avoid collision, which would prevent a dictator or transcriptionist from gaining access to the system. Immediate access for all users, whether dictating or transcribing, is critical to the system's success. When dictators call in, a digital channel selector automatically selects an available line without input from the dictator.

In addition, it is important to anticipate the amount of recording time necessary to meet current needs and to have sufficient space available to meet future needs. Recording time is often stored on two drives so that backup, or redundancy, is available in case one drive fails. Dictation/transcription systems need to interface with existing facility information systems (IS) personnel to ensure that a method exists to automatically download identification information from the master person index. Physicians or providers do not have to enter a great deal of information, and this promotes accuracy and consistency in patient identification. Password protection also needs to be in place to ensure that only authorized persons can access the system.

The facility must have vendor support to keep the system operational at all times. Transcription systems should be designed so that the transcriptionists can work independently if the general facility IS is not working. Although entering patient information without the connection will require greater effort, the work can continue to be generated.

Transcription systems may be designed to archive dictated information for any length of time. Some facilities archive for ninety days and others for six or more months. Long periods of storage may cause the system to work more slowly, but the advantage is continued access. Even when there are problems with nursing stations, clinics, and other areas not attaching dictated reports to the paper health records, the people who need the information for coding and billing purposes, quality studies, indexes, registries, and other operational needs can still access it.

Transcription can be centralized or decentralized. In a decentralized system, pathology, radiology, and other departments may have their own transcriptionists. Some HIM departments have centralized transcription areas that type reports for the whole facility or for all facilities in an integrated system. Moreover, some transcription departments perform work for physicians' offices in order to generate revenue. The transcription department must consider every possible customer and analyze every possible location for a dedicated dictation station, including nurses' stations, clinics, operative areas, and workrooms in the HIM department. Further, every acceptable format (for example, separate tapes of different sizes or downloads from PCs or handheld computers) must be determined and policies established for the types of recordings that are allowed. Using a variety of input devices will cause productivity problems and prevent full utilization of the word-processing system's capabilities. In physicians' offices and clinics, cassette tapes are used more often for dictation purposes than in larger facilities.

The HIM professional must fully understand the word-processing system application. A **certified medical transcriptionist** (CMT) may supervise the transcription area, but the manager of the HIM department is ultimately responsible for the work. Before purchasing any large system, the HIM professional should interview references and visit similar facilities to see the system in action. Often the vendor will arrange such visits. The HIM professional also might visit facilities that are using the equipment under consideration but have not been specifically recommended by the vendor. Further, he or she might attend trade shows and seminars and narrow the field to avoid confusion. In addition, he or she should include the people who will actually use the system in the decision-making process.

Finally, transcription equipment lasts five to seven years. Vendors play an important role in keeping the HIM professional aware of system upgrades and enhancements to ensure that the department gets as much use out of its system as possible.

Issues in the Management of Medical Word Processing

Although medical word processing, or transcription, is just one function of the HIM department, it often requires a great deal of the department's attention. A backlog of reports waiting to be word-processed cannot be tolerated because many, such as history and physical examination reports and operative reports, have accreditation and regulatory time limitations. Turnaround time from dictation to typed report is important because providers must be able to retrieve information when it is needed for patient care.

Recruitment and retention of qualified medical transcriptionists are major problems for HIM professionals. Word processing equipment is expensive to acquire and to maintain, and the equipment and technology are changing rapidly. Medical transcriptionists who can accurately transcribe dictation are in short supply, and the role of the medical transcriptionist is evolving. This evolution is discussed later in this chapter.

Internal versus Contract Word-Processing Systems

The facility must decide whether to handle transcription services in-house, to contract with word-processing or transcription companies outside the facility, or to use a combination of internal and contract services.

Outsourcing to transcription or word-processing service companies, or **contract services,** is on the rise. Some healthcare facilities routinely contract all or a portion of their workload; others use the contract service on an as-needed basis. The major advantage to a contract service is that it can save the facility money in terms of salaries, fringe benefits, equipment, depreciation, floor space, maintenance, workstations, supplies, and reference materials. Further, use of an outside service can eliminate problems associated with overloading the system with increased dictation prior to a JCAHO survey or at times when medical residents change clinical service rotations. However, although outsourcing transcription services is an attractive option, it must be analyzed carefully. The major disadvantages to outsourcing are the loss of control over the transcription service and the high cost of contract transcription services.

When selecting a contract service, the HIM professional should become as familiar with the company as possible. A growing number of offshore companies or U.S.-based companies send work via the Internet to transcription personnel in other countries. Such companies must provide assurance that their transcriptionists are bonded, trained in confidentiality, and well supervised.

The manner in which the company handles a sudden influx of work is important because this is one of the major reasons why healthcare facilities use outside transcription companies. The exact method and rationale for billing and counting the final product also is extremely important. The HIM professional should question the exact definitions of a line, word, page, keystroke, minutes, or bytes or whether style requirements such as capitalizing, boldface, or underlining are an additional charge.

The counting method should be fully explained in the contract. Most companies charge by the line, but the definition of a line may be sixty-five characters rather than as a physical line. For example, if physical lines are counted and the facility is paying $0.13 to $0.18 per line, the costs can add up in situations where one word on a line is considered a line. Using a smaller font to increase the amount of typing per line may be more costly because a smaller type may scan into an imaging system and or microfilm poorly. Some companies base their charge on turnaround time, with an increased cost per line when transcription is completed within a shorter time frame. For example, the charge for transcription within forty-eight hours would be $0.10 a line; within twenty-four hours, $0.12 a line; and within eight hours, $0.18 a line. In addition, the company may include disk storage costs of $2.00 to $6.00 per five minutes of dictation.

Billing can be complicated, and the HIM professional must determine the true cost of the outside contract company's service so that he or she can compare alternatives accurately. The distribution and delivery method and the number of copies provided by the company must be evaluated because reprints might cost as much as the original transcribed document. Some companies transmit information back to the facility to be printed by the facility or send information via the Internet, fax, overnight delivery service, or courier. The contract needs to state whether the facility or the company will pay for the service. In addition, there may be a additional charge for corrections. If the facility allows physicians or providers to dictate on devices other than directly into the dictation system, this may affect the cost.

The facility also must assess how the outside company's equipment will integrate with the facility's current system, for example, with regard to phone lines, software, and interface with the electronic record system, if one exists. If the printing is to be done in-house, responsibility for printer maintenance and supply costs must be determined. The quality of the work performed by the contract company must be evaluated in terms of content, proper abbreviation use, typing and spelling errors, general appearance, correction of grammatical errors, and correct spelling of physician names. Some companies provide several levels of proofreading, including by a physician. However, proofreading also must be performed by the healthcare facility, and the facility must maintain the dictation sound so that quality checks can be performed on the outside service's work to ensure that what was dictated was what was actually typed. The HIM professional must make sure the work is closely monitored.

Even with a contract service, the health information manager still has oversight responsibility for the outside contract service and quality control. Facility personnel must file the printed reports in the health record and distribute them to residents, referring physicians, and consultants, as appropriate. Further, contracts must be carefully reviewed to ensure that contract services provide for the security of patient information.

The HIM professional also must ensure fast and easy access to the system. If physicians and coders have the ability to listen to dictation prior to transcribing, this should not change when transcription is outsourced.

Staffing of the Word-Processing Area

When the healthcare facility chooses to do medical word processing internally, the staff must be carefully selected to ensure that transcription is of high quality. Each applicant for a transcription position should be tested using the kind of work to be performed to confirm that he or she can type from the dictated word. In addition, the applicant must have excellent concentration skills, excellent hearing skills, and excellent proofreading and editing skills.

Applicants who are CMTs are in great demand. The Medical Transcription Certification Commission grants certification upon the successful completion of an examination. The requirements for this voluntary examination are experience or formal education or both. The CMT must maintain currency and certification by earning continuing education hours. Proprietary business schools and community colleges offer formal educational programs and are excellent sources for transcriptionists. A healthcare facility's offer to allow students to obtain clinical experience at the facility is an excellent way to attract applicants. Some healthcare facilities train persons with excellent typing skills on the job.

The **American Association for Medical Transcription** (AAMT) has a model curriculum for formal educational programs. The curriculum includes the study of medical terminology, anatomy and physiology, medical science, operative procedures, instruments, supplies, laboratory values, reference use and research techniques, and English grammar. All applicants should have knowledge of the areas of the model curriculum.

In addition, the AAMT produces a bimonthly journal and has excellent reference materials. Continuing education (CE) opportunities are available for transcription professionals. Transcriptionists must be given the opportunity to participate in CE activities and to be updated in new medical procedures, tests, and terminology.

The AAMT has a model job description with three defined levels for the professional transcriptionist. Some facilities may use these levels as a guide for levels of classification of personnel and promotions.

Telestaffing, or telecommuting, is a growing alternative to transcriptionists working in-house. In telestaffing, personnel are allowed to work from home or some other remote location. This has been very successful for healthcare facilities, although remote transcriptionists require special supervisory attention. They need to feel that they are part of the HIM department. The supervisor must ensure ongoing communication with telestaffing employees via e-mail or by bringing them to the facility for CE meetings and interaction with other departmental personnel. Some healthcare facilities offer telecommuting only to employees who have been with them for a period of time, fully understand the system, and are known to be responsible and dependable. Transcriptionists working outside the healthcare facility use a telephone line or cable connection to access the system. The facility supplies the transcriptionist with the telephone line, the computer workstation, and reference materials. Transcriptionists working from home must be held to the same production and quality standards as in-house transcriptionists and must be fully trained in the security and confidentiality of healthcare information.

Determining the number of transcriptionists needed in relation to the number of providers dictating is challenging and depends on the types and amount of information typed, the specialties of the facility, whether the facility is a teaching hospital or a clinic, and the types of nontranscription duties, among other factors. In a clinic or physician's office, transcription may be done as part of a larger job. Vendors can be of assistance in determining the volume of work. The type and length of work also must be evaluated. A random sample of each type of work should be selected and counted. Some vendors suggest that lines be counted for ten reports of each type to determine an average number. A line is defined as sixty-five characters. Generally, the average transcriptionist on an eight-hour shift can produce 1,200 lines per day. There are approximately ten lines per one minute of dictation. These averages will assist the HIM professional in determining staffing needs.

Fluctuations in work flow may occur for numerous reasons depending on the healthcare facility. Hospitals have peak times, for example, before an accreditation survey, after notices are sent to physicians to complete charts, and when residents and medical students change service rotations. Teaching hospitals often have much longer hours of dictation to transcribe as medical students learn the art of taking histories and performing physical examinations. Medical students dictate much more detailed information than more experienced physicians.

Productivity Management

Pay for transcription varies depending on whether the transcriptionist works for a healthcare facility or a contract service. The AAMT estimates that the entry-level transcriptionist earns $10.00 to $16.00 per hour. Some contract services pay transcriptionists $25.00 to $30.00 an hour for straight production typing, but the transcriptionists may not have the benefits that are available to the employees of a healthcare facility. The AAMT has excellent current information about productivity on its Web site at www.aamt.org.

Quality is vitally important. The supervisor must review the quality of work produced on a regular basis. Among the items to review are punctuation errors, omitted dictation, misspelled words or medical terms, and formatting errors. An analysis of each transcriptionist's errors will target those areas that need improvement.

The facility may use numerous possible standards. For example, ten lines of typing produced for every one minute of dictation might be translated into three or four minutes of typing for every minute of dictation. There is a great deal of debate over what the standard production, or even the best unit of measurement, should be.

Incentive Programs

Because of the competition for CMTs, many healthcare facilities offer **incentive pay** plans to reward transcriptionists for high productivity. For example, a hospital may require a transcriptionist to type eight hours a day and produce 1,200 lines of typed output for a base monthly salary. Beyond 1,200 lines, the transcriptionist may earn a bonus of $0.06 per line, with the bonus cents per line increasing to the point where a transcriptionist typing 2,001 lines would receive a bonus of $0.12 per line. However, the quality of the work must remain at 98 percent accuracy based on regular quality review.

For fairness in the incentive system, work must be rotated so that each transcriptionist has the opportunity to perform different kinds of work from different providers. Providers for whom English is a second language may produce dictation that is more difficult to transcribe. Moreover, some providers are not careful in their dictation, which requires more listening and replaying.

The proponents of incentive pay plans believe that monetary incentives increase productivity, reduce turnover, provide fair and equitable pay, and motivate employees. Highly productive transcriptionists are paid for what they produce.

Evaluation of the Effectiveness and Efficiency of Medical Word-Processing Services

The effectiveness and efficiency of medical word-processing services are judged primarily by turnaround time and accuracy in typing the dictation. History and physical examinations and operative reports have time limitations set forth in JCAHO regulations. Discharge summaries are valuable sources of information for coding, billing, and reimbursement. With EMR systems, the dictated information and transcribed documents are accessible to all providers and healthcare personnel who need to refer to them. The success of the medical word processing depends on both the cooperation of the providers who dictate and the skills of the medical transcriptionists.

Check Your Understanding 8.4

Instructions: Answer the following questions on a separate sheet of paper.

1. What are the advantages of using a contract transcription system? What are the advantages of having transcription performed in-house?

2. What are the formal educational requirements for a certified medical transcriptionist?

3. How will voice recognition technology change the job of the medical transcriptionist?

4. What are the four benefits of an incentive pay plan?

5. What factors must be considered when determining the number of transcriptionists a healthcare facility needs?

Incomplete Record Control

Health records must be completed in order to provide all the information that is needed for patient care, billing, and reimbursement. The HIM department must verify that all records are received from the nursing floor, including any previous records that were on the floor. After the records arrive in the HIM department, their location must be carefully tracked until they reach final storage in the filing area.

The financial office notifies the HIM department of bills that are waiting for information from the physician so that the record can be coded and the bill prepared. The administration places a great deal of pressure on the HIM department to process bills in a timely manner so that revenue can be generated for the facility. In turn, the HIM professional must motivate physicians to provide the information the department needs to do its work. Incomplete records are a chronic problem in most healthcare facilities, and monitoring them is a constant challenge for the HIM professional.

Quantitative Analysis

Quantitative analysis, often called the **discharge analysis,** is a review of the health record for completeness and accuracy. It is generally conducted retrospectively, that is, after the patient's discharge from the facility or at the conclusion of treatment. Quantitative analysis also may be done while the patient is in the facility, in which case it is referred to as concurrent review or **concurrent analysis.**

One practice in the discharge analysis process is to rearrange the forms in the paper-based health record in a standard permanent sequence for filing. This order differs from the sequencing of forms while patients are under active treatment when convenient reference to certain information is needed. While in active use, the health record is arranged with the most current information on top as follows: orders, progress or clinic notes, operative notes, medications, graphic sheets, nursing notes, consultations, ancillary forms, consents, history and physical, demographic information, and face sheet. The order differs according to the facility, but the record forms the provider prepares and writes on most frequently are on top to allow for quick entry of orders and progress notes. Labeled tabs divide the chart into sections to assist in finding needed documents.

When the patient is discharged or treatment is terminated, the record arrives in the HIM department, where it is immediately rearranged in reverse order. The face sheet and demographic information are on top, followed by the history and physical examination, the discharge summary, ancillary reports, consents, operative reports, progress notes in date order with the earliest orders first, orders in date order, nursing notes in date order, and so forth. Many facilities leave the record in the order in which it arrives in the HIM department, rather than spending the time to rearrange it. This system is called **universal chart order** or uniform chart order. The benefits of the system are that time is saved in the HIM department and providers can more easily find the parts of the record they need because the arrangement remains the same.

A facility moving to universal chart order must involve nursing and physicians in the decisions about chart arrangement because they use the record as a reference for patient care every day. Labeled dividers and a standard table of contents help ensure that everyone who works with the chart knows the proper arrangement.

Quantitative analysis involves several additional steps. The record forms must be reviewed individually to make sure they belong in the record and belong to that particular patient. Organizing the paper forms is an important step. Forms are often intermingled and usually separated into a source-oriented format. Preliminary laboratory reports may be discarded when there is a final cumulative summary report.

Each facility must develop its own procedures for quantitative analysis. Responsibility for completion of the record must be assigned to each responsible provider. This is called deficiency assignment. The deficiencies, or parts of the record needing completion or signature, are entered into a computer software program or on paper worksheets attached to the incomplete, or deficient, health record.

Moreover, the record must be reviewed to ensure that certain basic reports that are common to all patient records are present, including the history and physical, progress notes, orders, nursing notes, and discharge summary. Other reports (for example, operative reports, diagnostic tests, consultations, and so on) may be included depending on the patient's course of treatment. Quantitative analysis also includes a review for authentication that may be done by written signature, rubber stamp facsimile, computer password, or initials, and must include the professional title of the responsible individual.

Any corrections to the record must be entered properly. The provider should draw a single line through the error, add a note explaining the error, initial and date the error with the date it was discovered, and make the correct entry in chronological order. The entry being replaced also must be indicated. For computer entries, a procedure should be followed that explains how to correct errors and make addenda to the health record.

Moreover, the record must be analyzed to ensure that symbols and abbreviations used in documentation have been approved by the medical staff and have only one clear meaning.

Criteria for Adequacy of Documentation

Documentation must reflect the care rendered to the patient and the patient's response. It must be timely and legible and signed by the person who wrote it. The health record is considered a legal document and a business record because it records events at or about the time they happen. Moreover, timeliness and legibility are two of the main areas of focus for accreditation and licensure bodies.

Concurrent analysis means that the record is analyzed during the patient's stay in the healthcare facility. It has the advantage of HIM or other personnel being present on the floors where the physicians see patients. HIM personnel can remind providers to complete items in the record and to sign orders and progress notes. Some facilities have HIM personnel physically located on the nursing floors to monitor record completion closely. Other facilities have HIM personnel visit patient care areas to obtain signatures and ensure that loose reports are placed in the health record.

After the patient is discharged, the record is brought to the HIM department by delivery or by HIM personnel who pick up records. Discharge analysis serves as an additional check to ensure that the record is complete and that all information belongs to the patient. Concurrent review and discharge analysis review the records for the same documentation.

Record Completion Policies and Procedures

The health record is not complete until all of its parts are assembled, organized, and authenticated. The HIM professional, the administration, and the medical staff must develop record completion policies and procedures and include them in the medical staff bylaws. Although the facility's governing body has overall responsibility for patient care, responsibility for the delivery and documentation of patient care is delegated to the medical staff. The medical staff and the individual physician have primary responsibility for completing the health record to document the process of care that was rendered.

Most facilities have a committee in place composed of members of the medical staff, the administration, nursing, and other provider disciplines with responsibility for ensuring that medical staff members follow the established rules and regulations for health records. This committee may be the health record committee, the quality committee, or some other committee responsible for ensuring compliance with rules and regulations. The HIM professional should serve on the committee and generally assist the physician or provider committee chair by preparing the agenda and minutes for meetings.

The HIM professional also assists the committee by preparing reports on the status of record completion and problems with the flow of the record through the facility. Reports regarding the percentage of records are important to ensure that accreditation standards are met on an ongoing basis. The findings from various types of record review, including concurrent reviews and retrospective reviews, are presented to the committee and discussed. The committee often plays a key role in the approval of forms so that the standard form and format of the record can be maintained.

The committee chair may communicate directly with physicians or other medical staff members to solve problems related to record completion. The committee can be a valuable resource to the HIM professional because it has representation from every area that documents in the patient record. Committee members can often assist the HIM department in acquiring equipment and personnel needed to properly perform its responsibilities. The committee generally reports to the executive committee of the medical staff and makes recommendations for executive staff action to improve patient record services.

Qualitative Analysis

In **qualitative analysis,** HIM personnel carefully review the quality and adequacy of record documentation and ensure that it is in accordance with the policies, rules, and regulations established by the facility, the standards of licensing and accrediting bodies, and government requirements. Like quantitative analysis, qualitative analysis may be done concurrently or retrospectively.

Qualitative analysis is a more in-depth review of health records than quantitative analysis is, although the processes may overlap somewhat, depending on the facility. When qualitative analysis is done while the patient is in the facility or under active treatment, it is called open-record review. The JCAHO requires an open-record review to ensure that its documentation standards are met at the point of care delivery. A specific format for open-record review covers all types of records. HIM personnel or case management personnel, nurses, physicians, and other providers should participate in the open-record review process. This review process looks at requirements such as presence of the history and physical examination prior to surgery, completion of the postoperative note, and many other aspects of the care process as documented in the health record. Open-record review should be done on an ongoing basis.

Qualitative review also is performed on **closed records. Closed-record review** means that the qualitative review is done retrospectively following discharge or termination of treatment. The benefit of open-record review is that problems in the care process that are revealed through the review can be corrected immediately. Closed-record review is an important way to obtain information about trends and patterns of documentation.

Role of Health Information Management Professionals

Medicare and state licensure standards require healthcare facilities to have an HIM department with administrative responsibility for health records. This includes having the staff, equipment, and policies and procedures to ensure that records are current and accurate and that information is accessible.

The HIM department works closely with the finance department regarding chart completion. The finance department and the entire organization depend on the HIM staff to work with physicians and other healthcare professionals to provide the necessary information so that bills can be finalized. Bills are usually sent within two to three days after discharge. The health information manager receives daily notification of accounts that need information, and procedures must be established to expedite the flow of information for payment purposes.

Role of the Medical Staff

Medical staff are responsible for developing bylaws governing their operation. The requirements for documentation and completion of health records as well as penalties for not adhering to them are included in the medical staff bylaws. Each member of the medical staff signs a statement that he or she will abide by the bylaws, and each is responsible for documentation.

Management of Incomplete Records

The HIM professional is responsible for ensuring that health records, whether manual or electronic, are readily accessible and that adequate equipment and personnel are available to facilitate record completion. No matter how well staffed and well organized the HIM department is, it can only facilitate the process. The providers are responsible for the documentation and must dictate, sign, and otherwise complete the patient health record.

Storage, Retrieval, and Tracking of Incomplete Records

Facilities provide access to incomplete records in various ways. Paper-based records needing completion are maintained in a file in the physician workroom. They may be arranged alphabetically by the last name of the responsible physician or filed in numerical order. Filing by physician name enables physicians to go directly to their own boxes to access and complete their own records.

One disadvantage is that completion is often delayed because the record may remain in one physician's box until it is completed and moved to the next box. In a facility with many specialists or many residents, maintaining incomplete records in numerical order by the patient's record number works well because the records are accessible to all providers who need to complete them. Other facilities file incomplete

records alphabetically by the patient's last name. Still other facilities immediately file the records into the general file area, using a combination of filing methods. When only one provider needs to work on a record, it is filed under that provider's name; when several physicians need to work on the records, a numerical system is used. The advantage is that records are all filed in one area for ease of location by the clerical staff.

In any of these arrangements, clerical staff must be available to assist providers and to ensure that the sections that need to be completed are actually done. When incomplete records are filed numerically, the facility might require physicians to call before arriving at the department so that the needed records can be pulled. Some HIM personnel speed up record completion by taking records to physicians' offices located on the hospital campus.

The completion time clock begins running when the patient is discharged or treatment is terminated. Records are considered deficient or incomplete immediately at discharge. Some facilities choose to begin the time clock after the records are reviewed quantitatively by the HIM staff and available to the providers; however, regulations and standards do not provide for "extra" time for analysis or transcription delays, computer system downtime, or physician unavailability. Healthcare facility policies and medical staff bylaws must define when incomplete records or deficient records become delinquent.

Delinquent health records are those records that are not completed within the specified time frame, for example, within fourteen days of discharge. The definition of a delinquent chart varies according to the facility, but most facilities require that records be completed within thirty days of discharge as mandated by Medicare regulations and JCAHO standards. Some facilities require a shorter time frame for completing records because of concerns about timely billing. **Chart tracking** of the location of incomplete and delinquent records as they move through the completion process is vital because many people need access to the records of recently treated patients.

Policies and Procedures on Completion of Records

When analyzing the record, HIM personnel list what needs to be done to complete it. This may be done by filling in a form listing the providers and items needing completion or signatures or by entering information into a computerized deficiency system. Physicians can then access the system to determine what they need to do.

Numerous other methods may be used to encourage the timely completion of records. The JCAHO specifies that the number of delinquent records cannot exceed 50 percent of the average number of discharges, so keeping the number of delinquent charts as low as possible is a constant challenge for HIM staff. Concurrent analysis by HIM personnel can help speed up completion time. Using case managers to work with physicians on chart completion issues while the patient is in the facility is also helpful in reducing the burden on the

HIM department. HIM professionals rely on medical staff committees, such as the health record committee; chiefs of medical services; and medical staff leaders to motivate providers to complete records. They and healthcare administrators are willing to try any creative ideas that will motivate physicians to complete patient health records.

Many facilities limit the retrospective checking and flagging of incomplete items in the HIM department to the discharge summary, history and physical examination, operative reports, consultations, and clinical reports. Nursing information is not reviewed nor are signatures on progress notes and orders checked. The reason why less detailed analysis is done after discharge is due to the increased emphasis on open-record review when patients are in the facility under active treatment. Requiring physicians to sign notes and orders retrospectively does not affect the process of patient care and treatment. The HIM department should continue to monitor a sample of notes and orders to ensure that signatures are present to comply with established facility policies, accreditation standards, and regulations. Corrective measures should be developed when there is a pattern of missing signatures.

As mentioned above, penalties for noncompletion of health records must be included in medical staff bylaws. Penalties such as suspension of admission privileges or surgical privileges for the individual physician and/or group and the levying of fines per incomplete chart or per day must be explained in the bylaws. Some hospitals make health record completion a condition of continued membership on the medical staff and suspend physicians who do not comply with the rules regarding completion. Suspended physicians must reapply for staff membership. Some states require that physicians suspended three times in a year be reported to the state medical board. However, in some small facilities or in facilities where the physician is responsible for many admissions, it is difficult to enforce the rules regarding suspension of admitting privileges.

The facility must have a policy in place for dealing with situations where records remain incomplete for an extended period. The HIM director can be given authority to declare that a record is complete for purposes of filing when a provider dies or has an extended illness that would prevent the record from ever being completed. Every effort should be made to have a partner or physician in the same specialty area work on the chart so that coding, billing, and statistical information is available. In teaching hospitals, residents sometimes leave before charts are completed and become difficult to locate. Thus, many facilities require departing residents to obtain clearance from the HIM department before the end of the residency period. The medical staff committee responsible for health record functions may review long-standing incomplete charts and direct that they be filed even though incomplete.

Physician Notification Processes

Most healthcare facilities notify physicians of charts that need completion on an escalating basis. For example, the first notice reminds the physician that records need completion; the second describes the penalties for noncompletion; the third limits the admission or operative privileges of the physician and his or her partners and might include suspension of even emergency admission privileges; and the fourth gives a warning regarding suspension or removal from the medical staff. Finally, the physician may be considered to have forfeited staff membership and would have to reapply for membership. Some teaching facilities withhold paychecks for residents or refuse to approve vacations until all of the physician's charts are complete.

The HIM department is responsible for counting incomplete charts and preparing lists of those providers who have delinquent records and those whose privileges have been suspended. Extensions are often granted when physicians are out of town, sick, have a death in the family, and so on. The handling of physician suspensions requires a great deal of cooperation among the HIM professional, the medical staff leadership, and the administration.

Authentication of Health Record Entries

Authentication means to prove authorship by signing a document and can be done in several ways. Signatures handwritten in ink are the most common method for signing paper-based health records. The JCAHO allows rubber-stamp facsimile signatures when there is a statement verifying that the physician is the only one who will use the stamp and will maintain control of it.

Autoauthentication is a policy that allows the physician or provider to state in advance that dictated and transcribed reports should automatically be considered approved and signed when the physician does not make corrections within a certain period of time. Another variation of autoauthentication is that physicians authorize the HIM department to send a weekly list of documents needing signatures. The list is then signed and returned to the HIM department. Some facilities use autoauthentication even though the JCAHO does not approve it. The objection is that evidence cannot be provided that the physician actually reviewed and approved each report. Facilities that use these methods of authentication state that the physicians' offices automatically receive copies of transcribed reports and thus providers have the ability to review the reports before the deadline or before signing the list of reports.

Electronic signature refers to a computer password affixed to a report or document. A statement ensuring that the password is controlled and used only by the responsible provider should be required to protect patient confidentiality and to ensure that others do not use it. Password security is critical. Electronic signatures will be used more frequently as more documents in the record are produced by, and remain in, the computer and do not become part of the paper record. Facilities that scan paper records of discharged patients into imaging systems must make it clear to physicians that these are images of papers that can be viewed, but not edited or signed.

Signatures in teaching hospitals are especially important to show that the attending physician responsible for the patient is actively involved in the patient's care. Signatures are generally required on all reports completed by residents and medical students. In electronic signature programs, the attending physician's co-signature should be entered after the resident has reviewed and signed the report to confirm the attending physician's participation.

Forms Design and Management

The management and design of forms used in the healthcare environment is a concern of all providers. Forms must be developed and approved in a careful, systematic process to ensure that they meet facility standards, are compatible with imaging and microfilming systems, and do not duplicate information on existing forms. (Examples of commonly used health record forms are provided in appendix A of this book.) HIM department personnel must be constantly vigilant to ensure that only approved forms become part of the permanent health record. Unapproved forms do not have the necessary form numbers or bar codes needed for imaging and indexing systems. Small forms and folded flowcharts create problems when records are handled and utilized. Oversize forms create problems in microfilming or optical imaging because special preparation is required to ensure that all information is filmed or scanned. As health records move toward a computer-based format, the forms design process becomes the process of designing computer views for entry of data, but the principles of control still apply.

Principles of Forms Design

A well-designed form improves the reliability of the data entered on it. A form should be designed to collect information in a consistent way and to remind providers of information that needs to be included. Many paper record forms consist of a single sheet. Other specialty forms, such as a unit-set form or a multipart form, have multiple-sheet forms preassembled in either carbon or carbonless sets. With spot carbons in unit-set forms, only part of the information on the original is visible on the copy. When the face sheet is the first page of a unit set and printed on the computer, the carbon can be positioned so that the copy for a clinical department would have only the patient identification information and not the financial information.

Continuous-feed forms use a series of forms separated with perforations that can be printed by a printer without having to load the paper for each form printed. The forms then can be separated and distributed. Continuous-feed forms can be used both for single sheets and multiset forms.

Most forms include similar basic components and at least a heading to describe the contents and purpose, instructions on how to fill out the form, and spaces to enter required and/or optional information. General guidelines to follow when designing forms include:

- The form should be easy to complete.
- Instructions on completion and use of the form should be included.

- The form should have a heading with a title that clearly identifies its purpose.
- The facility's name and address should appear on each page of the form.
- The name, patient identification number, and other identifying information should be present on each form. Most facilities now use **bar coding** as identifying information.
- Bar coding also should be included in indexing the form for random access in an optical scanner or microfilming system. Bar codes are generally printed directly on the document or on a label affixed to the document.
- The form number and date of revision should be included to ensure that the form being used is the correct and most current version.
- Outdated forms should be recalled and eliminated.
- The physical layout of the form should be logical. When a clerk is entering information as the patient gives it, the form should be organized to match the way the information is requested (for example, the patient's city, state, and zip code).
- Personal and address data and other items of information that relate to one another should be put together.
- Font selection should be standardized. Some experts recommend all capital letters.
- Margins should be left for hole punches to allow the document to be placed in folders or chart holders. The holes may be on the left-hand side of the form or at the top or both, depending on the types of folders or binders.
- Ruled lines may be used to outline sections of forms to allow for easy entry of data or to separate areas of the form.
- Shading can be used to separate and emphasize areas of the form.
- Check boxes and fields can be used to provide space for the collection of data.

Careful consideration also should be given to including information on the backs of forms. There is the possibility that another patient's information might be recorded on the back of the form. Facilities that are **scanning** and imaging paper records must have the bar-coded patient identification information on the back of the form to ensure proper indexing into the imaging system. Even though scanners can scan both sides of a document, the ability to index and thus access the information must be ensured.

Forms Control Systems

Facilities must develop strict guidelines and processes for forms control. Word-processing programs and programs specifically designed for forms design have made the process easier than in the past. Providers often design their own non-approved forms, which may appear in the paper record when it arrives in the HIM department. This affects procedures and the patient care process as well as procedures in the department. The person who designed the form may be unaware of the interrelated processes that are affected by changing a form.

Forms control systems must:

- Provide for the development of forms according to established guidelines
- Control the printing and use of forms
- Guide providers in designing forms according to established guidelines
- Prevent staff from changing or designing forms that duplicate existing forms or could be combined into other forms

Forms control is critical as the transition toward image- and computer-based record systems continues. The transition usually begins with using an imaging system to gather information about existing forms and to ensure that all forms can be properly scanned and indexed. Without indexing, the information cannot be retrieved. The forms control process also should establish processes for forms inventory, forms identification, forms analysis, and forms purchasing.

Forms Inventory

The first step in the forms control process is the forms inventory. This process involves gathering each form and all of its editions to ensure that the most current version is used. A subject file is a good idea for bringing together all the forms used by each of the areas, such as all admissions or registration forms, all operative forms, and all nursing forms. Organizing in this manner would prevent new forms from being developed when current forms have the needed information, assist in finding ways to combine forms with related information, and serve as a reminder that information changed on one form must be changed on related forms.

Forms Identification

The second part of the forms control process is forms identification. This involves assigning each form a distinct title that reflects its use. In paper systems, a forms number indicates that the form has been approved. The date and the source department are usually included with the number. Bar coding and labels with complete bar-coded information about the form are becoming more prevalent as facilities prepare for the eventual computerization of forms. A numerical listing of forms should be maintained.

Forms Analysis

Forms analysis involves the continuous review and revision of forms. The forms analysis process is often initiated because of procedural problems, for example, when providers are not receiving the information they need to do their work. Forms assist in guiding processes and ensuring that information is obtained and recorded. Flowcharting the development and distribution of the forms is helpful in determining whether a form is still useful, whether the information it contains is current, and whether it meets the current requirements of the facility.

Forms Purchasing

Purchasing and printing comprise the fourth part of the forms control process. A policy should be in place stating that forms cannot be ordered or reordered without approval of the forms committee or some other group or individual responsible for purchasing and printing approval.

Check Your Understanding 8.5

Instructions: Answer the following questions on a separate sheet of paper.

1. What are quantitative analysis and qualitative analysis? What purpose do they serve?
2. How does concurrent review facilitate record completion?
3. What is universal chart order, and why is it being adopted by healthcare facilities?
4. What is the difference between open- and closed-record review?
5. Why is the finance department concerned about the timely completion of records?
6. In what two ways do HIM departments store incomplete health records? How do the two storage systems work?
7. What is the difference between an incomplete record and a delinquent record?
8. How does the HIM professional help providers to complete health records?
9. What three methods do facilities use to authenticate health records? How does each method work?
10. Why have some facilities stopped notifying providers about orders and progress notes needing signatures?
11. Why is forms control a critical responsibility of the HIM professional?
12. What are the four parts of the forms control process?
13. Why is it important for those providers wanting a new form to go through the approval process?
14. How are bar codes and labels used in forms?

Creation, Storage, and Retention of Paper-Based Health Records

Healthcare organizations need policies covering the circulation and storage of health records to ensure that the records can be located quickly when they are needed for patient care and other uses. Controlling the storage of paper-based health records is critical to patient care. The image and reputation of the HIM department may depend on the speed with which patient health information can be retrieved.

Management of paper-based health records includes three processes: creation and identification, storage and retrieval, and retention and disposition.

Health Record Creation and Identification

As discussed earlier, the health record is created when the patient is first admitted to or treated in a healthcare facility. Every patient is assigned a specific identification number, and the health record is initiated with the collection of admission or registration information. As data and information about the patient's care and condition are documented, the record grows. The record remains in active use for the purposes of patient care, clinical coding, billing, statistical analysis, and other operational processes until the episode of care ends.

Health Record Identification Systems

In order that the correct health record can be quickly retrieved when it is needed, each record must be assigned a unique identifier. The choice of record identification system is tied to the organization's filing system.

Small healthcare facilities, such as physicians' offices, often use a simple alphabetical identifier: the patient's last and first names. Some experts suggest that alphabetical systems are most appropriate for facilities with fewer than 10,000 individual records. Other facilities use a straight numerical record identification system. Experts suggest that straight numerical systems can efficiently accommodate no more than 25,000 records. Most large organizations use a record identification system that assigns a multipart numerical identifier to each record.

Serial Numbering System

In a **serial numbering system,** each patient receives a new number at each visit, and numbers are assigned in straight numerical sequence to consecutive patients in the order in which they arrive for treatment. Each time a patient is treated by the facility, a new number is issued to link the patient to that particular visit or admission. This system is often used by clinics and physicians' offices.

Unit Numbering System

In a **unit numbering system,** the patient is assigned a number during the first encounter for care and keeps it for all subsequent encounters. The number may be assigned automatically by the computer system. Some facilities, such as Veterans Affairs facilities, use the patient's Social Security number as the unit number because it is a unique permanent number already assigned to the patient. Most large facilities use a unit numbering system.

Serial-Unit Numbering System

In a **serial-unit numbering system,** the patient is issued a different number for each admission or encounter for care and the records of past episodes of care are brought forward to be filed under the last number issued. This creates a unit record that contains information from all of the patient's encounters. Because this system requires a great deal of shifting of records and changing of numbers, it is not as commonly used as the unit numbering system.

When facilities change from a serial to a unit numbering system, it is important to pick a start date and move forward from that point. As patients are readmitted, they are assigned a new number that then becomes the permanent unit number and all records are brought forward and linked under the new number.

Family Numbering System

Family numbering is a type of unit numbering system. In this system, the entire family is assigned one number and all information on visits by any family member is filed in one location. This system may be appropriate for use in family practice settings.

Health Record Filing Systems

Most healthcare facilities use numerical filing systems for paper-based health records. Small facilities, such as physicians' offices and clinics, often use alphabetic filing; larger facilities generally use numerical filing systems.

Serial Filing System

In a **serial filing system,** records are filed according to the number assigned to a particular encounter or visit. The major shortcoming of serial filing is that the records for patients who received services multiple times at the facility would have different numbers and the different records would be filed in multiple places in the filing system. Therefore, a serial filing system requires more searching and more retrieval time than a unit filing system does.

Unit Filing System

A true **unit filing system** arranges the records for all inpatient and outpatient visits and procedures for a single patient together under a permanent unit number. The individual patient's unit record grows in size as additional information is added. There is only one record for the patient, and it is kept in one specific location in the file room.

Terminal-Digit Filing System

In a **terminal-digit filing system,** records are filed according to a three-part number made up of two-digit pairs. The basic terminal-digit filing system contains 10,000 divisions, with 100 sections ranging from 00–99 and 100 divisions within each section ranging from 00–99.

Terminal-digit filing is not difficult to learn, but it is different from straight numerical filing. In straight numerical filing, the first numbers (those farthest to the left) are considered first. The number itself can be a permanent unit number or a serial number.

In terminal-digit filing, the record number is placed into terminal-digit order when the health record is ready for filing. The number is broken down into two-digit pairs and is read from right to left. For example, the number 670187 would be written as 67-01-87. The first pair of digits on the right (87) is called the primary number or the terminal-digit number, the second pair of digits (01) is called the secondary number, and the third pair of digits (67) is called the tertiary or final number.

The primary number is considered first for filing. The primary numbers range from 00 to 99 and represent the 100 sections of the filing area. Because many records will be filed in each section, each section needs to be further subdivided, first according to the secondary number and then according to the tertiary number. As shown in figure 8.5, a record numbered 67-01-87 would be filed in section 87, in subsection 01, and then in numerical sequence for 67 (after 66-01-87 and before 68-01-87). All records with the tertiary and secondary numbers of 01-87 would be filed within this part of the file.

Consider three patients who were admitted to a facility and were issued the following numbers in sequence: 67-01-87, 67-01-88, and 67-01-89. In a terminal digit system, these records would be added to three different filing sections of the 100 sections of the file rather than all being filed at the end as in a straight numerical system. (See figure 8.6).

The advantage of terminal-digit filing is that filing shelves fill equally rather than at the end, as is the case with conventional straight numerical filing. There will be one record with the primary number 00, one with 01, and so on through 99 for every one hundred consecutive numbers issued to patients. For every one hundred records added to the file, each section of the file will be increased by only one record. The task of moving charts to alleviate overcrowding at the end of the file is reduced because consecutively numbered charts can be moved from each section periodically. One hundred consecutively numbered folders would be removed from 100 separate locations. Thus, the even distribution of records throughout the filing space can be maintained, and misfiles can be reduced because clerks need to remember only two numbers at a time.

Another advantage of terminal-digit filing is that the department's workload can be evenly distributed among filing personnel. Certain sections can be designated for each employee. For example, if a department has five file clerks, each could be given responsibility for a specific section, with clerk 1 responsible for section 00–19, clerk 2 responsible for section 20–39, and so on. In addition to maintaining each section, each clerk would file loose reports and keep the records in order, handle requests for information from patient records, and perform other duties.

Terminal-digit filing can be adapted to various types of numbering systems. A six-digit number is most common, but some facilities, such as Veterans Affairs facilities, use a longer number. The VA uses the Social Security number as the basis for terminal-digit filing. For example, number 401-80-1530 could be adapted to serve as a terminal digit by dividing it so that 30 is the primary number, 15 is the secondary number, and 40180 is the tertiary number. The files do not expand evenly because there is no facility control over the assignment of numbers to patients.

Generally, open-shelf filing is used for terminal-digit filing. The shelves are set up with guide tabs and folder tabs on the ends of the folders or guides so that they can easily be seen. In a standard terminal-digit filing area, there will be 10,000 guides to index the primary number sections and secondary number subdivisions so that behind each guide, all records will have the same final four digits. The guides are

Figure 8.5.   Filing of Patient Record 67-01-87 in a Terminal Digit System

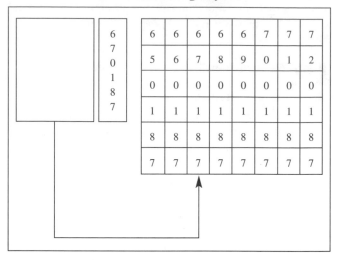

Figure 8.6.   Filing of Three Consecutive Patient Records under the Terminal Digit System

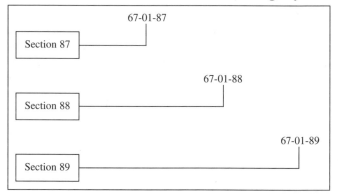

set up vertically with the digits above the line on the guide representing the division (secondary number) and the digits below the line representing the section (primary number). An index guide tab marked with 67 above the line and 80 below would indicate the 67 division of the 80 section.

Many facilities use different colors to represent each of the ten primary numbers 0 to 9, and the colors appear on the folders and guides. The records in a particular section are in blocks of color. This allows misfiles to be identified quickly. Vendors of file folders have endless possibilities of color-coding different pairs of numbers. The colors selected to represent particular digits must be permanent and continued when new folders are ordered or else the advantage of color-coding will be lost.

Even distribution of paper-based health records is difficult in today's environment. Patient records contain myriad information, including graphic tracings, photographs, and cumulative laboratory report printouts. Records are bulkier than in the past because of the large quantity of paper produced as documentation of care delivery.

Health Record Storage and Retrieval

The HIM department is responsible for ensuring that the paper record is available when needed by the provider for patient care. No matter how well organized and well managed the HIM department is, the timeliness of record delivery to providers is the measure of the quality of the department's services.

Health Record Storage

Storage is the application of efficient procedures for the use of filing equipment and storage media to keep records secure and available to those providers and other healthcare personnel authorized to access them. Record storage equipment can range from numerous types of file cabinets to open shelves of various heights and types.

Planning for record storage is a major responsibility for the HIM professional. He or she must maintain a leadership role in ensuring that sufficient conveniently accessible space is available for the storage of paper records. Ways must be provided to consistently maintain sufficient filing room by moving inactive records or by microfilming or imaging records.

Because space is expensive, administrators and facilities management personnel are always looking for ways to better use it. The HIM professional must make sure that records are not located in poor environmental conditions where they can be either damaged or difficult to locate. For example, health records should not be stored in areas where pipes and flammable substances are located.

Health Record Retrieval

Retrieval is concerned with locating requested records and information. It involves signing out or checking out records from the filing area and tracking those that are not returned within the specified time period. A number of excellent software systems are available for tracking patient records.

HIM personnel must be able to quickly determine the exact location of a specific health record at any time. Facilities should have strict policies and procedures in place that specify who is permitted to check out records from the filing area. Past records are generally requested when patients are readmitted or appear for appointments. Large clinics create a lot of activity in the filing area because records must be pulled in advance for patient appointments. Acute care facilities must provide past records for readmitted patients.

The filing area should be audited periodically to ensure that files are in correct order, regardless of the filing system used. Loose reports should be attached, and those awaiting attachment should be sorted and organized to facilitate retrieval. It should be possible to locate charts in emergency situations within fifteen minutes. The charge-out system should be reviewed to make sure the charged-out record is still under the responsibility of the person named in the system or on the charge-out form.

Statistics on the ratio of number of requests to number of records in the file should be maintained to demonstrate the activity in the filing area. Statistics on the ratio of the number of records located to number of records requested provide evidence of the filing function's accuracy and quality.

Health Record Filing and Storage Equipment

Filing equipment vendors are the HIM professional's best resource in planning a filing area that makes the best use of the available space. Open-shelf filing is the least expensive option for health record storage. Shelves are usually arranged back to back just as shelving in a library is. Shelving uses space more efficiently because only thirty to thirty-six inches are needed for each aisle. When standard file cabinets are used, aisles should be at least five feet wide to allow two facing file cabinets to be opened at the same time and to allow personnel who need to work in the same area to pass. Lateral files with drawers and doors also require sufficient aisle space for opening the individual drawers and allowing personnel to pass.

Many facilities use open-shelf files mounted on tracks to conserve valuable space. These are referred to as movable files, and many different styles are available. The main consideration is whether the files open electronically or manually. With movable files mounted on tracks, more sections of files can be installed because the floor space for many fixed aisles is not needed. The files in a mobile unit can be opened one aisle at a time. With permanently installed open shelves, there are fixed aisles between each shelf. Whatever type of shelving is selected, the shelves must be able to handle the heavy weight of paper-based health records.

Vendors estimate the amount of file shelves needed based on several factors. One consideration is the average size of individual records. The volume of patients and the number of repeat visits or readmissions will affect the potential expansion of each individual patient record. The type of facility also will affect the size of individual records. Acute care facilities with extensive ancillary services and more acutely ill patients will have larger individual patient records, as will facilities specializing in transplants, cancer, and other chronic diseases. When unit records are organized in a terminal-digit filing system, there must be adequate expansion space in each division of the filing area to allow for expansion of individual records.

It is the responsibility of the HIM professional to ensure that the vendors' estimates are adequate. The number of linear filing inches is the key factor. When there are existing records, the average size of the individual records can be easily calculated by measuring the number of files on a random sampling of shelves. The vendor should subtract for the side panels of the open-shelf filing units. The usable space must be measured from the inside of the panels, not from the outside of the shelves, so that the true number of linear filing inches is reflected. For example, one standard three-foot-wide shelf would have approximately thirty-three linear inches available for filing. Allowance also should be made for file guides, which also reduce the number of linear filing inches.

An example might be that of department expanding into another filing area. The department has selected eight-shelf open shelves that are thirty-six inches wide with thirty-three inches of actual filing space on each shelf. The department's present health records have been measured in random areas of the existing files and average two inches in thickness. With 5,000 discharges anticipated each year and a projection of five years, 25,000 records will need to be stored. Because records will average a two-inch thickness, 50,000 filing inches will be needed. Because each eight-shelf unit will have 264 linear filing inches available, the number of inches needed, 50,000, must be divided by 264 to determine the number of filing units that must be purchased, which will be 190.

Storage space is at a premium, and many facilities have several locations for storage of medical records. This can create retrieval problems when records are in distant locations or off-site. Much personnel time can be spent walking or driving to off-site locations. Some facilities contract with commercial storage companies to store inactive records; commercial storage companies can provide for transportation of records to the facility.

Health Record Retention and Disposition

Disposition involves determining the retention schedule to be followed to protect and preserve active and inactive records. Establishing policies that incorporate state and federal laws and maintaining a disaster plan are part of the disposition process. The transfer and destruction of records, optical scanning, and microfilming are all part of this stage. Facilities must be careful to monitor record maintenance so that records are continuously moved out of active storage as they become inactive or reach maximum retention periods. Records cannot be stored indefinitely because storage areas fill up. Older records may not be as useful in the patient care treatment process.

Accreditation and Legal Record Retention Requirements

The JCAHO asserts that the length of record retention depends on laws, regulations, and the use of health records for care and for other purposes such as research and education.

State laws, Medicare regulations, and other federal regulations, accreditation standards, and facility policies and procedures all must be reviewed when establishing a retention schedule. The HIM professional must adhere to the strictest time limit. In addition to the length of time for maintaining health records, the HIM professional must consider the required length of retention for immunization records, mammography records, X rays and radiographs, and the records of minors and incompetent patients.

Medicare requires records to be maintained for at least five years, according to 42 CFR 282.26(d). This includes committee reports, physician certification and recertification reports, radiologist records (printouts, films, scans, and other images), home health agency records, long-term care records, laboratory records, and any other records that document information about claims. When state laws or licensing standards require a longer retention period, the longer requirement must be followed. State law should be reviewed to determine the handling of other images. In many states, these are handled the same way that radiologist records are handled.

State agencies also may have retention requirements. The Occupational Safety and Health Administration (OSHA) requires records of employees with occupational exposure to be maintained for the duration of employment plus thirty years. The statutes of limitation (deadline for filing a lawsuit) in various types of legal actions are important considerations in developing a retention schedule.

The facility or provider is responsible for maintaining the record. When it cannot produce a record, it must be able to prove that the loss was unintentional and that there was no negligent treatment. The AHIMA recommends that retention of health information be based on the needs and requirements of the facility, such as legal requirements, continued patient care, research, education, and other legitimate uses. Primary records are the original records in whatever form they are kept; secondary records are by-products of the original information, such as indexes, physician profiles, databases, billing information, and other reports or queries. Other departments rely on the expertise of the HIM professional to assist them in developing record retention procedures.

Retention Requirements for Ancillary Materials

E-mail messages and faxes are used for instructions, information about appointments, and the reporting of information. These must be printed and attached to the health record folder.

Images, such as complete readouts or "strips" from EEGs, EKGs, fetal monitors, Holter monitors, treadmill tests, EMGs, echocardiograms, videotapes, and other imaging records, do not have to be kept within the physical health record but must be retrievable for as long as legally required. The original interpretations of the results must actually be part of the physical patient health record. Facilities may have computerized systems that directly feed the results of some systems into the imaging system so that the actual images are available to physicians and other providers. These scanned images are not always of diagnostic quality in some scanning systems, so ancillary departments should maintain the information for the appropriate retention period.

Fetal monitoring strips create storage problems for many HIM departments. They are part of the mother's record, but because the strips relate to the newborn, they should be maintained according to the length of time stipulated for a minor's records. Because these strips are not compatible with scanning systems, some facilities have specific computer software to maintain and store fetal monitoring strips within the labor and delivery area.

Magnetic tapes containing the digital versions of MRI and CT studies are not considered permanent health records as long as a hard copy of the final images (radiographic film) is placed in the patient's health record. The signed interpretation of the studies must be maintained in the record for the full retention period required by law. According to 21 CFR 900.12 (c)(4), mammograms must be maintained for five to ten years, depending on whether additional mammograms are performed. State laws may require a retention period for mammograms of twenty to thirty years. This is another example of the HIM professional having to ensure that the longer time period is followed when retention schedules are determined.

Microfilming or optical and electronic imaging technology is allowed by most state laws and is an acceptable method of maintaining patient health records. Because the images are of some documents, computerized results, and other test results, each type of work to be imaged must be carefully considered.

Destruction and Transfer of Health Records

The destruction of records after time limits for retention have been reached must ensure that records are burned, shredded, or destroyed in such a way that personal health information is not revealed. A retention plan must be carefully written and included in the departmental policy and procedure manual to ensure that record destruction is part of the normal course of business and that no one particular record or group of records is singled out for destruction.

When the facility is closed or sold, its health records are transferred to the successor provider, meaning the entity or individual that purchases the facility. In ambulatory care settings or physicians' offices, patients are informed of their options to transfer their records to another provider of choice before their records are transferred to the successor provider. When a physician leaves a group practice, patients should be given the choice to transfer their records and move with the physician or to have the records and the responsibility for care transferred to another provider in the group.

Development of a Record Retention Program

Figure 8.7 lists the objectives of a record retention program. The program must ensure that health records are retained; that inactive records are maintained; that retention is cost-effective in terms of storage space, equipment, and personnel; that a formal record destruction process is in place; and that retention periods are established. A task force or committee might be established with representation from administration, medical staff, health information services, risk management, and legal counsel to give consideration to the needs of all groups who use patient health information. Figure 8.8 lists some of the elements to consider. These include carefully looking at all of the record's uses and the cost of space.

Figure 8.7.   Objectives of a Record Retention Program

To ensure retention and preservation of all valued health records
To maintain noncurrent records of continuing value for uniform time periods and in designated locations
To ensure cost-effectiveness in record storage space, equipment, and personnel
To dispose of unnecessary records by developing an orderly, controlled, and confidential system of record destruction
To establish record retention periods consistent with patient care, regulatory requirements, and other legal considerations

Figure 8.8.   Elements to Consider in the Preservation of Records

Patient value for continued care
Record usage in the facility as guided by the patient population and activity of its medical staff
Legal value as determined by the statute of limitations
Research value
Historical value
Volume and cost to maintain hard-copy storage versus microfilm, optical disk, or remote storage
Storage and safety standards
Contractual arrangements with payers

The HIM director is generally responsible for implementing the retention program. However, other individuals may be charged with the shared responsibility of implementing the program in some facilities. Some facilities establish a task force to oversee the record retention program, sometimes chaired by an HIM professional.

The steps in developing a record retention program include:

1. Conducting an inventory of the facility's records
2. Determining the format and location of storage
3. Assigning each record a retention period
4. Destroying records that are no longer needed

Conducting an Inventory of Records

The first step in establishing a record retention program is to carefully and completely inventory the records or categories of records that are maintained. In this phase, it is important to determine all of the locations and formats of patient information, including images, videotapes, e-mails, tracings, computerized records, and other formats. The inventory also must include the records and registries maintained by all departments. A comprehensive list of all software and versions used also should be maintained so that records, documents, and images can be retrieved in the future. Specialized computer systems used by individual departments should be included.

Determining Storage Format and Location

Determining the format and location of storage is the second step in retention program development. Facilities may choose to retain records in paper format or on hard copy and store them either on-site or in off-site contract storage. Off-site contract storage should be located at a distance far enough away from the facility to ensure that a disaster affecting the facility will not also affect the storage location.

One storage mechanism for inactive records is microfilming. **Microfilming** is the process of recording miniaturized images of a patient health record on film. The images are usually filmed by a special camera onto rolls of 16-millimeter film. The microfilmed images may be stored permanently on the rolls, which may be either stored in boxes labeling the first and last patient numbers on a roll or inserted into special cartridges. Roll film contains information on many patients and cannot be changed. The images are often indexed at the time of filming to allow for quicker retrieval of information.

An alternative to storing microfilm rolls in cartridges is to store images in microfilm jackets. The roll film would be cut into strips and inserted into the channels of the jackets. The microfilm jacket has the advantage of serving as an individual folder for storing the records of one patient. Additional filmed images can be added to the jacket or changed. The jackets are usually four by six inches and have a strip at the top on which to record the patient's name and number. Because the strips can be color-coded, the jackets can be filed in filing cabinets or electric files using the same filing and numbering system the facility uses for paper records.

Microfilm cameras also can film directly onto a microfiche film format. Like the microfilm jacket, the microfiche has the advantage of having only one patient's information available on the fiche. However, its disadvantage is that patient information cannot be updated because the images are filmed directly onto the microfiche itself. The most common size of fiche is a four-by-six-inch sheet, with space for the patient's name and number.

The microfilming of records has many advantages, including:

- Microfilming saves space, which is the primary reason why facilities use it.
- Health records can be retrieved and retained for a long period of time.
- It is simple to duplicate microfilm records in order to provide security or backup copies, and paper copies can be printed from reader printer equipment.
- Microfilm is legally admissible as the original document.

Many facilities use a combination of microfilm formats to accommodate technology and equipment changes.

The facility must consider many issues when deciding whether to microfilm records. These issues include:

- Although microfilming saves a great deal of storage space, it is expensive. For example, preparing the records for filming is a major cost that involves removing staples, checking identification, adjusting oversized or overlapping forms for filming, repairing sheets, and other tasks.

- Special equipment is needed to read and copy microfilm.
- Personnel must be available in patient care areas or in the HIM department to find the microfilm jackets, microfiche, or roll microfilm and to locate the exact information needed.

Microfilming can be done on-site by facility personnel or under contract with a microfilming company. When the facility decides to have the microfilming done in-house, it must take into account the costs of labor and training, supplies, and maintenance.

On the other hand, when the facility decides to use an outside contract microfilming company, the contract should specify who performs the preparation and packs the boxes of records. After records have been transported to the outside contract company, the facility must be able to retrieve the patient's information at any time in case he or she is readmitted or appears for treatment. When records are to be indexed, the contract should fully explain the indexing procedure to ensure that needed documents are accessible. The contract also should specify the turnaround time for filming. Moreover, film returned to the facility must be carefully analyzed to ensure its quality and legibility before the original record is destroyed. The company microfilming the records usually handles their destruction after the facility has audited the returned film. The cost of microfilming is generally based on the number of images filmed.

A second storage mechanism is **optical scanning.** Records can be scanned into optical scanning equipment or digitally transferred. The imaging process converts paper or microfilm documents into a computer-readable digital format. The facility must determine what information can be fed directly into the imaging system, for example, registration and face sheet, discharge summary, and all other dictated and transcribed reports. Optical scanning produces an image of the record that can be indexed and quickly retrieved and simultaneously viewed by many providers. This is not a true electronic record because the image cannot be changed after it has been permanently archived.

Imaging involves preparing, or prepping, the documents, which must be done before the records are scanned. Staples must be removed, papers repaired, and each page checked to ensure the presence of a bar code on both the front and back of every form in the record. The scanning process involves inserting the paper into the optical scanner so that both the front and back pages are scanned at the same time. There are two types of scanners: flatbed scanners and automatic document-feed scanners. The type of scanner used depends on the volume to be scanned. Flatbed scanners are usually slower than automatic document-feed scanners but require less preparation of individual documents.

Indexing involves identifying each individual page. Indexing is critical. If the image is not indexed to the proper patient and the proper form for that admission, the information could not be retrieved. Image and indexing inspection is important to make sure the image is legible.

The scanner is the device that actually scans a human-readable document and uses optical character recognition software to convert the document into a machine-readable format. After being scanned, records must be verified and generally are not submitted to the final stored archive until the physician completes them. After records are archived in the imaging system, they cannot be changed. While waiting to be archived, images can be added or indexing changed.

Facilities assign several personnel to handle the tasks of preparation and scanning. Emergency department reports, outpatient reports, and reports submitted from physicians often do not have the proper patient numbers or encounter numbers, and all of this identifying information must be entered so that each form in the record can be properly indexed and retrieved. A concern for HIM professionals is that scanning equipment from one vendor may not work with equipment from another vendor. The long-term storage capability of optical disk has not been evaluated for long-term quality because the technology is still new and is changing quickly.

Beginning an imaging system requires detailed planning. Decisions must be made about converting existing records or whether only information from a certain date forward will be imaged. In addition, security backups of images should be available. Health records should be on the type of optical disk storage using WORM, "write once, read many," technology. This means that the data cannot be erased or altered. Rewritable or erasable optical disk technology is not appropriate for health records.

Although imaging has the advantages of rapid retrieval and simultaneous access, it is not an easy process to implement. Loose materials and late-arriving information still must be scanned and indexed. Moreover, problems still exist with recovering charts from the nursing areas after discharge and with unapproved forms being developed and included in the record that cannot be indexed because they do not have bar coding. The HIM department still must perform open-record review and check forms for signatures. In other words, the traditional functions of the HIM department do not change. While the patient is in the facility or in active treatment, the record is paper. The imaging system does not convert the paper into images until after patient discharge or termination of treatment.

Assigning a Retention Period

After all departments have been inventoried, the third step is to assign a retention period for each type of record. The retention period should be defined as time in active files, time in inactive storage, and total time before destruction.

As discussed previously, state and federal laws and regulations must be reviewed to ensure that records are maintained for the longest length of time required. Many states recommend that patient health records be retained for ten years following patient discharge or death. There are usually special requirements for minor patients. For example, the state of Tennessee requires that the records of minors or mentally disabled patients be maintained until the age of majority plus one year, or ten years, whichever is longer. Therefore, the record of a newborn in Tennessee would be maintained until the patient reaches the age of majority, which is eighteen plus one year or a total of nineteen years.

Analysis of the retention period should reflect the scope and needs of the facility, along with the preliminary costs associated with microfilming, imaging, and other methods of maintaining and storing records. Storage mechanisms should be selected that protect records and provide ease of access and employee safety. Humidity, lighting, hazard protection, and transportation of needed records are all considerations.

Commercial storage vendors should be selected carefully to ensure that records are protected from unauthorized access. Policies for security of all satellite record storage areas must be developed and agreements signed regarding timely access to, and retrieval of, records.

Destroying Unnecessary Records

Destroying records that are not needed is the fourth step in developing a record retention program. There must be a rule that no patient health information can be destroyed or thrown away without approval of the HIM director or other authorized committee or person according to facility policy. The HIM professional must be alert to changes in departmental administration or departmental relocation or remodeling because departments often use these events to clean out files, which could result in the destruction of needed patient information.

The destruction of patient records must be done as part of the facility's usual business. When the required retention schedule has been satisfied, a complete list of records to be destroyed should be compiled and submitted to the individual designated to authorize the destruction. Outsourcing of destruction to shredding companies should be carefully monitored to protect patient confidentiality. The destruction of computerized records should follow security guidelines to ensure that the information is destroyed permanently. Facilities must maintain basic information about the patient in the master patient index, which is maintained permanently even though the corresponding health record is destroyed.

The AHIMA recommends that records be destroyed in such a way that the information cannot possibly be reconstructed. The destruction should be documented, and the documentation should include:

- Date of destruction
- Method of destruction (shredding, burning, or other means)
- Description of the disposed record series of numbers or items
- Inclusive dates covered
- A statement that the records were destroyed in the normal course of business

- The signatures of the individuals supervising and witnessing the destruction

The AHIMA recommends that facilities maintain destruction certification documents permanently. Such certificates may be required as evidence that records were destroyed in the regular course of business. When facilities fail to apply destruction policies uniformly or when destruction is contrary to policy, courts may allow a jury to infer that the facility destroyed its records to hide evidence of its negligent care.

Check Your Understanding 8.6

Instructions: Answer the following questions on a separate sheet of paper.

1. What is the difference between a serial numbering system and a unit numbering system?

2. What are two advantages of terminal-digit filing over straight numerical filing?

3. What are the main factors in determining how long to maintain a health record?

4. What is the major advantage of microfilming health records?

5. What is the major advantage of optical imaging in the chart completion process?

6. What are the four primary steps in a record retention program?

Master Patient Index

The **master patient index** (MPI) is a permanent database including every patient ever admitted to or treated by the facility. Even though patient health records may be destroyed after legal retention periods have been met, the information contained in the MPI must be kept permanently. The MPI is also referred to as the master person index, the **master population index,** the master name file, the enterprisewide person or patient index (EMPI), and the master patient database. Whatever it is called, the MPI is an important key to the health record because it contains the patient's name and health record number.

The MPI can be a simple file containing cards with basic identification information about the patient or a computerized system. In a computer-based MPI, the database associates the patient with the particular number under which patient treatment information can be located. The index also helps to control number assignments to ensure that former patients are not inadvertently assigned an additional number.

The challenges are many. For example, patients may not remember previous admissions or may have been admitted under a different name. A person other than the patient may have provided incorrect information, resulting in a new number being assigned when the patient returns for an appointment or is readmitted to the hospital. Sometimes patients use different middle initials or a nickname rather than a given name, or their names may have many possible spellings or be hyphenated. In some cases, patients do not speak the same language as the clerk entering the information, resulting in miscommunication and incorrect data. Facilities that have either merged or separated must keep information on patients treated and often have problems combining information from two computer systems. Facilities may have manual card files that have been microfilmed in the past or may use a variety of formats, from index cards to microfilmed cards on rolls or microfiche to a computerized database.

The challenge for facilities is to maintain a correct and current MPI so that each patient has a unique identifier number. The goal is to have a true longitudinal record from birth to death, and the MPI serves as the link to information. There is movement toward a **universal patient identifier** that would be used nationwide, although there are concerns about compromising patient confidentiality.

Information contained in the MPI includes:

- The patient's full name and any other names the patient uses
- The patient's date of birth
- The patient's complete address
- The patient's health record number
- The patient's billing or account number
- The name of the attending physician
- The dates of the patient's admission and discharge or the date of the visit or encounter
- The patient's disposition at discharge or the conclusion of treatment
- The patient's date of death, if applicable
- The patient's marital status
- The patient's gender
- The patient's race
- The name of the patient's emergency contact

Other information may be included to further identify the patient and ensure that his or her name is linked to the proper record number. Some facilities include the mother's maiden name as another way to link the patient health record number and information to the proper patient.

Controls for accuracy include limiting access to the index and limiting the ability to make changes to the index to a few key personnel. The first key to maintaining an accurate index is to obtain the correct information in the beginning, but there are numerous problems, such as situations when the patient is unable to provide the correct information or when items are entered improperly. In the past, when only HIM personnel assigned numbers, there was more control; today, numbers are entered by many different personnel. The more people involved in entering data, the greater the potential for error.

When a patient's record cannot be located, his or her care may be compromised. Without prior information, the physician and other providers might duplicate tests or treatments. A second record for the same patient is then created under a new number, which adds to the problem of bringing the parts of the patient record together. Research to "clean up" duplicate numbers and other errors is among the HIM professional's responsibilities.

Check Your Understanding 8.7

Instructions: Answer the following questions on a separate piece of paper.

1. Why is the MPI considered the key index in the HIM department?

2. Why is accurate information critical for the MPI?

3. What are some of the reasons why incorrect information is obtained?

4. What is the consequence of a patient having duplicate health record numbers?

Real-World Case

A recently hired director of health information management is facing a difficult challenge. The hospital's inefficient record-tracking system has produced a tremendous backlog of incomplete records.

Three eight-shelf-high, open-filing shelves currently house the incomplete records of residents and attending physicians. The records are filed in straight numerical order because so many physicians are responsible for each record. The shelving cannot hold the vast number of delinquent records; thus, stacks of records are piled on the floor and in the dictation area booths. These piles of charts were not there when the new HIM director interviewed for the job.

Deficiencies are listed on index cards filed alphabetically by physician name and kept in a box on a table next to the shelving units. Physicians must ask someone in the department to pull their cards and then wait while the charts are pulled. Medicare charts or charts with high charges are filed in red folders to remind the physicians to do them first. The physicians complain about being unable to complete their charts unless a clerk is available to help them. The department is open from 8 a.m. until 4:30 p.m., Monday through Friday, and closed on weekends.

Mary Jones is responsible for the incomplete file. She counts charts that are two weeks old every two weeks and sends out cartoon notices she designs herself. For example, one card has a picture of a dog in a doghouse with the message, "Get out of the doghouse. Do your records." She also sends out seasonal messages. For example, at Thanksgiving, she sends out cards that say, "Don't be a turkey. You have 14 records to complete." There are over 4,500 delinquent records, which is well over the JCAHO rule for the number of discharges. The hospital definition of a delinquent record is one that is incomplete over fourteen days following discharge.

Mary suggests hiring two or three people to serve as runners to deliver health records directly to the physicians' offices for signature. This, she claims, would reduce the number of charts dramatically.

Several physicians on the Medical Record Committee commented that they find the notes irritating and offensive, especially when the service in the HIM department is so bad when they come in to do the charts. The chief of the medical staff claims that some hospitals in town do not make physi-

cians come in to sign charts that just need signatures on dictated reports. He wants to know why this facility cannot come up with an "automatic signature" policy like the one used at these facilities.

Discussion Questions

1. In order of priority, what are the major problems in this area of the department?

2. How would you address each of the identified problems?

3. What alternatives to sending cartoon notices could be developed to notify physicians about incomplete charts?

4. Should the definition of a delinquent record be changed?

5. How could an improved policy for signatures be designed?

6. How might the department improve service to physicians?

7. What type of filing system for incomplete charts would help physicians to complete charts?

8. Write a memorandum to the hospital administrator identifying the problems and how each might be addressed.

Summary

The patient health record is the foundation for most of the decisions made in any healthcare facility. Decisions relative to patient care and financial reimbursement depend on the quality of documentation in the health record. The record is the communication tool among the members of the patient's healthcare team. It is evidence of what was done for the patient, and the information it contains is used to evaluate the quality of care and to provide important information for research and public health needs. Moreover, the information in the health care record protects the legal interests of both the patient and the facility. The traditional saying, "If it wasn't documented, it wasn't done," is a reminder of how important the record is for the patient, the facility, and the numerous other users of the record and the information it contains.

Ensuring that the health record meets current regulatory, legal, accrediting, and licensing standards as well as the facility's bylaws and polices is an ongoing challenge for the HIM professional. He or she must continuously educate and update providers on changes affecting documentation. Records must be reviewed both while the patient is in active treatment and after treatment to ensure that they meet the current requirements. Analyzing and processing paper records efficiently is important to ensure that complete information is available for billing and reimbursement purposes. Facilitating the completion of records by providers is a key factor in ensuring that needed information can be provided to all authorized users.

Facilities use a variety of formats for storing patient records so that they are available for future use. As technology has changed, so have the methods of maintaining and storing patient records. Records may be copied onto different

types of microfilm stored in cabinets on rolls or on microfiche.

The patient index may be maintained partially on cards that
have been microfilmed and on different types of microfilm.
The facility may have a recently installed imaging system.
Healthcare information includes videotapes, graphic results,
videotapes, and images from specific computerized test results.

The HIM professional has been incrementally transitioning from managing paper health records to managing information in a variety of media and formats. The transition is
ongoing, and HIM professionals must take a leadership role
in ensuring that needed health information from the patient's
past continues to be available for use in the future. Chapter 9
describes the transition to computer-based patient records.

References

Abraham, P. R. 2001. *Documentation and Reimbursement for Home Care
and Hospice Programs.* Chicago: American Health Information Management Association.

American Health Information Management Association, Ambulatory Care
Section. 2001. *Documentation for Ambulatory Care,* revised edition.
Chicago: American Health Information Management Association.

The Centers for Medicare and Medicaid Services. Conditions of Participation for Hospitals. *Code of Federal Regulations,* 2001. 42 CFR, Chapter IV,
Part 482. Available online at www.access.gpo.gov/nara/cfr.

Dougherty, Michelle. 2001. Practice Brief: Verbal/telephone order authentication and time frames. *Journal of the American Health Information
Management Association* 72(2).

Fletcher, D. 1999. Practice Brief: Retention of health information. *Journal
of the American Health Information Management Association* 70(5).

Joint Commission on Accreditation of Healthcare Organizations. 2001.
Comprehensive Accreditation Manual for Hospitals. Oak Brook Terrace,
Ill.: Joint Commission on Accreditation of Healthcare Organizations.

Hughes, Gwen. 2001. Practice Brief: Destruction of patient health information. *Journal of the American Health Information Management
Association* 72(10).

Marrelli, T. M. 1996. *Nursing Documentation Handbook,* second edition.
St. Louis: Mosby/YearBook.

National Association for Home Care. 2001. Access online from www.nahc.org.

National Hospice and Palliative Care Organization. 2001. Access online
from www.nhpco.org.

Peden, A. 1998. *Comparative Records for Health Information Management.* Albany, N.Y.: Delmar Publishers.

Youmans, Karen G. 2000. *Basic Healthcare Statistics for Health Information Management Professionals.* Chicago: American Health Information
Management Association.

Application Exercises

1. Using a sample record for a patient who underwent an operative procedure, answer the following questions.

   History and Physical
   a. What was the chief complaint?
   b. List briefly the details of the present illness.
   c. List briefly relevant social and family history.
   d. What is included in the review of systems? (Remember, this will be
      in the history, not the physical.)
   e. What were the patient's vital signs?
   f. What abnormal findings are included in the physical?
   g. What is the provisional diagnosis?
   h. What is the plan?

   Pre- and Postanesthesia Documentation (This may be on a separate
   form or in the progress notes.)
   a. Who conducted the patient's preanesthesia evaluation?
   b. What type of information was included?
   c. What was the date of the postoperative anesthesia evaluation?

   Operative Report/Pathology (Be sure that there is an operative report
   and a pathology report in the record.)
   a. What is the preoperative diagnosis, and where is it located in the
      record if it was not listed on the operative report?
   b. What is the postoperative diagnosis?
   c. Who was the surgeon?
   d. What operation was done?
   e. What were the findings?
   f. What specimens were removed?
   g. Do the preoperative diagnosis, the microscopic pathologic
      diagnosis (on the pathology report), and the postoperative
      diagnoses agree? What are they?
   h. What does the operative progress note state? (This will be in the
      progress note section of the record.)

   Physician's Orders
   a. Is each order timed, signed, and dated?
   b. Is each verbal or telephone order signed by the physician?
   c. Look at the first day's admission orders. What types of services/
      medications and so on were ordered? Is there a corresponding
      report for each laboratory test, X ray, or procedure ordered? List
      exceptions.

   Progress Notes
   a. Is there an admission note? Summarize its content.
   b. What is included in the discharge progress note?
   c. Who else has written in the progress note section besides the
      attending physician? What type of information is included in these
      nonphysician notes?

   Discharge Summary
   a. What was the admitting or provisional diagnosis or reason for
      hospitalization?
   b. List briefly the significant (abnormal) findings.
   c. List briefly the operative procedures performed and other
      treatment.
   d. What was the patient's condition at discharge?
   e. What instructions were given to the patient and/or his family at
      discharge?
   f. What were the discharge diagnoses?

2. State where in an active patient record you would find documentation
   of the following:
   • Identification data
   • Reason for admission or treatment
   • Patient education
   • Clinical observations
   • Conclusions at the end of treatment
   • Discharge instructions
   • Notes on the patient's condition made by healthcare providers
   • Consent for surgery
   • Anesthesia plan
   • Name of surgeon/assistant

3. The hospital administrator wants you to investigate a proposal to bring transcription back in-house because of the high cost of using the outside contract service, Reports R Us. She asks you to estimate the costs involved. Telecommuting is a possibility.

At present, the hospital pays Reports R Us $0.15 per line and Reports R Us provides histories and physicals, discharge summaries, operative reports, and consultations.

Type of dictation	Number per day	Average number of lines	Total number of lines per day
History and physicals	50	25	1,250
Discharge summaries	20	30	600
Consultation reports	10	10	100
Operative reports	20	30	600

Calculate the total lines per day. The average transcriptionist can type 1,200 lines per day. How many full-time equivalents would be needed to staff the transcription area?

In addition to the salary of the transcriptionists, what other costs would you have to consider in reestablishing a transcription area in your facility?

4. You are responsible for writing the portion of the medical staff bylaws relating to patient health record documentation. Using three of the major healthcare providers in your facility, develop a list of rules for proper documentation in the patient health record.

5. Contrast the following three types of record formats in terms of advantages and disadvantages: source oriented, integrated, or problem oriented.

6. Your facility is moving to a new building in three years. The administrator tells you that he is not planning to include a filing area in the department because patient health records will be totally paperless by then. What is your response?

7. List and explain three items that the HIM professional must make sure are in a contract for outside microfilming.

8. Describe three measures of productivity and/or quality for the filing area of a HIM department.

Review Quiz

Instructions: Choose the most appropriate word or phrase to answer the following questions.

1. ___ Which professionals on the healthcare team are primarily responsible for documenting information in the patient record?
   a. Physicians and providers who direct patient care
   b. Administrators, medical director, and physicians
   c. Physicians, nurses, and health information professionals
   d. Surveyors and researchers who review records

2. ___ What is the traditional format for a hospital patient care record?
   a. Integrated
   b. Practice oriented
   c. Chronological
   d. Source oriented

3. ___ Which of the following is a governmental designation by the state that is necessary for the facility to offer services?
   a. Survey
   b. Licensure
   c. Certification
   d. Accreditation

4. ___ Which of the following is the goal of the quantitative analysis performed by HIM professionals?
   a. Ensuring that the record is legible
   b. Identifying deficiencies early so they can be corrected
   c. Verifying that health professionals are providing appropriate care
   d. Checking to ensure that bills are correct

5. ___ Which of the following is an acceptable means of authenticating a record entry?
   a. The physician's assistant signs for the physician.
   b. The HIM clerk stamps entries with the physician's signature stamp.
   c. The charge nurse signs the physician's name.
   d. The physician personally signs the entry.

6. ___ Which of the following is the primary goal of incentive pay plans for transcriptionists?
   a. Increased productivity
   b. Increased quality of transcribed reports
   c. Increased salary
   d. Increased competition among transcriptionists

7. ___ What is the primary purpose of the history and physical examination?
   a. To begin the record in proper chronological order
   b. To comply with JCAHO recommendations
   c. To assist registration personnel with room assignment
   d. To assist the physician in establishing a plan of care

8. ___ In which record numbering system is the patient assigned a health record number on the first visit that is kept for all subsequent visits?
   a. Unit numbering
   b. Index unit numbering
   c. Serial-unit numbering
   d. Serial numbering

9. ___ Which numerical filing system results in an even distribution of records and ensures activity throughout the filing area?
   a. Serial-unit filing system
   b. Serial filing system
   c. Unit filing system
   d. Terminal-digit filing system

10. ___ What is the advantage of the unit filing system?
    a. All records, both inpatient and outpatient, for a specific patient are filed together.
    b. The charts have to be split into volumes for filing.
    c. The hospital can accommodate a large outpatient clinic with many return visits.
    d. JCAHO approval is automatic because all parts of the record are filed together.

11. ___ What is the first consideration in determining how long records must be retained?
    a. The amount of space allocated for record filing
    b. The number of records
    c. The most stringent law or regulation in the state
    d. The cost of filing space

12. ___ Suppose that you are purchasing shelving units. The plan is to have units that are five shelves high, and each shelf is to be 36 inches wide and have 33 inches of actual filing space. From a sampling of records in the current files, you have determined that the average thickness of each record is 2 inches. You are planning to store ten years' worth of records, and the average discharge rate is 2,000 per year. How many shelving units would you need to purchase?
   a. 165
   b. 180
   c. 222
   d. 243

13. ___ What is a record arranged in strictly chronological order called?
   a. A sectional record
   b. An integrated record
   c. A consolidated record
   d. A source-oriented record

14. ___ Which of the following is a system in which the patient health record is kept in the same order on the nursing station and in the complete record?
   a. Standard
   b. Universal
   c. Source oriented
   d. Patient centered

15. ___ What is the primary reason that optical imaging is becoming more prevalent in HIM departments?
   a. It can cut personnel by a third.
   b. It represents the first step toward a computer-based patient record system.
   c. It is cheap to scan records.
   d. Accessibility to scanned records is improving.

16. ___ What must be done before authorization is given to destroy original records that have been microfilmed?
   a. Microfilm boxes should be marked with record numbers.
   b. Film should be packaged into cartridges.
   c. Specific documents should be indexed on the roll.
   d. Film should be audited for quality.

17. ___ Which microfilming system is best when you plan to file the film in a way to maintain a terminal-digit unit record system?
   a. Jackets
   b. Roll
   c. Cartridge
   d. Rotary

18. ___ In planning for implementing an optical disk imaging system, what is the first step the HIM should take?
   a. Standardize forms
   b. Buy equipment
   c. Develop physician interest
   d. Train personnel to scan documents

19. ___ Which of the following credentials is awarded to a person who passes the American Association for Medical Transcription examination?
   a. Accredited Medical Transcriptionist
   b. Certified Medical Transcriptionist
   c. Registered Medical Transcriptionist
   d. Licensed Medical Transcriptionist

20. ___ In which of the following systems is voice converted to computer-readable format and stored on a computer system?
   a. Discrete
   b. Digital
   c. Analog
   d. Voice recognition

21. ___ What or who is the best source of information about a particular word-processing system?
   a. Exhibitors at meetings and trade shows
   b. Vendors who sell the equipment
   c. Facilities with the equipment in place
   d. Professional journals

22. ___ To determine the number of transcriptionists needed, one must know all but which of the following?
   a. Work volume
   b. Other responsibilities of transcriptionists
   c. Competence of transcriptionists
   d. JCAHO staffing recommendations

23. ___ Which of the following statements best describes a unit record system?
   a. The charts generally have to be split into volumes for filing.
   b. All records, both inpatient and outpatient, for a specific patient are in one file.
   c. The hospital can accommodate a large outpatient clinic with many return visits.
   d. JCAHO approval is automatic because all parts of the record are filed together.

24. ___ When records are received in the HIM department after discharge or conclusion of the visit, what is the first thing that should be done?
   a. The records should be assembled in prescribed order.
   b. Someone should check to ensure that all records have been received.
   c. Record numbers should be entered in a chart locator system.
   d. Physicians' offices should be called for diagnoses.

25. ___ What type of record review is conducted while the patient is in the facility to ensure that items are completed and signatures are present?
   a. Closed review
   b. Qualitative review
   c. Concurrent review
   d. Delinquent review

Chapter 9
Computer-Based Patient Records

Margret Amatayakul, MBA, RHIA, FHIMSS

Learning Objectives

- To describe the evolution of the computer-based patient record and its supporting technologies
- To identify user needs and issues that must be addressed to achieve the benefits of computer-based patient records
- To evaluate how emerging technologies support and supplement computer-based patient records
- To describe the technical architecture required to create a computer-based patient record
- To establish a security program that addresses regulatory and business requirements of a computer-based patient record environment
- To develop an appreciation of the impact of environmental and technological change on the evolution of the computer-based patient record

Key Terms

Application service provider
Architecture
Clinical data repository (CDR)
Clinical decision support system (CDSS)
Computer-based patient record (CPR)
Confidentiality
Connectivity
Data exchange standards
Hospital information system (HIS)
Image processing
Integration
Integrity
Interface
Knowledge base
Message format standards
Patient care system
Risk analysis
Semantics
Syntax
Text processing
Vocabulary
Workstation

Introduction

Although the term *computer-based patient record* and its acronym *CPR* were coined in 1991, the concept of a fully integrated health information system to support healthcare has been around since the late 1960s. However, the concept has been difficult to achieve because there are many unique challenges in health information computing.

Health information computing is not just about quickly "crunching" a lot of numbers to produce a bank balance or to calculate an airplane weight for takeoff. Health information is largely textual. Narrative text is not as easy to manipulate by computer as numbers are. Moreover, health information is contextual. A given word may have different meanings when associated with other words; for example, red may indicate embarrassment when describing a face, or infection when describing a lesion.

Further, healthcare professionals who need to use computers are very mobile. They move to examining rooms, to the surgery suite, to a patient on a gurney, or even to patients in their homes. Although handheld devices have solved problems for the package delivery industry, healthcare professionals often need access to a large volume of information and may need to communicate data to other healthcare professionals in real time. Until recently, handheld devices have been limited in such capabilities.

Finally, most computerization has been built on the assumption that there are standard ways of doing things. However, the human body is anything but standard. Healthcare is as much an art as a science, although better data can contribute to creating standard protocols for diagnosing and treating patients.

This chapter focuses on the emergence of the computer-based patient record and its supporting technologies. It also discusses how CPRs are created and how patient information is managed in an electronic environment. Finally, the chapter looks at the future directions of information technologies.

Theory into Practice

Dr. Smith is at home having breakfast with his family. Before heading off to the hospital to check on patients and then to the office, a quick check via the home computer starts his day in real time.

The CPR Dr. Smith accesses provides an integrated in-box. The in-box reveals that one patient is deteriorating rapidly and that a colleague, Dr. Jones, has requested a consult for a patient with an especially severe condition. Dr. Smith decides to send Dr. Jones an e-mail attachment of the latest practice guidelines relative to the condition.

In addition, Dr. Smith's office is requesting a refill of a medication for a patient who is out of town. In responding to the refill request, an alert informs Dr. Smith that the patient is also due for a checkup, so this information is sent back to the office scheduling system for contacting the patient within the next ten days. Further checking today's schedule, Dr. Smith notes that a meeting with the local medical society is taking place this evening and there is an e-mail from another colleague wanting to chat before the meeting about a new treatment regime that appears promising. Not having seen literature on the new treatment regime, Dr. Smith checks the National Library of Medicine archives for any possible articles. Finding a few, he tags them for printing in the office.

Before logging off, Dr. Smith receives an instant message concerning the critical patient. Not wanting to wait until he arrives at the hospital, Dr. Smith engages the charge nurse in an exchange of information, including a streaming video of the patient's latest vital signs. Dr. Smith decides to move the patient to critical care and places a series of orders for the patient.

This scenario reflects the growing trends of remote connectivity; clinical messaging; integrating voice, data, and video; use of knowledge sources; and clinical decision support—all components of a CPR.

Evolution of the Computer-Based Patient Record

The **computer-based patient record** (CPR) is as much a concept as a product to buy or a system to build. In its landmark work, the Institute of Medicine (IOM) defined the CPR as an electronic record "that resides in a system specifically designed to support users by providing accessibility to complete and accurate data, alerts, reminders, clinical decision support systems, links to medical knowledge, and other aids" (1997, p. 55). In addition, The IOM provided the caveat that "merely automating the form, content, and procedures of current patient records will perpetuate their deficiencies and will be insufficient to meet emerging user needs" (p. 6).

As with any revolutionary system, the CPR has suffered somewhat from multiple different interpretations. When the IOM first released its report on CPRs, vendors rushed to market CPR systems. These systems typically were more vaporware than reality or were limited in true CPR functionality. In fact, some of them were so disappointing or cumbersome to use that they may have done more harm than good in achieving the Institute's goals. Some were nothing more than document imaging systems or clinical messaging systems. They made data more accessible, which was a good thing, but did not support data capture very well and had minimal decision support functionality.

There were also distinct differences between CPR systems designed for physician offices and those developed for hospitals. Although there certainly are distinct differences in work flow in these two environments, the result was that vendors developed either physician office products or hospital products. Some physicians bought and used the products for their offices but then found the products could not integrate well with the hospital. Hospitals have actually been slower to adopt full CPR systems. There are many reasons for this. First, hospitals have many more data in many different places. Some of these data are not currently automated at all. Some departments have nice departmental systems but do not "talk" to other systems in the hospital.

A first step toward achieving a CPR is to get a more integrated hospital information system. This ensures that all sources of data are at least automated, if not yet connected. Finally, getting clinicians of all types—physicians, nurses, therapists, and others—to enter data has been difficult. In most cases it is at least perceived to be faster to dictate or handwrite a note. In fact, in the case of order entry, the task is perceived to be clerical by many physicians. Very few vendors or providers have been successful in fully implementing a CPR in a hospital, let alone a CPR system that crosses the chasm between inpatient and outpatient (or acute care and ambulatory care).

However, many vendors and providers support the goals of a CPR and continue development work. Though not perfect, newer systems are making CPRs much more integrated and easier to use. There is also greater recognition that much more automation is needed in the core process of healthcare: managing health information to treat patients.

Technologies That Support the CPR

A CPR is not simply a computer software package or program. Unlike laboratory information systems or admitting systems that basically perform one major function or service one department, a CPR system may be viewed as the "engine" that integrates all other systems.

To serve its function of capturing data from multiple sources and converting them into timely, usable information, the CPR must embody many different technologies. These technologies include databases, data exchange standards, vocabulary standards, image processing, data retrieval technology, data capture technology, text processing, networks, workstations, and clinical decision support systems.

Databases and Database Management Systems

There are essentially two ways to integrate data for a CPR. One is to collect all the data needed in a central database and disperse them from there. This database needs very special indexing and management functions in order to capture, sort, process, and present information back to users—often in a split second! Such a database is called a **data repository.** To distinguish repositories that focus on clinical information (instead of financial and/or administrative data), the term **clinical data repository** (CDR) is used.

Database management systems (DBMS) help manage databases. The oldest form of DBMS is hierarchical, which is modeled from a treelike structure. Records at a branch level are sometimes referred to as parents, with records at the leaf level being children. A major constraint of the hierarchical DBMS is that to navigate through its branches, one must

follow the path from a child to a parent. As a result, this DBMS is referred to as a "flat file." Response time is slow and redundancies must be built into the structure in order to speed up processing. A network form of DBMS attempts to overcome the need for redundancies by supporting multiple paths to the same record; however, it remains a slow process to find the shortest path. The relational DBMS is the most common form today. This is constructed using tables that are easier and faster to navigate. A very recent approach is an object-oriented DBMS, which derives from object-oriented programming. There is no structure to this DBMS; rather, it relies on **integration** of data through programming.

Acquiring or building a CDR is the most common first step in developing a CPR, especially for hospitals. However, some hospitals have implemented a CDR without some of the other supporting technologies and have called it a CPR, when in reality it only serves as a data retrieval system to provide access to data from other systems. Not that a data retrieval system is not useful, but it has limited functionality. Furthermore, if data do not exist in an automated system, they cannot go into a repository and thus remain paper based. For example, most progress notes, original physician orders, and nursing notes in a hospital are not entered electronically into a computer and thus do not get stored in the repository. As a result, hospitals are essentially managing two medical record systems: the repository and the paper-based traditional record. Some hospitals attempt to print everything from the repository for the paper-based record to have a single, legal medical record. Others have deemed part of the repository to be a part of their legal medical record. As an aside, many hospitals have complained that they are not getting a good return on their investment for their "CPRs" (which are only CDRs) and this is surely true if they have to manage two systems.

Data Exchange Standards and Vocabulary Standards

The second way a CPR can be achieved is by retaining all the data in the various independent, departmental system databases and using **data exchange standards** to integrate the systems. Unless a hospital has very few systems from different vendors, this is generally not very successful. However, data exchange standards are still used to interconnect systems within hospital information systems and parts of CPR systems.

Data exchange standards have typically been called **message format standards.** Examples are Health Level Seven (HL7), American National Standards Institute (ANSI) Accredited Standards Committee (ASC) X12N, National Council for Prescription Drug Programs (NCPDP), and others. These standards make sure that the structure and format of data, as they are being transmitted from one system to another, are the same. This data structure and format is called **syntax.** Each proprietary system has its own syntax. For systems to exchange data or "talk" to one another, the syntax must be made the same. As an example, in figure 9.1, two different systems are attempting to convey the same information, but to use different field names (patient name versus individual name) and different element names (middle initial versus middle name) and to sequence the elements differently.

To make the syntax the same, system developers use message format standards. However, some of these standards, HL7 in particular, have a lot of optionality. As a result, even two systems that are HL7 compliant may not be fully interoperable. In this case, a program called an **interface** must be written to make them interoperable. The problem is compounded—and sometimes impossible to solve—when the vendors do not use HL7 at all. Although the syntaxes illustrated in figure 9.1 may seem subtle, they are sufficiently different as to render the two systems unable to communicate with one another without an interface.

The more standard the message format standards, the more easily systems using them can transmit data. NCPDP is a good example of this. NCPDP is used in over 90 percent of all retail pharmacies, and these pharmacies can very easily exchange data with insurance companies to verify coverage for a drug, calculate the patient's copay, and file a claim before the person ever leaves the pharmacy.

To date, message format standards have been limited to exchanging whatever data were sent from one system to another. There was no reconciliation that the terminology used in one system was the same in the other system. The data were not standardized. A common **vocabulary** was not used. Most recently, the industry has come to realize that for one clinical system to use another clinical system's data, terms must have the same meaning. **Semantics** is the term used to describe the fact that the content of a message has a common meaning. One of the most promising vocabularies is SNOMED. HL7 Version 3 has begun to embed SNOMED codes into its message format standard.

Image Processing, Storage, and Work Flow

Another technology that supports a CPR is **image processing.** In healthcare, there are document imaging systems and clinical imaging systems. Document imaging systems scan existing handwritten or printed documents and store them for viewing through a computer workstation. As documents are scanned, they are indexed, assigning a description of the document and key contents for later retrieval. The benefit of document imaging is greatly enhanced access to such documents. In fact, many document imaging systems add a "workflow" capability that directs documents to various systems for specific functions. For example, when paper medical record

forms are scanned, certain pages can be routed to coders and certain pages can be routed to billers simultaneously.

Clinical images are "pictures" generated by medical devices such as X rays, EKG monitors, and so on. Storage of these pictures is called PACS (picture archiving and communications systems). Clinical images from PACS can be viewed through standard monitors if great detail is not required. Diagnostic-quality viewing of such images requires special monitors with very high resolution and/or full-motion video capability.

Data Retrieval Technology

Because most information systems used today in hospitals are primarily data retrieval systems, technology to support this functionality is quite mature. Retrieval technology may be as basic as a lookup, where a query is made to access certain data from a specific system, for example, a lab result on a certain patient from the laboratory information system. The desired patient may be selected from a list or by entering his or her name and/or medical record number. Some navigational tools may be available to permit the user to select a specific data element, to make a customized table, or even to graph results.

More sophisticated retrieval technologies enable a user to access several different types of data from different source systems through a single application screen. Hence, a medication list may be viewed from the same application screen as the lab results. There may be windows for different types of data from different sources, or there may be predesigned or customizable screens that permit viewing a specific user's preferred set of data. The most sophisticated retrieval technology permits not only viewing of data by type, but also manipulation of several different types of data, such as plotting lab results on a graph against medication administration, vital signs, and so on.

The quality of retrieval technology is often measured by use of the screen's real estate. One disadvantage to using a computer to view information is the inability to "flip" quickly through multiple "pages" of data. Clinicians have been trained to rapidly scan a patient's record to both get an overall picture of the patient and find specific data. Although this capability is available through find features, color, and other navigational tools, they are not currently everyday tools used by clinicians. Eventually, everyone will use such tools as second nature, much as we recognize a nurse's progress note from a physician's progress note today. Now, however, they are still somewhat foreign to many users. Most users find it easier to use a printout of the electronically stored data to look at results. The key to achieving "scanability" of a CPR is to pack as much information on a single screen as possible. Although it may seem "cleaner" or user-friendlier to have fewer data on any given screen, the reverse has actually been proven to be true, although the layout of such a dense screen must be very carefully designed.

Thus, an important characteristic of retrieval technologies is that of screen layout and the ability to customize or tailor

Figure 9.1.   Different Systems Attempting to Convey the Same Information

System A	System B
Patient's Name: Last, First, Middle Initial	Individual's Name: First, Middle, Last

the layout to the preference of the user. Many CPR systems display a tailored screen based on the user's log-on. Thus, when Dr. Jones logs on, Dr. Jones's personally preferred screen layout is displayed. The ability to drill down to greater detail is also important; but, again, caution must be applied to avoid having so many pathways through data that the user gets lost and cannot effectively go back to an original screen. Research also has shown that three levels of screen layers are about the most anyone can use effectively.

A word about color, animation, icons, and sound is also appropriate in discussing retrieval technologies. Color can be very helpful in navigating a screen to find desired data, but the number of people (especially men) who are color-blind must be considered. Color should never be relied on solely for any critical alerts that are attempting to be conveyed; instead, it should be accompanied by a special icon, animation, or sound. Icons can be very effective in guiding users, but they must be large enough to see clearly and be very intuitive. Unfortunately, few standard symbols can be used in creating icons for health information systems. Of all the navigational elements available, sound may be the least used in healthcare because of the many medical devices that routinely emit sounds and have special sound alarms.

Data Capture Technology

If it is difficult to get clinicians to retrieve data from CPR systems, it is even more difficult to get them to enter data. With the exception of the most current generation of users, most clinicians have never learned to type and consider typing or any other form of keyboard use to be a clerical function. Even clinicians who are willing and able to type still often find data entry on a computer more challenging and time-consuming than handwriting or dictating.

Unfortunately, no ideal solution has yet been found to support data capture effectively for all users in all environments. However, there are a few key considerations. Most important, data entry must return value to the user. If the user can obtain decision support at the time of data entry that is valuable to the user, data entry will be more palatable. However, the decision support must be facilitating and not interfering with the flow of information processing. Clinicians are more inclined to do data entry when they can see that the direct result of their data entry is a benefit to their subsequent work (for example, it prompts for billing support data or automatically generates tailored instructions to the patient). However, if data entry is even perceived to take longer than traditional recording, even if its purpose is laudable (such as to have more legible data to improve patient safety), data entry will be a hard sell.

Technologies that can help make data capture easier include:

- *Structured data entry through point-and-click fields, pull-down menus, structured templates, or macros:* In addition to making data entry easier, structured data entry makes processing of the data easier. Devices supporting such data entry include the mouse, light pens, and touch screens. If the data are further codified to a standard vocabulary, that makes them much more valuable. However, many clinicians want to be able to convey more information than just that accommodated through such menus.

- *Speech recognition:* Speech recognition can be very effective for certain clinicians. It is not the panacea every clinician dreams of, but where data entry is fairly repetitive and the vocabulary used fairly limited, speech recognition devices can be effectively trained. Otherwise, speech recognition is essentially a more costly form of dictation, requiring "correctionists" to review and edit what has been entered. Handwriting recognition is a similar form of data entry with similar problems.

- *Handheld, wireless devices:* Such devices may be included in the discussion of data-entry devices. Although these still require some form of keying or picking from a list, they are easy for mobile professionals to have readily available. They are limited in terms of the volume of data they can store, their processing capabilities, the size of both the screen and the keypad, and the ability to communicate or link to primary information systems. However, they are ideal for certain limited functions, such as writing prescriptions or for use in capturing a home health data set.

- *Digital dictation:* Digital dictation is also a form of data entry. Although ultimately transcribed, digital dictation is available to other users by listening to the recorded dictation. Because we speak much more slowly than we read, however, listening to a long dictation can be very time-consuming. In using digital dictation, users should be trained to dictate the most pertinent data first so that they do not have to listen to an entire report to get key data.

- *Direct data capture from a medical device attached to a patient:* This is yet another important means of capturing certain kinds of data, such as vital signs. Special medical devices (such as a pacemaker) are even able to be connected to a standard telephone for capturing data or checking on the device's status.

- *Patient data entry:* Most clinicians are not yet very accepting of having a patient enter symptoms into a system for them to incorporate directly into the medical record. Still, limited patient entry is gaining momentum.

Text Processing

Text processing may actually be considered a special form of data entry. Text processing is the capability of a computer to apply very sophisticated mathematical and probabilistic formulas to narrative text and convert it to structured data. Although text processing is becoming more feasible, the technology has a long way to go before it will be able to be used routinely.

System Communication and Networks

The backbone of a CPR obviously is the hardware and software on which the system runs. The term **architecture** refers to the configuration, structure, and relationships of all components of a computer system. There are three main types of architecture used in creating a CPR:

- *Mainframe architecture* utilizes a single large computer to process data received from terminals into which data are entered. Mainframe systems tend to be considered legacy systems because they are the configuration of older applications. In general, mainframe architecture is limited in its ability to support extensive decision support capability at terminals.
- *Client/server architecture* is newer and uses a combination of smaller computers to process and capture data. Server computers are powerful processors. They supply service to multiple client computers. The clients have specialized data capture capabilities and some processing capability. Clients and servers are integrated into a network that affords **connectivity.**
- *Web-based architecture* uses the latest components of technology that draw from the Internet. Programs act as browsers to capture data and extensive networking to move data throughout an enterprise and beyond.

Network devices link computers and other networks, and direct network data traffic. Local area networks (LANs) transmit data at very high speeds through cables. Wide area networks (WANs) generally depend on telephone lines to transmit data. Depending on the type of phone service (analog or digital) and the number and type of lines leased from the telephone company, speeds can be slow or fast.

Workstations

CPRs depend not only on the architecture of the system overall, but also on the nature of the workstation and the software that makes workstations "intelligent." When software is applied to a hardware client such that the client can support highly complex processing and displays, the term **workstation** is used to describe the client computer. Workstations may include standard desktop personal computers, notebook computers, and even personal digital assistants (PDSPDAs). They may be connected directly to a power supply, use radio frequency or infrared technology to connect to the network, or require physical "docking" to a desktop workstation to download and upload data. Workstations may have standard monitors or flat-panel monitors. They may be mounted on walls or movable carts as well as located on desks. Additionally, they may include special devices such as printers and voice recognition systems.

Workstation software for a CPR system supports several general functions, including:

- *Results review:* Results review is generally the first function most clinicians want from a CPR. The difference between results review in a CPR and that from a mainframe application is that the results are integrated and can be manipulated at the workstation into graphics, tables, and so on.
- *Patient summary:* A patient summary may be as simple as a list of a patient's encounters or as complex as a problem list that includes current problems, medications, and diagnostic studies alerts.
- *Order-entry functionality:* Order-entry functionality should provide the ability not only to enter an order, but also to receive decision support, such as contraindications, cost of various alternative medications or tests, and reminders.
- *In-basket:* The in-basket function provides scheduling and reminders for a day's activities. It is often combined with e-mail capability or other forms of remote connectivity to integrate information from various sites of care.
- *Documentation:* Documentation is frequently the final function introduced in a CPR. This is the direct entry of notes and other data through one or more of the various forms of data capture discussed above.

Clinical Decision Support Systems

Clinical decision support depends on analytical tools that process data into useful information. When data for a single transaction such as data capture, editing, or storing are processed, the processing may be described as online transaction processing (OLTP). When processing is required on the data that are entered in order to return some form of analysis, the processing is often referred to as online analytical processing (OLAP). OLAP may include statistical analysis, search engines, or other special analytical tools. Special analytical tools include reminders and alerts, clinical guideline advice, benchmarking, expert system resources, and diagnostic or procedural investigative tools.

Clinical decision support systems often depend on an elaborate set of rules to trigger reminders or to direct data through a pathway. Figure 9.2 is a simplified model of how experts apply facts to data to create rules that are stored in a **knowledge base** and taped whenever a user has a query or enters data that trigger a reminder, alert, or pathway. A full discussion of decision support is provided in chapter 19.

Advantages and Disadvantages of CPR Systems

The greatest advantage of a CPR is its contribution to the quality of patient care. Greatly enhanced access to data is its current most important feature. Beyond the ability to retrieve data is the capability to use them. In the past, most clinicians did not truly value information, except for limited, short-term results data, as a tool to help them care for patients. For the most part, recording information about patient care was viewed as a necessary evil. If, however, such information could guide their work, communicable communicate to offers others better, and help avoid errors, the CPR should truly become the much- enhanced utility that the Institute of Medicine envisioned.

The greatest disadvantage of a CPR is directly related to its greatest advantage: Enhanced use and usability make the

Figure 9.2.   Simplified Model of a Knowledge Base

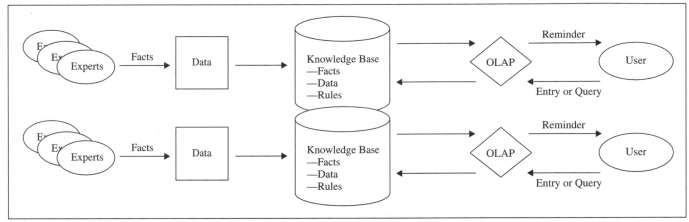

CPR a very costly application. As a result of lack of true marketability, low demand has kept costs high. Greater demand would contribute to economies of scale, in terms of both direct cost of production and contributing to product research and development to continually refine and produce even more usable and useful systems.

The impact of improved quality of patient care is virtually impossible to measure. Because it is so difficult to measure, the return on investment for a CPR is difficult to prove. And this return on investment is not only in real-dollar savings, but also in the level of effort to use the systems. Despite its costs, however, acquiring a CPR system remains the eventual goal of most providers.

Examples of CPR Systems

Over the years, many examples of CPRs have been developed. These include systems that have been homegrown, purchased, or developed through a vendor–provider partnership. There have been successes as well as failures.

First and foremost, the success of a CPR project relies on top- management commitment to its success, recognition of its value beyond pure return on investment, and willingness to support a long-term effort that significantly affects the organization.

Additionally, there must be strong clinician input every step of the way. The best CPR implementations are those where clinicians effectively created the project. There must be desire by end users for a CPR system: It is not something that the administration or the information systems department decides is now necessary and builds, buys, or leases and directs clinicians to use.

Further, there must be the understanding that the CPR changes fundamental practices. Not only does a CPR change how data are captured and information retrieved, but also how information is used in the practice of medicine. Clinical standards, guidelines, protocols, and pathways are key ingredients of the CPR. Clinicians must accept use of not only the system, but also its underlying standards; and these standards must be evidence based if they are to be accepted.

Functionality and technology are important to successful CPRs, but less so than the administrative and cultural issues.

Obviously, the CPR must provide the features that are needed to support patient care. Technology must be not only present and supportive of the applications, but also essentially pervasive. Technology rarely achieves success, but it can certainly create failure. Failures have resulted because there was inadequate technology—Many CPR projects have failed because of poor system performance, inadequate number of workstations, or connectivity issues.

A subset of technology is user training and support. Different users learn in different ways, and organizations must be prepared to support different learning styles. Unique to highly trained professionals, however, is also the need to learn in private. Learning how to use a device that most ten-year-olds are very proficient at using is not easy for someone who has devoted years in school. In fact, many clinicians learn CPR systems most effectively on their own, especially if the system is sufficiently intuitive. Many clinicians will spend hours exploring and tweaking, but no time in a classroom or dealing with a system problem.

Check Your Understanding 9.1

Instructions: Choose the best answer or answers for the following question.

1. ___ What makes a CPR difficult to achieve?
   a. Nature of data
   b. Lack of interest
   c. Vendor confusion
   d. Differences in work flow
   e. Mobility of healthcare professionals

Instructions: Match the following terms with their definitions.

a. Structure of a message
b. Means of integrating systems
c. Means of integrating data
d. System to manage data
e. Meaning of data

2. ___ Semantics

3. ___ Message format standards

4. ___ Data repository

5. ___ Syntax

6. ___ DBMS

Instructions: Indicate whether the following statements are true or false (T or F).

7. ____ Text processing is an easythe easiest way to convert narrative data into structured data.

8. ____ A workstation is the architecture of a CPR.

9. ____ The in-basket function often integrates data from multiple sources with e-mail.

10. ____ Most CPR systems are based on client/server architecture.

11. ____ Clinical decision support is essentially the application of a series of rules.

Instructions: Rank the following in order of importance to a successful CPR implementation.

12. a. ____ Acceptance of standards
    b. ____ Technology
    c. ____ Management commitment
    d. ____ User training
    e. ____ CliniciaIn input

User Needs and Issues

Clinician acceptance of computerization is changing and varies by type of clinician. In general, as clinicians become more used to computers, moving from some automation to a CPR is easier, as long as the "some automation" entails hands-on use. This is especially true for nurses, many of whom have suffered through some deplorable implementations of **hospital information systems** (HISs) or **patient care systems.** In general, allied health professionals also tend to adopt CPR systems more readily than other clinicians, perhaps because their application requirements are more moderate and they achieve so much more benefit from integrated information that they have not had in the past.

However, many clinicians still must overcome a number of issues before they will become completely comfortable using the CPR. For physicians, dealing with differences in office and hospital systems is a major issue. Security and privacy of health information are major concerns. Maintenance of the systems presents a number of problems. And finally, there is the question of the system's value in terms of dollars and cents.

System Issues

Physicians, it is interesting to note, tend to be more willing to adopt CPR systems in their own office practice than they are in the hospital or hospitals with which they are affiliated. There are several reasons for this. Perhaps foremost is the fact that the hospital system is just that—designed to support an institution, not necessarily an individual. There are significant differences between systems designed for physician offices and hospitals. These differences reflect the many differences in work flow between these two kinds of care. (See table 9.1.)

Table 9.1.   Differences in Hospital and Physician's Office Work Flow

	Hospital	Physician's Office
Work flow	Tightly coordinated	Loosely coordinated
Communication	Formal	Informal
Primary user	Nurse	Physician
Data content	Comprehensive	Fragmented
Data volume	High density	Low density
Data source	Multiple, disparate	Patient/provider generated
Information flow	Location centric	Geographically dispersed
Data input	Mobile	Stationary
I.S. decision making	Administration	Physicians

Copyright © 2001. Margret/A Consulting, LLC.

A physician views the office CPR from an ownership perspective and the hospital CPR from an indentured servant perspective. Couple that with the fact that the hospital system is different from the office system, representing a second system to learn, one can appreciate the challenge a physician has in using a hospital system. The most successful situation is one in which the office and hospital systems "look" and function very similarly. This, of course, can be aided by using a standard user interface (for example, Windows® based) and providing remote connectivity to accustom the physician to the look and feel of the hospital system.

All of this is not to suggest that the user interface is the only issue to be addressed. It also must be recognized that the entire discussion of clinician resistance will hopefully be a generational issue, with new generations of physicians coming into the profession as experienced computer-game users.

Security and Privacy Issues

Users are also concerned about security and privacy issues, as well as patient perception issues. Today's information systems have typically been secured by virtue of the fact that they contain minimal patient data, few people know how to use them, and they are closed systems. They do not connect to the outside world. As use and users expand, security must be enhanced to better protect privacy. On the other hand, however, security measures must not be so onerous as to make CPRs even more formidable to learn and use.

Some clinicians also have expressed concern about patient acceptance of computers. Will the patient perceive the computer to be a barrier between patient and clinician? Many clinicians are finding that patients actually expect them to use a computer, or at least are not surprised when they do. Many providers find computers add value to the patient encounter. Clinicians who make the computer a barrier because they do not use it well will surely create a barrier for their patients. However, the computer can be used to engage and provide the patient with instantaneous information and instructions.

Showing the patient a graph of personal data can be a powerful motivator. Instructions tailored specifically to the patient can improve his or her compliance with a treatment regime. Although its use is controversial and it must be specially secured, e-mail, or at least a patient portal to a secure Web site messaging system, can greatly contribute to patient–provider communications

Maintenance Issues

CPRs are a high-maintenance proposition. Virtually every component must be kept up to date. The formulary that supports prescription writing could potentially require daily updates, and clinical guidelines must be reviewed and updated periodically. There are ongoing advances in medicine where clinical decision support needs to be modified. These are just some of the ongoing efforts that require the attention of full-time staff.

Value Issues

The value proposition for a CPR is an issue for users and administrators alike. This has already been alluded to in the discussion of return on investment (ROI). Everyone believes there is value to a CPR, but proving it in actual dollars and cents is difficult.

First, the value of a CPR is primarily in improved patient care, or "clinical savings." Quality counts, but measuring quality is difficult. A number of efforts to prove ROI have been made. Several academic medical centers and large integrated delivery systems have conducted extensive research demonstrating that medication errors can be reduced, more accurate and quick diagnoses can be made, faster recovery can be achieved, and duplication of diagnostic studies can be reduced. All of these can be linked to savings in cost of care. For example, if one medication error during a hospitalization can be avoided, most hospitals believe the patient will have a shorter length of stay (LOS). Yet, a shorter LOS does not necessarily accrue to direct dollar savings. Instead, the hospital may only find indirect ROI through better managed care contracts as a result of its reduced medication error rate and shorter LOS.

There are potential operational savings as well as clinical savings from a CPR. Operational savings iIn physician offices that have gone paperless as a result of a CPR, there have beeninclude significant savings in personnel who pull, file, and transport charts. There has been a significant drop in transcription services when physician offices have adopted CPR systems (if they dictated many of their notes previously). In hospitals, these savings have not yet been fully realized because few, if any, hospitals are totally paperless. In fact, transcription costs have increased in cases where physicians have been given the option of dictation rather than direct data entry. Still, CPR systems have the potential for improved productivity in a number of areas. Some hospitals have demonstrated reduced nurse overtime as a result of better shift reporting or less time spent in documentation at end of shift. Physicians may complain that it takes longer to enter orders, but the orders are more legible and accurate and result in fewer follow-up calls from pharmacists. Quality assurance, utilization management, and other operational functions achieve enhanced support through a CPR. There may not be direct savings, but more accurate and timely information can produce more effective results.

In addition to the difficulty of costing out return on CPR investment, another interesting phenomenon occurs in healthcare: Everyone seems to believe they must prove their own ROI rather than accepting the studies of others. Although there are some unique attributes in different facilities, the idea that everyone is totally different is not true. Often the key difference is that some institutions are willing to conduct scientific studies on ROI, and others are not. For example, if an organization does not know its current medication error rate, it is impossible to determine what a change would be and thus impossible to identify true savings.

Check Your Understanding 9.2

Instructions: Answer *yes* or *no* to the following question. Which user needs and issues make CPRs difficult to implement?

1. ___ Clinician resistance
2. ___ Proving return on investment
3. ___ User interface
4. ___ Differences in work flow
5. ___ Scarcity of systems to choose from

Creation of Computer-Based Record Systems

A CPR is not a single product to buy. From a technical perspective, it is the integration of all systems that contain patient information and the adoption of software to support more robust processing of this information. This will certainly require additional software and hardware. There also are cultural and operational perspectives. It is getting users to integrate the computer into their daily activities and to adopt standards of care. Although technical issues cannot be minimized, the culture and operational issues are the most difficult to overcome. Chapter 6 provides a full discussion of systems planning and technology acquisition.

CPR System Planning

Healthcare organizations "create" CPR systems in a variety of ways. Some organizations build their own systems. This is especially true of more academic, research-based environments. Developing a system from scratch is becoming much less common as more sophisticated commercial products are introduced into the marketplace. Because it is difficult to hire and retain highly qualified information technology (IT) staff, this option is costly and time-consuming. Vendors can provide economies of scale that simply are not available to individual organizations.

Some organizations buy a fully integrated hospital information system and upgrade as the vendor supplies more functionality toward the ultimate goal of CPR. Many smaller hospitals and physician office practices find this to be a suitable solution. The advantage is that the vendor provides a tried-and-true solution. The disadvantage is that these systems generally are fairly basic, meeting minimum requirements of everyone rather than trying to address any special needs.

Some organizations lease systems. In leasing, the provider pays on a subscription, or lease, basis for the use of hardware, software, and support. Currently, this form of acquiring computer systems is referred to as an **application service provider** (ASP) model. For an organization with limited IT expertise and minimum functional requirements, this can be very advantageous. However, there are usually very limited customization capabilities and sometimes there are integration problems with systems that may already exist. Moreover, the total cost of leasing, over time, may exceed the cost of purchase.

Finally, some organizations plan a careful migration path toward achieving a CPR. This may include a combination of several of the above options. Key, however, is that these organizations understand their goal and undertake the process over a period of time in which management is stable. Organizations that have been most successful at this approach have chief information officers and physician champions who have long tenure with the organization. Executive management believes in a CPR and is willing to carry through on strategic investments rather than divert resources to short-term needs.

Organizational Goals for CPR Systems

However an organization acquires its CPR, it must establish goals for the CPR, put into place mechanisms to ensure that those goals are met, and conduct benefits realization studies to manage achievement of those goals. Every member of the organization must understand what a CPR is. There should be a common understanding and clearly stated definition. The expectation must be that all clinicians will use the system. The CPR is not an administrative or financial system; rather, it is a clinical system designed to support direct patient care. Clinicians who bypass the system for printouts or use clerical support for data entry are not achieving the benefit of the system and are undermining achievement of the system's goals. An organization that does not monitor achievement of goals to take corrective action is setting itself up for failure. CPRs can be powerful in helping an organization achieve its strategic initiatives, but they must be managed carefully.

After the organization establishes its CPR goals, it can better determine its overall approach to acquisition and select the best fit. Most organizations follow a well-defined approach to selecting the best vendor or ASP. The process may be looked upon as a funnel, in which the organization starts with a broad scope and narrows down to the final decision.

CPR Migration Path

CPR planning should begin as early as initial information systems are selected, although this rarely happens. Organizations that develop a migration path, however, are generally able to make support system selections that are more in line with their ultimate CPR requirements. (See figure 9.3.) If a migration path has not been established, CPR planning should include an assessment of current systems and their ability to support a CPR. Questions to consider include:

- What additional systems are needed?
- What changes to existing systems must be made?
- Are interfaces required? Is there a repository?
- Will the architecture support a CPR, or will a major investment in hardware need to be made first?
- Is the network sufficient to support all CPR users, or will this need to be enhanced?

Key selection criteria should be kept to a manageable number. The following prioritized list of criteria is a good starting point:

- Functionality
- Vendor viability
- Vendor support
- Training availability
- Implementation support
- Technology/architecture
- Vision (research and development momentum)
- Integration
- Vendor's clinical culture
- ROI potential

Except for the ROI potential, cost is not identified as a criterion for CPR selection. Although cost is undoubtedly important, it should not be used in the basic selection. Vendors have many ways to price products, and there are many financing options. The lowest bidder is likely to have the lowest ranking in most of the functionality. When the functionality does not support the user community, ROI will not be achieved.

Most organizations use a formal request for proposal process to solicit information from vendors on how they can meet the criteria. This may then be accompanied by product demonstrations. From there, most organizations are able to narrow their choice down to a finalist and backup. Due diligence in the form of site visits, corporate visits, reference checks, credit checks on owners, and other steps need to be

Figure 9.3.   Acquisition Model for CPR

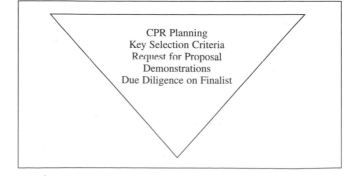

CPR Planning
Key Selection Criteria
Request for Proposal
Demonstrations
Due Diligence on Finalist

performed before a final contract is negotiated to ensure that the organization is getting the product it wants.

CPR System Implementation

After a system has been selected, installation and user training are the next critical steps in implementing a CPR. However, the CPR is an ongoing project rather than one with a definitive end point. Clinical processes are in a continual change mode; therefore, systems that support clinical processes can be expected to change as well. This, too, requires planning and careful attention.

System Installation

System installation should include operations analysis and work-flow redesign to support the CPR. Installations may be phased in a variety of ways—by special users, by department, by site, or by function. Often the vendor has the best recommendation and should be considered an important guide. This issue also should be evaluated during site visits and reference checks.

User Training

User training will require not only formal classroom instruction on use of the computer, but also considerable hand-holding and support. It is important to recognize that users learn in different ways. For example, nurses may do well in a classroom session where the experience can be shared. On the other hand, physicians often require one-on-one, private instruction. In fact, physicians often learn best when a system is intuitive and they can learn on their own. Sufficient online help is critical. However implementation is managed, training will be key to using the system and does not end at installation. Ongoing training of regular users hones their skills and helps them to learn new things on an ongoing basis. Finally, it also supports maintenance of the system.

Check Your Understanding 9.3

Instructions: Match the environment with the system or systems that represent the best fit.

1. ___ Physician's office
2. ___ Academic medical center
3. ___ Integrated delivery system undergoing mergers and acquisitions
4. ___ Well-established community hospital
5. ___ Small hospital

a. Acquire ASP
b. Plan system
c. Buy standard system
d. Build system

Information Management in an Electronic Environment

The Joint Commission on Accreditation of Healthcare Organizations (JCAHO) describes "the goal of the information management function is to obtain, manage, and use information to improve patient outcomes and individual and organi-

zational performance in patient care, governance, management, and support processes" (JCAHO 2000, p. IM–1). This involves:

- Ensuring timely and easy access to complete information throughout the facility
- Improving data accuracy
- Balancing requirements of security and ease of access
- Using aggregate and comparative data to pursue opportunities for improvement
- Redesigning information-related processes to improve efficiency
- Increasing collaboration and information sharing to enhance patient care

Although the JCAHO indicates that the principles of good information management apply to all forms of medical record keeping, it explicitly states that efficiency can be improved by computerization and other technologies.

Each of the major sections of the JCAHO's information management standard is supported by a CPR system. Planning and designing a CPR meets the requirement of planning and designing information management processes to meet internal and external information needs. CPR systems afford greater confidentiality, security, and integrity of data. They incorporate uniform data definitions and data capture methods that contribute to defining, capturing, analyzing, transforming, transmitting, and reporting patient-specific data and information related to care processes and outcomes. CPR systems serve not only as a repository of all health information content, but also as a reminder for users to document such information. Finally, CPR systems protect confidentiality and integrity of data through security measures.

Information Privacy, Security, and Confidentiality

Every individual has private information he or she does not share with anyone, including innermost thoughts, dreams, and feelings. When some of this information is shared with someone else in confidence, a condition is established that is called **confidentiality.** Sometimes this confidential information is written down or placed into a computer system. To ensure that confidential information can be accessed only by those to whom the individual has given permission, security measures are put into place. In healthcare, in addition to affording confidentiality to private information that has been shared with providers, security measures also protect the **integrity** of the information (so that it is not altered in any way) and ensure its availability (so that it is accessible when needed for subsequent care and other legitimate purposes). Because of the multiple types of protection needed for health information, the term *protected health information* is slowly replacing the term *confidential information,* and is being used to refer to individually identifiable health information that needs its confidentiality, integrity, and availability safeguarded.

A CPR system can afford better security for confidential information because access controls, audit trails, authentication systems, and other measures exist where they do not in a paper environment. Attention to security and privacy is not new. The Hippocratic Oath has directed physician protection of private information for centuries. Moreover, every provider has instituted security measures as part of his or her standard business practices. The Health Insurance Portability and Accountability Act (HIPAA) of 1996 now requires specific attention to security and privacy.

HIPAA Privacy Requirements

HIPAA privacy measures include specific policies and procedures on uses and disclosures of protected health information, individuals' rights with respect to their information (including the right to access, request restrictions, request amendment, and others), and privacy management. Although most of HIPAA's privacy requirements are accomplished through administrative and operational activities, CPR technology can assist in carrying out a number of the privacy standards. For example, because patients have the right to request restrictions on who may use and disclose protected health information, access controls need to be in place. In the paper environment, access control may be accomplished by putting a special note on the chart cover, which may not be very effective when many individuals are involved in treating a patient and may have access to parts of the medical record only. A CPR provides highly effective controls on specific categories of information for specific categories of people who may access the information. In another example, when patients request confidential communication, there needs to be a way to notify providers that an alternate address or phone number must be used to contact the patient concerning certain information. Again, a note on the chart cover may be the only available solution in the paper environment, but a flag that pops up on a computer screen or that automatically routes calls or letters would provide much greater assurance that the patient's request is being carried out. Many technical measures are available to help protect patient privacy. HIPAA privacy measures are also discussed in chapter 10.

HIPAA's security requirements are generally more technical than the privacy requirements, but they also require the establishment of policy to direct the type of technical tools that will be applied. For example, HIPAA requires access control technology. This special application limits the applications and/or information that a given person may access by means of an access profile that is associated with the individual's system user identification. Access profiles are established as a matter of policy. For example, some hospitals decide to control nurse access to patient information by the floor on which the nurse is working. Within nursing, there may be controls on who may view information and who may view and enter information. Laboratory technicians may be given access only to those patients for whom a laboratory test order has been placed. Their access may be limited to view-ing only certain information about the patient, such as diagnosis and current medications, and entering information only into the laboratory component of the information system.

HIPAA Security Requirements

HIPAA requires that every provider conduct a security analysis to determine its risks and to develop a security program that addresses those risks. A **risk analysis** is a systematic process of identifying security measures to afford protections given an organization's specific environment—where they are located, what level of automation they have, how sensitive the information is that needs protection, and many other factors.

Risk is the potential for harm. It is composed of vulnerabilities and threats. Vulnerabilities are potential avenues of attack. For example, in the paper environment, an unlocked back door to the file room is an avenue of attack. In a computer system, a vulnerability is not having a firewall on the network or not backing up a computer system.

Threats include targets, agents, and events. A *target* is what might be attacked. HIPAA identifies three targets: confidentiality, integrity, and availability (C-I-A). Many security experts include a fourth target—accountability. *Accountability* refers to the fact that a person who has accessed a system, entered data, or otherwise used a system is associated with that action and held responsible for it. HIPAA includes this as part of the other three forms of targets.

An *agent* is a means of attack. Frequently agents are individuals who have access to protected health information, knowledge of security weaknesses, and motivation to cause harm. However, it should be noted that there are other forms of agents that do not necessarily intend to do harm, do not result in harm, or are physical agents. For example, a person who has access to an information system may inadvertently do something that results in a breach of confidentiality, an integrity problem, or a lack of availability. Moreover, access, alteration, or unavailability could have resulted in harm but did not. Finally, there are acts of nature, such as fire or flood, that cause harm.

An *event* is the form of harm. Inappropriate access that causes a breach of confidentiality, modification of data that causes an integrity problem, denial of service that renders information unavailable, and repudiation that allows an individual to disavow responsibility for an action are forms of harm.

A risk analysis would study each vulnerability and determine its associated threats. Generally, when doing a risk analysis, the combination of threat and vulnerability is assigned a risk level to help determine what mitigation steps should be taken and in what priority order. The risk level may be a numeric score or a relative value statement, such as high, medium, and low. Obviously, those with the highest score or relative importance would receive the greatest resources and first attention. Table 9.2 provides a sample risk analysis tool using the HIPAA standards as a guide to identifying vulnerabilities.

Table 9.2.   Sample Risk Analysis Tool

HIPAA Standard	Vulnerability	Threat			Level of Risk	Mitigation	Resources and Time Line
		Target (C-I-A)	Agent	Event			
Certification	No system certification	C-I-A	Disgruntled employee	Files complaint w/HHS	Low	Develop criteria Self-certify	IS 6/3
Chain of trust	No contracts	C-I	Breach by business associate	Lawsuit filed by patient	Low	Use model chain-of-trust language for contracts	Contracts office 1/3
Contingency plan	No disaster recovery plan	A	Natural disaster Direct attack on power supply	Downtime	Medium	Backup daily Store backups off-site	IS 6/2

HIPAA security requirements are categorized into three sections: administrative procedures, physical safeguards, and technical security.

Administrative Procedures

Administrative procedures cover policies, procedures, contracts, and plans for security. HIPAA requires that systems be certified and that an internal audit practice be established to ensure that information systems meet minimum security requirements and that practices support those requirements. For example, if a minimum requirement is to have continual backups run and stored off-site daily, a system certification process would review systems for their capability to back up continuously and would ensure that such backups can be restored. An internal audit process would monitor backup tape storage and rotation policies.

Contingency planning is also an administrative security requirement. Applications should be categorized by criticality and backup plans, disaster recovery plans, and emergency mode operations plans developed in accordance with the criticality of the application and its information. These plans should be tested and revised routinely in accordance with the results of the tests. Configuration management refers to tracking system versions and other changes and ensuring that system maintenance is current.

Administrative procedures also address personnel security, security incident reporting and response, sanction policies, termination procedures, training, and assigned security responsibility. A specific individual should be assigned authority and responsibility for overseeing every aspect of information security. Training is a very large part of administrative procedures. It needs to include education (imparting knowledge), skill set development (so people know how to perform security activities), and awareness building (to ensure that security is "top of mind" at all times).

Physical Safeguards

Physical safeguards obviously have to do with protecting the environment, including ensuring that applicable doors have locks that are changed when needed and that fire, flood, and other natural disaster preparedness is in place (for example, fire alarms, sprinklers, smoke detectors, raised cabinets). Media control is also a very important part of physical safety. Many providers are evaluating whether they really need all the printers they have, how to dispose of confidential trash (including nonrecyclable containers with labels, paper awaiting shredding, and so on), and whether all workstations need floppy disk drives.

Other physical controls include badging and escorting visitors and other typical "security" functions such as patrolling the premises, logging equipment in and out, and camera-monitoring key areas. Finally, workstation location and use is an important physical safeguard. Workstation monitors should be out of view of those who do not have a need to know. Employees who use workstations also should know how to safeguard them, including ensuring that virus protection software is upgraded, that log-in failure is noticed, and so on.

Technical Security

HIPAA calls for two forms of technical security. *Technical security services* protect data in storage. *Technical security mechanisms* protect data during transmission.

Technical security services protect data at rest, that is, when data are stored whether in a database or even in temporary files. Access control technology requires use of access profiles and emergency mode access. Policies should be established that clarify what types of access different users require, who has authority to assign an access profile, how access is granted to a user (in person, after training, and based on acknowledgment of how access is to be used), and how access may be modified.

HIPAA permits organizations to select the strength of the access controls they adopt. For example:

- *User-based access control* basically gives a person access by who they are.

- *Role-based access control* is stronger. It establishes parameters by what role an individual plays (nurse, physician, pharmacist).
- *Context-based access control* is the strongest. It not only establishes a profile based on who the person is and what role he or she is playing, but also on what specific information may or may not be accessed.

Today, most hospitals have some form of role-based access control for most staff and generally user-based access control for physicians. As a result, most providers do not have emergency mode access controls (sometimes called "break glass" access). When physicians have only user-based access control, they have access to every patient's information and thus there is no need for emergency mode access. However, if physicians were given role-based access such that they could access only their own patients' information, they would need emergency-based access in the event of a true emergency. Emergency mode access permits access to information to which a user normally does not have access after a second level of password and/or justification is provided for the access. Such access is generally more closely monitored. Sometimes an emergency access will trigger a notification to the patient's attending physician of such access (or if it were a nurse, to the nursing supervisor).

Technical security services also include entity authentication, which is closely related to access controls. Entity authentication refers to unique user identification and one other level of proving identity. In most cases, this second level of authenticity is a password, although tokens, biometrics, callback procedures, and PINs also are permitted. Although not the strongest method of authentication, passwords can be strengthened through several means. First, they should never be shared and strong sanctions should be in place to enforce this. A strong password is one that is extremely difficult to guess. If the password is "strong," it does not need to be changed frequently. In fact, that will only encourage people to write a password down, making it accessible to others. Systems also should log off automatically after a period of inactivity to prevent anyone from seeing what is currently on a screen and to prevent others from using someone's log-on.

Technical security services also include data authentication. Data authentication is essentially data integrity. This is accomplished through technical measures, such as check-digits, hash totals, and other forms of edits that ensure that data are accurate and complete. Such measures ensure that data have not been altered during processing or transmission.

Finally, technical security services should include audit trails. Although some believe audit trails are not necessary with strong access controls, they do offer a way to ensure that access controls work, that everyone who should have been terminated from access is terminated, and that a manager is able to look for unusual, and possibly inappropriate, access by an authorized user. For example, if the provider only has user-based access control and there is a celebrity in-house, increased activity by users who have legitimate access to the system, but not necessarily to that celebrity, can be identified through audit trail. An audit trail also provides documentary evidence when a user needs to be sanctioned.

Technical security mechanisms guard data en route, that is, when they are transmitted within communications media and networks. In addition to the technical security services that also should be applied to data en route, there should be monitoring of network traffic and system alarms and event reporting when there are problems. Most providers use some form of firewall, which is a computer that controls access to an Internet-connected network. Such a computer should scan for and quarantine any files that appear to have viruses. Many providers also use firewalls to block inappropriate Web site access.

Check Your Understanding 9.4

Instructions: Match the following terms with their definitions.

a. Entity authentication
b. Configuration management
c. Target
d. Firewall
e. Access control
f. Threats
g. Security mechanisms
h. Vulnerability
i. Audit trail
j. Emergency mode plan

1. ___ Computer that monitors Internet traffic
2. ___ Avenue of attack
3. ___ Change or version control of systems
4. ___ Targets, agents, and events that cause computer attacks
5. ___ Contingency plan for when disaster strikes a system
6. ___ Availability of system for use
7. ___ Identification of a user to the system
8. ___ Profiles that limit what a person can do in a system
9. ___ Technical measures that protect data during transmission
10. ___ Provides evidence of who has accessed data

Future Directions of Information Technologies

This chapter represents both currently available technology and future directions. This is because all of the technology described here is in use somewhere, but not widely adopted and not necessarily adopted all in one place.

Today, it appears that information technology is beginning to be more broadly adopted for clinical information computing. Factors that are contributing to heightened interest and use of CPRs include a critical mass of support systems, the end of Y2K (preparation for potential year 2000 computer system breakdowns), more manageable technology, pervasive use of the Internet, the IOM patient safety report, and HIPAA.

A CPR depends on having a critical mass of support systems. All patient care areas, ancillary departments, and support services must be automated and supply data to a clinical data repository (or be fully integrated). More hospitals and physician offices are beginning to have all the necessary information systems in place to support a repository and eventually a CPR.

Before January 1, 2000, many information technology resources were diverted to efforts that would ensure that older systems would work, at a point when many providers were just starting to be ready to commit resources to finishing their CPR support automation efforts. Now that Y2K is over, providers should be able to focus resources on clinical computing over the next decade.

Perhaps the most critical precursor to CPR is the need for a user-friendly interface and other more manageable (and affordable) technologies. The healthcare industry has always been reactive rather than proactive to new technology. Even new medical technology undergoes years of testing before it is considered safe enough to use on patients. This reluctance to use new technology, coupled with the real lack of graphical user interfaces, mobile devices, data capture tools, and online application processing capabilities, truly have held back CPR adoption. Thanks to the Internet and e-commerce, many of these technologies are becoming more realistic for healthcare.

The explosion of Internet use and e-commerce has resulted in much more widespread use of computers in general and in particular by providers (who are realizing the value of enhanced communications through the Internet) and patients (who are demanding connectivity with their providers).

The biggest spurt of interest in CPR—and perhaps the most compelling for providers—is as a result of the IOM report on patient safety. As a result of this report that describes the extent of medical errors and their cause and potential cure, external pressure is being brought to bear on providers by employers and payer contracting groups. Caution must be applied, however, to recognize that many levels of automation can help reduce medical errors. Physician order entry can achieve greater legibility without a full CPR. A robust decision support system that is a component of a CPR, however, identifies contraindications, provides information on more efficacious medications, and offers best practice guidelines.

Yet to be fully realized is the impact HIPAA will have on achieving the CPR. The goal of HIPAA actually is to "encourage the development of a health information system." In fact, HIPAA really only started with privacy and security (and basic financial and administrative transactions, such as claims and eligibility verification). It also requires claims attachment standards and uniform data standards for electronic exchange of patient medical record information. Claims attachments standards permit data on ambulance

services, clinical reports, emergency department reports, laboratory results, medications, and rehabilitation services to be exchanged electronically with payers requiring such additional information. To take advantage of these claims attachments standards, providers need to have data automated and integrated with their patient accounting information system.

Patient medical record information (PMRI) standards also are just beginning to be addressed as part of HIPAA. The National Committee on Vital and Health Statistics (NCVHS) has been charged with developing recommendations relating to PMRI, and it is studying message format standards for achieving interoperability, standard vocabularies for data comparability, and data quality standards. Interoperability is critical to integrating data from disparate systems to support CPRs. Standard vocabularies ensure that content in disparate systems carries the same meaning. Data quality standards ensure internal consistency, accuracy, completeness, reliability, and timeliness.

Finally, electronic signature standards, although not a part of the final HIPAA security rule, are reaching maturity and can be expected to be required soon. This will further support the ability to exchange PMRI, which is critical to achieving a CPR.

There is every indication that the CPR's time has finally come. The future will include complete automation of support systems, use of Internet-based technology to make CPR adoption more affordable and easier to use, and, more than anything else, return on investment is finally beginning to be recognized.

All of this is not to say that CPRs are not expensive, complex to install, and demanding of clinical work-flow redesign. There are pitfalls at every turn. Few vendors truly have a CPR as described by the IOM report on patient records issued in 1991. No single vendor yet supports all components of integrated delivery networks. Clinician input into CPR selection and design is essential, and ongoing maintenance of a truly "mission-critical" system addressing the core business of healthcare—taking care of patients—is a basic requirement. For the value proposition to be realized, clinicians must use the CPR and use it to its full potential. Each user must see value to it personally. This means that, as the IOM report on patient records noted, the CPR must achieve the "broader view of the patient record than is current today, moving from the notion of a location or device for keeping track of patient care events to a resource with much enhanced utility in patient care, in management of the healthcare system, and in extension of knowledge" (IOM 1997, p. 47).

Real-World Case

The Leapfrog Group is a coalition of major employers, which started in the automotive industry, that contracts for healthcare services from hospitals and physician groups. It has begun to limit its contracts to providers who adopt methods to improve patient safety. As an example, one large integrated delivery network was required to improve its clinical computing capabilities to be granted a contract for services from one of the Leapfrog Group's member companies.

The main hospital already had a homegrown information system that included basic patient registration and billing functions. It also supported nursing personnel in order entry and ancillary departments in managing order communications. A laboratory information system was interfaced with the hospital information system so that laboratory results could be viewed from it. A special program had been developed recently to supply clinical guidelines for the treatment of diabetes and heart disease that were printed out by nursing personnel for each applicable patient and placed in his or her paper health record. Physicians in their offices had access to the hospital information system and also were able to maintain a patient problem list. The health information management department was scanning the contents of the medical record for archival purposes. However, the scanned documents could not be viewed through the hospital information system because the two systems did not communicate with one another. The hospital also had several other, smaller and independent information systems for its emergency department, nutrition services, and so on. Satellite hospitals had some very limited connectivity to the main hospital information system, but there was no enterprisewide master patient index.

In response to the Leapfrog Group, the hospital network decided to investigate the development or purchase of a CPR. It was important that whatever it planned for would reduce errors, would be as easy to use as the current system, could be tailored to meet network's specific needs, and would interface with other major systems.

Discussion Questions

1. What steps could be implemented to improve patient safety with the current system while the hospital network is investigating CPR systems?

2. Should the hospital network consider further self-development of a CPR? What are the advantages and disadvantages of buying a CPR?

3. What specific benefits should the hospital network be looking to achieve in a CPR?

4. If full connectivity is afforded the satellite hospitals, how can it be secured?

5. What can the hospital network expect to be its greatest hurdle in achieving success with a CPR?

Summary

A computer-based patient record (or whatever term may be used to describe a comprehensive information system that supports patient care) is both a reality today and a goal for tomorrow. Some providers are well on their way to achieving a CPR. Many other providers have many of the components

of a CPR that would make the next step of acquiring a data repository and clinical decision support, along with the necessary hardware upgrades and workstation expansion and enhancement, realistic. However, still many other providers do not yet have the supporting systems and have a long way to go. Although fewer hospitals than physician offices are using application service providers, this is beginning to be an attractive alternative to achieving core functionality for a CPR more rapidly.

A CPR is the integration of source information systems and the application of software that processes the data beyond simple retrieval to provide clinical decision support. For providers to achieve successful CPR implementation, adequate technology and functionality are important; but more critical are top-management commitment to a long-term investment and clinician input into planning, selection, design, and implementation so that clinicians actually use the system at the point of care. Ongoing system training, support, and maintenance are essential, as is a strong security program that safeguards the system's confidentiality, integrity, and availability.

References

Institute of Medicine. 1997. *The Computer-Based Patient Record: An Essential Technology for Health Care,* rev. ed. Washington, D.C.: National Academy Press.

Joint Commission on Accreditation of Healthcare Organizations. 2000. *2001 Comprehensive Accreditation Manual for Hospitals.* Oakbrook Terrace, Ill.: JCAHO.

Application Exercises

1. The Institute of Medicine has been a thought leader in improving health records in light of new technology. Review the National Academy Press Web site (www.nap.gov), where the IOM's reports are published for summaries of their contributions to CPR, the Internet, and patient safety. Write a brief summary of how these topics relate.

2. The National Committee on Vital and Health Statistics has been charged, under HIPAA legislation, to monitor implementation of HIPAA and to make recommendations for uniform data standards for electronic exchange of patient health record information. Visit the NCVHS Web site (www.ncvhs.hhs.gov) to review testimony the committee has heard, minutes of its deliberations, and reports it has produced. List the top five issues the NCVHS has addressed in the past year relating to patient health record information.

3. Conduct research about CPR using current literature or the Internet and compare your research to the status of CPR in healthcare organizations in your area. The Internet is one of the best sources of information about CPR and its various technologies. You may perform an Internet search on the term *computer-based patient record,* its acronym CPR, or any of the associated technologies. Alternatively, you may consult the several healthcare periodicals and publications that routinely survey the CPR market or publish articles about special implementations. Use these articles to learn more about CPR. Then, visit specific provider sites in your area to monitor the status of CPR (or EMR or EHR) implementations. Select three sites that have exemplary implementations of CPR systems and develop a brief report comparing their experiences.

Review Quiz

Instructions: Choose the most appropriate answer for the following questions.

1. ___ Which organization has had the most influence over defining the computer-based patient record?
   a. American Health Information Management Association (AHIMA)
   b. Health Level Seven (HL7)
   c. Institute of Medicine (IOM)
   d. U.S. Department of Health and Human Services (HHS)

2. ___ How can vendor readiness to supply CPR systems best be described?
   a Behind in research
   b. Continually in development
   c. Near the ultimate goal
   d. Ready to supply CPR

3. ___ What is a special database that integrates data from disparate vendor information systems called?
   a. Database management system
   b. Data repository
   c. Integration engine
   d. Interface standards

4. ___ Which of the following is an example of a data exchange standard that helps systems communicate with one another?
   a. CPT
   b. DBMS
   c. DICOM
   d. SNOMED

5. ___ What does the word *syntax* refer to?
   a. Common meaning of terms in a message
   b. Context of words in narrative form
   c. Structure of data elements in a message
   d. Text processing

6. ___ Which of the following is not available as an image through a CPR?
   a. Digitized signature
   b. Document
   c. PACS
   d. Work flow

7. ___ Which of the following is a data retrieval technology?
   a. Color
   b. Digital dictation
   c. Point-and-click
   d. Wireless device

8. ___ In which of the following applications would speech recognition be most successful?
   a. Family practice clinic
   b. Nursing unit
   c. Radiology department
   d. Surgery suite

9. ___ Most commercial CPR architecture today is what?
   a. Client/server
   b. Legacy
   c. Mainframe
   d. Web based

10. ___ Which of the following is generally not considered a CPR workstation?
    a. Desktop PC
    b. Notebook computer
    c. Personal digital assistant
    d. Terminal

11. ___ What do clinical decision support systems uniquely depend on?
    a. Database management system
    b. Expert rule development
    c. Online transaction processing
    d. Source system automation

12. ___ What is the greatest disadvantage of CPR systems?
    a. Communication capabilities
    b. Contribution to high-quality care
    c. Ease of use
    d. Security

13. ___ What is the most important element in achieving a successful CPR?
    a. Clinician training
    b. Help desk support
    c. Top-management commitment
    d. Vendor expertise

14. ___ What have most nursing documentation systems been called?
    a. Data retrieval systems
    b. Hospital information systems
    c. Nursing information systems
    d. Patient care systems

15. ___ Why have physicians had greater success implementing a CPR in their offices than hospitals have had?
    a. Hospitals have more complex communication problems.
    b. Physicians have made the purchase decision.
    c. Physicians do not view hospital systems as their own.
    d. All of the above

16. ___ Investments in CPR technology have had the most direct impact on which of the following areas?
    a. Patient care
    b. Quality assurance
    c. Transcription
    d. None of the above

17. ___ Which of the following is the least customizable way to acquire a CPR system?
    a. ASP
    b. Buy a vended product
    c. Plan a migration path
    d. Self-develop

18. ___ In purchasing a CPR system from a vendor, what does due diligence refer to?
    a. Checking references
    b. Conducting product demonstrations
    c. Financing the investment
    d. Negotiating the contract

19. ___ Which of the following is not a CPR selection criterion?
    a. Cost
    b. Functionality
    c. Implementation support
    d. Vendor vision

20. ___ Which of the following concepts best describe(s) confidentiality?
    a. Condition
    b. HIPAA requirement
    c. Target
    d. All of the above

21. ___ Which of the following is a systematic process of identifying security measures to afford protections given an organization's specific environment?
    a. Gap analysis
    b. Operations review
    c. Readiness assessment
    d. Risk analysis

22. ___ Which of the following events and targets do not match?
    a. Access—confidentiality
    b. Modification—availability
    c. Repudiation—accountability
    d. None of the above

23. ___ What are passwords a form of?
    a. Access control
    b. Data authentication
    c. Entity authentication
    d. All of the above

24. ___ What is the strongest form of access control?
    a. Context based
    b. Profile based
    c. Role based
    d. User based

25. ___ Which of the following controls external access to a network?
    a. Access controls
    b. Alarms
    c. Encryption
    d. Firewall

Chapter 10
Legal Issues in Health Information Management

Lynda A. Russell, EdD, JD, RHIA

Learning Objectives

- To define terms specific to civil litigation
- To diagram the state and federal court systems
- To describe the sources of law
- To explain the difference between civil law and criminal law
- To describe the process for a civil case and the process for a criminal case
- To discuss liability for a tort as it relates to healthcare
- To discuss liability for breach of contract as it relates to healthcare
- To discuss the legal aspects of a health record
- To discuss the purposes for retaining health records
- To outline the basic principles for releasing confidential health information with or without patient authorization
- To identify the required elements of an authorization for the release of confidential health information
- To analyze various requests for confidential health information and to determine whether patient authorization is required
- To elaborate on the role of the health record in medical staff appointments and privileges
- To explain the health information administrator's relationship with the risk manager in reducing facility liability

Key Terms

Administrative law
Civil law
Common law
Contract law
Controlled Substances Act
Court of appeals
Credentialing process
Criminal law
Default judgment
Defendant
Federal Register
Felony
Freedom of Information Act (FOIA)
Incident
Interrogatories
Jurisdiction
Licensure
Litigation
Misdemeanor
National Practitioner Data Bank
Negligence
Plaintiff
Privacy Act of 1974
Privacy rule
Privilege
Privileging process
Probate court
Prosecutor
Request for production
Restitution
Standard of care
Standards for Privacy of Individually Identifiable Health Information (privacy rule)
Statutory law
Tort
Trier of fact

Introduction

U.S. law consists of three systems: a legal system, a regulatory system, and an administrative system.

The legal system affords a person or entity the opportunity to bring a civil action against another person or entity believed to have caused harm to the original party. One can bring a wide variety of actions against an alleged wrongdoer. The legal system also affords a person or entity charged with criminal wrongdoing the opportunity to defend against those charges. In this way, the legal system provides an avenue for a wronged party to seek retribution or to clear one's name.

The regulatory system controls many activities related to industry, in particular the health care industry. These regulations exist as statutes or are derived from statutes. Often, the statutes set forth what action is required and the regulations set forth how that action is to be met.

The administrative system controls governmental administrative operations. Federal and state administrative agencies enact regulations that have the same force of law as statutory laws do.

Understanding the American legal, regulatory, and administrative systems gives an HIM professional an appreciation for the health record as a legal document and its role in each of these systems.

This chapter explains the basic workings of the U.S. legal system. It then identifies the legal principles that apply to healthcare in general and to health information administration in particular. Further, the chapter describes how health records are used in legal proceedings. Finally, medical staff appointments and privileging are discussed.

Because it is impossible to summarize the infinite variety of state laws, California statutes and codes are used throughout this chapter to provide examples. Health information management professionals must consult their individual state statutes, codes, and regulations for specific applications.

Theory into Practice

The Mid-America Medical Center (MAMC) is a 1000-bed acute care hospital located somewhere in America. A Level III trauma center, it has several critical care units for adults, children, and newborns; and offers a full range of services including heart, kidney, lung, and liver transplantation. In addition, it is a teaching hospital with residency programs in hand surgery, thoracic surgery, cardiac surgery, nephrology, internal medicine, orthopedics, general surgery, obstetrics, and pediatrics. MAMC has 7,500 staff members and 3,500 medical staff members, of which 2,500 are considered active.

The center's medical staff office (MSO) maintains all demographic, credentialing, and privileging information for every medical staff member in a physician database. The demographic information includes items such as the physician's name, educational degrees, professional license num-

ber, liability insurance information, office address, and office phone numbers, including any office facsimile (fax) numbers. The MSO has a policy and procedure for immediately updating the physician database upon receiving notice of any changed demographic information.

MAMC maintains all dictated medical reports, radiologic reports, lab/pathology reports, emergency department notes, and workers' compensation reports in a clinical data repository (CDR). It also maintains radiologic, EEG, and EKG images in digital format in the CDR. As the documents become available from medical transcription, they are uploaded immediately to the CDR and made available to caregivers. Further, as the digital images become available through the testing equipment, they likewise are uploaded immediately to the CDR and made available to caregivers. Upon loading into the CDR, the documents are autofaxed to the dictating physician and the attending physician, if different. The fax numbers in the CDR are updated on a real-time basis from the MSO physician database. This means that as soon as an MSO staff member updates the physician database with a new fax number, the number is automatically and immediately uploaded to the CDR for autofaxing purposes. The autofax cover sheet contains a confidentiality statement instructing anyone receiving material erroneously to call the director of the Health Information Management (HIM) Department.

On December 28, a situation arose regarding the physician database. The HIM director received a call from an individual who had never been a patient at MAMC, but who indicated that he had just received a faxed history and physical, operative report, and discharge summary on a patient with AIDS and related conditions. It turned out that the patient was the mayor of the city where MAMC was located. He had acquired AIDS from a blood transfusion three years earlier during open-heart surgery. The HIM director instructed the caller to mail the documents to her attention by certified mail, and the caller complied.

However, before mailing the documents, the caller copied them and sold the copies to a local tabloid press. The information in the reports was "revised," and a printed story gave sordid details about how the mayor had acquired AIDS. The mayor called the HIM director in a rage.

The HIM director immediately contacted the risk manager and the chief executive officer (CEO). The HIM director and the risk manager investigated the matter together and ascertained that the dictating physician had notified the MSO of a fax number change on December 21. The MSO staff had not followed policy and procedure for updating this information in the physician database because the fax number was not changed until December 30. Thus, the CDR was not updated and reports continued to be autofaxed to the old fax number. The fax number had actually been valid for the physician until December 27 at midnight. On December 28, the phone company assigned the number to the anonymous caller at his request. The physician database had a feature that allowed entering information such as a fax number and inputting an effective date. On that date, the updated information would automatically be in effect and uploaded to the CDR.

The mayor suffered significant harm from the misleading publication. He filed a lawsuit in the state trial court, suing the hospital, the MSO director, and the MSO data-entry clerk personally for breach of confidentiality. After considerable pretrial discovery was conducted, the case went to trial. The jury found in favor of the mayor against the hospital and the MSO director, stating that MAMC had breached the mayor's confidentiality by failing to follow its own policies and procedures for protecting his confidential health information. The jury based its decision on the tort of negligence.

The jury also found the data-entry clerk personally liable because pretrial discovery showed that she was angry with the mayor and intentionally had not entered the physician's updated fax number into the physician database. She knew that any reports regarding the mayor would continue to be automatically faxed to the old fax number, which her boyfriend had taken as of December 28. She shared in the money received from the tabloid for the information. The jury's decision was based on the intentional tort of invasion of privacy.

The hospital's liability insurance paid the $4 million judgment on behalf of the hospital and the MSO director. However, the hospital's insurance company refused to pay the $8 million judgment against the data-entry clerk, reasoning that her actions were intentional and not within her scope of work.

Introduction to the Legal System

To understand the role of the health information management (HIM) professional in protecting confidential health information, one must first understand the principles for disclosing such information. Because many disclosures are made as part of litigation, the HIM professional should be very comfortable with the legal process. The following sections present the basics about the sources of American law, the court system, the legal process, and the types of actions encountered in healthcare.

Sources of Law

The laws that rule all Americans' lives come from many sources, which results in a rather complex legal system. Overall, there is a federal legal system and fifty individual state legal systems. Regardless of the source, the legal system is a process through which members of society settle disputes. These disputes may be between private individuals and organizations or between either of these entities and the government, whether state, federal, or both.

Constitutional Law

Much of the law governing society is set out in the state and federal constitutions. The Constitution of the United States is the highest law in the land. It takes precedence over all conflicting state and local laws (Lewis 1988; Miller 1986). The Constitution sets up the federal government's general organization and grants powers to it (Lewis and Warden 1988; Miller 1986). It also places limits on what federal and state governments may do (Miller 1986).

Common Law

English common law is the primary source of many legal rules and principles and was based initially on tradition and custom. **Common law,** also known as judge-made or case law, is regularly referred to as unwritten law originating from court decisions where no applicable statute exists. Before the Norman Conquest in 1066, English laws primarily addressed violent crimes. After the Norman Conquest, a legal system began to develop that included a jury hearing complaints from the king's subjects (Pozgar 1999).

After the American Revolution, most states adopted all or part of the existing English common-law principles (Pozgar 1999). Louisiana is the exception because it bases much of its common law on the French (Code Civil des Francais) and Spanish civil law systems (Pozgar 1999). States continue to add to the body of common law through court decisions when existing statutes do not apply to the issue before the court. Because each state adds to the common laws within its boundaries, there is no body of national common law. Thus, a common-law principle established in one state has no effect in another state unless the second state also adopts the principle. Even then, it may be applied differently. After a court establishes a new common-law principle, that principle becomes a precedent for future cases addressing the same issues. The body of common law in a given state is continually evolving through being modified, overturned, abrogated, or created by court decisions.

Statutory Law

By contrast, **statutory** (legislative) **law** is written law established by federal and state legislatures. It may be amended, repealed, or expanded by the legislature. Statutory law also may be upheld or found by a court to violate or conflict with the state or federal constitution. Further, it may be found to conflict with a different state law or a federal law.

Courts also interpret laws in terms of how they apply to a given situation. Thus, statutory law may be "revised" by a court ruling in terms of its constitutionality and applicability. However, if the legislature disagrees with the court's interpretation, it can revise the statute. The legislative revision then becomes the law versus the court's revision based on its interpretation.

Administrative Law

Legislative bodies cannot possibly enact all necessary laws. Therefore, federal and state legislatures delegate this authority to appropriate federal and state administrative agencies. These agencies are thus empowered to enact regulations that have the same force of law that statutory law has (Lewis

1988). Accordingly, **administrative law** is the branch of law that controls governmental administrative operations (Pozgar 1999). Such administrative agencies include licensing and accrediting bodies, Medicare, Medicaid, and other federal government programs.

Federal administrative agencies function under the Administrative Procedures Act, which sets forth the following (Pozgar 1999):

- The procedures under which administrative agencies must operate
- The procedural responsibilities and authority of administrative agencies
- The legal remedies for individuals or entities harmed by agency actions

The act also requires administrative agencies to make agency rules, opinions, orders, records, and proceedings available to the public (Administrative Procedures Act, §552). The publication used to accomplish this is the ***Federal Register,*** which is issued by the U. S. Government Printing Office every business day. The information that agencies must publish includes their organizational structure and the location where the public can obtain information; formal and informal procedures; forms and instructions for using them; general statement of applicability; and amendments, revisions, or repeals of any of this information. Furthermore, agencies must publish proposed administrative rules and revisions to existing rules for which they are delegated the responsibility and authority to enact. These rules and/or revisions are published in the *Federal Register* for a comment period during which the public is invited to make comments on the applicability and impact of the proposed rules on a given person, group of persons, or entity. After the comment period ends, the applicable administrative agency may or may not finalize the rules. If the rules are finalized, the notice and the final rule are published in the *Federal Register*. The final rule is also codified and published in the appropriate code section. The Medicare Conditions of Participation regulations and the Administrative Simplification rules of the Health Insurance Portability and Accountability Act of 1996 (HIPAA) are examples of healthcare-related information published in the *Federal Register.*

The Court System

The American court system is composed of the state court system and the federal court system. The nature of the issue determines which court has **jurisdiction** over the issue. Matters in the following three categories belong only to federal courts: federal crimes, such as racketeering and bank robbery; constitutional issues; and civil actions where the parties do not live in the same state. Other civil and criminal cases are heard in the state court system.

State Court System

Typically, the state court system has several levels. In most states, the lowest level consists of specialty courts or local courts that hear cases involving traffic, small claims, and justice of the peace issues. State civil and criminal cases are initiated in the lower-level trial courts. These are referred to differently in different states, for example, as district trial courts or superior courts. Some trial courts at this level have limited jurisdiction and include courts such as probate, family, juvenile, surrogate, and criminal. Other trial courts at this same level have general jurisdiction. Decisions made in a court at this level may be appealed to the intermediate courts, usually known as the state appeals courts. State appellate courts have general jurisdiction.

State legal systems also include a court at the highest level. These courts also may be known by different terms in different states, for example, as the state supreme court. These higher courts also have general jurisdiction over all cases heard in the state's trial and appellate courts. Decisions coming from the state supreme court become the law of that state unless state legislative statute revisions override the court's decision.

Federal Court System

The trial-level federal courts are the U.S. district courts (trial courts). Included in the district courts are the bankruptcy courts. Special federal courts have jurisdiction over specific matters. These courts include the tax courts (hear cases involving federal tax matters only), the U. S. customs courts (review administrative decisions made by customs officials), the U.S. Court of Military Appeals, and the United States Court of Claims (hears certain claims against the government) (Pozgar 1999). The federal appellate level is composed of the U.S. **courts of appeals,** formerly known as circuit courts. The U.S. Supreme Court is the highest court in the U.S. legal system.

The Legal Process

The HIM professional can better serve patient privacy interests if he or she has an understanding of the legal process. This understanding should cover both the civil and criminal processes, even though healthcare facilities are rarely affected by criminal cases.

Civil Cases

Civil law involves relations between individuals, corporations, government entities, and other organizations. Most actions encountered in the healthcare industry are based in civil law. Typically, the remedy for a civil wrong is monetary in nature but also may include carrying out some action.

The party bringing the action or complaint in a civil case is the **plaintiff.** (In the Theory into Practice section of this chapter, the mayor was the plaintiff.) The plaintiff has the burden of proving the wrong, the harm from the wrong, and the expected **restitution.** The plaintiff presents evidence before a judge or a jury that must be more compelling than that of the opposing side, the **defendant.** The plaintiff or an attorney on the plaintiff's behalf begins the process by filing a complaint in the appropriate court. Hereafter in this discussion, "plaintiff" will refer collectively to the individual or entity bringing the action and that individual or entity's attorney. The plaintiff has a summons, including a copy of the filed complaint, served on the defendant. The defendant or an attorney on the defendant's behalf prepares an answer and files it in the same court where the original complaint was filed. Hereafter in this discussion, "defendant" will refer collectively to the person or entity against whom an action has been brought and that person or entity's attorney.

A case may be resolved in four ways:

1. A judge can dismiss the plaintiff's case for technical reasons. The plaintiff's complaint may not set forth a claim recognized by law or the summons and complaint may not have been properly served on the defendant. The judge may permit the plaintiff to correct the error and refile the case.
2. If the defendant fails to file a timely answer, the court will find in favor of the plaintiff and enter a **default judgment** against the defendant.
3. A case may be settled out of court before it goes to trial or at any time during trial before the **trier of fact** (judge or jury) announces the decision.
4. Presuming the case does not settle or is not dismissed or no default judgment is entered, the case will proceed with pretrial activities by both plaintiff and defendant. Such activities, known as pretrial discovery, include, but are not limited to, the taking of witnesses' depositions, the serving of **interrogatories** and **requests for production** on the opposing party, and the issuing of subpoenas, as necessary. The court (the judge assigned to the case) will set dates according to the law by which pretrial discovery must be completed. The case will then proceed to trial before a trier of fact. Upon conclusion of the trial, a verdict is given and a judgment rendered against the party determined to be wholly or partially liable for the harm. In civil cases, a verdict is more commonly referred to as being "liable" or "not liable." Either party may appeal the judgment to an appellate court and possibly even to the supreme court in that state.

Criminal Cases

Criminal law addresses crimes that are wrongful acts against public health, safety, and welfare. Criminal laws also include punishment for those persons violating the law. Criminal cases involve matters between individuals or groups of people and the government. Crimes are either a felony or a misdemeanor as defined by state statute. **Felonies** are the more serious crimes and include, among others, murder, larceny (thefts of large amounts of money), assault, and rape. **Misdemeanors** are lesser offenses and include disorderly conduct, thefts of small amounts of property, and breaking into an automobile.

When the police learn that a crime has or may have been committed, they begin an investigation. The state initiates a criminal action against those individuals or groups of people it believes have committed the crime based on the police investigation. When the **prosecutor** (prosecuting attorney), also known as the district or state attorney (depending on the state), determines sufficient evidence is present, he or she files charges against the defendant on behalf of the state. The court arraigns the charged person on the prosecutor's charge, and the prosecutor prosecutes those charges against the defendant. The prosecutor has the burden of proving the charges against the defendant. The type of crime and state laws determine the burden of proof the prosecuting attorney must meet—clear and convincing or beyond a reasonable doubt.

The accused defendant may plead guilty and be sentenced to probation or imprisonment and/or pay a fine. He or she also may plead not guilty, which results in a trial. Upon conclusion of the trial, a verdict of either guilty or not guilty is rendered. When a defendant is found not guilty, the charges are dismissed. A defendant found to be guilty is sentenced to probation or imprisonment and/or to pay a fine. Both the defendant who pleads guilty and the defendant who is found guilty at trial can proceed through the appellate process.

Actions Encountered in Healthcare

The healthcare industry is involved most often in civil cases and less often in criminal cases. Because government is increasing its investigations into and prosecutions for healthcare fraud and refusing to treat patients based on financial status, the healthcare industry will be faced with more criminal cases. However, this chapter focuses on civil actions. The types of civil legal actions that most typically affect the healthcare industry are torts and contracts. Many claims founded in tort and contract law are resolved without appearing in court.

Torts

A **tort** is an action brought when one party believes that another party caused harm through wrongful conduct and the party bringing the action seeks compensation for that harm. In addition to compensation, a second reason for bringing a tort action is to discourage the wrongdoer from committing further wrongful acts. Three categories of tort liability exist: negligent torts, intentional torts, and liability without fault (Pozgar 1999). Most healthcare incidents arise in the negligent tort category. (In the Theory into Practice section, the hospital and the MSO director were held liable for a negligent tort whereas the data-entry clerk was held liable for an intentional tort.)

Negligent Torts

Negligence results when a person does not act the way a reasonably prudent person would act under the same circumstances. A negligent tort may result from a person committing an act or failing to act as a reasonably prudent person would or would not in the given circumstances (Pozgar 1999). Typically, negligence is careless conduct that is outside the generally accepted standard of care. **Standard of care** is defined as what an individual is expected to do or not do in a given situation. Standards of care are established in a variety of ways: by professional associations, by statute or regulation, or by practice. Such standards are considered to represent expected behavior unless a court finds differently. Therefore, standards also are established by case law. Regulations are different from standards in that they have the force of law, whereas those standards established by other than statute or regulation do not.

In healthcare, the standard of care is the exercise of reasonable care by healthcare professionals having similar training and experience in the same or similar communities. However, some courts may define standards of care on a national level versus a community level.

Negligence also may occur in cases where an individual has evaluated the alternatives and the consequences of those alternatives and has exercised his or her best possible judgment. Thus, a person can be found negligent when he or she has failed to guard against a risk that he or she knew could happen. Furthermore, negligence can occur in circumstances where it is known, or should have been known, that a particular behavior would place others in unreasonable danger.

Negligence can further be categorized in other ways. For example, negligent torts can be categorized as (Pozgar 1999, p. 30):

- Mal*feasance:* The execution of an unlawful or improper act
- Mis*feasance:* The improper performance of an act
- Non*feasance:* The failure to act when there is a duty to act
- Mal*practice:* Negligence or carelessness of a professional person, such as a nurse, pharmacist, physician, or accountant
- *Criminal negligence:* Reckless disregard for the safety of another; the willful indifference to an injury that could follow an act

Applying this categorization to the Theory into Practice section, the hospital and MSO director would have committed nonfeasance and the data-entry clerk would have committed either malfeasance or misfeasance.

Further, negligence can be categorized by the degree of wrongdoing. *Ordinary negligence* is failure to do what a reasonably prudent person would do, or doing something that a reasonably prudent person would not do, in the same circumstances (Pozgar 1999). *Gross negligence* is intentionally omitting care that would be proper or providing care that would be substandard or improper (Pozgar 1999).

To recover damages caused by negligence, the plaintiff must show that all four elements of negligence are present:

1. There must be a *duty to use due care.* For this element to be present, a physician–patient, nurse–patient, therapist–patient, or other caregiver–patient relationship must exist at the time of the alleged wrongful act.

2. There must have been a *breach of the duty to use due care.* The plaintiff must present evidence that the defendant acted unreasonably under the circumstances.

3. The plaintiff must have *suffered an injury* as a result of the defendant's negligent act or failure to act. Injury includes not only physical harm, but also mental suffering and the invasion of a patient's rights and privacy.

4. The plaintiff must show that the defendant's conduct *caused* the plaintiff's harm. As an example, varying from a recognized procedure is insufficient to justify the plaintiff's recovery of damages. The plaintiff must show that the variance was unreasonable and that it caused the harm (Pozgar 1999).

Applying these elements to the Theory into Practice section, the MSO director had a *duty* to ensure that MSO staff followed policy. The director *breached that duty* by not ensuring that the data-entry clerk entered new physician information into the physician database immediately upon receipt. The mayor suffered *actual harm* from an inappropriate disclosure of confidential health information. And failure to change the fax number in the physician database *caused* the harm that the mayor suffered.

When no statute exists to define what is reasonable, the trier of fact determines what a reasonably prudent person would have done. The reasonably prudent person is generally defined in terms of the hypothetical person that a community believes exhibits ideal behavior in a given situation (Pozgar 1999). The trier of fact considers characteristics such as age, sex, training, education, mental capacity, physical condition, and knowledge in defining the reasonably prudent person. After the behavior of a reasonably prudent person is defined for the given circumstances, the trier of fact compares the defendant's behavior against that definition. If the defendant's behavior meets or exceeds the definition, no negligence has occurred. On the other hand, if the defendant's behavior does not meet the reasonably prudent person standard, negligence has occurred. In such a case, the trier of fact must determine whether:

- The harm that would result from the failure to meet the reasonably prudent standard could have been foreseen.
- The negligent act caused harm to the plaintiff.

Intentional Torts

Although most torts experienced in healthcare are based on negligence, an occasional intentional tort is committed that includes actions such as assault, battery, libel, slander, invasion of privacy, and false imprisonment. The element of intent is the difference between the intentional tort and the negligent tort. *Intent* means the person committed an act knowing that harm would likely occur. A quick review of several intentional torts gives the reader an idea of how they may occur in a healthcare setting. (In the Theory into Practice section, the data-entry clerk's conscious and intentional decision not to enter the new fax number into the physician database in a timely manner is an example of an intentional tort.)

Assault is a deliberate threat that is combined with the apparent ability to cause physical harm to another person (Pozgar 1999, p. 47). For example, a large male nurse in the emergency department tells a frail elderly woman that he will break her arm if she does not do what he tells her to do. His comment is a deliberate threat, and his size gives him the apparent ability to harm the woman. *Battery* is intentionally touching another person's body without that person's consent (Pozgar 1999, p. 47). In healthcare, laws regarding battery are especially important because of the requirement for consent for medical and surgical procedures. The hospital and the treating healthcare professionals may be held liable for harm caused by the lack of a proper patient consent. Even if the outcome of the procedure benefits the patient, touching the patient without proper consent may make the healthcare professional liable for battery.

False imprisonment is another intentional tort. A healthcare provider's efforts to prevent a patient from leaving a hospital may result in false imprisonment. This is not the case when a patient with a contagious disease or a mentally ill patient is compelled to remain in the hospital (Pozgar 1999). There are limits to the actions staff can take to compel a patient not to leave a hospital. For example, restraints can be used on mentally ill patients only to the extent necessary to protect them from harming themselves or others (Pozgar 1999). The patient's insistence on leaving the facility should be documented in his or her health record, and the patient should be asked to sign a discharge against medical advice form that releases the facility from responsibility. When excessive force is used to restrain a patient, the healthcare provider may be held liable for both false imprisonment and battery (Pozgar 1999).

Defamation of character is a communication about someone to a person other than the person defamed that tends to injure that person's reputation (Pozgar 1999). *Libel* is the written form of defamation, and *slander* is the spoken form. To recover in an action for libel, the plaintiff is *not* required to prove actual damage or harm. Yet, in cases involving slander, the plaintiff *must* show actual damage or harm to be compensated for that harm. However, there are four recognized exceptions to the general rule for slander. To recover damages for slander, the plaintiff is *not* required to show proof of actual harm to his or her reputation when the defendant allegedly performs one of the following acts (Pozgar 1999):

- Accuses the plaintiff of a crime
- Accuses the plaintiff of having a loathsome disease
- Uses words that affect the plaintiff's profession or business
- Calls a woman unchaste

With regard to the third exception, the professional is not required to show actual harm because slanderous references to a person's professional capacity are presumed to be damaging to that person's professional reputation (Pozgar 1999). As to the first and second exceptions, healthcare professionals are protected against claims of libel when complying with the law regarding the reporting of communicable diseases that the patient may consider loathsome (Pozgar 1999).

The defendant (the one being accused of defaming another) has two defenses available to a defamation action. The person making an alleged defamatory statement that harms another's reputation will not be liable for that statement if he or she shows that the statement was true (Pozgar 1999). The person making the allegedly defamatory communication can claim privilege if he or she is making the communication:

- In good faith
- On the proper occasion
- In the proper manner
- To persons who have a legitimate reason to receive the information

The defense of privilege is based on the person making the communication being charged with a higher duty. For example, in one case, a director of nurses wrote a letter to a nurse's professional registry stating that the hospital wanted to discontinue a particular nurse's services because narcotics were disappearing whenever the nurse was on duty (*Judge v. Rockford Memorial Hospital* 1958). The court found the communication to be privileged because the director of nurses had a legal duty to make the communication in the interests of society. Thus, the court denied the nurse's claim for damages.

Fraud is a prevalent concern in today's healthcare environment. It is defined as "a willful and intended misrepresentation that could cause harm or loss to a person or property" (Pozgar 1999, p. 57). For example, physicians can be held liable for fraud if they claim that a particular procedure will cure a patient's ailment when they know it will not.

Invasion of privacy is another major concern in healthcare. A person's right to privacy is the right to be left alone, to be free from unwarranted publicity and exposure to public view, and to live one's life without having one's name, picture, or private affairs made public against one's will (Pozgar 1999). The courts recognize that absolute privacy is not a reality in the medical or nursing care of a patient (Pozgar 1999). However, they hold healthcare providers liable for negligent disregard for patient right of privacy, especially when patients cannot adequately protect themselves because of unconsciousness or immobility (Pozgar 1999). One major actionable offense of concern in healthcare involving invasion of privacy is the release of health information without patient authorization in circumstances when it is required.

The *willful infliction of mental distress* for which a person can be held liable includes mental suffering resulting from such things as despair, shame, grief, and public humiliation (Pozgar 1999). If the plaintiff shows that the defendant (the one inflicting the distress) intended to cause mental distress and knew that his or her actions would do so, the plaintiff can recover damages even in the absence of physical harm (Pozgar 1999). To provide this relief, the courts are struggling with the fine line between negligent and intentional infliction of mental distress.

Liability without Fault

The principle of liability without fault, strict liability, is most prevalent in product liability wherein a manufacturer, seller, or supplier of equipment or supplies is liable to one with whom there is no contractual relationship and who suffers harm from the equipment or supplies. Recovery for product liability under the principle of strict liability can occur even in the absence of negligence by the manufacturer. The plaintiff must only show that he or she was injured while using the product in a proper manner. Recovery for product liability also can be based on negligence for an unsafe product design or breach of warranty. The plaintiff can recover from the manufacturer for injury caused by a device or supply even though he or she did not purchase the device or supply. The concepts of care, negligence, and ignorance are not defenses for the defendant.

Contract

Although on a more limited basis than torts, contracts are the second basis for a claim arising in the healthcare industry. A contract is an agreement, written or oral, that, in most cases, is legally enforceable through the legal system. Illegal contracts include those that courts view as against public policy, specific oral contracts that the law requires be in writing, and unconscionable contracts (Miller 1986). Unconscionable contracts are contracts that courts view as coercive (Miller 1986). **Contract law** is based on common law. However, some states have replaced common law with statutory law or administrative agency regulations. In those states, the statutes or administrative regulations control. A hospital contract with patients that attempts to limit their right to sue could be a contract to which a court would apply the unconscionable concept and hold the hospital liable. Another example of how contractual issues affect healthcare is a contract for services between the hospital and a contracting physician or physician group, such as pathologists, radiologists, anesthesiologists, and emergency medicine physicians.

The elements of a contract must be stated clearly and specifically. A contract cannot exist unless all the following elements exist. There must be an *agreement* between two or more persons or entities. The agreement must include a valid offer and acceptance—mutual consent. It must be supported by legal and bargained-for *consideration*. (Consideration is an inducement that may take the form of cause, reason, motive, or price.) The parties to a contract must have the *capacity* to enter into the agreement such as being a competent adult, being of age of majority, and not being incapacitated by medication or alcohol. Finally, the contract must be for a *legal purpose*. It must not be against public policy (Clarkson et al. 1992).

A contract action arises when one party claims that the other party has failed to meet an obligation set forth in the contract. Another way to state this is that the other party has breached the contract. The resolution available is either compensation (money damages) or performance of the obligation. The defendant can raise a variety of defenses to a breach of contract action including waiver and default, conduct of the parties, and waiving rights under the agreement.

Check Your Understanding 10.1

Instructions: Answer the following questions on a separate piece of paper.

1. What are the four sources of laws governing Americans?
2. What types of cases are typically heard in the federal court system?
3. Which court is the court of last resort in the U.S. legal system?
4. What are the two most common types of civil cases experienced in healthcare?
5. In a court, who is the trier of fact?
6. What is the result of a trial called?
7. What types of cases are covered by criminal laws?
8. What are the roles of prosecutor and defendant in a criminal case? Who has the burden of proof?
9. What are the possible outcomes of a criminal case?
10. What are the three categories of tort liability? From which category do most healthcare cases arise?
11. What is the definition of a negligent tort?
12. What are the four elements of negligence?
13. How might false imprisonment occur in a hospital?
14. What defenses are available to a defendant accused of defamation of character?
15. Privacy is difficult to achieve in a healthcare setting. However, courts will hold healthcare providers liable for what type of invasion of privacy?
16. What is a contract?
17. What action must occur for a contract case to arise?

Legal Aspects of Health Information Administration

The field of health information administration must recognize and treat the patient's health record as a legal document. Thus, the HIM professional must have an understanding of all the regulations and statutes that affect the creation and maintenance of the health record.

Form and Content of the Health Record

The health record is a complete, accurate, and current report of the medical history, condition, and treatment that a particular patient receives during an encounter with a healthcare provider. In a hospital, the encounter may be on either an inpatient or outpatient basis. Moreover, it may be defined as one episode of treatment or an accumulation of all episodes of treatment in any setting that is part of the organization.

The health record is composed of two sections: the demographic section and the clinical section. Most of the information in the *demographic section* is collected at the time of admission for treatment. It includes, among other items, the patient's name, sex, age, insurance information, and the person to contact in case of emergency. This information may be added to and changed throughout the patient's medical encounter. The *clinical section* comprises the patient's complaint, history of present illness, medical history, family history, social history, continuing documentation of ongoing medical care, report of diagnostic tests, X-ray reports, surgery and other procedure reports, consultant reports, nursing documentation, various graphs, and the final diagnoses. In some states, licensure regulations may specify the contents. In other states, the health record content is defined in broader terms.

Accrediting agency regulations or standards are one source for identifying health record content (see appendix C). The Joint Commission on Accreditation of Healthcare Organizations (JCAHO), the American Osteopathic Association (AOA), and other accrediting organizations include some level of requirements for health record content. The Medicare program's Conditions of Participation also include minimum requirements for health record content. However, some sources of regulations for health record content are more prescriptive than others are. For example, some regulations give details on the information to be retained, others specify the broad categories of information required, and still others state simply that the health record must be accurate, adequate, or complete. The HIM professional must be aware of the most stringent definition of the health record content to which his or her particular organization is subject.

It is also important to heed requirements of agencies and laws that regulate hospitals and have an impact on the process of creating and maintaining health records. The healthcare industry in general and hospitals in particular are extensively regulated by all levels of the government and by numerous agencies within each level of government. Additionally, they are regulated for accreditation purposes by nongovernment agencies. Quite often, hospitals are faced with conflicting requirements because of this multiple-regulation environment.

Regulatory (Licensure) Agencies

State legislatures have granted authority to a state administrative agency to:

- Develop standards hospitals must meet
- Issue licenses to those hospitals that meet the standards
- Monitor continuing compliance with the standards
- Penalize hospitals that violate the standards (Miller 1986)

Licensure is issued for the organization as a whole. It addresses policies and procedures, staffing, and hospital building integrity among many other facets of the organization. Some states require additional licenses for specific services in the hospital. For example, laboratory, radiology, renal dialysis, and substance abuse services may require separate licenses in addition to the facility license. Additional state and federal laws apply to the use of drugs and medical devices.

Hospitals cannot operate without a license. Those that violate the standards may lose their licenses or be penalized in other ways, such as fines. Thus, licensure is government regulation that is mandatory for hospitals.

Some states require separate licensure for hospital pharmacies whereas other states regulate hospital pharmacies through the general state hospital licensing system. Typically, the laws address dispensing and administering drugs to patients in the hospital and dispensing take-home drugs through an inpatient or outpatient hospital visit. Additionally, some regulations require sufficient staff members for the hospital pharmacy based on the hospital's size and scope of services.

Accreditation Agencies

Accreditation is offered through nongovernment agencies. One of the most important accrediting agencies for hospitals is the JCAHO. The JCAHO develops standards that hospitals must meet to be accredited. The healthcare organization applies to the JCAHO to be accredited, pays an accreditation fee, and submits to an extensive survey to ensure compliance with the JCAHO's published standards. Similarly, the AOA accredits osteopathic hospitals and functions in much the way that the JCAHO does.

Accreditation is considered voluntary and is not legally mandated, but it is very important to healthcare organizations. Some states accept JCAHO or AOA accreditation as a basis for partial or full licensure with limited or no additional survey by the state agency.

Whereas the JCAHO and the AOA focus on the entire hospital, other accrediting agencies focus on specific services of the hospital. For example, there is a separate accreditation process for laboratory and radiology services in addition to that of the JCAHO and the AOA.

The federal Medicare program also sets standards for hospitals in its Conditions of Participation. Although these are government regulations, participation in the Medicare program is considered voluntary. However, few, if any, hospitals elect not to participate in this program. Thus, a hospital must comply with these standards to receive payment from the Medicare program for covered services provided to Medicare beneficiaries. The Medicare program also recognizes organizations that have JCAHO or AOA accreditation as meeting most of the Conditions of Participation. A hospital would typically undergo an additional survey only if a special Medicare inspection finds noncompliance.

Statutory and Regulatory Law

The Comprehensive Drug Abuse Prevention and Control Act of 1970, the **Controlled Substances Act,** controls the use of narcotics, depressants, stimulants, and hallucinogens (Miller

1986; Pozgar 1999). Because this act affects the dispensing and administering of these specific drug categories, the pharmacy staff must be well versed in this law and how it interacts with state licensing and regulatory laws and accrediting standards. The controlled substances are classified into *schedules* according to the extent to which they are controlled. Schedule I drugs are subject to the tightest controls; schedule I–IV drugs may be dispensed only upon a practitioner's lawful order.

In the outpatient environment, a prescription that meets the requirements of the law is required. In the inpatient setting, an order in the health record satisfies this requirement for a lawful order. The practitioner signing the prescription or the order in the health record must be registered with the Drug Enforcement Administration (DEA) of the Department of Justice. State law determines which professionals may be classified as practitioners for this purpose.

The Food and Drug Administration (FDA) is a federal agency that controls the testing, manufacture, labeling, and distribution of drugs, cosmetics, and devices (Pozgar 1999). The FDA's regulations are published in the Food, Drug and Cosmetic Act, which includes the Medical Device Amendments of 1976. The drugs and devices covered under these regulations are very broad, thus requiring practitioners to review applicable statutes, regulations, and other reference materials to determine whether a particular drug or device is covered. Pursuant to this legislation, human blood is considered a drug (Miller 1986). Most equipment and supplies used in a hospital for patient care are regulated as devices under these regulations.

Public Health Reporting Requirements

Some health records contain information that is important to the public welfare. Such information must be reported to the state's public health service to ensure public safety. Public health reporting requirements vary from state to state. However, most, if not all, states have enacted laws requiring a healthcare provider to disclose health information for public health purposes. The type of health information that must be reported varies according to the government agency to which the information is being reported and the purpose of the reporting. Common examples of health information that is required to be released for public health purposes include:

- Vital statistics (births and deaths)
- Communicable diseases
- Child, adult, and elder abuse
- Wounds from stabs and gunshots
- Conditions affecting the ability to drive

The person(s) complying with reporting statutes are not considered to be making an unauthorized disclosure. Although the release of certain health information is statutorily mandated in these and other circumstances, a court may view the release to the wrong agency as a breach of confidentiality (Miller 1986). The **Standards for Privacy of**

Individually Identifiable Health Information (privacy rule) were promulgated and issued in December 2000 by the Department of Health and Human Services (HHS) pursuant to the Health Insurance Portability and Accountability Act of 1996 (HIPAA). These rules will become effective April 14, 2003, and will provide that the hospital or healthcare provider may disclose confidential health information to:

- Public health authority authorized to collect or receive information for preventing or controlling disease, injury, or disability
- Public health authority or other government authority authorized to receive reports of child abuse or neglect
- A person subject to the FDA
- A person who may have been exposed to a communicable disease or may be at risk of contracting or spreading a disease or condition (if the entity is authorized to notify such person [the privacy rule, section 164.512(b) (1)(i)-(iii)])

Retention of the Health Record

The health record serves several purposes and must be retained to meet those purposes. These purposes include:

- Most important, the health record is a tool used in the patient's continuing medical care because it provides complete and accurate information about the patient's previous care and treatment.
- It serves as a means of communication among the patient's healthcare providers—physicians, nurses, therapists, pharmacists, and technologists.
- It is used by the patient's healthcare providers as a basis for planning his or her course of treatment. Further, the health record may be reviewed after care is rendered to evaluate the quality of the care.
- It is a source of information for statistical, research, and educational purposes.
- It also serves as a source of billing and financial reports and information because billing records must be supported by the documentation in the health record.
- It is valuable in legal proceedings because it reflects the care given—the treatments, procedures, and medications that the patient received.

These varied purposes influence how long health records must be kept, or their retention period. Federal and state laws determine retention periods. In the absence of such laws, administrative policy and medical practice may determine them (Davis and McConnell 1997). For those periods determined by state law, the state defines what the minimum retention period will be. Some states are more specific than others are. For example, some states base the retention period, at least partially, on the statute of limitations for bringing a legal action. These regulations also may address standards for completing, maintaining, handling, signing, and filing health records. Specific retention requirements may be required for particular parts of the health record (for example, X rays) and may be based on patient type (for example, minors, mentally ill, deceased) (Davis and McConnell 1997).

The HIM professional must be aware of the retention statutes and retention periods in his or her state of employment. In some cases, the organization may define a retention period that is longer than the period required by the state. The organization should base its retention policy on hospital and medical needs and any applicable statutes and regulations.

Retention also includes the safeguarding of the confidential information maintained in health records. All hospital staff members with the right to access a patient's health record have an obligation to protect the confidentiality of patient information.

Ownership and Control of the Health Record

Patients often believe they own their health record. The HIM professional must be able to advise the patient regarding the actual ownership and control of the physical health record and the patient's rights to the information contained in it.

Ownership of the Physical Record

The physical health record is considered the property of the healthcare provider, the physician, or the hospital that maintains it because it is the healthcare provider's business record (Miller 1986). Yet, the patient and others have an interest in the information contained within the health record. The patient and others, as authorized, have the right to access the information but do not have a right to possess the physical record (Miller 1986).

Release and Disclosure of Patient Information

Unless otherwise specified by standards and regulations, most states permit competent patients to authorize their own access to their own health records. Some states also define the process patients are to follow to obtain access to their own record (Miller 1986). Additionally, some courts have recognized the common-law right of patients to access their own health records (Miller 1986). Further, some states have determined that releasing specific information, such as psychiatric information, to the patient would be against the patient's best interest (Miller 1986). Under these circumstances, courts have held that such information should be made available to the patient's representative, who may be another healthcare professional acting on the patient's behalf (Miller 1986).

Further, many third parties have a legitimate need to access the confidential health information contained in a health record. These include insurance companies for payment purposes, insurance companies when coverage has been applied for, government agencies to determine eligibility for healthcare programs, and so on. The patient controls access by all third parties except those to which the hospital is required to report information of a medical nature or as otherwise provided by law.

Elements of Patient Authorization

The **privacy rule** gives very detailed specifications for patient authorization to release confidential health information [Section 164.508(c)-(f)]. The authorization must include a specific description of the information to be used or disclosed. In addition, the name or other specific identification of the person(s) authorized to request and receive the requested information must be included. Further, the authorization must include the expiration date or event that relates to the individual or the purpose of the use or disclosure. The patient must be given the right to revoke the authorization in writing, the exceptions to this right, and a description of how he or she may revoke it. The authorization also must advise the patient that information released pursuant to the authorization may be subject to redisclosure by the recipient and no longer protected. Finally, the patient must sign and date the authorization.

If a personal representative signs the authorization, a description of his or her authority to act for the patient must be included in the authorization form. Further, the form must be written in plain language. The patient must be advised that the hospital will not condition treatment, payment, enrollment in a health plan, or eligibility for benefits on his or her providing authorization for the requested information. The authorization must include a description of each purpose for the requested information. Further, the authorization must contain a statement to the effect that the patient may inspect or copy the information and may refuse to sign it. The hospital must disclose to the patient whether the release of the information will result in direct or indirect remuneration to the facility from a third party. If there is remuneration, the authorization must state that such remuneration will result. Also, the patient is entitled to a copy of the signed authorization.

Authorizations for uses and disclosures of health information created for research that includes treatment of the patient must contain additional elements. For example, there must be a description of the extent to which the information will be used or disclosed to carry out treatment, payment, or healthcare operations. The authorization must further include a description of any health information that could be disclosed but will not be disclosed for facility directories or public health purposes. However, the facility may not include a limitation affecting its right to release information required by law.

If the facility has or intends to obtain a general consent or has provided or intends to provide the individual with a notice of privacy practices, the authorization must refer to that consent or notice and state that the statements made are binding.

Pursuant to Section 164.508(b)(2), if any of the following circumstances pertain to the authorization, it is considered "defective":

- The expiration date has passed or the expiration event has occurred.
- The authorization is not completely filled out.
- The authorization has been revoked.

- Any required elements are missing.
- The authorization is combined with any other document to create a "compound authorization" except where permitted.
- The facility knows that material information included in the authorization is false.

The California requirements for a valid patient authorization are fairly typical for such documents and contain many of the requirements addressed above in the privacy rule [California Civil Code Section 56.11(a)-(i)]. It does indicate specifically who can sign an authorization:

- A patient who is a competent adult (18 years old or over)
- A minor who could have consented to the treatment, was self-sufficient, emancipated, married, or in active military duty
- A patient who is seeking treatment for pregnancy, sexual assault/rape, communicable disease, mental health, or drug or alcohol abuse
- The patient's legal representative

For a minor, the legal representative is the parent, guardian, or person *in loco parentis*. For the incompetent adult, the conservator of the person (probate or psychiatric) or the attorney in-fact may serve as the legal representative. The patient's spouse or the person financially responsible for the patient may sign only for the limited purpose of enrolling the patient in a third-party payer plan. For a deceased patient, the beneficiary, legatee under a will or heir under intestacy laws, or the personal representative, executor, or administrator of the patient's estate may sign an authorization for the release of health information.

To be valid, the written authorization must state the limitations, if any, on the types of health information to be disclosed. Further, it must state the specific uses and limitations, if any, on the use of the health information by the recipients.

General Procedures for Release with Patient Authorization

The hospital must have clear policies and procedures for releasing confidential health information with patient authorization. These policies must provide for careful review of each request. They must provide for a careful review of the authorization to ensure that it meets all requirements stated in applicable state and federal statutes and regulations, depending on which requirements are more stringent. As provided in the privacy rule, the procedure must permit the opportunity for the patient to revoke an authorization at any time in writing, except to the extent that the hospital has relied on the authorization and taken action as a result of it [Section 164.508(b)(5)(i)]. It is a good practice to require a patient to sign an authorization for releasing confidential health information to the patient on whom the information is maintained. Finally, all policies and procedures for releasing confidential health information with

patient authorization must follow the guidelines established in the privacy rule discussed below.

General Procedures for Release without Patient Authorization

Although health information can be released without patient authorization in certain circumstances, such requests must be carefully scrutinized. Thus, healthcare facilities also must have clear policies and procedures for releasing confidential health information without patient authorization. Reporting required by statutes, whether federal or state, should be addressed. Information that can be released to the public without patient authorization should be specified. Typical mandatory disclosures that should be addressed in policies and procedures include those under court order and subpoena, whether served by a party to a suit or administrative proceeding, or by a government agency in the course of an investigation. Mandatory release pursuant to orders by a board, commission, or administrative agency engaged in formal adjudication of a dispute should be included in policies and procedures. Further, policies should address releasing health information pursuant to an order by an arbitrator or arbitration panel carrying out arbitration under the law. Also release without patient authorization can occur pursuant to a search warrant. This type of release should be detailed very carefully in policies and procedures. Release of health information in response to requests in workers' compensation cases is controlled by state law and should be included in hospital policies. Finally, policies also must identify the categories of internal staff needing confidential health information to carry out their job duties. Policies should also specify the types of information needed and the reasons for permitting access (Guidance). Policies and procedures should permit the opportunity for the patient to restrict how health information is used and disclosed to carry out treatment, payment, or healthcare operations [privacy rule, Section 164.506(c)(4)(i)]. All policies and procedures for releasing confidential health information without patient authorization must also follow the guidelines set in the privacy rule.

Types of Disclosures

There are numerous types of disclosures of confidential health information both with and without patient authorization. One of the most common and most important disclosures is for direct patient care purposes. Those involved with patient care must have timely access to health information. Some states, such as California, provide a statutory basis for this type disclosure. In California Civil Code Section 56.10(c)(1), information may be disclosed to healthcare providers and professionals, healthcare service plans, contractors, and facilities for the purpose of patient diagnosis or treatment. In emergency situations, California permits disclosure by radio transmission or other means between emergency medical personnel at the scene or in an emergency vehicle and emergency medical personnel at a licensed health facility [California Civil Code Section 56.10(c)(1)].

The privacy rule, in sections 164.506(a)(2)–(4), permits the facility and healthcare providers to use or disclose confidential information for patient treatment when:

- The healthcare provider has an indirect treatment relationship with the individual.
- The healthcare provider creates or receives the health information in the course of providing healthcare to an individual who is an inmate.
- In an emergency treatment situation, the healthcare provider attempts to obtain consent.
- The healthcare provider is required by law to treat the individual and attempts to obtain consent but is unable to do so.
- The healthcare provider attempts to obtain consent from the patient but is unable to do so because of substantial communication barriers and the provider determines, in the exercise of professional judgment, that the patient's consent to receive treatment is clearly inferred from the circumstances and thus documents the attempt to obtain the consent and the reason why it was not obtained.

Another important disclosure is for payment purposes. Again, using California as an example, the statutes permit disclosure of confidential health information to an insurer, employer, government authority, or any other person or entity responsible for paying for healthcare services rendered to the patient [California Civil Code §56.10(c)(2)]. This disclosure is limited to that information necessary to determine who is responsible for payment and for payment to be made. The California statute also permits the disclosure of health information to another healthcare provider, as necessary, to assist the other provider in obtaining payment for healthcare services rendered to the patient. Further, information may be disclosed to any person or entity that provides billing, claims management, medical data processing, or other administrative services for healthcare providers [California Civil Code §56.10(c)(3)]. The privacy rule permits the healthcare provider to use or disclose health information for payment purposes [Section 164.506(a)(1)].

One activity that is important to a hospital is quality monitoring. Quality monitoring is a standard healthcare operation and does not require patient authorization to use confidential health information. States such as California may statutorily provide for this disclosure of confidential health information. California's statutes specifically provide that information may be disclosed to a variety of entities reviewing the competence or qualifications of healthcare professionals or reviewing healthcare services with respect to medical necessity, level of care, quality of care, or justification of charges. Per California Civil Code Section 56.10(c)(4), these include:

- Organized committees and agents of professional societies or of medical staffs
- Professional standards review organizations

- Independent medical review organizations and their selected reviewers
- Utilization and quality control peer review organizations (now called quality improvement organizations) as established by Congress in Public Law 97-248 in 1982
- Contractors or persons or organizations insuring, responsible for, or defending professional liability that a provider may incur

Again, the privacy rule permits the use of confidential information to carry out healthcare operations [Section 164.506(a)(1)].

Many organizations participate in educational activities for their medical staff members and their clinical and non-clinical staff members. Some also participate in formalized training programs for physicians, nurses, and allied health professionals. All of these trainees require some level of access to confidential health information as part of their training. However, such access should be on a need-to-know basis. Typically, such use of confidential information does not require patient authorization.

Pursuant to Section 164.508(a)(2), the privacy rule addresses psychotherapy notes as a special circumstance. It states that the healthcare facility must obtain authorization for any use or disclosure of psychotherapy notes, except:

- To carry out treatment, payment, or healthcare operations
- To use or disclose in training programs in which students, trainees, or practitioners in mental health learn under supervision to practice or improve their skills in group, joint, family, or individual counseling

Research is another activity for which confidential health information is important. Hospital policy often requires that researchers' access to health information be documented as bona fide research. Such documentation may be provided through a recognized Institutional Review Board's approval of the research. California specifically addresses the use of health information for research purposes [California Civil Code §56.10(c)(7)]. Under the California statute, information may be disclosed to public agencies, clinical investigators, healthcare research organizations, and accredited public or private nonprofit educational or healthcare institutions for bona fide research purposes. The statute attempts to protect this information by stating that no information disclosed for research purposes is to be further disclosed by the recipient in any way that would identity the patient.

Many other states and the federal government have established regulations for the protection of human subjects, including protecting confidential information (Miller 1986). Any use of confidential health information for research purposes must comply with all such regulations including those set forth in the privacy rule. Under the privacy rule in Section 164.512(i), researchers may use or disclose health information, as necessary, to prepare a research protocol or for research purposes. This section also provides that researchers may use or disclose health information for the purpose of research on such information for decedents. The facility that creates confidential health information for research that includes treatment of the patient must obtain an authorization for the use or disclosure of that information.

Because health records are considered hospital business records, the information in them has many administrative uses. Hospital professional, technical, and administrative staff should have access to these records on a need-to-know basis. Administrative uses include, but are not limited to, auditing, billing, filing, replying to inquiries, and defending litigation (Miller 1986). As noted above, the privacy rule permits the facility to use or disclose health information for purposes of payment and healthcare operations [Section 164.506(a)].

Law enforcement agencies and officers may have a need to access health information. Issues surrounding whether law enforcement has the right to confidential health information without patient authorization usually arise when treatment and procedures are performed at the request of a law enforcement officer. The answer revolves on whether the request is (1) for a procedure merely to gather evidence, thus to the benefit of the law enforcement agency; or (2) to treat the patient for a condition, illness, or injury, thus to the benefit of the patient. For example, police officers may request hospital staff to perform a visual examination of an arrestee to determine whether he or she is under the influence of drugs. This is primarily for the benefit of the law enforcement officer, and the information probably may be released. By contrast, if the law enforcement officer requests treatment for an injury to the arrestee, such as a broken leg, the arrestee would benefit. Under these circumstances, the information regarding the treatment would most likely be considered confidential and not subject to disclosure without at least the patient's (arrestee's) authorization.

Under California criminal statutes, health records may only be disclosed to a state law enforcement official or agency by patient authorization, court order, or search warrant (California Penal Code Section 1543). Records in a sealed envelope addressed to the court may be given to law enforcement officials for delivery to the court. This is not considered a direct disclosure to the law enforcement officer.

Pursuant to the privacy rule in Section 164.512(f), the hospital may disclose health information to law enforcement officials without authorization for law enforcement purposes when one of the following conditions is met:

- The disclosure is required by law, including laws that require the reporting of certain types of wounds or other physical injuries.
- The disclosure is made in compliance with a court order, court-ordered warrant, subpoena, summons, or grand jury subpoena.

- The disclosure is made in response to an administrative request, that is, a subpoena or summons, a civil demand or an authorized investigative demand, or a similar process authorized under law.
- The purpose of the request is to identify or locate a suspect, fugitive, material witness, or missing person.
- The disclosure is made in response to a law enforcement official's request for such information about an individual who is, or is suspected to be, a victim of a crime.
- The purpose of the disclosure is to alert law enforcement of the suspicion that a patient's death may have resulted from criminal conduct.
- The hospital believes the health information is evidence of criminal conduct that occurred on its premises.

When providing healthcare in an emergency situation other than on the hospital's premises, the provider may disclose health information to law enforcement officials when it appears necessary to alert law enforcement to any of the following:

- Commission and nature of a crime
- Location of the crime or of the victim(s)
- Identity, description, and location of the perpetrator of the crime [the privacy rule, Section 164.512(f)(6)]

Another piece of federal legislation addressing a patient's right to privacy is the **Privacy Act of 1974.** This act gives individuals some control over the information collected about them by the federal government (AHIMA 2001a). Under this act, people have the right to:

- Learn what information has been collected about them
- View and have a copy of that information
- Maintain limited control over the disclosure of that information to other persons or entities (AHIMA 2001a)

This act also applies to federal government healthcare organizations such as the Veterans Health Administration (VHA) and Indian Health Services and to record systems operated pursuant to a contract with a federal government agency (AHIMA 2001a).

The healthcare provider also may release information to law enforcement if he or she believes the medical emergency is the result of abuse, neglect, or domestic violence of the individual in need of emergency healthcare.

As discussed earlier, patients are entitled to view and receive copies of their own health records. Although care should be taken in releasing all health information to a patient, particular care should be taken in releasing specialized information such as information related to mental health, drug and alcohol abuse, and sexually transmitted diseases. Federal and some state statutes address some or all of these types of specialized information. The privacy rule in Section 164.524(a)(1) provides the patient's right of access to inspect and obtain a copy of health information, except for psychotherapy notes and information compiled in reasonable anticipation of, or for use in, a civil, criminal, or administrative action or proceeding.

In Section 164.524(a)(2), the privacy rule gives the facility the opportunity to deny a patient's access to his or her health information without providing the patient the opportunity to have the denial reviewed when, among other circumstances, (1) the confidential health information is excluded from the right of access and (2) the health information was obtained from someone other than a healthcare provider under a promise of confidentiality.

Further, under the privacy rule, the hospital may deny access for other reasons, provided the patient is given a right to have such denials reviewed by a licensed healthcare professional designated by the hospital to act as a reviewing official and who did not participate in the original decision to deny. This reviewer must provide or deny access [Section 164.524(a)(3)].

The requirement for patient authorization typically extends to a request by a patient's family members, including the spouse. The physician may discuss general information about the patient's condition with family members without authorization unless the patient has instructed otherwise. If the patient is incapacitated, the physician and other caregivers may discuss health information and treatment plans with the next of kin or the patient's representative, however that is defined by a given state, to the extent necessary to make medical decisions on the incapacitated patient's behalf. The privacy rule permits the hospital to disclose to a family member, other relative, close personal friend, or any person identified by the patient health information directly relevant to that person's involvement in the patient's care or payment for healthcare [Section 164.510(b)(1)(i)]. Further, the hospital may use or disclose health information to notify or assist in notifying (identifying or locating) a family member, a personal representative, or some other person responsible for the individual's care, location, general condition, or death [Section 164.510(b)(1)(ii)].

Members of the news media are entitled to very limited health information about a patient. Unless otherwise authorized by the patient, the healthcare organization may only release information stating his or her general condition in terms of good, fair, or poor. No information may be released that reveals the patient's diagnosis. Further, only information may be released on those patients that the news media identifies by name.

Disclosing confidential health information in compliance with the legal process is typically provided for statutorily. Under the privacy rule in Section 164.512(e)(i)–(iv), a hospital may disclose health information in the course of any judicial or administrative proceeding in response to any of the following:

- Court or administrative tribunal order if the hospital discloses only the health information expressly authorized by such order

- Subpoena, discovery request, or other lawful process not accompanied by a court or administrative tribunal order if the hospital receives satisfactory assurance that reasonable efforts have been taken to give notice of the request to the person who is the subject of the requested information or to secure a qualified protective order that meets specific requirements

A hospital may disclose health information in response to lawful process without receiving the above-discussed satisfactory assurance when it makes reasonable efforts to provide notice to the individual or to seek a qualified protective order [Section 164.512(e)(vi)].

Use of the health record in legal proceedings is specifically discussed below.

Confidential health information may be disclosed in a number of circumstances. Statutes in some states covering workers' compensation cases permit the release of health information without patient authorization, but some states require patient authorization or a subpoena from an administrative agency or court for release. Some state courts have ruled that by filing a workers' compensation claim, the claimant is waiving the right to confidentiality of relevant health information (Miller 1986). It is important to be familiar with a particular state's laws before releasing any health information in workers' compensation cases. The privacy rule provides the hospital may disclose health information as authorized by, and to the extent necessary to comply with, laws relating to workers' compensation or other programs, established by law, to provide benefits for work-related injuries or illness without regard to fault [Section 164.512(l)].

Further, the **Freedom of Information Act** (FOIA) is a federal law through which individuals can seek access to information without the authorization of the person to whom the information applies. This act applies only to federal agencies. The Veterans Administration and Defense Department hospital systems are subject to this act, but few other hospitals are. The only protection of health information held by federal agencies exists when disclosure would "constitute a clearly unwarranted invasion of personal privacy" (Miller 1986).

A question that often arises is whether information should be released to a patient's employer. Under California Civil Code §56.10(c)(8), for example, health information created as a result of employment-related healthcare services pursuant to a specific written request and at the expense of the employer may be released to the employer provided that the information:

- Is relevant to a lawsuit, arbitration, grievance, or other claim to which employer and employee are parties and in which the employee has placed at issue his or her medical history
- Describes functional limitations of the patient that may entitle the patient to a leave from work for medical

reasons or limit the patient's fitness to perform his or her present employment, provided that no statement of medical cause is included in the information disclosed

Again, the privacy rule addresses such a release of health information in Section 164.512(b)(i)(v). The hospital may release information to an employer when one of the following conditions is met:

- The care provider is a member of the employer's workforce or provides healthcare to the patient at the employer's request.
- The care relates to a medical surveillance of the workplace or to a work-related illness or injury.
- The information that is disclosed consists of findings concerning a work-related illness or injury or a workplace-related medical surveillance.
- The employer needs the findings to comply with its obligations under federal and state laws.

The privacy rule also requires the hospital to provide written notice to the individual that health information relating to the workplace medical surveillance and work-related illnesses and injuries will be disclosed to the employer.

State statutes address the extent to which confidential health information relevant to the patient's condition, care, and treatment may be disclosed to a probate court investigator. For example, under California law, such information may be disclosed to a **probate court** investigator who is determining the need for an initial conservatorship or continuation of an existing conservatorship. This information may be released without patient authorization when the patient is unable to give authorization. The same standard applies to the release of information to a probate court investigator, probation officer, or domestic relations investigator engaged in determining the need for an initial guardianship or continuation of an existing guardianship [California Civil Code Section 56.10(c)(12)].

Health information may be disclosed to an organ procurement organization or a tissue bank processing the tissue of a decedent for transplantation into the body of another person. This only applies with respect to the donating decedent for the purpose of aiding the transplant [California Civil Code Section 56.10(c)(13)]. Section 164.512(h) of the privacy rule provides that a hospital may disclose health information to organ procurement organizations.

California specifically permits a private or public body responsible for licensing or accrediting the provider of healthcare to access confidential health information [California Civil Code §56.10(c)(5)]. However, this statute further specifies that no patient-identifying health information may be removed from the premises except as expressly permitted or required elsewhere by law. Under the privacy rule, the hospital may disclose confidential health information to an oversight agency responsible for activities such as audits; civil, administrative, or criminal investigations, proceedings, or

actions; inspections; licensure or disciplinary actions; or other activities necessary for appropriate oversight of any of the following entities:

- The healthcare system
- Government benefit programs for which health information is relevant to beneficiary eligibility
- Entities subject to government regulatory programs for which information is necessary for determining compliance with program standards
- Entities subject to civil rights laws for which health information is necessary for determining compliance [Section 164.412(d)]

In some cases, there is a common-law duty to disclose health information, for example, to warn persons of the presence of contagious disease. There is also a duty to warn an individual against whom the patient has made a credible threat to harm (*Tarasoff v. Board of Regents* 1976). In another case, a physician failed to warn his patient that she had contracted HIV through a blood transfusion. As a result, the hospital and the physician were sued three years later when the patient's sexual partner was exposed to the virus. The court held that the hospital was liable for the physician's failure to warn (Kadzielski and Hercz 2001; *Reisner v. Regents of the University of California* 1995). These cases should not be confused. *Reisner* involved the failure to warn a patient of a serious condition whereas *Tarasoff* involved the failure to warn a third party about potential harm from his patient.

Because most states have statutes that address many of the above circumstances, the HIM professional must be familiar with such statutes and regulations that permit or preclude disclosure of health information with or without patient authorization.

Redisclosure Issues

Redisclosure of health information is a significant concern to the healthcare industry. As such, the HIM professional must be alerted to state and federal statutes addressing this issue. As stated earlier, California, for example, permits the hospital to disclose information to any person or entity providing billing, claims management, medical data processing, or other administrative services for the hospital [California Civil Code §56.10(c)(3)]. However, the California statute specifically states that the recipient of such information may not redisclose it in any manner that would violate the statute. Further, California Civil Code §56.10(c)(5) provides that information used for licensing purposes may not be redisclosed by the recipient. A consent obtained by a hospital pursuant to the privacy rule in Section 164.506(a)(5) does not permit another hospital, healthcare provider, or clearinghouse to use or disclose information. However, the authorization content required in the privacy rule in Section 164.508(c)(i) must include a statement that the information disclosed pursuant to the authorization may be disclosed by the recipient and thus is no longer protected.

Legal Issues in Health Information Management 211

Legal Liability for Unauthorized Disclosure

Individuals are personally liable for their own acts of unauthorized disclosure of confidential health information. The individual's liability is based on fault because he or she did something wrong or failed to do something he or she should have done. Employers also may be held liable for any job-related acts of their employees or agents. It must be distinguished that the hospital is not liable for a breach of confidentiality by the members of its medical staff because they are not employees or agents of the hospital (Miller 1986). However, the organization may be liable for the consequences of any unauthorized disclosure, whether by employees, agents, or medical staff members, because of the breach of its duty to maintain information confidential (Miller 1986). The injured person benefits from these concepts of fault because he or she can sue the employer, the employee, or both.

Unauthorized release by various healthcare professionals also may be addressed in professional licensing and certifying laws or regulations. These provisions subject the professional to potential discipline by the licensing or certifying agency for breach of confidentiality because it is considered unprofessional conduct.

Statutory Provisions Mandating Privacy

There are many sources of the statutes mandating privacy of confidential health information. Some of these are discussed below.

Constitution

There is no right to privacy specifically stated in the U.S. Constitution. However, in 1965, the Supreme Court recognized the constitutional right of privacy in *Griswold v. Connecticut.* In this case, the court ruled that "the right to privacy limits governmental authority to regulate contraception, abortion, and other decisions affecting reproduction" (Miller 1986, pp. 6–7). Some states also have recognized the right to privacy in their state constitutions (California Constitution, Article 1 Declaration of Rights, Section 1; Arizona Constitution, 8 Right to privacy; Florida Constitution, Article I, Section 23, Right of privacy).

Federal Legislation

Despite the need for patient privacy, healthcare providers disclose health information to subsequent healthcare providers to the extent necessary to ensure continuity of patient care (AHIMA 2001b). Federal legislation that specifically provides for such disclosures includes, but is not limited to:

- The Medicare Conditions of Participation for Hospitals
- Conditions of Participation for Clinics, Rehabilitation Agencies, and Public Health Agencies as Providers of Outpatient Physical Therapy and Speech-Language Pathology
- Conditions of Participation for Home Health Agencies
- Confidentiality of Alcohol and Drug Abuse Patient Records

As to privacy rights, the Conditions of Participation for Hospitals rule states that hospitals must have procedures to protect the confidentiality of patient records (AHIMA 2001a). Under this rule, hospitals must protect records against unauthorized access and alteration. Further, original records may be removed from the facility only in accordance with federal and state laws (AHIMA 2001a).

The Conditions of Participation for Clinics, Rehabilitation Agencies, and Public Health Agencies as Providers of Outpatient Physical Therapy and Speech-Language Pathology regulations permit the physician to provide medical information to the receiving facility (AHIMA 2001b).

The Conditions of Participation for Home Health Agencies rule also requires facilities to have written policies and procedures to safeguard health information against loss or unauthorized use (AHIMA 2001a). Furthermore, the Requirements for States and Long-Term Care Facilities give the resident or his or her legal representative the right to access information about the resident. Additionally, these regulations give the resident the right to personal privacy and confidentiality of personal and clinical records (AHIMA 2001a).

The Confidentiality of Alcohol and Drug Abuse Patient Records rule is a federal rule that applies to information created for patients treated in a federally assisted drug or alcohol abuse program (AHIMA 2001a). This rule specifically protects the identity, diagnosis, prognosis, or treatment of these patients (AHIMA 2001a). The rule also specifies the circumstances under which information can be released without patient authorization and requires that language prohibiting redisclosure be attached to all released information (AHIMA 2001a).

The privacy rule is the most comprehensive federal rule to date that specifically sets forth standards for the privacy of individually identifiable health information.

HIPAA Privacy Provisions

As stated earlier, HHS promulgated the privacy rule pursuant to the Health Insurance Portability and Accountability Act (HIPAA). The privacy rule creates national standards to protect health information maintained by health plans, healthcare clearinghouses, and providers who transmit certain financial and administrative transactions electronically (AHIMA 2001a). In addition to the specific provisions discussed above regarding the release of information, the privacy rule requires that a notice of the organization's information practices be given to all patients. Patients have a right to know about the possible disclosures of health information that the facility may make, their rights regarding controlling these disclosures, and the facility's legal duties regarding health information [privacy rule, Section 164.520(a)]. The privacy rule gives the patient the right to request amendment of his or her health information [privacy rule, Section 164.526(a)]. It also sets forth a protocol for using protected health information for marketing and fundraising [privacy rule, Sections 164.514(e) and (f)]. One of the most striking features of this legislation is found in Section 164.528(I)] wherein it "establishes an individual's right to obtain an accounting of disclosures of his or her health information" (AHIMA 2001a).

Check Your Understanding 10.2

Instructions: Answer the following questions on a separate piece of paper.

1. What are the two sections of a health record? What type of information is contained in each section?

2. What is the primary difference between licensure and accreditation of healthcare organizations?

3. What are some common types of information that must be reported for public health purposes?

4. What, if any, circumstances might make a healthcare provider liable for breach of confidentiality when reporting public health information?

5. What national patient information confidentiality standards were promulgated in December 2000?

6. Who owns the physical health record?

7. In the HIPAA privacy rules, who may sign an authorization for the release of information?

8. Using California as an example, who may serve as a legal representative for a minor patient?

9. Using California as an example, who may serve as a legal representative for an incompetent adult?

10. What is one deciding factor affecting the release of health information to law enforcement agencies or officers?

11. Discuss the circumstances listed in the privacy rule under which a facility may deny a patient's request for access to his or her own health information without providing the patient the opportunity to have the denial reviewed.

12. Explain the access to health information available to the news media.

13. Under what circumstances does the privacy rule permit release of health information to a patient's employer?

14. On what basis can a plaintiff claim unauthorized disclosure of health information against a hospital?

15. What was the holding regarding privacy issued by the court in *Griswold v. Connecticut*?

16. What is the most striking feature of the privacy rule?

Use of Health Records in Litigation

This section discusses how the health record is used in **litigation.** The health record serves as documentation of care provided when the patient alleges wrongdoing against the hospital and healthcare providers in a lawsuit.

Admissibility of the Health Record

The health record may be valuable evidence in a legal proceeding. To be admissible, the court must be confident that the information contained in the record is complete, accurate, and timely (recorded at the time the event occurred). Further, the court must accept that the information was recorded as the result of treatment, not in anticipation of a legal proceed-

ing. Medical witnesses may refer to the health record to refresh their recollection. The custodian of records, typically the health information manager, may be called as a witness to identify the record as the one subpoenaed. He or she also may be called to testify as to policies and procedures relevant to the following:

- Creation of the record
- Maintenance of the record to prevent it from being altered
- Maintenance of the record to prevent it from being accessed without proper authorization

The actual admissibility as evidence depends on the facts and circumstances of the case and the applicable state and federal rules of evidence.

Privileges

Professional relationships between the patient and specific groups of caregivers further affect use of the record and its contents as evidence. These relationships are referred to as **privileges.** The information exchanged between patient and caregiver pursuant to a privilege is a confidential communication that the patient anticipates will be held confidential. Because there was no provision for privileges under common law, they only exist in states where the legislature or state courts have expressly provided for this relationship (Miller 1986).

One such widely recognized privilege is the physician–patient privilege. This privilege provides that the physician is not permitted to testify as a witness about certain information gained as a result of this relationship. However, this privilege applies only when a physician is being compelled to testify in a trial, a deposition, or an administrative proceeding. Further, it only applies when there is a true relationship between patient and physician. There are three methods by which a physician–patient relationship can be established by the physician:

- Contracting to care for a particular group of people and having a person from that group seek care
- Entering into an express contract with the patient or patient's representative for care
- Engaging in conduct from which a patient can imply that a contract exists (Miller 1986)

The information included in the physician–patient privilege is insulated from the discovery process when there is no patient authorization, waiver, or an overriding law or public policy (Davis and McConnell 1997). The physician–patient relationship usually does not apply to court-ordered examinations or other examinations completed on behalf of other third parties, such as insurance companies (Miller 1986). Depending on the state, similar privileges exist between psychotherapist and patient (California Evidence Code Section 1014), sexual assault victim and counselor (California Evidence Code Section 1035.8), and domestic violence victim and counselor (California Evidence Code Section 1037).

In states where these professional relationships are recognized, they apply when the caregiver is being compelled to testify as a witness concerning information obtained as a result of the relationship. However, these privileges do not preclude the caregiver from making reports as required by law.

Patient's Waiver of Privilege

The patient may release the caregiver from the privileges discussed through words or actions. This release is known as a *waiver of the privilege.* For example, a patient who placed his or her treatment at issue in a trial could not continue to claim a privilege to protect the information. The caregiver could then be compelled to testify regarding the information previously considered confidential.

Government's Right of Access to Health Records

The government, whether federal or state, has the right to access health information with and without patient authorization in certain circumstances. Healthcare providers must sign an agreement with the HHS to receive payments for care provided to patients covered under the Medicare program (Miller 1986). Medicaid is a joint federal and state program to provide medical care to individuals unable to pay for care. Healthcare providers apply to the responsible state agency for a contract with the state to provide services to Medicaid recipients in return for payment for services provided (Miller 1986). Both HHS and the state Medicaid agency may request information from the health record to support the healthcare provider's bill submitted for payment. By signing up with Medicare or Medicaid, the patient gives permission for the healthcare provider to release confidential health information to the appropriate agency without further authorization.

The government also may require access to health information for other investigative purposes such as pursuant to the federal fraud and abuse statutes that require information-sharing arrangements to be undertaken in an arm's-length transaction and pursuant to a written agreement (Kadzielski and Kogan 1997). Another important federal statute for which the government may need access to health information as part of an investigation is the Emergency Medical Treatment and Active Labor Act. This act involves the transfer of uninsured individuals from one hospital emergency department to another for financial reasons (Kadzielski and Kogan 1997).

Check Your Understanding 10.3

Instructions: Answer the following questions on a separate piece of paper.

1. What are the three methods by which a physician–patient privilege may be created?
2. What actions or requirements can release the care provider from the applicable privilege?
3. Give two examples of government access to health information with or without patient authorization.

Medical Staff Appointments, Privileges, and Peer Review

Patients expect the physicians who treat them in hospitals to have been evaluated for competency in their selected area of medical practice. Patients expect to receive treatment at or above the acceptable standard of care. Hospitals use the medical staff appointment process to accomplish this evaluation.

Duty to Use Reasonable Care in Granting Staff Appointments

The hospital governing board typically is composed of members from the community and sometimes includes medical staff members. This body has final responsibility for the operation of the hospital. Because of its responsibility for managing the hospital and upholding a satisfactory standard of care, it has the legal duty to select medical staff members. The governing board must use reasonable care in approving a physician's application to be a staff member and grant clinical privileges before the physician can treat patients in the hospital. Typically, after the physician is granted initial medical staff membership, he or she must reapply for membership and privileging every year or every two years. It must be noted that medical staff members are not employees or agents of the hospital. However, even though they are independent of the hospital, they are accountable individually and collectively to the board for the quality of care they provide.

In *Darling v. Charleston Community Memorial Hospital,* the court specifically held that the governing board has the "duty to establish mechanisms for the medical staff to evaluate, counsel, and when necessary, take action against an unreasonable risk of harm to a patient arising from the patient's treatment by a personal physician" (Pozgar 1999, p. 198). Further, the *Darling* court held that based on the hospital's obligation to select high-quality physicians to be medical staff members, the hospital may be held liable for a patient's injury caused by a physician who does not meet those standards but was given medical staff membership and privileges.

Darling involved an eighteen-year-old college football player studying to be a teacher and coach who suffered a broken leg during a game. He was taken to a small, accredited community hospital where the only physician on duty in the emergency department was a general practitioner who had not treated a severe leg fracture for three years. The physician ordered X rays that revealed fractures of both bones in the lower leg. The physician reduced the fractures and applied a full-leg plaster cast. The patient complained of pain, and the physician split the cast and visited the patient while in the hospital. However, the physician never called in a specialist because he thought it unnecessary. Two weeks later, the plaintiff was transferred to a larger hospital where he was treated by an orthopedic surgeon. The specialist found dead tissue in the fractured leg and removed dead tissue several times over the next two months. The specialist was unable to save the leg and amputated it eight inches below the knee.

The plaintiff's father rejected any settlement and filed suit against the hospital and the physician. The physician was eventually able to settle, but the case against the hospital continued to trial. A judgment was returned against the hospital and upheld in the Illinois Supreme Court.

The hospital's governing board relies on the medical staff structure to conduct the actual evaluation of physicians applying for medical staff membership and to make recommendations regarding a physician's suitability for membership. The mechanisms for selecting medical staff members pursuant to *Darling* and applicable state statutes indicate that peer review is the best system for monitoring physicians. Many states provide that peer review must be conducted in a reasonable and fair manner.

The Credentialing Process

The **credentialing process** is the screening process through which the medical staff evaluates a physician's application for medical staff membership. In this process, the medical staff validates a physician's credentials: medical education, including medical school, residencies, postdoctoral studies, and fellowships; license to practice; and medical practice experience. This process also includes reviewing and evaluating professional references and professional society membership.

One major step taken in this process is searching the **National Practitioner Data Bank** regarding judgments and settlements of claims of professional negligence regardless of the amount (Cohen 2001). Further, this process includes validating the physician's liability insurance. Having a license to practice medicine in a particular state does not give the physician the right to be a medical staff member in any hospital. It is merely one required criterion. Credentialing criteria should be related directly to patient care and based on objective factors such as education and experience (Kadzielski and Kogan 1997). In other words, no criteria for credentialing can be established that could result in discrimination on any basis (Miller 1986).

Federal laws in the form of the Medicare Conditions of Participation for Hospitals and for Long-Term Care Facilities set forth requirements for medical staff credentialing (Kadzielski and Kogan 1997). Most states typically address medical staff appointments in licensing statutes or statutes specific for the selection of medical staff members or both. Further accreditation standards, such as those published by the JCAHO, require physician credentialing prior to granting privileges to practice in a healthcare facility (Kadzielski and Hercz 2001).

The Privileging Process

After a physician is determined to meet the criteria to be a medical staff member in a particular hospital, the medical staff must evaluate his or her quality of medical practice and determine the services he or she is qualified to provide. This is known as the **privileging process.** A physician's clinical privileges determine the services he or she may provide, such as what operations he or she may perform. The medical staff must have established a written definition of what it means to be granted the privilege to provide a particular service. Some hospitals grant privileges for specific procedures; others grant privileges for categories of procedures. Still other hospitals grant privileges based on levels of care, such as privileges to care for critical care patients. Another approach is to grant privileges by medical specialty based on the services a particular specialty is permitted to perform.

To evaluate a physician for privileging, a hospital may require the physician to obtain a consultation before performing specific procedures. Physicians also may be required to have operative procedures proctored by an observing or assisting physician. A hospital may require certification beyond a license, such as board certification in a particular medical specialty, before granting privileges for a physician to practice in that specialty.

As stated above, physicians must periodically reapply for medical staff membership. As part of the reapplication process, the physician's privileges are reevaluated using established criteria. For example, the hospital may review, among other factors, the physician's blood usage patterns, lengths of stay, infection rates, complications and complication rates, health record documentation, and closed malpractice claims (Kurdwanowski and Schaedler 1997). The hospital also may review the outcome of focused studies, such as those discussed below. Moreover, physicians who have gained additional training since the last appointment may seek privileges not previously held. For any new privileges requested, the physician may be required to have consultation or proctoring performed. Most state statutes and the federal Health Care Quality Improvement Act require this collection and review of information in the privileging process (Davis and McConnell 1997).

The goal of privileging is to ensure that all physicians have the requisite training and experience to perform the requested services.

Accessibility and Confidentiality of Credentialing Files

In this discussion, *credentialing* is used as a collective term for the credentialing and privileging processes. In looking at accessibility to credentialing files, third parties, such as the JCAHO, and state and federal regulatory organizations, may review credentialing files as part of their accrediting and licensing functions. Some states statutorily protect credentialing files from discovery in legal proceedings. However, when a plaintiff alleges negligent credentialing against a hospital, whether the protection will hold up comes into question (Davis and McConnell 1997). In such a circumstance, the hospital finds itself in the situation of attempting to protect the information in the credentialing files while at the same time needing those very same documents to defend it (Davis and McConnell 1997). Although statutory protections may be in place for credentialing information, facilities should be reluctant to share such information "because any subsequent disclosure of peer review committee records could result in a loss of this protection" (Kadzielski and Kogan 1997, p. 98).

Confidentiality of Quality Improvement and Concurrent Review Activities

As noted above, outcomes of focused studies may be used to evaluate a physician's application for continued medical staff membership and privileges to practice. These studies are usually conducted as part of the hospital's quality improvement (QI) activities. Quality improvement is the process of improving medical care and potentially decreasing healthcare costs. (This process is discussed more fully in chapter 22.)

QI activities can be carried out on a concurrent review basis or on a retrospective basis. *Concurrent review* consists of evaluating medical care as it is being given. Concurrent review activities can be carried out in a variety of ways. One method is through case management (utilization review) that focuses on the appropriateness of the admission, the level of care, and length of stay (Miller 1986).

Retrospective review occurs after patient discharge. This review may take the form of a focused study based on a pattern of questionable care identified during concurrent review or other retrospective review activities. The questionable care leading to a focused study may be care provided by any caregiver, including physicians. The hospital has a responsibility to address any problems discovered through either review process. If a physician was the caregiver providing the questionable care and it is determined that he or she is not practicing at the expected level of care, an educational session may be conducted with the particular physician. If warranted, more stringent steps, such as suspension of the physician's medical staff privileges or medical staff membership termination, may be taken.

These review activities involve collecting outcomes and performance data on how a physician performed as a physician and may affect continued medical staff membership. Accordingly, the review files are considered confidential. Many states have statutes that specifically provide confidentiality to these types of files (Davis and McConnell 1997). California Evidence Code Section 1157 is an example of such a law. This statute protects from discovery the proceedings and records of organized peer review committees responsible for the evaluation and improvement of the quality of care.

Check Your Understanding 10.4

Instructions: Answer the following questions on a separate piece of paper.

1. After he or she completes an application, what is the process for granting a physician membership on the hospital medical staff?

2. What documentation is typically reviewed for the initial membership appointment?

3. What activities may a medical staff require of a physician in order to grant the physician privileges to provide a specific service?

4. As part of the reapplication process, what additional factors may the medical staff review in the privileges component?

5. Discuss circumstances in which confidential information in a credentialing file may be accessed.

6. Distinguish between concurrent and retrospective review activities.

7. What is the basis for maintaining quality improvement and concurrent review files confidential?

Other Liability Issues

Hospitals and other healthcare providers face other liability issues. Hospital staff members have a duty to advise an appropriate member of administration when they become aware of any action or failure to act that is below the standard of care. The standard of care does not just apply to direct patient care. By definition, it applies to the safeguarding of patient's personal belongings whether or not placed in the direct care of the facility. For patient and staff personal belongings not placed in the direct care of the facility, the facility must have policies and procedures for addressing questions of theft by staff.

The standard of care also applies to the physical safety of the premises for patients, staff, visitors, vendors, and members of the general public who come onto the premises. Physical safety means being free from physical defects in buildings and grounds and from being harmed by patients, nonstaff members, or staff members. Moreover, the hospital must address staff safety as it relates to treatment of violent or uncontrolled patients, for example, the patient who is under the influence of drugs or alcohol being treated in the emergency department.

Incident Reports

A happening that is inconsistent with the standard of care is generally defined as an **incident.** As discussed above, standards of care are not related only to direct patient care. Therefore, incidents do not relate only to patient care. Individual(s) witnessing or involved in an incident should complete an incident report as soon as possible after the incident as a way to capture the details of what happened. The incident report is one tool staff can use to report unusual incidents to administration. Data should be collected from the incident reports and analyzed to determine whether trends are developing.

Because incident reports contain facts, hospitals strive to protect their confidentiality. In some states, incident reports are protected under statutes protecting QI studies and activities (Davis and McConnell 1997; Vanagunas 1997). They also may be protected under the attorney–client privilege and the attorney work product doctrines (Vanagunas 1997; Youngblood 1990). Protection under both these doctrines may be based on whether the primary purpose of the incident report is to provide information to the hospital's attorney or liability insurer (Youngblood 1990).

To further ensure incident report confidentiality, no copies should be made and the original must not be filed in the health record nor removed from the files in the department responsible for maintaining them, typically risk management or quality improvement (Vanagunas 1997). Also no reference to the completion of an incident report should be made in the health record. Such a reference would likely render the incident report discoverable because it is mentioned in a document that is discoverable in legal proceedings.

Relationship to Risk Manager

The health information manager and the risk manager should work as a team. The risk manager depends on the health information manager to alert him or her to potentially compensible events. These are events that could result in a settlement or judgment against the facility, further resulting in a payout of funds whether through insurance or from facility internal funds. Such events can be identified through coding and abstracting, and various health record review activities conducted by health information department staff. The health information manager also can advise the risk manager when an attorney requests a copy of a health record. The risk manager can then review records identified by any of these methods to determine whether further action is necessary from a risk management standpoint.

Check Your Understanding 10.5

Instructions: Answer the following questions on a separate piece of paper.

1. Define *incident* as it relates to the healthcare environment.
2. Discuss at least two doctrines under which incident reports may be protected.
3. Why should incident reports be protected?
4. Discuss the relationship between the health information manager and the risk manager.

Real-World Case

Mary Beth Jones, RHIM professional, is the new director of the Health Information Department at a midsized hospital in California. The hospital has its own employment health service that maintains its own computerized employee health record database, and the records are maintained under a separate health record numbering system to the one used for hospital patients. Mary Beth has just determined that hospital managers have access to the database containing the computerized employee health records. Moreover, she has learned that hospital managers are routinely accessing information in the computerized employee health record database without the individual employee's authorization.

Further, Mary Beth has learned that various reports containing confidential health information are routinely printed out of the computerized employee health record database and placed in the applicable employee's personnel file. Often information from these personnel files is sent to subsequent employers.

Adapted from a recent publication on the Internet discussing the subject of employers' rights to obtain health information concerning their employees (Medical Investigations, available at http://smallbiz.hypermart.findlaw.com/employmentbook/HFXHP5_e.html).

Discussion Questions

1. Based on California law, as discussed in this chapter and through your additional Internet research on the particular California statute, is the managers' current practice for accessing employee health information appropriate? Thoroughly support your answer, including the bases on which an employer may have access to employee health information.

2. Based on the privacy rules, is the managers' current practice for accessing employee health information appropriate? Thoroughly support your answer, including the bases on which an employer may have access to employee health information

3. Presuming the managers' current practice is an invasion of privacy, identify and discuss the legal bases on which the employees could initiate a civil case against the hospital.

4. Do you see any problem with the practice of placing confidential employee health information in personnel files? Support your response with information from this chapter.

5. Discuss the duty, if any, the hospital has to its employees with regard to protecting their health information.

6. What actions should Mary Beth recommend be taken to correct the problems presented by the managers' current practices?

7. What actions should Mary Beth recommend be taken to correct the problems presented by the personnel file practices?

Summary

The basic court system is the same from one state to another. However, the HIM professional should become familiar with the differences that do exist for the state in which he or she works. This knowledge gives the HIM professional the ability to communicate effectively with legal counsel regarding health records and policies and procedures affecting health records when the inevitable lawsuit arises.

Knowledge that is more important and valuable to the HIM professional is of the statutes that control the release of confidential health information. These statutes are both federal and state in nature. This area of law is constantly in flux and requires the HIM professional to constantly review the many available resources pertaining to such statutes, including publications and seminars. These resources also address case law that may affect the continuing applicability of state and federal statutes.

Another body of knowledge the HIM professional should develop is a clear understanding of licensure and accreditation standards that affect the creation, completion, maintenance, and protection of health records.

The HIM professional must ensure that policies and procedures are in place and enforced and that they reflect all statutes, regulations, and standards pertaining to health records, particularly those pertaining to the release of confidential information.

Among the many members of the hospital staff with whom the HIM professional works, he or she must have a close relationship with the facility risk manager. The HIM professional can provide the risk manager tremendous assistance in identifying and addressing incidents that may place the facility at risk.

References

Administrative Procedures Act, 5 U.S.C.S. §§500-576 (Law. Co-op. 1989).

American Health Information Management Association. 2001a. Practice Brief: Laws and regulations governing the disclosure of health information. *Journal of the American Health Information Management Association* 72(5):64A–64C.

American Health Information Management Association. 2001b. Practice Brief: Transfer of patient health information across the continuum (updated). *Journal of the American Health Information Management Association* 72(6):64S–64Z.

Arizona Constitution, Section 8 Right to privacy. Available from www.azleg.state.az.us/const/2/8.htm.

California Constitution, Article 1 Declaration of rights, Section 1. Available from www.leginfo.ca.gov/cgi-bin/waisga.

Clarkson, K. W., R. L. Miller, G. A. Jentz, and F. B. Cross. 1992. *West's Business Law.* St. Paul, Minn.: West Publishing Company.

Cohen, M. 2001. Statutes, Standards and Regulations. In *Risk Management Handbook for Health Care Organizations,* third edition, edited by Roberta Carrol. San Francisco: Jossey-Bass.

Darling v. Charleston Community Memorial Hospital, 33 Ill.2d 326, 211 N.E. 2d, 253 (1965).

Davis, K. S., and J. C. McConnell. 1997. Data management. In *Risk Management Handbook for Health Care Organizations,* second edition, edited by Roberta Carrol. Chicago: American Hospital Publishing.

First Guidance on the final privacy rule (2001). Available from www.aspe.hhs.gov/admnsimp.

Florida Constitution, Article I, Section 23, Right of privacy. Available from www.leg.state.fl.us/State.../index.cfm?Mode=Constitution&Submenu=3&Tab=statute.

Griswold v. Connecticut, 381 U.SE. 479 (1965).

Health Care Financing Administration, Department of Health and Human Services. 2000. Conditions of Participation for Home Health Agencies. *Code of Federal Regulations* 42 CFR, Chapter IV, Part 484.

Health Care Financing Administration, Department of Health and Human Services. 2000. Conditions of Participation for Hospitals. *Code of Federal Regulations* 42 CFR, Chapter IV, Part 482.

Health Care Financing Administration, Department of Health and Human Services. 2000. Requirements for States and Long-Term Care Facilities. *Code of Federal Regulations* 42 CFR, Chapter IV, Part 483.

Health Care Financing Administration, Department of Health and Human Services. 2000. Standards for the Privacy of Individually Identifiable Health Information; Final Rule. 45 CFR Parts 160 through 164. *Federal Register* 65 (250) (December 28, 2000). Available from www.aspe://aspe.hhs.gov/admnsimp.

Health Insurance Portability and Accountability Act of 1996. Public Law 104-191.

Joint Commission on Accreditation of Healthcare Organizations. 2000. *Comprehensive Accreditation Manual for Hospitals: The Official Handbook.* Oakbrook Terrace, Ill.: Joint Commission on Accreditation of Healthcare Organizations.

Judge v. Rockford Memorial Hospital, 17 Ill. App. 2d 365, 150 N.E. 2d 202 (1958).

Kadzielski, M. A., and M. G. Hercz. 2001. Physician and allied health professional credentialing. In *Risk Management Handbook for Health Care Organizations,* third edition, edited by Roberta Carroll. San Francisco: Jossey-Bass.

Kadzielski, M. A., and E. I. Kogan. 1997. Physician and allied health professional credentialing. In *Risk Management Handbook for Health Care Organizations,* second edition, edited by Roberta Carroll. Chicago: American Hospital Publishing.

Kurdwanowski, F., and P. A. Schaedler. 1997. Internal and external relationships. In *Risk Management Handbook for Health Care Organizations,* second edition, edited by Roberta Carroll. Chicago: American Hospital Publishing.

Lewis, M. A., and C. D. Warden. 1988. *Law and Ethics in the Medical Office Including Bioethical Issues.* Philadelphia: F. A. Davis Company.

Miller, R. D. 1986. *Problems in Hospital Law.* Rockville, Md.: Aspen Publishers.

Pozgar, G. D. 1999. *Legal Aspects of Health Care Administration.* Gaithersburg, Md.: Aspen Publishers.

Public Health Service, Department of Health and Human Services. 2000. Confidentiality of Alcohol and Drug Abuse Patient Records. *Code of Federal Regulations* 42 CFR, Chapter I, Part 2.

Reisner v. Regents of the University of California, 37 Cal. Rptr2d 518 (1995).

Tarasoff v. Board of Regents, 17 Cal.3d 425, 551 P.2d 334 (Cal. 1976).

U.S. Department of Health and Human Services, Office for Civil Rights. 2001. Standards for Privacy of Individually Identifiable Health Information; Guidance (July 6, 2001).

Vanagunas, A. M. 1997. Systems for risk identification. In *Risk Management Handbook for Health Care Organizations,* second edition, edited by Roberta Carroll. Chicago: American Hospital Publishing.

Youngblood, B. J. 1990. *Essentials of Hospital Risk Management.* Gaithersburg, Md.: Aspen Publishers.

Application Exercises

1. Prepare a plan to analyze all policies and procedures in a health information department relating to maintaining the confidentiality of health information. List the specific steps you will take. Include how you will apply the standards in the privacy rule, JCAHO standards, and any applicable state licensure requirements.

2. Interview a privacy officer in a local hospital. Collect information on the approach being taken to implement the privacy rule. Determine the role the privacy officer expects of the director of the health information department in the implementation process. Be prepared to do an oral presentation in class. At the conclusion of all presentations, be prepared to outline similarities and differences among the privacy officer approaches presented by your classmates. Identify the approach you think would be the best and explain why.

3. Conduct a search using both the Internet and library resources for information on unauthorized release of health information. Attempt to find material that references a case, obtain a copy of it and review it. Be prepared to discuss the facts of the case. Identify the parties (plaintiff and defendant) and the end result of the case.

Review Quiz

Instructions: Choose the best answer for the following questions.

1. ___ Which of the four sources of law derives from the English common law and is also known as judge-made or case law?
   a. Constitutional law
   b. Statutory law
   c. Common law
   d. Administrative law

2. ___ Which of the four sources of law is the highest law of the land?
   a. U.S. Constitution
   b. Laws of the fifty states
   c. Common law
   d. Administrative law

3. ___ The party in a civil case that brings the action and has the burden of proof is the ___ and the party who allegedly committed the wrongdoing is the ___.
   a. Plaintiff
   b. Prosecutor
   c. Defendant

4. ___ In what ways might a civil case be resolved?
   a. Settlement
   b. Judgment
   c. Dismissal
   d. Default judgment
   e. All of the above
   f. None of the above

5. ___ How are standards of care established?
   a. By professional associations
   b. By statute or regulation
   c. By practice
   d. By case law
   e. All of the above
   f. None of the above

6. ___ What is the concept of a reasonably prudent person?
   a. A person who is polite
   b. A person who a community believes exhibits ideal behavior in a given situation
   c. A person who the court believes knows what should or should not be done in a given situation

7. ___ How is the prudent person concept derived for a given situation?
   a. By statute
   b. By the trier of fact
   c. Both of the above
   d. None of the above

8. ___ The difference between a negligent tort and an intentional tort is that the person committing the wrongful act does so knowing that harm will likely occur.
   a. True
   b. False

9. ___ If a person makes a deliberate threat with the apparent ability to cause physical harm (for example, a very large person threatening to hit a much smaller person), the wrongdoer has committed battery against the smaller person.
   a. True
   b. False

10. ___ An individual's liability for unauthorized disclosure of health information will be based on fault.
    a. True
    b. False

11. ___ To be valid, a contract must contain the following four elements: agreement, consideration, capacity, and legal purpose.
    a. True
    b. False

12. ___ Licensure and accrediting agency regulations and the Medicare Conditions of Participation are resources that can be used to determine the required content for health records.
    a. True
    b. False

13. ___ The benefit of accreditation to a hospital is that the Medicare program recognizes organizations having JCAHO and AOA accreditation as meeting most of the Conditions of Participation, which means the hospital does not have to go through a full Medicare survey.
    a. True
    b. False

14. ___ Which of the following are purposes for which health records are retained?
    a. As documentation of continuing medical care
    b. As a communication tool among healthcare providers
    c. As a basis for planning the course of treatment
    d. As a source of information for statistical, research, and educational purposes
    e. As a source of billing and financial reports and information
    f. As evidence in legal cases
    g. All the above
    h. a, c, d, and f only

15. ___ Except as provided by law, who controls access to a patient's health information by third parties such as insurance companies?
    a. The patient
    b. The patient's legal representative
    c. The physician
    d. All the above
    e. a and b
    f. c only

16. ___ HIPAA stands for Health Insurance Portability and Accountability Act.
    a. True
    b. False

17. ___ The privacy rule permits the caregiver to use protected health information for treatment, payment, and operations purposes.
    a. True
    b. False

18. ___ The record custodian typically can testify about which of the following when a party in a legal proceeding is attempting to admit a health record as evidence?
    a. Identification of the record as the one subpoenaed
    b. The care provided
    c. The qualifications of the treating physician
    d. Policies and procedures relevant to creation and maintenance of a record
    e. a and b only
    f. a and d only
    g. b and c only

19. ___ A privilege, as it relates to the relationship between physician and patient, means the physician is not permitted to testify as a witness about certain information gained as a result of the relationship.
   a. True
   b. False

20. ___ Circle the letter(s) of the conditions below under which the privacy rule permits disclosure of medical information to law enforcement agencies or officers.
   a. Required by law
   b. Pursuant to court order, court-ordered warrant, subpoena, summons, grand jury subpoena
   c. An administrative summons or subpoena, a civil or an authorized investigative demand
   d. For identifying or locating a suspect, fugitive, material witness, or missing person
   e. To respond to a law enforcement request about an individual suspected to be a victim of a crime
   f. To alert law enforcement of a suspicion that a patient's death may have resulted from criminal conduct
   g. Hospital's belief that the information is evidence of criminal conduct that occurred on its premises

21. ___ To what extent does the privacy rule permit a healthcare provider to release health information to a relative or friend?
   a. Not at all to either a relative or friend
   b. Only to a person identified by the patient, whether relative or friend
   c. Only that information relevant to the person's involvement in the patient's care or payment for healthcare
   d. c only
   e. b and c only

22. ___ The privacy rule provides that authorization must include a statement that the information disclosed pursuant to the authorization may be disclosed by the recipient and thus is no longer protected.
   a. True
   b. False

23. ___ Which of the following federal statutes or regulations provide the concept of patient privacy?
   a. Medicare Conditions of Participation for Hospitals
   b. Medicare Conditions of Participation for Home Health Agencies
   c. The Privacy Act of 1974
   d. The privacy rule pursuant to HIPAA
   e. All of the above
   f. a and c only

24. ___ What federal laws address the requirement for credentialing?
   a. Medicare Conditions of Participation for Hospitals
   b. Medicare Conditions of Participation for Home Health Agencies
   c. The Privacy Act of 1974
   d. Medicare Conditions of Participation for Long-Term Care Facilities
   e. All of the above
   f. a and b only
   g. a and d only

25. ___ The process through which the medical staff gives the physician the right to provide specific services to patients is called:
   a. Credentialing
   b. Privileging

26. ___ Reviewing medical care as it is being given is a:
   a. Concurrent review activity
   b. Retrospective review activity

27. ___ What entity in a hospital has final responsibility for granting medical staff membership and privileges?
   a. Credentialing committee
   b. Medical executive committee
   c. Chief executive officer of hospital
   d. Hospital board of directors

28. ___ What duty does the entity you identified in #27 above owe medical staff applicants?
   a. Prudent person
   b. Reasonable care
   c. Standard of care

29. ___ The basis for maintaining the confidentiality of credentialing review files is that these review activities involve collecting outcomes and performance data regarding how a physician performed as a physician and may have an impact on continued medical staff membership.
   a. True
   b. False

30. ___ What is(are) the liability issue(s) related to premises safety for nonstaff persons coming onto the premises? These persons include visitors, vendors, and members of the general public.
   a. Physical safety from defects in buildings and grounds
   b. Potential for being harmed by a patient, another nonstaff person, or a staff member
   c. a and b
   d. None of the above.

31. ___ By contrast, what is(are) the liability issue(s) pertaining to premises safety for staff?
   a. Physical safety from defects in buildings and grounds
   b. Potential for being harmed by a patient, a nonstaff person, or another staff member
   c. a and b
   d. None of the above

32. ___ What is the implication regarding the confidentiality of incident reports in a legal proceeding when a staff member documents in the health record that an incident report was completed about a specific incident.
   a. There is no impact.
   b. The person making the entry in the health record may not be called as a witness in trial.
   c. The incident report becomes discoverable because it is mentioned in a discoverable document.
   d. The incident report cannot be discovered because it is mentioned in a discoverable document

33. ___ The relationship between the health information manager and the risk manager includes:
   a. They work as a team.
   b. The risk manager depends on the health information manager to alert him or her to potentially compensible events.
   c. The health information manager can advise the risk manager when attorney requests a copy of a health record.
   d. All of the above
   e. None of the above

Chapter 11
Ethical Issues in Health Information Management

Laurinda B. Harman, PhD, RHIA

Learning Objectives

- To identify the major ethical principles that guide health information management decision making
- To identify professional values and obligations inherent in the Code of Ethics, including those important to patients, the healthcare team, employers, the public, peers and colleagues, and professional associations
- To understand how the steps in an ethical decision-making process arc used to resolve ethical issues
- To recognize some core health information ethical problems, including those related to the release of health information, fraud and abuse, coding, quality review, research and decision support, computerized health information systems, the management of sensitive information, and the emerging roles of entrepreneur and advocate

Key Terms

Autonomy
Beneficence
Blanket authorization
Bioethics
Confidentiality
Ethical decision making
Ethicist
Ethics
Justice
Morality
Need-to-know principle
Nonmaleficence
Privacy
Secondary release of information
Security

Introduction

The responsibilities of the health information administrator (HIA) include a wide range of functions and activities. Regardless of the employment site (healthcare facility, vendor, pharmaceutical company, research firm), the HIA's core ethical obligation is to protect patient privacy and confidential communication. This obligation is at the center of the decisions made on behalf of patients, the healthcare team, peer colleagues, the public, or the many other stakeholders who seek access to information.

Although most people probably have never undertaken a formal study of ethics, everyone is exposed to ethical principles, moral perspectives, and personal values throughout his or her lifetime. Individuals learn about basic moral values from families, religious leaders, teachers, government and community organizations, and other groups that influence our experiences and perspectives. **Ethical decision making** requires everyone to consider the perspectives of others, even when they have different values.

The terms introduced in this chapter are specific to the study of ethics. They describe principles most people already know, such as demonstrating respect for others and recognizing the importance of individuals deciding what happens to them, doing good, not harming others, and treating people fairly. In the terminology of ethics, **autonomy** means self-determination, **beneficence** means promoting good, **nonmaleficence** means not harming others, and **justice** means treating others fairly (Beauchamp and Childress 1994).

Theory into Practice

With regard to one of the HIA's primary functions, how might ethical principles apply in the case of deciding whether to release patient information?

- Autonomy would require the HIA to ensure that the patient, and not a spouse or third party, makes the decisions regarding access to his or her health information.
- Beneficence would require the HIA to ensure that the information is released only to individuals who need it to do something that will benefit the patient (for example, to an insurance company for payment of a claim).
- Nonmaleficence would require the HIA to ensure that the information is not released to someone who does not have authorization to access it and who might harm the patient if access were permitted (for example, a newspaper seeking information about a famous person).
- Justice would require the HIA to apply the rules fairly and consistently for all and not to make special exceptions based on personal or organizational perspectives.

This chapter discusses the role of ethical principles and professional values in HIM decision making. It also offers a step-by-step process that HIAs can use to make appropriate ethical choices and an analysis of what is and is not justified from an ethical perspective.

Key Responsibilities of the Health Information Administrator

Some of the HIA's core ethical responsibilities include (Harman 2001a):

- Working with vendors or his or her employer to build or maintain a patient database
- Coding for research and reimbursement and coding accurately to avoid fraud and abuse violations (for example, miscoding for the purpose of optimizing reimbursement)
- Designing and implementing the health information system to ensure completeness, accuracy, and timeliness
- Releasing patient information, with special attention to, and protections assigned for, genetic, adoption, drug treatment, alcohol treatment, sexual, and behavioral health issues
- Complying with regulations and standards from many sources, including the government, accreditation and licensure organizations, and the healthcare facility
- Reporting quality review outcomes honestly and accurately, even when the results might create conflict for an individual or an institution
- Ensuring that research and decision support activities are accurate and reliable
- Releasing accurate information for public health purposes for patients with communicable diseases, such as AIDS or venereal disease
- Supporting managed care managers by providing accurate, reliable information about patients, providers, and patterns of care
- Ensuring that the electronic patient record meets the standards of privacy and security
- Participating in software development and implementation to ensure that the needs of the healthcare facility's many stakeholders are met
- Participating in the development of integrated delivery systems so that patients can move through the continuum of care and the right information can be provided to the right people when needed
- Working in the emerging e-health systems to ensure that high-quality information is provided to patients and that patient privacy is protected in computerized information systems
- Serving as entrepreneur and advocate for patients, the healthcare team, and the communities with interests in the information system

Because the HIA works with individuals and departments throughout the healthcare organization and delivery system, his or her obligations extend into a variety of areas, as noted above. In fulfilling the responsibilities of the position, the HIA must apply ethical values when making decisions wherever he or she happens to be positioned within the organization.

Moral Values and Ethical Competencies

Morality is often described as actions that are either right or wrong. For example, some might consider it right to be nice to a neighbor and wrong to destroy the neighbor's property. However, these are not universal values. Others might consider it acceptable to be rude or mean to a neighbor and to destroy his or her property. Applying this language to health information management, it is right—and a moral obligation—to protect the neighbor's privacy when you learn about diseases and conditions while doing your job. It is wrong to share the neighbor's secrets with other neighbors, family, and friends.

Ethics is a process of reasoned discourse (discussion) among decision makers. They must carefully consider the shared and competing values and ethical principles that are important to the decision to be made. Ethical discussion provides a framework for resolving conflicts when competing values are at stake for the choices being considered. Ethical decision making requires people to explore options beyond the perspective of simple right or wrong (moral) options. According to Glover (2001, p. 25), "ethics is the formal process of intentionally and critically analyzing, with respect to clarity and consistency, the basis for one's moral judgments." When making health information decisions, HIA professionals must go beyond the right or wrong moral perspective and evaluate the many values and perspectives of others who are engaged in the decision to be made.

Ethical discussions in nonhealthcare contexts can be theoretical in nature, and the analysis of a problem does not necessarily result in action. For example, **ethicists** could discuss whether to require all citizens living in a certain community to donate ten hours a week as part of their civic duty. One ethicist might argue for a decision based on the ethical principle of beneficence, which would guide action to do good things for others. Another ethicist might argue for the same decision, but based on the principle of justice in which every citizen should contribute his or her fair share for the good of the whole. Neither argument is right or wrong, just different. These discussions and decisions would not require action but would help frame the ethical justification for a certain action.

In contrast, **bioethics** involves problems or issues regarding clinical care or the health information system that are never strictly theoretical in nature and must always result in a decision. HIAs cannot merely deliberate whether to release patient information. Rather, they must apply ethical principles and then perform an action—release the information requested or deny the request. In short, ethics applied in the work environment can never stay theoretical and always results in an action.

Moreover, HIAs should not make ethical decisions based solely on personal moral values or perspectives. Not everyone shares the same moral perspectives or values. When one individual sees only one solution to a problem and others have different solutions, ethics can help with making a decision.

Ethical Foundations in Health Information Management

Ethical principles and values have been important to the HIM profession since its beginning in 1928. The first ethical pledge was presented by Grace Whiting Myers in 1934. The HIM profession was launched with a recognition of the importance of privacy and the requirement of authorization for the release of health information:

> I pledge myself to give out no information from any clinical record placed in my charge, or from any other source to any person whatsoever, except upon order from the chief executive officer of the institution which I may be serving (Huffman 1972, p. 135).

The most important values embedded in this pledge are to protect patient privacy and confidential information and to recognize the importance of the moral agency of the HIM professional to protect patient information (Harman, DeWald, and Vollgraff-Rushton 2001, pp. 39–46).

The HIA has a clear ethical and professional obligation not to give any information to anyone unless its release has been authorized, regardless of employment site—direct patient care, facilities that need access to health information, or vendors, among others. Today, it is the patient who authorizes the release of information and not the chief executive officer (CEO), as stated in the original pledge.

Protection of Privacy, Maintenance of Confidentiality, and Assurance of Data Security

The terms *privacy, confidentiality,* and *security* are often used interchangeably. However, there are some important distinctions, including:

- **Privacy** is "the right of an individual to be let alone. It includes freedom from intrusion or observation into one's private affairs and the right to maintain control over certain personal and health information" (Harman 2001a, p. 376).
- **Confidentiality** carries "the responsibility for limiting disclosure of private matters. It includes the responsibility to use, disclose, or release such information only with the knowledge and consent of the individual" (Harman 2001a, p. 370). Confidential information may be written or verbal.
- **Security** includes "physical and electronic protection of the integrity, availability, and confidentiality of computer-based information and the resources used to enter,

store, process, and communicate it. The means to control access and protect information from accidental or intentional disclosure" (Harman 2001a, p. 372).

The HIA's responsibilities include ensuring that patient privacy and confidential information are protected and that data security measures are used to prevent unauthorized access to information. This responsibility includes ensuring that the release policies and procedures are accurate and up-to-date, that they are followed, and that all violations are reported to the proper authorities.

The Health Insurance Portability and Accountability Act of 1996 (HIPAA) is a "statute that establishes national standards for privacy and security of health information. It requires that health care plans, providers and clearinghouses adopt standards of safeguards to ensure the integrity and confidentiality of health information and protect against threats to the security or integrity of the information and against unauthorized uses of the information" (Harman 2001a, p. 374). This legislation includes administrative simplification standards and security and privacy standards. It will have a major impact on the collection and dissemination of information in the coming years. This legislation has an enforcement program, and the HIA will play an important role in ensuring compliance.

Health Information Management's Codes of Ethics

HIM professionals used the pledge as the basis for guiding ethical decision making until 1957, at which time the American Association of Medical Record Librarians' (AAMRL) House of Delegates passed the first Code of Ethics for the Practice of Medical Record Science. (See figure 11.1.) The first code of ethics combined ethical principles with a set of professional values to help support the decisions that HIM professionals had to make at work. The original Code of Ethics has been revised several times since 1957, and the ethical codes for 1957, 1978, 1988, and 1998 were examined and the professional values discussed below were derived from them. (See figures 11.2, 11.3, and 11.4, respectively.)

Upon being awarded the credential of RHIA (registered health information administrator) by the American Health Information Management Association (AHIMA), the HIM professional agrees to follow the principles and values discussed in this chapter and to base all professional actions and decisions on those principles and values. Even if federal or state laws did not require the protection of patient privacy, the HIM professional would be responsible for protecting it according to the AHIMA's Code of Ethics.

Professional Values and Obligations

Health information ethical and professional values are based on obligations to the patient, the healthcare team, the employer, the interests of the public, and oneself, one's peers, and one's professional associations (Harman 1999, 2001b).

Figure 11.1.   AAMRL Code of Ethics for the Practice of Medical Record Science

As a member of one of the paramedical professions he shall:

1. Place service before material gain, the honor of the profession before personal advantage, the health and welfare of patients above all personal and financial interests, and conduct himself in the practice of this profession so as to bring honor to himself, his associates, and to the medical record profession.

2. Preserve and protect the medical records in his custody and hold inviolate the privileged contents of the records and any other information of a confidential nature obtained in his official capacity, taking the due account of applicable statutes and of regulations and policies of his employer.

3. Serve his employer loyally, honorably discharging the duties and responsibilities entrusted to him and give due consideration to the nature of these responsibilities in giving his employer notice of intent to resign his position.

4. Refuse to participate in or conceal unethical practices or procedures.

5. Report to the proper authorities, but disclose to no one else, any evidence of conduct or practice revealed in the medical records in his custody that indicates possible violation of established rules and regulations of the employer or of professional practice.

6. Preserve the confidential nature of professional determinations made by the staff committee which he serves.

7. Accept only those fees that are customary and lawful in the area for services rendered in his official capacity.

8. Avoid encroachment on the professional responsibilities of the medical and other paramedical professions, and under no circumstances assume or give the appearance of assuming the right to make determinations in professional areas outside the scope of his assigned responsibilities.

9. Strive to advance the knowledge and practice of medical record science, including continued self-improvement in order to contribute to the best possible medical care.

10. Participate appropriately in developing and strengthening professional manpower and in representing the profession to the public.

11. Discharge honorably the responsibilities of any Association post to which appointed or elected, and preserve the confidentiality of any privileged information made known to him in his official capacity.

12. State truthfully and accurately his credentials, professional education, and experiences in any official transaction with the American Association of Medical Record Librarians and with any employer or prospective employer.

Copyright ©1957 by the American Association of Medical Librarians.

Obligations to the Patient and the Healthcare Team

With regard to the patient and the healthcare team, the HIA is obligated to:

- *Provide service to those who seek access to patient information:* Individuals who may request access to patient information include healthcare providers; insurance, research, or pharmaceutical companies; government agencies; and employers. The HIA must ensure the honor of the profession before personal advantage and the health and welfare of patients before all personal and financial interests. He or she also must balance the many competing interests of all the stakeholders who want patient information.

Figure 11.2.   1978 AMRA Code of Ethics

The medical record practitioner is concerned with the development, use, and maintenance of medical and health records for medical care, preventive medicine, quality assurance, professional education, administrative practices and study purposes with due consideration of patients' right to privacy. The American Medical Record Association believes that it is in the best interests of the medical record profession and the public which it serves that the principles of personal and professional accountability be reexamined and redefined to provide members of the Association, as well as medical record practitioners who are credentialed by the Association, with definitive and binding guidelines of conduct. To achieve this goal, the American Medical Record Association has adopted the following restated Code of Ethics:

1. Conduct yourself in the practice of this profession so as to bring honor and dignity to yourself, the medical record profession and the Association.

2. Place service before material gain and strive at all times to provide services consistent with the need for quality health care and treatment of all who are ill and injured.

3. Preserve and secure the medical and health records, the information contained therein, and the appropriate secondary records in your custody in accordance with professional management practices, employer's policies and existing legal provisions.

4. Uphold the doctrine of confidentiality and the individual's right to privacy in the disclosure of personally identifiable medical and social information.

5. Recognize the source of the authority and powers delegated to you and conscientiously discharge the duties and responsibilities thus entrusted.

6. Refuse to participate in or conceal unethical practices or procedures in your relationship with other individuals or organizations.

7. Disclose to no one but proper authorities any evidence of conduct or practice revealed in medical reports or observed that indicates possible violation of established rules and regulations of the employer or professional practice.

8. Safeguard the public and the profession by reporting to the Ethics Committee any breach of this Code of Ethics by fellow members of the profession.

9. Preserve the confidential nature of professional determinations made by official committees of health and health-service organizations.

10. Accept compensation only in accordance with services actually performed or negotiated with the health institution.

11. Cooperate with other health professions and organizations to promote the quality of health programs and advancement of medical care, ensuring respect and consideration for the responsibility and the dignity of medical and other health professions.

12. Strive to increase the profession's body of systematic knowledge and individual competency through continued self-improvement and application of current advancements in the conduct of medical record practices.

13. Participate in developing and strengthening professional manpower and appropriately represent the profession in public.

14. Discharge honorably the responsibilities of any Association position to which appointed or elected.

15. Represent truthfully and accurately professional credentials, education, and experience in any official transaction or notice, including other positions and duality of interests.

Figure 11.3.   1988 AMRA Code of Ethics

The medical record professional abides by a set of ethical principles developed to safeguard the public and to contribute within the scope of the profession to quality and efficiency in health care. This code of ethics, adopted by the members of the American Medical Record Association, defines the standards of behavior, which promote ethical conduct.

1. The Medical Record Professional demonstrates behavior that reflects integrity, supports objectivity, and fosters trust in professional activities.

2. The Medical Record Professional respects the dignity of each human being.

3. The Medical Record Professional strives to improve personal competence and quality of services.

4. The Medical Record Professional represents truthfully and accurately professional credentials, education, and experience.

5. The Medical Record Professional refuses to participate in illegal or unethical acts and also refuses to conceal the illegal, incompetent, or unethical acts of others.

6. The Medical Record Professional protects the confidentiality of primary and secondary health records as mandated by law, professional standards, and the employer's policies.

7. The Medical Record Professional promotes to others the tenets of confidentiality.

8. The Medical Record Professional adheres to pertinent laws and regulations while advocating changes which serve the best interest of the public.

9. The Medical Record Professional encourages appropriate use of health record information and advocates policies and systems that advance the management of health records and health information.

10. The Medical Record Professional recognizes and supports the association's mission.

- *Protect both medical and social information:* Clinical information (for example, diagnoses, procedures, pharmaceutical dosages, or genetic risk factors) must be protected as well as behavioral information (for example, use of drugs or alcohol, high-risk hobbies, sexual habits). These days, it is increasingly important to protect social information to avoid risks of discrimination.

- *Protect confidential information:* This involves ensuring that the information collected and documented in the patient information system is protected by all members of the healthcare team and by anyone with access to the information while performing his or her job. This responsibility also includes protection of verbal communications on behalf of a patient.

- *Preserve and secure health information:* This includes obligations to maintain and protect the medium that stores the information (computer, microfilm, CD-ROM) and to secure the information for both manual and computerized information systems. All databases and detailed secondary records and registries must be protected.

Figure 11.4.   AHIMA Code of Ethics

AHIMA's Mission

The American Health Information Management Association is committed to the quality of health information for the benefit of patients, providers and other users of clinical data. Our professional organization:

- Provides leadership in HIM education and professional development
- Sets and promotes professional practice standards
- Advocates patient privacy rights and confidentiality of health information
- Influences public and private policies including educating the public regarding health information
- Advances health information technologies

Guiding Principles

We are committed to the:

- Creation and utilization of systems and standards to ensure quality health information
- Achievement of member excellence
- Development of a supportive environment and provision of the resources to advance the profession
- Provision of the highest-quality service to members and healthcare information users
- Investigation and application of new technology to advance the management of health information

We value:

- The balance of patients' privacy rights and confidentiality of health information with legitimate uses of data
- The quality of health information as evidenced by its integrity, accuracy, consistency, reliability, and validity
- The quality of health information as evidenced by its impact on the quality of healthcare delivery

This Code of Ethics sets forth ethical principles for the health information management profession. Members of this profession are responsible for maintaining and promoting ethical practices. This Code of Ethics, adopted by the American Health Information Management Association, shall be binding on health information management professionals who are members of the Association and all individuals who hold an AHIMA credential.

I.   Health information management professionals respect the rights and dignity of all individuals.

II. Health information management professionals comply with all laws, regulations, and standards governing the practice of health information management.

III. Health information management professionals strive for professional excellence through self-assessment and continuing education.

IV. Health information management professionals truthfully and accurately represent their professional credentials, education, and experience.

V.   Health information management professionals adhere to the vision, mission, and values of the Association.

VI. Health information management professionals promote and protect the confidentiality and security of health records and health information.

VII. Health information management professionals strive to provide accurate and timely information.

VIII. Health information management professionals promote high standards for health information management practice, education, and research.

IX. Health information management professionals act with integrity and avoid conflicts of interest in the performance of their professional and AHIMA responsibilities.

Copyright ©1998 by the American Health Information Management Association.

- *Promote the quality and advancement of healthcare:* As an important member of the healthcare team, the HIA provides valuable expertise in the collection of health information that will help providers improve the quality of care they deliver. The HIA should develop expertise in clinical medicine, pharmacology, biostatistics, and quality improvement methodologies so as to interpret clinical information and support research.
- *Stay within the scope of responsibility and restrain from passing clinical judgment:* Sometimes healthcare data may indicate a problem with a provider of care, the treatment of a diagnosis, or some other problem. The HIA's obligation is to provide the data, no matter how often they are needed, but not to pass judgment on them. That obligation rests with the healthcare team that reviews the data. The HIA should repeatedly, consistently, and accurately results of studies.
- *Promote interdisciplinary cooperation and collaboration:* As an important member of the healthcare team, the HIA should work with others to analyze and address health information issues, facilitate conflict resolution, and recognize the expertise and dignity of his or her fellow team members.

Obligations to the Employer

With regard to the employer, the HIA is obligated to:

- *Demonstrate loyalty to the employer:* The HIA can do this by respecting and following the policies, rules, and regulations of employment unless they are illegal or unethical. This obligation includes giving the employer adequate notice when the HIA decides to change employment sites.
- *Protect committee deliberations:* The HIA should be as committed to protecting committee conversations and decisions as he or she is to protecting patient information. Examples of such committees include medical staff and employer committees.
- *Comply with all laws, regulations, and policies that govern the health information system:* The HIA should keep up-to-date with state and federal laws, accrediting and licensing standards, employer policies and procedures, and any other standards that affect the health information system.
- *Recognize both the authority and the power associated with the job responsibility:* This obligation rests with responsibilities to have a voice and be at the negotiation table. The HIA professional is the expert on privacy and

confidentiality and must be present at strategic meetings with clinical providers, administrative staff, financial and operations management personnel to be sure that HIM expertise is presented and understood. Unethical behaviors would be to hide and not be at the top-level strategic meetings, wait for the outcomes and then say "this decision is wrong but I wasn't asked." The HIA professional cannot remain quiet and let others have the power to decide what information is released, what software is installed or other important HIM decisions. HIA professionals do have both the power and the authority to say "no, that is not acceptable" or "this is appropriate action."

- *Accept compensation only in relationship to work responsibilities:* Increasingly, there are groups or individuals who could gain by having access to patient information and are willing to pay for such information. Access to databases with patient information on certain diagnoses such as AIDS or cancer could be sought by employers, commercial vendors, or others. The HIA must avoid the temptation to accept money for disclosing patient information or proprietary vendor secrets.

Obligations to the Public

With regard to the public interest, the IIIA is obligated to:

- *Advocate change when patterns or system problems are not in the best interests of the patients:* The HIA should be a change agent and lead initiatives to change laws, rules, and regulations that do not ensure the integrity of patient information, including the protection of privacy and confidentiality. Moreover, the HIA should be proactive about protecting patients, the healthcare team, the organization, the professional association, peers, and him- or herself.

- *Refuse to participate or conceal unethical practices:* The HIA should be accountable for identifying trends and potential problems related to provision of care, documentation, and billing practices. Further, he or she should refuse to conceal illegal, incompetent, or unethical behaviors of individuals or organizations.

- *Report violations of practice standards to the proper authorities:* The HIA should not share information learned at work with family or friends or discuss such information in public places. He or she should report the results of audits to the proper authorities only. Moreover, the HIA should bring potential or actual problems to the attention of those individuals responsible for the delivery and assessment of care and services.

Obligations to Self, Peers, and Professional Associations

With regard to self, peers, and professional associations, the HIA is obligated to:

- *Be honest about degrees, credentials, and work experiences:* The HIA should only report an acquired degree (such as a BS or MS) or successfully earned credentials

(such as an RHIA or a CCS). Work experiences must be reported accurately and honestly.

- *Bring honor to oneself, one's peers, and one's profession:* This obligation refers to personal competency and professional behavior (for example, at professional meetings). The HIA should try to ensure that peers and colleagues are proud to have him or her on the health information team.

- *Commit to continuing education and lifelong learning:* The HIA's education should not stop when he or she has earned a degree or a credential. Rather, the HIA should continue to attend educational sessions to keep abreast of changing laws, rules, and regulations that affect the health information system. The HIA should be a lifelong learner and contribute to improving the quality of healthcare service delivery. HIAs can keep their credentials by meeting the ongoing certification requirements of the AHIMA. Maintaining competency through self-improvement is an important directive that ensures the continuance of the profession.

- *Strengthen health information professional membership:* This obligation includes belonging to professional associations, actively participating on committees, making presentations, writing for publications, and encouraging others to seek health information management as a career.

- *Represent the health information profession to the public:* The HIA has a responsibility to advocate for the public interest in areas related to the principles and values of HIM practice.

- *Promote and participate in health information research:* When problems are discovered with the health information system, the HIA should conduct studies to clarify their sources and potential solutions.

Check Your Understanding 11.1

Instructions: Match the HIM professional's obligations to the following groups with the professional values expressed in the AHIMA's 1998 Code of Ethics (figure 11.1).

a. Patients and the healthcare team
b. Employer
c. Public interest
d. Oneself and one's peers and professional associations

1. ____ Accept compensation only in relationship to responsibilities
2. ____ Advocate change
3. ____ Preserve and secure health information
4. ____ Be honest
5. ____ Commit to continuing education and lifelong learning
6. ____ Promote interdisciplinary cooperation and collaboration
7. ____ Promote and participate in research
8. ____ Demonstrate loyalty to employer
9. ____ Discharge association duties honorably
10. ____ Protect committee deliberations
11. ____ Stay within the scope of responsibility and restrain from passing clinical judgment
12. ____ Bring honor to self, peers, and profession
13. ____ Protect medical and social information
14. ____ Promote the quality and advancement of healthcare

15. ___ Represent the profession to the public
16. ___ Comply with laws, regulations, and policies
17. ___ Report violations of practice standards to the proper authorities
18. ___ Refuse to participate in or conceal unethical practices
19. ___ Provide service
20. ___ Strengthen professional membership
21. ___ Recognize authority and power
22. ___ Promote confidentiality

Ethical Decision-Making Model

HIAs must factor several criteria into their decision making. These include, but are not limited to:

- *Cost:* Can the facility and the health information system afford the improvement in the system?
- *Technological feasibility:* Will the technological application provide accurate and reliable information for the decision-making process?
- *Federal and state laws:* Are there federal or state laws that must be considered before a change is made in the system?
- *Medical staff bylaws:* Are there rules or regulations unique to the facility that require or prohibit a decision?
- *Accreditation and licensing standards:* Which agencies have standards that are important to the decision being made? Do the standards allow or prohibit a certain action?
- *Employer policies, rules, or regulations:* Does the facility have policies, rules, or regulations that require or prohibit a decision?

Although these criteria must be assessed in the decision-making process, they cannot be used alone. Virtually every decision the HIA makes also must be based on ethical principles and professional values.

Ethicists provide assistance in this process. Glover (2001, pp. 27–30) has proposed a seven-step process to guide ethical decision making. When faced with an ethical issue, the HIA should ask and answer all of the following questions:

1. What is the ethical question?
2. What facts do you know, and what do you need to find out?
3. Who are the different stakeholders, what values are at stake, and what are the different obligations and interests of each of the stakeholders?
4. What options for action do you have?
5. What decision should you make, and what core HIM values are at stake?
6. What justifies the choice, and what are the value-based reasons to support the decision? What choice or choices cannot be justified?
7. What prevention options can be put into place so that this issue will not come up again?

The questions represent the steps in the decision-making process.

When a decision must be made about an issue and only one choice is identified, the decision most likely will be based on the narrow moral perspective of right or wrong. However, a decision based solely on right and wrong does not take into account the perspectives of competing stakeholders and their values. Decisions made without this model will not benefit from an ethical decision-making process that considers multiple options.

Check Your Understanding 11.2

Instructions: Using a, b, c, and so on, rearrange the steps of the ethical decision-making process in the correct order.

1. ___ What decision should you make, and what core HIM values are at stake?
2. ___ What facts do you know, and what do you need to find out?
3. ___ What options for action do you have?
4. ___ What is the ethical question?
5. ___ What justifies the choice, and what are the reasons to support the decision, based on values? What choice or choices cannot be justified?
6. ___ What prevention options can be put into place so that this issue will not happen again?
7. ___ Who are the different stakeholders, what values are at stake, and what are the different obligations and interests of each of the stakeholders?

Core Health Information Ethical Problems

Several problems face HIAs in today's complex world, including issues related to documentation, release of information, sources and uses of health information, coding, computerized health information systems, and the emerging roles of entrepreneur and advocate.

Ethical Issues Related to Documentation

Just a few years ago, only a few people created documentation in patient health records and fewer still wanted access to patient information after the episode of care was completed. However, those days are over. In today's healthcare system, many providers document their decision-making process and patient outcomes in the health information system and many more people want access to that information. The HIA plays a critical role in developing policies and procedures to ensure the integrity of patient information, including appropriate and authorized access.

In addition to writing policies and procedures to ensure compliance with federal and state laws, accrediting and licensing agencies, and the bylaws of the healthcare facility, the HIA can serve many functions that support the integrity of data and the protection of privacy. As a member of the HIM team, the HIA can design and deliver educational sessions to the healthcare team to make them aware of the documentation and access rules and regulations. Sometimes educational sessions address the issue of avoiding participation in fraudulent or retrospective documentation practices. Retrospective documentation practices are those where healthcare providers add documentation after care has been given for the purpose of increasing reimbursement or avoiding a medical legal action.

Unacceptable documentation practices include backdating progress notes or other documentation in the patient's record and changing the documentation to reflect the known outcomes of care (versus what was done at the time of the actual care). It is the HIA's responsibility to work with others to ensure that patient documentation is accurate, timely, and created by authorized parties. The professional Code of Ethics requires the HIA to assure accurate and timely documentation.

Ethical Issues Related to Release of Information

Three primary ethical problems are pertinent to the release of information (ROI):

- Violations of the **need-to-know principle**
- Misuse of **blanket authorizations**
- Violations of privacy that occur as a result of secondary release procedures

In the past, the standard for ROI was the need to know. If an insurance company had a patient request to pay for surgery, the request was sent to the healthcare facility and the HIM professional carefully examined it for legitimacy. He or she would:

- Compare the patient's signature to the one collected upon admission to the facility
- Check the date to ensure that the request was dated after the occurrence so that the patient was aware of what was being authorized and released
- Verify the insurance company as the one belonging to the patient
- Review the request for what was wanted and whether the requestor was entitled to the information

The HIA then reviewed the documentation and provided the information requested. For example, the admission and discharge dates, the diagnoses of cholecystitis and cholelithiasis, and the surgical procedure of cholecystectomy were provided to the insurance company so that the bill could be paid. The bottom line was: "Yes, insurance company, you can trust me as the health information professional. I reviewed the medical record, and you can pay for this surgery."

Today, the process of abstracting needed information is virtually nonexistent, except for disability cases, and documentation is copied above and beyond the criterion of need to know. For example, in response to the request to verify an admission for a cholecystectomy, the history and physical, the operative report, the discharge summary, and the laboratory report could be copied. That documentation could reveal social habits, genetic risks, and family history of disease that have nothing to do with the surgery. Patient privacy could be

violated as a result of the release of the information through subsequent discrimination by insurers.

Another common ethical problem is misuse of blanket authorizations. Patients often sign a blanket authorization, which authorizes the release of information from that point forward, without understanding the implications. The requestor of the information then could use the authorization to receive health information for many years. The problem with the use of blanket authorizations is that there is no way for the patient to know that the information is being accessed. How could patients authorize the release of information in 1994 for care that was not even provided until 2001? In 1994, they did not have AIDS, genetic risk to cancer, or a major psychiatric disorder, so how could they authorize release of the information?

A third problem is **secondary release** to others. This problem has increased in frequency since the computerization of health information. A legitimate request might be processed to pay for an insurance claim, but adequate safety and protections may not be in place for the information after it has been released. The initial requestor then could forward the information to others without patient authorization. An HIA cannot merely think about ROI within the context of the single request. The responsibility to "follow the information" is much more serious today than it was a few years ago. Does the HIA know who gains access to the information after it is released to an authorized requestor? If not, he or she may be contributing to the violations of patient privacy and a subsequent instance of discrimination by employers or insurance companies based on the information that was released.

Patients are increasingly expressing concerns about the use of blanket authorizations and secondary ROI by the initial requestor or receiving party. They fear that more information is being given out than is necessary and that they do not know of the many people and agencies that are gaining access to this information. HIPAA has been designed to address several issues related to patient privacy, including a return to the need-to-know principle. The HIA needs to participate in the development of computerized systems that can replicate the original human decisions regarding ROI—to release what is needed, but not more. Although it is easier to just photocopy the information, the HIA needs to carefully consider the implications of doing this within the context of patient privacy. This situation has created an opportunity for HIAs to participate with other HIM professionals in efforts to correct these problems.

Ethical Issues Related to Coding

In the past, coding was done almost exclusively for future clinical studies and quality assurance review processes. Although codes were provided for reimbursement purposes, the healthcare facility was reimbursed on the basis of usual, customary, and reasonable costs. The codes that were assigned became the basis of retrieval for clinical studies and the reimbursement system. Over time, healthcare facilities have continued to use the coding systems to retrieve information in health records for clinical and administrative studies but also began to use the codes for reimbursement purposes. After the codes became the basis for reimbursement, there were inherent incentives to code so that the greatest amount of reimbursement could be given. This placed the importance of accurate coding at the forefront of the ethical issues facing HIAs.

Figure 11.5.   AHIMA Standards of Ethical Coding

1. Coding professionals are expected to support the importance of accurate, complete, and consistent coding practices for the production of quality healthcare data.

2. Coding professionals in all healthcare settings should adhere to the *ICD-9-CM International Classification of Diseases, Ninth Revision, Clinical Modification,* coding conventions, official coding guidelines approved by the Cooperating Parties [AHIMA, Centers for Medicare and Medicaid Services, National Center for Health Statistics, and American Hospital Association], the CPT (Current Procedural Terminology) rules established by the American Medical Association, and any other official coding rules and guidelines established for use with mandated standard code sets. Selection and sequencing of diagnoses and procedures must meet the definitions of required data sets for applicable healthcare settings.

3. Coding professionals should use their skills, their knowledge of the currently mandated coding and classification systems, and official resources to select the appropriate diagnostic and procedural codes.

4. Coding professionals should only assign and report codes that are clearly and consistently supported by physician documentation in the health record.

5. Coding professionals should consult physicians for clarification and additional documentation prior to code assignment when there are conflicting or ambiguous data in the health record.

6. Coding professionals should not change codes or the narratives of codes on the billing abstract so that the meanings are misrepresented. Diagnoses or procedures should not be inappropriately included or excluded because the payment or insurance policy coverage requirements will be affected. When individual payer policies conflict with official coding rules and guidelines, these policies should be obtained in writing whenever possible. Reasonable efforts should be made to educate the payer on proper coding practices in order to influence a change in the payer's policy.

7. Coding professionals, as members of the healthcare team, should assist and educate physicians and other clinicians by advocating proper documentation practices, further specificity, resequencing, or inclusion of diagnoses or procedures when needed to more accurately reflect the acuity, severity, and the occurrence of events.

8. Coding professionals should participate in the development of institutional coding policies and should ensure that coding policies complement, not conflict with, official rules and guidelines.

9. Coding professionals should maintain and continually enhance their coding skills, as they have a professional responsibility to stay abreast of changes in codes, coding guidelines, and regulations.

10. Coding professionals should strive for the optimal payment to which the facility is legally entitled, remembering that it is unethical and illegal to maximize payment by means that contradict regulatory guidelines.

Ethical problems have risen in the past few years given the direct linkage between coding and payments for care. Increased pressure has been put on HIM professionals who are coding to transmit inaccurate information, creating problems that are legal and/or ethical in nature. Problems include pressure to code inappropriate levels of service, discovering misrepresentation in physician documentation, miscoding to avoid conflicts, discovering miscoding by other staff, lacking the tools and educational background to code accurately, and being required by employers to engage in negligent coding practices (Schraffenberger and Scichilone 2001, pp. 67–90). In response to these issues, the AHIMA passed standards that specifically address coding issues (figure 11.5).

Failure to heed the coding complexities can lead the HIA to problems with compliance and with fraud and abuse. If the HIA fails to establish adequate monitoring systems for accurate code assignment or submits a false claim, the consequences could include penalties, such as fees and prison. The HIA must know the laws and the penalties for failure to follow the laws and, most important, have the expertise to develop preventive programs to ensure that the false claim is a nonoccurrence. Fraud and abuse problems include documentation that does not justify the billed procedure, acceptance of money for information, fraudulent retrospective documentation on the part of the provider to avoid suspension, and code assignment without physician documentation. An important emerging role for the HIA is that of compliance officer (Hubbuch 2001, pp. 49–65).

Ethical Issues Related to Quality Management, Public Health, and Managed Care

Many factors contribute to the ethical problems faced by quality management professionals, including the rising cost of healthcare, limited resources, and concerns with patient safety. Some of the common quality outcome problems include (Spath 2001, pp. 91–112):

- Inaccurate performance data that are inappropriately shared with the public
- Negative care outcomes, such as infections that occur in the course of providing home health care
- Failure to check a physician's licensure status
- Incomplete health records hidden in preparation for accreditation or licensure surveys
- Patterns of inappropriate healthcare

The pressures to conceal information that could be potentially harmful to an employer and problems with patient safety require constant diligence and the courage to repeatedly report the truth.

Career opportunities for the HIA are growing in public health systems. Careers in this area require an understanding of the government's role in the collection and use of health information. The government's responsibility to protect the health of the public sometimes competes with the need to protect patient privacy, such as in the case of reporting HIV status. State and local mandatory reporting requirements exist for certain conditions, including infectious and communicable diseases. The government needs this information to monitor, investigate, and implement interventions, when necessary. Sometimes problems arise when the public's right to know or duty to one's employer conflicts with patient privacy (Neuberger 2001, pp. 131–54). The HIA can provide invaluable assistance with public health initiatives that will contribute to environmental and personal health. This role requires constant advocacy so that the interests of both the public and the individual patient can be served.

Another important role for the HIA is in working on behalf of managed care organizations that depend on high-quality information to meet commitments to the patients, clinicians, and communities they serve. As with other situations, access to information is key to the problems faced by the HIM professional as he or she helps with the organization's strategies regarding pricing, access to providers, and quality of care (Schick 2001, p. 159). Job responsibilities in this work context include providing information about provider practices, providing patient clinical and demographic information, and establishing policies and procedures that provide for patient privacy (Schick 2001, pp. 155–71).

Ethical Issues Related to Sensitive Health Information

All health information must be protected, but additional ethical issues have emerged around the release of sensitive information such as genetic, drug, and alcohol treatment, communicable disease, psychiatric, and adoption information. At least two levels of genetic information can be reported in an information system: presence of a disease, such as cystic fibrosis; and presence of a risk of disease, such as a genetic risk for breast cancer. Various state laws govern the use and release of genetic information, and the HIA must be aware of them. In recent years, there have been growing concerns about discrimination in employment and insurance based on the misuse of genetic information (Fuller and Hudson 2001, pp. 273–85). According to Fuller and Hudson, the HIA must be aware of the following issues related to genetic information:

(1) Genetic research and testing can give researchers, clinicians, and patients a means to prevent, treat, or screen for a disease. Often, however, individuals are reluctant to participate in genetic research and testing because they believe they can't be sure of the privacy of the genetic information that will be obtained from them and placed in their medical records or in research records.

(2) Insurers and employers may seek genetic information to identify at-risk individuals and deny them employment or insurance coverage, fire them, or raise their premiums. Genetic information may also be sought in custody battles or in cases of third-party liability. Even when this information is not used to discriminate, individuals may be concerned about its disclosure because of its possibility of causing psychosocial harm, such as harm to family relationships.

(3) It is difficult to provide special protections for genetic information as a category because it cannot be clearly separated from other med-ical information. Therefore, the best way to protect genetic information is to strengthen privacy and confidentiality protections for medical information in general and to enact antidiscrimination legislation.

(4) There are state laws to protect the confidentiality of health information, but, with few exceptions, federal laws do not address the privacy and confidentiality of medical records.

(5) The generation of experimental data by a research protocol is not specifically addressed by most state laws.

(6) HIM professions have the responsibility to ensure that their practices are guided by state and federal laws and regulations to protect genetic information and by the ethical imperative to protect the privacy and confidentiality of patients (p. 284).

One of the HIA's most important professional opportunities is to become involved in resolving the above-stated issues on behalf of patients and the healthcare system.

Federal and state laws also govern the use of behavioral health information and special concerns with its use. The HIA must respond to the government, the police, and other agencies that seek drug, alcohol, sexual, or other behavioral information. The inappropriate release of information can have serious discriminatory consequences, such as:

- The police officer presents an arrest warrant to a behavioral health facility. Do you confirm that the patient has been treated? What are the implications for patient privacy if you do (Randolph and Rinehart-Thompson 2001, p. 304)?
- A patient with schizophrenia and assaultive behavior is about to be released from a healthcare facility. Do you have a responsibility to inform the girlfriend, who has been assaulted in the past? What are your obligations to protect the privacy of the patient being released (Randolph and Rinehart-Thompson 2001, p. 307)?

The ROI dealing with substance abuse, sexually transmitted diseases, and mental health require extra caution on the part of the HIA when developing release policies and procedures. There are often competing interests between public safety and patient privacy. How does one deal with law enforcement officials within this context? Federal and state legislation can provide some guidance, but often additional legal counsel must be sought (Randolph and Rinehart-Thompson 2001, pp. 303–17).

The release of adoption information is another example of an issue in which the legal aspects are necessary, but insufficient, for solving the problems. The decisions cannot be made merely by following the legal rules. More and more, access to adoption information is being requested by adopted children seeking their biological parents, and vice versa. Biological parents often look for children who could be organ donors or for other assistance. This issue links with the complexities of releasing genetic and behavioral information because, increasingly, we define "self" within genetic parameters and biological heritage is becoming more important in defining self. Access to adoption information raises the larger issue of familial access to information, regardless of adoptive status. If biological children can gain access to health information for their biological parent(s), why cannot all children gain access to familial information? (Jones 2001, pp. 287–302). HIAs must be alert to these special needs and not process requests for adoption information without carefully considering the risks for violations of patient privacy, discrimination, or inappropriate access.

Ethical Issues Related to Technology

With a paper-based health record, access issues were relatively simple. Only one person at a time could access the information, and it was extremely difficult to collect and use data of an aggregate nature. With computerization, many requestors are allowed multiple, simultaneous access and it is relatively easy to share information across a continuum of care and with computerized systems well outside the boundaries of any individual care site. The advent of the computerized information system has presented complex challenges with regard to record integrity and information security, integrated linkage of information systems across a continuum of care, software development and implementation, and the protection of information in e-health systems (Harman 2001a, chapters 10–15).

As information systems became computerized and healthcare facilities began to link various health information systems, the temptation increased to sacrifice privacy and data integrity for the sake of business efficiency and timely access to information. There is an exponential increase in the risk to privacy and the protection of confidential information (Hanken and Murphy 2001, chapter 10). The HIA must do a thorough systems analysis of the independent systems and ensure that the merged systems meet the criteria of data integrity, information security, and ethical use of the information.

Information security carries additional burdens of ethical decision making. Many requestors, such as insurance companies, government agencies, managed care organizations, and employers, need health information to do their jobs. Unauthorized access to patient information becomes a constant challenge, given the need to balance the responsibility to protect information while giving others access to information within the context of job responsibilities. Internal requestors include, but are not limited to, patients, providers of care, financial agencies, and administrative and clinical personnel such as quality or risk management professionals. External stakeholders include other healthcare facilities, research institutes, accrediting and licensing agencies, and fiscal intermediaries (Czirr and Rosendale 2001, chapter 11). The HIA must develop a comprehensive information security policy, including detailed audit trails of access and actions. Moreover, the policy must be monitored with consequences for violations. Increasingly, HIAs are being designated as the information security officers within a healthcare facility or healthcare system.

Development and implementation of software systems are inherently interdisciplinary in nature, and the process requires collaboration and conflict resolution. The physicians, the HIA, the information technology experts, and administrative personnel often have competing interests. The HIA is often in the position of carefully delineating the details of competing interests so that appropriate decisions can be made. This role of being able to see the systems implications within the context of protecting privacy is invaluable (Fenton 2001, chapter 12). The HIA's role as interdisciplinary facilitator is crucial, which is why educational sessions on organizational development, team building, and conflict resolution are often key components of the HIA's continuing education program.

The expertise of the HIA includes data resource management because computerized information systems generate data repositories and huge amounts of health information of interest to many people. A primary focus of the HIPAA legislation is to ensure that systems are developed that protect privacy and threats against violations of integrity of the information and unauthorized access. Data resource managers must have both HIM technical expertise and information technology expertise so that they can design and monitor systems that ensure data security and patient privacy. These functions are accomplished through the use of many decision-making tools, including databases, clinical data repositories, and data-mining tools, among others. The primary ethical dilemma involves balancing the competing interests of access and appropriate use of information (Lee, White, and Wager 2001, pp. 229–44).

As HIM systems became computerized, the capacity for developing integrated delivery systems across a continuum of care became technologically possible. HIM systems relied on paper-based systems in which each facility had its own health record and the only way to transmit information from one site of care to another was through copying procedures. Now, information can follow the patient and be instantly and simultaneously shared and made available as needed. This is both good news and bad. The segregated, independent systems had some inherent protections of privacy. The integrated computerized systems require HIA diligence to ensure protection of information and access to only those who have a need to know. Information management policies, rules, and procedures for individual healthcare entities must be compatible with those of other facilities, and often the issues of competing interests can create major ethical conflicts as to the appropriate action.

The master patient index presents a major problem because there is often no consistency among facilities in terms of how and what information is collected. If the information is to follow the patient, the individual systems must be accurate and compatible. Data quality issues include accuracy, comprehensiveness, consistency, currency, granularity, precision, relevancy, and timeliness (AHIMA Data Quality Management Task Force 1998). Negotiation and problem-solving skills are an inherent requirement for the HIA working in an integrated delivery system (Olson, Grant, and Fletcher 2001, pp. 245–54). The HIA must lead the organization in addressing data quality issues associated with implementing integrated information systems.

Last, but not least, the HIA's ethical expertise is needed in the burgeoning e-health systems. Some of the ethical issues the HIA faces in the work environment include the quality of online information, privacy protections, and equity and privacy. The issue of equity is important to e-health systems because not everyone has access to the information on the electronic systems. There cannot be equity when one patient instead of another can easily gain access to invaluable and voluminous information about symptoms, diseases, pharmaceutical interventions, and treatment options. Privacy can be an issue when patients reveal sensitive information to a Web site and have no idea what will happen to the information or who will have access to it. The opportunities for the HIA are unlimited given the problems of consumer access to information, quality of information provided, and access to information. This nontraditional advocacy role for HIAs is important in this emerging technological advancement (Baur and Deering 2001, pp. 255–70.)

Emergent Roles of Entrepreneur and Advocate

As an entrepreneur, the HIA must understand the complexities of business practices intersecting with professional values and ethical principles. Common ethical dilemmas occur when establishing contracts, clarifying the roles of intrapreneur and entrepreneur, or acting as an independent contractor. Difficulties may arise when consulting for competitors (having access to sensitive information that might be of value to the competition), dealing with advertising, confronting unrealistic client expectations, or confusing profit versus not-for-profit motivations for decisions (Gardenier 2001, pp. 321–47).

HIAs have always been advocates for patients and providers, and the advocate role is important in today's healthcare delivery system. For the HIA, advocacy "is ethics in action: choosing to take a stand for and speak out for the rights or needs of a person, group, organization, or community to someone or some entity" (Helbig 2001, p. 349). HIM problems that require advocacy include:

- Protecting the privacy of prominent citizens
- Demonstrating compassion for drug-dependent peers
- Protecting the work environment for HIM employees
- Ensuring that consent forms are properly designed so that patients understand what they are signing and so that patient information is protected from unauthorized secondary disclosure

The advocacy role requires HIM expertise, ethical expertise, and an understanding of the patient's bill of rights (Helbig 2001, pp. 349–66).

Check Your Understanding 11.3

Instructions: Match the ethical principle with its definition.

1. ___ Autonomy
2. ___ Beneficence
3. ___ Nonmaleficence
4. ___ Justice
5. ___ Moral values
6. ___ Ethical decisions
7. ___ Privacy
8. ___ Confidentiality
9. ___ Data security
10. ___ HIPAA

a. Right or wrong
b. Reasoned discourse
c. Right to be let alone
d. Promote good
e. Self-determination
f. Healthcare communication
g. Do no harm
h. Fairness in applying rules
i. Establishes privacy and security standards
j. Electronic protection of information

Real-World Case

Health information management professionals frequently face ethical dilemmas on the job. Some of the many ethical challenges include situations similar to the following case (Harman 2001b):

You are responsible for the health record completion process and have identified several problems, including:

- There are more delinquent records than allowed by the accreditation standards. You are asked to report an inaccurate number to help the hospital avoid a citation.

- You have observed that physician signature stamps are being misused in violation of medical staff bylaws.

- Verbal orders are not signed on time.

- Several physicians are adding progress notes and other documentation to the health records and dating them as if they were written when the patient was in the hospital.

Discussion Questions

Name a few ethical dilemmas faced by HIA professionals in the following areas:

1. Release of information
2. Coding
3. Quality management
4. Public health
5. Managed care
6. Sensitive information: genetic, behavioral, and adoption-related
7. Technology
8. Electronic health records
9. Information security

Summary

Ethical decision making is one of the health information administrator's most challenging and rewarding job responsibilities. It requires courage because there will always be people who choose not tell the truth or do the right thing. HIAs must discuss these issues with their peer management professionals and other health information management professionals and seek the advice of the professional association when necessary.

The HIA's job responsibilities inherently require an understanding of ethical principles, professional values and obligations, and the importance of using an ethical decision-making matrix when confronting difficult challenges at work. With this knowledge, the informed HIA can move from understanding problems based on a moral perspective only to understanding the importance of applying an ethical decision-making process. Ethical decision making takes practice, and discussions with peers will help the HIA to build competency in this important area.

When making ethical decisions, the HIA must use the complete ethical decision-making matrix to consider all the stakeholders and their obligations and the important HIM professional values. More than one response can be given for any ethical issue as long as the complete matrix is applied. Just as there can be more than one "right" answer to a problem, there can be "wrong" answers, especially when an answer is based only on a moral value or the perspective of one individual or when the action violates ethical principles.

Bioethical decisions involving the use of health information require action, and such actions always require courage. The healthcare team, the patients, and the others who are served need to know that the HIA has the expertise and the courage to make the appropriate ethical decisions.

References

AHIMA's Data Quality Management Task Force. 1998. Practice Brief: Data quality management model. *Journal of the American Health Information Management Association* 69(6):72a–72h.

Beauchamp, T., and J. Childress. 1994. *Principles of Biomedical Ethics.* New York City: Oxford University Press.

Baur, C., and M. J. Deering. 2001. In *Ethical Challenges in the Management of Health Information,* edited by L. B. Harman. Gaithersburg, Md.: Aspen Publishers.

Czirr, K., and K. Rosendale. 2001. In *Ethical Challenges in the Management of Health Information,* edited by L. B. Harman. Gaithersburg, Md.: Aspen Publishers.

Fenton, S. H. 2001. Software development and implementation. In *Ethical Challenges in the Management of Health Information,* edited by L. B. Harman. Gaithersburg, Md.: Aspen Publishers.

Fuller, B. P., and K. L. Hudson. 2001. Genetic information. In *Ethical Challenges in the Management of Health Information,* edited by L. B. Harman. Gaithersburg, Md.: Aspen Publishers.

Gardenier, M. 2001. Entrepreneur. In *Ethical Challenges in the Management of Health Information,* edited by L. B. Harman. Gaithersburg, Md.: Aspen Publishers.

Glover, J. J. 2001. Ethical decision-making guidelines and tools. In *Ethical Challenges in the Management of Health Information,* edited by L. B. Harman. Gaithersburg, Md.: Aspen Publishers.

Hanken, M. A., and G. Murphy. 2001. Electronic patient record. In *Ethical Challenges in the Management of Health Information,* edited by L. B. Harman. Gaithersburg, Md.: Aspen Publishers.

Harman, L. B. 1999. HIM and ethics: confronting ethical dilemmas on the job, an HIM professional's guide. *Journal of the American Health Information Management Association* 71(5):45–49.

Harman, L. B., editor. 2001a. *Ethical Challenges in the Management of Health Information.* Gaithersburg, Md.: Aspen Publishers.

Harman, L. B. 2001b. Professional code of ethics and values. In *Ethical Challenges in the Management of Health Information,* L. B. Harman, editor. Gaithersburg, Md.: Aspen Publishers.

Harman, L. B. 2001c. *Instructor's Manual for the Ethical Challenges in the Management of Health Information.* Gaithersburg, Md.: Aspen Publishers.

Harman, L. B., L. A. DeWald, and D. Vollgraff-Rushton. 2001. Privacy and confidentiality. In *Ethical Challenges in the Management of Health Information,* edited by L. B. Harman. Gaithersburg, Md.: Aspen Publishers.

Helbig, S. 2001. Advocate. In *Ethical Challenges in the Management of Health Information,* edited by L. B. Harman. Gaithersburg, Md.: Aspen Publishers.

Hubbuch, A. 2001. Compliance, fraud, and abuse. In *Ethical Challenges in the Management of Health Information,* edited by L. B. Harman. Gaithersburg, Md.: Aspen Publishers.

Huffman, E. K. 1972. *Manual for Medical Record Librarians,* sixth edition. Chicago: Physician's Record Company.

Johns, M. L., and J. M. Hardin. 2001. Research and decision support. In *Ethical Challenges in the Management of Health Information,* edited by L. B. Harman. Gaithersburg, Md.: Aspen Publishers.

Jones, M. L. 2001. Adoption information. In *Ethical Challenges in the Management of Health Information,* edited by L. B. Harman. Gaithersburg, Md.: Aspen Publishers.

Lee, F. W., A. W. White, and K. A. Wager. 2001. Data resource management. In *Ethical Challenges in the Management of Health Information,* edited by L. B. Harman. Gaithersburg, Md.: Aspen Publishers.

Neuberger, B. J. 2001. Public health. In *Ethical Challenges in the Management of Health Information,* edited by L. B. Harman. Gaithersburg, Md.: Aspen Publishers.

Olson, B., K. G. Grant, and D. M. Fletcher. 2001. In *Ethical Challenges in the Management of Health Information,* edited by L. B. Harman. Gaithersburg, Md.: Aspen Publishers.

Randolph, S. J., and L. A. Rinehart-Thompson. 2001. Drug, alcohol, sexual, and behavioral health information. In *Ethical Challenges in the*

Management of Health Information, edited by L. B. Harman. Gaithersburg, Md.: Aspen Publishers.

Schick, I. C. 2001. Managed care. In *Ethical Challenges in the Management of Health Information,* edited by L. B. Harman. Gaithersburg, Md.: Aspen Publishers.

Schraffenberger, L. A., and R. A. Scichilone. 2001. Coding. In *Ethical Challenges in the Management of Health Information,* edited by L. B. Harman. Gaithersburg, Md.: Aspen Publishers.

Spath, P. L. 2001. Quality review. In *Ethical Challenges in the Management of Health Information,* edited by L. B. Harman. Gaithersburg, Md.: Aspen Publishers.

Application Exercises

1. The first example illustrates how to use the decision-making process to resolve an ethical dilemma.

> Kristin is both the HIM director and the privacy officer for her hospital. A large data warehouse company has approached the small hospital for which she works with a proposal to store and manage all of the hospital's clinical information using Web-enabled technology. The hospital's health record system is completely computerized. During negotiations, Kristin discovers that the data warehouse company has other business avenues in which it sells aggregate information derived from its various clients' data repositories. This is not illegal, since the data warehouses are not yet covered under federal or state laws. Kristin's hospital, like all others, publicly posts the various uses of its patient information so that patients and possible patients know about it. As Kristin discusses this further with the data warehouse company, she discovers that the company does not have clear criteria for the kind of entities that are entitled to buy this information.

> The data warehouse company is offering a substantial incentive to Kristin's hospital for every patient information sale it makes. There is no economically feasible way to monitor the security provisions that are written in the potential contract. On the basis of their calculation, the administration believes they will be able to cut overall staff by 15 percent, an outcome that is attractive to both the administration and the hospital board. Kristin is under pressure to sign off on her part of the contract. At this point in time, the committee believes that the records will be electronically transferred to the vendor six weeks after a patient is discharged as an inpatient and two weeks after a clinical visit. Kristin is a member of the committee that is researching the feasibility of changing the health information operations paradigm. This committee will make a recommendation to administration on whether to go forward with the proposal. The committee is led by the chief information officer and also includes the director of IT, the associate medical director for information, and the HIM systems project manager. It is a daunting project for all involved.

This scenario can be examined within the context of ethical decision making as shown in table 11.1 (Harman 2001c, pp. 73–75).

2. The following example illustrates a second application of ethics (Czirr and Rosendale 2001, p. 207):

> In a high-tech environment, patient care is expedited by real-time reports being generated immediately and directly from the laboratory, pathology, or radiology departments to the electronic record system. Physicians can pull these results up on their office PCs or at the nursing station immediately and make the changes needed for optimal patient care. The risk is, however, that in a rush to help these very patients, they may forget to log off of the systems, and others working in the vicinity of those PCs may deliberately or accidentally view patient information.

The ethical problem is analyzed by the application of the decision-making matrix in table 11.2, p. 237.

Table 11.1.   Decision-Making Matrix for the First Application Exercise

Decision-Making Matrix: The Data Warehouse Wants to Sell Patient Information		
Step 1	**Questions**	
What is the ethical question?	Should Kristin recommend going forward with the proposal?	
Step 2	**Known**	**To Be Gathered**
What are the facts?	The data warehouse company has a line of business in which it sells information from its clients' data repositories. The company does not have clear criteria for the kind of entities that are entitled to buy information.	Would the hospital be able to establish with the company a clear set of guidelines for the sale of information from its database? Could patient interests be harmed by the sale of information from the database? What are the opinions of the other members of the team? Could Kristen be held liable if patient confidentiality were violated? What are the customary practices in such cases? What does her boss expect her to do? What is the likely impact on self and family of changing jobs?
Step 3	**Stakeholder**	**Obligations/Interests**
What are the values at stake in this scenario?	Patient	Values confidentiality of medical information.
	HIM professional	Truth, integrity: Protect patient confidentiality. Demonstrate loyalty to employer. Avoid harm: Sharing patient information could harm the patient. Personal values: Promote welfare of self and family by avoiding loss of job.
	Administrators	Promote welfare of facility.
	Society	Protect confidentiality of health records.
Step 4		**Options**
What are the options in this case?		Gather more information. Recommend that the hospital move forward with the proposal. Recommend that the hospital insist that the company institute policies establishing clear criteria for the kind of entities entitled to purchase information.
Step 5	**Core HIM Values**	**Decision**
What should I do?	Be sure that all facts have been gathered. Be clear about values important to the case. Provide service. Protect medical and social information. Promote confidentiality. Preserve and secure health information. Demonstrate loyalty to employer. Comply with laws, regulations, and policies. Recognize authority and power. Advocate change. Refuse to participate or conceal unethical practices. Report violations of practice standards to the proper authorities. Represent profession to the public.	Recommend that the hospital insist that the company institute policies establishing clear criteria for the kind of entities entitled to purchase information.
Step 6	**Reasons to Support Based on Values**	**Not Justified**
What justifies my choice?	Obligation to protect patient confidentiality Obligation to protect security of computerized health record system Obligation to protect professional integrity	Recommend that the hospital move forward with the proposal. Jeopardize patient confidentiality. Jeopardize security of the computerized health record system. Jeopardize professional integrity.
Step 7		**Prevention Options**
How could this ethical problem have been prevented?		Determine whether system changes are needed. Discuss standards and the values that support them with colleagues. Learn more about confidentiality and security issues surrounding computerized data systems. Evaluate institutional integrity at job interview and subsequently as ethical problems arise.

Source: Harman, L. B. 2000c. *Instructor's Manual for Ethical Challenges in the Management of Health Information.* Gaithersburg, Md.: Aspen Publishers, pp. 140–42.

Table 11.2.   Decision-Making Matrix for the Second Application Exercise

Decision-Making Matrix: Failure to Log Off of the System		
Step 1	**Questions**	
What is the ethical question?	Does this system put patient confidentiality in jeopardy?	
Step 2	**Known**	**To Be Gathered**
What are the facts?	The system expedites patient care. Physicians must log off of the system to close access to the patient records.	What information is accessible via the system? Could the use of such a system increase the probability of confidentiality violations? Is it possible to implement a timed log-out if physicians forget to log out? What are the customary practices in such cases? What does your boss or supervisor expect you to do? What is the likely impact on self and family of changing jobs?
Step 3	**Stakeholder**	**Obligations/Interests**
What are the values at stake in this scenario?	Patient	Values privacy and confidentiality. Values protection of record integrity. Has an interest in prompt, accurate care.
	HIM professional	Integrity and accuracy: Preserve accuracy and confidentiality of records. Avoid harm: Sharing patient information could harm the patient. Personal values: Promote welfare of self and family by avoiding loss of job.
	Healthcare professionals	Value prompt, accurate patient care. Promote the welfare of patients through accurate documentation.
	Administrators	Promote welfare of facility. Benefit patients and keep from harm.
	Society	Preserve record integrity. Preserve confidentiality.
Step 4		**Options**
What are the options in this case?		Gather more information. Allow the system to operate as is. Require implementation of a timed automatic log-out system.
Step 5	**Core HIM Values**	**Decision**
What should I do?	Be sure that all facts have been gathered. Be clear about values important to the case. Provide service. Protect medical and social information. Promote confidentiality. Preserve and secure health information. Promote interdisciplinary cooperation and collaboration. Demonstrate loyalty to employer. Comply with laws, regulations, and policies. Recognize authority and power. Advocate change. Be honest. Bring honor to self, peers, and profession. Represent profession to the public.	Require implementation of a timed log-out system.
Step 6	**Reasons to Support Based On Values**	**Not Justified**
What justifies my choice?	Obligation to protect confidentiality Obligation to preserve record integrity Obligation to preserve professional integrity	Allow the system to operate as is. Jeopardize confidentiality. Jeopardize record integrity. Jeopardize professional integrity.
Step 7		**Prevention Options**
How could this ethical problem have been prevented?		Determine whether system changes are needed. Learn more about the issues surrounding the security of EMR systems. Discuss standards and the values that support them with colleagues.

Source: Harman, L. B. 2000c. *Instructor's Manual for Ethical Challenges in the Management of Health Information*. Gaithersburg, Md.: Aspen Publishers, pp. 140–42.

Review Quiz

Instructions: Choose the best answer to complete the following sentences.

1. ____ The health information administrator's core ethical obligation is to protect patient privacy and ____.
   a. Decision support activities
   b. Confidential communication
   c. Access to information
   d. Patient values

2. ____ In the terminology of ethics, ____ means self-determination.
   a. Justice
   b. Beneficence
   c. Nonmaleficence
   d. Autonomy

3. ____ In the past, the standard for release of information was the ____.
   a. Need to know
   b. Blanket authorization
   c. Patient request
   d. Expertise of the HIA

4. ____ Over time, healthcare facilities continued to use coding systems to retrieve information from health records for clinical and administrative studies but also began to use the codes for ____ purposes.
   a. ROI
   b. Security
   c. Reimbursement
   d. Ethical

5. ____ Ethics is a process of ____ discourse among decision makers.
   a. Shared
   b. Reasoned
   c. Acceptable
   d. Conflicting

6. ____ Ethics applied in the work environment can never stay theoretical and always results in ____.
   a. A decision
   b. An ethical pledge
   c. An action
   d. A principle

7. ____ The code of ethics combines ethical principles with ____ to help support the decisions that HIM professionals have to make at work.
   a. Professional values
   b. Ethical standards
   c. Moral perspectives
   d. Moral values

8. ____ With regard to the patient and the healthcare team, the HIM professional is obligated to promote ____ and advancement of healthcare.
   a. Expertise
   b. Research
   c. Interests
   d. Quality

9. ____ With regard to self, peers, and professional associations, the HIM professional is obligated to commit to continuing education and ____.
   a. Professional membership
   b. Lifelong learning
   c. Health information research
   d. Professional behavior

Part III

Aggregate Healthcare Data

Chapter 12
Secondary Records and Healthcare Databases

Elizabeth Bowman, MPA, RHIA

Learning Objectives

- To distinguish between primary and secondary data and between patient-identifiable and aggregate data
- To identify the internal and external users of secondary data
- To compare the facility-specific indexes commonly found in hospitals
- To describe the registries used in hospitals according to purpose, methods of case definition and case finding, data collection methods, reporting and follow-up, and pertinent laws and regulations affecting registry operations
- To define the terms pertinent to each type of secondary record or database
- To discuss agencies for approval and education and certification for cancer, immunization, trauma, birth defects, diabetes, implant, transplant, and immunization registries
- To distinguish among healthcare databases in terms of purpose and content
- To compare manual and automated methods of data collection and vendor systems with facility-specific systems
- To assess data quality issues in secondary records
- To recognize appropriate methods for ensuring data security and the confidentiality of secondary records
- To identify the role of the health information management professional in creating and maintaining secondary records

Key Terms

Abbreviated Injury Scale (AIS)
Abstracting
Accession number
Accession registry
Activities of daily living
Agency for Healthcare Research and Quality (AHRQ)
Aggregate data
Audit trail
Autodialing system
Case definition
Case finding
Claim
Clinical trial
Collaborative Stage Data Set
Computer virus
Credentialing
Data confidentiality
Data security
Database
Demographic information
Disease index
Disease registry
Edit
Encryption
Facility-based registry
Facility-specific system
Food and Drug Administration (FDA)
Health services research
Healthcare Integrity and Protection Data Bank (HIPDB)

Histocompatibility
Incidence
Index
Injury Severity Score (ISS)
Interrater reliability
Master population/patient index (MPI)
Medical Literature, Analysis, and Retrieval System Online (MEDLINE)
National Health Care Survey
National Practitioner Data Bank
National Vaccine Advisory Committee (NVAC)
Operation index
Patient-specific/identifiable data
Physician index
Population-based registry
Primary data source
Protocol
Public health
Secondary data source
Staging system
Traumatic injury
Unified Medical Language System (UMLS)
User groups
Vendor system
Vital statistics

Introduction

As a rich source of data about an individual patient, the health record fulfills the uses of patient care and reimbursement for individual encounters. However, it is not easy to see trends in a population of patients by looking at individual records. For this purpose, data must be extracted from individual records and entered into specialized databases that support analysis accross individual records. These data may be used in a facility-specific or population-based registry for research and improvement in patient care. In addition, they may be reported to the state and become part of state- and federal-level databases that are used to set health policy and improve healthcare.

The health information management (HIM) professional can play a variety of roles in managing secondary records and databases. He or she plays a key role in helping to set up databases. This task includes determining the content of the database or registry and ensuring compliance with the laws, regulations, and accrediting standards that affect the content and use of the registry or database. All data elements included in the database or registry must be defined in a data dictionary. In this role, the HIM professional may oversee the completeness and accuracy of the data abstracted for inclusion in the database or registry.

This chapter explains the difference between primary and secondary data sources and their users. It also offers an in-depth look at the types of secondary databases, including indexes and registries, and their functions. Finally, the chapter discusses how secondary databases are processed and maintained.

Theory into Practice

A hospital with a level I trauma center serving a tristate area had an ongoing problem. It was required to provide care to all major trauma cases from the three states within its service area regardless of the patients' ability to pay. However, one of the states (state X) was unwilling to pay for the care provided to its indigent patients. Because trauma care can be extremely intensive and costly, the hospital was losing a lot of money.

The American College of Surgeons requires certified trauma centers to maintain a trauma registry. To demonstrate the extent of the problem, the hospital administrator asked the trauma registrar to gather data on patients from state X. The trauma registrar easily identified these patients and provided information by zip code on their location and the type and severity of their injuries. After the patients had been identified, the business office was able to calculate the cost to the hospital of providing their care. The administrator then presented this information to state X's legislature to obtain the money to pay for the care the trauma center provided to the state's indigent patients.

Primary versus Secondary Data Sources and Databases

The health record is considered a **primary data source** because it contains information about a patient that has been documented by the professionals who provided care or services to that patient. Data taken from the primary health record and entered into registries and databases are considered a **secondary data source.**

Data also are categorized as either **patient-specific/ identifiable data** or aggregate data. The health record consists entirely of patient-identifiable data. In other words, every fact recorded in the record relates to a particular patient identified by name. Secondary data also may be patient identifiable. In some instances, data are entered into a database along with information such as the patient's name maintained in an identifiable form. Registries are an example of patient-identifiable data on groups of patients.

More often, however, secondary data are considered aggregate data. **Aggregate data** include data on groups of people or patients without identifying any particular patient individually. Examples of aggregate data are statistics on the average length of stay (ALOS) for patients discharged within a particular diagnosis-related group (DRG).

Purposes and Users of Secondary Data Sources

Secondary data sources consist of facility-specific indexes; registries, either facility or population based; and other healthcare databases. Healthcare organizations maintain those indexes, registries, and databases that are relevant to their specific operations.

Secondary data sources provide information that is not easily available by looking at individual health records. For example, if the HIM director doing a research study wanted to find the health records of twenty-five patients who had the principal diagnosis of myocardial infarction, he or she would have to look at numerous individual records to locate the number needed. This would be a time-consuming and laborious project.

Data extracted from health records and entered into disease-oriented databases can, for example, help researchers determine the effectiveness of alternate treatment methods. They also can quickly demonstrate survival rates at different stages of disease.

Internal users of secondary data are individuals located within the healthcare facility. For example, internal users include medical staff and administrative and management staff. Secondary data enable these users to identify patterns and trends that are helpful in patient care, long-range planning, budgeting, and benchmarking with other facilities.

External users of patient data are individuals and institutions outside the facility. Examples of external users are state data banks and federal agencies. States have laws that cases of patients with diseases such as tuberculosis and AIDS must be reported to the state department of health. Moreover, the federal government collects data from the states on vital events such as births and deaths.

The secondary data provided to external users is generally aggregate data and not patient-identifiable data. Thus, these data can be used as needed without risking breaches of confidentiality.

Check Your Understanding 12.1

Instructions: Answer the following questions on a separate piece of paper.

1. What is the difference between a primary data source and a secondary data source?
2. What is the difference between patient-identifiable data and aggregate data?
3. Why are secondary data sources developed?
4. What are the differences between internal users and external users of secondary data sources?

Facility-Specific Indexes

The most long-standing secondary data sources are those that have been developed within facilities to meet their individual needs. These **indexes** enable health records to be located by diagnosis, procedure, or physician. Prior to extensive computerization in healthcare, these indexes were kept on cards. They now are usually computerized reports available from data included in **databases** routinely maintained in the healthcare facility. Most acute care facilities maintain the following indexes:

- Master patient/population index
- Disease index
- Operation index
- Physician index

Master Population/Patient Index

The **master population/patient index** (MPI), which is sometimes called the master person index, contains patient-identifiable data such as name, address, date of birth, dates of hospitalizations or encounters, name of attending physician, and health record number. Because health records are filed numerically in most facilities, the MPI is an important source of patient health record numbers. These numbers enable the facility to quickly retrieve health information for specific patients.

Hospitals with a unit numbering system also depend on the MPI to determine whether a patient has been seen in the facility before and therefore has an existing medical record number. Having this information in the MPI avoids issuance of duplicate record numbers. Most of the information in the MPI is entered into the facility database at the time of the admission/preadmission or registration process.

Disease and Operation Indexes

In an acute care setting, the **disease index** is a listing in diagnosis code number order for patients discharged from the facility during a particular time period. Each patient's diagnoses are converted from a verbal description to a numerical code, usually using a coding resource such as the *International Classification of Diseases, Ninth Revision, Clinical Modification* (ICD-9-CM). In many cases, patient diagnosis codes are entered into the facility health information system as part of the discharge processing of the patient health record. The index always includes the patient's health record number as well as the diagnosis codes so that records can be retrieved by diagnosis. Because each patient is listed with the health record number, the disease index is considered patient-identifiable data. The disease index also may include other information such as the attending physician's name or the date of discharge. In nonacute settings, the disease index might be generated to reflect patients currently receiving services in the facility.

The **operation index** is similar to the disease index except that it is arranged in numerical order by the patient's procedure code(s) using ICD-9-CM or Current Procedural Terminology (CPT) codes. The other information listed in the operation index is generally the same as that listed in the disease index except that the surgeon may be listed in addition to, or instead of, the attending physician.

Physician Index

The **physician index** is a listing of cases in order by physician name or physician identification number. It also includes the patient's health record number and may include other information, such as date of discharge. The physician index enables users to retrieve information about a particular physician, including the number of cases seen during a particular time period.

Check Your Understanding 12.2

Instructions: Answer the following questions on a separate piece of paper.

1. How do HIM departments use facility-specific indexes?
2. What is the purpose of the master population/patient index? What types of information does it include?
3. What is the purpose of disease and operations indexes? What types of information do they include?
4. What is the purpose of the physician index? What types of information does it include?

Registries

Disease registries are collections of secondary data related to patients with a specific diagnosis, condition, or procedure. Registries are different from indexes in that they contain more extensive data. Index reports can usually be produced using data from the facility's existing databases. Registries often require more extensive data from the patient record. Each registry must define the cases that are to be included in it. This process is called **case definition.** In a trauma registry, for example, the case definition might be all patients admitted with a diagnosis falling into ICD-9-CM code numbers 800 through 959, the trauma diagnosis codes.

After the cases to be included have been determined, the next step in data acquisition is usually case finding. **Case finding** is a method used to identify the patients who have been seen and/or treated in the facility for the particular disease or condition of interest to the registry. After cases have been identified, extensive information is abstracted from the paper-based patient record into the registry database or extracted from other databases and entered into the registry database.

The sole purpose of some registries is to collect data from the patient health record and to make them available for users. Other registries take further steps to enter additional information in the registry database, such as routine follow-up of patients at specified intervals. Follow-up might include rate and duration of survival and quality of life issues over time.

Cancer Registries

Cancer registries have a long history in healthcare. According to the National Cancer Registrars Association (NCRA), the first hospital registry was founded in 1926 at Yale-New Haven Hospital (NCRA 2001). It has long been recognized that aggregate clinical information is needed to improve the diagnosis and treatment of cancer. Cancer registries were developed as an organized method to collect these data. The data may be facility based (for example, within a hospital or clinic) or population based (for example, information gathered from more than one facility within a state or region).

The data from **facility-based registries** are used to provide information for the improved understanding of cancer, including its causes and methods of diagnosis treatment. The data collected also may provide comparisons in survival rates and quality of life for patients with different treatments and at different stages of cancer at the time of diagnosis. In **population-based registries,** emphasis is on identifying trends and changes in the **incidence** (new cases) of cancer within the area covered by the registry.

The Cancer Registries Amendment Act of 1992 provided funding for a national program of cancer registries with population-based registries in each state. According to the law, these registries were mandated to collect data such as:

- Demographic information about each case of cancer
- Information on the industrial or occupational history of the individuals with the cancers (to the extent such information is available from the same record)
- Administrative information, including date of diagnosis and source of information
- Pathological data characterizing the cancer, including site, stage of neoplasm, incidence, and type of treatment

Case Definition and Case Finding in the Cancer Registry

As defined previously, case definition is the process of deciding what cases should be entered in the registry. In a cancer registry, for example, all cancer cases except skin cancer might meet the definition for the cases to be included.

In the facility-based cancer registry, the first step is case finding. One way to find cases is through the discharge process in the HIM department. During the discharge procedure, coders and/or discharge analysts can easily earmark cases of patients with cancer for inclusion in the registry. Another case-finding method is to use the facility-specific disease indexes to identify patients with diagnoses of cancer. Additional methods may include reviews of pathology reports and lists of patients receiving radiation therapy or other cancer treatments to determine cases that have not been found by other methods.

Population-based registries usually depend on hospitals, physicians' offices, radiation facilities, ambulatory surgery centers (ASCs), and pathology laboratories to identify and report cases to the central registry. The population-based registry has a responsibility to ensure that all cases of cancer have been identified and reported to the central registry.

Data Collection for the Cancer Registry

Data collection methods vary between facility-based registries and population-based registries. When a case is first entered in the registry, an **accession number** is assigned. This number consists of the first digits of the year the patient was first seen at the facility, and the remaining digits are assigned sequentially throughout the year. The accession number may be assigned manually or by the automated cancer database used by the organization. An **accession registry** of all cases can be kept manually or provided as a report by the database software. This listing of patients in accession number order provides a way to monitor that all cases have been entered into the registry.

In a facility-based registry, data are initially obtained by reviewing and collecting them from the patient's health record. Figure 12.1 shows an example of a data collection screen. In addition to **demographic information** (such as name, health record number, address), data in the registry about the patient include:

- Type and site of the cancer
- Diagnostic methodologies
- Treatment methodologies
- Stage at the time of diagnosis

The stage provides information on the size and spread of the tumor throughout the body. Historically, there have been several **staging systems** used. The American Joint Committee on Cancer (AJCC) has worked through its Collaborative Stage Task Force with other organizations with staging systems to develop a new standardized staging system, the **Collaborative Stage Data Set.** This new system is to be implemented in 2003 (AJCC 2001). After the initial information is collected at the patient's first encounter, information in the registry is updated periodically through the follow-up process discussed later.

Figure 12.1. Sample Data Collection Screen (IMPATH Cancer Registry™ Software)

Diagnosis Identification   Data Entry Screen from the IMPATH Cancer Registry™ software

C 2001/000001   123456   FULLER, JOHN M

Accession Year   2001

Site / Seq	C619	00	PROSTATE GLAND
Mor ICDO3	8140 / 3	MALIG-PRIMARY	ADENOCARCINOMA/ADENOMA
ICDO3 Flag	0	ORIGINALLY CODED ICD3	
Mor ICDO2	/		

Grade   1   WELL DIFFERENTIATED

Lateral   0   NOT A PAIRED SITE

0   NOT A PAIRED SITE
1   RIGHT: ORIGIN OF PRIMARY
2   LEFT: ORIGIN OF PRIMARY
3   ONLY ONE INVL R/L UNSPEC
4   BILATERL INVOL, LAT ORIGIN UNK
9   PAIRED SITE, LAT UNK: MIDLINE

Confirmation   1   POSITIVE HISTOLOGY

Rpt Src   1

Class   1   1ST DX AND ALL/PART 1ST THPY YOUR HOSP

1st Cnt   01/01/2001   I/O   1   INPATIENT ONLY

1st Pos Bx   01/01/2001   Admit   01/01/2001   Discharge   01/01/2001

Init Dx   01/01/2001

Prim Payer   31   MEDICAID

Family Hx   0   NO   Tobacco Hx   0   NEVER USED

Marital   2   MARRIED   Alcohol Hx   0   NO HISTORY ALCOHOL USE

Page Forward   Page Backward   QANote   Suspense   Record   Exit

245

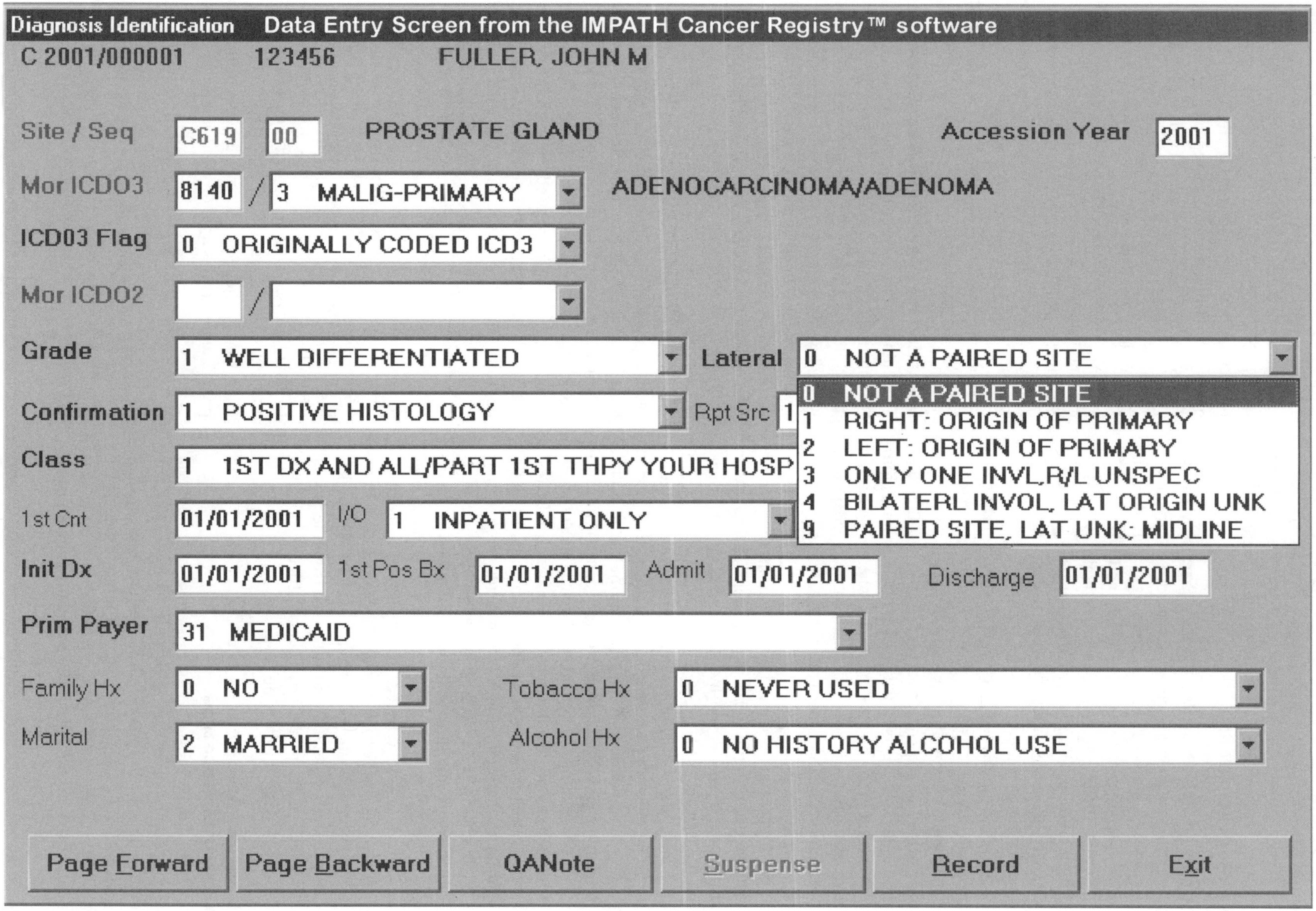

Frequently, the population-based registry only collects information when the patient is diagnosed. Sometimes, however, it receives follow-up information from its reporting entities. These entities usually submit the information to the central registry electronically.

Reporting and Follow-up for Cancer Registry Data

Formal reporting of cancer registry data is done through an annual report. The annual report includes aggregate data on the number of cases in the past year by site and type of cancer. It also may include information on patients by gender, age, and ethnic group. Often a particular site or type of cancer is featured with more in-depth data provided. Figure 12.2 shows an example of a cancer registry report.

Other reports are provided as needed. Data from the cancer registry are frequently used in the quality assessment process for a facility as well as in research.

Another activity of the cancer registry is patient follow-up. On an annual basis, the registry attempts to obtain information about each patient in the registry, including whether he or she is still alive, status of the cancer, and treatment received during the period. Various methods are used to obtain this information. For a facility-based registry, the facility's patient health records may be checked for return hospitalizations or visits for treatment. The patient's physician may be contacted to determine whether the patient is still living and to obtain information about the cancer.

When patient status cannot be determined through these methods, an attempt may be made to contact the patient directly using information in the registry such as address and telephone number of the patient and other contacts. In addition, contact information from the patient's health record may be used to request information from the patient's relatives. Other methods used include reading newspaper obituaries for deaths and using the Internet to locate patients through sites such as the Social Security Death Index and online telephone books. The information obtained through follow-up is important to allow the registry to develop statistics on survival rates for particular cancers and different treatment methodologies.

Population-based registries do not always include follow-up information on the patients in their databases. Those that do, however, usually receive the information from the reporting entities such as hospitals, physicians' offices, and other organizations providing follow-up care.

Standards and Agencies in the Approval Processes

Several organizations have developed standards or approval processes for cancer programs. (See table 12.1, p. 248.) The American College of Surgeons (ACS) Commission on Cancer has an approval process for cancer programs. One of the requirements of this process is the existence of a cancer registry as part of the program. The ACS standards are published in the *Standards of the Commission on Cancer Volume I: Cancer Program Standards and Volume II: Registry Operation and Data Standards* (ROADS). When the ACS surveys the cancer program, part of the survey process is a review of cancer registry activities.

The North American Association of Central Cancer Registries (NAACCR) has a certification program for state population-based registries. Certification is based on the quality of data collected and reported by the state registry. The NAACCR has developed standards for data quality and format and works with other cancer organizations to align their various standards sets.

The Centers for Disease Control and Prevention (CDC) also has national standards regarding completeness, timeliness, and quality of cancer registry data from state registries through the National Program of Cancer Registries (NPCR). The NPCR was developed as a result of the Cancer Registries Amendment Act of 1992. The CDC collects data from the NCPR state registries.

Education and Certification for Cancer Registrars

Traditionally, cancer registrars have been trained through on-the-job training and professional workshops and seminars. The National Cancer Registrars Association (NCRA) has worked with colleges to develop formal educational programs for cancer registrars. A cancer registrar may become certified as a certified cancer registrar (CTR) by passing an examination provided by the National Board for Certification of Registrars (NBCR).

Trauma Registries

Trauma registries maintain databases on patients with severe traumatic injuries. A **traumatic injury** is a wound caused by an external physical force such as an automobile accident, a shooting, a stabbing, or a fall. Information collected by the trauma registry may be used for performance improvement and research in the area of trauma care. Trauma registries may be facility based or may include data for a region or state.

Case Definition and Case Finding for Trauma Registries

The case definition for the trauma registry varies from registry to registry but frequently involves the inclusion of cases with diagnoses from ICD-9-CM sections 800 through 959, the trauma diagnosis codes. To find cases with trauma diagnoses, the trauma registrar may access the disease indexes looking for cases with codes in this section of ICD-9-CM. In addition, the registrar may look at deaths in services with frequent trauma diagnoses such as trauma, neurosurgery, orthopedics, and plastic surgery to find additional cases.

Data Collection for Trauma Registries

After the cases have been identified, information is abstracted from the health records of the injured patients and entered into the trauma registry database. The data elements collected in the abstracting process vary from registry to registry but usually include:

- Demographic information on the patient
- Information on the injury

Figure 12.2. Sample Cancer Registry Report (IMPATH Cancer Registry™ Software)

RPT 30 FREQUENCY REPORT - BODY SYSTEM FORMAT   PAGE 1
National Composite   SUMMARY BY LOCATION/SEX/CLASS/STATUS/AJCC   RUN-DATE 05/08/2002
CIRF: CASES ACCESSIONED IN 2000

| PRIMARY SITE | TOTAL | PERC | SEX | | CLASS OF CASE | | ALIVE | EXP | AJCC STAGE/ANALYTIC ONLY | | | | | | | |
			M	F	ANALY	N-ANALY			00	01	02	03	04	99	88	B/B
LIP	245	.2	174	71	245	0	227	18	12	165	20	2	14	30	2	0
TONGUE	909	.6	619	290	909	0	720	189	24	181	113	159	372	53	7	0
SALIVARY GLANDS	409	.3	226	183	409	0	552	57	0	203	34	24	111	22	15	0
FLOOR OF MOUTH	240	.2	163	77	240	0	185	55	15	59	44	23	84	14	1	0
GUM & OTHER MOUTH	517	.3	263	254	517	0	413	104	26	119	106	58	154	37	17	0
NASOPHARYNX	203	.1	144	59	203	0	168	35	0	14	41	36	82	23	7	0
TONSIL	505	.3	398	107	505	0	426	79	8	37	57	123	254	23	3	0
OROPHARYNX	172	.1	124	48	172	0	131	41	1	21	15	35	81	16	3	0
HYPOPHARYNX	311	.2	248	63	311	0	208	103	4	11	37	66	170	21	2	0
OTHER BUCCAL CAV & PHAR	83	.1	58	25	83	0	49	34	0	6	15	13	32	14	3	0
BUCCAL CAV & PHARYNX	3594	2.4	2417	1177	3594	0	2879	715	90	816	482	539	1354	253	60	0
ESOPHAGUS	1725	1.2	1342	383	1725	0	811	914	45	168	340	280	452	405	35	0
STOMACH	2257	1.5	1443	814	2257	0	1116	1141	33	342	218	383	725	387	169	0
SMALL INTESTINE	0	.0	0	0	0	0	0	0	0	0	0	0	0	0	0	0
CECUM	2854	1.9	1266	1588	2854	0	2166	688	170	598	723	698	479	146	40	0
APPENDIX	172	.1	86	86	172	0	142	30	2	17	33	15	38	5	62	1
ASCENDING COLON	2266	1.5	1064	1202	2266	0	1758	508	147	432	682	535	321	133	16	0
HEPATIC FLEXURE	664	.4	338	326	664	0	525	139	44	140	211	130	84	49	6	0
TRANSVERSE COLON	1123	.8	537	586	1123	0	861	262	65	234	348	239	173	52	12	0
SPLENIC FLEXURE	461	.3	256	205	461	0	335	126	20	73	142	110	80	32	4	0
DESCENDING COLON	732	.5	426	306	732	0	599	133	69	155	207	149	101	47	4	0
SIGMOID COLON	3925	2.6	2155	1770	3925	0	3314	611	458	972	905	759	532	275	24	0
LARGE INTESTINE, NOS	817	.5	446	371	817	0	559	258	81	133	121	125	213	125	19	0
COLON, EXCL RECTUM	13014	8.7	6574	6440	13014	0	10259	2755	1056	2754	3372	2760	2021	864	187	1
RECTOSIGMOID JUNCTION	1620	1.1	907	713	1620	0	1330	290	106	373	362	401	247	118	13	0
RECTUM	3854	2.6	2240	1614	3854	0	3293	561	342	1069	693	720	391	476	163	0
RECTUM & RECTOSIGMOID	5474	3.7	3147	2327	5474	0	4623	851	448	1442	1055	1121	638	594	176	0
ANUS, ANAL CANAL, ANORECT	535	.4	212	323	535	0	453	72	66	100	178	78	19	80	14	0
LIVER	1106	.7	825	281	1106	0	432	674	1	43	85	233	426	261	57	0
INTRAHEPATIC BILE DUCT	229	.2	118	111	229	0	78	151	1	8	13	34	64	94	15	0
LIVER & INTRAHEPATIC BI	1335	.9	943	392	1135	0	510	825	2	51	98	267	490	355	72	0
GALLBLADDER	0	.0	0	0	0	0	0	0	0	0	0	0	0	0	0	0
OTHER BILIARY	0	.0	0	0	0	0	0	0	0	0	0	0	0	0	0	0
PANCREAS	3156	2.1	1645	1511	3156	0	904	2252	16	241	243	329	1699	499	129	2
RETROPERITONEUM	0	.0	0	0	0	0	0	0	0	0	0	0	0	0	0	0
PERITONEUM, OMENTUM, MESE	0	.0	0	0	0	0	0	0	0	0	0	0	0	0	0	0
OTHER DIGESTIVE ORGANS	0	.0	0	0	0	0	0	0	0	0	0	0	0	0	0	0
DIGESTIVE SYSTEM	27496	18.4	15306	12190	27496	0	18686	8810	1666	5098	5504	5218	6044	3184	782	3

Table 12.1.   Standard-Setting or Approval Agencies for Cancer Registries

Agency	Type of Registry
American College of Surgeons (ACS)	Facility based
North American Association of Central Cancer Registries (NAACCR)	Population based
Centers for Disease Control and Prevention	Population based

- Care the patient received before hospitalization (such as care at another transferring hospital or care from an emergency medical technician who provided care at the scene of the accident and/or in transport from the accident site to the hospital)
- Status of the patient at the time of admission
- Patient's course in the hospital
- ICD-9-CM diagnosis and procedure codes
- Abbreviated Injury Scale
- Injury Severity Score

The **Abbreviated Injury Scale** (AIS) reflects the nature of the injury and the severity by body system. It may be assigned manually by the registrar or generated as part of the database from data entered by the registrar. The **Injury Severity Score** (ISS) is an overall severity measurement calculated from the AIS scores for the three most severe injuries of the patient (Chidley 2000, p. 23).

Reporting and Follow-up for Trauma Registries

Reporting varies among trauma registries. An annual report is often developed to show the activity of the trauma registry. Other reports may be generated as part of the performance improvement process, such as self-extubation (patients removing their own tubes) and delays in abdominal surgery or patient complications.

Trauma registries may or may not do follow-up of the patients entered in the registry. When follow-up is done, emphasis is frequently on the patient's quality of life after a period of time. Unlike cancer, where physician follow-up is crucial to detect recurrence, many traumatic injuries do not require continued patient care over time. Thus, follow-up is often not given the emphasis it receives in cancer registries.

Standards and Agencies for Approval of Trauma Registries

The American College of Surgeons (ACS) certifies levels I, II, III, and IV trauma centers. As part of its certification requirements, the ACS states that the level I trauma center must have a trauma registry (Garthe 1997, p. 26).

Education and Certification of Trauma Registrars

Trauma registrars may be registered health information technicians (RHITs), registered health information administrators (RHIAs), registered nurses (RNs), licensed practical nurses (LPNs), emergency medical technicians (EMTs), or other health professionals. Training for trauma registrars is accomplished through workshops and on-the-job training. The American Trauma Society (ATS), for example, provides core and advanced workshops for trauma registrars. It also provides a certification examination for trauma registrars through its Registrar Certification Board. Certified trauma registrars have earned the credential CSTR (certified specialist trauma registry).

Birth Defects Registries

Birth defects registries collect information on newborns with birth defects. Often population based, these registries serve a variety of purposes. For example, they provide information on the incidence of birth defects for the study of causes and prevention of birth defects, monitor trends in birth defects to improve medical care for children with birth defects, and target interventions for preventable birth defects such as folic acid to prevent neural tube defects.

In some cases, registries have been developed after specific events have put a spotlight on birth defects. After the Persian Gulf War, for example, some feared an increased incidence of birth defects among the children of Gulf War veterans. The Department of Defense subsequently started a birth defects registry to collect data on the children of these veterans to determine whether any pattern could be detected.

Case Definition and Case Finding for Birth Defects Registries

Birth defects registries use a variety of criteria to determine which cases to include in the registry. Some registries limit cases to those found within the first year of life. Others include those with a major defect that occurred in the first year of life and was discovered within the first five years of life. Still other registries include only children who were liveborn or stillborn babies with discernible birth defects.

Cases may be detected in a variety of ways, including review of disease indexes, labor and delivery logs, pathology and autopsy reports, ultrasound reports, and cytogenetic reports. In addition to information from hospitals and physicians, cases may be identified from rehabilitation centers and children's hospitals and from vital records such as birth, death, and fetal death certificates.

Data Collection for Birth Defects Registries

A variety of information is abstracted for the birth defects registry, including:

- Demographic information
- Codes for diagnoses
- Birth weight
- Status at birth, including liveborn, stillborn, aborted
- Autopsy
- Cytogenetics results
- Whether the infant was a single or multiple birth
- Mother's use of alcohol, tobacco, or illicit drugs
- Father's use of drugs and alcohol
- Family history of birth defects

Diabetes Registries

Diabetes registries collect data about patients with diabetes for the purpose of assistance in managing care as well as for research. Patients whose diabetes is not kept under good control frequently have numerous complications. The diabetes registry can keep up with whether the patient has been seen by a physician in an effort to prevent complications.

Case Definition and Case Finding for Diabetes Registries

There are two types of diabetes mellitus: insulin-dependent diabetes (type I) and non–insulin-dependent diabetes (type II). Registries sometimes limit their cases by type of diabetes. In some instances, there may be further definition by age. Some diabetes registries, for example, only include children with diabetes.

Case finding includes the review of health records of patients with diabetes. Other case-finding methods include the reviews of the following types of information:

- ICD-9-CM diagnostic codes
- Billing data
- Medication lists
- Physician identification
- Health plans

Although facility-based registries for cancer and trauma are usually hospital based, facility-based diabetes registries are often maintained by physicians' offices and clinics. The office or clinic is the main location for diabetes care. Thus, the data about the patient to be entered into the registry are available at these sites rather than at the hospital. Patient health records of diabetes patients in the physician practice may be identified through ICD-9-CM code numbers for diabetes, billing data for diabetes-related services, medication lists for patients on diabetic medications, or identification of patients as the physician sees them.

Health plans also are interested in optimal care for their enrollees because diabetes can have serious complications when not managed correctly. They may provide information to the office or clinic on enrollees in the health plan who are diabetics.

Data Collection for Diabetes Registries

In addition to demographic information about the cases, other data collected may include laboratory values such as HBA1c. This test is used to determine the patient's blood glucose for a period of approximately sixty days prior to the time of the test. Moreover, facility registries may track patient visits to follow up with patients who have not been seen in the past year.

Reporting and Follow-up for Diabetes Registries

A variety of reports may be developed from the diabetes registry. For facility-based registries, one report may keep up with laboratory monitoring of the patient's diabetes to allow intensive intervention with patients whose diabetes is not well controlled. Another report might be of patients who have not been tested within a year or have not had a primary care provider visit within a year.

Population-based diabetes registries might provide reporting on the incidence of diabetes for the geographic area covered by the registry. Registry data also may be used to investigate risk factors for diabetes.

Follow-up is aimed primarily at ensuring that the diabetic is seen by the physician at appropriate intervals to prevent complications.

Implant Registries

An implant is a material or substance inserted in the body, such as breast implants, heart valves, and pacemakers. Implant registries have been developed for the purpose of tracking the performance of implants, including complications, deaths, and defects resulting from implants, as well as longevity.

In the recent past, the safety of implants has been questioned in a number of highly publicized cases. In some cases, implant registries have been developed in response to such events. For example, there have been questions about the safety of silicone breast implants and temporomandibular joint implants. When such cases arise, it has often been difficult to ensure that all patients with the implant have been notified of safety questions. At one time, there was a national implant registry, but it was halted after several years because of minimal participation (Shelton 2001). It was felt that the legal implications of problem implants have prevented more interest in implant registries.

A number of federal laws have been enacted to regulate medical devices, including implants. These devices were first covered under Section 15 of the Food, Drug and Cosmetic Act. The Safe Medical Devices Act of 1990 was passed and then amended through the Medical Device Amendments of 1995. These acts required facilities to report deaths and severe complications thought to be due to a device to the manufacturer and the **Food and Drug Administration** (FDA). The 1995 Medical Device Amendments changed that requirement so that only a selected subset of user facilities would be required to report. Implant registries can help in complying with the legal requirement for reporting for the sample of facilities required to report.

Case Definition and Case Finding for Implant Registries

Implant registries sometimes include all types of implants but often are restricted to a specific type of implant such as cochlear, saline breast, or temporomandibular joint.

Data Collection for Implant Registries

Demographic data on patients receiving the implant are included in the registry. The FDA requires that all reportable events involving medical devices include information on the following (Center for Devices and Radiological Health 1996, p. 4):

- User facility report number
- Name and address of the device manufacturer
- Device brand name and common name
- Product model, catalog, and serial and lot number
- Brief description of the event reported to the manufacturer and/or the FDA

- Where the report was submitted (for example, to the FDA, manufacturer, or distributor)

Thus, these data items also should be included in the implant registry to facilitate reporting.

Reporting and Follow-up for Implant Registries

Data from the implant registry may be used to report to the FDA and the manufacturer when devices cause death or serious illness or injury. Follow-up is important to track the performance of the implant. When patients are tracked, they can be easily notified of product failures, recalls, or upgrades (Shelton 2001).

Transplant Registries

Transplant registries may have varied purposes. Some organ transplant registries maintain databases of patients who need organs. When an organ becomes available, a fair way then may be used to allocate the organ to the patient with the highest priority. In other cases, the purpose of the registry is to provide a database of potential donors for transplants using live donors, such as bone marrow transplants. Posttransplant information also is kept on organ recipients and donors.

Because transplant registries are used to try to match donor organs with recipients, they are often national or even international in scope. Examples of national registries include the Scientific Registry of the United Network for Organ Sharing (UNOS) and the registry of the National Marrow Donor Program (NMDP).

Data collected in the transplant registry also may be used for research, policy analysis, and quality control projects.

Case Definition and Case Finding for Transplant Registries

Physicians identify patients needing transplants. Information about the patient is provided to the registry. When an organ becomes available, information about it is matched with potential donors. For donor registries, donors are solicited through community information efforts similar to those carried out by blood banks to encourage blood donations.

Data Collection for Transplant Registries

The type of information collected varies according to the type of registry. Pretransplant data about the recipient include:

- Demographic data
- Patient's diagnosis
- Patient's status codes regarding medical urgency
- Patient's functional status
- Whether the patient is on life support
- Previous transplantations
- **Histocompatibility**

Information on donors varies according to whether the donor is living. For organs harvested from patients who have died, information is collected on:

- Cause and circumstances of the death
- Organ procurement and consent process

- Medications the donor was taking
- Other donor history

For a living donor, information includes:

- Relationship of the donor to the recipient (if any)
- Clinical information
- Information on organ recovery
- Histocompatibility

Reporting and Follow-up for Transplant Registries

Reporting includes information on donors and recipients as well as survival rates, length of time on the waiting list for an organ, and death rates. Follow-up information is collected for recipients as well as living donors. For living donors, the information collected might include complications of the procedure and length of stay in the hospital. Follow-up on recipients includes information on status at the time of follow-up (for example, living, dead, lost to follow-up), functional status, graft status, and treatment, such as immunosuppressive drugs. Follow-up is carried out at intervals throughout the first year after the transplant and then annually after that.

Immunization Registries

According to All Kids Count, an effort funded by the Robert Wood Johnson Foundation to encourage the development and operation of immunization registries, children are supposed to receive between eighteen and twenty-two immunizations during the first six years of life (All Kids Count 2001). These immunizations are so important that the federal government has set several objectives related to immunizations in Healthy People 2010, a set of health goals for the nation. These include increasing the proportion of children and adolescents that are fully immunized (Objective 14-24) and increasing the proportion of children in population-based immunization registries (Objective 14-26).

Immunization registries usually have the purpose of increasing the number of infants and children that receive proper immunizations at the proper intervals. To accomplish this goal, they collect information within a particular geographic area on children and their immunization status. They also help by maintaining a central source of information for a particular child's immunization history, even when the child has received immunizations from a variety of providers. This central location for immunization data also relieves parents of the responsibility of maintaining immunization records for their own children.

Case Definition and Case Finding for Immunization Registries

All children in the population area served by the registry should be included in the registry. Some registries limit their inclusion of patients to those seen at public clinics, excluding those seen exclusively by private practitioners. Although children are usually targeted in immunization registries, some registries do include information on adults for influenza and pneumonia vaccines.

Children are often entered in the registry at birth. Registry personnel may review birth and death certificates and adoption records to determine what children to include and what children to exclude because they died after birth. In some cases, children are entered electronically through a connection with an electronic birth record system.

Data Collection for Immunization Registries

The National Immunization Program at the CDC has worked with the **National Vaccine Advisory Committee** (NVAC) to develop a set of core immunization data elements to be included in all immunization registries. These data elements include (CDC National Immunization Program 2001):

- Patient's name (first, middle, and last)
- Patient's birth date
- Patient's sex
- Patient's birth state/country
- Mother's name (first, middle, last, and maiden)
- Vaccine type
- Vaccine manufacturer
- Vaccination date
- Vaccine lot number

Other items may be included, as needed, by the individual registry.

Reporting and Follow-up for Immunization Registries

Because the purpose of the immunization registry is to improve the number of children who receive immunizations in a timely manner, reporting should emphasize immunization rates, especially changes in rates in target areas. According to All Kids Count, immunization registries also can provide automatic reporting of children's immunization to schools to check the immunization status of their students (All Kids Count 2001).

Follow-up is directed toward reminding parents that it is time for immunizations as well as seeing whether the parents do not bring the child in for the immunization after a reminder. Reminders may include a letter or postcard or telephone calls. **Autodialing systems** may be used to call parents and deliver a prerecorded reminder. Moreover, registries must decide how frequently to follow up with parents who do not bring their children for immunization. Maintaining up-to-date addresses and telephone numbers is an important factor in providing follow-up. Registries may allow parents to opt out of the registry if they prefer not to be reminded.

Standards and Agencies for Approval of Immunization Registries

The CDC, through its National Immunization Program, provides funding for some population-based immunization registries. The CDC has identified twelve minimum functional standards for immunization registries (CDC National Immunization Program 2001), including:

- Electronically store data on all NVAC-approved core data elements.
- Establish a registry record within six weeks of birth for each newborn child born in the catchment area.
- Enable access to and retrieval of immunization information in the registry at the time of the encounter.
- Receive and process immunization information within one month of vaccine administration.
- Protect the confidentiality of healthcare information.
- Ensure the security of healthcare information.
- Exchange immunization records using Health Level Seven (HL7) standards.
- Automatically determine the routine childhood immunization(s) needed, in compliance with current ACIP [Advisory Committee on Immunization Practices] recommendations, when an individual presents for a scheduled immunization.
- Automatically identify individuals due/late for immunization(s) to enable the production of reminder/recall notifications.
- Automatically produce immunization coverage reports by providers, age groups, and geographic areas.
- Produce official immunization records.
- Promote the accuracy and completeness of registry data.

It has been proposed that CDC develop a certification program for immunization registries.

Other Registries

Registries may be developed for any type of disease or condition. Other types of registries that are commonly kept include HIV/AIDS and cardiac registries.

In addition, registries may be developed for administrative purposes. The National Provider Registry is an example of an administrative registry. Data collected for healthcare administrative purposes are discussed in the next subsection.

Check Your Understanding 12.3

Instructions: Answer the following questions on a separate piece of paper.

1. What is the difference between an index and a registry?
2. How is case definition different from case finding?
3. What is the difference between a facility-based registry and a population-based registry?

Answer questions 4 through 10 for each of the following registries: cancer, trauma, birth defects, diabetes, implant, transplant, and immunization.

4. What methods are used for case definition and case finding?
5. What methods of data collection are used?
6. What methods of reporting are used?
7. What methods of follow-up are used?
8. What standards are applicable and what agencies approve or accredit the registry?
9. What education is required for registrars?
10. What certification is available for registrars; what agency/organization provides certification, and what are the certification requirements?

Healthcare Databases

Databases also may be developed for a variety of purposes. The federal government, for example, has developed a wide variety of databases to enable it to carry out surveillance, improvement, and prevention duties. Health information managers may provide information for these databases through data abstraction or from data reported by a facility to state and local entities. They also may use these data to do research or work with other researchers on issues related to reimbursement and health status.

National Administrative Databases

Some databases are established for administrative rather than disease-oriented reasons. Data banks are developed, for example, for **claims** data submitted on Medicare claims. Other administrative databases assist in the **credentialing** and privileging of health practitioners.

Medicare Provider Analysis and Review File

The Medicare Provider Analysis and Review (MEDPAR) File is made up of acute care hospital and skilled nursing facility (SNF) claims data for all Medicare claims. It consists of the following types of data:

- Demographic data on the patient
- Data on the provider
- Information on Medicare coverage for the claim
- Total charges
- Charges broken down by specific types of services, such as operating room, physical therapy, and pharmacy charges
- ICD-9-CM diagnosis and procedure codes
- DRGs

The MEDPAR file is frequently used for research on topics such as charges for particular types of care and analysis by DRG. The limitation of the MEDPAR data for research purposes is that it only contains data about Medicare patients.

National Practitioner Data Bank

The **National Practitioner Data Bank** (NPDB) was mandated under the Health Care Quality Improvement Act of 1986 to provide a database of medical malpractice payments, sanctions taken by boards of medical examiners, and certain professional review actions (such as denial of medical staff privileges) taken by healthcare entities such as hospitals against physicians, dentists, and other healthcare providers. The problem that the NPDB was developed to alleviate was the lack of information on malpractice decisions, denial of medical staff privileges, or loss of medical license. Because these data were not widely available, physicians could move to another state or another facility and begin practicing again with the current state and/or facility unaware of the previous actions against the physician.

Information in the NPDB is provided through a required reporting mechanism. Entities making malpractice payments, including insurance companies, boards of medical examiners, and entities such as hospitals and professional societies must report to the NPDB. The information to be reported includes information on the practitioner, the reporting entity, and the judgment or settlement. Information on physicians must be reported, but information on other healthcare providers, though not mandatory, also will be accepted. Monetary penalties may be assessed for failure to report.

The law requires healthcare facilities to query the NPDB as part of the credentialing process when a physician initially applies for medical staff privileges and every two years thereafter.

Healthcare Integrity and Protection Data Bank

Part of the Health Insurance Portability and Accountability Act of 1996 (HIPAA) mandated the collection of information on healthcare fraud and abuse because there was no central place to obtain this information. As a result, the national **Healthcare Integrity and Protection Data Bank** (HIPDB) was developed. The types of items that must be reported to the data bank include reportable final adverse actions such as:

Actions related to provider, supplier, and practitioner practices that are inconsistent with accepted sound fiscal, business or medical practices, directly or indirectly resulting in: (1) unnecessary costs to the program; (2) improper payment; (3) services that fail to meet professionally recognized standards of care or that are medically unnecessary; or (4) adverse patient outcomes, failure to provide covered or needed care in violation of contractual arrangements, or delays in diagnosis or treatment (Office of Inspector General 1998, pp. 58341–58342).

These would include federal or state criminal convictions related to the delivery of healthcare, civil judgments related to the delivery of healthcare, exclusions from participation in federal or state healthcare programs such as Medicare and Medicaid, and other adjudicated actions or decisions. Civil judgments resulting in malpractice payments are not included because they are incorporated in the NPDB. There may be some overlap with the Healthcare Practitioner Data Bank, so a single report is made and then sorted to the appropriate data bank.

Information to be reported includes information on the healthcare provider, supplier, or practitioner that is the subject of the final adverse action, the nature of the act, and a description of the actions on which the decision was based. Only federal and state government agencies and health plans are required to report, and access to the data bank is limited to these organizations and to practitioners, providers, and suppliers who may only query about themselves.

National, State, and County Public Health Databases

Public health is the area of healthcare dealing with the health of populations in geographic areas such as states or counties. One of the duties of public health agencies is the surveillance of health status within their jurisdiction.

Databases developed by public health departments provide information on the incidence and prevalence of diseases, possible high-risk populations, survival statistics, and trends over time. Data for these databases may be collected using a variety of methods including interviews, physical examination of individuals, and review of health records. At the national level, the National Center for Health Statistics has responsibility for these databases.

National Health Care Survey

One of the major national public health surveys is the **National Health Care Survey.** To a large extent, it relies on data from patient health records. It consists of a number of databases, including:

- The National Discharge Survey
- The National Ambulatory Medical Care Survey
- The National Nursing Home Survey
- The National Health Provider Inventory
- The National Survey of Ambulatory Surgery
- The National Hospital Ambulatory Medical Care Survey
- The National Home and Hospice Care Survey
- The National Employer Health Insurance Survey

Table 12.2 lists the component databases of the National Health Care Survey, along with their corresponding data sources.

Data in the National Discharge Survey are abstracted manually from a sample of acute care hospitals or from discharged inpatient records or are obtained from state or other discharge databases. Items collected follow the Uniform Hospital Discharge Data Set (UHDDS), including demographic data, admission and discharge dates, and final diagnoses and procedures.

Table 12.2.   Databases Included in the National Health Care Survey

Database	Data Source
National Discharge Survey	Abstracted discharged patient records
	State discharge databases
National Ambulatory Medical Care Survey	Office-based physician records
National Nursing Home Survey	Interview with administrator
	Interview with nurse caregiver
National Health Provider Inventory	Facility inventory
National Survey of Ambulatory Surgery	Abstracts of ASC records
National Hospital Ambulatory Medical Care Survey	Abstracts of hospital emergency department and outpatient clinic records
National Home and Hospice Care Survey	Interview with administrator
	Interview with caregiver
National Employer Health Insurance Survey	Data on employer health insurance plans

The National Ambulatory Medical Care Survey includes data collected by a sample of office-based physicians and their staffs from the records of patients seen in a one-week reporting period. Data included are demographic data, the patient's reason for visit, the diagnoses, diagnostic/screening services, therapeutic and preventive services, ambulatory surgical procedures, and medications/injections, in addition to information on the visit disposition and time spent with the physician.

The National Nursing Home Survey provides data on the facility, current residents, and discharged residents. Information is gathered through an interview process. The administrator or designee provides information about the facility. For information on the residents, the nursing staff member most familiar with the resident's care is interviewed. The staff member uses the resident's health record for reference in the interview. Data collected on the facility includes information on ownership, size, certification status, admissions, services, full-time equivalent employees, and basic charges. Both the current and discharged resident interviews provide demographic information on the resident as well as length of stay, diagnoses, level of care received, **activities of daily living,** and charges.

In the past, data have been collected on nursing homes and board and care homes as well as home health agencies and hospices for the National Provider Inventory. This was an inventory of these facilities, not a sample. For home health agencies and hospices, data included the number of current and discharged clients, services provided, and state and county FIPS codes. (Federal information processing standards codes are uniform geographic codes issued by the National Institute of Standards and Technology.) For nursing homes and board and care homes, information includes ownership, number of beds and residents, resident ages, as well as sex of residents and state and county FIPS codes.

The National Survey of Ambulatory Surgery collects data on freestanding and hospital-based ambulatory surgery centers. Data are abstracted from the patient health records of ambulatory surgery patients, and data elements include most of the UHDDS data items included in the National Discharge Survey. Elements included are patient demographic data, payment data, information about the surgical visit, and the final diagnoses and procedures.

Data for the National Hospital Ambulatory Medical Care Survey are collected on patient visits to hospital-based emergency departments and outpatient clinics. Information is obtained through an abstracting process from the patient health record. Different abstracting forms are used for the emergency department records and the outpatient clinics. The emergency department abstract includes demographic data on the patient, expected source of payment, how soon the patient should be seen, the patient's complaints or reason for visit, diagnoses, diagnostic/screening services, procedures, medications/injections, providers seen, and visit disposition. The outpatient department abstract includes similar information. Facility personnel do the abstracting.

For the National Home and Hospice Care Survey, data are collected on the home health or hospice agency as well as on their current and discharged patients. For the facility, data collected include the agency identifier, the number of current patients, type of ownership, certification status (for example, Medicare or Medicaid), number of staff, and services available. For current and discharged patients, data include patient demographic information, current living arrangements, source of referral, diagnoses, type of care received, primary caregiver, vision and hearing status, activities of daily living, and expected sources of payment. Facility data are obtained through an interview with the administrator or designee. Patient information is obtained from the caregiver who is most familiar with the patient's care. The caregiver may use the patient's health record in answering the interview questions.

The National Employer Health Insurance Survey includes data on health insurance plans sponsored by employers, including businesses, governments, and self-employed individuals with no employees.

Other national public health databases include the National Health Interview Survey and the National Immunization Survey.

State and local public health departments also develop databases, as needed, to perform their duties of health surveillance, disease prevention, and research. An example of a state database is infectious/notifiable disease databases. Each state has a list of diseases that must be reported to the state, such as AIDS, measles, and syphilis, so that containment and prevention measures may be taken to avoid large outbreaks of these diseases. As mentioned previously, there also may be statewide databases/registries that collect extensive information on particular diseases and conditions such as birth defects, immunization, and cancer registries.

Vital Statistics

Vital statistics include data on births, deaths, fetal deaths, marriages, and divorces. Responsibility for the collection of vital statistics rests with the states. The states share information with the National Center for Health Statistics (NCHS). The actual collection of the information is carried out at the local level. For example, birth certificates are completed at the facility where the birth occurred. They are then sent to the state. The state serves as the official repository for the certificates and provides vital statistics information to the NCHS. From the vital statistics collected, states and the national government develop a variety of databases.

One database at the national level is the Linked Birth and Infant Death Data Set. In this database, the information from birth certificates is compared to death certificates for infants under one year of age who die. This database provides data to conduct analyses for patterns of infant death. Other national programs that use vital statistics data include the National Maternal and Infant Health Survey, the National

Mortality Followback Survey, the National Survey of Family Growth, and the National Death Index (CDC National Center for Health Statistics 2001). In some of these databases, such as the National Maternal and Infant Health Survey and the National Mortality Followback Survey, additional information is collected on deaths originally identified through the vital statistics system.

Similar databases using vital statistics data as a basis are found at the state level. Birth defects registries, for example, frequently use vital records data with information on the birth defect as part of their data collection process.

Clinical Trials

A **clinical trial** is a research project in which new treatments and tests are investigated to determine whether they are safe and effective. The trial proceeds according to a protocol. A **protocol** is the list of rules and procedures to be followed. Clinical trials databases have been developed to allow physicians and patients to find clinical trials. A patient with cancer or AIDS, for example, might be interested in participating in a clinical trial but not know how to locate one applicable to his or her type of disease. Clinical trials databases provide the data to enable patients and practitioners to determine what clinical trials are available and applicable to the patient.

The Food and Drug Administration Modernization Act of 1997 mandated that a clinical trials database be developed. The National Library of Medicine has developed the database, called ClinicalTrials.gov, which is available on the Internet for use by both patients and practitioners (NLM 2001). Information in the database includes:

- Study identification number
- Study sponsor
- Brief title
- Brief summary
- Location of trial
- Recruitment status
- Contact information
- Eligibility criteria
- Study type
- Study design
- Study phase
- Condition
- Intervention
- Data provider
- Date last modified

Each data element has been defined. For example, the study sponsor is the organization carrying out the clinical trial. The brief summary gives an overview of the treatments being studied and types of patients to be included. The location of the trial tells where the trial is being carried out so that patients can select trials in convenient locations. Recruitment status indicates whether subjects are currently being entered in the trial or will be in the future or whether the trial is closed to new subjects. Eligibility criteria include information on the type of condition to be studied, in some cases the stage of the disease, and what other treatments are allowed during the trial or must have been completed before entering the trial. Age is also a frequent eligibility criterion. Study types include diagnostic, genetic, monitoring, natural history, prevention, screening, supportive care, training, and treatment (McCray and Ide 2000, p. 316). Study design includes the research design being followed.

A clinical trial consists of four study phases. Phase I studies research the safety of the treatment in a small group of people. In phase II studies, emphasis is on determining the treatment's effectiveness and further investigating safety. Phase III studies look at effectiveness and side effects and make comparisons to other available treatments in larger populations. Phase IV studies look at the treatment after it has entered the market.

Some clinical trials databases concentrate on a particular disease. The Department of Health and Human Services, for example, has developed ACTIS, the AIDS Clinical Trials Information Service. The National Cancer Institute sponsors PDQ, a database for cancer clinical trials. These databases contain information similar to ClinicalTrials.gov.

Although ClinicalTrials.gov has been set up for use by both patients and health practitioners, some databases are more oriented to practitioners. Moreover, some efforts have been made to develop databases of published articles and proceedings from meetings on the subject of clinical trials. The Cochrane Controlled Trials Register, for example, is a bibliographic database of literature on clinical trials developed by the Cochrane Library, an electronic library.

Health Services Research Databases

Health services research is research concerning healthcare delivery systems, including organization and delivery and care effectiveness and efficiency. Within the federal government, the organization most involved in health services research is the **Agency for Healthcare Research and Quality** (AHRQ). The AHRQ looks at issues related to the efficiency and effectiveness of the healthcare delivery system, disease protocols, and guidelines for improved disease outcomes.

A major initiative for the AHRQ has been the Healthcare Cost and Utilization Project (HCUP). HCUP uses data collected at the state level from either claims data from the UB-92 or discharge-abstracted data, including the Uniform Hospital Discharge Data Set (UHDDS) items reported by individual hospitals and, in some cases, by freestanding ambulatory care centers. Which data are reported depends on the individual state. Data may be reported by the facilities to a state agency or to the state hospital association, depending on state regulations. The data are then reported from the state to the AHRQ where they become part of the HCUP databases.

HCUP consists of a set of databases, including:

- The Nationwide Inpatient Sample (NIS), which consists of inpatient discharge data from a sample of approximately a thousand hospitals throughout the United States
- The State Inpatient Database (SID), which includes data collected by states on hospital discharges
- The State Ambulatory Surgery Database (SASD), which includes information from a sample of states on hospital-affiliated ASCs and, from some states, data from freestanding surgery centers
- The Kids Inpatient Database (KID), which is made up of inpatient discharge data on children younger than nineteen years old

These databases are unique because they include data on inpatients whose care is paid for by all types of payers including Medicare, Medicaid, and private insurance as well as by self-paying and/or uninsured patients. Data elements include demographic information, information on diagnoses and procedures, admission and discharge status, payment sources, total charges, length of stay, and information on the hospital or freestanding ambulatory surgery center. Researchers may use these databases to look at issues such as those related to the costs of treating particular diseases, the extent to which treatments are used, and differences in outcomes and cost for alternative treatments.

National Library of Medicine

The National Library of Medicine produces two databases of special interest to the HIM professional: MEDLINE and UMLS.

Medical Literature, Analysis, and Retrieval System Online

Medical Literature, Analysis, and Retrieval System Online (MEDLINE) is the best-known database from the National Library of Medicine. It includes bibliographic listings for publications in the areas of medicine, dentistry, nursing, pharmacy, allied health, and veterinary medicine. HIM professionals use MEDLINE to locate articles on HIM issues as well as articles on medical topics necessary to carry out quality improvement and medical research activities.

Unified Medical Language System

The Unified Medical Language System (UMLS) provides a way to integrate biomedical concepts from a variety of sources to show their relationships. This process allows links to be made between different information systems for purposes such as the computer-based patient record. The UMLS is of particular interest to the HIM professional because medical classifications such as ICD-9-CM, CPT, and HCPCS (Healthcare Common Procedure Coding System) are among the items included.

Processing and Maintenance of Secondary Databases

Several issues surround the processing and maintenance of secondary databases. Health information professionals are often involved in decisions concerning these issues.

Manual versus Automated Methods of Data Collection

Although registries and databases are almost universally computerized, data collection is commonly done manually. The most frequent method is abstracting. **Abstracting** is the process of reviewing the patient health record and entering the required data elements into the database. In some cases, the abstracting may initially be done on an abstract form. The data then would be entered into the database from the form. In many cases, it is done directly from the primary patient health record into a data collection screen in the computerized database system.

Not all data collection is done manually. In some cases, data can be downloaded directly from other electronic systems. Birth defects registries, for example, often download information on births and birth defects from the vital records system. In some cases, providers such as hospitals and physicians send information in electronic format to the registry or database. The National Discharge Survey from the National Center for Health Statistics uses information in electronic format from state databases.

Vendor Systems versus Facility-Specific Systems

A **vendor system** is an information system developed by an outside company and sold to a variety of organizations. A **facility-specific system** is an information system developed within the facility for its own use.

One clear advantage to using vendor systems is that they have been used at a variety of sites. Thus, the vendor likely has developed expertise in the system based on past experience. When investigating possible systems, purchasers can find out about the performance of vendor systems from other users. As changes in healthcare occur, such as the recent Health Insurance Portability and Accountability Act (HIPAA) privacy and security regulations, it is often easier for a vendor to make the necessary changes because its entire business is related to a limited number of products. In addition, **user groups** are often developed from organizations that have purchased the system and can be helpful in maximizing the system's performance.

One disadvantage to a vendor system is that the vendor may be unable to modify it to meet all of the organization's needs. Moreover, the level of training and problem-solving support varies from vendor to vendor. In some cases, vendors are unavailable to help with system problems after the initial start-up period.

One advantage to a facility-specific system is that it can be developed to meet the specific information needs of the healthcare facility. Because the system's developers are on-site, training and problem solving are always available.

However, if the system is not well documented when it is developed, it will be difficult to sustain maintenance in the event the original developers leave the facility. Moreover, in-house developers may not have the broad experience in the type of product developed that a vendor is likely to have. The ability of facility personnel to undertake the development and maintenance of the system should be considered very carefully before deciding to develop a system in-house.

Data Quality Issues

Indexes, registries, and databases are only helpful when the data they contain are accurate. Decisions concerning new treatment methods, healthcare policy, and physician credentialing and privileging are made based on these databases. Incorrect data will likely result in serious errors in decision making.

Several factors must be addressed when assessing data quality, including data validity, reliability, completeness, and timeliness.

Validity of the Data

Validity refers to the accuracy of the data. For example, in a cancer registry, the **stage of the neoplasm** must be recorded accurately because statistical information on survival rates by stage is commonly reported.

Several methods may be used to ensure validity. One method is to incorporate edits in the database. An **edit** is a check on the accuracy of the data, such as setting data types. When a particular data element, such as admission date, is set up with a data type of date, the computer will not allow other types of data to be entered in that field. Other edits may use comparisons between fields to ensure accuracy. For example, an edit might check to see that all patients with the diagnosis of prostate cancer are listed as males in the database.

Reliability of the Data

Another factor to be considered in looking at data quality is reliability. *Reliability* refers to the consistency of the data. For example, all patients in a trauma registry with the same level, severity, and site of injury should have the same Abbreviated Injury Score. Reliability is frequently checked by having more than one person abstract data for the same case. The results are then compared to identify any discrepancies. This is called an **interrater reliability** method of checking. Several different people may be used to do the checking, for example, a supervisor within the area. In the cancer registry, physician members of the cancer committee are called on to check the reliability of the data.

The use of uniform terminology is an important way to improve data reliability. This has been evident in case definition for registries. The criteria for including a patient in a registry must have a clear definition. Definitions for terms such as *race,* for example, must include the categories to be used in determining race. When uniform terms are not used, the data will not be consistent. Also, it will be impossible to make comparisons between systems when uniform terms have not been used for all data. A data dictionary in which all data elements are defined helps ensure that uniform data definitions are being followed.

Completeness of the Data

Completeness is another factor to be considered in data quality. Missing data may prevent the database from being useful for research or clinical decision making. To avoid missing data, some databases will not allow the user to move to the next field without making an entry in the current one, especially for fields considered crucial. Looking at a variety of sources in case finding is one way to avoid omitting patients who should be included in a registry.

Timeliness of the Data

Another concept important in data quality is timeliness. Data must be available within a time frame helpful to the user. Factors that influence decisions may change over time, so it is important that the data reflect up-to-date information.

Data Security and Confidentiality Issues

Data security usually refers to efforts to control access to health information. **Data confidentiality** usually refers to efforts to guarantee the privacy of personal health information.

Data Security

A number of methods may be used to ensure that only authorized people have access to patient data in the facility's computer system. One common method is the use of passwords. Other methods may involve using retinal scans or fingerprints. Tokens such as identification badges also may be used.

Moreover, the facility may establish levels of access to the computer system. In this case, each user would be allowed access to only certain parts of the system. Only those parts of the system to which the users have access appear on the screen. In addition, a record of all transactions in the system, called an **audit trail,** should be maintained and reviewed for instances of unauthorized access.

Loss of data is another important consideration in data security. Although data sometimes are lost as a result of unauthorized access, more often they are lost in more routine ways. For example, a computer malfunction can cause data to be erased or lost. Backing up the data on electronic media such as tapes or disks is commonly done to avoid such losses. The backup must be done frequently, and the backup media must be kept away from the site where the main system is kept. Moreover, when the backup is kept on-site, it is vulnerable to destruction affecting the main system from sources such as fire and flood.

Computer viruses constitute yet another threat to data security. These are computer programs that attack systems and reproduce themselves. They may alter or destroy data. Facilities must use antivirus software to combat viruses. Moreover, they must keep the antivirus software up-to-date because new viruses appear regularly.

Physical security of the system is another consideration. Computer terminals must be kept in areas that are not physically accessible to unauthorized people. Reports and printouts from the system should not be left where they can be seen. When they are no longer needed, they should be destroyed.

Finally, it may be necessary for sensitive data to be encrypted. **Encryption** is a method of scrambling data so that they cannot be read without first being decoded. An AIDS registry, for example, might want to use an encryption method to protect patient-identifiable information.

Data Confidentiality

Maintaining the confidentiality of health data is a traditional role of HIM professionals. When looking at methods to protect secondary records, patient-specific information requires more control than aggregate data because individual patients cannot be identified in aggregate data. Policies on who may access the data provide the basic protection for confidentiality.

The type of data maintained also may affect policies on confidentiality. For many of the government databases discussed earlier, the information is aggregate and the data are readily available to any interested users. For example, public health data are frequently published in many formats, including printed reports, Internet access, and direct computer access.

Employees working with the data should receive training on confidentiality. Further, they should be required to sign a yearly statement indicating that they have received the training and understand the implications of failure to maintain confidentiality of the data.

Trends in the Collection of Secondary Data

The main trend in collecting secondary data seems to be the increased use of automated data entry. Registries and databases are more commonly using data already available in electronic form rather than manually abstracting all data. As the computerized health record becomes more common, separate databases for various diseases and conditions such as cancer, diabetes, and trauma will become unnecessary. The patient health record itself will be a database that can be queried for information currently obtained from specialized registries.

Check Your Understanding 12.5

Instructions: Answer the following questions on a separate piece of paper.

1. What factors must be considered when determining the quality of data?
2. Which errors in registries and other secondary databases can cause serious problems?
3. What methods and systems can be used to ensure the quality of secondary healthcare data?
4. What is the difference between security and confidentiality?
5. What methods might be used to control access to a health information system?
6. How can a potential loss of data be avoided?
7. Which factors should be considered when developing a physical security program?
8. What types of data should be encrypted?
9. What methods can be used to ensure data confidentiality?
10. What trends are evident in the collection of secondary data?

Real-World Case

In an article entitled "Benchmarking with National ICD-9-CM Coded Data," Carol Osborn, PhD, RHIA (1999, p. 59), stated that:

> As HIM professionals, we want to be assured that we are providing the highest quality data for reimbursement and research and research purposes. We can review coded data internally, but this does not give us a clear picture of the total information that is being submitted to the Health Care Financing Administration (HCFA) [now called the Centers for Medicare and Medicaid Services, CMS]. . . . Recently a new tool has come out that helps HIM professionals evaluate the quality of coded data. This tool, *DRG Resource Book: Data for Benchmarking and Analysis,* is published by the Center for Healthcare Industry Performance Studies in Columbus, OH. The book con-

tains comparative information for the top 50 medical and the top 25 surgical DRGs for the Medicare population, so HIM professionals can compare their coded data to a national database. The source of this information is the HCFA Medicare Provider and Review File (MEDPAR file) for the federal fiscal year 1995, which consists of data compiled from UB-92 data submitted by hospitals for inpatient Medicare discharges.

> This resource reports DRG summary information, cost analysis information, state-specific profiles of charges per discharge and by department, utilization and quality indicators, and clinical coding analysis—all by DRG. This article [analyzes] the ICD-9-CM codes reported for the 75 medical and surgical DRGs.

Discussion Questions

1. From the description of the data used in the article, indicate whether the data are primary or secondary. Explain your answer.
2. Do these data represent aggregate or patient-identifiable information? Explain your answer.
3. What is the purpose of the MEDPAR database? What data would it lack that might be helpful in looking at the quality of coded data?
4. What other national database would be useful in evaluating the quality of coded data? Which data would it include that the MEDPAR database does not?

Summary

Health records contain extensive information about individual patients but are difficult to use when attempting to perceive trends in care or quality. For that reason, secondary records were developed. One type of secondary record is the index. An index is a report from the database that provides information on patients and supports retrieval by diagnosis, procedure, or physician. Health information management departments routinely produce indexes.

Disease registries are developed when extensive information is needed about specific diagnoses, procedures, or conditions. They are commonly used for research and to improve patient care and health status. From the database created through the data collection process, reports can be developed to answer questions regarding patient care or issues such as rates of immunization and birth defects. In some cases, patient follow-up is done to assess survival rates and quality of life after a disease or accident.

HIM professionals perform a variety of roles in relation to registries. In some cases, they work on setting up the registry. Moreover, they may work in data collection and management of registry functions. HIM professionals are well suited to such positions because of their background and education in management, health record content, regulatory and legal compliance, and medical science and terminology.

Today, organizations and institutions of all types commonly maintain databases pertaining to healthcare. At the federal level, some administrative databases provide data and information for decisions regarding claims and practitioner credentialing. Other databases focus on the public health area, using data collected at the local level and shared with states and the federal government. These databases assist in government surveillance of health status in the United States. Some databases, such as the clinical trials database, are mandated by law and help patients and providers to locate clinical trials regardless of source or location.

Registries and databases raise a number of managerial issues. Data collection is often time-consuming, so some databases now use automated entry methods. In addition, decisions must be made between vendor and facility-specific products. Finally, the quality of the data is an important issue because the decisions made based on data in registries and databases depend on the data's validity, reliability, accuracy, and timeliness.

Another important issue related to registries and databases is data security. Facilities must adopt methods that will ensure controlled access to data as well as prevent the loss of data. Confidentiality is always of concern to the HIM professional, and steps must be taken to protect it.

In the future, separate registries and databases may become less common with the advent of the computer-based patient record. Essentially a large database, the CPR can be queried directly rather than having to first abstract data from the primary record into a secondary record.

References

All Kids Count. 2001. Accessed online from www.allkidscount.org.

American Joint Committee on Cancer. 2001. Accessed online from www.cancerstaging.org.

Center for Devices and Radiological Health. 1996. Medical device reporting for user facilities. Accessed online November 2001 from www.fda.gov/cdrh/mdruf.pdf.

Centers for Disease Control, National Immunization Program. 2001. Accessed online from www.cdc.gov/nip/registry/factsht.htm.

Centers for Disease Control, National Center for Health Statistics. 2001. Accessed online from www.cdc.gov/nchs/nvss.htm.

Chidley, Elise. 2000. Revisiting the Abbreviated Injury Scale. *For the Record* 12(4):20–23.

Garthe, Elizabeth. 1997. Overview of trauma registries in the United States. *Journal of the American Health Information Management Association* 68(7):26, 28, 30–31.

McCray, Alexa, and Nicholas C. Ide. 2000. Design and implementation of a national clinical trials registry. *Journal of the American Medical Informatics Association* 7:313–23.

National Cancer Registrars Association. 2001. Accessed online from www.ncra-usa.org.

National Library of Medicine. 2001. Accessed online from www.clinicaltrials.gov.

Office of Inspector General. 1998. Health Care Fraud and Abuse Data Collection Program: Reporting of Final Adverse Actions, Notice of proposed rulemaking. *Federal Register* 63(210):58341-58342.

Osborn, Carol E. 1999. Benchmarking with national ICD-9-CM coded data. *Journal of the American Health Information Management Association* 70(4):59–69.

Shelton, Deborah L. 2001. Retrieved implants could be a source of important data. *American Medical News,* February 14.

Application Exercises

1. Check the Web site for your state department of health. Determine whether your state has a statewide cancer or immunization registry. If so, determine the source of the data included in the registries. Then find out what diseases are on the notifiable/reportable list for your state.

2. Visit a cancer registry in your area. Review the annual report. Describe the types of information included in the report and how the information is used within the facility. Then find out whether the facility uses a vendor or a facility-specific system. Find out why the particular system was chosen and its advantages and disadvantages. Determine what data security methods are used for the system. What measures are taken to ensure confidentiality of the data?

3. Visit the credentialing office of a local hospital. Discuss how it queries the National Practitioner Data Bank for credentialing and recredentialing purposes.

4. On the Internet, access ClinicalTrials.gov and find a clinical trial in your city or state. Give the title, condition under study, and location of the trial. Summarize the recruitment status, eligibility criteria, and phase of the clinical trial.

5. Access the HCUP Web site (www.ahrq.gov/data/hcup) and find out whether your state participates in the HCUP program. If so, determine who the state contact is for the HCUP program.

6. Using MEDLINE, find an article on the disease registry of your choice. Summarize the article.

Review Quiz

Instructions: Choose the most appropriate answer for each of the following questions.

1. ___ Which of the following indexes and databases includes patient-identifiable information?
   a. MEDLINE
   b. Clinical trials database
   c. Master population/patient index
   d. UMLS

2. ___ Which of the following is an external user of data?
   a. Public health department
   b. Medical staff
   c. Hospital administrator
   d. Director of the clinical laboratory

3. ___ Review of disease indexes, pathology reports, and radiation therapy reports is part of which function in the cancer registry?
   a. Case definition
   b. Case finding
   c. Follow-up
   d. Reporting

4. ___ What is information identifying the patient (such as name, health record number, address, and telephone number) called?
   a. Accession data
   b. Indicator data
   c. Reference data
   d. Demographic data

5. ___ Cancer registries receive approval as part of the facility cancer program from which of the following agencies?
   a. American Cancer Society
   b. National Cancer Registrars Association
   c. National Cancer Institute
   d. American College of Surgeons

6. ___ Which national database includes data on all discharged patients regardless of payer?
   a. Healthcare Cost and Utilization Project
   b. Medicare Provider Analysis and Review file
   c. Unified Medical Language System
   d. Uniform Hospital Discharge Data Set

7. ___ Two clerks are abstracting data for a registry. When their work is checked, discrepancies are found. Which data quality component is lacking?
   a. Completeness
   b. Validity
   c. Reliability
   d. Timeliness

8. ___ What does an audit trail check for?
   a. Unauthorized access to a system
   b. Loss of data
   c. Presence of a virus
   d. Successful completion of a backup

9. ___ Which of the following laws requires the reporting of deaths and severe complications resulting from the use of medical devices?
   a. Medical Implantation and Transplantation Act of 1986
   b. Medical Devices Reporting Act of 1972
   c. Food and Drug Modernization Act of 1997
   d. Safe Medical Devices Act of 1990

10. ___ Which of the following is a database from the National Health Care Survey that uses the health record as a data source?
   a. National Health Provider Inventory
   b. National Ambulatory Medical Care Survey
   c. National Employer Health Insurance Survey
   d. National Infectious Disease Inventory

Chapter 13
Clinical Classifications and Terminologies

Susan H. Fenton, MBA, RHIA

Learning Objectives

- To differentiate among, and to identify the correct uses of, classifications, nomenclatures, and terminologies
- To discuss the strengths and weaknesses of the classification systems currently required in the United States
- To describe a quality assessment procedure for coding
- To differentiate between encoding and automated coding and to describe how each can be used in the coding process
- To analyze corporate compliance policies and procedures for appropriateness
- To discuss emerging healthcare terminologies
- To identify data retrieval needs and to select a terminology most likely to meet them
- To understand the need for a terminology in a computer-based patient record

Key Terms

Classification
Clinical TERMS Version 3 (CTV3)
Coding
Compliance
Concept
Context
Digital Imaging and Communications in Medicine (DICOM)
Encoder
Lexicon
Logical Observation Identifier Names and Codes (LOINC)
Metathesaurus
Nomenclature
Nosology
Read Codes
Reference terminology
Relationship
Systemized Nomenclature of Medicine (SNOMED)
Systemized Nomenclature of Medicine Clinical Terms (SNOMED CT)
Systemized Nomenclature of Medicine Reference Terminology (SNOMED RT)
Terminology
Terminology standard
Unified Medical Language System (UMLS)
Upcoding
Vocabulary

Introduction

Healthcare is faced with many challenges, including an aging population, the need to conserve resources, medical knowledge that is increasing exponentially, and a consumer population with Internet access. To meet these challenges, healthcare organizations must have the ability to operate effectively and efficiently using the latest medical data and knowledge. Unfortunately, the healthcare industry in the United States has yet to agree on a common terminology that would allow healthcare facilities and practitioners throughout the country to exchange and use information reliably.

It is difficult to believe that the quest to classify morbidity and mortality is quite old. London parishes first began to keep death records in 1532. In 1662, John Graunt, a merchant, wrote *Natural and Political Observations . . . Made upon the Bills of Mortality.* His friend, Sir William Petty, was able to extrapolate from mortality rates an estimate of community economic loss caused by deaths. Two hundred years later, Florence Nightingale, in *Notes on a Hospital,* wrote, "In attempting to arrive at the truth, I have applied everywhere for information, but in scarcely an instance have I been able to obtain hospital records fit for any purposes of comparison. If they could be obtained . . . they would show subscribers how their money was being spent, what amount of good was really being done with it, or whether the money was not doing mischief rather than good" (Barnett et al. 1993, p. 1046).

Many of the same issues remain in healthcare today. It is vitally important to be able to compare data for outcomes measurement, quality assurance, resource utilization, best practices, and medical research. These tasks can be accomplished only when healthcare has a common terminology that is easily integrated into the computer-based patient record.

This chapter examines the history and current practices of classification in the healthcare industry, including the focus on compliance. It also considers various emerging terminologies and the desired characteristics of a terminology.

Theory into Practice

Dr. French walks into his clinic in the morning and activates his personal digital assistant (PDA). It immediately connects to the organizational database via wireless technology and downloads all of his appointments for the day, as well as e-mail and other items requiring his attention. His schedule shows that his first appointment is a clinic patient. After accessing the organizational computer-based patient record (CPR), he downloads the patient information and begins reviewing it. As he reads, he has a question about one of the patient's conditions. He indicates on the screen that he would like more information on the specified condition, and within two minutes, the latest relevant abstracts have been down-loaded into his PDA. Upon review, he finds an article that will answer his questions and downloads it.

When Dr. French meets with the patient, he recommends a particular course of treatment. The patient's first question is "How have other patients responded to this treatment?" Using recently developed software, Dr. French searches many healthcare organization databases to determine how patients with similar characteristics have responded to the recommended treatment and shares his findings with the patient. This gives the patient the information he needs to make an informed decision.

As Dr. French finishes documenting the patient's condition and the agreed-upon treatment, the administrative components of the system analyze the documentation. If necessary, it alerts Dr. French to any required components that may be missing or ambiguous. If the documentation is determined to be complete, the appropriate billing codes are assigned and the required data are instantly transmitted to the third-party payer.

Development of Classifications Systems for Healthcare Data

As the discussion of classification systems for healthcare data begins, it is important to have a common understanding of how **classifications, nomenclatures,** and **terminologies** are defined. Unfortunately, it is difficult to get complete agreement in even this area. The most widely accepted **terminology standard** is the International Standards Organization (ISO) Standard 1087 (Terminology-Vocabulary) (Hammond and Cimino 2000, p. 224). AHIMA's Coding Policy and Strategy Committee has defined the entity *classification* (AHIMA 1999, p. 72). Its definition is essentially equivalent to the ISO's definition of a nomenclature.

AHIMA's Coding Policy and Strategy Committee also defines a clinical **vocabulary** as a list or collection of clinical words or phrases with their meanings. In the committee's opinion, a clinical terminology provides for the proper use of clinical words as names or symbols. The committee equated a clinical terminology with a nomenclature (AHIMA 1999, p. 72). It is important to recognize that this problem of multiple definitions and names is endemic in the field of healthcare terminology. Standardized terms can be efficiently mapped to broader classifications for administrative, regulatory, oversight, and fiscal requirements (Chute 2000, p. 301).

Because all these definitions can be confusing, the illustration in figure 13.1 may be helpful. The terms *classification* and *nomenclature* are often used interchangeably. Chute (2000, p. 298) stated that "classifications and nomenclatures can be more helpfully regarded as lying along a continuum, where the first categorizes and aggregates while the second supports detailed descriptions." Further down from the apex of the pyramid is a terminology, which is the whole set of terms representing the system of concepts of a particular

Figure 13.1.   Comparative Level of Detail in Nomenclatures, Terminologies, and Languages

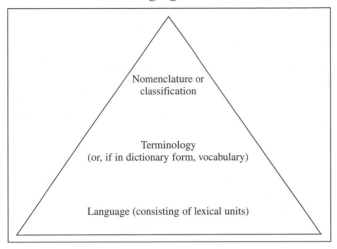

Nomenclature or classification

Terminology (or, if in dictionary form, vocabulary)

Language (consisting of lexical units)

subject field. So, while a classification or nomenclature categorizes and aggregates, a terminology represents the whole of a subject field. The pyramid in figure 13.1 illustrates how a nomenclature can be less specific than a terminology, which is less specific than a language.

Check Your Understanding 13.1

Instructions: Answer the following questions on a separate piece of paper.

1. What are the general functions of classifications and nomenclatures? Give examples of each.

2. What is one of the most significant problems in the field of healthcare terminology and vocabulary standards today? Explain the problem's significance.

Current Systems of Classification and Nomenclature

Systems for classifying diseases have progressed through various stages since the first classification system was developed in the late nineteenth century. The following sections describe past, current, and near-future developments.

International Classification of Diseases

The *International Classification of Diseases* began as the *Bertillion Classification of Diseases* in 1893. In 1900, the French government convened an international meeting to update the Bertillion classification to the *International List of Causes of Death.* The goal was to develop a common system for describing the causes of mortality. The latest version of the *International Classification of Diseases* is the tenth edition (ICD-10), which was released in 1992. According to the Centers for Disease Control (CDC), the current purpose of ICD-10 is to promote international comparability in the collection, classification, processing, and presentation of mortality statistics.

In 1999, the United States began using ICD-10 to report mortality statistics under its agreement with the World Health Organization (WHO). The U.S. Department of Health and Human Services (HHS) reports that WHO currently has no plans to issue an ICD-11. WHO has established a procedure for updating ICD-10 regularly. The National Center for Health Statistics (NCHS) is the WHO Collaborating Center for the Classification of Diseases for North America.

International Classification of Diseases, Ninth Edition, Clinical Modification

Developed by the NCHS, the *International Classification of Diseases, Ninth Revision, Clinical Modification* (ICD-9-CM) is a derivative work of the *International Classification of Diseases, Ninth Revision,* as developed by the WHO. ICD-9-CM is used in the United States only to code and classify diagnoses from inpatient and outpatient records, as well as inpatient procedures. Although diagnostic and procedural coding were the original functions of the system, ICD-9-CM also has been used to communicate provider reimbursement information on healthcare services since 1983. Today, coding for reimbursement is a vital part of healthcare operations. The official ICD-9-CM coding guidelines are published quarterly in *Coding Clinic for ICD-9-CM* by the Central Office on ICD-9-CM Coding of the American Hospital Association.

Changes and updates to ICD-9-CM are managed by the ICD-9-CM Coordination and Maintenance Committee, a federal committee cochaired by representatives from the NCHS and the Centers for Medicare and Medicaid Services, or CMS (formerly known as the Health Care Financing Administration, or HCFA). The NCHS is responsible for volumes 1 and 2 (diagnoses), and the CMS is responsible for volume 3 (procedures). Both the public and private sectors are invited to make suggestions for modifications to ICD-9-CM, and meetings are open to the public. Modifications are implemented on October 1 of each year, the beginning of the federal government's fiscal year. Figure 13.2 (p. 264) is an example of a section of an entry in the Tabular Listing of Diseases (ICD-9-CM, volume 1).

International Classification of Diseases, Tenth Revision, Clinical Modification

As with ICD-9, the U.S. government modified ICD-10 for the reporting of morbidity data. Between December 1997 and February 1998, the NCHS posted a draft of the ICD-10-CM Tabular List of Diseases on its Web site for public comment. Originally targeted for release in late 2001, ICD-10-CM is still undergoing revision and, as of this writing, has not yet been released.

ICD-10-CM contains substantial increases in content over ICD-9-CM. Improvements in the content and format of the draft include:

- Additional information relevant to ambulatory and managed care encounters

- Expanded injury codes
- New combination diagnosis/symptom codes to reduce the number of codes needed to fully describe a condition
- New six-digit codes
- Additional four- and five-digit subclassification codes
- Laterality (right and left)
- Greater specificity in code assignment

Figure 13.2.   Example of Volume 1 ICD-9-CM Entry

TUBERCULOSIS (010–018)

Includes: infection by Mycobacterium tuberculosis
(human) (bovine)

| Excludes: | congenital tuberculosis (771.2) |
| | late effects of tuberculosis (137.0–137.4) |

The following fifth-digit subclassification is for use with categories 010–018:

0   unspecified
1   bacteriological or histological examination not done
2   bacteriological or histological examination unknown (at present)
3   tubercle bacilli found (in sputum) by microscopy
4   tubercle bacilli not found (in sputum) by microscopy, but found by bacterial culture
5   tubercle bacilli not found by bacteriological examination, but tuberculosis confirmed histologically
6   tubercle bacilli not found by bacteriological or histological examination but tuberculosis confirmed by other methods [inoculation of animals]

§ 010   Primary tuberculous infection

010.0   **Primary tuberculous infection**

Excludes:	nonspecific reaction to tuberculin skin test
	without active tuberculosis (795.5)
	positive:
	PPD (795.5)
	tuberculin skin test without active
	tuberculosis (795.5)

010.1   **Tuberculous pleurisy in primary progressive tuberculosis**

010.8   **Other primary progressive tuberculosis**

| Excludes: | tuberculous erythema nodosum (017.1) |

010.9   **Primary tuberculous infection, unspecified**

§ 011   **Pulmonary tuberculosis**

Use additional code to identify any associated silicosis (502)

011.0   **Tuberculosis of lung, infiltrative**
011.1   **Tuberculosis of lung, nodular**
011.2   **Tuberculosis of lung with cavitation**
011.3   **Tuberculosis of bronchus**

| Excludes: | isolated bronchial tuberculosis (012.2) |

011.4   **Tuberculous fibrosis of lung**
011.5   **Tuberculous bronchiectasis**
011.6   **Tuberculous pneumonia [any form]**
011.7   **Tuberculous pneumothorax**
011.8   **Other specified pulmonary tuberculosis**
011.9   **Pulmonary tuberculosis, unspecified**
        Respiratory tuberculosis NOS
        Tuberculosis of lung NOS

§ Requires fifth-digit. See codes and definitions.

The original target for releasing ICD-10-CM was late 2001, but as of this writing, no official implementation date has been set. Because the Health Insurance Portability and Accountability Act (HIPAA) of 1996 dictates standards for code sets, implementation of ICD-10-CM will conform to HIPAA standards.

International Classification of Diseases, Tenth Revision, Procedural Coding System

In the mid-1990s, HCFA (now known as the CMS) awarded a contract to the 3M Health Information Systems group to develop a new procedural coding system to replace the Tabular List of Procedures, volume 3 of ICD-9-CM. The objectives of the project were to:

- Improve the accuracy and efficiency of coding
- Reduce training efforts
- Improve communication with physicians

The *International Classification of Diseases, Tenth Revision, Procedural Coding System* (ICD-10-PCS), is based on a seven-character alphanumeric code with the following four essential characteristics:

- *Completeness:* All substantially different procedures have a unique code.
- *Expandability:* The structure of the system allows incorporation of new procedures as unique codes.
- *Standardized terminology* (or definitions): Each term is assigned a specific meaning.
- *Multiaxial structure:* Each code character has the same meaning with the specific procedure section and across procedure sections to the extent possible.

ICD-10-PCS is divided into sixteen sections, each of which covers a specific diagnostic area (for example, medical and surgical, chiropractic, and so on). Depending on the requirements of each section, the seven characters are assigned different meanings. For example, in the medical and surgical section, the fourth character represents the body part or region involved in the procedure; in the placement section, it represents the body region or orifice; and in the chiropractic section, it represents the body region.

As of this writing, the CMS has not published information on implementation of ICD-10-PCS. The ICD-9-CM Coordination and Maintenance Committee has indicated that implementation will not occur before October 2003.

Current Procedural Terminology

The American Medical Association (AMA) publishes the *Current Procedural Terminology* (CPT). According to the AMA, the purpose of CPT is "to provide a uniform language that accurately describes medical, surgical, and diagnostic services, and thereby serves as an effective means for reliable nationwide communication among physicians, patients and third parties." CPT was first developed and published by the AMA in 1966. In 1983, the system was adopted by

HCFA (now called the CMS) as level I of the Healthcare Common Procedure Coding System (HCPCS). Since that time, CPT has become widely used as a standard for outpatient and ambulatory care procedural coding in **contexts** related to reimbursement.

Like ICD-9-CM, CPT is updated every year (CPT on January 1 and ICD-9-CM on October 1). The 2001 version of CPT contained 7,928 codes and descriptors. The codebook is organized into chapters by specialty, body system, or service provided. The codes themselves consist of five digits, and the descriptions of the codes are often accompanied by inclusion and exclusion notes. Modifiers to the five-digit codes also are used extensively.

CPT is maintained by the CPT Editorial Panel, which is authorized to revise, update, and modify CPT. The majority (eleven of sixteen) of the panel's members are physicians, with the rest coming from industry and government. Supporting the work of the CPT Editorial Panel is the CPT Health Care Professionals Advisory Committee (HCPAC). The HCPAC includes participation in the CPT process from organizations representing limited-license medical practitioners and allied health professionals.

The AMA is responsible for developing and publishing the official guidelines for CPT. The association provides support in several ways. It publishes *CPT Assistant,* a monthly newsletter, and offers CPT Information Services, a telephone service that provides users with expert advice on code use. The association also conducts an annual CPT coding symposium.

The AMA is currently revising the fourth edition of CPT. The fifth edition project represents an effort to respond to emerging user needs and HIPAA confidentiality and security requirements. The AMA's stated intent for the project is to "ensure that CPT meets all the requirements of, and is unambiguously selected by the Secretary of HHS as the standard for reporting physicians' services under HIPAA." All enhancements and modifications will occur gradually through the usual CPT editorial process. The fifth edition of CPT is scheduled for publication by 2003. Some of the changes outlined on the AMA Web site include:

- The elimination of ambiguous terms
- Codes for home health services
- A new section for performance measurement codes
- A new section for investigational service codes
- Codes for evaluation and assessment services performed by health professionals who are not physicians
- Counseling or preventive medicine services codes/core concept extenders
- Code combinations for included and excluded services
- Web-based communication to enhance the editorial process, including code change requests
- Development of a terminology model
- XML-enabled, browser-based versions of CPT
- An annual list of deleted codes

It remains to be seen whether these changes will be enough for the secretary of HHS to determine that CPT should continue to be the coding standard for physician and ambulatory care services. For detailed information on the background of the fourth and current edition of CPT and on the proposed fifth edition, readers should refer to the AMA Web site at ama.association.org.

Healthcare Common Procedure Coding System

The Healthcare Common Procedure Coding System (HCPCS) is used to report physicians' services provided to Medicare recipients. HCPCS is administered by the CMS and includes three levels of codes. Level I is made up entirely of CPT codes as published by the AMA. Level II includes alphanumeric procedure and modifier codes established by the CMS's Alphanumeric Editorial Panel. Level II codes primarily represent items, supplies, and nonphysician services not covered by the AMA's CPT codes. The codes are used in reimbursement claims processing.

Except for temporary codes (those beginning with G, K, or Q), HCPCS codes are updated every year on January 1. The HCPCS level II codes can be downloaded from the HCPCS Web site; however, the file does not include the Current Dental Terminology codes (HCPCS codes beginning with D) as published by the American Dental Association. HCPCS level III codes (W to Z) are used by Medicare carriers and fiscal intermediaries as local procedure and modifier codes. Figure 13.3 shows an example of HCPCS codes.

HCPCS was included in the HIPAA final rule on transaction and code sets, with the exception of the level III codes. The presence of level III codes is not consistent with HIPAA's national standards goal. The future of HCPCS beyond the first HIPAA implementation is unclear.

Figure 13.3.   Example of HCPCS Codes

Code	Long Description
A0428	AMBULANCE SERVICE, BASIC LIFE SUPPORT, NON-EMERGENCY TRANSPORT (BLS)
A0429	AMBULANCE SERVICE, BASIC LIFE SUPPORT, EMERGENCY TRANSPORT (BLS-EMERGENCY)
A0430	AMBULANCE SERVICE, CONVENTIONAL AIR SERVICES, TRANSPORT, ONE WAY (FIXED WING)
A0431	AMBULANCE SERVICE, CONVENTIONAL AIR SERVICES, TRANSPORT, ONE WAY (ROTARY WING)
A0432	PARAMEDIC INTERCEPT (PI), RURAL AREA, TRANSPORT FURNISHED BY A VOLUNTEER
A0432	AMBULANCE COMPANY WHICH IS PROHIBITED BY STATE LAW FROM BILLING THIRD PARTY
A0432	PAYERS
A0433	ADVANCED LIFE SUPPORT, LEVEL 2 (ALS 2)
A0434	SPECIALTY CARE TRANSPORT (SCT)
A0435	FIXED WING AIR MILEAGE, PER STATUTE MILE
A0436	ROTARY WING AIR MILEAGE, PER STATUTE MILE

International Classification of Diseases for Oncology

The *International Classification of Diseases for Oncology* (ICD-O) is currently in its third edition. This classification is used for coding diagnoses of neoplasms in tumor and cancer registries and in pathology laboratories. The topography code describes the site of origin of the neoplasm and uses the same three- and four-character categories as in the neoplasm section of the second chapter of ICD-10. The morphology code describes the characteristics of the tumor itself, including cell type and biologic activity. The topography codes remain the same as in the previous edition, but the morphology codes have been thoroughly reviewed and revised where necessary.

To the greatest extent possible, ICD-O uses the nomenclature published in the WHO series, *International Histological Classification of Tumors*. ICD-O is under the purview of the heads of the WHO Collaborating Centres for Classification of Disease. The International Association of Cancer Registries (IACR) is an additional resource. (The information in this section is taken from the WHO Web site at www.who.inst.)

Diagnostic and Statistical Manual of Mental Diseases

The *Diagnostic and Statistical Manual of Mental Diseases* was first published by the American Psychiatric Association (APA) in 1952. The fourth and most recent complete revision was introduced in 1994. In 2000, the APA introduced DSM-IV-TR (Text Revision), which is the most current version available.

DSM is a multiaxial coding system with five axes. Axis I includes the mental disorders or illnesses comparable to general medical illnesses. Axis II includes personality disorders. Axis III includes general medical illnesses. Axis IV covers life events or social problems that affect the patient. Axis V is the overall level of the patient's functioning, usually as determined by the Global Assessment of Functioning (GAF). Figure 13.4 provides an example of DSM-IV-TR codes and instructions.

The APA Web site states two general uses for DSM: as a source of diagnostic information that enhances clinical practice, research, and education and as a language for communicating diagnostic information to other parties, such as government agencies and insurance companies. Theoretically, DSM can be used for reimbursement purposes because all of the diagnostic codes in DSM-IV are also valid ICD-9-CM codes. The APA updates the DSM to correspond to ICD-9-CM each year. According to the APA Web site (www.psych.org), the DSM will be updated to ICD-10-CM when it is implemented in the United States.

Check Your Understanding 13.2

Instructions: Answer the following questions on a separate piece of paper.

1. What was the original purpose of ICD-9-CM?
2. What are the four essential characteristics of ICD-10-PCS? Describe them.
3. What is the primary function of CPT?
4. What does the topography code in ICD-O describe?

Figure 13.4.   Example of DSM-IV-TR Codes

Diagnostic Criteria for Mental Retardation

A. Significantly subaverage intellectual functioning: an IQ of approximately 70 or below on an individually administered IQ test (for infants, a clinical judgment of significantly subaverage intellectual functioning).

B. Concurrent deficits or impairments in present adaptive functioning (i.e., the person's effectiveness in meeting the standards expected for his or her age by his or her cultural group) in at least two of the following areas: communication, self-care, home living, social/interpersonal skills, use of community resources, self-direction, functional academic skills, work, leisure, health, and safety.

C. The onset is before age 18 years.

Code based on degree of severity reflecting level of intellectual impairment:

317 Mild Mental Retardation: IQ level 50–55 to approximately 70
318.0 Moderate Mental Retardation: IQ level 35–40 to 50–55
318.1 Severe Mental Retardation: IQ level 20–25 to 35–40
318.2 Profound Mental Retardation: IQ level below 20 or 25
319 Mental Retardation, Severity Unspecified: when there is strong presumption of Mental Retardation but the person's intelligence is untestable by standard tests

Copyright 1994, American Psychiatric Association.

Coding

Traditionally, health information management (HIM) professionals have been responsible for the process of **coding,** or clinical code assignment, in healthcare organizations. Historically, the coding function has served two primary purposes: to create secondary records (for example, diagnostic and procedural indexes) and to create documentation for reimbursement purposes.

Standards of Ethical Coding

In the U.S. healthcare system, the majority of expenses are reimbursed by third-party payers such as government programs and insurance companies rather than by the patients themselves. As healthcare costs have risen over the past thirty years, third-party payers have searched for ways to contain costs. With the implementation of prospective payment systems based on coded clinical data, procedural reviews of documentation to substantiate code assignment have become routine. In other words, accurate coding has become central to the financial survival of healthcare provider organizations.

The coding professional's first responsibility is to ensure the accuracy of coded data. To this end, the American Health Information Management Association (AHIMA) has established a code of professional ethics by which coders must abide. (See figure 13.5.) Coders also need to balance the following three competing responsibilities:

- To perform their tasks using established guidelines and their best professional judgment
- To safeguard the viability of their hospitals in order to serve their communities
- To remain employed and able to support themselves and their families (Fox 1992, p. 34)

Figure 13.5. Standards of Ethical Coding

In this era of payment based on diagnostic and procedural coding, the professional ethics of health information coding professionals continue to be challenged. A conscientious goal for coding and maintaining a quality database is accurate clinical and statistical data. The following standards of ethical coding, developed by AHIMA's Coding Policy and Strategy Committee and approved by AHIMA's Board of Directors, are offered to guide coding professionals in this process.

1. Coding professionals are expected to support the importance of accurate, complete, and consistent coding practices for the production of quality healthcare data.

2. Coding professionals in all healthcare settings should adhere to the ICD-9-CM *(International Classification of Diseases, Ninth Revision, Clinical Modification)* coding conventions, official coding guidelines approved by the Cooperating Parties,* the CPT *(Current Procedural Terminology)* rules established by the American Medical Association, and any other official coding rules and guidelines established for use with mandated standard code sets. Selection and sequencing of diagnoses and procedures must meet the definitions of required data sets for applicable healthcare settings.

3. Coding professionals should use their skills, their knowledge of currently mandated coding and classification systems, and official resources to select the appropriate diagnostic and procedural codes.

4. Coding professionals should only assign and report codes that are clearly and consistently supported by physician documentation in the health record.

5. Coding professionals should consult physicians for clarification and additional documentation prior to code assignment when there is conflicting or ambiguous data in the health record.

6. Coding professionals should not change codes or the narratives of codes on the billing abstract so that meanings are misrepresented. Diagnoses or procedures should not be inappropriately included or excluded because payment or insurance policy coverage requirements will be affected. When individual payer policies conflict with official coding rules and guidelines, these policies should be obtained in writing whenever possible. Reasonable efforts should be made to educate the payer on proper coding practices in order to influence a change in the payer's policy.

7. Coding professionals, as members of the healthcare team, should assist and educate physicians and other clinicians by advocating proper documentation practices, further specificity, and resequencing or inclusion of diagnoses or procedures when needed to more accurately reflect the acuity, severity, and occurrence of events.

8. Coding professionals should participate in the development of institutional coding policies and should ensure that coding policies complement, not conflict with, official coding rules and guidelines.

9. Coding professionals should maintain and continually enhance their coding skills, as they have a professional responsibility to stay abreast of changes in codes, coding guidelines, and regulations.

10. Coding professionals should strive for optimal payment to which the facility is legally entitled, remembering that it is unethical and illegal to maximize payment by means that contradict regulatory guidelines.

*The Cooperating Parties are the American Health Information Management Association, American Hospital Association, Health Care Financing Administration, and National Center for Health Statistics. All rights reserved. Reprint and quote only with proper reference to AHIMA's authorship.

Elements of Coding Quality

The quality of coded clinical data depends on a number of factors, including:

- Adequate training for everyone involved in the coding process, including coders, coding supervisors, clinicians, and financial personnel
- Adequate references and support resources, including up-to-date coding books, as well as subscription publications that communicate official guidelines (namely, *Coding Clinic for ICD-9-CM* and *CPT Assistant*) and, in some cases, encoders or other support software
- Accurate and complete clinical documentation that includes every pertinent condition and service provided to the patient
- The support of senior managers, who must understand how important the coding function is to the organization's continued existence
- A performance improvement plan for the coding function that ensures continuous quality improvement processes

When all of these components are present, the quality of coded clinical data can be evaluated according to the following elements:

- *Reliability:* the extent to which the data can be reproduced by subsequent measurements or tests (for example, coded clinical data are considered reliable when multiple coders assign the same codes to a record)
- *Validity:* The extent to which the coded data accurately reflect the patient's diagnoses and procedures (Bowman 2001, p. 250)
- *Completeness:* The extent to which the coded data represent all of the patient's relevant diagnoses or procedures
- *Timeliness:* The extent to which the coded data are available within the time frames required for billing purposes, decision support, and other uses

Coding Policies and Procedures

As with other organizational policies and procedures, coding policies and procedures are needed to promote consistency. Items to be included in coding policies and procedures include:

- Directions for reviewing the record
- Instructions on how to address incomplete or conflicting documentation
- Instructions for communicating with physicians and developing physician queries and for clarification and recording health record addenda
- Instructions on the actions to be taken when an appropriate code cannot be located
- Use of codes not required for reimbursement (optional codes)

- Standardized definitions or codes sets (for example, HIPAA requirements)
- Use of reference materials and books and instructions for updating
- Computerized data entry or other processes (Bowman 2001, p. 251)

These items must be specified in policies and procedures so that coders know what is expected of them and so that the healthcare organization can ensure its compliance with government and payer requirements.

Steps in the Coding Process

Although the coding process may vary from organization to organization, or even within an organization between care settings, certain steps are usually followed when codes are assigned either manually or with an encoder. Initially, the coder should review the relevant documentation, whether it is a complete patient record for an inpatient stay or a short note for an ambulatory care encounter. Using their knowledge of the applicable definitions such as principal diagnosis, primary diagnoses, principal procedure, and so on, the coder then should select the conditions, treatment, and procedures that need to be coded. The definitions are important because they determine the order (or sequence) in which the codes are submitted to the third-party payer. After selecting the applicable conditions, treatments, or procedures, the coder should use the required coding system or nomenclature and select the most appropriate code, again, based on the guidelines.

After the code assignments and the order of the codes have been determined, it is imperative to use the correct reimbursement classification or grouping system. For example, in ambulatory care, ambulatory payment classifications (APCs) are used. (See chapter 14 for more information on reimbursement systems.) Services in each APC are similar clinically and in terms of the resources they require. A payment rate has been established for each APC. The APC is determined by a combination of ICD-9-CM diagnosis and CPT procedure codes. In most cases, a computerized software program called a grouper is used for this function. It is common for all of the coding and grouping data to be entered into and stored in a computerized information system. When the codes and other data provided by the coders are deemed complete, they are often transmitted or otherwise communicated to the billing personnel for reimbursement purposes. Figure 13.6 shows the steps in the coding process.

Figure 13.6.   Steps in the Coding Process

1. Review relevant documentation.
2. Select conditions, treatments, and procedures to be coded.
3. Select most appropriate codes.
4. Utilize the appropriate reimbursement classification system.
5. Enter or abstract data into the computer.

Quality Assessment for the Coding Process

Quality assessment for the coding process is also referred to as performance improvement for the coding process. It involves looking at more than just the assigned codes. As stated previously, accurate coding is essential to the economic survival of the healthcare organization; hence, ongoing efforts to improve the coding process should yield better economic benefits.

Most important to improving any coding process is to first document and understand the current coding process. The preceding section can be used as a guide for documenting that process, remembering that the actual process is different in every organization. One of the most important items in the coding process is the quality of the clinical documentation. Even though HIM professionals have little to no direct control over the documentation, they should work with the clinicians and other personnel to continue to improve its quality.

After the current coding process has been documented, quality measurement points should be established at specific stages in the process. Baseline measurements need to be taken, and benchmarks for improvement should be set up. For example, if the current process results in records being coded an average of ten work-hours after arriving in the HIM department, a benchmark for improvement might be to code records in under eight hours. To establish valid internal coding data monitors, comparative data will be necessary. Comparative data can be obtained from a variety of sources, including state data organizations, hospital associations, peer review organizations, and the Medicare MedPar data, which can be obtained from the Centers for Medicare and Medicaid Services (CMS). The National Health Information Resource Center (www.nhirc.org) and the National Association of Health Data Organizations (www.nahdo.org) are additional sources of information on health data.

Quality assessment of a process is generally ongoing. Even when the most ambitious goals for the most important measures have been accomplished, the measures should continue to be monitored. In addition, management should continually search for ways to improve the coding process through computerization or other methods.

Check Your Understanding 13.3

Instructions: Answer the following questions on a separate piece of paper.

1. What is the coder's primary responsibility?
2. What is the main factor in ensuring the quality of clinical coding?
3. Why is it important for organizations to establish and follow specific coding policies and procedures?
4. Describe the quality assessment process for coding.

Application of Technology to the Coding Process

Recent technologies are having a considerable impact on the coding process, and new technologies hold promise for the future. Some of the most significant advances are discussed below.

Encoders

An **encoder** is a computer software program designed to assist coders in assigning appropriate clinical codes to words and phrases expressed in natural human language (Slee and Slee 1991). Initially developed during the era of paper-based health records, the principal purpose of encoders was to help ensure accurate reporting for reimbursement (Beinborn 1999).

Encoders come in two distinct categories: logic-based and automated codebook formats. A *logic-based encoder* prompts the user through a variety of questions and choices based on the clinical terminology entered. The coder selects the most accurate code for a service or condition (and any possible complications or comorbidities).

An *automated codebook* provides screen views that resemble the actual format of the coding system. This allows the coder to review code selections, notes, look-up tables, edits, and various other automated notations that help him or her to choose the most accurate code for a condition or service. Although encoders can cite official coding guidelines and provide code optimization guidance, they require user interaction. Encoders promote accuracy as well as consistency in the coding of diagnoses and procedures.

A number of companies currently market encoder products. An up-to-date list of these products can be found in the annual coding issue of the *Journal of the American Health Information Management Association*.

Automated Code Assignment

Rather than prompting the user to make various selections on the basis of patient record documentation, automated code assignment uses data that have been entered into the computer to automatically assign codes (Beinborn 1999). Automated code assignment uses natural language processing (NLP) technology to read the data contained in a CPR. The natural language processing technology used might be algorithmic (rules based) or statistical. Schnitzer (2000) has stated that statistical approaches that can predict how an experienced coder might code a record and use machine learning techniques are superior to rigid rule sets. This opinion is congruent with the oft-heard argument that "coding is subjective."

According to Schnitzer, the advantages to using automated code assignment include:

- *Consistency:* Automated code assignment is consistently correct and consistently incorrect; thus, errors, once detected, are easier to locate and fix.
- *Accuracy:* As with medical knowledge, the amount of information that must be synthesized to correctly code patient records has increased substantially. Expert computer software programs can apply these rules and guidelines accurately.

- *Speed:* The computational power of computers can apply the many coding rules and guidelines efficiently.

It is important to note, however, that automated code assignment is not a magic bullet. For example, it cannot address the major obstacle facing today's human coder: the lack of accurate, complete clinical documentation. As Schnitzer (2000) put it, "If a service isn't appropriately documented, there's no way for NLP to find it, assume it, or infer it." In addition, automated code assignment has not developed to the point where it can operate without substantial human interaction (Warner 2000). Finally, the most effective automated code assignment system will need to accommodate any weaknesses and deficiencies in the classification and coding systems it uses (Beinborn 1999).

As automated code assignment continues to evolve, so, too, will the role of the coding professional. In its Vision 2006, the AHIMA (1996) pictures a clinical data specialist in the future and predicts that this individual will manage data in a number of areas, including clinical coding, outcomes measurement, specialty registries, and research databases. Beinborn (1999) stated that coders will be essential to the implementation and maintenance of automated code assignment systems as well as of decision support systems, data interpretation, and other evolving areas that rely on healthcare data.

Emerging Technologies

As is apparent from the preceding subsection, the status quo will not continue for coding. A number of emerging technologies will likely be used to support the coding function.

Speech recognition is one candidate for improving the coding process as well as coding accuracy. As speech recognition improves and has the ability to accurately document what the clinician is saying, the ease of completely documenting healthcare services also improves. Schwager (2000, p. 64) has maintained that "speech recognition, combined with technology designed to extract and structure medical information (natural language processing) contained in narrative text, can automate the coding process used in reimbursement." He also has discussed the possibility that the computerized patient record software could analyze the record in an interactive fashion, prompting the clinician for higher-quality documentation.

Handheld computers or personal digital assistants (PDAs) also are becoming commonplace. Many physicians and other healthcare professionals find them helpful. As computer systems continue to develop, it will only be a matter of time before these small units are used for data entry and other functions in healthcare organizations.

A discussion of emerging technologies to support coding would not be complete without a discussion of clinical terminologies. The currently emerging vocabularies and classifications, as well as the characteristics necessary in a clinical terminology and considerations when selecting a clinical terminology, are discussed later in this chapter.

Coding and Corporate Compliance

The federal government, through the HHS Office of the Inspector General, has initiated efforts to investigate healthcare fraud and to establish guidelines to ensure corporate compliance with the government guidelines. Part of the initiative involved providing healthcare organizations with guidelines for developing comprehensive compliance programs with specific policies and procedures.

History of Corporate Compliance in Healthcare

Probably the most pertinent fact in the history of corporate **compliance** related to healthcare organizations is that the federal government, specifically the HHS, is the largest purchaser of healthcare in the United States. Because one of the federal government's duties is to use the taxpayers' monies wisely, federal agencies must ensure that the healthcare provided to enrollees in federal healthcare programs is appropriate and is actually provided.

The federal government began to investigate fraud in the Medicare program in 1977 with passage of the Anti-Fraud and Abuse Amendments of 1977 to Title XIX of the Social Security Act. However, detecting, preventing, and prosecuting fraud and abuse did not reach true prominence until the Health Insurance Portability and Accountability Act (HIPAA) of 1996 established Sections 1128C and 1128D of the Social Security Act. Sections 1128C and 1128D authorized the HHS Office of the Inspector General (OIG) to conduct investigations, audits, and evaluations related to healthcare fraud.

HIPAA expanded the OIG's duties to include:

- The coordination of federal, state, and local enforcement efforts targeting healthcare fraud
- The provision of industry guidance concerning fraudulent healthcare practices
- The establishment of a national data bank for reporting final adverse actions against healthcare providers

Significantly, HIPAA authorizes the OIG to investigate cases of healthcare fraud that involve private healthcare plans as well as federally funded programs, although, according to information on the OIG Web site, present policies restrict the OIG's investigative focus to cases of fraud that affect federally funded programs.

From February 1998 until the present, the OIG continues to issue compliance guidance for various types of healthcare organizations. The OIG Web site (www.oig.hhs.gov) posts the documents that most healthcare organizations need to develop fraud and abuse compliance plans.

Elements of Corporate Compliance

In the February 23, 1998, *Federal Register* (p. 8989), the OIG outlined the following seven elements as the minimum necessary for a comprehensive compliance program:

1. The development and distribution of written standards of conduct, as well as written policies and procedures that promote the hospital's commitment to compliance and that address specific areas of potential fraud, such as claims development and submission processes, code gaming, and financial relationships with physicians and other healthcare professionals
2. The designation of a chief compliance officer and other appropriate bodies, for example, a corporate compliance committee, charged with the responsibility for operating and monitoring the compliance program, and who report directly to the CEO and the governing body
3. The development and implementation of regular, effective education and training programs for all affected employees
4. The maintenance of a process, such as a hotline, to receive complaints and the adoption of procedures to protect the anonymity of complainants and to protect whistleblowers from retaliation
5. The development of a system to respond to allegations of improper/illegal activities and the enforcement of appropriate disciplinary action against employees who have violated internal compliance policies, applicable statutes, regulations, or federal healthcare program requirements
6. The use of audits and/or other evaluation techniques to monitor compliance and assist in the reduction of identified problem areas
7. The investigation and remediation of identified systemic problems and the development of policies addressing the nonemployment or retention of sanctioned individuals

The OIG believes that a compliance program conforming to these elements above will not only "fulfill the organization's legal duty to ensure that it is not submitting false or inaccurate claims to government and private payers," but will also result in additional potential benefits, including, among others:

- Demonstration of the organization's commitment to responsible conduct toward employees and the community
- Provision of a more accurate view of behavior relating to fraud and abuse
- Identification and prevention of criminal and unethical conduct
- Improvements in the quality of patient care

(For additional resources on compliance and fraud and abuse, see figure 13.7.)

Figure 13.7.   Online Compliance Resources

Department of Health and Human Services, Office of the Inspector General	www.oig.hhs.gov
American Health Information Management Association	www.ahima.org
Health Care Compliance Association	www.hcca-info.org
National Health Care Anti-Fraud Association	www.nhcaa.org
Centers for Medicare and Medicaid Services	www.cms.hhs.gov
CMS Fraud Page	www.medicare.gov

Relationship between Coding Practice and Corporate Compliance

The first element of the OIG's basic seven elements of compliance mentions coding. Because the accuracy and completeness of the assignment of ICD-9-CM diagnostic and procedure codes determine the provider payment, the reference to coding is not surprising. Although the Department of Justice has stated that it does not intend to assess fines and penalties for honest billing mistakes, it also has stated that organizations must establish adequate internal procedures to ensure the accuracy of claims submissions (Averill 1999). Disregard for the requirements of the law can turn an honest mistake into a false claim, which can be subject to penalties that include a base fine plus three times the amount of the claim (Averill 1999). Thus, it is essential that healthcare organizations have a strong coding compliance program.

Unfortunately, some healthcare organizations practice upcoding. **Upcoding** is the practice of assigning a reimbursement code specifically for the purpose of obtaining a higher level of payment. It is most often found when reimbursement-grouping systems are used. It is because of these and other documented instances of healthcare fraud and abuse that the government began to require healthcare organizations to have corporate compliance programs. (See chapter 14 for more information on reimbursement systems.)

Policies and Procedures for Corporate Compliance

OIG compliance guidelines require that each compliance program be supported by written policies and procedures. In addition, the OIG states that it is important that all individuals affected by a policy or procedure, including the hospital's agents and independent contractors, receive a copy of the policy or procedure. Organizations should develop specific policies and procedures in the following areas as well as other areas, as necessary:

- *Conduct:* Policies on the conduct of the coding program should state the organization's mission, goals, and ethical requirements, in addition to its commitment to comply with federal and state standards and to prevent fraud and abuse.
- *Risk areas:* At the beginning of each fiscal year, the OIG publishes guidance on its "special areas of concern" for

the upcoming year. The OIG publishes its work plan in the *Federal Register* and posts it on its Web site. The table of contents for the HHS/OIG Fiscal Year 2002 Work Plan is shown in figure 13.8 (p. 272). More details are available on the OIG Web site (www.oig.hhs.gov). The OIG recommends that policies and procedures be coordinated with education and training programs to address organizational activities in these areas. Compliance personnel should monitor the OIG Web site for changes in the special areas of concern.

- *Claim development and submission process:* Claim development and submission policies and procedures should address documentation practices, claims preparation and submission, coding processes, and related areas.
- *Medical necessity (reasonable and necessary services):* Policies on medical necessity must ensure that claims are submitted only for those services that have been deemed reasonable and necessary and that a clear, comprehensive summary of medical necessity rules and definitions must be prepared and distributed to the appropriate personnel.
- *Antikickback and self-referral:* Organizational policies and procedures should comply with federal and state antikickback statutes, as well as the Stark physician self-referral law. According to the Stark physician self-referral law, when a physician or a member of a physician's immediate family has a financial relationship with a health care entity, the physician may not make referrals to that entity for the furnishing of certain designated health services (DHS) under the Medicare program, unless a specified exception applies (*Federal Register* 2001, p. 856).
- *Bad debts:* The organization should have a mechanism in place to review its bad-debt practices on an annual basis.
- *Credit balances:* The organization should have procedures in place to track and monitor the status of accounts with credit balances.
- *Retention of records:* Policies and procedures should be established to address the creation, distribution, retention, storage, retrieval, and destruction of clinical records, medical records, and claims documentation as well as the records necessary to protect the integrity of the organizational compliance process and to confirm its effectiveness.
- *Compliance as an element of staff performance planning:* Managers and supervisors should adhere to and promote their organizations' compliance programs. Moreover, compliance should become a part of their performance plan.

When corporate compliance is performed diligently, it can benefit the healthcare organization both economically and culturally. In the September 2001 *Journal of the American Health*

Figure 13.8.   HHS/OIG Fiscal Year 2002 Work Plan—Centers for Medicare and Medicaid Services

Medicare Hospitals
  Medicare Payment Error Prevention Program
  Medicare Education Payments
  Hospital Privileging Activities
  One-Day Hospital Stays
  Hospital Discharges and Subsequent Readmissions
  Consecutive Inpatient Days
  Payments to Acute Care Prospective Payment System Hospitals
  Implementation of Critical Access Hospital Program
  Satellite Hospitals
  Prospective Payment System Transfers during Hospital Mergers
  Diagnosis-Related Group Payment Limits
  Outlier Payments for Expanded Services
  Periodic Interim Payments
  Uncollected Beneficiary Deductibles and Coinsurance
  Diagnosis-Related Group Payment Window—Part B Providers
  Expansion of Diagnosis-Related Group Payment Window
  Hospital Reporting of Restraint-Related Deaths
  Reporting of Restraint and Seclusion Use in Psychiatric Hospitals
  Outpatient Prospective Payment System
  Outlier Payments under Outpatient Prospective Payment System
  Outpatient Services on Same Day as Discharge and Readmission
  Outpatient Pharmacy Services at Acute Care Hospitals
  Outpatient Medical Supplies at Acute Care Hospitals
  Procedure Coding of Outpatient and Physician Services
  Peer Review Organization Sanction Authority

Home Health
  Oversight of Home Health Care Quality
  Home Health Compliance Programs
  Home Health Payment System Controls
  Coding of Home Health Resource Groups

Nursing Home Care
  Quality Assessment and Assurance Committees
  Nurse Aide Training
  Family Experience with Nursing Home Care
  Three-Day Stay Requirement
  Consolidated Billing Requirements
  Survey and Certification Process
  Use of Penalties

Hospice Care
  Plans of Care
  Hospice Payments to Nursing Homes

Physicians
  Beneficiary Access to Preventive Services
  Advance Beneficiary Notices
  Physicians at Teaching Hospitals
  Billing for Residents' Services
  Physician Evaluation and Management Codes
  Consultations
  Inpatient Dialysis Services
  Bone Density Screening
  Services and Supplies Incident to Physicians' Services
  Reassignment of Benefits

Medical Equipment and Supplies
  Medical Necessity of Durable Medical Equipment
  Medicare Pricing of Equipment and Supplies

Laboratory Services
  Clinical Laboratory Improvement Amendments Certifications
  Medicare Billings for Cholesterol Testing
  Clinical Laboratory Proficiency Testing

End-Stage Renal Disease
  Utilization Service Patterns of Beneficiaries
  Medicare Payments for EPOGEN®
  Method II Billing

Drug Reimbursement
  Medicare Coverage of Prescription Drugs
  Drug Prices Paid by Medicare versus Other Sources
  Medicare Billings for Nebulizer Drugs

Other Medicare Services
  Beneficiaries' Experiences with Medigap Insurance
  Rural Health Clinics
  Medicare Payments for Clinical Trials
  Medicare Mental Health National Error Rate

Medicare Managed Care
  Adjusted Community Rate Proposals
  General and Administrative Costs
  Cost-Based Managed Care Plans
  Enhanced Managed Care Payments
  Managed Care Organization Profits
  Managed Care Additional Benefits
  Educating Beneficiaries about Medicare+Choice
  Physician Perspectives on Managed Care Organizations

Medicaid Hospitals
  Medicaid Graduate Medical Education Payments
  Hospital-Specific Disproportionate-Share Payment Limits
  Medicaid Hospital Patient Transfers
  Outpatient Clinical Diagnostic Laboratory Services
    under Ambulatory Procedure Group Systems
  Credit Balances in Inpatient Accounts

Medicaid Managed Care
  Marketing and Enrollment Practices
  Public-Sponsored Managed Care Health Plans
  Managed Care Payments as Part of the Fee-for-Service
    Upper-Payment-Limit Calculation
  Medicaid Fee-for-Service and Managed Care Duplicate Payments
  Pharmacy Benefit Managers
  HIV/AIDS Antiretroviral Drug Therapy
  Cost Containment of Medicaid Mental Health Drugs

Medicaid/State Children's Health Insurance Program
  Adolescent Enrollment in Medicaid/State Children's Health
    Insurance Program
  Educating Families of Children Newly Enrolled in Medicaid
    Managed Care
  Disenrollment from State Children's Health Insurance Program

Other Medicaid Services
  Mutually Exclusive Procedure Claims
  Payments for Services to Dually Eligible Beneficiaries
  Medicaid Fee-for-Service Payments for Dually Eligible Medicare
    Managed Care Enrollees
  Upper-Payment-Limit Calculations
  Intergovernmental Transfers
  Nursing Facility Administrative Costs
  Medicaid Services for the Severely Mentally Ill
  Medicaid Benefits for the Severely Mentally Ill
  Claims for Residents of Institutions from Mental Disorders
  Payments for Inmates of Public Institutions
  Restraints and Seclusion in Residential Treatment Centers
  Discharge Planning: Intermediate-Care Facilities/Institutions
    for the Mentally Retarded
  Durable Medical Equipment Reimbursement Rates
  Follow-up on Clinical Laboratory Services
  Average Wholesale Drug Prices Reported to Medicaid
  Medicaid Outpatient Prescription Drug Pricing

Information Management Association, Meaney reported that the most successful approach to compliance emphasizes positive organizational ethics and values as well as legal and regulatory compliance. He reported that employees respond best to a program that stresses the importance of shared values, ethical corporate culture, and behavioral compliance.

Check Your Understanding 13.5

Instructions: Answer the following questions on a separate piece of paper.

1. Which function of the HHS Office of the Inspector General is discussed in this chapter?

2. Describe some of the benefits of effective corporate compliance programs for healthcare organizations.

3. What roles do individual coders play in corporate compliance?

Emerging Vocabularies and Classifications

A number of vocabularies and classifications have been developed in recent years, some of which will have a significant impact on the role of the HIM professional in the future. The following sections examine some of these recent and emerging vocabularies and classifications.

Systematized Nomenclature of Medicine

The **Systematized Nomenclature of Medicine** (SNOMED) is developed, maintained, and distributed by the College of American Pathologists (CAP). SNOMED was originally built on the Systematized Nomenclature of Pathology (SNOP), which was introduced in 1965. Like SNOP, SNOMED uses an alphanumeric, multiaxial coding scheme (Kudla and Blakemore 2001).

In 1997, the CAP worked with a team of physicians and nurses from Kaiser Permanente to begin development of the **Systematized Nomenclature of Medicine Reference Terminology** (SNOMED RT) (Kudla and Blakemore 2001). In 1997, Spackman, Campbell, and Cote defined a **reference terminology** for clinical data as "a set of concepts and relationships that provides a common reference point for comparison and aggregation of data about the entire health care process, recorded by multiple different individuals, systems or institutions." One of the ways that SNOMED RT does this is by including an elementary mapping to ICD-9-CM (Kudla and Blakemore 2001). SNOMED also is working with the Digital Imaging and Communications in Medicine (DICOM) community, the Logical Observation Identifier Names and Codes (LOINC) system, and the various nursing vocabularies to further expand its content.

Released in 2000, SNOMED RT is a concept-based terminology consisting of more than 110,000 concepts with linkages to more than 180,000 terms with unique computer-readable codes. The following illustration shows why there would be a different number of concepts and terms:

CONCEPT	D2-04610 Paralysis of glottis
TERMS	D2-04610 01 Paralysis of glottis
	D2-04610 02 Paralysis of vocal cords
	D2-04610 03 Vocal cord paralysis

Table 13.1 is an example of a SNOMED RT concept table. Instead of being deleted, certain **concepts** and codes are retired so that they cannot be used for new code assignments.

In addition to the numerous concepts and terms, more than 260,000 relationships exist between and among the terms. A **relationship** is a type of connection between two terms. Examples of types of relationships are "assoc-etiology," "is a," and so on. SNOMED has an average of seven levels of hierarchy per concept, allowing the retrieval of a case on numerous criteria arranged hierarchically (for example, Diabetes, anatomic relationships—leg injuries). Table 13.2 shows an example of a SNOMED RT relationship table. This table illustrates how the same concept code, "DE-11200," can have multiple relationships with multiple parent codes.

The content coverage in SNOMED RT is expanded from version 3 with the addition of oncology. SNOMED is mapped to version 2 of ICD-O. It includes living organisms, drug ingredients and brand names, and laboratory medicine. It also addresses LOINC and forensics.

The folowing are the major sections of SNOMED RT:

- Findings, conclusions, and/or assessments
- Procedures
- Body structures
- Biological functions
- Living organisms
- Substances (drugs and chemicals)
- Physical agents, activities, and/or forces
- Occupations
- Social context
- Modifiers/linkage terms and/or qualifiers

Table 13.1.   Example of a SNOMED RT Concepts Table

Concept Code	Fully Specified Name	Status
DE-11200	Anthrax	OK
DE-11207	Anthrax septicemia	OK
DE-11208	Other specified anthrax manifestations	RET
DE-11312	Toxicoinfectious botulism	OK

Table 13.2.   Example of a SNOMED RT Relationship Table

Concept Code	Relationship	Parent Concept Code
DE-11200	ISA	DE-00000
DE-11200	ISA	DE-10000
DE-11200	ASSOC-ETIOLOGY	L-12200
DE-11200	ASSOC-ETIOLOGY	L-12202

Because SNOMED RT has a tremendous amount of content and is concept based, it has the potential to standardize medical terms, enabling accurate communication among diverse systems. In addition, it allows healthcare personnel and organizations to collect and analyze data more effectively, to compare the quality of healthcare being administered, to develop effective treatment guidelines, and to conduct outcomes research (Kudla and Blakemore 2001).

However, because of its tremendous amount of content, SNOMED RT would be difficult to use as a reimbursement classification system (although it could be used in the underlying clinical information system). It is highly likely that numerous systems, potentially working in concert, would be required to both support an efficient and effective clinical information system (IS) and handle the reimbursement needs of a healthcare organization. In addition, because SNOMED RT is not published in a paper format, organizations that are not technologically advanced would have difficulty using it.

However, keeping in mind the definition of a reference terminology and assuming that SNOMED RT qualifies as one, SNOMED RT would have great utility in a computerized system. Full use of its relationships would enable healthcare organizations to better support their employees. It would also allow them to glean new knowledge from their information systems.

The future for SNOMED is ambitious. In 2002, the CAP, in alliance with the National Health Service of the United Kingdom, is planning to release **SNOMED Clinical Terms** (SNOMED CT) (Kudla and Blakemore 2001). SNOMED CT will be the result of merging SNOMED RT with the National Health Service (NHS) vocabulary, Clinical Terms Version 3, or CTV3 (formerly known as the Read Codes). SNOMED CT will incorporate all of the content from both SNOMED RT and CTV3 into a data structure that will have between 250,000 and 300,000 concepts, 400,000 terms, and more than a million relationships to add meaning. Moreover, SNOMED CT will retain the SNOMED RT and CTV3 identifiers for longitudinal reporting purposes. (See figure 13.9 for an illustration of the core structure of SNOMED CT.)

Clinical Terms Version 3 (Read Codes)

In the 1980s, James Read, a family practice physician in England, developed the **Read Codes** for recording and retrieving computerized primary care patient data (Kudla and Blakemore 2001). The Read Codes, now known as **Clinical Terms, Version 3** (CTV3), are covered by Crown Copyright. The British National Health Service (NHS) Information Authority distributes the codes on behalf of the U.K. Department of Health (www.coding.nhisa.nhs.uk).

First distributed in July 1994, CTV3 now is used in the majority of the primary care practices in the United Kingdom. Use of CTV3 in the United States is becoming—and will continue to become—more widespread as a result of the agreement described above to combine CTV3 with SNOMED-RT to create SNOMED CT.

The features of CTV3 include:

- *File structure:* Although previously hierarchical, CTV3 has implemented a parent–child relationship table that allows for polyhierarchy.
- *Qualifiers:* Qualifiers were added in 1995–1996 to add extra information and clinical detail. They are linked to core terms. This is called compositionality. Instead of having all of the possible variations, they are created as needed.
- *Natural terms:* "Other specified" and NEC are marked as optional, and long, complex terms have been kept to a minimum, with qualifiers being used instead. Read codes will never be deleted; rather, they are indicated with an asterisk as optional.

CTV3 chapters include:

- Clinical findings
  —History and observations
  —Disorders
  —Morphology findings
- Operations, procedures, and interventions
  —Operations and procedures
  —Clinical examinations
  —Psychotherapeutic, behavioral, and communication procedures
  —Activities of daily living procedures and interventions
  —Indirect care procedures (for example, care plans)
  —Regimes and therapies (hormone therapy, contraception, art therapy, special diets, etc.)
  —Investigations
- Causes of injury and poisoning
- Administration
- Occupations
- Drugs
- Appliances and equipment

Following are the partial results for a search done on the term *cough:*

Coughs
Coughing
Cough
Difficulty coughing
Cough suppressants
Cough reflex impaired
H/O: whooping cough

Figure 13.9.   Core Structure of SNOMED CT

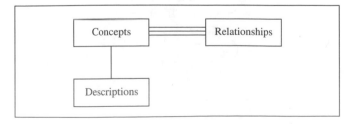

A request for details on *coughs* results in the following display:

READ Code: <u>Xa4N4</u>   Term ID: <u>YaQrY</u>
Does cough

<u>Terms</u>
Does cough
Coughs

In examining the operations, procedures, and interventions chapter, items such as health education, counseling, and screening are among those listed. The presence of these items shows that the primary care focus of CTV3 combined with the specialty focus of SNOMED RT will result in a formidable terminology.

Because many of the characteristics of SNOMED RT also are found in CTV3, the advantages and disadvantages are similar. One significant difference is that CTV3 has been widely implemented in computerized systems, thus demonstrating its applicability in healthcare information systems.

Logical Observation Identifier Names and Codes

The work on **Logical Observation Identifier Names and Codes** (LOINC) began in February 1994. Today, LOINC is generally accepted as the exchange standard for laboratory results, enabling standards to be developed and adopted relatively quickly to meet a desperate need.

The goal for LOINC is not to replace the laboratory fields in facility databases but, rather, to provide a mapping mechanism. The LOINC committee hoped that laboratories would create fields in their master files for storing LOINC codes and names as attributes of their own data elements.

The LOINC committee first established a rule for creating LOINC names. "If a test has its own column on a clinical report, or has a reference range that is significantly different from other tests, or has clinical significance distinct from other closely related tests, it should be assigned a separate name" (Forrey et al. 1996, p. 82). Thus, each LOINC name identifies a distinct laboratory observation.

Each LOINC name is structured and can contain up to six parts, including:

- Analyte/component (for example, potassium, hemoglobin)
- Kind of property measured or observed (for example, mass, mass concentration, enzyme concentration)
- Time aspect of the measurement or observation (a point in time versus an observation integrated over time)
- System/sample type (for example, urine, blood, serum)
- Type of measurement or observation scale (quantitative [a number] versus qualitative [a trait such as cloudy])
- Type of measurement or observation method used (for example, clean catch or catheter)

After the names were established, unique codes were simply assigned to the names. The codes have no inherent meaning; they were designed for use by computers, not humans. LOINC has rules for using each part of the LOINC name. That detail can be accessed on the LOINC Web site at www.regenstrief.org/loinc. Table 13.3 provides an example of LOINC codes and names.

The LOINC database contains twenty-three fields in addition to the six named ones. Finally, records that should no longer be used are tagged as such rather than removed.

The primary disadvantage to LOINC is that it may require significant modifications to work with a current laboratory information system. As with SNOMED RT and CTV3, LOINC is usable only in computerized systems.

A distinct advantage to using LOINC is that it enables the standardized communication of laboratory results. Large integrated delivery systems that have very diverse laboratory processing systems (the machines that perform the tests) will find it easier to maintain and use a CPR with valid laboratory results.

Nursing Classifications

The care delivered by nurses is very different from the care delivered by other healthcare professionals. In an effort to research, teach, practice, and create public policy for nursing, the nursing profession, under the leadership of the American Nurses Association (ANA), has developed nursing classifications. The purpose of these classifications is to describe the nursing process, document nursing care, and facilitate aggregation of data for comparisons at the local, regional, national, and international levels (Henry et al. 1998).

The ANA established the Steering Committee on Databases to Support Clinical Nursing Practice (SCD) to monitor and support the development and evolution of the use of multiple vocabularies and classification schemes (Henry et al. 1998). Out of that initiative came the creation of the Nursing Information and Data Set Evaluation Center (NIDSEC). The purpose of the NIDSEC is to review, evaluate against defined criteria, and recognize IS developers and manufacturers that support nursing care documentation with automated Nursing Information Systems (NIS) or within CPR systems (www.nursingworld.org/nidsec). Figure 13.10 (p. 276) lists the ANA criteria for recognition of nursing classifications (Henry et al. 1998).

Through the NIDSEC, the ANA has recognized a total of twelve classifications for nursing. Figure 13.11 (p. 276) lists the classifications along with their Web sites, where applicable.

Currently, nursing professionals are working with SNOMED RT and other vocabulary system developers to

Table 13.3.   LOINC Codes and Names

Code	Name
11-7	AMIKACIN:SUSC:PT:ISLT:QN:MBC
2603-9	MALONATE:MCNC:PT:SER:QN
5874-3	RESPIRATORY SYNCYTIAL VIRUS AG:ACNC:PT:THRT:SQ:EIA

create classifications that will meet the needs of nursing. As Henry states in the May 1998 *Journal of the American Health Information Management Association,* "In this era of numerous requests for data and information from multiple accrediting, governing, and quality monitoring agencies, it is vital that the HIM professional be aware of classification sys-

Figure 13.10.   ANA Criteria for the Recognition of Nursing Classifications

1. The classification must be clinically useful for making diagnostic, intervention, and/or outcome decisions.
2. The classification must go beyond an application or synthesis/adaptation of vocabulary/classification schemes currently recognized by the ANA or present an explicit rationale why it should also be recognized.
3. The classification must be stated in clear and unambiguous terms, with the terms precisely defined.
4. The classification must have been tested for reliability of the vocabulary terms.
5. The classification must have been validated as useful for clinical purposes.
6. The classification must be accompanied by documentation of a systematic methodology for development.
7. The classification must be accompanied by evidence of process for periodic review and provision for addition, revision, and deletion of terms.
8. The classification must have a taxonomic structure that is conceptually coherent.
9. The classification must have terms that are associated with a unique identifier or code.
10. The classification must leave a machine-readable audit trail.
11. The classification must include defining characteristics, especially for nursing diagnoses.

Figure 13.11.   ANA-Recognized Nursing Classifications

North American Nursing Diagnosis Association (NANDA)
www.nanda.org

Nursing Interventions Classifications
www.nursing.uiowa.edu/cnc

Nursing Outcomes Classification
www.nursing.uiowa.edu/cnc

Home Health Care Classification (HHCC)
www.sabacare.com

Omaha System
www.con.ufl.edu/omaha

Nursing Management Minimum Data Set (NMMDS)

Patient Care Data Set (PCDS)

Perioperative Nursing Dataset
www.aorn.org

SNOMED RT
www.snomed.org

Nursing Minimum Data Sets (NMDA)

International Classification for Nursing Practice (ICNP)
www.icn.ch/icnp.htm

ABCcodes
www.alternativelink.com

tems and related national efforts, beyond those that are typically physician-centric in nature (for example, ICD-9-CM and CPT). Without reliable and valid data concerning the contributions of the entire healthcare team, it is truly impossible to engage in the practice of evidence-based healthcare delivery."

Unified Medical Language System

The **Unified Medical Language System** (UMLS) is a government-funded project from the National Library of Medicine (NLM). The UMLS has been in development since 1986. According to the UMLS Fact Sheet, "The purpose of the UMLS is to aid the development of systems that help health professionals and researchers retrieve and integrate electronic biomedical information from a variety of sources and to make it easy for users to link disparate information systems, including computer-based patient records, bibliographic databases, factual databases, and expert systems." This goal is achieved through the three knowledge sources found in the UMLS: (1) the UMLS Metathesaurus®, (2) the SPECIALIST **Lexicon,** and (3) the UMLS Semantic Network. (More information on the UMLS can be obtained from the NLM Web site at www.nlm.nih.gov/research/umls.) When looking in-depth at the UMLS, it is important to keep in mind that it has been designed for computer use; its layouts and so on are meant for machines.

UMLS Metathesaurus

The UMLS Metathesaurus contains information on biomedical concepts and terms from more than sixty controlled vocabularies and classifications used in health records, administrative health data, bibliographic and full-text databases, and expert systems. It preserves the names, meanings, hierarchical contexts, attributes, and interterm relationships present in its source vocabularies; adds certain basic information to each concept; and establishes new relationships among terms from different source vocabularies. Its source vocabularies include terminologies designed for use in health record systems; large disease and procedure classifications used for statistical reporting and billing; more narrowly focused vocabularies used to record data related to psychiatry, nursing, medical devices, adverse drug reactions, and so on; disease and finding terminologies from expert diagnostic systems; and some thesauri used in information retrieval.

Computer programs can use information in the Metathesaurus to interpret user inquiries, interact with users to refine their questions, identify the databases that contain information relevant to particular inquiries, and convert the users' terms into the vocabulary used by relevant information sources. The scope of the Metathesaurus is determined by the combined scope of its source vocabularies.

The Metathesaurus is produced by the automated processing of machine-readable versions of its source vocabularies, followed by human review and editing by subject experts. It is intended primarily for use by system developers but also can be a useful reference tool for database builders, librarians, and other information professionals.

SPECIALIST Lexicon

The SPECIALIST Lexicon is an English-language lexicon containing many biomedical terms. It has been developed in the context of the SPECIALIST natural language processing project at the National Library of Medicine (NLM). The current version includes some 108,000 lexical records, with more than 186,000 strings (concept names).

The lexicon entry for each word or term records syntactic, morphological, and orthographic information. (*Syntactic* refers to the formal properties of language; *morphological* refers to the study and description of word formation in a language, including inflection, derivation, and compounding; and *orthographic* refers to the correctness of spelling or the representation of the sounds of a language by written or printed symbols.) Lexical entries may be single-word or multiword terms. Entries that share their base form and spelling variants, if any, are collected into a single lexical record. The base form is the uninflected form of the lexical item—the singular form in the case of a noun, the infinitive form in the case of a verb, and the positive form in the case of an adjective or adverb.

UMLS Semantic Network

The Semantic Network, through its 134 semantic types, provides a consistent categorization of all concepts represented in the UMLS Metathesaurus. The fifty-four links between semantic types provide the structure for the network and represent important relationships in the biomedical domain. All information on specific concepts is found in the Metathesaurus; the network provides information on the basic semantic types assigned to these concepts and defines their possible relationships.

Digital Imaging and Communications in Medicine

Through a cooperative effort between the American College of Radiology and the National Electronic Manufacturers Association, **Digital Imaging and Communications in Medicine** (DICOM) was originally created to permit the interchange of biomedical image wave forms and related information. These organizations define the health record to include not only textual, coded, and numeric information (linguistic), but also a detailed, structured record of image-related information (Bidgood 1997).

The information associated with each image is the standard administrative and billing information used today—patient name, procedure code, and so on. Combined with the open protocol, this only provides for data interchange, not data understanding. The people who developed the exchange standard now have taken another step and suggested a mapping/terminology resource to index the content of biomedical images in a clinically relevant manner (Bidgood 1997).

Nosology

Nosology is the branch of medical science that deals with classification issues. Practically, nosology is different from coding in that it is about all classification issues, whether they are related to reimbursement or other purposes.

As the need grows to formalize (classify in some manner) all health record data in any medium (text, image, voice) for purposes of outcomes research, decision support, and knowledge management, HIM professionals will have to expand their coding classification horizons to become nosologists.

Check Your Understanding 13.6

Instructions: Answer the following questions on a separate piece of paper.

1. A connection between two terms is called a relationship. Explain some uses of relationships in a terminology?

2. What is the future goal of DICOM?

3. Name the three knowledge sources found in the UMLS.

4. Define the term nosology.

5. Name the main advantage and the main disadvantage to using the LOINC system.

Evaluation of Clinical Terminologies and Classification Systems

As HIM professionals search for ways to formalize the myriad types of data contained in CPRs, it helps to be able to evaluate the different classifications and terminologies. Certain characteristics are desirable. The first twelve characteristics listed below are taken from Cimino (1998). The second six are taken from Campbell (Campbell et al. 1999), who presented additional requirements after his experience with implementing a terminology for Kaiser Permanente. The characteristics are:

1. *Content:* The content of clinical classifications and terminologies should be determined by their intended use. It is wise to assume that the first identified need will never be the last or only need. It is far better to have too much content initially than to have too little to meet subsequent needs.

2. *Concept orientation:* The content of terminologies and classifications should be oriented toward concepts rather than terms or code numbers.

3. *Concept permanence:* Terminologies and classifications must be permanent if they are to be useful for longitudinal reporting. Concepts may be inactivated but must never be deleted.

4. *Nonsemantic concept identifier:* No implicit or explicit meaning can be associated with the code numbers used in a classification system. Because primary healthcare systems are now computerized, the human ability to use a classification system without a computer is no longer necessary.

5. *Polyhierarchy:* Multiple relationships should exist for every concept. For example, bacterial pneumonia is both a pulmonary disease and an infectious disease.

6. *Formal definitions:* Standardized definitions are necessary to ensure comparability among terminologies and classifications.

7. *Reject Not Elsewhere Classified (NEC):* Not Elsewhere Classified is not the same as Not Otherwise Specified (NOS). NOS means that there is no additional information. NEC means you have more information but no place to put it. It also means that any additional information will be lost forever if it is assigned the NEC label (for example, Pneumonia, NEC).

8. *Multiple granularities:* Because classifications and terminologies must fulfill multiple purposes, the information in them may be specific or general so that all needs can be met.

9. *Multiple consistent views:* Classifications and terminologies must accommodate more than one viewpoint to allow them to be multipurpose as well as to ensure continuity of care. When caring for the same patient, nurses want to use nurse speak and physicians want to use physician speak.

10. *Context representation:* Words have different meanings when used in different contexts or as different grammatical parts of language. Context is determined by how the concepts relate to each other. For example, consider the term "cold." In the phrase "the patient is cold," cold is how the patient feels. In the phrase, "the patient has a cold," cold is a disease. The difference between the two phrases reflects the two different contexts of the word "cold."

11. *Graceful evolution:* The days of yearly updates need to end soon. Future updates will have to be made monthly or, more likely, weekly. The growth of medical knowledge is exponential; classification systems and terminologies must to be able to keep up.

12. *Recognized redundancy:* Classifications and terminologies need to accommodate redundancy.

13. *Licensed and copyrighted:* Terminologies and classifications need to be copyrighted and licensed to control local modifications, which result in semantic drift and produce incomparable data.

14. *Vendor neutral:* Classifications and terminologies must be vendor neutral so that they can be readily used as national standards by all vendors without conferring a competitive advantage to any one of them.

15. *Scientifically valid:* Terminologies and classifications should be understandable, reproducible, and useful and should reflect the current understanding of the science.

16. *Adequate maintenance:* A central authority that provides a rapid response to requests for new terms is essential to minimize the need for local enhancements and to keep terminologies and classifications current.

17. *Self-sustaining:* Classifications and terminologies should be supported by public or endowment funding. Alternatively, licensing fees should be proportional to the value the system provides to users.

18. *Scalable infrastructure and process control:* The tools and processes for maintaining a terminology or classification should be scalable, especially for a nationally standardized terminology.

In addition to following the preceding criteria, HIM professionals should use all of their system analysis and data management skills when evaluating the appropriateness of a clinical terminology for a particular function or need. Another helpful reference for evaluating the quality of a clinical terminology is the American Society for Testing and Materials (ASTM) Standard E 2087-00: Standard Specification for Quality Indicators for Controlled Health Vocabularies. (The standard is available from ASTM at www.astm.org.)

Check Your Understanding 13.7

Instructions: Answer the following questions on a separate piece of paper.

1. Why is concept of permanence important in clinical terminologies and classifications?

2. What is another name for *context representation*? What does the term mean?

Real-World Case

Matthew Greene, RHIA, CCS is one of about twenty-five people currently working on a health data repository (HDR) for the entire Veterans Health Administration (VHA) healthcare system. The overall goal of the HDR is to have one place to store a patient's healthcare data. Initially, this will be VHA-only data, though VHA is coordinating its efforts with the Department of Defense and even envisions a time when they will exchange data with nongovernmental entities.

Matthew's official title is health data repository functional analyst/health information management specialist. Earlier in his career, he held the following positions:

- Coder and analyst at Buffalo VAMC for ten years
- Senior coding specialist at VA Salt Lake City Healthcare System for one year
- Coding supervisor/assistant chief, HIM, at VA Salt Lake City Healthcare System for four years

In his current position he is particularly responsible for working with clinicians and other domain experts to determine the content or what will be stored in the HDR. It is important to note that the VHA Office of Information created this position specifically for a person with an HIM background.

Given Matthew's main duties of determining the content of the HDR, he must not only possess up-to-date knowledge of the current legal requirements and standards for a clinical record; he must also be aware of what is new in the field. This can include anything from retention requirements to required fields to use the LOINC laboratory standard to the ASTM content standards. Matthew also maintains a wish list of data elements that people would want to see in the HDR in the future. Examples of this might include cardiac ejection fraction or the DICOM data fields. Matthew has to keep in mind that this database will be used for research and forecasting, as well as for clinical care.

Other persons on the database design team of the HDR include Michael Lincoln, MD, the database design team leader, a clinician and vocabulary expert who has performed research in this area for a number of years. Ferdinand Frankson is the software system engineer responsible for the health data dictionary, and Ann Miles is the senior business services analyst who addresses the mapping issues. There is also a quality assurance tester, Lee Ann Hulet, to ensure the excellence of the project.

In relation to terminology and vocabulary efforts, VHA already has firm plans in place to utilize SNOMED and the UMLS. Specifically, they intend to use SNOMED to:

- Code complex history and physical exam information, for example, to code "right-sided substernal chest pain," so that it is retrievable
- Code surgical pathology or cytology diagnoses and anatomic body parts
- Provide the ability to produce more specific patient queries for their peer review program
- Describe meaningful "IS_A" relationships for decision support, data aggregation, and forecasting purposes
- Code diagnoses, problems, surgical procedures and other pertinent conditions into the problem list

They plan to use the UMLS as a metadictionary to cross-link across coding systems, as well as to their own VA Lexicon Utility Version 2.0, which will be included in the VHA enterprise terminology.

When asked which characteristic is most helpful to his position, Matthew answers quickly, "being detail oriented." The requirements for both the terminology and the data elements are very detailed—little things can mean a lot. While his knowledge of traditional coding systems is excellent, Matthew did have to learn a lot about the terminologies that are being developed and used in healthcare today. Matthew also feels that his HIM background helped him with the broad understanding of the data and how it interrelates, as well as the details necessary to make the data useful. He also states that his biggest weakness at the beginning of this project was a lack of knowledge about terminologies and record standards in general.

Matthew feels that one of the biggest benefits to a standardized terminology will be improving communication among organizations. Even in an organization as standardized as VHA, one will still find clinicians using terminology in an inconsistent manner. He also states that the terminology will allow VHA to analyze data across the system without the limiting factors of ICD-9-CM and CPT. The organization will be able to analyze with much more detail and specificity. The terminology will also help VHA further develop their clinical decision support with health factors (treatments that currently resist coding).

Discussion Question

List two ways VHA wants to utilize a terminology and give an example of each. Compare and discuss your answers with fellow students.

Summary

The coding and classification systems currently used in the healthcare industry are inadequate to support today's standards of patient care, but they are necessary for reimbursement. The technologies to support healthcare information needs will continue to develop at a phenomenal rate. As with other industries, healthcare requires information systems that can not only facilitate its current work but also assist in managing the knowledge explosion. These systems are impossible to develop without a "language for healthcare." HIM professionals must participate in the development, implementation, and maintenance of information systems that use standard vocabulaties, nomenclatures, and classification systems.

References

American Health Information Management Association. 1999. Clarification of clinical data sets, vocabularies, terminologies, and classifications. *Journal of the American Health Information Management Association* 70(2):72–73.

American Health Information Management Association. 2000. *Evolving HIM Careers: Seven Roles for the Future.* Chicago: AHIMA.

American Health Information Management Association. 2000. Standards of Ethical Coding.

American Hospital Association, Coding Resource Center. Accessed online from www.ahacentraloffice.org.

American Medical Association, Current Procedural Terminology. Accessed online from www.ama-assn.org.

American Psychiatric Association, DSM-IV Questions and Answers. Accessed online from www.psych.org.

Averill, R. F. 1999. Honest mistakes or fraud: meeting the coding compliance challenge. *Journal of the American Health Information Management Association* 70(5).

Barnett, O. G., et al. 1993. The computer-based clinical record: where do we stand? *Annals of Internal Medicine* 119(10):1046–48.

BehaveNet, Clinical Capsule. Accessed online from www.behavenet.com.

Beinborn, J. 1999. Automated coding: the next step. *Journal of the American Health Information Management Association* 70(7).

Bidgood, W. D., Jr. 1997. Documenting the information content of images. *Proceedings of the AMIA Annual Fall Symposium,* pp. 424–28.

Bowman, E. 2001. Coding, classification, and reimbursement systems. In *Health Information: Management of a Strategic Resource,* second edition, edited by M. Abdelhak et al. Philadelphia: W. B. Saunders Company.

Campbell, K. E., B. Hochhalter, J. Slaughter, and J. Mattison. 1999. Enterprise issues pertaining to implementing controlled terminologies. IMIA Conference.

Centers for Medicare and Medicaid Services. Accessed online from www.cms.gov.

Chute, C. G. 2000. Clinical classification and terminology: some history and current observations. *Journal of the American Medical Informatics Association* 7(3):298–303.

Cimino, J. J. 1998. Desiderata for controlled medical vocabularies in the twenty-first century. *Methods of Information in Medicine* 37:394–403.

Department of Health and Human Services, Centers for Disease Control, National Center for Health Statistics. *International Classification of Diseases, 10th Revision.* Document downloaded from Web site.

Department of Health and Human Services. Administrative Simplification Transaction and Code Sets, Frequently Asked Questions. Accessed online from aspe.os.dhhs.gov.

Department of Health and Human Services, Office of Inspector General. History document. Accessed online from ois.hhs.gov.

Encyclopaedia Britanica Online. Accessed online from www.eb.com.

Federal Register 66, no. 3, January 4, 2001.

Forrey, A. W., C. J. McDonald, G. DeMoor, and others. 1996. Logical Observation Identifier Names and Codes (LOINC) Database: a public use set of codes and names for electronic reporting of clinical laboratory results. *Clinical Chemistry* 42:1:81–90.

Fox, L .A. 1992. An ethical dilemma: coding medical records for reimbursement. *Journal of the American Health Information Management Association* 63(1):34–37.

Hammond, W. E., and J. J. Cimino. 2000. Standards in medical informatics. In *Medical Informatics: Computer Applications in Health Care and Biomedicine,* second edition, edited by Edward H. Shortliffe and Leslie E. Perreault, pp. 212–56. New York City: Springer.

Health Care Financing Administration, ICD-10-PCS Speaker Slides. Accessed online from www.cms.gov.

Health Care Financing Administration, HCPCS. Accessed online from www.cms.gov.

Henry, S. B., et al. 1998. Nursing data, classification systems, and quality indicators: what every HIM professional needs to know. *Journal of the American Health Information Management Association* 69(5):48–54.

ICD-9-CM Coordination and Maintenance Committee. May 17, 2001. Minutes. Accessed online from www.cms.gov.

Kudla, K. M., and M. Blakemore. SNOMED takes the next step. *Journal of the American Health Information Management Association* 72(7):62–68.

LOINC. Accessed online from www.regenstrief.org.

Meaney, M. E. 2001. A blue-ribbon approach to compliance. *Journal of the American Health Information Management Association* 72(8):24–25.

National Center for Health Statistics, ICD-9. Accessed online from www.cdc.gov/nchs.

National Center for Health Statistics, ICD-10-CM. Accessed online from www.cdc.gov/nchs.

National Health Service Information Center. Accessed online from www.coding.nhisa.nhs.uk.

National Health Service Information Centre, NHS Centre for Coding and Classification. 1999. *The READ Codes.* Demonstration CD.

Nursing Information & Data Set Evaluation Center. Accessed online from www.nursingworld.org/nidsec.

Schnitzer, G. L. 2000. Natural language processing: a coding professional's perspective. *Journal of the American Health Information Management Association* 71(9).

Schwager, R. 2000. Speech recognition propels transcription revolution. *Journal of the American Health Information Management Association* 71(9).

Slee, V. N., and D. A. Slee. 1991. *Health Care Terms,* second edition. St. Paul, Minn.: Tringa Press.

SNOMED. Accessed online from www.snomed.org.

Spackman, K. A., K. E. Campbell, and R. A. Cote. 1997. SNOMED RT: a reference terminology for health care. *Proceedings of the American Medical Informatics Association Annual Symposium,* pp. 640–44.

Warner, H. R., Jr. 2000. Can natural language processing aid outpatient coders? *Journal of the American Health Information Management Association* 71(8).

World Health Organization. Accessed online from www.who.int.

Application Exercises

1. Choose a clinical classification or vocabulary and evaluate it against the characteristics presented in this chapter.

2. Using an Internet search or after discussions with your instructor, fellow students, or HIA professionals, locate a clinical classification or vocabulary that is not described in this chapter. Find out who and how it was developed, its current purpose and use, an overview of the structure, its advantages and disadvantages, and its applicability in a computerized system. Present your findings to the class.

3. Describe how an encoder and an automated coder would be used for different purposes.

Review Quiz

Instructions: Choose the best word or phrase to complete the following statements.

1. ____ Healthcare organizations and practitioners throughout the country need a common terminology to____.
   a. Read tests more accurately
   b. Exchange and use information reliably
   c. Prepare secondary records
   d. Track population mortality

2. ____ The most widely accepted standard about terminology is____.
   a. The AMIA Board of Directors editorial
   b. ASTM Standard E 2087-00
   c. ISO Standard 1087
   d. ANSI Standard X12N

3. ____ Classifications and nomenclatures____.
   a. Categorize and aggregate
   b. Represent the whole of a subject field
   c. Assign code numbers to concepts
   d. Help with computerized patient records

4. ____ The International Classification of Diseases was originally developed to promote the international collection and processing of____.
   a. Morbidity statistics
   b. Healthcare service utilization
   c. Procedure statistics
   d. Mortality statistics

5. ____ ICD-10 began to be used in the United States for mortality reporting in____.
   a. 1990
   b. 1999
   c. 1995
   d. 2001

6. ____ New coding system standards for the United States will be adopted via the process set forth by____.
   a. HCFA
   b. The ICD-9-CM Coordination and Maintenance Committee
   c. The Health Insurance Portability and Accountability Act of 1996
   d. WHO

7. ____ True or false: ICD-10-PCS is based on a seven-character alphanumeric code. The meanings of each individual character changes according to the needs of the clinical section.
   a. True
   b. False

8. ____ The first level of HCPCS consists of ____.
   a. CPT
   b. CDT
   c. NDC
   d. DSM

9. ____ The two primary purposes of historical coding systems have been____.
   a. Knowledge management and patient care
   b. Decision support and quality assurance
   c. Reimbursement and the creation of secondary records
   d. Research and utilization review

10. ____ The extent to which an experiment, test, or measuring procedure yields the same results in repeated trials is____.
    a. Validity
    b. Reliability
    c. Timeliness
    d. Completeness

11. ____ Technology that "reads" the data contained in a CPR is____.
    a. Encoding
    b. Speech recognition
    c. Image processing
    d. Natural language processing

12. ____ Investigations, audits, and evaluations conducted by the HHS OIG relating to healthcare fraud have resulted in ____.
    a. Compliance programs
    b. The Social Security Act
    c. Terminology standardization
    d. Peer review programs

13. ____ The most successful approach to compliance is____.
    a. Complete discipline
    b. No discipline, completely voluntary
    c. Combining ethics and values with legal compliance
    d. None of the above

14. ____ SNOMED RT is a ____-based terminology.
    a. Term
    b. Code
    c. Classification
    d. Concept

15. ____ The merger between SNOMED RT and CTV3 is posited to be successful because it combines ____.
    a. Primary and specialty care systems
    b. American and United Kingdom terms
    c. Their code numbers
    d. Their distribution systems

16. ____ The goal of LOINC is to ____.
    a. Replace the laboratory fields in everyone's database
    b. Provide a mapping mechanism
    c. Standardize laboratory testing machines
    d. Limit the types of laboratory tests

17. ____ Nosology is____.
    a. An advanced form of coding and classification
    b. The classification of images
    c. A type of natural language processing
    d. A branch of medical science dealing with classification issues

18. ____ Not Elsewhere Classified should not be present in a clinical terminology because it results in____.
    a. Imprecise data
    b. Difficult data entry
    c. Reimbursement denials
    d. Data warehouse problems

Chapter 14
Reimbursement Methodologies

Michelle A. Green, MPS, RHIA, CMA

Learning Objectives

- To understand the historical development of healthcare reimbursement in the United States
- To describe current reimbursement processes, forms, and support practices for healthcare reimbursement
- To understand the difference between commercial health insurance and employer self-insurance
- To describe the purpose and basic benefits of the following government-sponsored health programs: Medicare Part A, Medicare Part B, Medicare+Choice, Medicaid, CHAMPVA, TRICARE, HIS, TANF, PACE, SCHIP, Workers' Compensation, and FECA

- To understand the concept of managed care and to provide examples of different types of managed care organizations
- To identify the different types of fee-for-service reimbursement methods
- To understand ambulatory surgery center rates
- To describe prospective payment systems
- To understand the purpose of the fee schedules, chargemasters, and auditing procedures that support the reimbursement process

Key Terms

Accept assignment
Accounts receivable
Accredited Standards Committee, Electronic Data Interchange (ASC X12)
Acute care prospective payment system (PPS)
Administrative services only (ASO) contracts
All Patient DRGs (AP-DRGs)
All Patient Refined DRGs (APR-DRGs)
Ambulatory payment classification (APC) system
Ambulatory surgery center (ASC)
American National Standards Institute (ANSI)
Attending Physician Statement (APS) (or COMB-1)
Audit trail
Auditing
Balance billing
Balanced Budget Refinement Act (BBRA)
Blue Cross and Blue Shield (BC/BS)
Blue Cross and Blue Shield Federal Employee Program (FEP)
Bundled payments
Capitation
Carrier (Medicare)
Case mix
Case-mix groups
Case-mix group payment rates
Case-mix group relative weights
Categorically needy eligibility groups (Medicaid)
Centers for Medicare and Medicaid Services (CMS)
Chargemaster
Civilian Health and Medical Program—Veterans Administration (CHAMPVA)
Civilian Health and Medical Program of the Uniformed Services (CHAMPUS)

Claim
CMS-1500
Code of Federal Regulations (CFR)
Coinsurance
Comorbidity
Compliance
Compliance program guidance
Complication
Conversion factor (CF)
Coordinated care plans
Coordination of benefits (COB) transaction
Correct Coding Initiative (CCI)
Cost outlier
Cost outlier adjustment
CPT (Current Procedural Terminology)
Department of Health and Human Services (HHS)
Diagnosis-related groups (DRGs)
Discharge planning
Discounting
DRG grouper
Electronic data interchange (EDI)
Electronic remittance advice (ERA)
Emergency Maternal and Infant Care Program (EMIC)
Employer-based self-insurance
Episode-of-care (EOC) reimbursement
Exclusive provider organization (EPO)
Explanation of benefits
External reviews (audits)
Federal Employees' Compensation Act (FECA)
Federal poverty level (FPL)
Fee schedule
Fee-for-service basis

Fiscal intermediary (FI)
Fraud and abuse
Geographic practice cost index (GPCI)
Global payment
Global surgery payment
Group health insurance
Group model health maintenance organization
Group practice without walls (GPWW)
CMS-1500
HCPCS (Healthcare Common Procedure Coding System)
Health Care Financing Administration (HCFA)
Health information management (HIM) professionals
Health maintenance organization (HMO)
Health Plan Employer Data and Information Set (HEDIS®)
Health Resources and Services Administration (HRSA)
Healthcare claims (HCC) and payment/advise transaction
Healthcare provider
Home Assessment Validation and Entry (HAVEN)
Home health agency (HHA)
Home health prospective payment system (HH PPS)
Home health resource group (HHRG)
Hospice
Hospitalization insurance (HI) (Medicare Part A)
ICD-9-CM (International Classification of Diseases,
    Ninth Revision, Clinical Modification)
Indemnity plans
Independent practice association (IPA)
Indian Health Service (IHS)
Inpatient coding compliance
Inpatient rehabilitation facility (IRF)
Inpatient Rehabilitation Validation and Entry (IRVEN)
Insured
Insurer
Integrated delivery system (IDS)
Integrated provider organization (IPO)
Interim payment system (IPS)
Low-utilization payment adjustment (LUPA)
Major medical insurance (catastrophic coverage)
Managed care
Managed fee-for-service reimbursement
Management service organization (MSO)
Medicaid
Medical foundation
Medical Group Management Association (MGMA)
Medical savings account (MSA) plans
Medically needy option (Medicaid)
Medicare
Medicare Economic Index (MEI)
Medicare fee schedule (MFS)
Medicare+Choice (Medicare Part C)
Medigap
Minimum Data Set 2.0 (MDS)
Minimum Data Set for Post Acute Care (MDS-PAC)
National Committee for Quality Assurance (NCQA)
National conversion factor (CF)
National Uniform Billing Committee (NUBC)
National Uniform Claim Committee (NUCC)
Network model health maintenance program
Network provider
Nonparticipating providers
Omnibus Budget Reconciliation Act (OBRA)

Outcome and Assessment Information Set (OASIS)
Out-of-pocket expenses
Outpatient
Outpatient and emergency department coding compliance
Outpatient code editor (OCE)
Outpatient prospective payment system (OPPS)
Packaging
Payer of last resort (Medicaid)
Payment status indicator (PSI)
Per diem reimbursement
Per member per month (PMPM)
Per patient per month (PPPM)
Physician-hospital organization (PHO)
Point-of-service (POS) plan
Policyholder
Preferred provider organization (PPO)
Premium
Primary care manager (PCM)
Primary care physician (PCP)
Principal diagnosis
Principal procedure
Professional component (PC)
Programs of All-Inclusive Care for the Elderly (PACE)
Prospective payment system (PPS)
Public assistance
Qualified disabled and working individuals (QDWls)
Qualified Medicare beneficiaries (QMBs)
Qualifying individuals (QIs)
Relative value unit (RVU)
Remittance advice (RA)
Resident Assessment Instrument (RAI)
Resident Assessment Validation and Entry (RAVEN)
Resource Utilization Groups, Version III (RUG-III)
Resource-based relative value scale (RBRVS)
Respite care
Retrospective payment system
Revenue codes
Skilled nursing facility (SNF)
Skilled nursing facility prospective payment system
    (SNF PPS)
Social Security Act
Specified low-income Medicare beneficiaries (SLMBs)
Staff model health maintenance organization
State Children's Health Insurance Program (SCHIP)
State workers' compensation insurance funds
Supplemental medical insurance (SMI) (Medicare Part B)
Tax Equity and Fiscal Responsibility Act of 1982
    (TEFRA)
Technical component (TC)
Temporary Assistance for Needy Families (TANF)
Third-party payer
Traditional fee-for-service reimbursement
TRICARE
TRICARE Extra
TRICARE Prime
TRICARE Prime Remote
TRICARE Senior Prime
TRICARE Standard
UB-92 (CMS-1450)
Usual, customary, and reasonable (UCR) charges
Workers' compensation

Introduction

In the United States, the systems used to pay healthcare organizations and individual healthcare professionals for the services they provide are very complex. This complexity is due in part to the variety of reimbursement methods in use today as well as to strict requirements for detailed documentation to support medical claims. The government and other third-party payers also are concerned about potential fraud and abuse in claims processing. Therefore, ensuring that bills and claims are accurate and correctly presented is an important focus of healthcare compliance.

A reimbursement **claim** is a statement of services submitted by a healthcare provider (for example, a physician or a hospital) to a **third-party payer** (for example, an insurance company or Medicare). The claim documents the medical services that were provided to a specific patient during a specific episode of care. Accurate reimbursement is critical to the operational and financial health of healthcare organizations. In most healthcare organizations, health insurance specialists process reimbursement claims. **Health information management (HIM) professionals** also play an important role in healthcare reimbursement by:

- Ensuring that health record documentation supports services billed
- Assigning diagnostic and procedural codes according to patient record documentation
- Appealing insurance claims denials

This chapter reviews the history of healthcare reimbursement in the United States and explains the different reimbursement systems commonly used since the advent of the various types of prospective payment systems. It then discusses a variety of healthcare reimbursement methodologies with a focus on Medicare prospective payment systems. Finally, it explains how reimbursement claims are processed and the support processes involved.

Theory into Practice

It is not uncommon to hear the phrase "if it wasn't documented, it wasn't done" in reference to health record documentation. In the context of reimbursement, this phrase means that when a **healthcare provider** (for example, a hospital) provides a service to a patient but fails to document the service in the patient's health record, that provider has no documentation to support a claim for the service. As a result, the third-party payer may deny the claim.

For example, suppose that a hospital submitted a claim for **outpatient** services totaling $1,950. When the third-party payer reviewed the claim, it might disallow $200 in charges for which there was no health record documentation. The payer then would recalculate the claim for a total payment of $1,750. The hospital would have lost $200 in revenue on this one case. However, if the hospital were underpaid $200 on every case because of incomplete documentation and the hospital discharged 36,500 patients per year, the potential revenue loss for one year would be $7,300,000!

History of Healthcare Reimbursement in the United States

Healthcare reimbursement in the United States has a long and complex history. Until the late 1800s, Americans paid their own healthcare expenses. Many people without the means to pay for care received charity care or no care at all. Over the past 100 years, a number of groups have attempted to develop systems that would ensure adequate healthcare for every American. But the development of prepaid insurance plans and third-party reimbursement systems did not follow a straight path. The result is the complicated reimbursement system in place today.

Campaigns for National Health Insurance

The American Association of Labor Legislation (AALL) began the campaign for health insurance in the United States with the creation of a committee on social welfare. The committee held its first national conference in 1913 and drafted model health insurance legislation in 1915. The proposed legislation limited coverage to the working class and others who earned less than $1,200 a year, including their dependents. Coverage included the services of physicians, nurses, and hospitals; sick pay; maternity benefits; and a death benefit of $50 to pay for funeral expenses. Although the plan was supported by the American Medical Association (AMA), it was never passed into law.

During the 1930s, expanding access to medical care services became the focus of healthcare reforms. Hospital costs increased as the middle class used more hospital services. Medical care, especially hospital care, became a bigger item in family budgets. The Committee on the Cost of Medical Care (CCMC) was formed to address concerns about the cost and distribution of medical care. The committee was funded by eight philanthropic organizations, including the Rockefeller, Millbank, and Rosenwald foundations. It first met in 1926 and stopped meeting in 1932. The CCMC's published research findings demonstrated the need for additional healthcare services. The committee recommended that national resources be allocated for healthcare and that voluntary health insurance be provided as a means of covering medical costs. Like the AALL's earlier efforts, however, nothing came of the CCMC initiative.

In 1937, the Tactical Committee on Medical Care was formed. It drafted the Wagner National Health Act of 1939. The act supported a federally funded national health program to be administered by states and localities. The Wagner Act evolved from a proposal for federal grants-in-aid to a plan for national health insurance. The proposal called for compulsory national health insurance and a payroll tax. Although the proposed legislation generated extensive national debate, it was not passed into law by Congress.

In 1945, the healthcare issue received the support of an American president for the first time when Harry Truman introduced a plan for universal comprehensive national health insurance. Proposed compromises included a system of private insurance for those who could afford it and public welfare services for the poor. Truman's plan died in a congressional committee in 1946.

After the Second World War, private insurance systems expanded and union-negotiated healthcare benefits served to protect workers from the impact of unforeseen healthcare expenses. The Hill-Burton Act (formally called the Hospital Survey and Construction Act) was passed in 1946. This health facility construction program was instituted under Title VI of the Public Health Service Act. The program was designed to provide federal grants for modernizing hospitals that had become obsolete due to a lack of capital investment during the Great Depression and the Second World War (1929 to 1945). The program later evolved to address other types of infrastructure needs. In return for federal funds, facilities agreed to provide medical services free or at reduced rates to patients who were unable to pay for their own care.

Congress first introduced a bill to fund coverage of hospital costs for the Social Security beneficiaries in 1948. In response to criticism from the AMA, the proposed legislation was expanded to cover physician services. The concept of federal health insurance programs for the aged and the poor was highly controversial. It was not until 1965 that President Lyndon Johnson signed the law that created federal healthcare programs for the elderly and poor as part of his Great Society legislation (also called the War on Poverty).

Title XVIII of the **Social Security Act,** or Health Insurance for the Aged and Disabled, is commonly known as Medicare. Medicare legislation was enacted as one element of the 1965 amendments to the Social Security Act. **Medicare** is a health insurance program designed to complement the retirement, survivors, and disability insurance benefits enacted under Title II of the Social Security Act. Medicare covered most Americans over the age of sixty-five when it was first implemented in 1966. In 1973, several additional groups became eligible for Medicare benefits, including those entitled to Social Security or Railroad Retirement disability cash benefits for at least twenty-four months, most persons with end-stage renal disease (ESRD), and certain individuals over sixty-five who were not eligible for paid coverage but elected to pay for Medicare benefits.

Medicaid was designed as a cost-sharing program between the federal and state governments. It pays for the healthcare services provided to many low-income Americans. The program became effective in 1966 under Title XIX of the Social Security Act. It allowed states to add health coverage to their **public assistance** programs for low-income groups, families with dependent children, the aged, and the disabled. Because Medicaid eligibility is based on meeting criteria other than income, today the program covers only about 40 percent of the population living in poverty.

The Medicare and Medicaid programs were originally the responsibility of the Department of Health, Education, and Welfare (predecessor to the **Department of Health and Human Services** [HHS]). The Social Security Administration (SSA) administered the Medicare program, and the Social and Rehabilitation Service (SRS) administered the Medicaid Program. In 1977, administration of Medicare and Medicaid was transferred to a newly created administrative agency within HHS, the **Health Care Financing Administration** (HCFA). HCFA's name was changed in 2001, and the agency is now called the **Centers for Medicare and Medicaid Services** (CMS).

The demand for medical services grew tremendously during the 1970s and early 1980s. As a result, health insurance premiums and the cost of funding Medicare and Medicaid programs skyrocketed. By the mid-1980s, both private and government-sponsored healthcare programs had instituted cost-cutting programs.

Since 1983, HCFA (now called CMS) has developed **prospective payment systems** to manage the costs of the Medicare and Medicaid programs. The prospective payment system for inpatient acute care was the first to be implemented. The prospective payment systems for outpatient care provided to Medicare beneficiaries was the most recent. (Medicare and Medicaid reimbursement is discussed in more detail later in the chapter.)

Private and self-insured health insurance plans also have implemented a number of cost-containing measures, most notably, managed care delivery and reimbursement systems. Managed care has virtually eliminated traditional fee-for-service reimbursement systems in just two decades. The implementation of managed care systems has had far-reaching effects on healthcare organizations and providers in every setting. However, hospitals have experienced the greatest financial pressure. (Managed care is discussed in detail later in this chapter.)

Development of Prepaid Health Plans

In 1860, Franklin Health Assurance Company of Massachusetts became the first commercial insurance company in the United States to provide private healthcare coverage for injuries that did not result in death. Within twenty years, sixty other insurance companies offered health insurance policies. By 1900, both accident insurance companies and life insurance companies were offering policies. These early policies covered loss of income and provided benefits for a limited number of illnesses (such as typhus, typhoid, scarlet fever, and smallpox).

Modern health insurance was born in 1929 when Baylor University Hospital in Dallas, Texas, agreed to provide healthcare services to Dallas schoolteachers. The hospital agreed to provide room, board, and certain ancillary services to the teachers for a set monthly fee of fifty cents. This plan is generally considered to be the first Blue Cross plan. Such plans were attractive to consumers and hospitals alike because they provided a way to ensure that patients would be able to pay for hospital services when they needed them. Payment was made directly to the hospital, not to the patient. In addition, coverage usually included a hospital stay for a specified number of days or for specific hospital services.

The Blue Cross plans contrasted with standard **indemnity plans** (insurance benefits provided in the form of cash payments) offered by private insurance companies that reimbursed (or indemnified) the patient for covered services up to a specified dollar limit. It was then the responsibility of the hospital to collect the money from the patient. Blue Shield plans were eventually developed by physicians. The plans were similar to Blue Cross plans except that they offered coverage for physicians' services.

Starting in the 1930s and continuing through the Second World War, traditional insurance companies added health insurance coverage for hospital, surgical, and medical expenses to their accident and life insurance plans. During the Second World War, **group health insurance** was offered as a way to attract scarce wartime labor. Group health insurance plans provide healthcare benefits to full-time employees of a company. This trend was strengthened by the favorable tax treatment for fringe benefits. Unlike monetary wages, fringe benefits were not subject to income or Social Security taxes. Therefore, a pretax dollar spent on health insurance coverage was worth more than an after-tax dollar spent directly on medical services. After the war, the Supreme Court ruled that employee benefits, including health insurance, were a legitimate part of the labor–management bargaining process. Health insurance quickly became a popular employee benefit.

Although early health insurance policies covered expenses associated with common accidents and illnesses, they were inadequate for coverage of extended illnesses and lengthy hospital stays. To correct this deficiency, insurance companies began offering **major medical insurance** coverage for catastrophic illnesses and injuries during the early 1950s. Major medical insurance provides benefits up to a high-dollar limit for most types of medical expenses. However, it usually requires patients to pay large deductibles. It also may place limits on charges (for example, room and board) and require patients to pay a portion of the expenses. **Blue Cross and Blue Shield** soon followed by offering similar plans.

Typically, the major medical insurance **policyholder** (or **insured**) paid a specified deductible (the amount the insured pays before the insurer assumes liability for any remaining costs of covered services). After the deductible had been paid, insured and **insurer** (third-party payer) shared covered losses according to a specified ratio, and the insured paid a coinsurance amount. **Coinsurance** refers to the amount the insured pays as a requirement of the insurance policy. For example, an insurance company may require the insured to pay a percentage of the daily costs for inpatient care.

According to the Washington Insurance Council (a nonprofit association of insurance companies and insurance professionals), by 1955, health insurance coverage continued to expand, and eventually 77 million Americans were covered by either an indemnity plan or a major medical plan. In subsequent years, insurance companies introduced high-benefit-level major medical plans, which limited out-of-pocket expenses. **Out-of-pocket expenses** are the healthcare expenses the insured is responsible for paying. After the insured has paid an amount specified in the insurance plan (that is, the deductible plus any copayments), the plan pays 100 percent of covered expenses. Such health insurance plans are common today and have been expanded to include coverage for advanced medical technology.

According to the U.S. Census Bureau, the percentage of people covered by health insurance in 2000 increased to 86 percent (from 84.5 percent in 1999). (See table 14.1.) One explanation for this increase may be that more people are getting health insurance coverage through their employers.

The lack of health insurance for so many Americans, however, continues to be a serious concern. Because of the financial constraints brought about by changes in Medicare/Medicaid and managed care reimbursement, many hospitals are no longer able to provide charitable services. As a result, underfunded and overcrowded public hospitals are struggling to provide services to uninsured patients who cannot pay for their own care. In addition, many uninsured patients delay seeking medical treatment until they are extremely ill, with long-term consequences for their own health and for the healthcare system. Thousands of patients with chronic diseases such as diabetes and asthma are brought to hospital emergency departments every day because they do not have access to basic healthcare services.

Table 14.1.   Health Insurance Coverage Status: 1987–2000 (numbers in thousands)

Year	Total U.S. Population	Number Covered	Percentage Covered
2000	276,540	237,812	86.0
1999	274,087	231,533	84.5
1998	271,743	227,462	83.7
1997	269,094	225,646	83.9
1996	266,792	225,077	84.4
1995	264,314	223,733	84.6
1994	262,105	222,387	84.8
1993	259,753	220,040	84.7
1992	256,830	218,189	85.0
1991	251,447	216,003	85.9
1990	248,886	214,167	86.1
1989	246,191	212,807	86.4
1988	243,685	211,005	86.6
1987	241,187	210,161	87.1

Source: Based on U.S. Census Bureau information (www.census.gov/hhes/hlthins/historic/hihistt4.html).

One solution to the problem may be to expand government-sponsored healthcare programs. Another may be to create tax incentives to help individuals and small employers purchase private health insurance. (For example, tax deductions could be offered to low-income people who buy their own insurance, or tax credits could be offered to small employers that offer health insurance coverage to employees.)

Check Your Understanding 14.1

Instructions: Answer the following questions on a separate piece of paper.

1. How did the uninsured pay for healthcare services prior to implementation of government programs (for example, Medicare)?

2. Why did the Centers for Medicare and Medicaid Services (formerly the Health Care Financing Administration) develop prospective payment systems?

3. Using table 14.1, calculate the percentage change in health insurance coverage status from 1999 to 2000.

4. Which government agency administers the Medicaid and Medicare programs?

5. During the Second World War, what did employers do to try to increase wartime labor?

Healthcare Reimbursement Systems

Before the widespread availability of health insurance coverage, individuals were assured access to healthcare only when they were able to pay for the services themselves. They paid cash for services on a retrospective **fee-for-service basis,** in which the patient was expected to pay the healthcare provider after a service was rendered. Until the advent of managed care, **capitation,** and other prospective payment systems, private insurance plans and government-sponsored programs also reimbursed providers on a retrospective fee-for-service basis.

Fee-for-service reimbursement is now rare for most types of medical services. Today, most Americans are covered by some form of health insurance and most health insurance plans compensate providers according to predetermined discounted rates rather than fee-for-service charges. However, some types of care are not covered by most health insurance plans and are still paid for directly by patients on a fee-for-service basis. Cosmetic surgery is one example of a medical service that is not considered medically necessary and so is not covered by most insurance plans. Many insurance plans also limit coverage for psychiatric services, substance abuse treatment, and the testing and correction of vision and hearing.

Commercial Insurance

Most Americans are covered by private group insurance plans tied to their employment. Typically, employers and employees share the cost of such plans. Two types of commercial insurance are commonly available: private insurance and **employer-based self-insurance.**

Private Health Insurance Plans

Private commercial insurance plans are financed through the payment of **premiums.** Each covered individual or family pays a preestablished amount (usually monthly), and the insurance company sets aside the premiums from all the people covered by the plan in a special fund. When a claim for medical care is submitted to the insurance company, the claim is paid out of the fund's reserves.

Before payment is made, the insurance company reviews every claim to determine whether the services described on the claim are covered by the patient's policy. The company also reviews the documentation provided with the claim to ensure that the services provided were medically necessary. Payment then is made to either the provider or the policyholder.

When purchasing an insurance policy, the policyholder receives written confirmation from the insurance company when the insurance goes into effect. This confirmation document usually includes a policy number and a telephone number to be called in case of medical emergency. An insurance policy represents a legal contract for services between the insured and the insurance company.

Most insurance policies include the following information:

- What medical services the company will cover
- When the company will pay for medical services
- How much and for how long the company will pay for covered services
- What process is to be followed to ensure that covered medical expenses are paid

Employer-Based Self-Insurance Plans

During the 1970s, a number of large companies discovered that they could save money by self-insuring their employee health plans rather than purchasing coverage from private insurers. Large companies have large workforces, and so aggregate (total) employee medical experiences and associated expenses vary only slightly from one year to the next. The exception to this is during periods of rapid inflation in healthcare charges. The companies understood that it was in their best interest to self-insure their health plans because yearly expenses could be predicted relatively accurately.

The cost of self-insurance funding is lower than the cost of paying premiums to private insurers because the premiums reflect more than the actual cost of the services provided to beneficiaries. Private insurers build additional fees into premiums to compensate them for assuming the risk of providing insurance coverage. In self-insured plans, the employer assumes the risk. By budgeting a certain amount to pay its employees' medical claims, the employer retains control over the funds until such time as medical claims need to be paid.

Employer-based self-insurance has become a common form of group health insurance coverage. Many employers enter into **administrative services only** (ASO) **contracts** with private insurers and fund the plans themselves. The private insurers administer self-insurance plans on behalf of the employers.

Blue Cross and Blue Shield Plans

Blue Cross and Blue Shield (BC/BS) plans, also known as the Blues, were the first prepaid health plans in the United States. Originally, Blue Cross plans covered hospital care and Blue Shield plans covered physicians' services. The Blues are different from commercial health insurance companies in that they are nonprofit organizations.

The first Blue Cross plan was created in 1929. In 1939, a commission of the American Hospital Association (AHA) adopted the Blue Cross national emblem for plans that met specific guidelines. The Blue Cross Association was created in 1960, and the relationship with the AHA ended in 1972.

The first Blue Shield plan was created in 1939, and the Associated Medical Care Plans (later known as the National Association of Blue Shield Plans) adopted the Blue Shield symbol in 1948. In 1982, the Blue Cross Association and the National Association of Blue Shield Plans merged to create the Blue Cross and Blue Shield Association.

Today, the Blue Cross and Blue Shield Association includes forty-eight independent, locally operated companies with plans in fifty states, the District of Columbia, and Puerto Rico. The Blues offer health insurance to individuals, small businesses, seniors, and large employer groups. In addition, federal employees are eligible to enroll in the **BC/BS Federal Employee Program** (FEP) (also called the BC/BS Service Benefit Plan). The plan offers the two products to federal employees:

- A **preferred provider organization** (PPO) plan (in which healthcare providers provide healthcare services to members of the plan at a discounted rate)
- A **point-of-service plan** (in which subscribers are encouraged to select providers from a prescribed network but are allowed to seek healthcare services from providers outside the network at a higher level of copay)

Government-Sponsored Healthcare Programs

The federal government administers several healthcare programs. The best known are Medicare and Medicaid. The Medicare program pays for the healthcare services provided to Social Security beneficiaries sixty-five years old and older as well as permanently disabled people, people with end-stage renal disease, and certain other groups of individuals. State governments work with the federal Medicaid program to provide healthcare coverage to low-income individuals and families

In addition, the federal government offers three health programs to address the needs of military personnel and their dependents as well as native Americans. The **Civilian Health and Medical Program—Veterans Administration** (CHAMPVA) provides healthcare services for dependents and survivors of disabled veterans, survivors of veterans who died from service-related conditions, and survivors of military personnel who died in the line of duty. **TRICARE** (formerly CHAMPUS, the Civilian Health and Medical Program–Uniformed Services) provides coverage for the dependents of armed forces personnel and retirees receiving care outside a military treatment facility. The **Indian Health Service** (IHS) provides federal health services to American Indians and Alaska natives.

Medicare

The original Medicare program was implemented on July 1, 1966. In 1973, Medicare benefits were expanded to include individuals of any age who suffered from a permanent disability or end-stage renal disease.

For Americans receiving Social Security benefits, Medicare automatically provides **hospitalization insurance** (HI) **(Medicare Part A).** It also offers voluntary **supplemental medical insurance** (SMI) **(Medicare Part B)** to help pay for physicians' services, medical services, and medical–surgical supplies not covered by the hospitalization plan. Enrollees pay extra for Part B benefits. To fill gaps in Medicare coverage, most Medicare enrollees also supplement their Medicare benefits with private insurance policies. These private policies are referred to as **Medigap** insurance. **Medicare Part C** (or **Medicare+Choice**) was established by the Balanced Budget Act of 1997 to expand the options for participation in private healthcare plans.

According to the CMS, approximately 19 million Americans were enrolled in the Medicare program in 1966. In 2000, approximately 40 million people were enrolled in Parts A and/or B of the Medicare program, and 6.4 million of the enrollees participated in a Medicare+Choice plan.

Medicare Part A

Medicare Part A is generally provided free of charge to individuals age sixty-five and over who are eligible for Social Security or Railroad Retirement benefits. Individuals who do not claim their monthly cash benefits are still eligible for Medicare. In addition, workers (and their spouses) who have been employed in federal, state, or local government for a sufficient period of time qualify for Medicare coverage beginning at age sixty-five.

Similarly, individuals who have been entitled to Social Security or Railroad Retirement disability benefits for at least twenty-four months and government employees with Medicare coverage who have been disabled for more than twenty-nine months are entitled to Part A benefits. This coverage also is provided to insured workers (and their spouses) with end-state renal disease as well as to children with end-stage renal disease. In addition, some otherwise-ineligible aged and disabled beneficiaries who voluntarily pay a monthly premium for their coverage are eligible for Medicare Part A.

The following healthcare services are covered under Medicare Part A: inpatient hospital care, long-term care, **skilled nursing facility** (SNF) care, home health care, and **hospice** care. (See table 14.2.) Inpatient hospital care and long-term care are paid for under Medicare Part A when such care is medically necessary. An initial deductible payment is required for each hospital admission, plus copayments for all hospital days following day sixty within a benefit period.

Each benefit period begins the day the Medicare beneficiary is admitted to the hospital and ends when he or she has not been hospitalized for a period of sixty consecutive days. Inpatient hospital care is usually limited to ninety days during each benefit period. There is no limit to the number of benefit periods covered by Medicare hospital insurance during a beneficiary's lifetime. However, copayment requirements apply to days sixty-one through ninety. When a beneficiary exhausts the ninety days of inpatient hospital care available during a benefit period, a nonrenewable lifetime reserve of up to a total of sixty additional days of inpatient hospital care can be used. Copayments are required for such additional days.

Skilled nursing facility (SNF) care is covered when it occurs within thirty days of a three-day-long or longer hospitalization and is certified as medically necessary. The number of SNF days provided under Medicare is limited to 100 days per benefit period, with a copayment required for days 21 through 100. Hospital insurance does not cover SNF care when the patient does not require skilled nursing care or skilled rehabilitation services.

Care provided by a **home health agency** (HHA) may be furnished part-time in the residence of a homebound beneficiary when intermittent or part-time skilled nursing and/or certain other therapy or rehabilitation care is needed. Certain medical supplies and durable medical equipment (DME) also may be paid for under the Medicare home health benefit.

The Medicare program requires the HHA to develop a treatment plan that is periodically reviewed by a physician. Home health care under Medicare Part A has no limitations on duration, no copayments, and no deductibles.

For DME, beneficiaries must pay 20 percent coinsurance, as required under Medicare Part B. The Balanced Budget Act of 1997 requires that home health care services not associated with an inpatient stay at a hospital or SNF must be covered by Medicare Part B instead of by Part A as in the past. This transition to Part B coverage is being phased in over a six-year period through 2003. Over this period, beneficiaries also will pay an increasing portion of Part B premiums. Part A will continue to cover the first 100 visits following a three-day stay in a hospital or a stay in an SNF.

Terminally ill persons whose life expectancies are six months or less may elect to receive hospice services. To qualify for Medicare reimbursement for hospice care, patients must elect to forgo standard Medicare benefits for treatment of their illnesses and agree to receive only hospice care. When a hospice patient requires treatment for a condition that is not related to his or her terminal illness, however, Medicare does pay for all covered services necessary for that condition. The Medicare beneficiary pays no deductible for hospice coverage but does pay coinsurance amounts for drugs and inpatient **respite care.** (Respite care is any inpatient care provided to the hospice patient for the purpose of providing primary caregivers a break from their care-giving responsibilities.)

Medicare Part B

Medicare Part B (supplemental medical insurance) covers the following services and supplies:

- Physicians' and surgeons' services, including some covered services furnished by chiropractors, podiatrists, dentists, and optometrists; and services provided by the

Table 14.2.   Medicare Part A Benefit Period, Beneficiary Deductibles and Copayments, and Medicare Payment Responsibilities According to Health Care Setting

Healthcare Setting	Benefit Period	Patient's Responsibility	Medicare Payments
Hospital (Inpatient)	First 60 days	$792 annual deductible	All but $792
	Days 61–90	$198 per day	All but $198/day
	Days 91–150 (these reserve days can be used only once in the patient's lifetime)	$396 per day	All but $396/day
	Beyond 150 days	All costs	Nothing
Skilled Nursing Facility	First 20 days	Nothing	100% approved amount
	Days 21–100	$99 per day	All but $99 per day
	Beyond 100 days	All costs	Nothing
Home Health Care	For as long as patient meets Medicare medical necessity criteria	Nothing for services, but 20% of approved amount for durable medical equipment (DME)	100% of the approved amount, and 80% of the approved amount for DME
Hospice Care	For as long as physician certifies need for care	Limited costs for outpatient drugs and inpatient respite care	All but limited costs for outpatient drugs and inpatient respite care
Blood	Unlimited if medical necessity criteria are met	First 3 pints (if previously paid under Part B, does not have to pay again under Part A)	All but first 3 pints per calendar year

following Medicare-approved practitioners who are not physicians: certified registered nurse anesthetists, clinical psychologists, clinical social workers (other than those employed by a hospital or an SNF), physician assistants, and nurse practitioners and clinical nurse specialists working in collaboration with a physician

- Services in an emergency department or outpatient clinic, including same-day surgery and ambulance services
- Home health care not covered under Medicare Part A
- Laboratory tests, X rays, and other diagnostic radiology services, as well as certain preventive care screening tests
- **Ambulatory surgery center** (ASC) services in Medicare-approved facilities
- Most physical and occupational therapy and speech pathology services
- Comprehensive outpatient rehabilitation facility services and mental health care provided as part of a partial hospitalization psychiatric program when a physician certifies that inpatient treatment would be required without the partial hospitalization services
- Radiation therapy, renal dialysis and kidney transplants, and heart and liver transplants under certain limited conditions
- Durable medical equipment approved for home use, such as oxygen equipment, wheelchairs, prosthetic devices, and surgical dressings, splints, and casts
- Drugs and biologicals that cannot be self-administered, such as hepatitis B vaccines and immunosuppressive drugs (plus certain self-administered anticancer drugs)

To be covered, all Medicare Part B services must be either documented as medically necessary or covered as one of several prescribed preventive benefits. Part B services also are generally subject to deductibles and coinsurance payments. (See table 14.3.) Certain medical services and related care are subject to special payment rules, for example:

- Deductibles for administration of blood and blood products
- Maximum approved amounts for Medicare-approved physical or occupational therapy services performed in settings other than hospitals
- Higher cost-sharing requirements, such as those for outpatient psychiatric care

It should be noted that the following healthcare services are not covered by Medicare Part A or B and are only covered by private health plans under the Medicare+Choice program:

- Long-term nursing care
- Custodial care
- Dentures and dental care
- Eyeglasses

Table 14.3. Medicare Part B Benefit Deductibles and Copayments, and Medicare Payment Responsibilities According to Type of Service

Type of Service	Benefit	Deductible and Copayment	Medicare Payment
Medical Expenses	Physicians' services, inpatient and outpatient medical and surgical services and supplies, and durable medical equipment (DME)	$100 annual deductible, plus 20% of approved amount after deductible has been met, except in outpatient setting	80% of approved amount (after patient has paid $100 deductible)
	Mental health care	50% of most outpatient care	50% of most outpatient care
	Occupational, physical, and speech therapy	20% of the first $1500 and all charges thereafter	80% of first $1500
Clinical Laboratory Services	Blood tests, urinalysis, and more	Nothing	100% of approved amount
Home Health Care	Intermittent skilled care, home health aide services, DME and supplies, and other services	Nothing for home care service / 20% of approved amount for DME	100% of approved amount / 80% of approved amount for DME
Outpatient Hospital Services	Services for diagnosis and/or treatment of an illness or injury	$100 annual deductible, plus a coinsurance amount for *each service* received during an outpatient visit. For *each* outpatient service received, the coinsurance amount cannot be greater than the Medicare Part A inpatient hospital deductible. The coinsurance amount is based on 20% of the national median charge for services in the ambulatory payment classification associated with the service. / Charges for items or services that Medicare does not cover	Payment based on ambulatory patient classifications/outpatient prospective payment system
Blood	Unlimited if medical necessity criteria are met	First 3 pints (if met under Part B, does not have to be met again under Part A)	All but first 3 pints per calendar year

- Hearing aids
- Most prescription drugs

Medicare Part C

Medicare Part C (Medicare+Choice) provides expanded coverage of many healthcare services. Although any Medicare beneficiary may receive benefits through the original fee-for-service program, most beneficiaries enrolled in both Parts A and B can choose to participate in a Medicare+Choice plan instead. Organizations that offer Medicare+Choice plans must meet specific requirements as determined by the CMS (formerly the HCFA).

Primary Medicare+Choice products include the following types of plans:

- **Coordinated care plans,** which include **health maintenance organizations** (HMOs), provider-sponsored organizations (PSOs), preferred provider organizations (PPOs), and other certified coordinated care plans and entities that meet Medicare standards
- Private, unrestricted, fee-for-service plans, which allow beneficiaries to select a provider from a list of private providers who have agreed to accept the plan's payment terms and conditions
- **Medical savings account** (MSA) **plans,** which provide benefits after a single high deductible has been paid by the beneficiary

MSAs are currently being offered as part of a pilot program for a limited number of Medicare beneficiaries. In the pilot program, Medicare makes an annual deposit to the MSA and the beneficiary is expected to use the money in the MSA to pay for medical expenses.

Except for MSA plans, all Medicare+Choice plans are required to provide at least the current Medicare benefit package, excluding hospice services. Plans may offer additional covered services and are required to do so (or return excess payments) when the cost of providing services under the plan is lower than the Medicare payments received by the plan.

Out-of-Pocket Expenses and Medigap Insurance

Medicare beneficiaries who elect the fee-for-service option are responsible for charges not covered by the Medicare program and for various cost-sharing aspects of Parts A and B. These liabilities may be paid by the Medicare beneficiary; by a third party, such as an employer-sponsored health plan or private Medigap insurance; or by Medicaid, when the person is eligible.

Medigap is private health insurance that pays, within limits, most of the healthcare service charges not covered by Medicare Parts A and/or B. These policies, which must meet federal standards, are offered by Blue Cross and Blue Shield and various commercial health insurance companies.

For beneficiaries enrolled in Medicare+Choice plans, their payment share is based on the cost-sharing structure of the specific plan they select. Most plans have lower deductibles and coinsurance than are required of Medicare fee-for-service

beneficiaries. Such beneficiaries pay the monthly Part B premium and may pay an additional plan premium, depending on the plan.

For hospital care covered under Medicare Part A, a fee-for-service beneficiary's payment share includes a one-time deductible amount payable at the beginning of each benefit period. In 2001, the deductible was $792. This deductible covers the beneficiary's part of the first sixty days of each inpatient hospital stay. When continued inpatient care is needed beyond the sixty days, additional coinsurance payments ($198 per day in 2001) are required through the ninetieth day of a benefit period. Each Part A beneficiary also has a lifetime reserve of sixty additional hospital days that may be used when the covered days within a benefit period have been exhausted. Lifetime reserve days may be used only once, and coinsurance payments ($396 per day in 2001) are required.

For SNF care covered under Part A, Medicare fully covers the first twenty days in a benefit period. For days 21 through 100, a copayment ($99 per day in 2001) is required. Medicare benefits expire after the first 100 days of SNF care during a benefit period.

Home health care services require no deductible or coinsurance payment by the beneficiary. For any Part A service, the beneficiary is responsible for paying fees to cover the first three pints or units of nonreplaced blood per calendar year. The beneficiary has the option of paying the fee or arranging for the blood to be replaced by family and friends.

Most beneficiaries covered by Medicare Part A pay no premiums. Eligibility is generally earned through the work experience of the beneficiary or of his or her spouse. In addition, most individuals over sixty-five who are otherwise ineligible for Medicare Part A coverage can enroll voluntarily by paying a monthly premium when they also enroll in Part B. For people with fewer than thirty quarters of coverage as defined by the Social Security Administration, the 2001 Part A monthly premium rate is $300. For those with thirty to thirty-nine quarters of coverage, the monthly premium is reduced to $165. Voluntary coverage paid for with a Part A premium, with or without enrollment in Part B, is also available to disabled individuals who earn too much money to qualify for Social Security cash benefits.

For Part B (table 14.3), the beneficiary's payment share includes:

- One annual deductible ($100 in 2001)
- Monthly premiums ($50 per month in 2001)
- Coinsurance payments for Part B services (usually 20 percent of medically allowable charges)
- Any deductibles for blood products
- Certain charges above approved charges (for claims not on assignment)
- Payment for any services that are not covered by Medicare
- Fifty percent of approved charges for outpatient psychiatric services

Medicaid

Title XIX of the Social Security Act enacted Medicaid in 1965. The Medicaid program pays for medical assistance provided to individuals and families with low incomes and limited financial resources. Individual states must meet broad national guidelines established by federal statutes, regulations, and policies to qualify for federal matching grants under the Medicaid program. Individual state medical assistance agencies, however, establish the Medicaid eligibility standards for residents of their states. The states also determine the type, amount, duration, and scope of covered services; calculate the rate of payment for covered services; and administer local programs.

Medicaid policies on eligibility, services, and payment are complex and vary considerably among states, even among states of similar size or geographic proximity. Therefore, an individual who is eligible for Medicaid in one state may not be eligible in another. In addition, the amount, duration, and scope of care provided vary considerably from state to state. Moreover, Medicaid eligibility and/or services within a state can change from year to year.

Medicaid Eligibility Criteria

Low income is only one test for Medicaid eligibility. Other financial resources also are compared against eligibility standards. These standards are determined by each state according to federal guidelines.

Generally, each state is allowed to determine which groups Medicaid will cover. Each state also establishes its own financial criteria for Medicaid eligibility. However, to be eligible for federal funds, states are required to provide Medicaid coverage to certain individuals. These individuals include recipients of federally assisted income maintenance payments, as well as related groups of individuals who do not receive cash payments. The **categorically needy eligibility groups** include:

- Individuals eligible for Medicaid when they meet requirements for Temporary Assistance for Needy Families (TANF), which replaced the Aid to Families with Dependent Children program in effect in their state
- Children below age six whose family income is at or below 133 percent of the **federal poverty level** (FPL) (the income threshold established by the federal government)
- Pregnant women whose family income is below 133 percent of the FPL (services are limited to those related to pregnancy, complications of pregnancy, delivery, and postpartum care)
- Supplemental Security Income (SSI) recipients in most states
- Recipients of adoption or foster care assistance under Title IV of the Social Security Act
- Special protected groups (typically individuals who lose their cash assistance due to earnings from work or from increased Social Security benefits, but who may keep Medicaid for a period of time)

- All children born after September 30, 1983, who are under age nineteen and living in families with incomes at or below the FPL (this process phases in coverage so that by the year 2002 all such poor children under age nineteen will be covered)
- Certain Medicare beneficiaries

States also have the option of providing Medicaid coverage to other categorically related groups. Categorically related groups share the characteristics of the eligible groups (that is, they fall within defined categories), but the eligibility criteria are somewhat more liberally defined. A **medically needy option** also allows states to extend Medicaid eligibility to persons who would be eligible for Medicaid under one of the mandatory or optional groups except that their income and/or resources are above the eligibility level set by their state. Individuals may qualify immediately or may "spend down" by incurring medical expenses that reduce their income to or below their state's income level for the medically needy.

In 1996, Congress passed the Personal Responsibility and Work Opportunity Reconciliation Act (also known as welfare reform). The act made restrictive changes in the eligibility requirements for SSI coverage. These changes also affected eligibility for participation in the Medicaid program.

According to the provisions of the act, for example, legal resident aliens and other qualified aliens who entered the United States on or after August 22, 1996, are not eligible for Medicaid for five years. States have the option of providing Medicaid coverage for most aliens who entered the country before that date and for aliens eligible after the five-year moratorium. However, coverage for emergency medical services is mandatory for both groups. For aliens who lose their SSI benefits because of the new restrictions, Medicaid can continue only when the individuals affected can be covered for Medicaid under some other eligibility status.

The welfare reform act also affected a number of disabled children. Many lost their SSI benefits as a result of the restrictive changes. However, their eligibility for Medicaid was reinstituted by the Balanced Budget Act of 1997.

In addition, the welfare reform act repealed the open-ended federal entitlement program known as Aid to Families with Dependent Children (AFDC). **Temporary Assistance for Needy Families** (TANF) replaced AFDC. TANF provides states with grant money to be used for time-limited cash assistance. A family's lifetime cash welfare benefits are generally limited to a maximum of five years. Individual states also are allowed to impose other eligibility restrictions.

Medicaid Services

To be eligible for federal matching funds, each state's Medicaid program must offer medical assistance for the following basic services:

- Inpatient hospital services
- Outpatient hospital services
- Prenatal care

- Vaccines for children
- Physicians' services
- Nursing facility services for persons aged twenty-one or older
- Family planning services and supplies
- Rural health clinic services
- Home health care for persons eligible for skilled nursing services
- Laboratory and X-ray services
- Pediatric and family nurse practitioner services
- Nurse–midwife services
- Federally qualified health center (FQHC) services and ambulatory services performed at an FQHC that would be available in other settings
- Early and periodic screening and diagnostic and therapeutic services for children under age twenty-one

States also may receive federal matching funds to provide the following optional services:

- Diagnostic services
- Clinic services
- Intermediate care facility services for the mentally retarded
- Prescription drugs and prosthetic devices
- Optometric services and eyeglasses
- Nursing facility services for children under age twenty-one
- Transportation services
- Rehabilitation and physical therapy services
- Home care and community-based care services for persons with chronic impairments

The Balanced Budget Act of 1997 also called for the implementation of a state option called **Programs of All-Inclusive Care for the Elderly** (PACE). PACE provides an alternative to institutional care for individuals fifty-five years old or older who require a level of care usually provided at nursing facilities. It offers and manages all of the health, medical, and social services needed by a beneficiary and mobilizes other services, as needed, to provide preventive, rehabilitative, curative, and supportive care.

PACE services can be provided in day healthcare centers, homes, hospitals, and nursing homes. The program helps its beneficiaries to maintain their independence, dignity, and quality of life. PACE also functions within the Medicare program. Individuals enrolled in PACE receive benefits solely through the PACE program.

Medicaid–Medicare Relationship

Medicare beneficiaries who have low incomes and limited financial resources also may receive help from the Medicaid program. For persons eligible for full Medicaid coverage, Medicare coverage is supplemented by services that are available under their state's Medicaid program according to their eligibility category. Additional services may include, for example, nursing facility care beyond the 100-day limit

covered by Medicare, prescription drugs, eyeglasses, and hearing aids. For those enrolled in both programs, any services covered by Medicare are paid for by the Medicare program before any payments are made by the Medicaid program because Medicaid is always the **payer of last resort.**

Certain other Medicare beneficiaries may receive help with Medicare premium and cost-sharing payments through their state Medicaid program. **Qualified Medicare beneficiaries** (QMBs) and **specified low-income Medicare beneficiaries** (SLMBs) are the best-known categories and the largest in number. QMBs include those Medicare beneficiaries who have resources at or below twice the standard allowed under the Supplementary Security Income program and incomes at or below 100 percent of the federal poverty level (FPL). For qualified Medicare beneficiaries, Medicaid pays Parts A and B premiums along with the Medicare coinsurance and deductibles, subject to limits that states may impose on payment rates. SLMBs include Medicare enrollees who have resources similar to the QMBs, but higher incomes, although still less than 120 percent of the federal poverty level. Medicaid pays only Part B premiums for SLMBs.

A third category of Medicare beneficiaries eligible for assistance includes disabled and working people who previously qualified for Medicare because of their disability but lost their entitlement because of their return to work. They are allowed to purchase Medicare Parts A and B coverage. When their income falls below 200 percent of the FPL (and they do not meet any other Medicaid assistance category), Medicaid also may pay their Medicare Part A premiums under the program for **qualified disabled and working individuals** (QDWIs).

For Medicare beneficiaries whose incomes are 120 percent above, but less than 175 percent of the FPL, the Balanced Budget Act of 1997 established a capped allocation to states for payment of all or some of the premiums for Medicare Part A. These beneficiaries are known as **qualifying individuals** (QIs) and cannot be otherwise eligible for medical assistance under a state plan. Payment of this QI benefit is federally funded up to the state's allocation. Table 14.4 provides a comparison of Medicare and Medicaid programs.

State Children's Health Insurance Program

The **State Children's Health Insurance Program** (SCHIP) (Title XXI of the Social Security Act) is a new program initiated by the Balanced Budget Act of 1997. SCHIP (sometimes referred to as the Children's Health Insurance Program, or CHIP) allows states to expand existing insurance programs. It provides additional federal funds to states so that Medicaid eligibility can be expanded to include a greater number of children.

SCHIP became available on October 1, 1997. It will provide $24 billion in federal matching funds over five years to help states expand healthcare coverage to as many as five

Table 14.4.   Comparison of Medicare and Medicaid Programs

Medicare	Medicaid
Health insurance for people age 65 and older, or people under 65 who are entitled to Medicare because of disability or are receiving dialysis for permanent kidney failure	Health assistance for people of any age
Administered through fiscal intermediaries, insurance companies under contract to the government to process Medicare claims	Administered by the federal government through state and local governments following federal and state guidelines
Medicare regulations are the same in all states	Medicaid regulations vary from state to state
Financed by monthly premiums paid by the beneficiary and by payroll tax deductions	Financed by federal, state and county tax dollars
For people age 65 and over, eligibility is based on Social Security or Railroad Retirement participation. For people under age 65, eligibility is based on disability. For people who undergo kidney dialysis, eligibility is not dependent on age	Eligibility based on financial need
Beneficiary responsible for paying deductibles, coinsurance or copayments, and Part B premiums	Medicaid can help pay Medicare deductible, coinsurance or copayment, and premiums
Hospital and medical benefits; preventive care and long-term care benefits are limited	Comprehensive benefits include hospital, preventive care, long-term care, and other services not covered under Medicare such as dental work, prescriptions, transportation, eyeglasses, and hearing aids

million of the nation's uninsured children. The CMS (formerly the HCFA) and the **Health Resources and Services Administration** (HRSA) administer SCHIP. Following broad federal guidelines, states establish eligibility and coverage guidelines and have flexibility in the way they provide services. Recipients in all states must meet three eligibility criteria:

- They must have low incomes.
- They must be otherwise ineligible for Medicaid.
- They must be uninsured.

States are required to offer the following services:

- Inpatient hospital services
- Outpatient hospital services
- Physicians' surgical and medical services
- Laboratory and X-ray services
- Well-baby/child care services, including immunizations

TRICARE

TRICARE is a healthcare program for active-duty members of the military and other qualified family members. CHAMPUS-eligible retirees and their family members as well as eligible survivors of members of the uniformed services also are eligible for TRICARE.

The idea of medical care for the families of active-duty members of the uniformed military services dates back to the late 1700s. It was not until 1884, however, that Congress directed Army medical officers and contract surgeons to care for the families of military personnel free of charge.

There was very little change in the provision of medical care to members of the military and their families until the Second World War, when the military was made up mostly of young men who had wives of childbearing age. The military medical care system could not handle the large number of births or the care of young children. So, in 1943, Congress authorized the **Emergency Maternal and Infant Care Program** (EMIC). The program provided maternity and infant care to dependents of service members in the lowest four pay grades.

During the early 1950s, the Korean conflict also strained the capabilities of the military healthcare system. As a result, the Dependents Medical Care Act was signed into law in 1956. Amendments to the act created the **Civilian Health and Medical Program of the Uniformed Services** (CHAMPUS) in 1966.

During the 1980s, the search for ways to improve access to top-quality medical care and at the same time control costs led to implementation of CHAMPUS demonstration projects in various parts of the country. The most successful of these projects was the CHAMPUS Reform Initiative (CRI) in California and Hawaii. Initiated in 1988, the CRI offered military service families a choice in the way their military healthcare benefits could be used. Five years of successful operation and high levels of patient satisfaction persuaded Department of Defense officials that they should extend and improve the CRI concepts as a uniform program nationwide.

The new program, known as TRICARE, was phased in nationally by 1998. Expansion to overseas military bases will soon be complete. TRICARE offers three options: TRICARE Prime, TRICARE Extra, and TRICARE Standard.

TRICARE Prime

Of the three options, **TRICARE Prime** provides the most comprehensive healthcare benefits at the lowest cost. Military treatment facilities (for example, military base hospitals) serve as the principal source of healthcare, and a **primary care manager** (PCM) is assigned to each enrollee.

Two specialized programs supplement TRICARE Prime. **TRICARE Prime Remote** provides healthcare services to active-duty military personnel stationed in the United States in areas not served by the traditional military healthcare system. (Active-duty personnel include members of the Army, Navy, Marine Corps, Air Force, Coast Guard, and active National Guard.) **TRICARE Senior Prime** is a managed care demonstration program designed to serve the medical needs of military retirees who are sixty-five years old or over and their dependents and survivors.

TRICARE Extra

TRICARE Extra is a cost-effective preferred provider network (PPN) option. Healthcare costs in TRICARE Extra are lower than for TRICARE Standard because beneficiaries must select physicians and medical specialists from a network of civilian healthcare professionals working under contract with TRICARE. The healthcare professionals who participate in TRICARE Extra agree to charge a preestablished discounted rate for the medical treatments and procedures provided to participants in the plan.

TRICARE Standard

TRICARE Standard incorporates the services previously provided by CHAMPUS. TRICARE Standard allows eligible beneficiaries to choose any physician or healthcare provider. It pays a set percentage of the providers' fees, and the enrollee pays the rest. This option permits the most flexibility but may be the most expensive for the enrollee, particularly when the provider's charges are higher than the amounts allowed by the program.

CHAMPVA

The Civilian Health and Medical Program-Veterans Administration (CHAMPVA) is a healthcare program for dependents and survivors of permanently and totally disabled veterans, survivors of veterans who died from service-related conditions, and survivors of military personnel who died in the line of duty. CHAMPVA is a voluntary program that allows beneficiaries to be treated for free at participating VA healthcare facilities, with the VA sharing the cost of covered healthcare services and supplies. Because of the similarity between CHAMPVA and TRICARE (which replaced CHAMPUS), people sometimes confuse the two programs. However, CHAMPVA is separate from TRICARE and there are distinct differences between them.

Indian Health Service

The provision of health services to native Americans originally developed from the relationship between the federal government and federally recognized Indian tribes. This relationship was established in 1787. It is based on Article I, Section 8, of the U.S. Constitution. It has been given form and substance by numerous treaties, laws, Supreme Court decisions, and executive orders.

The Indian Health Service (IHS) is an agency within the Department of Health and Human Services (HHS). It is responsible for providing healthcare services to American Indians and Alaska natives. The American Indians and Alaska natives served by the IHS receive preventive healthcare services, primary medical services (hospital and ambulatory care), community health services, substance abuse treatment services, and rehabilitative services. Secondary medical care, highly specialized medical services, and other rehabilitative care are provided by IHS staff or by private healthcare professionals working under contract with the IHS.

A system of acute and ambulatory care facilities operates on Indian reservations and in Indian and Alaska native communities. In locations where the IHS does not have its own facilities or is not equipped to provide a needed service, it con-

tracts with local hospitals, state and local healthcare agencies, tribal health institutions, and individual healthcare providers.

Workers' Compensation

Most employees are eligible for some type of **workers' compensation** insurance. Workers' compensation programs cover healthcare costs and lost income associated with work-related injuries and illnesses. Federal government employees are covered by the Federal Employees' Compensation Act (FECA). Individual states pass legislation that addresses workers' compensation coverage for nonfederal government employees. Some states exclude certain workers (for example, business owners, independent contractors, farm workers, and so on). (Texas employers are not required to provide workers' compensation coverage.)

Federal Workers' Compensation Funds

In 1908, President Theodore Roosevelt signed legislation to provide workers' compensation for certain federal employees in unusually hazardous jobs. The scope of the law was narrow, and its benefits were limited. The 1908 law represented the first workers' compensation program to pass the test of constitutionality applied by the U.S. Supreme Court.

The **Federal Employees' Compensation Act** (FECA) replaced the 1908 statute in 1916. Under FECA, civilian employees of the federal government are provided medical care, survivors' benefits, and compensation for lost wages. The Office of Workers' Compensation Programs (OWCP) administers FECA as well as the Longshore and Harbor Workers' Compensation Act of 1927 and the Black Lung Benefits Reform Act of 1977.

FECA also provides vocational rehabilitation services to partially disabled employees. Employees who fully or partially recover from their injuries are expected to return to work. FECA does not provide retirement benefits.

State Workers' Compensation Funds

According to the American Association of State Compensation Insurance Funds (AASCIF), state workers' compensation insurance was developed in response to the concerns of employers. Before state workers' compensation programs became widely available, employers faced the possibility of going out of business when insurance companies refused to provide coverage or charged excessive premiums. Legislators in most states have addressed these concerns by establishing **state workers' compensation insurance funds** that provide a stable source of insurance coverage and serve to protect employers from uncertainties about the continuing availability of coverage. Because state funds are provided on a nonprofit basis, the premiums can be kept low. In addition, the funds provide only one type of insurance: workers' compensation. This specialization allows the funds to concentrate resources, knowledge, and expertise in a single field of insurance.

State workers' compensation insurance funds do not operate at taxpayer expense because, by law, the funds support themselves through income derived from premiums and investments. As nonprofit departments of the state or as independent nonprofit companies, they return surplus assets to policyholders as dividends or safety refunds. This system reduces the overall cost of state-level workers' compensation insurance. Numerous court decisions have determined that the assets, reserves, and surplus of the funds are not public funds but, instead, the property of the employers insured by the funds.

In states where state funds have not been mandated, employers purchase workers' compensation coverage from private carriers or provide self-insurance coverage.

Managed Care

Healthcare costs in the United States rose dramatically during the 1970s and 1980s. As a result, the federal government, employers, and other third-party payers began investigating more cost-effective healthcare delivery systems. The federal government decided to move toward prospective payments systems for the Medicare program in the mid-1980s. (Prospective payment as a reimbursement methodology is discussed later in this chapter.) Commercial insurance providers looked to managed care.

Managed care is the generic term for prepaid health plans that integrate the financial and delivery aspects of healthcare services. In other words, managed care organizations work to control the cost of, and access to, healthcare services at the same time that they strive to meet high-quality standards. Managed care organizations manage healthcare costs by negotiating discounted providers' fees and controlling patients' access to expensive healthcare services. In managed care plans, services are carefully coordinated to ensure that they are medically appropriate and needed. The cost of providing appropriate services also is continuously monitored to determine whether the services are being delivered in the most efficient and cost-effective way possible.

Since 1973, several pieces of federal legislation have been passed with the goal of encouraging the development of managed healthcare systems. (See table 14.5.) The Health Maintenance Organization Assistance Act of 1973 authorized federal grants and loans to private organizations that wished to develop HMOs. Another important advancement in managed care was development of the **Health Plan Employer Data and Information Set** (HEDIS®) by the **National Committee for Quality Assurance** (NCQA).

Table 14.5.   Federal Legislation Relevant to Managed Care

Year	Legislative Title	Legislative Summary
1973	Federal Health Maintenance Organization Assistance Act of 1973 (HMO Act of 1973)	• Authorized grants and loans to develop HMOs under private sponsorship • Defined a federally qualified HMO (certified to provide healthcare services to Medicare and Medicaid enrollees) as one that has applied for and met federal standards established in the HMO Act of 1973 • Required most employers with more than 25 employees to offer HMO coverage when local plans were available
1974	Employee Retirement Income Security Act of 1974 (ERISA)	• Mandated reporting and disclosure requirements for group life and health plans (including managed care plans) • Permitted large employers to self-insure employee healthcare benefits • Exempted large employers from taxes on health insurance premium
1982	Tax Equity and Fiscal Responsibility Act of 1982 (TEFRA)	• Modified the HMO Act of 1973 • Created Medicare risk programs, which allowed federally qualified HMOs and competitive medical plans that met specified Medicare requirements to provide Medicare-covered services under a risk contract • Defined risk contract as an arrangement among providers to provide capitated (fixed, prepaid basis) healthcare services to Medicare beneficiaries • Defined competitive medical plan (CMP) as an HMO that meets federal eligibility requirements for a Medicare risk contract but is not licensed as a federally qualified plan
1981	Omnibus Budget Reconciliation Act of 1981 (OBRA)	• Provided states with flexibility to establish HMOs for Medicare and Medicaid programs • Resulted in increased enrollment
1985	Preferred Provider Health Care Act of 1985	• Eased restrictions on preferred provider organizations • Allowed subscribers to seek healthcare from providers outside the PPO
1985	Consolidated Omnibus Budget Reconciliation Act of 1985 (COBRA)	• Established an employee's right to continue healthcare coverage beyond scheduled benefit termination date (including HMO coverage)
1988	Amendment to the HMO Act of 1973	• Allowed federally qualified HMOs to permit members to occasionally use non-HMO physicians and be partially reimbursed
1989	Health Plan Employer Data and Information Set (HEDIS)—developed by National Committee for Quality Assurance (NCQA)	• Created standards to assess managed care systems in terms of membership, utilization of services, quality, access, health plan management and activities, and financial indicators
1994	HCFA's Office of Managed Care established	• Facilitated innovation and competition among Medicare HMOs

The NCQA is a private, not-for-profit organization that accredits, assesses, and reports on the quality of managed care plans in the United States. It worked with public and private healthcare purchasers, health plans, researchers, and consumer advocates to develop HEDIS in 1989. HEDIS is a set of standardized measures used to compare managed care plans in terms of the quality of services they provide. The standards cover areas such as plan membership, utilization of and access to services, and financial indicators. The goals of the program include:

- To help beneficiaries make informed choices among the numerous managed care plans available
- To improve the quality of care provided by managed care plans
- To help the government and other third-party payers make informed purchasing decisions

CMS (formerly HCFA) offers several managed care options to Medicare and Medicaid enrollees. It began collecting HEDIS data from Medicare managed care plans in 1996.

Several kinds of managed care plans are available in the United States, including:

- Health maintenance organizations (HMOs)
- Preferred provider organizations (PPOs)
- Point-of-service (POS) plans
- Exclusive provider organizations (EPOs)
- Integrated delivery systems (IDSs)

Health Maintenance Organizations

An HMO is a prepaid voluntary health plan that provides healthcare services in return for the payment of a monthly membership premium. HMO premiums are based on a projection of the costs that are likely to be involved in treating the plan's average enrollee over a specified period of time. If the actual cost per enrollee were to exceed the projected cost, the HMO would experience a financial loss. If the actual cost per enrollee turned out to be lower than the projection, the HMO would show a profit. Because most HMOs are for-profit organizations, they emphasize cost control and preventive medicine.

Today, most employers and insurance companies offer enrollees some type of HMO option. The benefit to third-party payers and enrollees alike is cost savings. Most HMO enrollees have significantly lower out-of-pocket expenses than enrollees of traditional fee-for-service and other types of managed care plans. The HMO premiums shared by employers and enrollees also are lower than the premiums for other types of healthcare plans.

HMOs can be organized in several different ways, including the group model HMO, the independent practice association (IPA), the network model HMO, and the staff model HMO.

Group Model HMOs

In the **group model HMO,** the HMO enters into a contract with an independent multispecialty physician group to provide medical services to members of the plan. The providers usually agree to devote a fixed percentage of their practice time to the HMO. Alternatively, the HMO may own or directly manage the physician group, in which case the physicians and their support staff would be considered its employees.

Group model HMOs are closed-panel arrangements. In other words, the physicians are not allowed to treat patients from other managed care plans. Enrollees of group model HMOs are required to seek services from the designated physician group.

Independent Practice Associations

Independent practice associations (IPAs) are sometimes called individual practice associations. In the IPA model, the HMO enters into a contract with an organized group of physicians who join together for purposes of fulfilling the HMO contract but retain their individual practices. The IPA serves as an intermediary during contract negotiations. It also manages the premiums from the HMO and pays individual physicians as appropriate. The physicians are not considered employees of the HMO. They work from their own private offices and continue to see other patients. The HMO usually pays the IPA according to a prenegotiated list of discounted fees. Alternatively, physicians may agree to provide services to HMO members for a set prepaid capitated payment for a specified period of time. (Capitation is discussed later in this chapter.)

The IPA is an open-panel HMO, which means that the physicians are free to treat patients from other plans. Enrollees of such HMOs are required to seek services from the designated physician group.

Network Model HMOs

Network model HMOs are similar to group model HMOs except that the HMO contracts for services with two or more multispecialty group practices instead of just one practice. Members of network model HMOs receive a list of all the physicians on the approved panel and are required to select providers from the list.

Staff Model HMOs

Staff model HMOs directly employ physicians and other healthcare professionals to provide medical services to members. Members of the salaried medical staff are considered employees of the HMO rather than independent practitioners. Premiums are paid directly to the HMO, and ambulatory care services are usually provided within the HMO's corporate facilities. The staff model HMO is a closed-panel arrangement.

Preferred Provider Organizations

Preferred provider organizations (PPOs) represent contractual agreements between healthcare providers and a self-insured employer or a health insurance carrier. Beneficiaries of PPOs select providers (physicians or hospitals, for example) from a list of participating providers who have agreed to furnish healthcare services to the covered population. Beneficiaries may elect to receive services from nonparticipating providers but must pay a greater portion of the cost (in other words, higher deductibles and copays). Providers are usually reimbursed on a discounted fee-for-service basis.

Point-of-Service Plans

Point-of-service (POS) plans are similar to HMOs in that subscribers must select a **primary care physician** (PCP) from a network of participating physicians. (The PCP is usually a family or general practice physician or an internal medicine specialist.) The PCP acts as a service gatekeeper to control the patient's access to specialty, surgical, and hospital care as well as expensive diagnostic services.

POS plans are different from HMOs in that subscribers are allowed to seek care from providers outside the network. However, the subscribers must pay a greater share of the charges for out-of-network services. POS plans were created to increase the flexibility of managed care plans and to allow patients more choice in providers.

Exclusive Provider Organizations

Exclusive provider organizations (EPOs) are similar to PPOs except that EPOs provide benefits to enrollees only when the enrollees receive healthcare services from **network providers.** In other words, EPO beneficiaries do not receive reimbursement for services furnished by nonparticipating providers. In addition, healthcare services must be coordinated by a primary care physician. EPOs are regulated by state insurance departments. (In contrast, HMOs are regulated by state departments of commerce or departments of incorporation.)

Integrated Delivery Systems

An **integrated delivery system** (IDS) is a healthcare provider made up of a number of associated medical facilities that furnish coordinated healthcare services. Most IDSs include a number of facilities that provide services along the continuum of care, for example, ambulatory surgery centers, physicians' office practices, outpatient clinics, acute care hospitals, skilled nursing facilities, and so on.

Integrated delivery systems can be structured according to several different models, including:

- Group practices without walls
- Integrated provider organizations
- Management service organizations
- Medical foundations
- Physician–hospital organizations

Group Practices without Walls

A **group practice without walls** (GPWW) is an arrangement that allows physicians to maintain their own offices, but to share administrative services (for example, medical transcription and billing) for the purpose of fulfilling contracts with managed care organizations.

Integrated Provider Organizations

An **integrated provider organization** (IPO) manages and coordinates the delivery of healthcare services performed by a number of healthcare professionals and facilities. IPOs typically provide acute care (hospital) services, physicians' services, ambulatory care services, and skilled nursing services. The physicians working in an IPO are salaried employees. IPOs are sometimes referred to as delivery systems, horizontally integrated systems, health delivery networks, accountable health plans, integrated service networks (ISNs), vertically integrated plans (VIPs), and vertically integrated systems.

Management Service Organizations

Management service organizations (MSOs) provide practice management (administrative and support) services to individual physicians' practices. MSOs are usually owned by a group of physicians or a hospital.

Medical Foundations

Medical foundations are nonprofit organizations that enter into contracts with physicians to manage the physicians' practices. The typical medical foundation owns clinical and business resources and makes them available to the participating physicians. Clinical assets include medical equipment and supplies, and treatment facilities. Business assets include billing and administrative support systems.

Physician–Hospital Organizations

A **physician–hospital organization** (PHO) provides healthcare services through a contractual arrangement between physicians and hospital(s). PHOs were previously known as medical staff–hospital organizations (MeSHs). PHO arrangements make it possible for the managed care market to view the hospital(s) and physicians as a single entity for the purpose of establishing a contract for services.

Check Your Understanding 14.2

Instructions: Answer the following questions on a separate piece of paper.

1. What is fee-for-service reimbursement? Why is it rarely used today as a reimbursement method?

2. How are private commercial insurance plans financed?

3. What process do most insurance companies use to reimburse healthcare services?

4. What are administrative services only contracts?

5. What federal program pays for healthcare services provided to financially needy individuals?

6. For which populations of individuals do TRICARE (formerly CHAMPUS) and CHAMPVA reimburse healthcare services?

7. Why is Medicare Part B referred to as supplemental medical insurance?

8. What federal legislation expanded Medicare options by creating Medicare+Choice?

9. What private health insurance pays (within limits) for most healthcare services not covered by Medicare Part A?

10. How did the Medicare and Medicaid programs come into effect? How are the two programs different?

11. How are Medicaid eligibility standards established?

12. What is the difference between a preferred provider organization and a point-of-service plan?

13. What is the purpose of the State Children's Health Insurance Program?

14. What type of Medicare coverage applies to inpatient hospitalization? To prescription eyeglasses? To emergency department visits? To dental care? To ambulatory surgery center service? To hospice care?

15. What is the difference between TRICARE Extra and TRICARE Prime?

16. How does State Workers' Compensation coverage differ from Federal Workers' Compensation coverage?

17. What type of HMO model employs physicians and other healthcare professionals to provide healthcare services to members?

18. What is the difference between an independent practice association and a staff model HMO?

19. Define managed care and describe the various types of managed care programs available in the United States?

20. What do management service organizations do?

Healthcare Reimbursement Methodologies

As mentioned earlier in this chapter, about 85 percent of Americans are covered by some type of private prepaid health plan or federal healthcare program. Therefore, most healthcare expenses in the United States are reimbursed through third-party payers rather than by the actual recipients of the services. (The recipients can be considered the "first parties" and the providers the "second parties.") Third-party payers include commercial for-profit insurance companies, nonprofit Blue Cross and Blue Shield organizations, self-insured employers, federal programs (Medicare, Medicaid, SCHIP, TRICARE, CHAMPVA, and IHS), and workers' compensation programs.

The type of reimbursement methodology used depends on the type of third-party payer. For example, commercial insurance plans usually reimburse healthcare providers under some type of **retrospective payment system.** The federal Medicare program uses prospective payment systems (PPSs). In retrospective payment systems, the exact amount of the payment is determined after the service has been delivered. In a PPS, the exact amount of the payment is determined before the service is delivered.

Fee-for-Service Reimbursement Methodologies

Fee-for-service reimbursement methodologies issue payments to healthcare providers on the basis of the charges assigned to each of the separate services that were performed for the patient. In fee-for-service arrangements, healthcare facilities develop **chargemasters** that list the individual charges for every element entailed in providing a service (for example, surgical supplies, surgical equipment, room and board, nursing care, respiratory therapy, pharmaceuticals, medical equipment, and so on). The total bill for an episode of care represents the sum of all of the itemized charges for

every element of the care provided. Independent clinical professionals such as physicians and psychologists who are not employees of the facility issue separate itemized bills to cover their services after the services are completed or on a monthly basis when the services are ongoing.

Before prepaid insurance plans became common in the 1950s and the Medicare and Medicaid programs were developed in the 1960s, healthcare providers sent itemized bills directly to their patients. Patients were held responsible for paying their own medical bills. When prepaid health plans and the Medicare/Medicaid programs were originally developed, they also based reimbursement on itemized fees.

Traditional Fee-for-Service Reimbursement

In **traditional fee-for-service** (FFS) **reimbursement** systems, third-party payers and/or patients issue payments to healthcare providers after the services have been provided. Payments are based on the specific services delivered. The fees charged for services vary considerably by the type of services provided, the resources required, and the type and number of healthcare professionals involved.

For example, the charges for a typical visit to a physician's office might include a fee for the physician's consultation and examination and a charge for the blood tests performed by the laboratory personnel in the physician's office. The physician's overhead expenses (rent, equipment, utilities, payroll, taxes, and so on) are included in the physician's fee schedule.

Obviously, the charges for heart transplantation surgery would be much higher. They would include the professional fees of the individual surgeons, the surgeons' assistants, and the anesthesiologist as well as hospital charges for surgical supplies and equipment, nursing care, postoperative and rehabilitative services, room and board, drugs and surgical dressings, and a lot more. As for the physician's charges, the hospital's overhead expenses would be built in to the hospital's fee schedule. In these examples, the total charges for the trip to the physician's office might be less than $125, but the total charges for the heart surgery might be well over $150,000, depending on the geographic location of the facilities that provided the services.

Payments can be calculated on the basis of actual billed charges, discounted charges, prenegotiated rate schedules, or the usual or customary charges in a specific community. Usual or customary charges represent the amount a third-party payer will reimburse a provider for a particular service or procedure. **Usual, customary, and reasonable charges** (UCR) are based on the amount considered to represent reasonable compensation for the service or procedure in a specific area of the country. For example, the charge for a particular service would likely be higher in a large northern city than in a rural southern farm town.

Typically, in the traditional FFS payment methodology, the third-party payer reimburses providers according to charges that are calculated after the healthcare services have been rendered (for example, after the patient has been discharged from the hospital). First, an employee of the healthcare facility analyzes the patient's health record and assigns appropriate diagnostic and procedural codes to represent the facts as documented in the health record. (In hospitals, diagnostic and procedural codes are assigned by HIM personnel. In other settings, coding may be performed by nurses, physicians, trained administrative staff, and/or HIM professionals. Facilities also may enter into contracts with coding vendors.)

After the codes have been assigned, the billing department takes over the process, following these general steps:

1. The provider's billing department itemizes the services provided to the patient as represented by the procedural codes assigned to the case.
2. The billing department assigns a fee to each service from the provider's standard fee schedule or chargemaster.
3. The billing department applies the charges to the patient's account.
4. The billing department transmits the detailed claim to the patient's third-party payer and sends an itemized account of the billed services to the patient.

The amount to be paid by the third-party payer is based on the payer's reimbursement policy and the terms of the plan. For example, some third-party payers pay only the maximum allowable charges as determined by the plan. Maximum allowable charges may be significantly lower than the provider's billed charges. Some payers issue payments on the basis of usual and customary charges. Commercial insurance and Blue Cross/Blue Shield plans often issue payments based on prenegotiated discount rates and contractual cost-sharing arrangements with the patient.

For many plans, the health plan and the patient share costs on an 80:20 percent arrangement. The portion of the claim covered by the patient's insurance plan would be 80 percent of allowable charges. After the third-party payer transmits its payment to the provider, the provider's billing department issues a final statement to the patient. The statement shows the amount for which the patient is responsible (in this example, 20 percent of allowable charges).

The traditional FFS reimbursement methodology is still used by many commercial insurance companies for visits to physicians' offices.

Managed Fee-for-Service Reimbursement

Managed fee-for-service (FFS) **reimbursement** is similar to traditional FFS reimbursement except that managed care plans control costs primarily by managing their members' use of healthcare services. Most managed care plans also negotiate with providers to develop discounted fee schedules. Managed FFS reimbursement is common for inpatient hospital care. In some areas of the country, however, it also is applied to outpatient and ambulatory services, surgical procedures, high-cost diagnostic procedures, and physicians' services.

Utilization controls include the prospective and retrospective review of the healthcare services planned for, or provided to, patients. For example, a *prospective utilization review* of a plan to hospitalize a patient for minor surgery might determine that the surgery could be safely performed less expensively in an outpatient setting. Prospective utilization review is sometimes called precertification.

In a *retrospective utilization review,* the plan might determine that part or all of the services provided to a patient were not medically necessary or were not covered by the plan. In such cases, the plan would disallow part or all of the provider's charges, and the patient would be responsible for paying the provider's outstanding charges.

Discharge planning also can be considered a type of utilization control. The managed care plan may be able to move the patient to a less intensive (and therefore less expensive) care setting as soon as possible by coordinating his or her discharge from inpatient care.

Episode-of-Care Reimbursement Methodologies

Plans that use **episode-of-care** (EOC) **reimbursement** methods issue lump-sum payments to providers to compensate them for all of the healthcare services delivered to a patient for a specific illness and/or over a specific period of time. EOC payments also are called bundled payments. **Bundled payments** cover multiple services and also may involve multiple providers of care. EOC reimbursement methods include capitated payments, global payments, global surgery payments, Medicare ambulatory surgery center rates, and Medicare prospective payment systems.

Capitation

Capitation is based on per-person premiums or membership fees rather than on itemized per-procedure or per-service charges. The capitated managed care plan negotiates a contract with an employer or government agency representing a specific group of individuals. According to the contract, the managed care organization agrees to provide all of the contracted healthcare services that the covered individuals need over a specified period of time (usually one year). In exchange, the individual enrollee and/or third-party payer agrees to pay a fixed premium for the covered group. Like other insurance plans, a capitated insurance contract stipulates as part of the contract exactly which healthcare services are covered and which ones are not.

Capitated premiums are calculated on the projected cost of providing covered services **per patient or member per month** (PPPM or PMPM). The capitated premium for an individual member of a plan includes all of the services covered by the plan, regardless of the number of services actually provided during the period or their cost. If the average member of the plan actually used more services than originally assumed in the PPPM calculation, the plan would show a loss for the period. If the average member actually used fewer services, the plan would show a profit.

The purchasers of capitated coverage (usually the member's employer) pay monthly premiums to the managed care plan. (The individual enrollees usually pay part of the premium as well.) The plan then compensates the providers who actually furnished the services. In some arrangements, the managed care plan accepts all of the risk involved in the contract. In others, some of the risk is passed on to the primary care physicians who agreed to act as gatekeepers for the plan.

The capitated managed care organization may own or operate some or all of the healthcare facilities that provide care to members and directly employ clinical professionals. Staff model HMOs operate in this way. Alternatively, the capitated managed care organization may purchase services from independent physicians and facilities, as do group model HMOs. For example:

> The ABC HMO awarded a capitated contract to the XYZ Medical Center for a total compensation of $3,600,000 in the year 2000. According to the terms of the contract, the medical center agreed to provide comprehensive healthcare services to all 500 enrollees covered under the contract for twelve months. The medical center received lump-sum payments of $300,000 per month over the twelve-month period. A large, multispecialty physician–hospital organization owned by the hospital acted as primary care gatekeepers and provided medical services to the enrollees. Inpatient and outpatient services were provided directly by the medical center.

Global Payment

Global payment methodology is sometimes applied to radiological procedures and similar types of procedures that involve professional and **technical components. Global payments** are lump-sum payments distributed among the physicians who performed the procedure or interpreted its results and the healthcare facility that provided the equipment, supplies, and technical support required. The procedure's **professional component** is supplied by physicians (for example, radiologists), and its technical component (for example, radiological supplies, equipment, and support services) is supplied by a hospital or freestanding diagnostic or surgical center. For example:

> Larry Timber underwent a scheduled carotid angiogram as a hospital outpatient. He had complained of ringing in his ears and dizziness, and his physician scheduled the procedure to determine whether there was a blockage in one of Larry's carotid arteries. The procedure required a surgeon to inject radiopaque contrast material through a catheter into Larry's left carotid artery. A radiological technician then took an X ray of Larry's neck. The technician was supervised by a radiologist (both were employees of the hospital).
>
> *Professional component:* Injection of radiopaque contrast material by the surgeon
>
> *Technical component:* X ray of the neck region
>
> *Global payment:* The facility received a lump-sum payment for the procedure and paid for the services of the surgeon from that payment.

Global Surgery Payments

A single **global surgery payment** covers all of the healthcare services entailed in planning and completing a specific surgical procedure. In other words, every element of the procedure from the treatment decision through normal postoperative patient care is covered by a single bundled payment. For example:

> Tammy Murdock received all of the prenatal, perinatal, and postnatal care involved in the birth of her daughter from Dr. Thomas Michaels. She received one bill from the physician for a total of $2,200. The bill represented the total charges for the obstetrical services associated with her pregnancy.
>
> However, the two-day inpatient hospital stay for the normal delivery was not included in the global payment nor were the laboratory services she received during her hospital stay. Tammy received a separate bill for these services. In addition, if she had suffered a postdelivery complication (for example, a wound infection) or an unrelated medical problem, the physician and hospital services required to treat the complications would not have been covered by the global surgical payment.

Medicare Ambulatory Surgery

The CMS (formerly the HCFA) defines an ambulatory surgery center (ASC) as a state-licensed, Medicare-certified supplier (not a provider) of surgical healthcare services. ASCs must **accept assignment** on Medicare claims, which means the supplier accepts as payment in full whatever Medicare reimburses. Because payments are subject to Medicare Part B deductible and coinsurance requirements, reimbursement is 80 percent of the prospectively determined rate (adjusted for regional wage variations). The CMS replaced the ASC rates (which categorized approximately 2,500 surgical procedures into eight payment groups) with the **ambulatory payment classification** (APC) **system** and the **outpatient prospective payment system** (OPPS) in 2000 for hospital-based outpatient services and procedures.

To qualify as a Medicare-certified ASC, the surgical center must be a separate entity distinguishable from any other entity or type of facility. This means that the ASC must be separate from any other organization with respect to licensure, accreditation, governance, professional supervision, administrative functions, clinical services, record keeping, financial and accounting systems, and national identifier or supplier number. The ASC can be physically located within the space of another entity and still be considered separate for Medicare payment purposes when the preceding criteria are met.

Medicare pays a prospectively determined fee for ASC services that are included on the approved list. The services that fall within the scope of ASC services include, but are not limited to, services performed by nurses and technicians, supplies, drugs and biologicals, surgical dressings, housekeeping services, and use of the facility.

The professional services of physicians and other practitioners do not fall within the scope of ASC facility services. Therefore, the ASC facility fee does not include payment for the professional services of physicians and other practitioners. ASCs should not bill for the following physicians' services: anesthesiology, surgery, or assistance at surgery services. The anesthesiologist, surgeon, and assistant surgeon submit separate claims.

The CMS's ASC rates are categorized into eight separate payment groups. (See table 14.6.) The payment groups are based on the complexity of the surgical procedures involved. The CMS also updates and publishes the rate-setting methodology and establishes wage index (WI) tables for use in urban and rural areas.

Special rules apply when more than one surgical procedure is performed during the same operative session. The ASC is reimbursed at 100 percent for the procedure classified in the highest payment group, and any other procedure performed during the same session is reimbursed at 50 percent of the procedure's applicable group rate. Bilateral procedures are reimbursed at 150 percent of the applicable rate. The reimbursement of physicians for ASC-approved procedures is subject to 20 percent coinsurance and deductible provisions. Payment is made at 80 percent of the Medicare physician fee schedule. Fees for approved procedures in an ASC setting are noted on the fee schedule as a facility fee.

Prospective Payment

In 1983, the HCFA (now called the CMS) implemented a prospective payment system (PPS) for inpatient hospital care provided to Medicare beneficiaries. The PPS is called **diagnosis-related groups** (DRGs). The DRG system was implemented as a way to control Medicare spending. It reimburses hospitals a predetermined amount for each Medicare inpatient stay. Payments are determined by the DRG to which each case is assigned according to the patient's diagnosis at the time of discharge from the hospital.

After DRG implementation in 1983, expenditures for Medicare post–acute care benefits quickly escalated. According to the Department of Health and Human Services, post-acute expenditures totaled approximately $2.5 billion in 1986, but more than $30 billion in 1996. This drastic increase in spending alarmed Medicare policy makers. In response, the Balanced Budget Act of 1997 mandated PPS implementation for non–acute care services, including care in skilled nursing facilities, outpatient services and procedures, home health care, and rehabilitation care. In addition, the act included a legislative proposal on a PPS for long-term care.

Table 14.6. Ambulatory Surgery Center Payment Groups and Rates—2001

ASC Group	Reimbursement Rate
Group 1 Procedure	$320
Group 2 Procedure	$429
Group 3 Procedure	$491
Group 4 Procedure	$606
Group 5 Procedure	$690
Group 6 Procedure	$800 ($650 + $150 for intraocular lenses)
Group 7 Procedure	$957
Group 8 Procedure	$942 ($792 + $150 for intraocular lenses)

Source: DHHS HCFA Program Memorandum, Intermediaries/Carriers, Transmittal AB-00-82, September 1, 2000.

Check Your Understanding 14.3

Instructions: Answer the following questions on a separate piece of paper.

1. What type of payment system is in place when the amount of payment is determined before the service is delivered?

2. What is a chargemaster, and why do healthcare facilities develop chargemasters?

3. What are usual, customary, and reasonable (UCR) charges based on?

4. Many insurance plans require patients to share costs for healthcare services. What is the most typical cost share ratio?

5. Which utilization control is most closely associated with managed fee-for-service reimbursement?

6. What would a managed care plan likely show when a group of patients uses more services than the plan originally calculated in its contract with the group?

7. What are bundled payments? What is another name for bundled payments?

8. Describe the concept of capitation and explain how capitated payments are calculated.

9. How are ambulatory surgery center rates calculated?

10. How is reimbursement limited when multiple ambulatory surgery center procedures are performed on the same patient during the same visit?

11. How did the first prospective payment system implemented by HCFA (now called CMS) affect inpatient reimbursement?

12. What are diagnosis-related groups? What was the effect of DRG implementation in 1983 on Medicare expenditures?

13. What are the general steps taken by the billing department after codes have been assigned?

Medicare's Prospective Payment Systems

As discussed briefly in the preceding section, Congress enacted the first Medicare PPS in 1983 as a cost-cutting measure. Implementation of the acute care PPS resulted in a shift of clinical services and expenditures away from the inpatient hospital setting to outpatient settings. As a result, spending on nonacute care exploded.

Congress responded by enacting legislation that required implementation of Medicare PPSs for other types of healthcare services provided to Medicare beneficiaries. Although the legislation was passed in 1987, development and implementation of nonacute care PPSs have proved complex.

Medicare's Acute Care Prospective Payment System

As mentioned previously, prior to 1983, Medicare Part A payments to hospitals were determined on a traditional FFS reimbursement methodology. Payment was based on the cost of services provided, and reasonable cost and/or per-diem costs were used to determine payment.

During the late 1960s, just a few years after the Medicare and Medicaid health programs were implemented, Congress authorized a group at Yale University to develop a system for monitoring quality of care and utilization of services. This system was known as diagnosis-related groups (DRGs). DRGs were implemented on an experimental basis by the New Jersey Department of Health in the late 1970s as a way to predetermine reimbursement for hospital inpatient stays.

At the conclusion of the New Jersey DRG experiment, Congress passed the **Tax Equity and Fiscal Responsibility Act of 1982** (TEFRA). TEFRA modified Medicare's retrospective reimbursement system for inpatient hospital stays by requiring implementation of the DRG PPS in 1983. Medicare now pays most hospitals for inpatient hospital services according to a predetermined rate for each discharge under DRGs.

Under the **acute care prospective payment system,** a predetermined rate based on the DRG(s) assigned to each case is used to reimburse hospitals for inpatient care provided to Medicare beneficiaries. Hospitals determine DRGs by assigning **ICD-9-CM** codes to each patient's principal diagnosis, comorbidities, complications, principal procedure, and/or secondary procedures. These code numbers and other information on the patient (age, gender, and discharge status) are entered into a DRG grouper. A **DRG grouper** is a computer software program that assigns appropriate DRGs according to the information provided for each episode of care.

Reimbursement for each episode of care is based on the DRGs assigned. Different diagnoses require different levels of care and expenditures of resources. Therefore, each DRG is assigned a different level of payment that reflects the average amount of resources required to treat a patient assigned to that DRG. A single episode of care may represent more than one DRG when the patient has complex medical needs and comorbid conditions. Each DRG is associated with a description, a relative weight, a geometric mean length of stay (LOS), and an arithmetic mean LOS.

For example, DRG 1, organized within major diagnostic category (MDC) 01, is described as SURG CRANIOTOMY AGE >17 EXCEPT FOR TRAUMA and has a relative weight of 3.0970, a geometric mean length of stay (LOS) of 6.3, and an arithmetic mean LOS of 9.1.

At this time, several types of hospitals are excluded from Medicare acute care PPS. The following facilities are still paid on the basis of reasonable cost, subject to payment limits per discharge:

- Psychiatric and rehabilitation hospitals and psychiatric and rehabilitation units within larger medical facilities
- Long-term care hospitals, which are defined as hospitals with an average length of stay of twenty-five days or more
- Children's hospitals
- Cancer hospitals

The CMS adjusts the Medicare DRG list and reimbursement rates every year. For fiscal year 2002, the list includes 511 DRGs (including one for a diagnosis that is invalid as a

discharge diagnosis and one for ungroupable diagnoses) organized within twenty-five major diagnostic categories (MDCs). Most MDCs are based on a particular organ system of the body (for example, MDC 6, Diseases and Disorders of the Digestive System). (See figure 14.1.) However, some MDCs are not constructed on this basis because they involve multiple organ systems (for example, MDC 22, Burns).

In general, cases are assigned to an MDC according to the patient's principal diagnosis before a DRG is assigned. However, at this time, there are five DRGs to which cases are directly assigned on the basis of procedural codes: the DRGs for liver, bone marrow, and lung transplants (DRGs 480, 481, and 495, respectively) and the two DRGs for tracheostomies (DRGs 482 and 483).

Within most MDCs, cases are divided into surgical DRGs (based on a surgical hierarchy that orders individual procedures or groups of procedures by resource intensity) and medical DRGs. Medical DRGs generally are differentiated on the basis of diagnosis and age. Some surgical and medical DRGs are further differentiated on the basis of the presence or absence of complications or comorbidities.

The DRG system allows a hospital to relate its **case mix** (types or categories of patients treated by the hospital) to the costs incurred for inpatient care. This information allows the hospital to make administrative decisions about services to be offered to its patient population. For example:

> The hospital's case-mix report indicated that a small population of patients was receiving obstetrical services, but that the costs associated with providing such services was disproportionately high. This report (along with other data) might result in the hospital's administrative decision to discontinue its obstetrical services department.

The **principal procedure** is (1) a procedure performed for therapeutic rather than diagnostic reasons, (2) a procedure performed to treat a complication, or (3) the procedure that is most closely related to the principal diagnosis. The **principal diagnosis** is the condition established after study to have resulted in the inpatient admission. **Comorbidities** are coexisting conditions (for example, hypertension) that affect the inpatient stay, and complications are conditions that arise during the hospitalization (for example, postoperative wound infection). The definition of principal procedure has three parts. For example:

> The patient was admitted to the hospital with chest pain. After study, it was determined that the patient had pneumonia. The principal diagnosis is pneumonia, not chest pain.

In some cases, the DRG payment received by the hospital may be lower than the actual cost of providing Medicare Part A inpatient services. In such cases, the hospital must absorb the loss. In other cases, the hospital may receive a payment for more than its actual cost and, therefore, makes a profit. It is expected that, on average, hospitals will be reimbursed for their total costs in providing services to Medicare patients.

Special circumstances also can apply to inpatient cases and result in an outlier payment to the hospital. An outlier case results in exceptionally high costs when compared with

Figure 14.1.   Portion of Major Diagnostic Category, Diseases and Disorders of the Digestive System

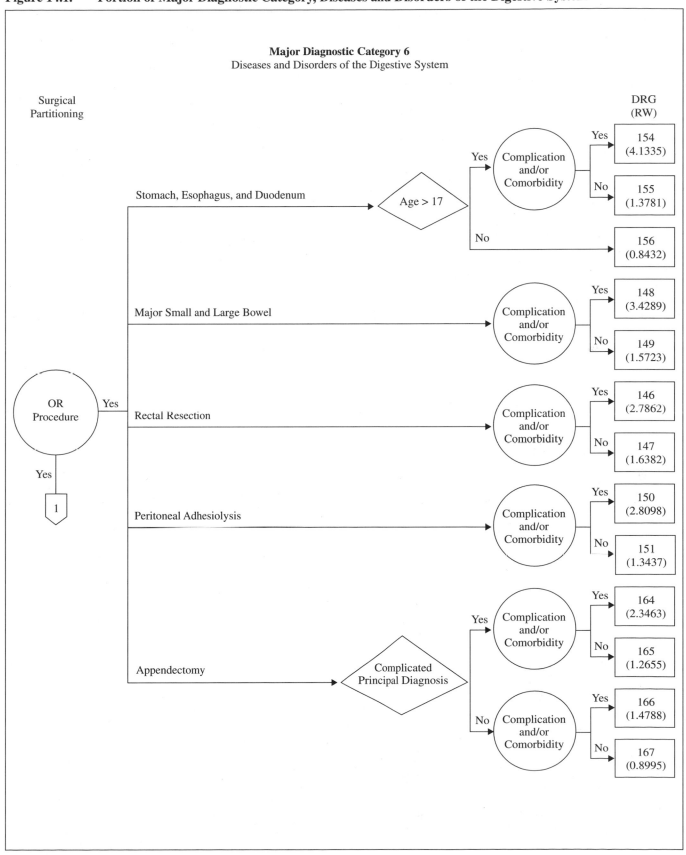

other cases in the same DRG. For fiscal year (FY) 2002, to quality for a **cost outlier,** a hospital's charges for a case (adjusted to cost) must exceed the payment rate for the DRG by $21,025. The additional payment amount is equal to 80 percent of the difference between the hospital's entire cost for the stay and the threshold amount.

An All Patient DRG (AP-DRG) system was developed in 1988 by 3M Health Information Systems as the basis for New York's hospital reimbursement program for non-Medicare discharges. AP-DRGs are still used in a number of states as a basis for payment of non-Medicare claims. AP-DRGs use the patient's age, sex, discharge status, and ICD-9-CM diagnoses and procedure codes to determine a DRG which, in turn, determines reimbursement. 3M has also developed All Patient Refined DRGs (APR-DRGs as an extension of the DRG concept. APR-DRGs adjust patient data for severity of illness and risk of mortality, help to develop clinical pathways, are used as a basis for quality assurance programs, and are used in comparative profiling and setting capitation rates (3M 2002).

Resource-Based Relative Value Scale (RBRVS) System

In 1992, the HCFA (now called the CMS) implemented the **resource-based relative value scale** (RBRVS) system for physician's services (for example, office visits) covered under Medicare Part B. The system reimburses physicians according to a fee schedule based on predetermined values assigned to specific services. A **fee schedule** is a complete list of fees paid to physicians and other clinical professionals for specific services. The **Medicare fee schedule** (MFS) is a feature of the RBRVS system and is revised annually.

To calculate fee schedule amounts, Medicare uses a formula that incorporates the following factors:

- **Relative value units** for physician work (RVUw)
- Practice expenses (RVUpe)
- Malpractice costs (RVUm)

Payment localities are adjusted according to three **geographic practice cost indices** (GPCIs):

- Physician work (GPCIw)
- Practice expenses (GPCIpe)
- Malpractice costs (GPCIm)

A **national conversion factor** (CF) converts the RVUs into payments. In 2001, the CF was $38.2581.

The RBRVS fee schedule uses the following formula:

$$[(RVUw \times GPCIw) + (RVUpe \times GPCIpe) + (RVUm \times GPCIm)] \times CF = Payment$$

As an example, the payment for performing a biopsy of a skin lesion in Birmingham, Alabama, in 2001, can be calculated. RVU values include:

- Work RVU (RVUw) = 0.81
- Practice expense RVU (RVUpe) = 0.51
- Malpractice RVU (RVUm) = 0.04

GPCI values include:

- Work GPCI (GPCIw) = 0.994
- Practice expense GPCI (GPCIpe) = 0.912
- Malpractice GPCI (GPCIm) = 0.927
- National CF = $38.2581

The calculation is as follows:

$$(0.81 \times 0.994) + (0.51 \times 0.912) + (0.04 \times 0.927) \times \$38.2581$$
$$0.81 + 0.47 + 0.04 \times \$38.2581$$
$$1.32 \times \$38.2581$$
$$\text{Fee schedule payment} = \$50.50$$

Medicare Skilled Nursing Facility Prospective Payment System

The Balanced Budget Act (BBA) of 1997 mandated implementation of a **skilled nursing facility prospective payment system** (SNF PPS). The system was to cover all costs (routine, ancillary, and capital) associated with covered SNF services furnished to Medicare Part A beneficiaries. Certain educational activities were exempt from the new system.

The SNF PPS was implemented on July 1, 1998. Under the PPS, SNFs are no longer paid under a system based on reasonable costs. Instead, they are paid according to a per-diem prospective system based on case mix–adjusted payment rates.

Medicare Part A covers posthospital SNF services and all items and services paid under Medicare Part B before July 1, 1998 (other than physician and certain other services specifically excluded under the BBA). Major elements of the SNF PPS include rates, coverage, transition, and consolidated billing.

The **Omnibus Budget Reconciliation Act of 1987** required the HCFA (now called the CMS) to develop an assessment instrument to standardize the collection of SNF patient data. That instrument is known as the **Resident Assessment Instrument** (RAI) and includes the **Minimum Data Set 2.0** (MDS).

The MDS is the minimum core of defined and categorized patient assessment questions that serves as the basis for documentation and reimbursement in an SNF. The MDS form contains a face sheet for documentation of resident identification information, demographic information, and the patient's customary routine.

Resource Utilization Groups

SNF reimbursement rates are paid according to **Resource Utilization Groups, Version III** (RUG-III) (a resident classification system) based on the MDS resident assessments.

The RUG-III classification system uses resident assessment data from the MDS collected by SNFs to assign residents to one of forty-four groups. SNFs complete MDS assessments according to a schedule specifically designed for Medicare payment (that is, on the fifth, fourteenth, thirtieth, sixtieth, and ninetieth days after admission to the SNF). For Medicare billing purposes, specific codes are associated with each of the forty-four RUG-III groups, and each assessment applies to specific days within a resident's SNF stay. SNFs that fail to perform timely assessments are paid a default payment for the days they are not in compliance with this schedule.

Resident Assessment Validation and Entry

The HCFA (now called the CMS) developed a computerized data-entry system for long-term care facilities that offers users the ability to collect MDS assessments in a database and transmit them in CMS-standard format to their state database. The data-entry software is entitled **Resident Assessment Validation and Entry** (RAVEN). RAVEN imports and exports data in standard MDS record format; maintains facility, resident, and employee information; enforces data integrity via rigorous edit checks; and provides comprehensive online help. It includes a data dictionary and a RUG calculator.

Consolidated Billing Provision

The BBA includes a billing provision that requires an SNF to submit consolidated Medicare bills for its residents for services covered under either Part A or Part B. In addition, SNFs report **Healthcare Common Procedure Coding System** (HCPCS) codes on all Part B bills.

Medicare/Medicaid Outpatient Prospective Payment System

The Balanced Budget Act of 1997 authorized implementation of a Medicare PPS for outpatient services. The outpatient prospective payment system (OPPS), implemented in October 2001, applies to the following services:

- Services provided by hospital outpatient departments, including partial hospitalization services
- Certain Part B services provided to hospital inpatients who have no Part A coverage
- Partial hospitalization services provided by community mental health centers (CMHCs)
- Vaccines, splints, casts, and antigens provided by home health agencies that provide medical and health-related services
- Vaccines provided by comprehensive outpatient rehabilitation facilities (CORFs)
- Splints, casts, and antigens provided to hospice patients for the treatment of nonterminal illnesses

The OPPS does not apply to critical access hospitals (CAHs) or hospitals in Maryland that are excluded because they qualify under the Social Security Act for payment under the state's payment system. In addition, IHS hospitals and hospitals located in Saipan, American Samoa, and Guam were initially excluded but will be included in the future.

Implementation of the OPPS resulted in the discontinuation of the blended payment method for radiology and other diagnostic services and for ASC services provided in hospital-based outpatient departments. In addition, the following provisions are associated with the OPPS:

- Payments are established in a budget-neutral manner based on estimates of amounts payable in 1999 from the Medicare Part B Trust Fund and the beneficiary coinsurance in effect prior to implementation of the OPPS.
- OPPS payment weights, rates, payment adjustments and groups, and annual consultation are reviewed and updated annually by an expert provider advisory panel.
- Budget-neutral outlier adjustments are based on charges, adjusted to costs, for all OPPS services included on outpatient bills submitted before January 1, 2002, and, thereafter, based on individual services billed.
- Provisions for transitional passthroughs are related to additional costs of new and current medical devices, drugs, and biologicals for at least two years, but not more than three years.
- Provisions are in place for OPPS payment for implantable devices, including durable medical equipment, prosthetics, and implantable devices used in diagnostic testing.
- Transitional payments limit provider losses under the OPPS. (Additional payments continue for three and a half years for CMHCs and most hospitals and are permanent for the ten cancer hospitals.)
- The amount of the beneficiary's coinsurance payment is limited for an individual service paid under the OPPS to that which equals the inpatient hospital deductible.

The OPPS is not applicable to clinical diagnostic laboratory services, orthotics, prosthetics, and take-home surgical dressings. These services are paid on the basis of a fee schedule. Chronic dialysis is reimbursed under the composite rate, but acute dialysis (for example, for treatment of poisonings) is paid under the OPPS. Reimbursement for screening mammographies is based on current payment limitations. Outpatient rehabilitation services (physical, speech–language–pathology, and occupational therapy) are reimbursed under the Medicare physician fee schedule.

The calculation of payment for services under the OPPS is based on the categorization of outpatient services into ambulatory payment classification (APC) groups. The more than 450 APCs are categorized into significant procedure APCs, radiology and other diagnostic APCs, medical visit APCs, and a partial hospitalization APC. Services within an APC are similar, both clinically and with regard to resource consumption, and each APC is assigned a fixed payment rate for the facility fee or technical component of the outpatient visit. Payment rates are then adjusted according to the hospital's wage index.

Medicare has assigned **payment status indicators** (PSIs) (figure 14.2) to HCPCS/CPT codes to indicate whether a service/procedure is to be reimbursed under the OPPS.

OPPS payments will be made for clinical diagnostic laboratory tests and radiology and other diagnostic services in addition to the payment for a surgical procedure or medical visit performed on the same day. However, the OPPS also incorporates the **packaging** of certain items, such as anesthesia, supplies, certain drugs, and the use of recovery and observation rooms.

Figure 14.2.   OPPS Payment Status Indicators and Description of Payment under OPPS

PSI A	Services paid under some other method (such as a fee schedule): • Pulmonary rehabilitation clinical trial (not paid under OPPS) • Durable medical equipment, prosthetics, and orthotics (paid according to the DMEPOS fee schedule) • Physical/occupational/speech therapy (paid according to the rehabilitation fee schedule) • Ambulance services (paid according to the ambulance fee schedule) • Erythropoitin services for end-stage renal disease (ESRD) patients (paid according to the national rate) • Clinical diagnostic laboratory services (paid according to the laboratory fee schedule) • Physician services for ESRD patients (not paid under OPPS) • Screening mammography (paid according to charges or national rate, whichever is lower)
PSI C	Inpatient procedures (billed on an inpatient basis)
PSI E	Noncovered items and services (not paid under OPPS)
PSI F	Corneal tissue acquisition costs, which are paid separately (paid on a reasonable cost basis)
PSI G	Current drug or biological passthrough (eligible for additional payment under OPPS)
PSI H	Device passthrough (eligible for additional payment under OPPS)
PSI J	New drug or biological pass-through (eligible for additional payment under OPPS)
PSI N	Incidental services, packaged into APC rate
PSI P	Partial hospitalization (paid on a per diem APC basis)
PSI S	Significant procedure, not discounted when multiple (paid under OPPS)
PSI T	Significant procedure, multiple procedure discounting applies (paid under OPPS)
PSI V	Visits to clinic or emergency department (paid under OPPS)
PSI X	Ancillary service (paid under OPPS)

Discounting applies to multiple surgical procedures furnished during the same operative session. For discounted procedures, the full APC rate is paid for the surgical procedure with the highest weight, and other surgical procedure(s) performed at the same time are reimbursed at 50 percent of the APC rate. Similar discounting occurs under the physician fee schedule and the payment system for ASCs.

Surgical procedures terminated after a patient is prepared for surgery, but before induction of anesthesia, are paid for at 50 percent of the APC rate. In addition, when multiple surgical procedures are performed during the same operative session, the beneficiary's coinsurance is discounted in proportion to the APC payment.

Note: Services that Medicare has identified as "inpatient-only" services are not reimbursed by Medicare when they are provided on an outpatient basis.

Home Health Prospective Payment System

The Balanced Budget Act of 1997 was amended by the Omnibus Consolidated and Emergency Supplemental Appropriations Act (OCESAA) of 1999. The BBA of 1997 called for the development and implementation of a **home health prospective payment system** (HH PPS) for reimbursement of services provided to Medicare beneficiaries. An **interim payment system** (IPS) that consisted of cost-based reimbursement was in place until the HH PPS could be phased in starting on October 1, 2000.

OASIS and HAVEN

Home health agencies (HHAs) use the OASIS data set and HAVEN data-entry software to conduct all patient assessments (not just the assessments for Medicare beneficiaries). OASIS stands for **Outcome and Assessment Information Set.** It consists of data elements that (1) represent core items for the comprehensive assessment of an adult home care patient and (2) form the basis for measuring patient outcomes for the purpose of outcome-based quality improvement (OBQI). OASIS is a key component of Medicare's partnership with the home care industry to foster and monitor improved home health care outcomes. It has been proposed that OASIS will become an integral part of the revised *Conditions of Participation* for Medicare-certified HHAs.

The HCFA (now called the CMS) also developed the OASIS data-entry system called HAVEN (**Home Assessment Validation and Entry).** HAVEN is available to HHAs at no charge through the CMS's Web site or on CD-ROM. HAVEN offers users the ability to collect OASIS data in a database and transmit them in a standard format to state databases. The data-entry software imports and exports data in standard OASIS record format; maintains agency, patient, and employee information; maintains data integrity through rigorous edit checks; and provides comprehensive online help.

Home Health Resource Groups

Home health resource groups (HHRGs) represent the classification system established for the prospective reimbursement of covered home care services to Medicare beneficiaries during a sixty-day episode of care. Covered services include skilled nursing visits, home health aide visits, therapy services (for example, physical, occupational, and speech therapy), medical social services, and nonroutine medical supplies. Durable medical equipment (DME) is excluded from the episode-of-care payment. DME is reimbursed under the DME fee schedule.

The classification of a patient into one of eighty HHRGs is based on OASIS data, which establish the severity of clinical and functional needs and services utilized. Grouper software is used to establish the appropriate HHRG. The HHRG is a six-character alphanumeric code that represents severity levels in three domains: clinical, functional, and service utilization. (See table 14.7.)

Episode-of-care reimbursements vary from $1,000 to almost $6,000 and are affected by treatment level and regional wage differentials. The initial episode is reimbursed under a 60:40 split, with 60 percent paid at the start of treatment and the remainder paid at the end of the episode. Additional episodes are paid under a 50:50 split. There is no limit to the number of sixty-day episodes of care that a patient may receive as long as Medicare coverage criteria are met. For example:

> OASIS data collected on a seventy-six-year-old male home care patient resulted in an HHRG of C3F4S3. This HHRG is interpreted as a clinical domain of high severity, a functional domain of high severity, and a service utilization domain of high utilization.

Low Utilization and Outlier Payments

When a patient receives fewer than four home care visits during a sixty-day episode, an alternate (reduced) payment, or **low-utilization payment adjustment** (LUPA), is made instead of the full HHRG reimbursement rate. Home care agencies are eligible for a **cost outlier adjustment,** which is a payment for certain high-cost home care patients based on the loss-sharing ratio (a percentage) of costs in excess of a threshold amount for each HHRG. The threshold is the sixty-day episode payment plus a fixed-dollar loss that is constant across the HHRGs.

ICD-9-CM Diagnostic Coding

Accurate ICD-9-CM diagnostic coding for home care patients is essential because the codes reported for HHRG purposes affect the payment level in the HH PPS. HHAs must enter the complete ICD-9-CM code for the principal diagnosis. Up to eight additional codes can be entered for conditions that co-existed at the time the plan of care was established.

Ambulance Fee Schedule

A new Medicare payment system for medically necessary transports effective for services provided on or after January 1, 2001, was included as part of the Balanced Budget Act of 1997. The new payment system requires the reporting of HCPCS codes and establishes new payment methods and claim requirements. The CMS will no longer pay for ambulance services based on reasonable charges or reasonable costs. Instead, payment will be made from a fee schedule that applies to all ambulance services, including volunteer, municipal, private, independent, and institutional providers (hospitals, critical access hospitals, SNFs, and HHAs).

Ambulance services will be reported on claims using HCPCS codes that reflect the seven categories of ground service and two categories of air service. Mandatory assignment will be required for all ambulance services after the fee schedule has been phased in over a four-year period. When fully implemented, the fee schedule will replace the current retrospective reasonable cost reimbursement system for providers and the reasonable charge system for ambulance suppliers.

The seven categories of ground (land and water) ambulance services include:

- Basic life support
- Basic life support—emergency
- Advanced life support, level 1
- Advanced life support, level 1—emergency
- Advanced life support, level 2
- Specialty care transport
- Paramedic intercept

The air service categories include fixed-wing air ambulance (airplane) and rotary-wing air ambulance (helicopter).

Inpatient Rehabilitation Facility Prospective Payment System

The Balanced Budget Act of 1997 (as amended the **Balanced Budget Refinement Act** of 1999) authorized implementation of a per-discharge PPS for care provided to Medicare

Table 14.7.   HHRG Severity Levels in Three Domains: Clinical, Functional, and Service Utilization

Domain	Score	Points	Severity Level
Clinical	C0	0–7	Minimal severity
	C1	8–19	Low severity
	C2	20–40	Moderate severity
	C3	41+	High severity
Functional	F0	0–2	Minimal severity
	F1	3–15	Low severity
	F2	16–23	Moderate severity
	F3	24–29	High severity
	F4	30+	Maximum severity
Service utilization	S0	0–2	Minimum utilization
	S1	3	Low utilization
	S2	4–6	Moderate utilization
	S3	7	High utilization

beneficiaries by inpatient rehabilitation hospitals and rehabilitation units, referred to as inpatient rehabilitation facilities (IRFs). The CMS began phasing in the IRF PPS on April 1, 2001.

CMS has implemented IRVEN, the Inpatient Rehabilitation Validation and Entry system, for computerized data entry for IRFs. IRVEN allows user to collect the IRF Patient Assessment Instrument (IRF-PAI) in a database that can be electronically transmitted to the IRF-PAI national database. This data is used in assessing clinical characteristics of patients in rehabilitation settings. It will ultimately be used to provide survey agencies with a means to objectively measure and compare facility performance and quality and to allow researchers to develop improved standards of care (CMS 2001).

The IRF PPS uses information from a patient assessment instrument to classify patients into distinct groups on the basis of clinical characteristics and expected resource needs. Separate payments are calculated for each group, including the application of case- and facility-level adjustments. Major elements of the IRF PPS include:

- **Minimum Data Set for Post Acute Care** (MDS-PAC): A patient assessment instrument that is to be completed for every Medicare patient. The MDS-PAC is a patient-centered assessment instrument that emphasizes the patient's care needs instead of the provider's characteristics. The MDS-PAC classifies patients for Medicare payment and contains an appropriate quality of care-monitoring system, including the use of quality indicators.
- **Case-mix groups** (CMGs): Ninety-seven function-related groups into which patient discharges are to be classified. The groups are based on the patient's level of impairment, age, comorbidities, and functional capability as well as other factors. CMGs also predict the resources needed to furnish patient care to various types of patients. Data used to construct the CMGs include rehabilitation impairment categories, functional status (both motor and cognitive), age, comorbidities, and other factors deemed appropriate to improve the explanatory power of the groups. Data elements from the MDS-PAC are used to classify a patient into a CMG.
- **CMG relative weights:** Weights that account for the variance in cost per discharge and resource utilization among CMGs. Reimbursement is based on a national formula that adjusts for case mix.
- **CMG payment rates:** A predetermined, per-discharge reimbursement amount for each CMG that includes all of the operating and capital costs involved in furnishing covered inpatient rehabilitation services (that is, routine, ancillary, and capital costs), but not costs associated with bad debts, approved educational activities, and other costs not paid for under the PPS.

Processing of Reimbursement Claims

Understanding payment mechanisms is an important foundation for accurately processing claims forms. However, it is not enough just to understand payment mechanisms.

A facility's patient accounts department is responsible for billing third-party payers, processing **accounts receivable** (payments received from third-party payers), and verifying insurance coverage. Medicare carriers and **fiscal intermediaries** (FIs) contract with the CMS (formerly the HCFA) to serve as the financial agent between providers and the federal government to locally administer Medicare's Part A and Part B.

Third-Party Payers

Depending on the services provided to patients, either the CMS-1500 or **UB-92** (CMS-1450) claim form will be submitted to the third-party payer for reimbursement purposes. The CMS-1500 is used to bill third-party payers for provider services (for example, physician's office visit), and the UB-92 is submitted for inpatient, outpatient, home health care, hospice, and long-term care services.

CMS-1500

In 1958, the Health Insurance Association of America (HIAA) and the American Medical Association (AMA) originally created a standardized insurance claim form called the **Attending Physician Statement** (APS) (or COMB-1). However, some third-party payers did not accept its use. In April 1975, the AMA and HCFA (now called the CMS) cochaired the Uniform Claim Form Task Force, which approved a universal claim form now known as **CMS-1500** (figure 14.3, p. 312). CMS-1500 is used for processing both group and individual healthcare claims.

In 1995, the Uniform Claim Form Task Force was replaced by the **National Uniform Claim Committee** (NUCC). The NUCC developed a standard data set to be used in the transmission of noninstitutional provider claims to (and from) third-party payers. NUCC membership includes representation from the following organizations:

- Alliance for Managed Care
- American Association of Health Plans
- American Medical Association
- ANSI ASC X12N
- Blue Cross and Blue Shield Association
- Centers for Medicare and Medicaid Services (formerly HCFA)
- Health Insurance Association of America
- **Medical Group Management Association**
- National Association of Insurance Commissioners
- National Association of Medical Equipment Services
- National Association of State Medicaid Directors
- National Uniform Billing Committee

The CMS-1500 was revised in 1990 and printed in red ink to meet optical scanning guidelines. In May 1992, Medicare required that all services delivered to patients by physicians and suppliers (except for ambulance services) be billed on this scannable form. CMS-1500 contains thirty-five blocks that are completed according to third-party payer guidelines. Noninstitutional providers and suppliers submit it in accordance with these guidelines. It is important to follow payer guidelines when completing the claim form. Otherwise, reimbursement will be delayed until the form is corrected.

UB-92 (CMS-1450)

Healthcare facilities, such as hospitals, submit the UB-92 (figure 14.4, p. 313), or Uniform Bill, to third-party payers for reimbursement of patient services. The data elements and design of the UB-92 are the responsibility of the **National Uniform Billing Committee** (NUBC), which includes representation from the following organizations:

- American Association of Health Plans
- American Health Care Association
- American Hospital Association
- AHA's state hospital association representatives
- Alliance for Managed Care
- American National Standards Institute Accredited Standards

- Committee X12N—Insurance Subcommittee (ANSI ASC X12N)
- Blue Cross and Blue Shield Association
- Center for Healthcare Information Management
- Federation of American Health Systems
- Centers for Medicare and Medicaid Services: Medicare
- Centers for Medicare and Medicaid Services: Medicaid
- Health Insurance Association of America—National Association for Home Care
- National Association of State Medicaid Directors
- National Uniform Claim Committee
- Public Health/Health Services Research: national
- Public Health/Health Services Research: state
- TRICARE (CHAMPUS)

The UB-92 form and instructions are used by institutional and other selected providers to complete a Medicare, Part A, paper claim for submission to Medicare FIs (and other third-party payers). The UB-92 contains eighty-six form locators (FLs) (figure 14.5, p. 314), which are completed according to third-party payer guidelines. FLs of particular importance are those that require entry of **revenue codes,** which identify services provided to patients as reported on the UB-92. The types of organizations that submit the UB-92 include:

- Ambulance companies
- Ambulatory surgery centers
- Home health agencies
- Hospice organizations
- Hospitals (emergency department and inpatient and outpatient services)
- Psychiatric and drug/alcohol treatment facilities (inpatient and outpatient services)
- Skilled nursing facilities
- Subacute facilities
- Stand-alone clinical/laboratory facilities
- Walk-in clinics

Medicare Carriers

Medicare **carriers** process Part B claims for services by physicians and medical suppliers. Examples of carriers might include a Blue Shield plan in a state or commercial insurance companies or other organizations under contract with Medicare. Carriers are responsible for performing the following functions:

- Determining the charges allowed by Medicare
- Maintaining the quality of performance records
- Assisting in fraud and abuse investigations
- Assisting both suppliers and beneficiaries as needed
- Making payments to physicians and suppliers for Part B–covered services

Figure 14.3.   CMS-1500 Claim Form

PLEASE
DO NOT
STAPLE
IN THIS
AREA

CARRIER →

HEALTH INSURANCE CLAIM FORM

| PICA | | PICA |

PICA | | | PICA

1. MEDICARE   MEDICAID   CHAMPUS   CHAMPVA   GROUP HEALTH PLAN   FECA BLK LUNG   OTHER
   (Medicare #)   (Medicaid #)   (Sponsor's SSN)   (VA File #)   (SSN or ID)   (SSN)   (ID)

1a. INSURED'S I.D. NUMBER   (FOR PROGRAM IN ITEM 1)

2. PATIENT'S NAME (Last Name, First Name, Middle Initial)

3. PATIENT'S BIRTH DATE
   MM   DD   YY   SEX
   M   F

4. INSURED'S NAME (Last Name, First Name, Middle Initial)

5. PATIENT'S ADDRESS (No., Street)

6. PATIENT RELATIONSHIP TO INSURED
   Self   Spouse   Child   Other

7. INSURED'S ADDRESS (No., Street)

CITY   STATE

8. PATIENT STATUS
   Single   Married   Other

CITY   STATE

ZIP CODE   TELEPHONE (Include Area Code)
   (   )

Employed   Full-Time Student   Part-Time Student

ZIP CODE   TELEPHONE (INCLUDE AREA CODE)
   (   )

9. OTHER INSURED'S NAME (Last Name, First Name, Middle Initial)

10. IS PATIENT'S CONDITION RELATED TO:

11. INSURED'S POLICY GROUP OR FECA NUMBER

a. OTHER INSURED'S POLICY OR GROUP NUMBER

a. EMPLOYMENT? (CURRENT OR PREVIOUS)
   YES   NO

a. INSURED'S DATE OF BIRTH
   MM   DD   YY   SEX
   M   F

b. OTHER INSURED'S DATE OF BIRTH
   MM   DD   YY   SEX
   M   F

b. AUTO ACCIDENT?   PLACE (State)
   YES   NO

b. EMPLOYER'S NAME OR SCHOOL NAME

c. EMPLOYER'S NAME OR SCHOOL NAME

c. OTHER ACCIDENT?
   YES   NO

c. INSURANCE PLAN NAME OR PROGRAM NAME

d. INSURANCE PLAN NAME OR PROGRAM NAME

10d. RESERVED FOR LOCAL USE

d. IS THERE ANOTHER HEALTH BENEFIT PLAN?
   YES   NO   *If yes*, return to and complete item 9 a-d.

READ BACK OF FORM BEFORE COMPLETING & SIGNING THIS FORM.
12. PATIENT'S OR AUTHORIZED PERSON'S SIGNATURE I authorize the release of any medical or other information necessary to process this claim. I also request payment of government benefits either to myself or to the party who accepts assignment below.

SIGNED _____   DATE _____

13. INSURED'S OR AUTHORIZED PERSON'S SIGNATURE I authorize payment of medical benefits to the undersigned physician or supplier for services described below.

SIGNED _____

PATIENT AND INSURED INFORMATION →

14. DATE OF CURRENT: ILLNESS (First symptom) OR
    MM   DD   YY   INJURY (Accident) OR
                          PREGNANCY(LMP)

15. IF PATIENT HAS HAD SAME OR SIMILAR ILLNESS.
    GIVE FIRST DATE   MM   DD   YY

16. DATES PATIENT UNABLE TO WORK IN CURRENT OCCUPATION
    MM   DD   YY   MM   DD   YY
    FROM   TO

17. NAME OF REFERRING PHYSICIAN OR OTHER SOURCE

17a. I.D. NUMBER OF REFERRING PHYSICIAN

18. HOSPITALIZATION DATES RELATED TO CURRENT SERVICES
    MM   DD   YY   MM   DD   YY
    FROM   TO

19. RESERVED FOR LOCAL USE

20. OUTSIDE LAB? $ CHARGES
    YES   NO

21. DIAGNOSIS OR NATURE OF ILLNESS OR INJURY. (RELATE ITEMS 1,2,3 OR 4 TO ITEM 24E BY LINE)

1. |____.__   3. |____.__

2. |____.__   4. |____.__

22. MEDICAID RESUBMISSION
    CODE   ORIGINAL REF. NO.

23. PRIOR AUTHORIZATION NUMBER

24. A				B	C	D	E	F	G	H	I	J	K
DATE(S) OF SERVICE				Place of Service	Type of Service	PROCEDURES, SERVICES, OR SUPPLIES (Explain Unusual Circumstances)	DIAGNOSIS CODE	$ CHARGES	DAYS OR UNITS	EPSDT Family Plan	EMG	COB	RESERVED FOR LOCAL USE
From MM DD YY	To MM DD YY					CPT/HCPCS MODIFIER							
1													
2													
3													
4													
5													
6													

PHYSICIAN OR SUPPLIER INFORMATION →

25. FEDERAL TAX I.D. NUMBER   SSN EIN

26. PATIENT'S ACCOUNT NO.

27. ACCEPT ASSIGNMENT? (For govt. claims, see back)
    YES   NO

28. TOTAL CHARGE
    $

29. AMOUNT PAID
    $

30. BALANCE DUE
    $

31. SIGNATURE OF PHYSICIAN OR SUPPLIER INCLUDING DEGREES OR CREDENTIALS
    (I certify that the statements on the reverse apply to this bill and are made a part thereof.)

SIGNED   DATE

32. NAME AND ADDRESS OF FACILITY WHERE SERVICES WERE RENDERED (If other than home or office)

33. PHYSICIAN'S, SUPPLIER'S BILLING NAME, ADDRESS, ZIP CODE & PHONE #

PIN#   GRP#

(APPROVED BY AMA COUNCIL ON MEDICAL SERVICE 8/88)   **PLEASE PRINT OR TYPE**   APPROVED OMB-0938-0008 FORM CMS-1500 (12-90),   FORM RRB-1500
APPROVED OMB-1215-0055 FORM OWCP-1500,   APPROVED OMB-0720-0001 (CHAMPUS)

Figure 14.4.   UB-92 (CMS-1450) Claim Form

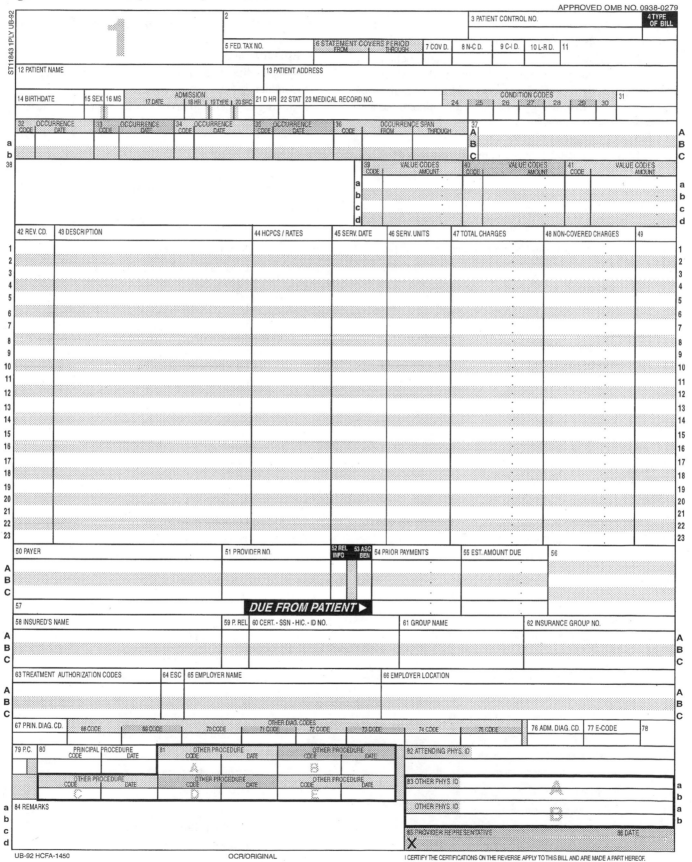

Medicare Fiscal Intermediaries

Medicare FIs process Part A claims and hospital-based Part B claims for institutional services, including inpatient hospital claims, skilled nursing facilities, home health agencies, and hospice services. They also process outpatient claims for supplemental medical insurance (Medicare Part B). Examples of FIs include Blue Cross and Blue Shield organizations and commercial insurance companies under contract with Medicare.

FIs are responsible for performing the following functions:

- Determining costs and reimbursement amounts
- Maintaining records
- Establishing controls
- Safeguarding against fraud and abuse or excess use
- Conducting reviews and audits
- Making payments to providers for covered services
- Assisting both providers and beneficiaries, as needed

Figure 14.5.   UB-92 Form Locators and Brief Description of Information to Be Entered into Each

Form Locator	Brief Description	Form Locator	Brief Description
1	Provider's Name, Address, and Telephone Number	46	Units of Service
2	Unlabeled Field—State Use	47	Total Charges (by Revenue Code Category)
3	Patient's Control Number (Account Number)	48	Noncovered Charges
4	Type of Bill	49	Unlabeled Field—National Use
5	Federal Tax Number	50A-C	Payer Identification
6	Statement Covers Period	51A-C	Provider Number
7	Covered Days	52A-C	Release of Information Certification Indicator
8	Noncovered days	53A-C	Assignment of Benefits Certification Indicator
9	Coinsurance Days	54A-C, P	Prior Payments—Payers and Patient
10	Lifetime Reserve Days	55A-C, P	Estimated Amount Due
11	Unlabeled Field—State Use	56	DRG Number and Grouper ID
12	Patient Name	57	Unlabeled Field—National Use
13	Patient Address	58A-C	Insured's Name
14	Patient Birthdate	59A-C	Patient's Relationship to Insured
15	Patient Sex	60A-C	Health Insurance Claim Identification Number
16	Patient Marital Status	61A-C	Insured Group Name
17	Admission Date	62A-C	Insurance Group Number
18	Admission Hour	63A-C	Treatment Authorization Code
19	Type of Admission	64A-C	Employment Status Code
20	Source of Admission	65A-C	Employer Name
21	Discharge Hour	66A-C	Employer Location
22	Patient Status	67	Principal Diagnosis Code
23	Medical/Health Record Number	68-75	Other Diagnosis Codes
24-30	Condition Codes	76	Admitting Diagnosis
31	Unlabeled Field—National Use	77	External Cause of Injury Code (E-Code)
32-35a,b	Occurrence Codes and Dates	78	Not Titled
36a,b	Occurrence Span Codes and Dates	79	Procedure Coding Method Used
37	Internal Control Number (ICN)	80	Principal Procedure Code and Date
38	Responsible Party Name and Address	81A-E	Other Procedure Codes and Dates
39-41a-d	Value Codes and Amounts	82	Attending Physician ID
42	Revenue Code	83a-b	Other Physician ID
43	Revenue Description	84a-d	Remarks
44	HCPCS/Rates	85	Provider Representative Signature
45	Service Date	86	Date Bill Submitted

Electronic Data Interchange

Health claims data is frequently transmitted electronically between a healthcare organization and a third party payer using electronic data interchange (EDI), which is addressed in chapter 7.

The **healthcare claims transaction** is the transmission of a request to obtain payment for healthcare, along with the necessary accompanying information from a healthcare provider to a health plan. If no direct claim is transmitted because the reimbursement contract is based on a mechanism other than charges or reimbursement rates for specific services (for example, managed care capitation contract), the transaction is the transmission of encounter information for the purpose of reporting healthcare.

A **coordination of benefits** (COB) transaction is an electronic transmission from a healthcare provider to a health plan for the purpose of determining (1) relative payment responsibilities for healthcare claims and/or (2) payment information.

A **healthcare claim and payment/advise transaction** is an electronic transmission provided by a health plan to a healthcare provider's financial institution for the purpose of determining payment, information about the transfer of funds, or payment-processing information. In addition, a health plan submits electronic transmissions to healthcare providers to communicate an explanation of benefits.

An **explanation of benefits** is a statement sent to the healthcare provider and the patient to explain services provided, amounts billed, and payments made by the health plan. Medicare replaced its Part A and Part B Explanation of Medicare Benefits (EOMB) with a newly designed Medicare Summary Notice (MSN). (See figure 14.6 [p. 316] for a sample Part A MSN.)

An RA (figure 14.7, p. 317) explains payments made by third-party payers (for example, reports claims denials). Prior to the availability of the ANSI ASC X12 835, commonly known as the **electronic remittance advice** (ERA), providers used either paper and/or tape transmissions to post payments to their Medicare accounts. Tape transmissions are no longer an option. The ERA is currently available in three different versions, and many providers still use a paper remittance to process Medicare payments.

Check Your Understanding 14.5

Instructions: Answer the following questions on a separate piece of paper.

1. What is CMS-1500 used for? What is another name for this form?

2. What entity is responsible for the data elements and design of CMS-1450?

3. What types of organizations submit the UB-92 form?

4. What kinds of codes are associated with CMS-1450?

5. What is the difference between a Medicare carrier and a fiscal intermediary? What functions is each responsible for performing?

6. What does the electronic data interchange (EDI) allow entities within healthcare organizations to do?

7. What is a COB transaction, and what is its purpose?

Reimbursement Support Processes

Reimbursement support processes are routinely reviewed and revised by third-party payers to control payments to providers. Healthcare facilities also conduct reimbursement support processes to make sure that they are receiving the level of reimbursement to which they are entitled. Third-party payers revise fee schedules, and healthcare facilities revise chargemasters, evaluate the quality of documentation and coding, conduct internal audits, and implement compliance programs.

Management of Fee Schedules

Third-party payers that reimburse providers on a fee-for-service basis, where providers receive payment based on billed charges for services provided, generally update fee schedules on an annual basis. A fee schedule is a list of healthcare services and procedures (usually **CPT/HCPCS** codes) and charges associated with each. (See table 14.8, p. 317.) The fee schedule (sometimes referred to as a table of allowances) represents the approved payment levels for a given insurance plan (for example, Medicare, Medicaid, and BC/BS).

Physicians, practitioners, and suppliers must notify Medicare by December 31 of each year whether they intend to participate in the Medicare program during the coming year. Medicare participation means that the provider or supplier agrees to accept assignment for all covered services provided to Medicare patients. To accept assignment means the provider or supplier accepts, as payment in full, the allowed charge (from the fee schedule). The provider or supplier is prohibited from **balance billing,** which means the patient cannot be held responsible for charges in excess of the Medicare fee schedule. Medicare does reimburse participating providers who deliver services and supplies (for example, drugs and biologicals) incidental to professional services at 5 percent above the fee schedule amount. The 5 percent increase also applies to outpatient physical and occupational therapy services, diagnostic tests, and radiology services.

Nonparticipating providers do not sign a participation agreement with Medicare and are not obligated to accept assignment on Medicare claims. This means the patient can be balance billed at a rate limited to 15 percent above the allowed charge for nonparticipating physicians.

Management of the Chargemaster

The chargemaster (table 14.9, p. 317), also called the charge description master, contains information about healthcare services (and transactions) provided to a patient. It includes a charge code (often linked to an HCPCS code), the associated charge, and any additional information necessary to process reimbursement. Services, supplies, and procedures included on the chargemaster generate reimbursement for almost 75 percent of UB-92 claims submitted for outpatient services alone.

Figure 14.6.   Sample Medicare Part A Summary Notice

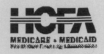 **Medicare Summary Notice**

BENEFICIARY NAME
STREET ADDRESS
CITY, STATE   ZIP CODE

HELP STOP FRAUD: Beware of "free" medical services or products. If it sounds too good to be true, it probably is.

CUSTOMER SERVICE INFORMATION

Your Medicare Number: 111-11-1111A

If you have questions, write or call:
Medicare
555 Medicare Blvd.
Suite 200
Medicare Building
Medicare, US XXXXX-XXXX

Local: (XXX) XXX-XXXX
Toll-free: 1-800-XXX-XXXX
TTY for Hearing Impaired: 1-800-XXX-XXXX

This is a summary of claims processed from 5/15/2000 through 6/10/2000.

PART A: HOSPITAL INSURANCE—PATIENT CLAIMS

Dates of Service	Benefit Days Used	Noncovered Charges	Deductible and Coinsurance	You May Be Billed	See Notes Section
Claim number 12345-84956-84556-45621 Care Hospital, 123 Sick Lane, Dallas, TX 75555 Referred by: Paul Jones, M.D.					
4/25/00–5/09/00	14 days	$0.00	$776.00	$776.00	a,b
Claim number 12345-84956-84556-45622 Continued Care Hospital, 124 Sick Lane, Dallas, TX 75555 Referred by: Paul Jones, M.D.					
5/09/00–6/20/00	11 days	$0.00	$0.00	$0.00	

PART B: MEDICAL INSURANCE—OUTPATIENT FACILITY CLAIMS

Dates of Service	Services Provided	Amount Charged	Noncovered Charges	Deductible and Coinsurance	You May Be Billed	See Notes Section
Claim number 1235-8056-8458 Medicare Hospital, 123 Medicare Lane, Dallas, TX 75209 Referred by: Paul Jones, M.D.						
4/02/00	I.V. Therapy (Q0081)	$33.00	$0.00	$6.60	$6.60	
	Lab (88104)	1,140.50	0.00	228.10	228.10	
	Operating Room (31628)	786.50	0.00	157.30	157.30	
	Observation Room (99201)	293.00	0.00	58.60	58.60	
	Claim Total	$2,253.00	$0.00	$450.60	$450.60	

(continued)

THIS IS NOT A BILL—Keep this notice for your records.

Figure 14.7.   Sample Single-Claim Remittance Advice

```
Medicare National Standard Intermediary Remittance Advice
FPE:                                    07/30/01
PAID:                                   01/25/01
CLM#                                    2
TOB:                                    111
-----------------------------------------------------------------------------------
PATIENT:      JOHN DOE                                    PCN:    235617
HIC:          123456           SVC FROM:    01/05/01      MRN:    124767
PAT STAT:     01    CLAIM STAT:    1    THRU:    01/06/01  ICN:    987654
-----------------------------------------------------------------------------------
CHARGES:                     PAYMENT DATA: 140=DRG    0.000    =REIM RATE
1939.90      =REPORTED        2741.69   =DRG AMOUNT    0.00    =MSP PRIM PAYER
0.00         =NONCOVERED      2497.26   =DRG/OPER      0.00    =PROF COMPONENT
0.00         =DENIED          244.43    =DRG/CAPITAL   0.00    =ESRD AMOUNT
1939.90      =COVERED         0.00      =OUTLIER       0.00    =HCPCS AMOUNT
DAYS/VISITS:                  0.00      =CAP OUTLIER   0.00    =ALLOWED AMOUNT
1            =COST REPT       768.00    =CASH DEDUCT   0.00    =G/R AMOUNT
1            =COVD/UTIL       0.00      =BLOOD DEDUCT  0.00    =INTEREST
0            =NONCOVERED      0.00      =COINSURANCE   -801.79 =CONTRACT ADJ
0            =COVD VISITS     0.00      =PAT REFUND    675.00  =PER DIEM AMT
0            =NCOV VISITS     0.00      =MSP LIAB MET  1973.69 =NET REIM AMT
ADJ REASON CODES:     CO  A2 -801.79
                      PR        1
                      768
REMARK CODES:         MA02
-----------------------------------------------------------------------------------
```

Table 14.8.   Partial 2001 Physician Fee Schedule Payment Amounts for Services Covered by the Medicare Physician Fee Schedule—Western New York State Region

Carrier Number	Locality Code	HCPCS Code	Nonfacility Fee Schedule Amount	Facility Fee Schedule Amount
00801	99	10040	0000092.75	0000062.55
00801	99	10060	0000086.71	0000131.26
00801	99	10061	0000157.46	0000131.26
00801	99	10040	0000092.75	0000062.55
00801	99	10060	0000086.71	0000067.06
00801	99	10061	0000157.46	0000131.26
00801	99	10080	0000107.02	0000068.82
00801	99	10081	0000185.79	0000148.32
00801	99	10120	0000101.95	0000071.39
00801	99	10121	0000194.20	0000164.36

Source: CPT codes and descriptions only are copyright 2000 by the American Medical Association. All rights reserved.

Table 14.9.   Sample Portion of a Facility's Chargemaster

Service Code	Service Description	CPT/HCPCS Code	UB-92 Revenue Code	Charge
56215978	IV Infusion Therapy—Medicare	Q0081	260	26.00
56231577	Medical/Surgical Supplies—General		270	19.00
56251359	Blood Pressure Monitor in ED		450	26.00
56235948	Cardiac Monitor in ED		450	62.00

Facilities use computer software to generate the chargemaster. Ongoing maintenance includes input and review of billing, financial, and health information personnel. Billing and financial personnel are responsible for the accuracy of revenue codes and associated charges that appear on the chargemaster. In addition, they should monitor billing and reimbursement problems. HIM personnel are responsible for ensuring the accuracy of the ICD-9-CM and HCPCS codes that appear on the chargemaster and verifying that documentation supports the codes selected.

An inaccurate chargemaster adversely affects facility reimbursement, compliance, and data quality. According to a 1999 AHIMA Practice Brief (Rhodes 2002), negative effects that may result from an inaccurate chargemaster include overpayment, undercharging for delivery of healthcare services, claims rejections, and fines/penalties. Chargemaster programs are automated and involve the billing of numerous services for high volumes of patients, often without human intervention. Therefore, it is highly likely that a single error on the chargemaster could result in multiple errors before it is identified and corrected.

Management of Documentation and Coding Quality

According to Deborah Elder, RHIA, CPC, manager of inpatient and outpatient coding services, Medical Management Plus, Inc., Birmingham, Alabama:

> The importance of complete and accurate coding cannot be underestimated. ICD-9-CM and CPT-4 coding drives reimbursement and also presents a mechanism by which external and internal agents evaluate utilization of services, quality of care, and the hospital's patient acuity level. This numerically abbreviated medical information is only as complete as the physician documentation and is only as accurate as the coder's translation. Coders have a monumental impact on the hospital and this impact will broaden as other health care services are converted to a prospective payment method of reimbursement, including Outpatient Services, Extended Care Facilities and Home Health Agencies (Elder 2000).

The HCFA (now known as the CMS) implemented the **Correct Coding Initiative** (CCI) in 1996 to develop correct coding methodologies to improve the appropriate payment of Medicare Part B claims. CCI policies are based on:

- Coding conventions defined in the CPT codebooks
- National and local policies and coding edits
- Coding guidelines developed by the CMS
- Analysis of standard medical and surgical practice
- Review of current coding practices

Portions of the CCI are incorporated into the **outpatient code editor** (OCE). The OCE applies a set of logical rules to determine whether various combinations of codes are correct and appropriately represent services provided. The OCE contains more than 65,000 edits based on the CCI, and billing issues result because CCI/OCE edits produce line item rejections from fiscal intermediaries. For example:

The CCI identifies mutually exclusive pairs of procedures that cannot be performed on the same day. The following codes are considered mutually exclusive if reported on the same patient, for the same date, and on the same UB-92:

23330	Removal of foreign body, shoulder; subcutaneous
23331	Removal of foreign body, shoulder; deep (for example, NEER hemiarthroplasty removal)

The foreign body removal, shoulder, must be documented as either subcutaneous or deep. When both codes are reported, the facility must be reimbursed for just one (the less costly) of the procedures. Note that when two foreign bodies were removed from the shoulder (one at the subcutaneous level and the other at the deep level), assignment of modifier -51 (multiple procedures) to code 23330 would override the CCI edit, and reimbursement would be generated for both procedures.

Internal Audits

Ongoing evaluation is critical to successful coding and billing for third-party payer reimbursement. In the past, the goal of internal audit programs was to increase revenues for the provider. Today, their goal is to protect providers from sanctions or fines. Healthcare organizations can implement monitoring programs by conducting regular, periodic audits of (1) ICD-9-CM and CPT/HCPCS coding and (2) claims development and submission. In addition, audits should be conducted to follow up on previous reviews that resulted in the identification of problems (for example, poor coding quality or errors in claims submission).

Auditing involves the performance of internal and/or **external reviews** to identify variations from established baselines (for example, review outpatient coding as compared with CMS outpatient coding guidelines). Internal reviews are conducted by facility-based staff (for example, HIM professionals), and external reviews may be conducted by either consultants hired for this purpose (for example, corporations that specialize in such reviews and independent health information consultants) or third-party payers.

Significant variations from baselines should prompt an investigation to determine cause(s). When variations are caused by improper procedures or a misunderstanding of rules, including fraud and systemic problems, the healthcare organization should take immediate action to correct the problem. In addition, overpayments discovered as a result of review should be returned promptly to the affected payer, with appropriate documentation and a thorough explanation of the reason for the refund. The investigation into the cause(s) of variations can include interviews of coding and claims development/submission personnel and reviews of medical and financial records and other source documents that support claims for reimbursement and Medicare cost reports. An example of a claim with a coding compliance problem is shown in figure 14.8 (Averill 1999).

Suppose the erroneous coding in this example was an honest mistake. The Department of Justice (DOJ) has stated that it is not its policy to assess fines and penalties for honest

Figure 14.8.   Claim with a Probable Coding Compliance Problem

ICD-9-CM Code		Diagnosis/Procedure
Principal diagnosis:	807.01	Fracture one rib, closed
Secondary diagnosis:	874.10	Open wound of the larynx and trachea, complicated
Procedure:	31.1	Temporary tracheostomy

Discussion: The claim containing ICD-9-CM codes as reported above would be assigned DRG 483 (Tracheostomy, except for face, mouth, and neck diagnoses), with a payment weight of 16.3395. However, the traumatic injury that necessitated the hospital admission was the complicated open wound of the larynx and trachea (not the closed rib fracture).

If the complicated open wound of the larynx and trachea is reported as the principal diagnosis, DRG 482 (Tracheostomy for face, mouth, and neck diagnoses) is assigned, with a much lower payment weight of 3.6031. The original coding of the claim results in a higher payment weight because the DRG logic assumes that the tracheostomy is being performed on a patient who is in respiratory failure and needs long-term mechanical ventilation, as opposed to treatment of the open wound of the larynx and trachea. The payment amount associated with the claim as originally coded would be approximately $75,000.

If this claim were determined to be fraudulent, the health care facility would be penalized a base fine in the range of $5,000 to $10,000 plus an additional fine of three times the amount of the claim (approximately $230,000). Thus, this single coding error would have substantial financial consequences.

Source: Based on Averill 1999.

billing mistakes. However, it also says that facilities must establish adequate internal procedures to ensure the accuracy of claims submissions. Failure to establish such procedures represents a disregard for the requirements of the law and can turn an honest billing mistake into a false claim that is subject to penalties. Intent to defraud is not required for a claim to be considered a false claim. The lack of adequate safeguards can turn any coding error into a false claim. Ignorance of the law is not a defense against a false claim. Because some ambiguity exists in determining the precise circumstances under which an honest mistake becomes a false claim, the best policy is to assume that when it comes to coding compliance, there are no honest mistakes.

Coding Compliance Program

The goal of **compliance** programs is to prevent accusations of fraud and abuse, make operations run more smoothly, improve services, and contain costs (Anderson 2000). The Office of Inspector General (OIG) of the Department of Health and Human Services (HHS) published a **compliance program guidance** for healthcare organizations to assist in the development of internal controls that promote adherence to applicable federal and state laws and program requirements of federal, state, and private health plans. (Figure 14.9 [p. 320] illustrates the components of a coding compliance program.)

The adoption and implementation of voluntary compliance programs significantly advance the prevention of fraud,

abuse, and waste in these healthcare plans and at the same time further the fundamental mission of all hospitals, which is to provide high-quality care to patients. Specifically, compliance programs guide a hospital's governing body, chief executive officer, managers, other employees, and physicians and other healthcare professionals in the efficient management and operation of a hospital. Compliance programs are especially critical as an internal control in the reimbursement and payment areas, where claims and billing operations are often the source of fraud and abuse and, therefore, historically have been the focus of government regulation, scrutiny, and sanctions.

The compliance issue that most affects the HIM department is related to ICD-9-CM and CPT/HCPCS coding for inpatients, outpatients, and emergency department patients. **Inpatient coding compliance** involves the accurate and complete assignment of ICD-9-CM diagnosis and procedure codes, along with appropriate sequencing (for example, identification of principal diagnosis and so on) to determine the DRG and resultant payment. **Outpatient and emergency department coding compliance** involves the accurate and complete assignment of ICD-9-CM diagnosis codes and CPT/HCPCS procedure/service codes, along with appropriate sequencing (for example, identification of the principal diagnosis).

Coding compliance programs involve staff employed by the facility as well as outside consultants to perform coding functions. The steps in a coding compliance program completed internally by healthcare facility coding staff may include:

1. The coder initially codes diagnoses and procedures documented in the patient record and inputs the codes into the facility's coding compliance program database system. Specially designed software generates a coding compliance worksheet that identifies potential problems and provides guidance, and the coder makes necessary coding changes based on feedback from the worksheet.
2. A coding supervisor reviews the record when the coder cannot resolve coding compliance issues identified on the worksheet.
3. The codes assigned after the coding compliance review is completed are sent to billing and stored in the coding compliance system database.

Coding compliance functions performed by an independent auditor (consultant) may include the following steps:

1. The coder completes the initial coding of the record, and this set of codes is stored in the coding compliance database system.
2. Coding compliance worksheets are generated by audit software and sent to the independent auditor who makes necessary coding changes. This set of codes is sent to billing and also is stored in the coding compliance database system.

Figure 14.9.   Components of a Coding Compliance Program

Component	Description of Activity
Detection	Identify patient records that contain potential coding compliance problems by monitoring ICD-9-CM and CPT/HCPCS codes for accuracy and completeness.
	• Perform random chart audits on samples of records. For example, review patient records that contain documentation of procedures to ensure that a diagnosis that justifies the procedure has been documented.
	• Implement computerized edits of coding, clinical information, and resource consumption by:
	—Performing edit checks to ensure adherence to coding guidelines.
	—Evaluating clinical consistency as related to the diagnoses, procedures, age, sex, and discharge status of patients.
	—Evaluating lengths of stay and charges to ensure consistency with patients' conditions.
	For example, note that the review of the record of an acute myocardial infarction patient who was discharged alive after a one-day length of stay would reveal the probability of a compliance problem (resource consumption).
Correction	Perform comprehensive chart audits, and make necessary corrections.
	• Once a record has been identified by a computerized audit as having a probable compliance problem, review the record to make necessary corrections to coding/sequencing errors.
	• Complete the correction process prior to billing third-party payers to avoid resubmissions (sending claim information to an insurer a second time), which may trigger external audits by government agencies and private insurers.
	• Emphasize that coding is done for reasons other than reimbursement (for example, statistical analysis, resource consumption, and so on).
	For example, provider report cards are published in many states to compare hospital performance in terms of resource use and outcomes (based on severity adjustments, which are detailed distinctions based on the presence of specific combinations of comorbid conditions). To accurately report severity adjustments, a greater level of coding completeness and accuracy is required (than is necessary just for reimbursement purposes). Poor performance on a report card as the result of inaccurate severity adjustments (due to undercoding) can have a substantial negative financial impact on the hospital—patients may not seek health care services from the hospital, thus reducing the hospital's patient volume.
Prevention	Educate coders to prevent future coding compliance problems.
	• Conduct in-service education programs, based on problems identified during audits.
	• Provide funding for attendance at coding workshops and seminars.
	• Encourage coders to pursue formal education (for example, college-level courses in medical terminology, anatomy/physiology, pathophysiology, and coding).

Component	Description of Activity
Verification	Provide an audit trail of all coding compliance actions.
	• Maintain a detailed audit trail of all code changes and coding compliance-related actions.
	• Maintain three complete sets of codes for each admission within the coding compliance system:
	—*Original version:* final set of codes assigned prior to the first computerized audit.
	—*Billed version:* final set of codes at the time of the initial bill, reflecting any code changes made after computerized audit and any chart audit.
	—*Post-billed version:* final set of codes after claim submission, reflecting internal or external audits, fiscal intermediary adjudication, and any other reasons for rebilling.
	• Generate reports documenting the results of coding compliance activities, maintain a record of the nature of all code changes (for example, missing secondary diagnosis), and the reason the code changes were necessary (for example, insufficient physician documentation, coder error); detail in the coding compliance database makes it easier to identify patterns in coding compliance problems and take corrective actions.
Comparison	Compare coding patterns over time and to external norms.
	• The comparison function provides a benchmark to external coding norms so a hospital can determine how its coding practices compare to those of other hospitals.

Example of Coding Compliance Benchmark Comparison Report

Acute Cardiac Cluster Comparison

	Hospital 1997	Hospital 1998	National
AMI	58.2%	60.1%	48.9%
Angina	18.6%	16.9%	22.4%
Chest Pain	23.2%	23.0%	28.7%
Test of Significance	P(<0.05)	P(<.01)	

The table above is an example of a coding compliance benchmark comparison report that contains data about three clinically-related diagnoses: acute myocardial infarction (AMI), angina, and chest pain.

The three diagnoses represent an acute cardiac cluster and the percentage of Medicare medical admissions in 1997 and 1998 are listed, along with national percentages (each column totals to 100 percent).

The percentage of hospital admissions with AMI within the acute cardiac cluster increased between 1997 and 1998 from 58.2 percent to 60.1 percent (overall, much higher than the national average of 48.9 percent).

The statistical test of significance (P-value) indicates that the distribution of admissions in the acute cardiac cluster in the hospital is significantly different statistically than the national distribution in both years.

This suggests that AMI diagnosis codes are being incorrectly assigned. The hospital should review AMI coding to ensure that a compliance problem does not exist (for example, perhaps cases should be assigned angina or chest pain codes instead).

Source: Based on Averill 1999.

Coding compliance programs involve updating the database system so that copies of both sets of codes—those originally assigned by the coder and those assigned after the coding compliance worksheet is reviewed and changes are made—are maintained to trend data and identify patterns. Thus, an **audit trail** of coding compliance actions is maintained, verifying an active coding compliance program that identifies and corrects problems.

Check Your Understanding 14.6

Instructions: Answer the following questions on a separate piece of paper.

1. How often do third-party payers update fee schedules?

2. What does the term *accept assignment* mean?

3. How might an inaccurately generated chargemaster affect facility reimbursement?

4. What are the CCI policies implemented in 1996 to develop correct coding methodologies to improve appropriate payment of Medicare Part B claims based on?

5. What do coding compliance programs concentrate on preventing? Which federal agency has established the precise steps that each healthcare facility must follow in establishing its compliance program?

Real-World Case

Itemized charges on the UB-92 that are not supported by patient record documentation are unlikely to be reimbursed by a third-party payer. Examples of charges that would not be paid upon review of the patient record in comparison to the UB-92 include:

- Duplicate charges (for example, multiple charges for same service, such as surgery)
- Laboratory panel tests for which there should be a single charge
- Medications and diagnostic tests not prescribed by a physician
- Medications that a patient did not receive
- Tests repeated because of hospital error
- Services listed for dates after the patient was discharged from the facility
- Professional services performed by nurses or technicians (for example, equipment monitoring)

Discussion Question

For each inappropriate charge above, what report in the patient record would the third-party payer representative review to justify denial of reimbursement?

Summary

From its very beginnings, financial reimbursement for healthcare services has followed several paths. Among these are private pay, commercial insurance, employer self-insurance, and various government programs. The mixture of payment mechanisms has made healthcare reimbursement very complex in the United States.

As a consequence, the processing of medical claims can be complicated. How a claim is processed, what documentation is required, and how much reimbursement will be paid depend on the payer and the type of claim. Many attempts have been made to create a uniform healthcare claim that would accommodate all payment mechanisms. Claims processed for payment under Medicare have been consolidated in a uniform bill.

Healthcare organizations have developed several tools to help manage the billing and reimbursement process, including development of fee schedules and chargemasters. The HIM professional is frequently called on to provide expertise in the development, management, and auditing of these tools. In addition, organizations have recognized that ongoing evaluation of the entire billing process is essential to ensure accurate payment as well as to avoid fraud and abuse sanctions or fines. The HIM professional's work is likely to involve helping to develop such audit programs in addition to conducting the audits themselves.

Over the past two decades, the billing and reimbursement process has become an integral part of the job functions of many HIM professionals. The expertise brought to bear on the process to ensure accurate and timely claims submission is critical to the operations of any healthcare organization.

Payments for the delivery of healthcare services increased from $27 billion in 1960 to more than $1.1 trillion in 1998. In response, private insurers introduced managed care programs and the federal government implemented prospective payment systems to replace the costly per-diem (or traditional fee-for-service) reimbursement methods. The federal government also incorporated managed care into its healthcare programs.

Health claims reimbursement processing has evolved from the submission of handwritten CMS-1500 and UB-92 forms to specially designed forms to be used for optical scanning purposes to electronic data interchange. EDI was greatly affected by HIPAA legislation passed in 1996. Of recently enacted federal legislation affecting claims reimbursement processing, the CCI and the OIG coding compliance programs have had the most effect on HIM professionals.

References

3M Health Information Systems. www.3Mhis.com.

Abraham, Prinny Rose. 2001. *Documentation and Reimbursement for Home Health and Hospice Programs.* Chicago: American Health Information Management Association.

American Medical Association. 2001. *Current Procedural Terminology,* 2002 edition. Chicago: AMA.

Anderson, S. 2000. Audit outpatient bills to get all the money you deserve. 2000. *Medical Records Briefing* 15(12):6.

Averill, Richard F. 1999. Honest mistake or fraud? Meeting the coding compliance challenge. *Journal of the American Health Information Management Association* 70(5):16–21.

Campbell, Claudia, Homer Schmitz, and Linda Waller. 1998. *Financial Management in a Managed Care Environment.* Albany, N.Y.: Delmar Thomson Learning.

Centers for Medicare and Medicaid Services. 2001. IRVEN: CMS's IRF-PAI data entry software. Available online from www.cms.gov.

Coder's Desk Reference. 2002. Salt Lake City: Ingenix.

Davis, James B. 2000. *Reimbursement Manual for the Medical Office: A Comprehensive Guide to Coding, Billing and Fee Management.* Los Angeles: Practice Management Information Corporation.

Davison, Jan, and Maxine Lewis. 2000. *Working with Insurance and Managed Care Plans: A Guide for Getting Paid.* Los Angeles: Practice Management Information Corporation.

Dougherty, Michelle. 2000. New home care PPS brings major changes. *Journal of the American Health Information Management Association* 71 (10):78–82.

Elder, D. 2000. Coding: The key to compliance. Birmingham, Ala.: Medical Management Plus, Inc. Available online from www.mmplusinc.com.

Gannon, Edmund J. HCFA outlines new PPS for rehabilitation facilities. Available on-line from www.mxcity.com.

Green, Michelle A., and Joann C. Rowell. 2002. *Understanding Health Insurance: A Guide to Professional Billing.* Albany, N.Y.: Delmar Thomson Learning.

Harkins, Patrick D. 2000. The alphabet soup of Medicare reimbursement. *Advance for Health Information Professionals,* October 16, p. 25.

Hazelwood, Anita, and Carol Venable. 2002. *ICD-9-CM Diagnostic Coding for Physician Services.* Chicago: American Health Information Management Association.

Health Care Financing Administration. HHS announces electronic standards to simplify health care transactions. 2000. Available online from www.hhs.gov.

Johnson, Sandra L. 2000. *Understanding Medical Coding: A Comprehensive Guide.* Albany, N.Y.: Delmar Thomson Learning.

Jones, Lolita J., editor. 2001. *Reimbursement Methodologies for Healthcare Services.* Chicago: American Health Information Management Association.

Lewis, Maxine. 2000. *Medicare Rules and Regulations.* Los Angeles: Practice Management Information Corporation.

Make sure that your APC claim makes it through the OCE. 2000. *Medical Records Briefing* 15(9):1.

Medicare Hospital Outpatient Payment System Quick Reference Guide. 2002. Available online at www.cms.gov.

National Committee for Quality Assurance. www.ncqa.org.

Palmer, Karen. 1999. A brief history: universal health care efforts in the US: late 1800s to Medicare. Available online from www.pnhp.org.

Rhodes, Harry. 2002. Practice Brief: The care and management of charge masters. Chicago: American Health Information Management Association.

Rizzo, Christina D. 2000. *Uniform Billing: A Guide to Claims Processing.* Albany, N.Y.: Delmar Thomson Learning.

Role of the physician in the home health prospective payment system. 2000. Medicare Newsroom, November 7. Available online from www.hgsa.com.

Schraffenberger, Lou Ann. 2003. *Basic ICD-9-CM Coding.* Chicago: American Health Information Management Association.

Smith, Gail. 2002. *Basic CPT/HCPCS Coding.* Chicago: American Health Information Management Association.

State funds: their role in workers' compensation. Available online from www.aascif.org.

Stewart, Margaret. 2001. *Coding and Reimbursement under the Outpatient Prospective Payment.* Chicago: American Health Information Management Association.

Wieland, LaVonne, and Lynn Kuehn. 2002. *CPT/HCPCS Coding and Reimbursement for Physician Services.* Chicago: American Health Information Management Association.

Application Exercises

1. Under the new outpatient prospective payment system, Medicare decides how much a hospital or a community mental health center will be reimbursed for each service rendered. Depending on the service, the patient pays either a coinsurance amount (20 percent) or a fixed copayment amount, whichever is less. For each case below, determine whether the patient will pay the coinsurance or copayment amount.

   a. Mr. Smith was charged $85 for a minor procedure performed in the hospital outpatient department. The fixed copayment amount for this type of procedure, adjusted for wages in the geographic area, is $15. Mr. Smith has already paid his annual Medicare Part B deductible of $100.

   b. Mr. Jones and Mrs. Day live in the same area of the country. They are having the same outpatient procedure done, but at different hospitals. Mr. Jones's hospital charges $250 for the procedure, but Mrs. Day's hospital charges $150. The national median charge for this procedure is $225 (adjusted for wages in their area) with a fixed copayment of $54. Both patients have already paid their $100 yearly Medicare Part B deductible.

2. Alfred State Medical Center's charges/payments/adjustments from third-party payers for the month of July are represented in table 14.10.

   a. Calculate the percentage of charges, payments, and adjustments for each third-party payer and enter the percentages in the percentages columns of table 14.10.

   b. Based on the percentages calculated in the charges column, identify the payer the facility does the most business with and the payer it does the least business with.

   c. Based on the percentages calculated in the payment column, identify the payers that reimburse the facility the most and the least.

   d. Based on the percentages calculated in the adjustments column, identify the payers that proportionately reimburse the facility the most and the least.

Table 14.10.   Sample Charges, Payments, and Adjustments for Application Exercise 2

Payer	Charges	Payments	Adjustment	Charges	Payments	Adjustments
BC/BS	$450,000	$360,000	$90,000	%	%	%
Commercial	$250,000	$200,000	$50,000	%	%	%
Medicaid*	$350,000	$75,000	$275,000	%	%	%
Medicare	$750,000	$495,000	$255,000	%	%	%
TRICARE*	$150,000	$50,000	$100,000	%	%	%
Totals	$1,950,000	$1,180,000	$770,000	100%	100%	100%

*Managed care capitated payment for period.

Review Quiz

Instructions: Select the best answer for questions 1–11.

1. ___ Which of the following plans reimburses patients up to a specified amount?
   a. Health insurance
   b. Coinsurance
   c. Indemnity
   d. Major medical plan

2. ___ The number of days Medicare will cover skilled nursing facility inpatient care is limited to which of the following?
   a. 21
   b. 60
   c. 30
   d. 100

3. ___ Under what circumstances is hospital insurance included under Medicare?
   a. Only for those who pay a monthly premium
   b. For those who do not receive Social Security
   c. For beneficiaries enrolled in Medicare Part A
   d. For beneficiaries enrolled in Medicare Part B

4. ___ On which criterion is Medicaid eligibility based?
   a. Income
   b. Whether a person is Medicare eligible
   c. Age
   d. Health status

5. ___ Which term is used for retrospective reimbursement charges submitted by a provider for each service rendered?
   a. Fee-for-service
   b. Deductible
   c. Actuarial
   d. Prospective

6. ___ Which of the following programs is funded by the federal government to provide medical care to people on public assistance?
   a. CHAMPUS
   b. Medicare
   c. Medicaid
   d. Medigap

7. ___ Which of the following reimbursement methods pays providers according to charges that are calculated before the healthcare services are rendered?
   a. Fee-for-service reimbursement method
   b. Prospective payment method
   c. Retrospective payment method
   d. Resource-based payment method

8. ___ Which of the following payment methods reimburses healthcare providers in the form of lump sums for all healthcare services delivered to a patient for a specific illness?
   a. Managed fee-for-service
   b. Capitation
   c. Episode of care
   d. Point of service

9. ___ Which of the following classification systems uses resident assessment data to assign residents to one of forty-four groups, with each assessment applying to specific days within a resident's stay?
   a. DRGs
   b. APCs
   c. RUGs
   d. HH PPS

10. ___ Which of the following terms is used in reference to the transfer of health claims using electronic media?
    a. ANSI
    b. ASC X12
    c. EDI
    d. Optical scanning

11. ___ What is the list of healthcare services/procedures and charges called?
    a. Explanation of benefits
    b. Fee schedule
    c. Table of allowances
    d. a and c

Instructions: Match the following definitions with the terms they represent.

   a. Condition established after study to be the reason for hospitalization
   b. Categories of patients treated
   c. Coexisting condition
   d. Condition arising during hospitalization

12. ___ Case mix

13. ___ Principal diagnosis

14. ___ Complication

15. ___ Comorbidity

Part IV

Comparative Data

Chapter 15
Healthcare Statistics

Carol E. Osborn, PhD, RHIA

Learning Objectives

- To identify various ways in which statistics are used in healthcare
- To differentiate between descriptive and inferential statistics
- To define hospital-related statistical terms
- To calculate hospital-related inpatient and outpatient statistics
- To define community-based morbidity and mortality rates
- To calculate community-based morbidity and mortality rates
- To define and calculate measures of central tendency and variability
- To describe the characteristics of the normal distribution
- To identify the relationships of measures of central tendency and variation to the normal distribution
- To display healthcare data using tables, charts, and graphs, as appropriate
- To calculate the case-mix index
- To locate healthcare-related state and federal databases on the Internet
- To use healthcare data collected from online databases in comparative statistical reports

Key Terms

Acute care
Ambulatory surgery center (ASC)
Average daily census
Average length of stay (ALOS)
Bar chart
Bed count (complement)
Bed count day
Bed turnover rate
Case fatality rate
Case mix
Case-mix index (CMI)
Cause-specific death rate
Census
Consultation rate
Crude birth rate
Crude death rate
Daily inpatient census
Descriptive statistics
Discrete variables
Encounter
Fetal autopsy rate
Fetal death (stillborn)
Fetal death rate
Frequency distribution
Frequency polygon
Gross autopsy rate
Gross death rate
Histogram
Hospital autopsy
Hospital autopsy rate
Hospital death rate
Hospital inpatient autopsy
Hospital newborn inpatient
Incidence rate
Infant mortality rate
Inferential statistics
Inpatient bed occupancy rate (percentage of occupancy)
Inpatient service day
Length of stay (LOS)

Line graph
Maternal death rate (hospital based)
Maternal mortality rate (community based)
Mean
Measures of central tendency
Median
Mode
National Vital Statistics System (NVSS)
Neonatal mortality rate
Net autopsy rate
Net death rate
Newborn (NB)
Newborn autopsy rate
Newborn death rate
Normal distribution
Nosocomial (hospital-acquired) infection
Nosocomial infection rate
Notifiable disease
Occasion of service
Pie chart
Population-based statistics
Postneonatal mortality rate
Postoperative infection rate
Prevalence rate
Proportion
Proportionate mortality ratio (PMR)
Range
Rate
Ratio
Referred outpatient
Standard deviation
Table
Total length of stay (discharge days)
Variability
Variance

Introduction

Complete and accurate information is at the heart of good decision making. The health information management (HIM) professional has responsibility for ensuring that the data collected are accurate and organized into information that is useful to healthcare decision makers.

The primary source of clinical data in a healthcare facility is the health record. To be useful in decision making, data taken from the health record must be as complete and accurate as possible. Data are compiled in various ways to help in making decisions about patient care, the facility's financial status, and/or facility planning, to name a few.

This chapter discusses common statistical measures and types of data used by organizations in different healthcare settings. Methods and tools for graphically displaying data are then discussed. In the last part of the chapter, data collection and reporting on a community, regional, and national basis are discussed.

Theory into Practice

The Department of Quality Improvement at Community Hospital asks the HIM director to provide the hospital's C-section rate for the previous year for benchmarking purposes. It is recommended that the C-section rate for any hospital not exceed 15 percent. For the previous year, the hospital performed 556 C-sections out of 4,233 deliveries. Its C-section rate is 13.1 percent ([556/4,233] $\times$ 100). The quality improvement coordinator is pleased that the hospital's C-section rate falls within national guidelines.

In another hospital, the administration is evaluating the appropriateness of an expansion program. The associate administrator in charge of facility planning asks the HIM director for the bed occupancy rate for the hospital and its major services for the past five years and the number of outpatient and emergency department visits for the same time period. The director's findings are displayed in table 15.1 and figure 15.1.

Table 15.1.   Bed Occupancy Rates, Community Hospital, 1996–2000

Hospital/Service	1996	1997	1998	1999	2000
Total	85%	88%	90%	92%	95%
Medicine	90%	90%	92%	92%	95%
Surgery	80%	85%	85%	88%	90%
Obstetrics	65%	70%	72%	77%	79%
Pediatrics	85%	88%	88%	86%	89%

Figure 15.1.   Bed Occupancy Rates, Community Hospital, 1996–2000

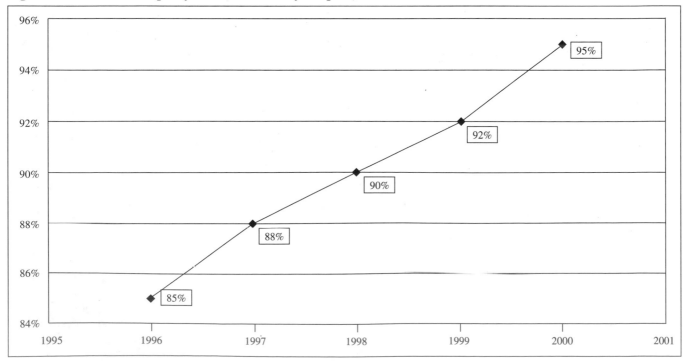

Common Statistical Measures Used in Healthcare

Healthcare data are collected to describe the health status of groups or populations. The data reported about healthcare facilities and communities describe the occurrence of illnesses, births, and deaths for specific periods of time. Data that are collected may be either facility based or population based. The sources of facility-based statistics are **acute care** facilities, long-term care facilities, and other types of healthcare organizations. The population-based statistics are gathered from cities, counties, states, or specific groups within the population, such as individuals affected by arthritis.

Reporting statistics for a healthcare facility is similar to reporting statistics for a community. Rates for healthcare facilities are reported as per 100 cases or percent; a community rate is reported as per 1,000, 10,000, or 100,000 people. For example, if a hospital experienced two deaths in a given month and 100 patients were discharged in the same month, the death rate would be 2 percent ($2 \times 100/100$). If there were 200 deaths in a community of 80,000 for a given period of time, the death rate would be reported as 25 deaths per 10,000 population ($[200 \times 10,000]/80,000$) for the same period of time.

Ratios, Proportions, and Rates

Many healthcare statistics are reported in the form of a **ratio, proportion,** or **rate.** These measures are used to report morbidity (illness), mortality (death), and natality (birthrate) at the local, state, and national levels. Basically, these measures indicate the number of times something happened relative to the number of times it *could have* happened. All three measures are based on formula 15.1. In this formula, x and y are the quantities being compared and x is divided by y. 10^n is 10 to the nth power. The size of 10^n may equal 10, 100, 1,000, 10,000, and so on, depending on the value of n:

$$10^0 = 1$$
$$10^1 = 10$$
$$10^2 = 10 \times 10 = 100$$
$$10^3 = 10 \times 10 \times 10 = 1,000$$

Ratios

In a ratio, the quantities being compared, such as patient discharge status (x = alive, y = dead), may be expressed so that x and y are completely independent of each other, or x may be included in y. For example, the outcome of patients discharged from Community Hospital could be compared in one of two ways:

Alive/dead, or x/y

Alive/(alive + dead), or $x/(x + y)$

In the first example, x is completely independent of y. The ratio represents the number of patients discharged alive compared to the number of patients who died. In the second example, x is part of the whole ($x + y$). The ratio represents the number of patients discharged alive compared to all patients discharged. Both expressions are considered ratios.

Proportions

A proportion is a particular type of ratio in which x is a portion of the whole ($x + y$). In a proportion, the numerator is always included in the denominator. Figures 15.2 and 15.3 describe the procedures for calculating ratios and proportions.

Rates

Rates are often used to measure events over a period of time. Sometimes they also are used in performance improvement studies. Like ratios and proportions, rates may be reported daily, weekly, monthly, or yearly. This allows for trend analysis and comparisons over time. The basic formula for calculating a rate is shown in formula 15.2.

Formula 15.1.   General Formula for Calculating Rates, Proportions, and Ratios

Ratio, proportion, rate = $x/y \times 10^n$

Figure 15.2.   Calculation of a Ratio, Discharge Status of Patients Discharged on May 20xx

1. Define x and y:
   x = number of patients discharged alive
   y = number of patients who died

2. Identify x and y:
   $x = 235$
   $y = 22$

3. *Set up the ratio x/y:*
   235/22

4. Reduce the fraction so that either x or y equals 1:
   10.68/1

There were 10.68 live discharges for every patient who died.

Figure 15.3.   Calculation of a Proportion, Discharge Status of Patients Discharged on May 20xx

1. Define x and y:
   x = number of patients discharged alive
   y = number of patients who died

2. Identify x and y:
   $x = 235$
   $y = 22$

3. Set up the proportion $x/x + y$:
   235/(235 + 22) = 235/257

4. Reduce the fraction so that either x or y equals 1:
   0.91/1

The proportion of patients discharged alive was 0.91.

Formula 15.2.   Formula for Calculating Risk for Contracting a Disease

$$\text{Risk rate} = \frac{\text{Number of cases occurring during a given time period}}{\text{Total number of cases or population at risk during the same time period}}$$

Healthcare facilities calculate many types of morbidity and mortality rates. For example, the cesarean section (C-section) rate is a measure of the proportion, or percentage, of C-sections performed during a given period of time. C-section rates are closely monitored because they present more risk to the mother and baby and because they are more expensive than vaginal deliveries. In calculating the C-section rate, the number of C-sections performed during the specified period of time is counted and this value is placed in the numerator. The number of cases, or the population at risk, is the number of women who delivered during the same time period. This number is placed in the denominator. By convention, inpatient hospital rates are reported as the rate per 100 cases ($10^n = 10^2 = 10 \times 10 = 100$) and are expressed as percentages.

Figure 15.4 shows the procedure for calculating a rate. In the example, 33 of the 263 deliveries at hospital X during the month of May were C-sections. In the formula, the numerator is the number of C-sections performed in May (given period of time) and the denominator is the total number of deliveries including C-sections (the population at risk) performed in the same time frame. In calculating the rate, the numerator is always included in the denominator. Also, when calculating a facility-based rate, the numerator is first multiplied by 100 and then divided by the denominator.

Because hospital rates rarely result in a whole number, they usually must be rounded. The hospital should set a policy on whether rates are to be reported to one or two decimal places. The division should be carried out to at least one more decimal place than desired.

When rounding, if the last number is five or greater, the preceding number should be increased one digit. In contrast, if the last number is less than five, the preceding number remains the same. For example, when rounding 25.56 percent to one decimal place, the rate becomes 25.6 percent because the last number is greater than five. When rounding 1.563 percent to two places, the rate becomes 1.56 percent because the last digit is less than five. Rates of less than one percent are usually carried out to three decimal places and rounded to two. For rates less than one percent, a zero should precede the decimal to emphasize that the rate is less than 1 percent, for example, 0.56 percent.

Check Your Understanding 15.1

Instructions: Identify the following statements as a rate, ratio, or proportion.

1. ____ Female discharges outnumber male discharges 3 to 1.

2. ____ Of the 100 discharges on October 1, 60 were female and 40 were male. Therefore, 0.60 of the discharges were women.

3. ____ Of the 100 patients discharged on October 1, 99 percent were discharged alive.

Measures of Central Tendency

Measures of central tendency and variability also can be used to describe populations. The measures of central tendency discussed in this subsection are the mean, the median, and the mode. The measures of variability discussed in the next subsection are the range, the variance, and the standard deviation.

Measures of central tendency are measures of location. They indicate the typical value of a frequency distribution. A frequency distribution shows the values that a variable can take and the number of observations associated with each value. For example, for the variable **length of stay** (LOS), five patients were discharged with the following lengths of stay:

Patient	LOS
1	2 days
2	3 days
3	4 days
4	2 days
5	3 days

The data displayed in the table above are referred to as a frequency distribution. A **frequency distribution** displays the number of times a particular observation occurs for the variable being measured. In this example, the number of times a certain LOS occurs is the variable of interest. The frequency distribution for LOS, in ascending order, is 2, 2, 3, 3, and 4 days.

In a frequency distribution, variables may be either continuous or discrete. With continuous variables there are no gaps in the measurement data. For example, an individual's weight may be 120 or 121 or any weight between 120 and 121. Continuous variables include fractions. Arithmetic operations—addition, subtraction, multiplication, and division—may be performed on continuous variables.

Discrete variables are variables that fall into categories. For example, the variable "sex" has two categories: male and female. The variable "third-party payer" has a number of categories, depending on the healthcare facility. Examples of payers include Medicare, Medicaid, commercial insurance, and private or self-pay.

Figure 15.4.   Calculation of a Rate, C-Section Rate for May 20xx

During May, 263 women delivered; of these, 33 deliveries were by C-section. What is the C-section rate for May?

1. Define the numerator (number of times an event occurred) and the denominator (number of times an event could have occurred):

   Numerator = total number of C-sections performed during the time period

   Denominator = total number of deliveries, including C-sections, in the same time period

2. Identify the numerator and the denominator:

   Numerator = 33
   Denominator = 263

3. Set up the rate:
   33/263

4. Multiply the numerator by 100 and then divide by the denominator:
   $([33 \times 100]/263) = 12.5\%$

The C-section rate for May is 12.5 percent.

To construct a frequency distribution, the collected data must be continuous. As an example, Community Hospital wants to construct a frequency distribution showing the LOS of patients who were discharged on May 10. The hospital wants to see how many of these patients were in the hospital for a particular LOS (for example, four days). The variable is the LOS, and the frequency is the number of times that a particular LOS occurred among the patients discharged on May 10.

To construct a frequency distribution, list all the values that the particular LOS can take, from the lowest observed value to the highest. Then enter the number of times a discharged patient had that particular LOS. Table 15.2 shows a frequency distribution for LOS on May 10. Notice that the frequency distribution lists all the values for LOS between the lowest and the highest, even when there are no observations for some of the values. For example, there are no observations of patients spending three days in the hospital. Six patients have LOS of four days. The data in table 15.2 can be used to calculate measures of both central tendency and variability.

The Mean

The **mean** is the arithmetic average of a frequency distribution. The symbol for the mean is $\overline{X}$ (pronounced ex bar). The formula for calculating the mean in a frequency distribution is:

$$\overline{X} = \sum_{i}^{n} X_i / N$$

where Σ is summation, X_i is each successive observation from the first one in the frequency distribution, $i = 1$, to the last observation (n), and N is the total number of observations.

To calculate the **average length of stay** (ALOS) for the data in table 15.2, substitute the appropriate figures into the following formula:

$$\overline{X} = \sum_{i}^{n} X_i / N$$

$$\overline{X} = \frac{\begin{array}{c} 1 + 1 + 2 + 2 + 4 + 4 + 4 + 4 + 4 + 4 \\ + 5 + 5 + 5 + 5 + 5 + 5 \\ + 6 + 6 + 6 + 6 + 6 + 6 + 6 + 6 + 6 + 6 + 6 \\ + 7 + 7 + 7 + 7 + 7 + 7 \\ + 8 + 8 + 8 + 8 + 8 + 9 + 9 + 9 + 10 \end{array}}{42}$$

$$\overline{X} = 245/42$$

$$\overline{X} = 5.8$$

The ALOS for patients discharged from Community Hospital on May 10 is 5.8 days (rounded).

Two disadvantages are associated with using the mean as the most typical value in a frequency distribution. First, in this example, the lengths of stay for the 42 patients are integers (whole numbers). However, the ALOS is fractional (5.8), even though there is no fractional LOS. Fractional values are considered more a problem of interpretation than a result that is not meaningful. In this case, the ALOS is interpreted as, "On average, the ALOS for the patients discharged from the Community Hospital on May 10 is between 5 and 6 days."

Table 15.2. **Frequency Distribution for Length of Stay, Community Hospital**

Patient Discharges, May 10	
LOS in Days	**Number of Patients (frequency)**
1	2
2	2
3	0
4	6
5	6
6	11
7	6
8	5
9	3
10	1
Total	42

Second, the mean is sensitive to extreme measures. That is, it is strongly influenced by outliers. For example, if the 10-day LOS were actually a 25-day LOS, the ALOS would increase to 6.2 days.

Thus, the average or arithmetic mean may not always be the most appropriate way to summarize the most typical value of a frequency distribution. The measure of central tendency selected to describe the typical value of a frequency distribution should be based on the characteristics of that particular frequency distribution.

The Median

The **median** is the midpoint of a frequency distribution. It is the point at which 50 percent of the observations fall above and 50 percent fall below. If an odd number of observations is in the frequency distribution, the median is the middle number. In the following frequency distribution, the median is 13. Three observations fall above the value of 13, and three fall below it:

$$10 \quad 11 \quad 12 \quad \boxed{13} \quad 14 \quad 15 \quad 16$$

If an even number of observations is in the frequency distribution, the median is the midpoint between the two middle observations. It is found by averaging the two middle scores ([$x + y$]/2). In the following example, the median is 13.5 ([13 + 14]/2):

$$10 \quad 11 \quad 12 \quad \boxed{13 \quad 14} \quad 15 \quad 16 \quad 17$$

If the two middle observations take on the same value, the median is that value. When determining the median, it does not matter whether there are duplicate observations in the frequency distribution. Consider the following frequency distribution:

$$10 \quad 11 \quad 11 \quad 12 \quad \boxed{13 \quad 13} \quad 14 \quad 15 \quad 16 \quad 17$$

In this frequency distribution, the median falls between the fifth and sixth observations. Therefore, the median is 13 ([13 + 13]/2).

Table 15.2 records LOS data for 42 patients. In this example, the median falls between the twenty-first and twenty-second observations. Placed in order from lowest to highest, the distribution is:

1 1 2 2 4 4 4 4 4 4 5 5 5 5 5 5 6 6 6 6 $\boxed{6\ 6}$
6 6 6 6 6 7 7 7 7 7 7 7 8 8 8 8 9 9 9 10

The median is 6 ([6 + 6]/2).

The median offers the following three advantages:

- It is relatively easy to calculate.
- It is based on the whole distribution and not just a portion of it, as is the case with the mode.
- Unlike the mean, it is not influenced by extreme values or unusual outliers in the frequency distribution.

The Mode

The **mode** is the simplest measure of central tendency. It is used to indicate the most frequent observation in a frequency distribution. The mode offers several advantages, including:

- It is easy to obtain and interpret.
- It is not sensitive to extreme observations in the frequency distribution.
- It is easy to communicate and explain to others.

However, there are also disadvantages, including:

- It may not be descriptive of the distribution when the most frequent observation does not occur very often, especially when the number of observations is large.
- It may not be unique. That is, more than one mode may be in a distribution. A frequency distribution may be unimodal, bimodal, or multimodal. When each observation occurs an equal number of times, the distribution does not have a mode.
- It does not provide information about the entire distribution, only the observation that occurs most frequently.

In table 15.2, the mode is 6 because 11 patients had lengths of stay of 6 days. To summarize, for the LOS data in table 15.2, the measures of central tendency are similar. The mean is 5.8 days, the median is 6 days, and the mode is 6 days.

Measures of Variability

In addition to measures of central tendency, the hospital can use measures of **variability** to describe frequency distributions. These measures indicate how widely the observations are spread out around the measures of central tendency. The measures of spread increase with greater variation in the frequency distribution. The spread is equal to zero when there is no variation. This subsection discusses the following measures of spread: the range, the variance, and the standard deviation.

The Range

The **range** is the simplest measure of spread. It is the difference between the smallest and largest values in a frequency distribution:

$$\text{Range} = X_{\max} - X_{\min}$$

The range for the LOS data in table 15.2 is 9 (10 − 1 = 9).

One disadvantage of the range is that it can be affected by extreme values, or outliers, in the distribution. Also, the range varies widely from sample to sample. Only the two most extreme observations in the distribution affect its value, so it is not sensitive to other observations in the distribution.

Two frequency distributions may have the same range but differ greatly in variation. For example, the range for the following frequency distributions is 9 (10 − 1 = 9):

Distribution 1: 1 2 3 4 5 6 7 8 9 10
Distribution 2: 1 1.5 3 3.5 3.7 7 8 8.26 10 10

However, when the two distributions are compared, the second distribution has more variation than the first distribution. This is demonstrated when the variance is calculated. The variance for the first distribution is 3.03, and the variance for the second distribution is 3.44.

The Variance

The **variance** of a frequency distribution is the average of the squared deviations from the mean. The variance of a sample is symbolized by s^2. The variance of a distribution is larger when the observations are widely spread. The formula for calculating the variance is:

$$s^2 = \sum_i^n (X_i - \overline{X})^2 / N - 1$$

The squared deviations of the mean are calculated by subtracting the mean of the frequency distribution from each value in the distribution. The difference between the two values is squared, $(X - \overline{X})^2$. The squared differences are summed and divided by $N - 1$. The calculations for the variance for the LOS data in table 15.2 are shown in figure 15.5.

In the calculations for the variance, the sum of $(X - \overline{X})$ is equal to zero. This is because the mean is the balance point in the distribution. When a value is less than the mean, the difference is negative (1 − 5.8 = −4.8); and when the value is greater than the mean, the difference is positive (6 − 5.8 = +0.2). Therefore, the sum of the differences from the mean is equal to zero. In this example, the sum approximates zero because the actual mean of 5.8333 was rounded to 5.8 for ease in calculation.

The Standard Deviation

The variance for the LOS data is 4.39, but what does this mean? The interpretation of the variance is not meaningful at the descriptive level because the original units of measure—the lengths of stay—are squared to arrive at the variance. By calculating the square root of the variance, the data are returned to the original units of measurement. This is called the **standard deviation,** which is symbolized by s. The formula for the standard deviation is:

$$s = \sqrt{\sum_i^n (X_i - \overline{X})^2 / N - 1}$$

The standard deviation for the LOS data is 2.09.

Figure 15.5.   Calculation of the Variance, LOS Data

LOS	LOS − Mean (5.8) ($X - \overline{X}$)	(LOS − Mean)² ($X - \overline{X}$)²
1	−4.8	23.04
1	−4.8	23.04
2	−3.8	14.44
2	−3.8	14.44
4	−1.8	3.24
4	−1.8	3.24
4	−1.8	3.24
4	−1.8	3.24
4	−1.8	3.24
4	−1.8	3.24
5	−0.8	0.64
5	−0.8	0.64
5	−0.8	0.64
5	−0.8	0.64
5	−0.8	0.64
5	−0.8	0.64
6	0.2	0.04
6	0.2	0.04
6	0.2	0.04
6	0.2	0.04
6	0.2	0.04
6	0.2	0.04
6	0.2	0.04
6	0.2	0.04
6	0.2	0.04
6	0.2	0.04
6	0.2	0.04
7	1.2	1.44
7	1.2	1.44
7	1.2	1.44
7	1.2	1.44
7	1.2	1.44
7	1.2	1.44
8	2.2	4.84
8	2.2	4.84
8	2.2	4.84
8	2.2	4.84
8	2.2	4.84
9	3.2	10.24
9	3.2	10.24
9	3.2	10.24
10	4.2	17.64
Total	0*	179.88

*rounded

$$s^2 = \sum_{i}^{n} (X_i - \overline{X})^2 / N - 1$$
$$= 179.88/44$$
$$= 4.39$$

The standard deviation is the most widely used measure of variability in **descriptive statistics.** Because it is easy to interpret, it is the preferred measure of dispersion for frequency distributions. Most handheld calculators include features for calculating the variance and the standard deviation.

Check Your Understanding 15.2

Instructions: Fifteen infants were born at Community Hospital during the week of December 1. Using a handheld calculator, determine the measures of central tendency and variability for the following infant birth weights (in grams):

2,450	2,750	2,600
2,540	2,815	2,540
2,300	1,735	1,720
2,715	1,800	2,780
2,400	2,485	2,640

1. ___ Mean
2. ___ Median
3. ___ Mode
4. ___ Range
5. ___ Variance
6. ___ Standard deviation

Normal Distribution

Measures of central tendency and variation are interpreted as they relate to the normal distribution. The **normal distribution** is actually a theoretical family of distributions that may have any mean or any standard deviation. It is bell-shaped and symmetrical about the mean. Because it is symmetrical, 50 percent of the observations fall above the mean and 50 percent fall below it. In a normal distribution, the mean, median, and mode are equal. The values of the normal distribution range from minus infinity ($-\infty$) to plus infinity ($+\infty$).

In the normal distribution, the standard deviation indicates how many observations fall within a certain range of the mean. Typically, 68 percent of the observations fall within one standard deviation of the mean, 95 percent fall within two standard deviations, and 99.7 percent fall within three standard deviations.

Figure 15.6 (p. 334) shows an example of a normal distribution superimposed on a histogram. The center of the distribution, or mean, is 6. (The median and the mode also are 6.) The standard deviation is 2.45. This means that 68 percent of the observations in the frequency distribution fall within 2.45 standard deviations of 6 (6 ± 2.45). Thus, 68 percent fall between 3.55 and 8.45; 95 percent fall between 1.1 and 10.9; and 99.7 percent fall between −1.35 and 13.35.

As shown in the figure, a characteristic of the normal distribution is that each tail of the curve approaches the *x*-axis but never touches it, no matter how far from center the line is.

A histogram of the frequency distribution for the LOS data in table 15.2 is shown in figure 15.7 (p. 334). The distribution is kurtotic. *Kurtosis* is the vertical stretching of a distribution. The distribution is more peaked than the normal distribution and so is considered kurtotic.

A skewed distribution is asymmetrical. *Skewness* is the horizontal stretching of a frequency distribution to one side or the other so that one tail is longer than the other. The longer tail has more observations. Because the mean is sensitive to extreme observations, it moves in the direction of the long tail when a distribution is skewed. When the direction of the tail is off to the right, the distribution is positively skewed, or skewed to the right. When the direction of the tail is off to the left, the distribution is negatively skewed, or skewed to the left. When the mean and the median approximate one another (as with the LOS data), the distribution is not significantly skewed.

The measures of central tendency and variation may be calculated using a handheld calculator. Also, statistical packages such as SPSS are available for performing these and other descriptive and **inferential statistics.** The histograms were prepared using SPSS. The SPSS output for the LOS data appears in figure 15.8. The slight differences between the handheld calculator results and the SPSS results in the mean, variance, and standard deviation are because of rounding.

Check Your Understanding 15.3

Instructions: Answer the following questions on a separate piece of paper.

1. What are the characteristics of a normal distribution?
2. What is the definition of the term *skewness*?

Figure 15.6.   Histogram Showing Normal Distribution

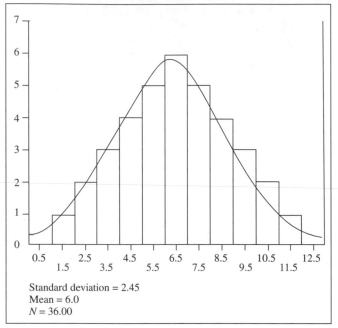

Standard deviation = 2.45
Mean = 6.0
N = 36.00

Basic Statistical Data Used in Acute Care Facilities

In the daily operations of any organization, whether in business, manufacturing, or healthcare, data are collected for decision making. To be effective, the decision makers must have confidence in the data collected. Confidence requires that the data collected be accurate, reliable, and timely. The types of data collected in the acute care setting are discussed in the following section.

Administrative Statistical Data

Hospitals collect data on both inpatients and outpatients on a daily basis. They use these statistics to monitor the volume of patients treated daily, weekly, monthly, or within some other specified time frame. The statistics give healthcare decision makers the information they need to plan facilities and to monitor inpatient and outpatient revenue streams. For these

Figure 15.7.   Histogram Showing the Normal Distribution of LOS Data

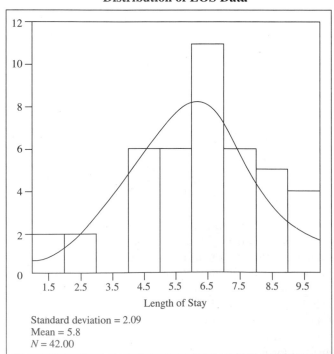

Length of Stay

Standard deviation = 2.09
Mean = 5.8
N = 42.00

Figure 15.8.   SPSS Output for LOS Data

Statistics			
Length of Stay			
N		Valid	42
		Missing	0
Mean			5.8333
Median			6.0000
Mode			6.00
Standard deviation			2.0943
Variance			4.3862
Range			9.00
Sum			245.00

reasons, the HIM professional must be well versed in data collection and reporting methods.

Standard definitions have been developed to ensure that all healthcare providers collect and report data in a consistent manner. The *Glossary of Healthcare Terms,* developed by the American Health Information Management Association (AHIMA), is a resource commonly used to describe the types of healthcare events for which data are collected. (The glossary is currently published as an appendix in *Basic Statistics for Health Information Management Professionals* [Youmans 2000].) The glossary includes definitions of terms related to healthcare corporations, health maintenance organizations (HMOs), and other health-related programs and facilities. Some basic terms that HIM professionals should be familiar with include:

- **Hospital inpatient:** A patient who is provided with room, board, and continuous general nursing service in an area of the hospital where patients generally stay at least overnight.
- **Hospital newborn inpatient:** A patient who is born in the hospital at the beginning of the current inpatient hospitalization. **Newborns** are usually counted separately because their care is so different from that of other inpatients. Infants born on the way to the hospital or at home are considered hospital inpatients, not hospital newborn inpatients.
- **Inpatient hospitalization:** A period in a person's life during which he or she is an inpatient in a single hospital without interruption, except by possible intervening leaves of absence.
- **Inpatient admission:** The formal acceptance by a hospital of a patient who is to be provided with room, board, and continuous nursing service in an area of the hospital where patients generally stay overnight.
- **Inpatient discharge:** The termination of a period of inpatient hospitalization through the formal release of the inpatient by the hospital. The term includes patients who are discharged alive (by physician's order), who are discharged against medical advice (AMA), or who died while hospitalized. Unless otherwise indicated, inpatient discharges include deaths.
- **Hospital outpatient:** A hospital patient who receives services in one or more of the outpatient facilities when he or she is not currently an inpatient or home care patient. An outpatient may be classified as either an emergency outpatient or a clinic outpatient. An emergency outpatient is admitted to the emergency department of a hospital for diagnosis and treatment of a condition that requires immediate medical, dental, or other emergency services. A clinic outpatient is admitted to a clinical service of the clinic or hospital for diagnosis and treatment on an ambulatory basis.

Inpatient Census Data

Even though much of the data collection process has been automated, an ongoing responsibility of the HIM profes-sional is to verify the census data that are collected daily. The census reports patient activity for a 24-hour reporting period. Included in the census report is the number of inpatients admitted and discharged for the previous 24-hour period as well as the number of intrahospital transfers. An *intrahospital transfer* is a patient who is moved from one patient care unit (for example, the intensive care unit) to another (for example, the surgical unit). The usual 24-hour reporting period begins at 12:01 a.m. and ends at 12:00 midnight. In the census count, adults and children (A&C) are reported separately from newborns.

Before compiling census data, however, it is important to understand their related terminology. The **census** is the number of hospital inpatients present at any one time. For example, the census in a 300-bed hospital may be 250 patients at 2:00 p.m. on May 1, but 245 an hour later. Because the census may change throughout the day as admissions and discharges occur, hospitals designate an official census-taking time. In most facilities, the official count takes place at midnight. The result of the official count taken at midnight is called the **daily inpatient census.** This is the number of inpatients present at the official census-taking time each day. Also included in the daily inpatient census are any patients who were admitted and discharged that same day. For example, if a patient were admitted to the cardiac care unit (CCU) at 1:00 p.m. on May 1 and died at 4.00 p.m. on May 1, he would be counted as a patient who was both admitted and discharged the same day.

Because patients admitted and discharged the same day are not present at the census-taking time, the hospital must account for them separately. If it did not, credit for the services provided these patients would be lost. The daily inpatient census reflects the total number of patients treated during the 24-hour period. Figure 15.9 displays a sample daily inpatient census report.

A unit of measure that reflects the services received by one inpatient during a 24-hour period is called an **inpatient service day.** The number of inpatient service days for a 24-hour period is equal to the daily inpatient census, that is, one service day for each patient treated. In figure 15.9, the total number of inpatient service days for May 2 is 230.

Figure 15.9.   Daily Inpatient Census Report, Adults and Children

May 2	
Number of patients in hospital at midnight, May 1	230
+ Number of patients admitted May 2	+ 35
− Number of patients discharged, including deaths, May 2	− 40
Number of patients in hospital at midnight, May 2	225
+ Number of patients both admitted and discharged, including deaths	+5
Daily inpatient census at midnight, May 2	230
Total inpatient service days, May 2	230

Inpatient service days are compiled daily, weekly, monthly, and annually. They reflect the volume of services provided by the healthcare facility: the greater the volume of services, the greater the revenues to the facility. Daily reporting of the number of inpatient service days is an indicator of the hospital's financial condition.

As previously mentioned, the daily inpatient census is equal to the number of inpatient service days provided for that day as shown below:

Daily Inpatient Census		Inpatient Service Days
Day 1	240	240
Day 2	253	253
Day 3	237	237
Total		730

Thus, the total number of inpatient service days for a week, a month, and so on can be divided by the total number of days in the period of interest to obtain the **average daily census.** In the preceding example, 730 inpatient service days is divided by three days to obtain an average daily census of 243.3. The average daily census is the average number of inpatients treated during a given period of time. The general formula for calculating the average daily census is shown in formula 15.3.

In calculating the average daily census for adults and children (A&C), the average daily census for newborns is reported separately. This is because the intensity of services provided to adults and children is greater than it is for newborns. To calculate the average daily census for adults and children, the general formula is modified as shown in formula 15.4.

The formula for the average daily census for newborns is shown in formula 15.5. For example, the total number of inpatient service days provided to adults and children for the week of May 1 is 1,729, and the total for newborns is 119. Using the formulas, the average daily census for adults and children is 247 (1,729/7) and for newborns it is 17 (119/7).

Formula 15.3.   Formula for Calculating Average Daily Census

$$\text{Average daily census} = \frac{\text{Total number of inpatient service days for a given period}}{\text{Total number of days in the same period}}$$

Formula 15.4.   Formula for Calculating Average Daily Census for Adults and Children

$$\text{Average daily census for A\&C} = \frac{\text{Total number of inpatient service days for A\&C for a given period}}{\text{Total number of days for the same period}}$$

Formula 15.5.   Formula for Calculating Average Daily Census for Newborns

$$\text{Average daily census for NBs} = \frac{\text{Total number of inpatient service days for NBs for a given period}}{\text{Total number of days for the same period}}$$

The average daily census for all hospital inpatients for the week of May 1 is 264 ([1,729 + 119]/7). Table 15.3 compares the various formulas for calculating the average daily census.

Check Your Understanding 15.4

Instructions: Using the information given, answer the following questions on a separate piece of paper.

1. The inpatient census for Community Hospital at midnight on August 1 was 268; the daily inpatient census for August 1 was 270. On August 2, 16 patients were admitted, 9 were discharged, and 2 were admitted and discharged on the same day. Calculate the following statistics for August 2.

   a. ____ Inpatient census
   b. ____ Daily inpatient census
   c. ____ Inpatient service days
   d. ____ Total inpatient service days for August 1 and 2

2. Nine patients were in the intensive care unit (ICU) at midnight on August 1. On August 2, two patients were admitted, one was transferred from 3N to the ICU, one died, one was transferred from the ICU to the cardiology service, and two who were admitted on August 2 died on August 2. Calculate the following statistics for the ICU on August 2.

   a. ____ Inpatient census
   b. ____ Daily inpatient census

Inpatient Bed Occupancy Rate

Another indicator of the hospital's financial position is the inpatient bed occupancy rate, also called the percentage of occupancy. The **inpatient bed occupancy rate** is the percentage of official beds occupied by hospital inpatients for a given period of time. In general, the greater the occupancy rate, the greater the revenues to the hospital. For a bed to be included in the official count, it must be set up, staffed, equipped, and available for patient care. The total number of inpatient service days is used in the numerator because it is equal to the daily inpatient census or the number of patients treated daily. The occupancy rate compares the number of patients treated over a given period of time to the total number of beds available for the same period of time.

For example, if 200 patients occupied 280 beds on May 2, the inpatient bed occupancy rate would be 71.4 percent ([200/{280 × 1}] × 100). If the rate were for more than one day, the number of beds would be multiplied by the number of days in that particular time frame. For example, if 1,729 inpatient service days were provided during the week of May 1, the inpatient bed occupancy rate for that week would be 88.2 percent ([1,729/{280 × 7}] × 100).

The denominator in this formula is actually the total possible number of inpatient service days. That is, if every available bed in the hospital were occupied every single day, this would be the maximum number of inpatient service days that could be provided. This is an important concept, especially when the official **bed count** changes for a given reporting period. For example, if the bed count changed from 280 beds to 300, the bed occupancy rate would reflect the change. The total number of inpatient beds times the total number of days in the period is called the total number of **bed count days.** The general formula for the inpatient bed occupancy rate is shown in formula 15.6.

For example, in May the total number of inpatient service days provided was 7,582. The bed count for the month of May changed from 280 beds to 300 on May 20. To calculate the inpatient bed occupancy rate for May, the total number of bed count days must be determined. There are 31 days in May; therefore, the total number of bed count days is calculated as:

Number of beds, May 1–May 19 = 280 × 19 days = 5,320 bed count days
Number of beds, May 20–May 31 = 300 × 12 days = 3,600 bed count days
5,320 + 3,600 = 8,920 bed count days

The inpatient bed occupancy rate for the month of May is 85.0 percent ([7,582/8,920] × 100).

As with the average daily census, the inpatient bed occupancy rate for adults and children is reported separately from that of newborns. To calculate the total number of bed count days for newborns, the official count for newborn bassinets is used. Table 15.4 reviews the formulas for calculating inpatient bed occupancy rates.

It is possible for the inpatient bed occupancy rate to be greater than 100 percent. This occurs when the hospital faces an epidemic or disaster. In this type of situation, hospitals set up temporary beds that usually are not included in the official bed count. As an example, Community Hospital experienced an excessive number of admissions in January because of an outbreak of influenza. In January, the official bed count was 150 beds. On January 5, the daily inpatient census was 156. Therefore, the inpatient bed occupancy rate for January 5 was 104 percent ([156/150] × 100).

Bed Turnover Rate

The **bed turnover rat**e is a measure of hospital utilization. It includes the number of times each hospital bed changed occupants. The formula for the bed turnover rate is shown in formula 15.7 (p. 338). For example, Community Hospital experienced 2,060 discharges and deaths for the month of April. Its bed count for April averaged 677. The bed turnover rate is 3.04 (2,060/677). The interpretation is that, on average, each hospital bed had three occupants during April.

Check Your Understanding 15.5

Instructions: Using the information provided, answer the following questions on a separate piece of paper.

1. What is the inpatient bed occupancy rate for each of the following patient care units for the month of August?

Unit	Inpatient Service Days	Average Bed Count	Bed Count Occupancy Rate
Medical	2,850	100	_____
Surgical	988	34	_____
Pediatric	422	15	_____
Orthopedic	502	18	_____
Obstetric	544	20	_____
Newborn	524	18	_____
Total	___	___	_____

2. In 1999, Community Hospital had 67,120 inpatient service days for adults and children and 4,850 inpatient service days for newborns. The bed count for adults and children was 220, and the bed count for newborn bassinets was 22.

   a. ___ What was the average daily inpatient census for adults and children?

   b. ___ What was the average daily inpatient census for newborns?

   c. ___ What was the inpatient bed occupancy rate for adults and children?

   d. ___ What was the inpatient bed occupancy rate for newborns?

Table 15.3.   Calculation of Census Statistics

Indicator	Numerator	Denominator
Average daily inpatient census	Total number of inpatient service days for a given period	Total number of days for the same period
Average daily inpatient census for adults and children (A&C)	Total number of inpatient service days for A&C for a given period	Total number of days for the same period
Average daily inpatient census for newborns	Total number of inpatient service days for NBs for a given period	Total number of days for the same period

Formula 15.6.   Formula for Calculating Inpatient Bed Occupancy Rate

$$\text{Inpatient bed occupancy} = \frac{\text{Total number of inpatient service days for a given period}}{\text{Total number of inpatient bed count days for the same period}} \times 100$$

Table 15.4.   Calculation of Inpatient Bed Occupancy Rates

Rate	Numerator	Denominator
Inpatient bed occupancy rate	Total number of inpatient service days for a given period × 100	Total number of inpatient bed count days for the same period
Inpatient bed occupancy rate for adults and children (A&C)	Total number of inpatient service days for A&C for a given period × 100	Total number of inpatient bed count days for A&C for the same period
Newborn (NB) bed occupancy rate	Total number of NB inpatient service days for a given period × 100	Total number of bassinet bed count days for the same period

Length of Stay Data

Length of stay (LOS) is calculated for each patient after he or she is discharged from the hospital. The LOS is the number of calendar days from the day of patient admission to the day of patient discharge. When the patient is admitted and discharged in the same month, the LOS is determined by subtracting the date of admission from the date of discharge. For example, the LOS for a patient admitted on May 12 and discharged on May 17 is five days ($17 - 12 = 5$).

When the patient is admitted in one month and discharged in another, the calculations must be adjusted. One way to calculate the LOS in this case is to subtract the date of admission from the total number of days in the month the patient was admitted and then to add the total number of hospitalized days for the month in which the patient was discharged. For example, the LOS for a patient admitted on May 28 and discharged on June 6 is nine days ([May 31–May 28 = 3 days] + June 1–6 = 6 days; LOS = 9 days).

When a patient is admitted and discharged on the same day, the LOS is one day. A partial day's stay is never reported as a fraction of a day. The LOS for a patient discharged the day after admission also is one day. Thus, the LOS for a patient who was admitted to the ICU on May 10 at 9:00 a.m. and died at 3:00 p.m. on the same day is one day. Likewise, the LOS for a patient admitted on May 12 and discharged on May 13 is one day.

When the LOS for all patients discharged for a given period of time is summed, the result is the **total length of stay.** As an example, five patients were discharged from the pediatric unit on May 9. The LOS for each patient was as follows:

Patient	LOS
1	5
2	3
3	1
4	8
5	10
Total LOS	27

In the preceding example, the total length of stay is 27 days ($5 + 3 + 1 + 8 + 10$). The total LOS is also referred to as the number of days of care provided to patients who were discharged or died (discharge days) during a given period of time.

The average length of stay (ALOS) is calculated from the total length of stay. The total LOS divided by the number of patients discharged is the ALOS. Using the data in the preceding example, the ALOS for the five patients discharged from the pediatric unit is 5.4 days (27/5).

The general formula for calculating the ALOS is shown in formula 15.8. As with the measures already discussed, the ALOS for adults and children is reported separately from the ALOS for newborns. Table 15.5 reviews the formulas for ALOS. Table 15.6 displays an example of a hospital statistical summary prepared by the HIM department using census and discharge data.

Check Your Understanding 15.6

Instructions: Complete the following exercise on a separate piece of paper.

1. Calculate the total length of stay for all patient discharges and the average length of stay.

Number of Patients Discharged	Length of Stay	Total Discharge Days
10	2	_____
7	3	_____
2	4	_____
1	7	_____
1	9	_____
1	10	_____
1	16	_____

  a. Total length of stay _____

  b. Average length of stay _____

Formula 15.7.   Formula for Calculating Bed Turnover Rate

$$\text{Bed turnover rate} = \frac{\text{Total number of discharges, including deaths, for a given time period}}{\text{Average bed count for the same time period}}$$

Formula 15.8.   Formula for Calculating Average Length of Stay

$$\text{Average length of stay} = \frac{\text{Total length of stay for a given period}}{\text{Total number of discharges, including deaths, for the same period}}$$

Table 15.5.   Calculation of LOS Statistics

Indicator	Numerator	Denominator
Average length of stay	Total length of stay (discharge days) for a given period	Total number of discharges, including deaths, for the same period
Average length of stay, adults and children (A&C)	Total length of stay for A&C, including deaths (discharge days), for a given period	Total number of discharges, including deaths, for A&C for the same period
Average newborn (NB) length of stay	Total length of stay for all NB discharges and deaths (discharge days) for a given period	Total number of NB discharges, including deaths, for the same period

Table 15.6.   Statistical Summary, Community Hospital for the Period Ending July 20xx

Admissions	July 20xx		Year-to-Date 20xx	
	Actual	Budget	Actual	Budget
Medical	728	769	5,075	5,082
Surgical	578	583	3,964	3,964
OB/GYN	402	440	2,839	3,027
Psychiatry	113	99	818	711
Physical Medicine & Rehab	48	57	380	384
Other Adult	191	178	1,209	1,212
Total Adult	2,060	2,126	14,285	14,380
Newborn	294	312	2,143	2,195
Total Admissions	2,354	2,438	16,428	16,575

Average Length of Stay	July 20xx		Year-to-Date 20xx	
	Actual	Budget	Actual	Budget
Medical	6.1	6.4	6.0	6.1
Surgical	7.0	7.2	7.7	7.7
OB/GYN	2.9	3.2	3.5	3.1
Psychiatry	10.8	11.6	10.4	11.6
Physical Medicine & Rehab	27.5	23.0	28.1	24.3
Other Adult	3.6	3.9	4.0	4.1
Total Adult	6.3	6.4	6.7	6.5
Newborn	5.6	5.0	5.6	5.0
Total ALOS	6.2	6.3	6.5	6.3

Patient Days	June 20xx		Year-to-Date 20xx	
	Actual	Budget	Actual	Budget
Medical	4,436	4,915	30,654	30,762
Surgical	4,036	4,215	30,381	30,331
OB/GYN	1,170	1,417	10,051	9,442
Psychiatry	1,223	1,144	8,524	8,242
Physical Medicine & Rehab	1,318	1,310	10,672	9,338
Other Adult	688	699	4,858	4,921
Total Adult	12,871	13,700	95,140	93,036
Newborn	1,633	1,552	12,015	10,963
Total Patient Days	14,504	15,252	107,155	103,999

Other Key Statistics	June 20xx		Year-to-Date 20xx	
	Actual	Budget	Actual	Budget
Average Daily Census	485	492	498	486
Average Beds Available	677	660	677	660
Clinic Visits	21,621	18,975	144,271	136,513
Emergency Visits	3,822	3,688	26,262	25,604
Inpatient Surgery Patients	657	583	4,546	4,093
Outpatient Surgery Patients	603	554	4,457	3,987

Patient Care/Clinical Statistical Data

Thus far, this chapter has discussed statistical measures that are indicators of volume of services and utilization of services. The collection of data related to morbidity and mortality also is an important aspect of evaluating the quality of hospital services. Morbidity/mortality rates are reported for all patient discharges within a certain time frame. They also may be reported by service or by physician or other variable of interest in order to identify trends or problems that require corrective action. The most frequently collected morbidity/mortality rates are presented in this section.

Hospital Death (Mortality) Rates

The **hospital death rate** is based on the number of patients discharged, alive and dead, from the hospital. Deaths are considered discharges because they are the end point of a period of hospitalization. In contrast to the rates discussed in the preceding section, newborns are not counted separately from adults and children.

Gross Death Rate

The **gross death rate** is the proportion of all hospital discharges that ended in death. It is the basic indicator of mortality in a healthcare facility. The gross death rate is calculated by dividing the total number of deaths occurring in a given time period by the total number of discharges, including deaths, for the same time period. The formula for calculating the gross death rate is shown in formula 15.9.

As an example, Community Hospital experienced 21 deaths (A&C and NBs) during the month of May. There were 633 total discharges, including deaths. The gross death rate is 3.3 percent ([21/633] $\times$ 100).

Net Death Rate

The **net death rate** is an adjusted death rate. It is calculated in the belief that certain deaths should not "count against the hospital." The net death rate is an adjusted rate because it does not include patients who die within 48 hours of admis-

sion. The reason for excluding these deaths is that 48 hours is not enough time to positively affect patient outcome. In other words, the patient was not admitted to the hospital in a manner timely enough for treatment to have an effect on his or her outcome. However, in view of currently available technology, some people believe that the net death rate is no longer a meaningful indicator. The formula for calculating the net death rate is shown in formula 15.10.

Continuing with the preceding example, of the 21 patients who died at Community Hospital, three died within 48 hours of admission. Therefore, the net death rate is 2.9 percent ([{21 − 3}/{633 − 3}] $\times$ 100 = 2.9%). The fact that the net death rate is less than the gross death rate is favorable to Community Hospital because lower death rates may be an indicator of better care.

Newborn Death Rate

Even though newborn deaths are included in the hospital's gross and net death rates, the newborn death rate can be calculated separately. Newborns include only infants born alive in the hospital. The **newborn death rate** is the number of newborns who died in comparison to the total number of newborns discharged, alive and dead. To qualify as a newborn death, the newborn must have been delivered alive. A stillborn infant is not included in either the newborn death rate or the gross or net death rate. The formula for calculating the newborn death rate is shown in formula 15.11.

Fetal Death Rate

In hospital terminology, the death of a stillborn baby is called a fetal death. A **fetal death** is a death prior to the fetus's complete expulsion or extraction from the mother in a hospital facility, regardless of the length of the pregnancy. Thus, stillborns are neither admitted nor discharged from the hospital. A fetal death occurs when the fetus fails to breathe or show any other evidence of life, such as a heartbeat, a pulsation of the umbilical cord, or a movement of the voluntary muscles.

Formula 15.9.   Formula for Calculating Gross Death Rate

$$\text{Gross death rate} = \frac{\text{Total number of inpatient deaths (including NBs) for a given period}}{\text{Total number of discharges, including A\&C and NB deaths, for the same period}} \times 100$$

Formula 15.10.   Formula for Calculating Net Death Rate

$$\text{Net death rate} = \frac{\text{Total number of inpatient deaths (including NBs) minus deaths} < 48 \text{ hours for a given period}}{\text{Total number of discharges (including A\&C and NB deaths) minus deaths} < 48 \text{ hours for the same period}} \times 100$$

Formula 15.11.   Formula for Calculating Newborn Death Rate

$$\text{Newborn death rate} = \frac{\text{Total number of NB deaths for a given period}}{\text{Total number of NB discharges (including deaths) for the same period}} \times 100$$

Fetal deaths also are classified into categories based on length of gestation or weight. (See table 15.7.) To calculate the **fetal death rate,** divide the total number of intermediate and late fetal deaths for the period by the total number of live births and intermediate and late fetal deaths for the same period. The formula for calculating the fetal death rate is shown in formula 15.12. For example, during the month of May, Community Hospital experienced 269 live births and 13 intermediate and late fetal deaths. The fetal death rate is 4.6 percent ($[13/\{269 + 13\}] \times 100$).

Maternal Death Rate

Hospitals also calculate the **maternal death rate.** A maternal death is the death of any woman from any cause related to, or aggravated by, pregnancy or its management, regardless of the duration or site of the pregnancy. Maternal deaths that result from accidental or incidental causes are not included in the maternal death rate.

Maternal deaths are classified as either direct or indirect. A *direct maternal death* is the death of a woman resulting from obstetrical (OB) complications of the pregnancy state, labor, or puerperium (the period including the six weeks after delivery). Direct maternal deaths are included in the maternal death rate. An *indirect maternal death* is the death of a woman from a previously existing disease or a disease that developed during pregnancy, labor, or the puerperium that was not due to obstetric causes, although the physiologic effects of pregnancy were partially responsible.

The maternal death rate may be an indicator of the availability of prenatal care in a community. The hospital also may use it to help identify conditions that could lead to a maternal death. The formula for calculating the maternal death rate is shown in formula 15.13. For example, during the month of May, Community Hospital experienced 275 maternal discharges. Two of these patients died. The mater-

nal death rate for May is 0.73 percent ($[2/275] \times 100$). Table 15.8 (p. 342) summarizes hospital-based mortality rates.

Check Your Understanding 15.7

Instructions: Using the data provided on deaths and discharges at Community Hospital for the past calendar year, answer the following questions.

Total discharges, including deaths (A&C)	754
Total deaths (A&C)	14
Deaths less than 48 hours after admission (A&C)	6
Fetal deaths	3
Live births	140
Newborn deaths	3
Newborn deaths, including discharges	122
Maternal deaths (direct)	2
OB discharges, including deaths	133

1. ___ What is the gross death rate for adults and children?
2. ___ What is the net death rate for adults and children?
3. ___ What is the fetal death rate?
4. ___ What is the newborn death rate?
5. ___ What is the gross death rate for adults and children and newborns combined?
6. ___ What is the maternal death rate (direct)?

Autopsy Rates

An autopsy is an examination of a dead body to determine the cause of death. Autopsies are very useful in the education of medical students and residents. In addition, they can alert family members to conditions or diseases for which they may be at risk.

Two categories of hospital autopsies are conducted in acute care facilities: hospital inpatient autopsies and hospital autopsies. A **hospital inpatient autopsy** is an examination of the body of a patient who died while being treated in the hospital. The patient's death marked the end of the patient's stay in the hospital. A pathologist or some other physician on the medical staff performs this type of autopsy in the facility.

A **hospital autopsy** is an examination of the body of an individual who at some time in the past had been a hospital patient and was not a hospital inpatient at the time of death. A pathologist or some other physician on the medical staff performs this type of autopsy.

The following sections describe the different types of autopsy rates calculated by acute care hospitals.

Table 15.7.   Classifications of Fetal Death

Classification	Length of Gestation	Weight
Early fetal death	Less than 20 weeks' gestation	500 grams or less
Intermediate fetal death	20 weeks' completed gestation, but less than 28 weeks	501 to 1,000 grams
Late fetal death	28 weeks' completed gestation	Over 1,000 grams

Formula 15.12.   Formula for Calculating Fetal Death Rate

$$\text{Fetal death rate} = \frac{\text{Total number of intermediate and late fetal deaths for a given period}}{\text{Total number of live births plus total number of intermediate and late fetal deaths for the same period}} \times 100$$

Formula 15.13.   Formula for Calculating Maternal Death Rate

$$\text{Maternal death rate} = \frac{\text{Total number of direct maternal deaths for a given period}}{\text{Total number of maternal (OB) discharges, including deaths, for the same period}} \times 100$$

Gross Autopsy Rates

A **gross autopsy rate** is the proportion or percentage of deaths that are followed by the performance of autopsy. The formula for calculating the gross autopsy rate is shown in formula 15.14. For example, during the month of May, Community Hospital experienced 21 deaths. Autopsies were performed on four of these patients. The gross autopsy rate is 19.0 percent ([4/21] × 100).

Net Autopsy Rates

The bodies of patients who have died are not always available for autopsy. For example, a coroner or medical examiner may claim a body for an autopsy for legal reasons. In these situations, the hospital calculates a **net autopsy rate.** In calculating the net autopsy rate, bodies that have been removed by the coroner or medical examiner are excluded from the denominator. The formula for calculating the net autopsy rate is shown in formula 15.15. Continuing with the example in the preceding section, the medical examiner claimed three of the patients for autopsy. The numerator remains the same because four autopsies were performed by the hospital pathologist. However, because three of the deaths were identified as medical examiner's cases and removed from the hospital, three is subtracted from 21. The net autopsy rate is 22.2 percent ([4/{21 − 3}] × 100).

Hospital Autopsy Rates

A third type of autopsy rate is called the **hospital autopsy rate.** This is an adjusted rate that includes autopsies on anyone who may have once been a hospital patient. The formula for calculating the hospital autopsy rate is shown in formula 15.16. The hospital autopsy rate includes autopsies performed on any of the following:

- Bodies of inpatients, except those removed by the coroner or medical examiner. When the hospital pathologist or other designated physician acts as an agent in the performance of an autopsy on an inpatient, the death and the autopsy are included in the percentage.
- Bodies of other hospital patients, including ambulatory care patients, hospital home care patients, and former hospital patients who died elsewhere, but whose bodies have been made available for autopsy to be performed by the hospital pathologist or other designated physician. These autopsies and deaths are included in computations of the percentage.

Generally, it is impossible to determine the number of bodies of former hospital patients who may have died in a given time period. In the formula, the phrase *available for hospital autopsy* involves several conditions, including:

- The autopsy must be performed by the hospital pathologist or a designated physician on the body of a patient treated at some time at the hospital.
- The report of the autopsy must be filed in the patient's health record and in the hospital laboratory or pathology department.
- The tissue specimens must be maintained in the hospital laboratory.

Table 15.8.   Calculation of Hospital-Based Mortality Rates

Rate	Numerator	Denominator
Gross death rate	Total number of inpatient deaths, including NBs, for a given period × 100	Total number of discharges, including A&C and NB deaths, for the same period
Net death rate (institutional death rate)	Total number of inpatient deaths, including NBs, minus deaths < 48 hours for a given period × 100	Total number of discharges, including A&C and NB deaths, minus deaths < 48 hours for the same period
Newborn death rate	Total number of NB deaths for a given period × 100	Total number of NB discharges, including deaths, for the same period
Fetal death rate	Total number of intermediate and late fetal deaths for a given period × 100	Total number of live births plus total number of intermediate and late fetal deaths for the same period
Maternal death rate	Total number of direct maternal deaths for a given period × 100	Total number of maternal (obstetric) discharges, including deaths, for the same period

Formula 15.14.   Formula for Calculating Gross Autopsy Rate

$$\text{Gross autopsy rate} = \frac{\text{Total inpatient autopsies for a given period}}{\text{Total number of inpatient deaths for the same period}} \times 100$$

Formula 15.15.   Formula for Calculating Net Autopsy Rate

$$\text{Net autopsy rate} = \frac{\text{Total number of autopsies on inpatient deaths for a period}}{\text{Total number of inpatient deaths minus unautopsied coroners' or medical examiners' cases for the same period}} \times 100$$

Figure 15.10 explains how to calculate the hospital autopsy rate.

Newborn Autopsy Rates

Autopsy rates usually include autopsies performed on newborn infants unless a separate rate is requested. The formula for calculating the **newborn autopsy rate** is shown in formula 15.17 (p. 344).

Fetal Autopsy Rates

Hospitals sometimes also calculate the **fetal autopsy rate.** Fetal autopsies are performed on stillborn infants who have been classified as either intermediate or late fetal deaths. This is the proportion or percentage of autopsies done on intermediate or late fetal deaths out of the total number of intermediate or late fetal deaths. The formula for calculating the fetal autopsy rate is shown in formula 15.18 (p. 344). Table 15.9 (p. 344) summarizes the different hospital autopsy rates.

Check Your Understanding 15.8

Instructions: Read the scenario below and answer the questions that follow.

In October, Community Hospital experienced 44 deaths. Three of them were coroner's cases, and one was autopsied by the hospital pathologist. Twenty-one autopsies were performed on the remaining deaths.

1. ___ What is the gross autopsy rate for Community Hospital for the month of October?

2. ___ What is the net autopsy rate for Community Hospital for the month of October?

Hospital Infection Rates

The most common morbidity rates calculated for hospitals are related to hospital-acquired infections, or **nosocomial infections.** The hospital must monitor the number of infections that occur in its various patient care units continuously. Infection can adversely affect the course of a patient's treatment and possibly result in death. The Joint Commission on Accreditation of Healthcare Organizations (JCAHO) requires hospitals to follow written guidelines for reporting all types of infections. Examples of the different types of infections are respiratory, gastrointestinal, surgical wound, skin, urinary tract, septicemias, and infections related to intravascular catheters.

Nosocomial Infection Rates

Nosocomial infection rates may be calculated for the entire hospital or for a specific unit in the hospital. They also may be calculated for the specific types of infections. Ideally, the hospital should strive for an infection rate of 0.0 percent. The formula for calculating the nosocomial infection rate is shown in formula 15.19 (p. 344). For example, Community Hospital discharged 725 patients during the month of June. Thirty-two of these patients experienced hospital-acquired infections. The nosocomial infection rate is 4.4 percent ($[32/725] \times 100$).

Formula 15.16.   **Formula for Calculating Hospital Autopsy Rate**

$$\text{Hospital autopsy rate} = \frac{\text{Total number of hospital autopsies for a given period}}{\text{Total number of deaths of hospital patients whose bodies were available for autopsy for the same period}} \times 100$$

Figure 15.10.   **Calculation of the Hospital Autopsy Rate**

In June, 33 inpatient deaths occurred. Three of these were medical examiner's cases. Two of the bodies were removed from the hospital and so were not available for hospital autopsy. One of the medical examiner's cases was autopsied by the hospital pathologist. Fourteen other autopsies were performed on hospital inpatients who died during the month of June. In addition, autopsies were performed in the hospital on:

- A child with congenital heart disease who died in the emergency department
- A former hospital inpatient who died in an extended care facility and whose body was brought to the hospital for autopsy
- A former hospital inpatient who died at home and whose body was brought to the hospital for autopsy
- A hospital outpatient who died while receiving chemotherapy for cancer
- A hospital home care patient whose body was brought to the hospital for autopsy
- A former hospital inpatient who died in an emergency vehicle on the way to the hospital

Calculation of total hospital autopsies:

```
  1 autopsy on medical examiner's case
+14 autopsies on hospital inpatients
+ 6 autopsies on hospital patients whose bodies were available for autopsy
```
 21 autopsies performed by the hospital pathologist

Calculation of number of deaths of hospital patients whose bodies were available for autopsy:

```
 33 inpatient deaths
− 2 medical examiner's cases
+ 6 deaths of hospital patients
```
 37 total bodies available for autopsy

Calculation of the hospital autopsy rate:

$$\frac{\text{Total number of hospital autopsies for the period}}{\text{Total number of deaths of hospital patients with bodies available for hospital autopsy for the period}} \times 100$$

$$(21 \times 100)/37 = 56.8\%$$

Postoperative Infection Rates

Hospitals often track their postoperative infection rate. The **postoperative infection rate** is the proportion or percentage of infections in clean surgical cases out of the total number of surgical operations performed. A clean surgical case is one in which no infection existed prior to surgery. The postoperative infection rate may be an indicator of a problem in the hospital environment or of some type of surgical contamination.

The individual calculating the postoperative infection rate must know the difference between a surgical procedure and a surgical operation. A *surgical procedure* is any separate, systematic process on or within the body that can be complete in itself. A physician, dentist, or some other licensed practitioner performs a surgical procedure, with or without instruments, to:

- Restore disunited or deficient parts
- Remove diseased or injured tissues
- Extract foreign matter
- Assist in obstetrical delivery
- Aid in diagnosis

A surgical operation involves one or more surgical procedures that are performed on one patient at one time using one approach to achieve a common purpose. An example of a surgical operation is the resection of a portion of both the intestine and the liver in a cancer patient. This involves two procedures, but one operation using one approach for a common purpose. In contrast, a tonsillectomy followed by an appendectomy performed at the same time is an example of two operations and two procedures. In this case, the two procedures do not have a common approach or purpose. The formula for calculating the postoperative infection rate is shown in formula 15.20.

Consultation Rates

A consultation occurs when two or more physicians collaborate on a particular patient's diagnosis or treatment. The attending physician requests the consultation and explains his or her reason for doing so. The consultant then examines the patient and the patient's health record and makes recommendations in a written report. The formula for calculating the **consultation rate** is shown in formula 15.21.

Formula 15.17.   Formula for Calculating Newborn Autopsy Rate

$$\text{Newborn autopsy rate} = \frac{\text{Total number of autopsies on NB deaths for a given time period}}{\text{Total number of NB deaths for the same period}} \times 100$$

Formula 15.18.   Formula for Calculating Fetal Autopsy Rate

$$\text{Fetal autopsy rate} = \frac{\text{Total number of autopsies on intermediate and late fetal deaths for a given period}}{\text{Total number of intermediate and late fetal deaths for the same period}} \times 100$$

Table 15.9.   Calculation of Hospital Autopsy Rates

Rate	Numerator	Denominator
Gross autopsy rate	Total number of autopsies on inpatient deaths for a given period × 100	Total number of inpatient deaths for the same period
Net autopsy rate	Total number of autopsies on inpatient deaths for a given period × 100	Total number of inpatient deaths minus unautopsied coroner or medical examiner cases for the same period
Hospital autopsy rate	Total number of hospital autopsies for a given period × 100	Total number of deaths of hospital patients whose bodies are available for hospital autopsy for the same period
Newborn (NB) autopsy rate	Total number of autopsies on NB deaths for a given period × 100	Total number of NB deaths for the same period
Fetal autopsy rate	Total number of autopsies on intermediate and late fetal deaths for a given period × 100	Total number of intermediate and late fetal deaths for the same period

Formula 15.19.   Formula for Calculating Nosocomial Infection Rate

$$\text{Nosocomial infection rate} = \frac{\text{Total number of nosocomial infections for a given period}}{\text{Total number of discharges, including deaths, for the same period}} \times 100$$

Formula 15.20.   Formula for Calculating Postoperative Infection Rate

$$\text{Postoperative infection rate} = \frac{\text{Number of infections in clean surgical cases for a given period}}{\text{Total number of surgical operations for the same period}} \times 100$$

Formula 15.21.   Formula for Calculating Consultation Rate

$$\text{Consultation rate} = \frac{\text{Total number of patients receiving consultations for a given period}}{\text{Total number of discharges and deaths for the same period}}$$

Case-Mix Statistical Data

Case mix is a method of grouping patients according to a predefined set of characteristics. Diagnosis-related groups (DRGs) are often used to determine case mix in hospitals.

When calculating case mix using DRGs, the **case-mix index** (CMI) is the average DRG weight for patients discharged from the hospital. The CMI is a measure of the relative costliness of treating the patients in each hospital or group of hospitals. It may be calculated for all patients discharged, Medicare discharges, and/or the discharges of a particular physician.

Table 15.10 provides an example of a case-mix calculation for ten DRGs at Community Hospital. The CMI is calculated by multiplying the number of cases for each DRG by the relative weight of the DRG, summing the results (2206.4701) and dividing by the total number of cases (1,631).

The CMI can be used to indicate the average reimbursement for the hospital. In this example, the reimbursement is approximately 1.35 times the hospital's base rate. It also is a measure of the severity of illness of Medicare patients and the intensity of the resources required to treat them. A hospital's annual CMI for all Medicare patients is compared to the national CMI for the same year.

Other data analyzed by DRG include LOS and mortality rates. LOS and mortality data are benchmarked against the hospital's peer group and national data. The process of benchmarking is comparing the hospital's performance to an external standard or benchmark. An excellent source of information for benchmarking purposes is the Healthcare Cost Utilization Project database (HCUPnet), which is available online at http://hcup.ahrq.gov/HCUPnet. A comparison of hospital and national data for DRG 127 appears in table 15.11.

Gross analysis of the data indicates that Community Hospital's ALOS and mortality rate are better than the national average. But, at the same time, the average charges are somewhat higher than the national average.

Statistical Data Used in Ambulatory Care Facilities

Ambulatory care includes healthcare services provided to patients who are not hospitalized (that is, who are not considered inpatients or residents and do not stay in the healthcare facility overnight). Such patients are referred to as outpatients. Most ambulatory care services today are provided in freestanding physicians' offices, emergency care centers, and ambulatory diagnostic surgery centers that are not owned or operated by acute care organizations. Hospitals do, however, provide many hospital-based healthcare services to outpatients. Hospital outpatients receive services in one or more areas within the hospital, including clinics, same-day surgery departments, diagnostic departments, and emergency departments.

Outpatient statistics include records of the number of patient visits and the types of services provided. Many different terms are used to describe outpatients and ambulatory care services, including:

- *Hospital ambulatory care:* Hospital-directed preventive, therapeutic, and rehabilitative services provided by physicians and their surrogates to patients who are not hospital inpatients or home care patients
- *Outpatient:* A patient who receives care without being admitted for inpatient or residential care
- *Hospital outpatient:* A patient who receives services in one or more of the facilities owned and operated by a hospital
- *Emergency outpatient:* A patient who is admitted to the emergency department or equivalent service of a hospital for diagnosis and treatment of a condition that requires immediate medical services, dental services, or related healthcare services

Table 15.10.   Calculation of Case-Mix Index for Community Hospital

DRG	Number (N)	DRG Weight	$N \times$ DRG Weight
127	287	1.0265	294.6055
89	104	1.1156	116.0224
88	120	0.9846	118.1520
14	115	1.1999	137.9885
209	162	2.2606	366.2172
79	67	1.6300	109.2100
143	71	0.5223	37.0833
182	60	0.7789	46.7340
462	542	1.4298	774.9516
174	103	1.9952	205.5056
	1,631		2206.4701
CMI			**1.3528**

Table 15.11.   Benchmark Data, Community Hospital versus National Average for DRG 127, Heart Failure and Shock

	ALOS	Mortality Rate	Average Charges
Community Hospital	4.6	0.3%	$12,042
National average	5.4	5.0%	$9,694

- *Clinic outpatient:* A patient who is admitted to a clinical service of a clinic or hospital for diagnosis or treatment on an ambulatory basis
- *Referred outpatient:* A patient who is provided special hospital-based diagnostic or therapeutic services on an ambulatory basis; the services are ordered by a referring physician and the responsibility for medical care remains with that physician rather than with the hospital
- *Outpatient visit:* A provision of services to an outpatient in one or more units or facilities located in or directed by the provider maintaining the outpatient healthcare services
- *Encounter:* A contact between a patient and a healthcare professional who has primary responsibility for assessing and treating a patient at a given contact and for exercising independent medical judgment
- *Occasion of service:* A specified, identifiable service involved in the care of a patient or consumer that is not an encounter; occasions of service may be the result of an encounter, for example, to fulfill physicians' orders for tests or procedures ordered as part of an encounter
- *Ambulatory surgery centers:* Hospital-based or freestanding surgical facilities that perform elective surgical procedures on patients who are classified as outpatients and who are typically released from the facility on the same day the surgery was performed; also referred to as short-stay surgery, one-day surgery, same-day surgery, or come-and-go surgery services

Presentation of Statistical Data

Collected data are often more meaningful when presented in graphic form. Tables, charts, and graphs offer the opportunity to analyze data sets and to explore, understand, and present distributions, trends, and relationships in the data. Methods of displaying data in graphic form are discussed in the following subsections.

Graphic Presentations

After data have been summarized in aggregate form, it is often useful to display them in a graphic form such as a table, chart, or graph. Graphic forms are effective ways of presenting large quantities of information. The purpose of tables, charts, and graphs is to communicate information about the data to the user of the data.

Whatever type of graphic form is used, it should:

- Display the data
- Allow the user to think about the meaning of the data
- Avoid distortion of the data
- Encourage the user to make comparisons
- Reveal data at several levels, from a broad overview to the fine detail

Tables

A **table** is an orderly arrangement of values that groups data into rows and columns. Almost any type of quantitative information can be organized into a table. Tables are useful for demonstrating patterns and other kinds of relationships. In addition, they may serve as the basis for more visual displays of data, such as charts and graphs, where some of the detail may be lost. However, because tables are not very interesting, they should be used sparingly.

A useful first step is to prepare a table shell that shows how the data will be organized and displayed. A table shell is the outline of a table with everything in place except for the data. (See table 15.12.) A table should contain all the information the reader needs to understand the data in it. It should have the following characteristics:

Table 15.12.   Table Shell

TITLE							
		Sex				Total	
		Male		Female			
Box Head	*Age*	**Number**	**%**	**Number**	**%**	**Number**	**%**
Stub	*Row Variable*		→→→→→	→→→→→	→→→→→	→→→→→	→→→→→
	<45			*Column Variable*			
↓	45–54			↓			
↓	55–64			↓			
↓	65–74			↓			
↓	75+			↓			

Source: Adapted from *Self-Instructional Manual for Cancer Registries, Book 7: Statistics and Epidemiology for Cancer Registries.* U.S. Department of Health and Human Services, Public Health Service, NIH Publication No. 94-3766. 1994.

- It is a logical unit.
- It is self-explanatory and can stand on its own when photocopied and/or removed from its context.
- All sources are specified.
- Specific, understandable headings are provided for every column and row.
- Row and column totals are checked for accuracy.
- Blank cells are not left empty. When no information is available for a particular cell, the cell should contain a zero or a dash.
- Categories are mutually exclusive and exhaustive.

The data contained in tables should be aligned. Guidelines for aligning text and numbers include:

- Text in the table should be aligned at left.
- Text that serves as a column label may be centered.
- Numeric values should be aligned at right.
- When numeric values contain decimals, the decimals should be aligned.

The essential components of a table are summarized in figure 15.11.

Tables may contain information on one, two, or three variables. Tables 15.13 and 15.14 are examples of one- and two-variable tables, respectively.

Charts and Graphs

Charts and graphs of various types are the best means for presenting data for quick visualization of relationships. They emphasize the main points and analyze and clarify relationships among variables.

Several principles are involved in the construction of charts and graphs. When constructing charts and graphs, the following points should be considered:

- *Distortion:* To avoid distorting the data, the representation of the numbers should be proportional to the numerical quantities represented.
- *Proportion and scale:* Graphs should emphasize the horizontal. It is easier for the eye to read along the horizontal axis from left to right. Also, graphs should be greater in length than height. A useful guideline is to follow the three-quarter-high rule. This rule states that the height (*y*-axis) of the graph should be three-fourths the length (*x*-axis) of the graph.
- *Abbreviations:* Any abbreviations should be spelled out in notes.
- *Color:* Colors may be used to highlight groupings that appear in the graph.
- *Print:* Both upper- and lowercase letters should be used in titles; the use of all capital letters can be unfriendly to the eyes.

Bar Charts

Bar charts are used to display data from one or more variables. The bars may be drawn vertically or horizontally. The simplest bar chart is the one-variable bar chart. In this type of

Figure 15.11.   Essential Components of a Table

Title	The title should be as complete as possible and should clearly relate to the content of the table. It should answer the following questions: • What are the data (e.g., counts, percentages)? • Who (e.g., white females with breast cancer; black males with lung cancer)? • Where are the data from (e.g., hospital, state, community)? • When (e.g., year, month)? A sample title might be: Site Distribution by Age and Sex of Cancer Patients upon First Admission to Community Hospital
Box Head	The box head contains the captions or column headings. The heading of each column should contain as few words as possible but should explain exactly what the data in the column represent.
Stub	The row captions are known as the stub. Items in the stub should be grouped to make it easy to interpret the data, for example, ages grouped into five-year intervals.
Cell	The cell is the box formed by the intersection of a column and a row.
Optional Items:	
Note	Notes are used to explain anything in the table that the reader cannot understand from the title, box head, or stub. They contain numbers, preliminary or revised numbers, or explanations of any unusual numbers. Definitions, abbreviations, and/or qualifications for captions or cell names should be footnoted. A note usually applies to a specific cell(s) within the table, and a symbol (e.g., ** or #) may be used to key the cell to the note. If several notes are used, it is better to use small letters than symbols or numbers. Note any numbers that may be confused with the numbers within the table.
Source	If data are used from a source outside the research, the exact reference to the source should be given. The source lends authenticity to the data and allows the reader to locate the original information if he or she needs it.

Source: Adapted from *Self-Instructional Manual for Cancer Registries, Book 7: Statistics and Epidemiology for Cancer Registries.* U.S. Department of Health and Human Services, Public Health Service, NIH Publication No. 94-3766. 1994.

Table 15.13.   One-Variable Table, Community Hospital Admissions, by Sex

Sex	Number	%
Male	3,546	42.4
Female	4,825	57.6
Total	8,371	100.0

Table 15.14.   Two-Variable Table, Community Hospital Admissions by Race and Sex, 1999

	Sex		
Race	**Male**	**Female**	**Total**
White	2,908	3,860	6,768
Nonwhite	638	965	1,603
Total	3,546	4,825	8,371

chart, a bar represents each category of the variable. For example, if the data in table 15.13 were displayed in a bar chart, "sex" would be the variable and "male and female" would be the variable categories. Figure 15.12 displays the data from table 15.13 as a bar chart. The length or height of each bar is proportional to the number of males and females discharged. Presentation of the data in a bar chart makes it easy to see that more females than males were admitted to Community Hospital in 1999.

Figure 15.13 displays the two-variable data from table 15.14 as a two-variable or grouped-variable bar chart in a three-dimensional format. Computer software makes it easy to present data in this way. However, presenting data in a three-dimensional format can be tricky. The reader may not always be able to estimate the true height of the bar. In a three-dimensional bar chart, the back edges of the bar appear higher than the front edge, as in figure 15.13. To make sure

the reader correctly interprets the chart, the bars should include the actual values for each category.

Figure 15.14 presents guidelines for constructing bar charts.

Pie Charts

A **pie chart** is an easily understood chart in which the sizes of the slices of the pie show the proportional contribution of each part. Pie charts can be used to show the component parts of a single group or variable.

To calculate the size of each slice of the pie, first determine the proportion that each slice is to represent. Multiplying the proportion by 360 (the total number of degrees in a circle) will give the size of each slice of the pie in degrees.

Figure 15.15 shows data collected on admissions to Community Hospital by religion. The summary data for one year show that 50 percent of the patients were Protestant, 20 per-

Figure 15.12.   One-Variable Bar Chart, Community Hospital Admissions by Sex, 1999

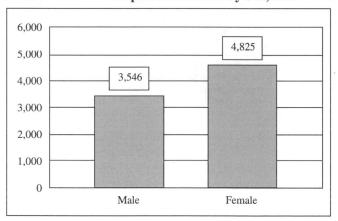

Figure 15.14.   Guidelines for Constructing a Bar Chart

When constructing a bar chart, keep the following points in mind:

- Arrange the bar categories in a natural order, such as alphabetical order, order by increasing age, or an order that will produce increasing or decreasing bar lengths.
- The bars may be positioned vertically or horizontally.
- All bars should be the same width.
- The length of the bars should be proportional to the frequency of the event.
- Avoid using more than one three bars (categories) within a group of bars.
- Leave a space between adjacent groups of bars, but not between bars within a group.
- Code different categories of variables by differences in bar color, shading, and/or cross-hatching. Include a legend that explains the coding system.

Source: Adapted from U.S. Department of Health and Human Services, Public Health Service. 1992. *Principles of Epidemiology: An Introduction to Applied Epidemiology and Biostatistics.* Atlanta: USDHHS.

Figure 15.13.   Two-Variable Bar Chart, Community Hospital Admissions by Race and Sex, 1999

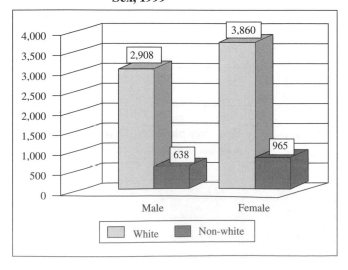

Figure 15.15.   Pie Chart, Community Hospital Admissions by Religion, 1999

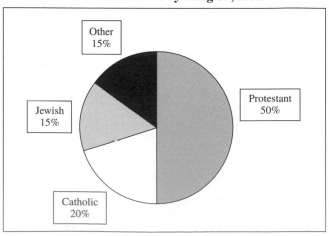

cent were Catholic, 15 percent were Jewish, and 15 percent fell into the "other" category. With 50 percent of the pie chart, the Protestant category equals 180° (360° × .50 = 180°). The Jewish and "other" categories each equal 54° (360° × .15 = 54°). Finally, the Catholic category equals 72° (360° × .20 = 72°). Taken together, the four slices equal 360° (180° + 54° + 54° + 72° = 360°).

The slices of the pie should be arranged in some logical order. By convention, the largest slices begin at twelve o'clock. Computer software is available to make the construction of pie charts easy. The pie chart in figure 15.15 was prepared using Excel™.

Line Graphs

A **line graph** may be used to display time trends. The x-axis shows the unit of time from left to right, and the y-axis measures the values of the variable being plotted. A line graph does not represent a frequency distribution.

A line graph consists of a line connecting a series of points. Like all graphs, a line graph should be constructed so that it is easy to read. Selection of the proper scale, a complete and accurate title, and an informative legend is important. When a graph is too long and narrow, either vertically or horizontally, it has an awkward appearance and may exaggerate one aspect of the data.

A line graph is especially useful for plotting a large number of observations. It also allows several sets of data to be presented on one graph.

Either actual numbers or percentages may be used on the y-axis of the graph. Percentages should be used on the y-axis when more than one distribution is to be shown. A percent-age distribution allows comparisons among groups where the actual totals are different.

When two or more sets of data are plotted on the same graph, the lines should be made different—solid or broken—for each set. However, the number of lines should be kept to a minimum to avoid confusion. Each line then should be identified in a legend located on the graph.

There are two kinds of time-trend data: point data and period data. *Point data* reflect an instant in time. Figure 15.16 displays point data—the total number of admissions for each year represented in the graph. *Period data* are averages or totals over a specified period of time, such as a five-year time frame. Table 15.15 (p. 350) summarizes period data for survival rates of patients diagnosed with kidney cancer. Figure 15.17 (p. 350) displays these period data in a line graph.

Histograms

As mentioned earlier, a **histogram** is used to display a frequency distribution. It is different from a bar graph in that a bar graph is used to display data that fall into groups or categories. The categories are noncontinuous, or discrete. In a bar chart, the bars representing the different categories are separated. (See figures 15.12 and 15.13.) On the other hand, histograms are used to illustrate frequency distributions of continuous variables, such as age or LOS. A continuous variable can take on a fractional value (for example, 75.345°F). With continuous variables, there are no gaps between values because the values progress fractionally.

In a histogram, the frequency distribution may be displayed as a number or a percentage. The histogram consists of a series of bars. Each bar has one class interval as its base

Figure 15.16.   Line Graph with Point Data, Community Hospital Admissions, 1995–1999

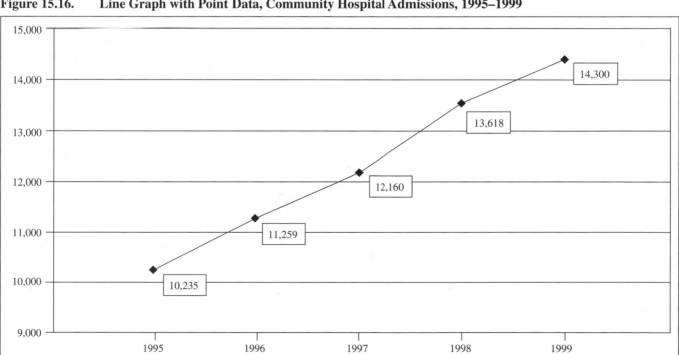

Table 15.15.   Sample Five-Year Survival Rates for Kidney Cancer, by Stage, for Patients Diagnosed between 1990 and 1997

Year of Diagnosis	Midpoint of Interval	Survival Rate (%)		
		Localized	Regional	Distant
1990–1992	1991	80	71	28
1993–1995	1994	84	71	29
1996–1998	1997	85	74	31

and the number (frequency) or percentage of cases in that class interval as its height. A class interval is a type of category. It can represent one value in a frequency distribution (for example, three years of age) or a group of values (for example, ages three to five).

In histograms, there are no spaces between the bars. (See figure 15.18.) The lack of spaces between bars depicts the continuous nature of the distribution. The sum of the heights of the bars represents the total number, or 100 percent, of the cases. Histograms should be used when the distribution of the data needs to be emphasized more than the values of the distribution.

Frequency Polygons

A **frequency polygon** is an alternative to a histogram. Like a histogram, it is a graph of a frequency distribution, but in line form rather than bar form. The advantage of frequency polygons is that several of them can be placed on the same graph to make comparisons. Another advantage is that frequency polygons are easy to interpret.

When constructing a frequency polygon, the *x*-axis should be made longer than the *y*-axis to avoid distorting the data. The frequency of observations is always placed on the *y*-axis and the scale of the variable on the *x*-axis. The frequency polygon in figure 15.19 plots the same data that appear in the histogram in figure 15.18. Because the *x*-axis represents the entire frequency distribution, the line starts at zero cases and ends with zero cases.

Spreadsheets and Statistical Packages

Electronic spreadsheets, such as Microsoft Excel, and statistical packages, such as SPSS or SAS, can be used to facilitate the data collection and analysis processes. The advantage of using one of these tools is that charts and graphs may be formulated at the time the data are being analyzed. Because instruction in the use of these tools is beyond the scope of this chapter, it is strongly recommended that the reader become well versed in the use of the available microcomputer software.

Check Your Understanding 15.9

Instructions: Fill in the blanks in the following sentences.

1. A presentation of data in rows and columns is a ___.
2. A graphic display technique used to display parts of a whole is a ___.
3. A graphic display technique used to show trends over time is a ___.
4. A graphic display technique used to display categories of a variable is a ___.
5. A graphic display technique that may be used to show the age distribution of a population is a ___.

Figure 15.17.   Period Data Trend Line: Survival Rates for Kidney Cancer by Stage for Patients Diagnosed from 1990 through 1997

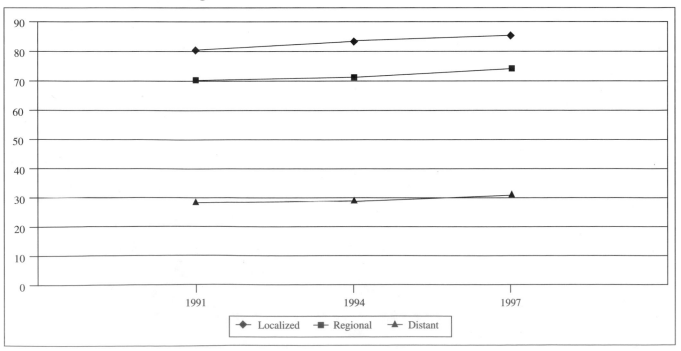

Public Health Statistics and Epidemiological Information

Just as statistics are collected in the healthcare organizational setting, they also are collected on a community, regional, and national basis. Vital statistics are an example of data collected and reported at these levels. The term *vital*

Figure 15.18. **Histogram, Community Hospital Length of Stay of Patients Discharged from DRG 127, 1997**

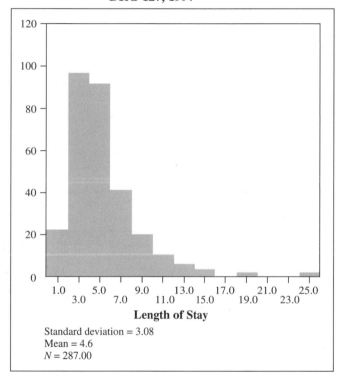

Standard deviation = 3.08
Mean = 4.6
$N = 287.00$

statistics refers to the collection and analysis of data related to the crucial events in life: birth, death, marriage, divorce, fetal death, and induced terminations of pregnancy. These statistics are used to identify trends. For example, a higher-than-expected death rate among newborns may be an indication of the lack of prenatal services in a community. A number of deaths in a region due to the same cause may indicate an environmental problem.

These types of data are used as part of the effort to preserve and improve the health of a defined population—the public health. The study of factors that influence the health status of a population is called epidemiology.

National Vital Statistics System

The **National Vital Statistics System** (NVSS) is responsible for maintaining the official vital statistics of the United States. These statistics are provided to the federal government by state-operated registration systems. The NVSS is housed in the National Center for Health Statistics (NCHS) of the Centers for Disease Control (CDC).

To facilitate data collection, standard forms and model procedures for the uniform registration of events are developed and recommended for state use through cooperative activities of the individual states and the NCHS. The standard certificates represent the minimum basic data set necessary for the collection and publication of comparable national, state, and local vital statistics data. The standard forms are revised about every ten years, with the last revision being done in 1989.

The *certificate of live birth* is used for registration purposes and is composed of two parts. The first part contains the information related to the child and the parents. The second part is used to collect data about the mother's pregnancy. This information is used for the collection of aggregate data

Figure 15.19.   Frequency Polygon, Community Hospital Length of Stay of Patients Discharged from DRG 127, 1997

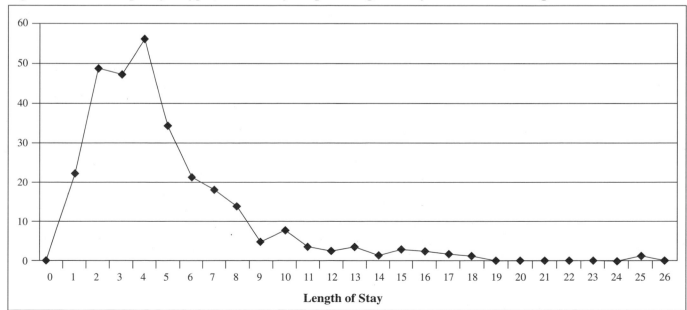

only. No identification information appears on this portion of the certificate nor does it ever appear on the official certificate of birth. Pregnancy-related information includes complications of pregnancy, concurrent illnesses or conditions affecting pregnancy, and abnormal conditions and/or congenital anomalies of the newborn. Lifestyle factors such as use of alcohol and tobacco also are collected. Thus, the birth certificate is the major source of maternal and natality statistics. A listing of pregnancy-related information appears in figure 15.20.

Data collected from *death certificates* are used to compile causes of death in the United States. The certificate of death contains decedent information, place of death information, medical certification, and disposition information. Examples of the content of death certificates appear in figure 15.21.

A *report of fetal death* is completed when a pregnancy results in a stillbirth. This report contains information on the parents, the history of the pregnancy, and the cause of the fetal death. Information collected on the pregnancy is the same as that recorded on the birth certificate. To assess the effects of environmental exposures on the fetus, the parents' occupational data are collected. Data items related to the fetus include:

- Cause of fetal death, whether fetal or maternal
- Other significant conditions of the fetus or mother
- When fetus died—before labor, during labor or delivery, or unknown

The *report of induced termination of pregnancy* records information on the place of the induced termination of preg-

nancy, the type of termination procedure, and the patient. (See figure 15.22.)

A tool for monitoring and exploring the interrelationships between infant death and risk factors at birth is the linked birth and infant death data set. This is a service provided by the NCHS. In this data set, the information from the death

Figure 15.21.   Content of the U.S. Certificate of Death, 1989

Decedent Information:	Medical Certification:
Name	Immediate cause of death—
Sex	interval between onset and
Race	death:
Hispanic origin	Due to—
Age in years and months	Due to—
Date of birth	Due to—
Birthplace	Other significant conditions
Marital status	Was autopsy performed?
Surviving spouse (if wife, give	Were autopsy findings available
maiden name	prior to completion of cause
Was decedent ever in U.S.	of death?
armed forces?	For deaths from external causes:
Social Security number	Date of injury
Usual occupation	Time of injury
Business or industry	How injury occurred
Residence	Injury at work?
Education	Place of injury
Father's name	Location of injury
Birthplace of father	
Mother's maiden name	**Disposition Information:**
Birthplace of mother	Method of disposition
	Name of cemetery or crematory
Place of Death Information:	and location
County	Name of funeral director
City, town, or location	Name of funeral home
Name of facility	Address of funeral home
If hospital or institution,	
indicate whether dead on	
arrival, outpatient or	
emergency room, or inpatient	
If not in hospital or institution,	
give street address of location	

Figure 15.22.   Content of the U.S. Certificate of Termination of Pregnancy, 1989

Place of Induced Termination:	Patient Information:
Name of facility	Patient identification
Address (city, town, state,	Age
county)	Marital status
	Residence (city, state, county,
Induced Termination	ZIP code)
Information:	Race
Date of pregnancy termination	Education
Previous pregnancies:	Hispanic origin
Live births, now living	
Live births, now dead	
Other terminations	
(spontaneous)	
Other terminations (induced)	
Date last normal menses began	
Physician's estimate of	
gestation	
Clinical estimate of gestation	
Type of termination procedures	
Procedure that terminated	
pregnancy	
Additional procedures used	

Figure 15.20.   Content of the U.S. Certificate of Live Birth, 1989

Birth Information	Pregnancy History
Name of child	Live births, now living
Sex	Live births, now dead
Date of birth	Other terminations
Time of birth	(spontaneous and induced at
Place of birth (name of	any time after conception)
hospital)	Date of last live birth
Birth weight	Date of last other termination
Single, twin, triplet, etc.	Clinical estimate of gestation
Apgar scores—1 and 5 minutes	Date last normal menses began
	Month prenatal care began
Mother's Information	Number of prenatal visits
Maiden surname	Medical risk factors for
Full name	pregnancy
Date of birth	Other risk factors for pregnancy
Birthplace (state or country)	(smoking, alcohol use, weight
Residence	gain)
Mother's mailing address	Complications of labor and/or
Hispanic origin	delivery
Race	Obstetric procedures
Education	Method of delivery
Mother married?	Abnormal conditions of the
	newborn
Father's Information	Congenital anomalies of child
Name	
Date of birth	
Birthplace	
Hispanic origin	
Race	
Education	

certificate (such as age and underlying or multiple causes of death) is linked to the information in the birth certificate (such as age, race, birth weight, prenatal care usage, maternal education, and so on) for each infant who dies in the United States, Puerto Rico, the Virgin Islands, and Guam. The purpose of the data set is to use the many additional variables available from the birth certificate to conduct a detailed analysis of infant mortality patterns.

Birth, death, fetal death, and termination of pregnancy certificates provide vital information for use in medical research, epidemiological studies, and other public health programs. In addition, they are the source of data for compiling morbidity, birth, and mortality rates that describe the health of a given population at the local, state, or national level. Because of their many uses, the data on these certificates must be complete and accurate.

Population-Based Statistics

Population-based statistics are based on the mortality and morbidity rates from which the health of a population can be inferred. The entire defined population is used in the collection and reporting of these statistics. The size of the defined population serves as the denominator in the calculation of these rates.

Birth Rates and Measures of Infant Mortality

Two community-based rates that are commonly used to describe a community's health are the crude birth rate and measures of infant mortality. The official international definition of a live birth is the delivery of a product of conception that shows any sign of life after complete removal from the mother. A sign of life may consist of a breath or cry, any spontaneous movement, a pulse or heartbeat, or pulsation of the umbilical cord.

Rates that describe infant mortality are based on age. Therefore, the definitions for the various age groups must be strictly followed. Table 15.16 summarizes the calculations for community-based birth and infant mortality rates.

Crude Birth Rate

As shown in formula 15.22, the **crude birth rate** is the number of live births divided by the population at risk. As the formula shows, community rates are calculated using the multiplier 1,000, 10,000, or 100,000. The purpose is to bring the rate to a whole number, as discussed earlier in the chapter. The result of the formula would be stated as the number of live births per 1,000 population. For example, if there were 7,532 live births in a community of 600,000 in 1999, the crude birth rate for that year would be 12.6 per 1,000 population ([7,532/600,000] × 1000).

Neonatal Mortality Rate

The **neonatal mortality rate** can be used as an indirect measure of the quality of prenatal care and/or the mother's prenatal behavior (for example, alcohol, drug, or tobacco use). The neonatal period is the period from birth up to, but not including, 28 days of age. In the formula for calculating the neonatal mortality rate, the numerator is the number of deaths of infants under 28 days of age during a given time period and the denominator is the total number of live births during the same time period.

Postneonatal Mortality Rate

The **postneonatal mortality rate** is often used as an indicator of the quality of the home or community environment of infants. The postneonatal period is the period from 28 days up to but not including one year of age. In the formula for calculating the postneonatal mortality rate, the numerator is the number of deaths among infants from age 28 days up to but not including one year during a given time period and the denominator is the total number of live births less the number of neonatal deaths during the same time period.

Infant Mortality Rate

The **infant mortality rate** is the summary of the neonatal and postneonatal mortality rates. In the formula for calculating the infant mortality rate, the numerator is the number of deaths

Table 15.16.   Calculation of Community-Based Birth and Infant Death (Mortality) Rates

Measure	Numerator (x)	Denominator (y)	10^n
Crude birth rate	Number of live births for a given community for a specified time period	Estimated population for the same community and the same time period	1,000
Neonatal death rate	Number of deaths under 28 days up to but not including one year of age during a given time period	Number of live births during the same time period	1,000
Postneonatal death rate	Number of deaths from 28 days up to but not including one year of age during a given time period	Number of live births during the same time period less neonatal deaths	1,000
Infant death rate	Number of deaths under one year of age during a given time period	Number of live births during the same time period	1,000

Formula 15.22.   Formula for Calculating Crude Birth Rate

$$\text{Crude birth rate} = \frac{\text{Number of live births for a given community for a specified time period}}{\text{Estimated population for the same community and the same time period}} \times 1,000$$

among infants under one year of age and the denominator is the number of live births during the same period. The infant mortality rate is the most commonly used measure for comparing health status among nations. All the rates are expressed in terms of the number of deaths per 1,000.

Death (Mortality) Rates

Other measures of mortality with which the HIM professional should be familiar include the crude death rate, the cause-specific death rate, the case fatality rate, the proportionate mortality rate, and the maternal death rate. Table 15.17 summarizes the calculations for these rates.

Crude Death Rate

The **crude death rate** is a measure of the actual or observed mortality in a given population. Crude death rates apply to a population without regard to characteristics such as age, race, and sex. They measure the proportion of the population that has died during a given period of time (usually one year) or the number of deaths in a community per 1,000 for a given period of time. The formula for calculating the crude death rate is shown in formula 15.23.

Cause-Specific Death Rate

As its name indicates, the **cause-specific death rate** is the rate of death due to a specified cause. It may be calculated for an entire population or for any age, sex, or race. In the formula, the numerator is the number of deaths due to a specified cause for a given time period and the denominator is the estimated population for the same time period.

Table 15.18 displays cause-specific death rates for men and women due to pneumonia for the year 1995. The cause-specific death rates for each age group are consistently higher for men than for women. This information could lead to an investigation of why men are more susceptible to death from pneumonia than women.

Case Fatality Rate

The **case fatality rate** measures the probability of death among the diagnosed cases of a disease, most often acute illness. In the formula for calculating the case fatality rate, the numerator is the number of deaths due to a specific disease that occurred during a specific time period and the denominator is the number of diagnosed cases during the same time period. The higher the case fatality rate, the more virulent the infection.

Table 15.17.   Calculation of Community-Based Death (Mortality) Rates

Rate	Numerator (x)	Denominator (y)	10^n
Crude death rate	Total number of deaths for a population during a specified time period	Estimated population for the same time period	1,000 or 10,000 or 100,000
Cause-specific death rate	Total number of deaths due to a specific cause during a specified time period	Estimated population for the same time period	100,000
Case fatality rate	Total number of deaths due to a specific disease during a specified time period	Total number of cases due to a specific disease during the same time period	100
Proportionate mortality (ratio)	Total number of deaths due to a specific cause during a specified time period	Total number of deaths from all causes during the same time period	NA
Maternal mortality rate	Total number of deaths due to pregnancy-related conditions during a specified time period	Total number of live births during the same time period	100,000

Formula 15.23.   Formula for Calculating Crude Death Rate

$$\text{Crude death rate} = \frac{\text{Total number of deaths for a population during a specified time period}}{\text{Estimated population for the same time period}} \times 10^n$$

Table 15.18.   Cause-Specific Mortality Rates due to Pneumonia (ICD-9-CM Codes 480–486.9), Age 65+, United States, 1995

Age Group	Men			Women		
	Population	Deaths	Rate/100,000	Population	Deaths	Rate/100,000
65–74	8,342,094	6,223	74.60	10,417,069	1,385	13.30
75–84	4,329,706	13,154	303.81	6,815,274	12,696	186.29
85+	1,016,875	13,000	1,278.43	2,611,279	24,275	929.62
	13,688,675	32,377	236.52	19,843,622	38,356	193.29

Source: Centers for Disease Control and Prevention, CDC Wonder Data Base. Information from http://wonder.cdc.gov.

Proportionate Mortality Rate

The **proportionate mortality ratio** (PMR) is a measure of mortality due to a specific cause for a specific time period. In the formula for calculating the PMR, the numerator is the number of deaths due to a specific disease for a specific time period and the denominator is the number of deaths from all causes for the same time period. Table 15.19 displays the PMRs for pneumonia in the United States in 1995.

Maternal Mortality Rate

The **maternal mortality rate** measures the deaths associated with pregnancy for a specific community for a specific period of time. It is calculated only for deaths that are directly related to pregnancy. In the formula for calculating the maternal mortality rate, the numerator is the number of deaths attributed to causes related to pregnancy during a spe-

cific time period for a given community and the denominator is the number of live births reported during the same time period for the same community. Because the maternal mortality rate is very small, it is usually expressed as the number of deaths per 100,000 live births.

Check Your Understanding 15.10

Instructions: Review the mortality data in table 15.20 and then answer the following questions on a separate piece of paper.

1. ___ What is the AIDS crude death rate per 1,000,000 for men?
2. ___ What is the AIDS crude death rate per 1,000,000 for women?
3. ___ What is the AIDS crude death rate per 1,000,000 for the entire group?
4. ___ What is the AIDS crude death rate per 1,000,000 for men ages 35–44?
5. ___ What is the AIDS crude death rate per 1,000,000 for women ages 35–55?

Measures of Morbidity

Two measures are commonly used to describe the presence of disease in a community or specific location (for example, a nursing home): incidence and prevalence rates. *Disease* is defined as any illness, injury, or disability. Incidence and prevalence measures can be broken down by race, sex, age, or other characteristics of a population.

Incidence Rate

An **incidence rate** is used to compare the frequency of disease in populations. Populations are compared using rates instead of raw numbers because rates adjust for differences in population size. The incidence rate is the probability or risk of illness in a population over a period of time.

The formula for calculating the incidence rate is shown in formula 15.24 (p. 356). The denominator represents the population from which the case in the numerator arose, such as a nursing home, school, or organization. For 10^n, a value is selected so that the smallest rate calculated results in a whole number.

Table 15.19.   Proportionate Mortality Ratios for Pneumonia (ICD-9-CM Codes 480–486.9), United States, 1995

Age Group	Pneumonia Deaths	All Deaths	PMR
0–4	634	35,976	.018
5–14	121	8,596	.014
15–24	201	34,244	.006
25–34	621	57,745	.011
35–44	1,466	102,270	.014
45–54	2,061	143,000	.014
55–64	3,427	235,512	.015
65–74	10,657	480,890	.022
75–84	25,850	652,177	.040
85+	37,275	561,259	.066
Total	82,313	2,311,669	.036

Source: Centers for Disease Control and Prevention, CDC Wonder Data Base. Information from http://wonder.cdc.gov.

Table 15.20.   Data for Check Your Understanding 15.10

Age Group	Deaths due to AIDS (ICD-9 Code 042), by Age and Sex, United States, 1997			
	Males		Females	
	Deaths due to AIDS	Total Population	Deaths due to AIDS	Total Population
<20 years	102	39,531,297	89	37,548,585
20-34 years	2,950	28,789,715	1,038	28,331,602
35-44 years	5,277	21,882,825	1,387	22,115,103
45-54 years	2,683	16,456,766	592	17,175,868
55-64 years	818	10,390,590	168	11,422,400
65-74 years	262	8,268,823	50	10,229,727
75-84 years	38	4,628,816	19	7,076,897
85+ years	3	1,111,910	2	2,759,438
Total	12,133	131,060,742	3,345	136,659,620

Source: Centers for Disease Control and Prevention, CDC Wonder Data Base. Information from http://wonder.cdc.gov.

Prevalence Rate

The **prevalence rate** is the proportion of persons in a population who have a particular disease at a specific point in time or over a specified period of time. The formula for calculating the prevalence rate is shown in formula 15.25. The prevalence rate describes the magnitude of an epidemic and can be an indicator of the medical resources needed in a community for the duration of the epidemic.

It is easy to confuse incidence and prevalence rates. The distinction is in the numerators of their formulas. The numerator in the formula for the incidence rate is the number of *new* cases occurring in a given time period. The numerator in the formula for the prevalence rate is all cases present during a given time period. In addition, the incidence rate includes only patients whose illness began during a specified time period whereas the prevalence rate includes all patients from a specified cause regardless of when the illness began. Moreover, the prevalence rate includes a patient until he or she recovers.

National Notifiable Diseases Surveillance System

In 1878, Congress authorized the U.S. Marine Hospital Service to collect morbidity reports on cholera, smallpox, plague, and yellow fever from U.S. consuls overseas. This information was used to implement quarantine measures to prevent the spread of these diseases to the United States. In 1879, Congress provided for the weekly collection and publication of reports of these diseases. In 1893, Congress expanded the scope to include weekly reporting from states and municipalities. To provide for more uniformity in data collection, Congress enacted a law in 1902 that directed the Surgeon General to provide standard forms for the collection, compilation, and publication of reports at the national level. In 1912, the states and U.S. territories recommended that infectious disease be immediately reported by telegraph. By 1928, all states, the District of Columbia, Hawaii, and Puerto Rico were participating in the national reporting of twenty-nine specified diseases. In 1961, the CDC assumed responsibility for the collection and publication of data concerning nationally notifiable diseases.

A **notifiable disease** is one for which regular, frequent, and timely information on individual cases is considered necessary to prevent and control disease. The list of notifiable diseases varies over time and by state. The Council of State and Territorial Epidemiologists (CSTE) collaborate with the CDC to determine which diseases should be reported. State reporting to the CDC is voluntary. However, all states generally report the internationally quarantinable diseases in accordance with the World Health Organization's International Health Regulations. Completeness of reporting varies by state and type of disease and may be influenced by any of the following factors:

- The type and severity of the illness
- Whether treatment in a healthcare facility was sought
- The diagnosis of an illness
- The availability of diagnostic services
- The disease-control measures in effect
- The public's awareness of the disease
- The resources, priorities, and interests of state and local public health officials

Information that is reported includes date, county, age, sex, race/ethnicity, and disease-specific epidemiologic information; personal identifiers are not included. A strict CSTE Data Release Policy regulates the dissemination of the data. A list of nationally notifiable infectious diseases appears in figure 15.23.

National morbidity data are reported weekly. Public health managers and providers use the reports to rapidly identify disease epidemics and to understand patterns of disease occurrence. Case-specific information is included in the reports. Changes in age, sex, race/ethnicity, and geographic distributions can be monitored and investigated as necessary.

Check Your Understanding 15.11

Instructions: Answer the following questions on a separate piece of paper.

1. Define incidence and prevalence.

2. Calculate the incidence rate, per 100,000, for the following hypothetical data: In 2000, 41,595 new cases of AIDS were reported in the United States. The estimated population for 2000 was 248,710,000.

Formula 15.24.   Formula for Calculating Incidence Rate

$$\text{Incidence rate} = \frac{\text{Total number of new cases of a specific disease during a given time period}}{\text{Total population at risk during the same time period}} \times 10^n$$

Formula 15.25.   Formula for Calculating Prevalence Rate

$$\text{Prevalence rate} = \frac{\text{All new and preexisting cases of a specific disease during a given time period}}{\text{Total population during the same time period}} \times 10^n$$

Figure 15.23.   Nationally Notifiable Infectious Diseases, United States, 2001

Acquired immunodeficiency syndrome (AIDS)	Malaria
	Measles
Anthrax	Meningococcal disease
Botulism	Mumps
Brucellosis	Pertussis
Chancroid	Plague
Chlamydia trachomatis, genital infections	Poliomyelitis, paralytic
	Psittacosis
Cholera	Q fever
Coccidioidomycosis	Rabies, animal
Cryptosporidiosis	Rabies, human
Cyclosporiasis	Rocky Mountain spotted fever
Diphtheria	Rubella
Ehrlichiosis	Rubella, congenital syndrome
Encephalitis	Salmonellosis
Enterohemorrhagic *Escherichia coli*	Shigellosis
	Streptococcal disease, invasive, group A
Gonorrhea	
Haemophilus influenzae, invasive disease	Streptococcal toxic shock syndrome
Hanson disease (leprosy)	*Streptococcus pneumoniae,* drug-resistant, invasive disease
Hantavirus pulmonary syndrome	
Hemolytic uremic syndrome, postdiarrheal	*Streptococcus pneumoniae,* invasive in children <5 years old
Hepatitis A	
Hepatitis B	Syphilis
Hepatitis B virus infection, perinatal	Syphilis, congenital
	Tetanus
Hepatitis C, non-A, non-B	Toxic shock syndrome
HIV infection, adult (≥13 years old)	Trichinosis
	Tuberculosis
HIV infection, pediatric (<13 years old)	Tularemia
	Typhoid fever
Legionellosis	Varicella (deaths only)
Listeriosis	Yellow fever
Lyme disease	

Source: Centers for Disease Control. Division of Public Health Surveillance and Informatics. Nationally Notifiable Diseases: 2001. Information from www.cdc.gov/epo/dphsi/phs/infdis.htm.

Real-World Case

The quality improvement committee of Community Hospital wanted to study DRG 320, Kidney and urinary tract infections age >17 with CC, because of wide variations in LOS and total charges. The committee asked the HIM director to prepare a profile of patients discharged from DRG 320. A summary of the patients discharged from DRG 320 at Community Hospital was prepared using information found in the hospital's online database (table 15.21, p. 358). The committee also had specific questions regarding DRG 320, namely:

1. What was the average length of stay?
2. What was the modal length of stay?
3. What was the median length of stay?
4. What were the variance and the standard deviation?
5. What percentage of discharges was male? Female?
6. What was the average gross charge?
7. What was the average age?
8. What was the average age of patients discharged to skilled nursing facilities?
9. What was the average age of patients discharged home?

Discussion Question

Calculate the statistics requested by the quality improvement committee. Then prepare a pie chart showing patient discharges by discharge status. Next, prepare a histogram of the age distribution of patients discharged from DRG 320. Prepare a bar graph of the principal diagnosis codes. Finally, discuss the results of your analysis with classmates.

Summary

Rates, ratios, and proportions, and statistics are commonly used to describe community and hospital populations. They are considered to be descriptive statistics because they portray the characteristics of a group or population. Public health officials use community-based rates, ratios, and proportions to evaluate the general health status of a community. Morbidity and morality rates are used as indicators of the accessibility and availability of healthcare services in a community.

Hospital-based rates are used for a variety of purposes. First, they describe the general characteristics of the patients treated at the facility. Hospital administrators use the data to monitor the volume of patients treated monthly, weekly, or within some other specified time frame. The statistics give healthcare decision makers the information they need to plan facilities and to monitor inpatient and outpatient revenue streams.

Graphic techniques are often used to summarize and clarify data. Data may be displayed in a variety of ways, for example, as charts, graphs, and/or tables. Graphic forms are effective ways to present large quantities of information.

The health information management professional is in a position to serve as a data broker for the healthcare organization. To do this, he or she must fully understand the clinical data that are collected and their application to the decision-making process. In addition, he or she must know what information is needed and how to provide it in a timely manner. With this knowledge, the HIM professional can become an invaluable member of the healthcare team.

References

Agency for Health Care Policy and Research. 2000. HCUPnet, Healthcare Cost and Utilization Project. Rockville, Md.: Agency for Health Care Policy and Research. Information from http://www.ahcpr.gov/data/hcup/hcupnet.htm.

Agency for Healthcare Research and Quality. 2000. *AHRQ Profile: Quality Research for Quality Healthcare* (AHRQ Publication No. 00-P005). Rockville, Md.: Agency for Healthcare Research and Quality. Information from http://www.ahrq.gov/about/provile.htm.

Centers for Disease Control and Prevention. CDC Wonder Data Base. Information from http://wonder.cdc.gov.

Table 15.21.   Data for Real-World Case Discussion

Case	PDX	DX1	DX2	DX3	DX4	Discharge Status	Race	Sex	Age	LOS	Total Gross Charges
1	5990	4270	4254	3591	V461	Discharged to SNF	White	M	33	7	$19,734.00
2	5990	20280	78820	5640		Discharged home	White	M	73	1	$1,798.00
3	5990	42731	2900	2859	04111	Discharged to other type of institution	White	M	80	4	$9,612.00
4	5990	496	4359	41401	27800	Discharged home	White	M	88	4	$12,680.00
5	5990	25001	4240	0414	4019	Discharged home	White	M	83	5	$10,188.00
6	5990	496	5997	57420	2859	Discharged home	White	M	85	3	$10,170.00
7	5990	496				Discharged home	White	F	82	1	$2,323.00
8	5959	5997	6011			Discharged home	White	M	78	2	$7,009.00
9	5990	7803	2761	3320	2449	Discharged to other type of institution	White	M	79	4	$9,415.00
10	5990	494	0414			Discharged home	White	F	85	3	$7,745.00
11	5990	2765	586			Discharged to ICF	White	M	81	3	$10,527.00
12	5990	7070	11289	25000	0414	Discharged to other type of institution	White	F	61	6	$11,312.00
13	5902	2839	04111	5990	04104	Discharged to SNF	Black	F	85	3	$8,743.00
14	5990	5997	78820	496	5789	Discharged to SNF	White	M	90	6	$19,086.00
15	5990	0414	2765	25001	71590	Discharged to SNF	Black	F	86	2	$7,610.00
16	59080	5997	591	4019	5990	Discharged home	White	F	74	3	$7,987.00
17	5990	5849	78039	45111	2888	Discharged home	Black	M	53	6	$9,598.00
18	5990	2765	4019	2859		Discharged home	White	F	87	6	$13,096.00
19	5990	42731	7802	41401	3320	Discharged to other type of institution	Black	F	85	4	$10,194.00
20	5990	2765	4019	25000	2720	Discharged home	White	F	71	5	$13,116.00
21	5990	3481				Discharged to SNF	White	F	59	3	$6,450.00
22	5990	2765	2639	7809	3310	Discharged to SNF	White	F	82	8	$17,064.00
23	59080	5997	591	56210		Discharged home	Black	F	37	6	$13,887.00
24	5990	5789	2800	2761	7802	Discharged to home care	White	F	74	4	$12,153.00
25	5959	5997	78820	2800	7802	Discharged home	White	F	74	4	$8,824.00
26	59010	5950	5921	59781	53081	Discharged home	White	F	47	3	$11,076.00
27	5990	4512	185	27800	4439	Discharged home	White	M	80	6	$14,462.00
28	5990	2765	78039	99665	43820	Discharged to SNF	Black	M	53	7	$14,315.00
29	5990	42731	496	2113	0414	Discharged home	White	F	75	2	$11,509.00
30	5990	2875	4139	04111	V090	Discharged to SNF	White	M	87	4	$5,806.00
31	5990	25001	2765	3310	0414	Discharged to SNF	White	F	92	5	$8,937.00
32	5990	25001	4280	2765	2859	Discharged home	White	M	68	11	$19,889.00
33	5990	25003	7070	3441	0414	Discharged home	White	M	43	2	$6,397.00

SNF = Skilled nursing facility

ICF = Intermediate care facility

Cofer, Jennifer, editor. 1994. *Health Information Management,* tenth edition. Berwyn: Ill.: Physicians' Record Company.

National Center for Health Statistics. 2000. Centers for Disease Control and Prevention. Information from http://www.cdc.gov/nchs.

Osborn, Carol E. 2000. *Statistical Applications for Health Information Management.* Gaithersburg, Md.: Aspen Publications.

Youmans, Karen. 2000. *Basic Statistics for Health Information Management Professionals,* revised edition. Chicago: American Health Information Management Association.

Application Exercises

1. For the month of August, Community Hospital, a 425-bed hospital, provided 12,220 days of service to hospital inpatients. Calculate the average daily census and the inpatient bed occupancy rate for the month.

2. For the month of August, Community Hospital provided 1,015 days of service to newborns. There are 35 beds in the newborn nursery. Calculate the average daily census for newborns and the inpatient bed occupancy rate for newborns for the month.

3. For the month of March, Community Hospital experienced 19 deaths, nine of which occurred within 48 hours of admission. It also experienced 522 live discharges. Calculate the gross death rate and the net death rate for the month.

4. For the month of March, Community Hospital experienced 150 deliveries, 7 of which were C-sections. Calculate the C-section rate.

5. Beginning January 1, 2000, Community Hospital had 175 inpatient beds. On June 15, the bed count was increased to 200. There were 67,106 inpatient service days provided to hospital inpatients and 68,012 days of service provided to discharged patients. The hospital experienced 9,601 admissions and 9,488 discharges. Calculate the average daily census for the year. Also calculate the ALOS and the bed occupancy rate for the year.

6. During 1999, Community Hospital experienced 31 late and intermediate fetal deaths and 1,000 live births. Calculate the fetal death rate.

7. Table 15.22 shows a comparative report for Community Hospital for June 20aa and June 20bb. Calculate the following statistics for June 20aa and 20bb:

   - Average daily inpatient census: total, A&C, and NB
   - ALOS: total, A&C, and NB
   - Inpatient bed occupancy rate: total, A&C, and NB
   - Hospital death rate
   - Net death rate
   - Newborn death rate
   - Fetal death rate

8. There were 8,302 deaths in Republic County in 2000 out of a population of 248,239. Calculate the crude death rate per 1,000 population for Republic County in 2000.

9. In 1999, 76,550 people died from pneumonia in the United States. The total number of deaths from all causes was 2,150,466, and the total population was 248,239,000. Calculate the cause-specific death rate for pneumonia per 10,000 population.

10. In 1999, 46,833 people died from diabetes mellitus in the United States. The total number of deaths from all causes was 2,150,466, and the total population was 248,239,000. Calculate the proportionate mortality ratio for diabetes mellitus.

11. For one year in the 1990s, 4,040,958 deaths occurred in the United States, of which 2,069,490 were male and 1,971,468 were female. Review the additional data for that year provided in tables 15.23, 15.24 (p. 360), and 15.25 (p. 360), and answer the following questions.

Table 15.22. Data for Application Exercise #7

Comparative Report for Community Hospital for June 20aa and June 20bb		
Hospital Statistic	June 20aa	June 20bb
Bed Count	292	280
Adults and children	257	240
Newborns	35	40
Admissions	935	850
Adults and children	819	765
Newborns	116	75
Discharges (including deaths)	903	833
Adults and children	790	746
Newborns	113	87
Inpatient Service Days	7,645	7,226
Adults and children	6,685	6,416
Newborns	960	810
Total Length of Stay	6,241	6,156
Adults and children	5,939	5,876
Newborns	302	280
Deaths	25	28
<48 hours	11	12
≥48 hours	14	16
Adults and children	21	25
Newborns	4	3
Fetal	7	4

Table 15.23. Data for Application Exercise #11

Estimated Population (× 1,000), by Age and Sex, United States, July 1, 19xx			
Age Group	Male	Female	Total
<1 year	2,020	1,925	3,945
1–4 years	7,578	7,229	14,807
5–9 years	9,321	8,891	18,212
10–14 years	8,689	8,260	16,949
15–19 years	9,091	8,721	17,812
20–24 years	9,368	9,334	18,702
25–29 years	10,865	10,834	21,699
30–34 years	11,078	11,058	22,136
35–39 years	9,731	9,890	19,621
40–44 years	8,294	8,588	16,882
45–49 years	6,601	6,920	13,521
50–54 years	5,509	5,866	11,375
55–59 years	5,121	5,605	10,726
60–64 years	5,079	5,788	10,867
65–69 years	4,631	5,538	10,169
70–74 years	3,464	4,549	8,013
75–79 years	2,385	3,648	6,033
80–84 years	1,306	2,422	3,728
85+ years	850	2,192	3,042
Total	120,981	127,258	248,239

Table 15.24.   Data for Application Exercise #11

Age Group	Male	Female	Total
Deaths by Age and Sex, United States, 19xx			
	Sex		
	Male	**Female**	**Total**
<28 days	14,059	11,109	25,168
28 days–11 months	8,302	6,185	14,487
1–4 years	4,110	3,182	7,292
5–9 years	2,510	1,803	4,313
10–14 years	2,914	1,687	4,601
15–19 years	11,263	4,307	15,570
20–24 years	15,902	5,016	20,918
25–29 years	19,932	6,998	26,930
30–34 years	24,222	9,372	33,594
35–39 years	26,742	11,120	37,862
40–44 years	28,586	14,471	43,057
45–49 years	32,718	18,139	50,857
50–54 years	42,105	25,304	67,409
55–59 years	62,981	38,493	101,474
60–64 years	96,628	61,956	158,584
65–69 years	129,847	89,250	219,097
70–74 years	148,559	113,568	262,127
75–79 years	157,090	144,135	301,225
80–84 years	135,580	162,401	297,981
85+ years	150,140	307,780	457,920
Total	1,114,190	1,036,276	2,150,466

a. Using the data from the population table, answer the following questions:

- Of the total population, what was the ratio of women to men?
- Of the total population, what was the proportion of men?
- What proportion of the total population was 65 years old or older?
- What was the proportion of the women under age 65?
- What was the ratio of boys to girls for the age group under one year?
- What was the ratio of women to men in the age group 40–44?

b. What was the crude birth rate per 1,000?

c. What was the crude death rate per 1,000?

d. What was the crude death rate for men per 1,000?

e. What was the crude death rate for women per 1,000?

f. What is the infant death rate per 1,000?

g. What was the postneonatal death rate per 1,000?

h. What was the ratio of deaths, men to women, for the age groups 40–44 and 45–49?

i. What was the cause-specific death rate for (1) motor vehicle injuries per 10,000, (2) heart disease per 10,000, (3) pneumonia per 10,000, (4) HIV per 100,000, and (5) diabetes per 10,000?

j. What was the proportionate mortality rate for (1) motor vehicle injuries, (2) heart disease, (3) pneumonia, (4) HIV, and (5) diabetes?

12. Prepare a bar graph and a pie chart of the selected causes of death, total, for 19xx.

13. Prepare a grouped bar graph comparing male and female populations, by age, grouped in ten-year intervals.

14. Review the data in table 15.26. Prepare a line graph displaying deaths due to AIDS, by sex, for the years 1987–1998.

Table 15.25.   Data for Application Exercise #11

Age Group	Heart Disease	Pneumonia	Motor Vehicle Injuries	Diabetes Mellitus	HIV	All Other	Total
Deaths by Age and Selected Causes of Death, United States, 19xx							
<1	776	636	216	6	120	37,901	39,655
1–4	281	228	1,005	15	112	5,651	7,292
5–14	295	122	2,266	32	64	6,135	8,914
15–24	938	271	12,941	136	626	21,589	36,488
25–34	3,462	881	10,269	687	7,759	37,466	60,524
35–44	11,782	1,415	6,302	1,432	8,563	51,425	80,919
45–54	30,992	1,707	3,879	2,784	3,285	75,689	118,266
55–64	81,351	3,880	3,408	6,942	1,144	163,333	260,058
65–74	165,787	10,418	3,465	13,168	327	288,059	481,224
75–84	234,318	24,022	2,909	14,160	70	323,727	599,206
85+	203,885	32,970	915	7,471	12	212,584	457,920
Total	733,867	76,550	47,575	46,833	22,082	1,223,559	2,150,466

Table 15.26.   Data for Application Exercise #14

Deaths due to AIDS, by Year and Sex, United States, 1987–1998			
Year	Sex		Total
	Male	Female	
1987	11,829	1,322	13,151
1988	14,495	1,715	16,210
1989	19,224	2,228	21,452
1990	21,621	2,668	24,289
1991	25,021	3,269	28,290
1992	28,131	3,973	32,104
1993	30,789	4,886	35,675
1994	34,131	6,169	40,300
1995	34,525	6,863	41,388
1996	24,139	5,558	29,697
1997	12,137	3,346	15,483
1998	9,581	2,878	12,459
Total	265,623	44,875	310,498

Source: Centers for Disease Control and Prevention, CDC Wonder
Mortality Data Base. Information from http://wonder.cdc.gov.

Review Quiz

Instructions: Choose the most appropriate answer to the following questions.

1. ___ What is the number of inpatients present at the census-taking time each day plus the number of inpatients who were both admitted and discharged after the census-taking time the previous day?
   a. Inpatient census
   b. Daily inpatient census
   c. Inpatient service day
   d. Inpatient bed occupancy ratio

2. ___ Which of the following is not a type of inpatient hospital discharge?
   a. Death
   b. Intrahospital transfer from MICU to medicine
   c. Discharge against medical advice
   d. Discharge transfer to a long-term care facility

3. ___ Which of the following is a unit of measure denoting the services received by one inpatient during a 24-hour period?
   a. Inpatient census
   b. Inpatient service day
   c. Daily inpatient census
   d. Average daily inpatient census

4. ___ What does the hospital gross death rate include?
   a. Deaths of inpatients only
   b. All inpatient deaths and stillborn infants
   c. Deaths of all inpatients and deaths occurring in the emergency department
   d. Deaths of all inpatients, DOAs, and deaths occurring in the emergency department

5. ___ When computing the C-section rate, the denominator is the total number of what?
   a. Births
   b. Deliveries
   c. Obstetric discharges
   d. Newborns

6. ___ What is a measure of the actual observed mortality in a community called?
   a. Crude death rate
   b. Sex-specific death rate
   c. Cause-specific death rate
   d. Age-adjusted death rate

7. ___ At midnight December 1, the inpatient census at Watson Hospital was 378. On December 2, 18 patients were discharged alive, 1 patient died, 22 patients were admitted, and 2 patients were admitted and discharged the same day. How many inpatient service days were provided on December 2?
   a. 375
   b. 377
   c. 381
   d. 383

8. ___ At Community Hospital, 238 operations were performed in January. Fifteen of these patients developed infections within ten days of surgery. During January, 432 patients were admitted and 470 patients were discharged. What is the postoperative infection rate for the month?
   a. 0.06%
   b. 3.19%
   c. 3.47%
   d. 6.3%

9. ___ On December 1, Community Hospital had a bed capacity of 520; on December 15, 45 beds were closed. During the month of December, there were 13,050 inpatient service days, 15,450 days rendered to discharged patients, and 945 discharges and deaths. What is the inpatient bed occupancy rate for December?
   a. 80.9%
   b. 84.5%
   c. 84.7%
   d. 85.0%

Instructions: For questions 10 and 11, refer to the following information. In August, Community Hospital discharged 1,575 patients and admitted 1,650 patients. The hospital provided 10,215 days of service to inpatients and 9,763 days of service to discharged patients.

10. ___ What is the average daily census at Community Hospital for the month of August?
    a. 315
    b. 323
    c. 330
    d. 334

11. ___ What is the average length of stay at Community Hospital for the month of August?
    a. 5.9 days
    b. 6.2 days
    c. 6.5 days
    d. 6.8 days

12. ___ In a community of 38,000, there were 230 deaths in 2000. What is the crude mortality rate?
    a. 23 per 100
    b. 6.1 per 1,000
    c. 8.6 per 1,000
    d. 6.1 per 10,000

13. ___ You want to graph the average length of stay by sex and service for the month of April. Which graphic tool would you use?
    a. Bar graph
    b. Histogram
    c. Line graph
    d. Pie chart

14. ___ You want to graph the number of deaths due to prostate cancer for 1990 through 1999. Which graphic tool would you use?
    a. Frequency polygon
    b. Histogram
    c. Line graph
    d. Pie chart

15. ___ A pie chart may be used to display what kind of data?
    a. Average length of stay by year
    b. Percentage of discharges by third-party payer
    c. Number of discharges per year and third-party payer
    d. Number of patients discharged by sex and service

16. ___ What information would a histogram be used to display?
    a. Discharges by age
    b. Discharges by sex
    c. Discharges by third-party payer
    d. Discharges by service

17. ___ There were 40 students in section I of a medical terminology class and 20 students in section II. The mean score on a midterm exam for section I was 60, and the mean score for section II was 70. What was the mean score for the two classes combined?
    a. 50
    b. 63.3
    c. 65
    d. 65.5

18. ___ In a frequency distribution, the lowest score is 25 and the highest score is 50; the mean is 37.5. What is the range?
    a. 11
    b. 12.5
    c. 24
    d. 25

19. ___ Which of the following is a measure of spread?
    a. Mean
    b. Median
    c. Mode
    d. Standard deviation

20. ___ The standard deviation of a frequency distribution is 10. What is the variance?
    a. 20
    b. 50
    c. 75
    d. 100

21. ___ For the two observations 8 and 12, what is the $\Sigma (X - \bar{X})^2$?
    a. 2
    b. 4
    c. 8
    d. 12

22. ___ In a normal distribution, 99.7 percent of the observations fall within which of the following standard deviations?
    a. ± 1 s.d. of the mean
    b. ± 2 s.d. of the mean
    c. ± 3 s.d. of the mean
    d. ± 1.5 s.d. of the mean

23. ___ Which of the following words/phrases best describes the normal distribution?
    a. Continuous
    b. A family of distributions
    c. Symmetrical about the mean
    d. All of the above

24. ___ Which entity prepares model procedures for the preparation of vital records such as birth and death certificates?
    a. The registrar for each state
    b. National Center for Health Statistics
    c. County departments of health
    d. Hospital departments of health information management

25. ___ Which entity is responsible for the weekly collection and publication of notifiable diseases in the United States?
    a. Public Health Service
    b. Centers for Disease Control
    c. National Center for Health Statistics
    d. World Health Organization

Chapter 16
Research Methods

Elizabeth Layman, PhD, RHIA, CCS, FAHIMA

Learning Objectives

- To describe basic research designs and methods used in the practice of health information management
- To formulate research problems in terms of research questions
- To plan research projects appropriate to the research questions
- To conduct research projects using standard and suitable tools and techniques
- To present research findings in formats consistent with the purpose of the research
- To critically evaluate research studies in health-related fields

Key Terms

Alternative hypothesis
Applied research
Basic research
Bivariate
Case study
Case-control (retrospective) study
Categorical data
Causal-comparative research
Causal relationship
Census survey
Clinical (medical) research
Clinical trial
Cluster sampling
Confounding (extraneous, secondary) variable
Construct validity
Content analysis
Content validity
Continuous data
Control group
Convenience sample
Correlational research
Cross-sectional
Deductive reasoning
Dependent variable
Descriptive research
Descriptive statistics
Discrete data
Double-blind study
Empiricism
Ethnography

Evaluation research
Experimental (study) group
Experimental research
External validity
Focused studies
Generalizability
Heterogeneity
Historical research
Hypothesis
Independent variable
Inductive reasoning
Inferential statistics
Institutional Review Board (IRB)
Instrument
Internal validity
Interrater reliability
Interval data
Intervention
Interview guide
Interview survey
Intrarater reliability
Level of significance
Literature review
Longitudinal
Meta-analysis
Model
Mortality (attrition)
Multivariate
Naturalism
Naturalistic observation
Negative (inverse) relationship

Nominal data
Nonparametric (distribution-free) technique
Nonparticipant observation
Nonrandom sampling
Null hypothesis
Observational research
One-tailed hypothesis
Ordinal data
Paradigm
Parametric technique
Participant observation
Peer review
Peer-reviewed (refereed) journal
Pilot study
Placebo
Positive (direct) relationship
Positivism
Primary analysis
Primary source
Protocol
Purposive sampling
Qualitative approach
Quantitative approach
Questionnaire survey
Random sampling
Randomization
Randomized clinical trial (RCT)
Ratio data
Reliability
Research

Research method
Research methodology
Retrospective
Sample
Sample size
Sample size calculation
Sample survey
Scientific inquiry
Secondary analysis
Secondary source
Semistructured question
Simple random sampling
Simulation observation
Stratified random sampling
Structured (close-ended) question
Survey
Systematic sampling
Target population
Test statistics
Theory
Treatment
Two-tailed hypothesis
Type I error
Type II error
Univariate
Unstructured (open-ended) question
Validity
Variable

Introduction

Health information management is an intersection of many different fields of study, and health information managers are businesspeople in a health-related profession. Thus, health information managers draw on the theories from the many fields associated with both business and healthcare, including management, organizational behavior, sociology, psychology, medical sciences, computer science, and decision support. In this chapter, research concepts are applied to healthcare settings and the role of the HIM professional in research is explored.

Research is a way to create knowledge. It answers questions and provides solutions to everyday problems. Unfortunately, people wrongly believe that research is some vague, mysterious activity for geniuses. Rather, it is a step-by-step method that ordinary people can use to collect reliable and accurate facts in order to generate valuable information.

Generally, there are two types of research: basic and applied. These two types are ends of a continuum, not separate entities. Therefore, the distinction between them is sometimes unclear. In essence, **basic research** focuses on the development of theories and their refinement. **Applied research** focuses on the implementation of the theories in practice. For example, as applied researchers, some HIM professionals study questions they believe will improve health information practices in the continuum of care. Another way to differentiate basic and applied research is that basic research answers the question "why" and applied research answers the questions "what" and "how" (Gay 1987).

Research into medicine and healthcare has greatly enhanced the quality and length of people's lives. For example, antibiotics, endoscopic surgery, and the Medicare inpatient prospective payment system, among many others, all are the result of research. Moreover, continued advances in effective treatments and efficient methods of healthcare delivery depend on future research.

This chapter overviews the role of research in medicine and healthcare and the development of theories and models. It also presents a step-by-step process for conducting research. Finally, the chapter addresses the practical matters of research techniques used to conduct library and data searches and to access data.

Theory into Practice

At a large Midwestern teaching hospital, research studies was a functional unit within the Department of Health Information Services (HIS). Several of the department's activities were aligned with the hospital's research mission. For example, one of the HIS director's responsibilities was to represent the department on the hospital's Institutional Review Board (IRB). With their jurisdiction specified in both federal regulations and institutional policies, IRBs provide oversight for the research studies conducted within institutions and thus have the authority to review and approve or reject them. In this way, IRBs protect the rights and welfare of human research subjects recruited to participate in research activities.

Because the HIS director provided expert information on the content of the hospital's paper-based patient records, computer-based patient records, and other databases maintained by the department and because she was in a position to explain the impact on the department of researchers' protocols, she was a key member of the IRB. She was assisted in these tasks by the supervisor of research studies, who was responsible for evaluating and summarizing research proposals that were related to data in the HIS department's databases and to the use of the hospital's paper patient records. The supervisor submitted her evaluations and summaries to the HIS director.

One day, the supervisor of research studies received a letter from a graduate student working on a master's thesis in sociology requesting the hospital's participation in a research study. The student explained that he was investigating the effect of the state's recently enacted parental notification statute, which required that a minor's parents be notified prior to an abortion. He wanted to know how many abortions had been performed in the hospital each year for the past five years and specifically requested data from ICD-9-CM categories 634 through 638. His letter included a table for the hospital worker to complete and return as part of the study. (See table 16.1.)

After reviewing the student's request, the supervisor advised the HIS director to reject it, stating that it did not merit the IRB's consideration. Moreover, she recommended that the request be returned to the student with a brief explanation of the ICD-9-CM codes and the suggestion to consult with a health information management (HIM) professional about coding.

The supervisor based her decision on the following points:

- The student had specifically requested information on abortions performed in the hospital. This excluded abortions attempted outside the hospital, such as self-induced, illegal abortions. He did not note that the only possible use of code 636, Illegally induced abortion, in the inpatient setting was for externally performed abortions to ensure their completeness or to treat a complication. Obviously, the hospital did not perform illegal abortions.

Table 16.1.   Number of Hospital Abortions by Year

Code	Year 1	Year 2	Year 3	Year 4	Year 5
634					
635					
636					
637					
638					

- He had not asked an HIM professional to review his codes before submitting his request. An HIM professional would have told him that ICD code 636 was incorrect in his scenario.
- Finally, he had not conducted a **pilot study** (trial run) with a small group of hospitals prior to beginning his research, which would have revealed the error related to ICD code 636.

The supervisor was concerned that these flaws in the design of the student's research signaled others that would result in a study with questionable findings. In her opinion, complying with the student's request for information would be a waste of an HIS staff member's time.

In this case, the supervisor used two bodies of knowledge to assist the director: her knowledge of coding, an area unique to health information management; and her knowledge of research methods. An understanding of research methods aids professionals whenever they use data or information to answer a question or to make a decision.

Research in Medicine and Healthcare

The history of research in medicine and healthcare parallels the history of civilization. The tradition of proposing rational explanations for the causes of disease dates back to 3500 BC. The Egyptians recorded symptoms and cures for illnesses, and the Greeks continued the tradition. Indeed, Hippocrates, practicing medicine in about 400 BC, wrote more than fifty books on health and disease. Similar advances occurred in India and China. Scientists and philosophers continued to advance knowledge about medicine and health through the Middle Ages and the Renaissance.

In the United States, research in medicine and healthcare and interest in the research university evolved together. The present form of the research university emerged in the 1860s (Rudolph 1990). Yale awarded the first doctoral degrees in the United States in 1861 (Rudolph 1990). Cornell University was chartered in 1865; the Johns Hopkins University was founded in 1867. In the 1890s, national learned societies and journals were established (Jencks and Riesman 1977). The university structure of departments, such as biology, philosophy, and history, also were established in the 1890s. By 1914, the two dozen leading U.S. universities had been established (Jencks and Riesman 1977).

During the early 1900s, Flexner (1910) investigated the quality of medical education and recommended that many shoddy medical schools be closed. He also described the ideal organization of medical education. Flexner recommended that medical schools be located in leading universities with associated hospitals. He identified outstanding examples such as the Johns Hopkins University, the University of Michigan, and the University of Minnesota. Today's, academic health center was born from the union of medical schools, hospitals, and research universities.

Academic health centers became especially important after the federal government increased its funding for research in the 1950s. These federal research grants became important sources of revenue for universities. As conduits for federal dollars, academic health centers became increasingly prominent in their universities. One major source of federal funding for medical research is the National Institutes of Health (NIH). Today, the NIH supports 35,000 grants related to medical research. Thus, research, as means to raise funds, became an integral part of the academic enterprise.

Theory and Research

A **theory** is the systematic organization of knowledge that predicts or explains behavior or events. Theories and research have a chicken-and-egg relationship. Theories are both the result and the foundation of research. Researchers begin with informed predictions or raw theories of what they believe will happen. As they collect observations and data, they refine their theories. Over time, the refined theories become more predictive of subsequent events than their previous embryonic versions.

Theories are practical and efficient. They help people understand their world. Without theories, people are merely speculating. Although speculation may be informed by experiences and some facts, it is nevertheless speculation.

Apparent in all fields of study, theories explain what people have observed. In addition, they provide definitions, relationships, and boundaries. In other words, theories systematically organize everything people know about a concept. Amatayakul and Shah (1992) formally defined theories as:

- Concepts that are abstract ideas generalized from particular instances
- Interrelationships that are assumed to exist among these concepts
- Consequences that are assumed to follow logically from the relationships proposed in the theory

The best theories simplify the situation, explain the most facts in the broadest range of circumstances, and most accurately predict behavior (Singleton, Straits, and Straits 1993). Thus, research theories are practical and efficient because they help researchers explain and predict many events in simple and precise terms. In other words, theories organize knowledge. When knowledge is organized, ordinary people can access and use it. Everyone benefits.

Clinical Research and Clinical Trials

Clinical (medical) research is a specialized area of research that primarily investigates the efficacy of preventive, diagnostic, and therapeutic procedures. Efficacy involves both safety and effectiveness. Because clinical means "at the bedside," the focus of clinical research is the individual patient.

Clinical trials are the specific, individual studies within the field of clinical research. Each trial investigates a new therapy, such as a new drug or a new treatment regimen. Because clinical trials involve patients, they can begin only after the researcher has shown promising results in the laboratory or on research animals.

Researchers conduct clinical trials using protocols. **Protocols** are sets of strict procedures that specify the language of informed consent, the types of subjects, the timing of treatments, the period of participation, and the evaluation of efficacy. For example, in **randomized clinical trials** (RCTs), researchers must follow strict rules in assigning patients to groups. The rules ensure that both known and unknown risk factors will occur in approximately equal numbers between the group of patients receiving the treatment and the group of patients not receiving it.

The NIH supports thousands of clinical trials (Clinical trials.gov). Private organizations such as drug companies and health maintenance organizations also support clinical trials. Trial sites are teaching and community hospitals, physician group practices, or health departments.

Clinical trials consist of four stages: Phase I, Phase II, Phase III, and Phase IV (table 16.2). The four phases represent continued development of a drug or treatment (Clinical trials.gov). For example, in Phase I clinical trials, researchers test a new drug or treatment for the first time on a small group of participants. The researchers evaluate the safety of the new drug or treatment, determine safe procedures, and identify side effects or complications. On the other hand, Phase IV clinical trials occur after the drug or treatment has been marketed. In Phase IV clinical trials, the researchers determine whether the drug or treatment has particular effects for certain groups (populations) or whether side effects develop after long-term use.

A clinical trial is a systematic way to introduce, evaluate, and monitor new drugs, treatments, and devices prior to their dissemination throughout the healthcare system. In so doing, clinical trials protect the public's health. Finally, clinical trials have proved to be effective means of advancing knowledge about medicine and health and, thus, improving the quality of healthcare in the United States.

Health Record Data in Research

Just as the history of medicine follows the history of civilization, so too does the use of the data in health records. With the development of writing, ancient physicians and scribes could record diseases and their treatments. For example, in 3000 BC, it was recorded that an Egyptian physician "healed the king's nostrils" (BBC Education 2001).

More recently, medical records became an integral part of the hospital standardization program of the American College of Surgeons (ACS). In 1918, the ACS began to evaluate the quality of care that a hospital provided by evaluating its patient records. Since then, researchers have used patient records as a way to both log data during research and access existing data for their research. For example, many protocols of clinical trials state that specific data will be obtained from patient records. Such data include medical histories, glucose levels, body mass indexes, pulmonary function tests, audiograms, utilization of services, and so on.

A recently published study illustrates the use of data from health records. Bell and Hudson (2001) investigated the treatment of patients who presented to the emergency department with chest pain. From 379 health records, the researchers collected data on admitting and discharge diagnoses, coexisting diseases, race, gender, age, health insurance status, and diagnostic and therapeutic procedures performed. They found statistically significant differences between races for time to the first electrocardiogram and for the percentage of patients receiving echocardiography and cardiac catheterization.

This study's findings were based totally on the retrospective review of data in health records. Thousands of studies have followed methods similar to this study. The fact that researchers have conducted their studies entirely through reviews of health records demonstrates the importance of health record data in research.

Research Models

A **model** is a representation of a theory in a visual format. Models can portray theories with objects, can be smaller-scaled versions, or can be graphic representations. A popular synonym for model is **paradigm.**

A model includes all of a theory's known properties. The American Health Information Management Association (AHIMA), for example, has a theory about what defines data quality. Experts at the AHIMA have identified collection, analysis, application, and warehousing as the functions of data quality management and hypothesize that data quality

Table 16.2.   Phases of Clinical Trials

Phase	I	II	III	IV
Number of Subjects	20–80	100–300	1000 3000	Multitudes postmarketing
Purpose	Evaluate safety Determine dosage Identify side effects	Evaluate safety Determine effectiveness	Collect more information about safe usage Confirm effectiveness Monitor side effects Compare to alternatives	Collect data on effect on specific groups (populations) Monitor long-term side effects

will result if practitioners follow proper procedures within these activities. (See figure 16.1 for a model of the AHIMA theory.)

Research methodology is the study and analysis of research methods and theories. At a higher and more general level, researchers in research methodology have described two overarching approaches to research: the quantitative approach and the qualitative approach. These two approaches are models on a grand scale. Within each approach, researchers make certain basic assumptions.

Within the **quantitative approach,** researchers assume that they can:

- Find the single truth
- Apply that single truth across time and place
- Adopt a neutral, unbiased stance
- Identify a chronological sequence of causes

Another name for the quantitative approach is **positivism.** A classic example of quantitative research is the human genome project.

Within the **qualitative approach,** researchers believe that:

- Multiple truths exist simultaneously.
- Truths are bound to place and time (contextual).
- Neutrality is impossible because researchers choose their topics of investigation.
- Influences interact within one another to color researchers' views of the past, present, and future.

Another name for the qualitative approach is **naturalism.** A classic example of qualitative research is Margaret Mead's anthropological study of the Polynesian culture of American Samoa in the early 1920s.

The purpose of the research determines the approach. Research that is exploratory and preliminary often begins with a qualitative investigation; research that investigates numerically measurable observations or tests a hypothesis is often quantitative. Scientific inquiry, for example, is quantitative.

Some large topics require both approaches with many researchers conducting complementary studies. For example, anthropological studies of other cultures are often qualitative (specifically, ethnographic). Examples in medicine involve studies of near-death experiences, dying, and being a patient. Without qualitative research, healthcare personnel would not have learned that elderly, married patients cut their pills in half in order to share their prescriptions when they run out of money.

Most advances in medicine have been the result of quantitative research. Quantitative research is based on scientific inquiry and empiricism. **Scientific inquiry** involves making predictions, collecting and analyzing evidence, testing alternative theories, and choosing the best theory. **Empiricism** means "based on observed and validated evidence." For example, research based on experiments is empirical. Quantitative research, with its scientific and evidence-based approach, is also the approach that HIM researchers select.

Within both the quantitative and the qualitative approaches, researchers use inductive and deductive reasoning. **Inductive reasoning,** or induction, involves drawing conclusions based on a limited number of observations. For example, during his professional practice experience, a student might observe that all coders in the coding department at XYZ hospital had the RHIT credential. Thus, he might conclude that all coders have the RHIT credential. **Deductive reasoning,** or deduction, involves drawing conclusions based on generalizations. For example, all coders have the RHIT credential. Jane Doe is a coder. Therefore, Jane Doe must have the RHIT credential.

As the examples demonstrate, neither induction nor deduction alone is completely satisfactory. Used together, however, they are very effective and are the basis of the research.

Figure 16.1.   AHIMA's Model of Data Quality

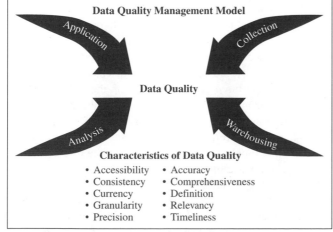

Source: AHIMA Data Quality Management Task Force. 1998. Practice Brief: Data quality management model. *Journal of the American Health Information Management Association* 69(6).

Check Your Understanding 16.1

Instructions: Answer the following questions on a separate piece of paper.

1. What is research?

2. What are the basic steps of research?

3. Why is the research conducted by HIM professionals considered applied research?

4. What are the three characteristics of a theory?

5. How does the phrase "keep it simple" apply to theories?

6. How does clinical research differ from epidemiology, which focuses on populations?

7. Why are health records important in clinical research?

8. What are the advantages of models?

9. How do inductive reasoning and deductive reasoning differ?

10. Why is knowing their purpose so important for researchers?

Research Process

Conceptually, there are five major activities in which researchers participate:

1. Defining the research question (problem)
2. Summarizing prior pertinent knowledge
3. Gathering data
4. Analyzing the data
5. Interpreting and presenting findings

However, because these major activities are so broad, most researchers divide them into more manageable components. Thus, the research process becomes orderly problem solving. In the verbal shorthand of researchers, these basic components are:

1. Defining the research question (problem)
2. Performing a literature review
3. Determining a research design and method
4. Selecting an instrument
5. Gathering data
6. Analyzing the data
7. Presenting results

Defining the Research Question (Problem)

Research begins with defining the problem. Other language for defining the problem is specifying the research question. Whichever phrase is used, both mean that researchers must be crystal clear about what they are investigating. Vague notions lead to shoddy research, which is a waste of time, effort, and energy for both researchers and participants.

The importance of investing time and effort in developing the research question cannot be overstated. Experts "agree that the key element, the starting point and the most important issue in developing research, is the *research question*" (Metz 2001, p. 13).

According to Metz (2001), the criteria for a well-developed research question are:

- The question is clearly and exactly stated.
- The question has theoretical significance, practical worth, or both.
- The question has obvious and explicit links to a larger body of knowledge, such as a theory or a research model.
- The research's results advance knowledge in a definable way.
- The answer to the question or the solution to the problem is worthwhile.

The first step in developing the research question is to identify a general problem in an area of interest and expertise. Three excellent sources of meaningful problems exist:

- *Research models:* Research models show all the factors and relationships in a theory. Researchers can select one or two factors that other researchers have raised questions about or have found problematic. An added

benefit is that the model suggests the relationships among the factors. For example, researchers in health information management could use the AHIMA's Model of Data Quality to develop a research problem (figure 16.1). These hypothetical researchers could investigate the relationship between collection and data quality. Finally, research models explicitly link to a larger body of knowledge, one of the criteria for a well-developed research question.

- *Recommendations of earlier researchers:* In journal articles, researchers specifically make recommendations for future research. Their research raises yet more questions that later researchers can answer.

- *Gaps in the body of knowledge:* A comprehensive review of the literature related to the problem or question will identify gaps or problematic areas. For example, researchers will often identify unintentional flaws in their own study that later researchers could correct in a replication study. Correcting the flaw in the subsequent study could produce more accurate and predictive results than were found in the original study. Researchers make similar recommendations in master's theses and doctoral dissertations. Therefore, a careful and thoughtful reading of journal articles, master's theses, doctoral dissertations, and literature reviews can identify meaningful research problems.

The next step is to narrow the focus of the question to a manageable and researchable issue. Researchers clearly state the research problem or question in their article or paper in order to draw the reader into the topic. A helpful metaphor is the funnel. Researchers begin with a broad, general question and then gradually pinpoint the topic to their precise problem or question.

Moreover, an effective problem statement delimits or sets the boundaries of the problem. By clearly stating the study's area of investigation, researchers also specify the aspects of the problem that are beyond or outside the scope of their research. Finally, they state their assumptions and the limitations of their research. For example, the researcher might begin the problem statement with a general societal concern. Supporting citations would come from the popular literature and opinion articles. Then, he or she would concentrate the discussion by explaining how this problem or question affects the field of health information management. A researcher describing a questionnaire study might add that one assumption is that people are honest and that one limitation is that the study only reflects one point in time. Finally, he or she would state the research problem or question succinctly and accurately.

The last step in developing the research question or problem is to ensure that the issue has merit. Similar to shoddy research, research on a trite issue that no one cares about is a waste of time, effort, and energy. Therefore, the key to defining the problem statement is to find a meaningful problem that needs a solution or a significant question that needs an answer.

Performing a Literature Review

A **literature review** is a systematic investigation of all the knowledge about a topic. After completing this orderly and organized approach to the literature, researchers know the following about a topic:

- Mainstream and lesser-known theories, theorists, and factors
- Key turning points in the development of ideas about the topic
- Typical research methods
- Major research instruments
- Appropriate analytical approaches

Researchers will be able to assess the competency of research studies and to identify gaps or holes in the field's body of knowledge. As previously noted, these gaps or holes are excellent areas for new research.

The literature comprises journal articles, theses, and dissertations. Literature is classified in two ways: type of journal and source of material. Each classification affects the quality of the literature review.

Journals may be peer reviewed (also called research, **refereed,** and professional) or non–peer reviewed (also called popular). In **peer-reviewed journals,** the articles are evaluated in manuscript form by experts in the field (peers) for quality prior to publication. The process is called **peer review.**

Both print and electronic journals are peer reviewed. Examples of peer-reviewed journals are the *Journal of the American Medical Association,* the *New England Journal of Medicine, Science,* and the *Journal of the American Medical Informatics Association.* In the field of health information management, the major peer-reviewed journals are *Educational Perspectives in Health Information Management,* the *Journal of the American Health Information Management Association,* and *Topics in Health Information Management.* Thus, researchers must make a distinction between research (professional) literature and popular literature. In a properly conducted literature review, the bulk of the discussion focuses on research literature.

The literature is based on primary and/or secondary sources. **Primary sources** are the original works of the researchers who conducted the investigation; **secondary sources** are summaries of the original works. Encyclopedias and textbooks are familiar secondary sources. Other examples of secondary sources are annual reviews. Annual reviews summarize and synthesize current and recent knowledge on a topic. They may be special issues of print or electronic journals or entire books. (Examples of annual reviews can be found at www.annualreviews.org.) For literature reviews, primary sources are preferable to secondary sources.

Literature review has three meanings. In the first meaning, it is the *process* of reading, analyzing, summarizing, and synthesizing the writings of other researchers and thinkers. In the second meaning, the literature review is a *product*—the portion of a manuscript or an article in which researchers record their analysis and summary of the literature they have read. Finally, the third meaning is an expanded and more sophisticated version of the product in the second meaning. In this meaning, the literature review is a specialized form of research that results in an analysis and summary of the current status of knowledge on a topic. The annual reviews mentioned above are examples of the third meaning of literature review.

Purpose of the Literature Review

As mentioned above, the first meaning of the literature review is a process. Its purpose is to identify, analyze, summarize, and synthesize knowledge and research on the topic and related topics. The process of a literature review consists of four steps:

1. Determining the literature to review
2. Obtaining the literature
3. Analyzing the research questions, methods, and results presented in the literature
4. Synthesizing the information in the literature

In the course of the literature review, the researcher comes to a complete understanding of the topic. This means that he or she can:

- Determine applicable theories, pertinent factors, and appropriate research designs and methods
- Assess the thoroughness of literature reviews in published studies
- Relate theorists and researchers with their ideas and findings
- Differentiate between accepted theories and those outside the mainstream
- Discriminate between relevant and irrelevant factors
- Clarify concepts, recognize trends, and identify confounding factors
- State advantages and disadvantages of various research methods
- Cite the strengths and weaknesses of various instruments
- Select appropriate techniques for analysis
- Identify competently conducted research and inadequately conducted research
- Detect the holes in the body of knowledge that his or her research can fill

Thus, when viewed as a process, the literature review results in the researcher "owning" this particular slice of the body of knowledge. He or she knows the theories; the names of the researchers, theorists, and collaborators; the sources of the data; common research designs; and gaps in the body of knowledge.

Sources of Information

As a process, the well-developed literature review begins with a systematic plan to identify, categorize, organize, and obtain the literature. This subsection begins with the first step of the plan: identifying sources of information. A later subsection on the subject of techniques for searching details addresses the remaining steps of categorizing, organizing, and obtaining the literature.

Sources of information include periodicals; books, brochures, and book chapters; technical and research reports; proceedings of conferences; doctoral dissertations and master's theses; unpublished works; reviews; audiovisual media; and electronic media (figure 16.2). The gold standard for a literature review is primary research in peer-reviewed journals. Therefore, this discussion focuses on databases that access the articles in these journals.

Because health information management combines theories from many academic fields, HIM researchers must search the databases that include the literature related to management, organizational behavior, sociology, psychology, medical sciences, computer science, and decision support (table 16.3).

Development of Literature Review

In the second and third meanings of the literature review, literature reviews are written products. In the second meaning, these are parts within journal articles or papers; in the third meaning, they are entire articles or papers. Therefore, in reality, the third meaning is an amplified and enhanced version of the second meaning. It is a specialized form of research that results in an exhaustive analysis and summary of the current status of knowledge on a topic. However, in both meanings, a well-developed literature review concisely and logically states what is known and unknown about a topic.

In the second meaning, the literature review is a written portion of the research study. Its purpose is to persuade the reader of the necessity of the study. A secondary purpose is to assure the reader that the researcher has conducted a thorough and diligent review of all aspects of the topic. The thoroughness of the literature review lends credibility to both the researcher and the entire investigation.

In a complex or broad topic, researchers should briefly describe the strategy they used to identify literature. In addition, they should explain the scope of the literature review by explicitly stating both their inclusion and exclusion criteria. For example, a researcher could state, "The topic of health information systems is broad. This literature review focused on research articles related to mental health."

Researchers should make a conscious effort to identify, consider, and use an organizing function or factor for the literature review. Using the research model is one organizing function; chronology is another. Explicitly stating the order helps to guide and direct the reader. A coherent and logical order clarifies the topic.

Figure 16.2.   Sources of Information

Periodicals	**Books, Brochures, and Book Chapters**	**Technical and Research Reports**
Abstract	Book	Government bulletin
Annual review	Book chapter	Government report
Cartoon	Brochure	Industry report
Journal	Dictionary	Issue brief
Magazine	Encyclopedia	Monograph
Monograph	Legal citation	Nongovernment agency report
Newsletter	Manual	Position paper
Newspaper	Map or chart	Reference report
Press release	Pamphlet	University report
	Product insert	White paper
	Published or archived letter	Working paper
Proceedings of Meetings	**Doctoral Dissertations and Master's Theses**	**Unpublished Works**
Conference	Abstract of dissertation	Submitted manuscript
Meeting	Abstract of thesis	Unpublished letter
Poster session	Dissertation	Unpublished manuscript
Symposium	Thesis	Unpublished raw data
Unpublished proceeding paper		
Reviews	**Audiovisual Media**	**Electronic Media**
Book	Address	Abstract on CD-ROM
Film	Audiotape	CD-ROM
Video	Chart	Computer program
	Film	Computer software
	Lecture	Electronic database
	Music recording	Internet Web site
	Performance	On-line abstract
	Published interview	On line book
	Recorded interview	On-line journal
	Slide	Software manual
	Speech	
	Television broadcast and transcript	
	Television series and transcript	
	Unpublished interview	
	Work of art	

Table 16.3.   Databases for Literature Searches

Database	Description	Areas of Content					
		Business	Education	Gov't & Law	Health & Medicine	Science & Technology	Social Sciences
ABI/INFORM Global	Abstracts from more than 1,000 business and management publications, including 600 in full text	X				X	X
Academic Abstracts™	950 publications, including 400 peer-reviewed journals	X			X	X	
Academic Search™ Elite	2,720 scholarly journals, including 1,700 peer-reviewed journals	X			X	X	X
Academic Search™ Premier	4,150 scholarly journals, many dating back to 1984		X		X	X	X
Academic Universe	6,000 journals in full text	X		X	X		
ACM Digital Library	Database of publications of the Association for Computing Machinery (ACM), including journals, magazines, and conference proceedings, most in full text					X	
AGRICOLA	Bibliographic citations for agriculture and life science, compiled by the U.S. National Agricultural Library				X	X	
Alt-Health Watch	170 international journals, many peer-reviewed, related to complementary, holistic, and integrated approaches to health				X		
Alternative Medicine (AMED)	Bibliographic record from over 400 journals, books, newspapers, and conference proceedings; provided by the British Lending Library				X		
Applied Science & Technology Abstracts	Bibliographic database of abstracts					X	
arXiv.org	Over 100,000 papers on physics, mathematics, nonlinear sciences, and computer science					X	
BioethicsLine	Materials on ethical, legal, and public policy issues of healthcare and biomedical research			X	X	X	X
Biological Abstracts®	Complete collection of bibliographic references to international journals related to life sciences				X	X	
BioMed Central	Peer-reviewed research of biology and medicine				X	X	
BioMedical FullTEXT Collection	550 full-text journals				X	X	
BioOne	Full text of 40 peer-reviewed bioscience journals and bulletins from SPARC (Scholarly Publishing & Academic Resources Coalition)				X	X	
BIOSIS	350 common publications in the life sciences, including reports, reviews, newspapers, and trade publications				X	X	
Business Source®	Cumulative full text for 2,260 business publications of which 800 are peer reviewed	X					
CANCERLIT®	Over 4,000 sources of information about cancer therapy				X		
CARL UnCover	Database of citations to 8.8 million articles from 18,000 journals	X	X	X	X	X	X
Child Abuse, Child Welfare & Adoption	Database of over 31,000 citations and abstracts of journals, government reports, conference papers, state annual reports, curricula, and unpublished papers			X	X		X

(Continued on next page)

Table 16.3.   (Continued)

Database	Description	Areas of Content					
		Business	Education	Gov't & Law	Health & Medicine	Science & Technology	Social Sciences
CINAHL™ (Cumulative Index of Nursing and Allied Health Literature)	Journals and publications in nursing, biomedicine, health sciences librarianship, consumer health, and 17 allied health disciplines				X		
Computer Source	135 full-text periodicals					X	
Congressional Universe	Indexing, abstracts, and some full text of publications from and about U.S. Congress, including congressional bills, testimony, reports, documents, Congressional Record, U.S. Code, Federal Register, and Code of Federal Regulations			X			
Criminal Justice Abstracts	Criminology and related disciplines, including journals, books, and reports			X			
CSA Life Sciences Collection	Abstracts related to life sciences, from Cambridge Scientific Abstracts				X	X	
Current Citations™	International primary research materials, including 14,000 journals and 360,000 published proceedings	X		X	X	X	
Digital Dissertations	Citations for dissertations and master's theses, beginning with the first U.S. dissertation accepted in 1861 and representing over 1,000 North American graduate schools and European universities	X	X	X	X	X	X
EconLit	Database of the American Economic Association, including over 350,000 records such as articles, books, working papers, and dissertations	X					X
Emerald (Electronic Management Research Library Database)	Over 130 journals related to management and human resources	X					X
e-psyche	Documents related to psychology and associated behavioral disciplines; includes dissertations, newsletters, technical reports, proceedings, and 3,600 journals						X
ERIC®	980 journals in education and full text of more than 2,200 digests		X				
Family and Society Studies Worldwide	Database of 1,000 professional journals, books, popular literature, conference papers, government reports, and other sources				X		X
Government Periodicals Universe	170 U.S. government periodicals			X			
GPO Access	Free electronic access to information products of the U.S. government, including Federal Register; Code of Federal Regulations; U.S. Code; Congressional Record; Commerce Business Daily,; congressional bills, documents and reports; GAO blue books, and Economic Indicators	X		X			
Health Business	Over 420 journals, including 410 in full text	X			X	X	
Health Reference Center—Academic	General-interest articles from a variety of health periodicals				X		

Table 16.3.   (Continued)

Database	Description	Areas of Content					
		Business	Education	Gov't & Law	Health & Medicine	Science & Technology	Social Sciences
Health Source®: Consumer	Over 170 general health, nutrition, and professional healthcare publications				X		
Health Source®: Nursing/Academic	Over 500 scholarly full-text journals, many focused on nursing and allied health	X			X		
HealthSTAR (Ovid)—Defunct June 2001, Combined with MEDLINE	Over 3 million citations addressing health services technology, administration, and research, published from 1975 to present, from the National Library of Medicine and the American Hospital Association. Both clinical and nonclinical aspects of healthcare delivery are featured in sources such as journal articles, government documents, newspaper articles, monographs, book chapters, technical reports, and meeting abstracts and papers.	X		X	X	X	X
ICON	Over 70,000 reports on international business data	X					
IDEAL	Full text of 174 academic press journals and other selections	X		X	X	X	X
InfoTrac Expanded Academic ASAP	1,500 full-text scholarly, trade, and general-interest publications (1,400 peer-reviewed), plus indexing and abstracts from an additional 1,200 publications	X	X		X	X	X
International Pharmaceutical Abstracts	Includes records on over 750 pharmaceutical, medical, and health-related journals and on state pharmacy journals with regulations and laws			X	X		
LegalTrac	1,875 publications, including major law reviews, legal newspapers, bar association journals, international legal journals, and law-related articles from business and general interest	X		X			
MasterFILE Premier	Abstracts for over 2,780 general periodicals, over 1,810 in full text	X			X	X	X
MEDLINE®	Authoritative source of information on medicine, nursing, allied health, dentistry, veterinary medicine, healthcare systems, and preclinical sciences	X			X	X	
NTIS (National Technical Information Service)	Database of research sponsored by the U.S. and some foreign governments					X	
OVID	Over 90 databases, including BIOSIS; CINAHL; EBM Reviews-ACP Journal Club, Cochrane, & Dare; EMBASE; HealthSTAR; and MEDLINE®	X		X	X	X	X

(Continued on next page)

Table 16.3.   (Continued)

Database	Description	Areas of Content					
		Business	Education	Gov't & Law	Health & Medicine	Science & Technology	Social Sciences
PAIS International	Indexes and abstracts from journal articles, government documents, selected books, and conference proceedings in public affairs, public administration, business, economics, international relations, and social studies	X		X			X
POPLINE	Indexes and abstracts of published and unpublished international population literature, including family planning, population law and policy, demography, sexually transmitted diseases, and maternal and child health			X	X		X
Project Muse	115 academic journals in full text					X	X
PsycInfo®	Database provided by American Psychological Association includes dissertations, book chapters, books, reports, and over 1,500 international journals	X	X	X	X		X
PubMed Central	NIH repository for peer-reviewed primary research reports in life science				X	X	
Science Citation Index Expanded	5,700 journals across 164 scientific disciplines				X	X	
Science Direct	800 journals in full text	X			X	X	X
Social Science Abstracts	518 periodicals	X		X	X		X
Social Science Source®	Over 580 journals, 130 in full text	X			X		X
Sociological Collection	Comprehensive database with over 560 full-text journals and over 500 peer-reviewed journals	X					X
SPORTDiscus	Over 500,000 bibliographic citations for research literature related to physical fitness and health				X		X
STAT!Ref	Full text of Medical Letter on Drugs and Therapeutics and other medical references				X		
Statistical Universe	Three databases for materials containing international, federal, and state statistics			X			
STAT-USA	U.S. Department of Commerce delivers vital economic, business, and international trade information, including analyses and market research	X					
THOMAS	Full-text legislative information, including congressional bills, public laws, roll call votes, Congressional Record, and committee reports			X			
TOXNET	Several databases on toxicology, hazardous chemicals, and related topics from the National Library of Medicine				X	X	
U.S. Census of Population and Housing	1990 U.S. census data			X			
Web of Science	Three databases with more than 8,000 peer-reviewed journals, produced by the Institute for Scientific Information (ISI)	X			X	X	X

In the literature review, the researcher identifies the key points or turning points in the development of knowledge about a topic. The literature included should be the research studies that either moved the topic forward or added new factors to the topic. However, important studies with contradictory findings also should be included. Otherwise, readers could perceive the absence of contradictory studies as bias. Evidence of bias detracts from the credibility of the literature review. Explanations of the contradictory findings, based on evaluation and analysis, might be suggested.

Moreover, the studies included in the research study should be pertinent. When tangential studies are included, their relevance should be explicitly stated. Generally, the least-related studies should be discussed first and the most-related studies discussed last.

Research studies that either were conducted inadequately or resulted in gaps or conflicting results should be included, especially if the researcher is rectifying the errors. Again, the researcher should specifically point out the inadequacies, gaps, or conflicting results.

Key research studies or turning-point studies should be described in greater detail than replication or duplicative studies. Enough information about the key studies (design, time frame, method, sample, response rate, statistical techniques, and findings) should be included so that the reader can evaluate their quality. Research that has the same findings with the same factors should be bundled. For example, the author could state, "Research (citation one, citation two, citation three, and so on) has shown that smoking is bad for skin tone."

Tradition and logic demand that researchers pay close attention to verb tense when they write the literature review. The tense of the verb situates the event or idea in time. Present tense expresses truths, accepted theories, and facts. Recent, valid studies also are explained in the present tense. For example:

- *Accepted theory:* Specific goals motivate employees more than vague goals.
- *Recent study:* Johnson's results illustrate the importance of specific goals.

Past studies with continued historical value can be described in the past tense. Including the date to situate the study is a common practice. For example:

- *Study of historical importance:* In 1972, the study of Smith et al. showed the importance of expectancy in motivation.

However, the easiest and safest rule is to use present tense for published studies and theories.

A table that briefly highlights the important features of the studies in the literature review is an effective tool. Readers can quickly see trends and gaps in the literature. Bell (1999) created a table in his review of the literature on the use of computer-assisted instruction. His table listed each study in a row, with columns displaying each study's summary, advantages, and disadvantages. Another possible structure for the table would be to use rows for the studies, but substitute features of the studies in the columns (table 16.4).

In short, the literature review should guide the reader to reach the same conclusions the researchers reached and the same question or problem. Moreover, the reader should conclude that the logical and necessary next step is the research proposed by the researchers. Finally, the literature review should conclude with a clear and exact statement of the hypothesis.

In the third meaning of the literature review, the review is a special form of scholarly work. Like the second meaning, this type of literature review must be thorough, logical, and follow an explicit order.

Researchers write this form of literature review as an overview that analyzes, summarizes, and synthesizes the current status of knowledge on particularly important and topical issues. Also, in these overviews, the researchers identify gaps or discrepancies in the body of knowledge. Journals publish such overviews as separate, independent articles.

Because overviews identify gaps or discrepancies in a field's knowledge, they are excellent sources of problems or research questions that researchers can investigate. Literature reviews in health information management have covered a wide range of subjects, including:

- Case mix and data quality (Siemon 1982)
- Legal aspects of patient records (Kennedy and Jacobs 1981)
- Quality management (Grove 1980)
- Cost containment in the management of departments of health information services (Lewis 1980)

Table 16.4.   Summary of the Literature

Author	Year	Design	Time Frame	Method	Sample	Rate	Statistical Techniques	Findings
X and Y	1980	Descriptive	One-shot	Survey	20 patients, convenience	100%	Means and percentages	More smokers in dermatology clinic
A and B	1995	Correlational	One-shot	Survey	70 random subjects	30%	Bivariate correlation	Relationship between smoking and skin tone
L, M, and N	2001	Quasi-experimental	1 year	Static Group Comparison	40 subjects	100%	ANOVA	Skin tone of nonsmokers significantly more toned than skin tone of smokers

- Use of computer-aided system engineering tools in the development of healthcare information systems (Lee 1996)
- Hospital information systems (Abdelhak 1982; Abelhak, Firouzan, and Ullman 1993)

More information on performing literature reviews is available in *Health Sciences Literature Review Made Easy* (Garrard 1999), which focuses on literature reviews in the health sciences.

Check Your Understanding 16.2

Instructions: Answer the following questions on a separate piece of paper.

1. What are five characteristics of a well-developed research question?
2. What are three rich sources of meaningful research questions?
3. Why would the director of health information services select the productivity standard recommended in a peer-reviewed journal rather than the productivity standard recommended in a popular magazine?
4. Why is conducting a literature review important for a researcher?
5. Why should studies with contradictory results be included in the review of the literature?
6. In the review of the literature, what information about key studies should readers expect?

Determining a Research Design and Method

Researchers can investigate the same broad question or problem using several different research designs. The design chosen depends on the purpose of the research. An important point to remember is that how the problem or question is defined in the problem statement indicates the appropriate research design.

Researchers can choose from among many research designs. Moreover, different disciplines, such as history, medicine, and anthropology, tend to emphasize and use different designs. Certain designs are better suited to answer certain types of questions or to solve certain types of problems than other designs are. (See table 16.5.)

Similarly, certain research methods are more associated with one design than another. However, there is considerable overlap among the methods and their designs. Again, the purpose of the research determines the appropriate research method. Thus, the choice of both the research design and the research method depends on the research question or problem.

Table 16.5.   Designs of Research and Their Applications

Design	Application	Method	Example in Healthcare
Historical	Understand past events	Case study	What factors led to the enactment of Medicare legislation?
		Biography	How did events in the history of the American College of Surgeons affect the development of the field of health information management?
Descriptive	Describe current status	Survey	What barriers prevent healthcare personnel from using computers during the delivery of patient care?
		Observation	How do coders use references and help screens when they code?
Correlational	Determine existence and degree of relationship	Survey	How are credential and performance related?
		Secondary Analysis	What is the relationship between provider satisfaction and EMR systems?
Evaluation	Evaluate effectiveness	Case Study	How has implementation of an EMR system affected the enterprise's ability to deliver healthcare to underserved populations?
			How has EDI reduced the costs of delivery of healthcare to Medicare patients?
Causal-Comparative (Quasi-Experimental)	Detect causal relationship	One-Shot Case Study	What is the effect of a coder training program on the case mix index?
		One-Group Pretest–Posttest	What is the effect of having a working mother on childhood obesity?
		Static Group Comparison	
		Nonparticipant Observation	
Experimental	To establish cause and effect	Randomized, Double-Blind, Clinical Trial	Which group of molecules with innate immunity affects the risk and severity of invasive Blastomycosis dermatitidis infection?
		Pretest–Posttest Control Group Method	Which dosage level of the medication is more efficacious and safer for immunocompromised patients with uncomplicated herpes zoster?
		Solomon Four-Group Method	
		Posttest-Only Control Group	

Research Designs

There are six common research designs: historical, descriptive, correlational, evaluation, causal-comparative, and experimental (Gay 1987). These designs are particularly well suited to research in topics related to healthcare and, specifically, health information management. Which design is appropriate depends on the problem and the researcher's definition of the problem.

Historical Research

Historical research investigates the past. Researchers examine primary and secondary sources such as wills, charters, reports, minutes, eyewitness accounts, letters, and e-mail records. Primary sources are superior to secondary sources. An example of historical research in healthcare would be an investigation of the development of health insurance in the United States. Examining both primary and secondary sources, researchers in health information management could explore the founding of the professional association, the development of the code of ethics, or the establishment of the technical level and the various specialty credentials.

Descriptive Research

Descriptive research determines and reports the current status of topics and subjects. Common tools used to collect descriptive data are surveys, interviews, and observations. The shortcomings of descriptive research include the lack of standardized questions, trained observers, and high response rates. Examples of descriptive studies include polls of Americans' opinions concerning abortion, the patient's bill of rights, stem-cell research, and bioengineering.

In health information management, researchers also conduct descriptive studies. A very limited list of examples includes studies on the status of the composition of the HIM work force, employee morale in HIS departments, coding accuracy, the extent of electronic medical record (EMR) implementation, and the types of tasks that HIM technicians and administrators perform.

Correlational Research

Correlational research determines the existence and degree of relationships among factors. For example, HIM professionals have conducted correlational studies on factors related to burnout among directors of HIM departments (Brodnik 1993; Layman and Guyden 1999). Other correlational studies in health information management might investigate relationships between credential and coding accuracy, job satisfaction and educational level, and increased patient volumes and the level of organizational computerization.

The factors in correlational research and other research designs are called **variables.** The degree or strength of the relationship can range from .00 to 1.00 (or −1.00). A strength of .00 means absolutely no relationship; a strength of 1.00 (or −1.00) means a perfect relationship. For example, a **positive (direct) relationship** (.5332) exists between confidence and feelings of personal accomplishment (Layman and Guyden 1999). A positive relationship means that the more confident the person, the higher his or her feelings of personal accomplishment. Conversely, **a negative (inverse) relationship** (−.3993) exists between confidence and emotional exhaustion (Layman and Guyden 1999). An inverse relationship means that the more confident the person, the lower his or her emotional exhaustion. Strongly related variables allow researchers to make predictions. In prediction studies, the predictor variables suggest scores on criterion variables. For example, the predictor variable of a mother's smoking predicts a low birth weight (criterion variable) in her baby.

However, correlational research can only detect the existence and degree of relationship. For example, in the Layman and Guyden study mentioned above, the researchers could not state whether confidence causes feelings of personal accomplishment or whether feelings of personal accomplishment cause confidence. Adding to the researchers' difficulties, a third unlisted factor, such as self-esteem, could produce feelings of both personal accomplishment and confidence. This third, unlisted factor is called a **confounding (extraneous, secondary) variable** because it confounds (confuses) interpretation of the data.

Researchers conducting correlational studies use surveys, standardized tests, observations, and secondary data. The important point to remember is that correlational research never establishes causal relationships.

Evaluation Research

Evaluation research examines the effectiveness of policies, programs, or organizations. Researchers examine several aspects of programs or organizations, such as conceptualization, design, implementation, impact, and generalizability (Shi 1997). For example, researchers might investigate the effectiveness of a new agency for rehabilitation services. Educational programs also are often the focus of evaluation research. Often grants supporting public services require an evaluation of a service's effectiveness. Case studies are often associated with evaluation research.

In health information management, leaders of an integrated health delivery system could evaluate the effectiveness of aspects of different information systems (IS). For example, leaders of the health systems of the Veterans Administration (VA) evaluated the effectiveness of both the different IS designs and the results of different encoding software applications (Lloyd and Layman 1997). Eight VA medical centers tested encoding software applications from three vendors. The research found that the IS design was the crucial element in increasing coding speed.

Causal-Comparative Research

Causal-comparative research is a type of quasi-experimental design. Quasi means resembling or having some of the characteristics. Therefore, causal-comparative research resembles experimental research by having many, but not all, of the characteristics of experimental research. However, causal-comparative research lacks two key characteristics of experimental research: random assignment to a group and manipulation of treatment.

Choosing causal-comparative research is correct when one of the three following situations exist:

- The variables cannot be manipulated (gender, age, race, birthplace).
- The variables should not be manipulated (accidental death or injury, child abuse).
- The variables represent differing conditions that have already occurred (medication error, heart catheterization performed, smoking).

This research design is also called "ex post facto," meaning retrospective. Examples of quasi-experimental research are case-control (retrospective) studies, field experiments, and natural experiments.

Epidemiologists investigating the development of disease often use **case-control (retrospective) studies.** In case-control studies, the epidemiologists look for characteristics and occurrences that are related to the subsequent development of a disease. In these studies, epidemiologists collect masses of data from health records and through interviews with both persons with the disease (cases) and persons without it (controls). HIM professionals are often involved with case-control studies because they are experts on the content of health records, at finding cases using ICD-9-CM codes, and at finding controls using health information systems.

Researchers investigating the sociology of medicine often conduct field experiments by going into the site (field) and observing activities. The strength of this type of research is that the participants will tend to act more naturally in their real setting. An outstanding example of field research is the research on health practitioners' conversations overheard in elevators. Researchers rode hospital elevators all day listening and recording conversations. They found that patient confidentiality was severely breached.

Researchers conducting natural experiments wait for the event to occur *naturally*. For example, researchers interested in the effectiveness of triage in emergencies would wait for a disaster. Prior to the disaster, they would establish baseline data and tools for data collection. When the disaster occurred, they would record their observations of the actions and results.

In case-control studies, field experiments, and natural experiments, researchers relinquish control of the situations. For purists, however, the lack of randomization and control of treatment lessens the value of causal-comparative (quasi-experimental) research. The research only weakly determines causation. However, as the examples illustrate, in some situations, causal-comparative research is the only design that is logistically and ethically feasible. Causal-comparative research, then, determines the possibility of causal relationships.

Experimental Research

Experimental research establishes causal relationships. A **causal relationship** shows cause and effect. For example,

smoking (the cause) results in lung cancer (the effect). The key characteristic of experimental research is control. Experimental research is the gold standard.

Researchers conducting experimental research select both independent and dependent variables. **Independent variables** are the factors that researchers manipulate directly; **independent variables** are antecedent or prior factors. Dependent variables are the measured variables; they depend upon the independent variables. The dependent variables reflect the results that the researcher theorizes. They occur subsequently or after the independent variables. Therefore, the independent variable causes an effect in the dependent variable.

The independent variables that researchers manipulate are also called **interventions** or **treatments.** Researchers use the term treatment generically or broadly, beyond its usual meaning of therapy. Therefore, treatment could mean a physical conditioning program, a computer training program, a particular laboratory medium, or the timing of prophylactic medications.

In experimental research, researchers select subjects for comparison groups. The **experimental group** comprises the research subjects. Another group, the **control group,** comprises the control subjects. The experimental subjects undergo the intervention of the research study. For comparison, the control subjects do not.

Important elements of experimental research are random sampling and randomization. Although the terms are similar, they represent two different procedures. **Random sampling** is the unbiased selection of subjects from the population of interest. (Random sampling is discussed in greater detail in a subsection on gathering data.) **Randomization** is the random allocation of subjects between experimental groups and control groups. Thus, step one is to select subjects from the population using random sampling and step two is to randomly assign the randomly selected subjects to experimental or control groups.

Random sampling and randomization characterize double-blind studies. A **double-blind study** is an extremely rigorous form of experimental research in which neither the researcher nor the subject knows to which group the subject belongs. The random selection and the random allocation eliminate the effects of expectations and perceptions. For instance, a participant receiving a new heart medication may expect to have more energy and actually believe that he or she does. In addition, the researcher who knows the participant is receiving the new heart medication may perceive that the participant's color has improved. Thus, double-blind studies control biasing because of false expectations and perceptions.

Double-blind studies are often used in the investigation of new drugs. When experimental and control groups are created, neither the participants nor the researchers know to which group the individual participants belong. In order to receive what appears to be the new drug, the participants in the control group are given a placebo. A **placebo** looks exactly like the new drug but, instead, contains harmless ingredients (sometimes called a sugar pill). Therefore, the expectations of the researchers and the participants do not bias the results.

Time Frame as an Element of Research Design
Another element of design cuts across all six types of design. This element is the time frame of the study. The three time frames are retrospective, cross-sectional, and longitudinal.

Studies within a **retrospective** time frame look back in time. For example, many early research studies of stress were retrospective. In these retrospective studies, the researchers measured the participant's level of stress and then asked the participant to reconstruct events that had occurred in a past period of time. Leadership studies in which the researcher asked the leader to list factors that led to his or her success are another example of a retrospective time frame. For some types of questions, such as those related to historic events, a retrospective design is the only possible design.

Research studies with a **cross-sectional** design collect data at one point in time. Cross-sectional studies are snapshots and, as such, may collect data at an entirely unrepresentative point in time. The great advantage of cross-sectional studies is that they are efficient.

Longitudinal studies collect data from the same participants at multiple points in time. Cancer registries that collect data on cancer patients throughout their lifetimes are prime examples of longitudinal studies. Other longitudinal studies include studies of breast cancer and cardiovascular disease. For example, the Nurses' Health Study has followed the health of over 120,000 nurses for more than twenty years (Giovannucci et al. 1998).

The six types of research designs are not rigid boxes. Researchers often combine designs to address their particular research questions or problems. For instance, many studies include both descriptive and correlational findings. In describing their study, researchers also will often state its time frame. Thus, a researcher would state that the study was descriptive, correlational, and cross-sectional. However, the key to classifying the design is to understand the purpose of the research.

Check Your Understanding 16.3

Instructions: Answer the following questions on a separate piece of paper.

1. What determines a researcher's choice of a research design?

2. Which research design would a researcher use to investigate the relationship between a supervisor's level of stress and the number of his or her subordinates?

3. What would be a direct relationship between the supervisor's level of stress and the number of his or her subordinates?

4. How does quasi-experimental research differ from experimental research?

5. What is the key characteristic of experimental research?

6. How do independent variables and dependent variables differ?

7. In a double-blind study, who knows which subjects are in the study group and which subjects are in the control group?

8. Why would a researcher choose a longitudinal study rather than a cross-sectional study?

Research Methods

A **research method** is the particular strategy that a researcher uses to collect, analyze, and present data. Particular methods are associated with certain designs, although considerable overlap exists. For example, researchers can use surveys in both descriptive and correlational designs.

Surveys
A **survey** is a common research method. Surveys are a form of self-report research in which the individuals themselves are the source of data. They collect data about a population to determine its current status with regard to certain factors (Gay 1987). Surveys that collect from all the members of the population are **census surveys;** surveys that collect data from representative members of the population are **sample surveys.**

HIM professionals conduct both types of surveys. For example, when surveying the members of the local HIM association, the past president of the association surveyed every member (Garvin 2001). On the other hand, when information about the members of the national association (a population of more than 40,000) is needed, researchers conduct only a sample survey. A census survey of a large population is generally beyond the resources of a solitary researcher or a small research team. For example, Brodnik (1993) surveyed a representative group of 700 directors of HIM departments to ascertain their level of burnout and then estimated the level of burnout for all directors of HIM departments.

Survey research is further categorized as interview or questionnaire. Researchers conduct **interview surveys** by personally questioning the members of the target population. In **questionnaire surveys,** researchers create electronic or paper forms that include the questions.

In both categories, the questions can be structured, semistructured, or unstructured. **Structured (closed-ended) questions** list all the possible responses; **unstructured (open-ended) questions** allow free-form responses. In **semistructured questions,** researchers first ask structured questions and then follow with open-ended questions to clarify. The disadvantage of unstructured questions is that they are more difficult to quantify, tabulate, and analyze than structured questions are. The advantages of unstructured questions are that they allow in-depth questions and may uncover aspects of a problem unknown to the researcher.

For example, researchers (Lippin et al. 2000) investigated the effect of a training program on safety practices. They conducted a semistructured, telephone interview with 362 workers and managers using both structured questions from a written list and unstructured questions. For the analysis of the structured questions, the researchers calculated percentages to compare responses across the various job classes, such as hospital manager of public-sector blue-collar workers. However, in order to analyze the responses to the open-ended questions, the researchers first had to transcribe them verbatim and code them. The greater time commitment for open-ended questions is demonstrated.

Interviews

In interview surveys, researchers orally question the members of the population. Examples of interview surveys are telephone surveys, exit polls, and focused studies. Researchers can question members of the population individually or as a group using a written list of questions called an **interview guide.** Use of an interview guide ensures that all members of the group are asked the same questions. In **focused studies,** the researcher and the group members have a group discussion. Researchers can strictly control the questions and responses or can allow a free-flowing conversation. They often record sessions and then transcribe the comments.

For example, Monsen (1999) conducted a study in which she asked the mothers of children with spina bifida to describe their experiences. She audiotaped the interviews, transcribed them, and then analyzed the texts using a specialized software program and multiple readings of the text to interpret the mothers' comments. The data revealed themes that helped nurses to understand the lives of mothers of children with disabilities.

Questionnaires

Questionnaire surveys also query members of the population. Rather than asking questions orally, researchers mail participants an electronic or print form to complete and return. Questionnaire studies are efficient because they require less time and money than interview studies do and because they allow the researchers to collect data from many more members of the target population. Moreover, questionnaire studies that are Internet based further enhance efficiency because the subjects' answers are entered directly into the database, which eliminates a step for the researchers.

For example, Garvin (2001) used a questionnaire to conduct her census survey of the members of the local HIM association (figure 16.3). The leadership of the local association used this study to investigate its memberships' current knowledge of coding skills. Then, from the information the questionnaire provided, the leadership could project the future educational needs of the local members and plan appropriate workshops and seminars to meet those needs. In another example, Osborn (2000a) investigated managerial practices in HIM departments. She randomly selected 1,000 directors of acute care facilities from the membership roster of the AHIMA and mailed them questionnaires; 200 directors responded. The questionnaire collected data about record turnaround time; discharge analysis procedures; inpatient coding productivity; assembly, analysis, and electronic storage; outsourcing; and other electronic functions. The data from this study describe current practices in health information management. Health information managers can use its findings to assess their own practices.

Observational Research

In o**bservational research,** researchers obtain data by observing rather than by asking. Observational research is used in

Figure 16.3.   Excerpt from Survey Questionnaire

Questionnaire on Coding Skills Contained in AHIMA's Vision 2006

On a scale of 1 to 5, 5 being the most capable, please designate how capable you feel in the following areas:

1. Understanding the current clinical coding systems relevant to the organization:

A.	ICD-9-CM	5	4	3	2	1
B.	CPT	5	4	3	2	1
C.	DSM-IV	5	4	3	2	1
D.	SNOMED	5	4	3	2	1
E.	ICD-O	5	4	3	2	1
F.	ICD-10	5	4	3	2	1

2. Ability to gather clinical data from primary data sources   5 4 3 2 1

3. Understanding of the elements required for research and outcomes   5 4 3 2 1

4. Ability to participate in the design of studies   5 4 3 2 1

Source: Garvin, Jennifer Hornung. 2001. Building on the vision: exploratory research in future skill areas of the clinical data specialist as described in evolving HIM careers. *Educational Perspectives in Health Information Management* 4(1):19–32.

many designs. For example, sociologists used a descriptive design to describe the culture of medical students (Becker et al. 1961). There are three common types of observational research: nonparticipant observation, participant observation, and ethnography.

Nonparticipant Observation

In **nonparticipant observation,** researchers act as neutral observers who neither intentionally interact with nor affect the actions of the population being observed. Of the three types of observational research, HIM professionals are more likely to encounter nonparticipant observation. This method takes three common forms: naturalistic observation, simulation observation, and case study.

Researchers use **naturalistic observation** for certain behaviors and events that are best observed as they occur naturally. The researchers observe, record, and analyze the behaviors and events. To record the behaviors and events, they typically use check sheets, audiotapes, or videotapes. For the audiotapes and videotapes, they must insert the additional step of transcription. Then, the researchers use coding systems to transform all the recorded observations into analyzable data. For example, researchers investigated the language development of children with compensatory articulation disorder (CAD), a common condition associated with cleft palate (Pamplona et al. 2000). The researchers observed and videotaped fifty-eight children as they played and read stories over a two-week period. They coded the transcribed videotapes using the Situational-Discourse-Semantic Model. Using naturalistic observation, the researchers found that, in all contexts, the children with CAD had delays in language development. Thus, the researchers were able to improve the treatment of patients.

Simulation observation is very similar to naturalistic observation except that the researchers stage the events rather than allowing them to occur naturally. Researchers can invent their own simulations or use standardized vignettes to stage the events. For example, researchers in occupational therapy (Brown et al. 1996) investigated the congruence among therapists' assessments of patients' independence. Measures of independence are achievements of activities of daily living, such as making a purchase in a store and taking a bus. The researchers compared therapists' assessments on simulations and their assessments on tasks in the natural setting. They found that the assessments in the natural setting were more accurate. Therefore, this research assisted occupational therapists in their practice.

The **case study** is another type of nonparticipant observation. Case studies are in-depth investigations of one person, one group, or one institution. Researchers conduct these studies to determine characteristics associated with the person, group, or institution. The characteristics then can shed light on similar persons, groups, or institutions. Often case studies suggest hypotheses that researchers subsequently investigate using other methods. Case studies are intensive, and researchers amass extensive details. Sources of data include administrative records, financial records, policy and procedure manuals, legal documents, government documents, surveys, and interviews. These many sources result in layer upon layer of detailed data, often called rich data.

Sigmund Freud conducted case studies at the individual person level (Borg and Gall 1989). This type of case study is called a clinical case study. Early research in medicine comprised clinical case studies. From a physician's presentation of detailed information about an individual patient, other physicians learned about similar patients.

Other case studies are at the group level and the institutional level. For example, at the group level researchers could investigate the influence that AIDS action groups have had on funding practices of the National Institutes of Health. At the institutional level, Meyer and Blumenthal (1996) investigated the effects of changes in Medicaid policies on two academic medical centers in Tennessee.

Participant Observation

In **participant observation,** researchers are also participants in the observed actions. They can participate overtly (openly) or covertly (secretly). For example, researchers in Australia (van de Mortel and Heyman 1995) wanted to know the incidence of hand washing postpatient contact. The researchers covertly observed the incidence of hand washing to establish a baseline and overtly observed the action to assess the effect of their intervention. On the positive side, participant observation presents the insiders' perspectives. On the negative side, the deception of covert observation undermines human relationships and breaches ethics (Johnson 1992). Moreover, as participants, researchers can reflect the biases and narrow view of insiders. Therefore, in participant observation, researchers attempt to maintain neutrality while in the "thick of the action."

Ethnography

Ethnography is observational research that came to the life sciences from anthropology. It includes both qualitative and quantitative approaches and both participant and nonparticipant observation. Ethnographers typically investigate aspects of culture in naturalistic settings. For example, an HIM professional could choose ethnography to investigate how the culture of a nursing unit or clinic affects the timeliness and comprehensiveness of provider documentation. Are areas of the unit or clinic set aside for documentation, indicating that the culture of the unit or clinic values accurate and comprehensive documentation? Or, do providers attempt to document in health records in corners or on ledges of the unit or clinic, indicating less attention to documentation?

Two key differences exist between ethnography and other types of research. First, in ethnography, the literature review results in working or tentative hypotheses rather than testable hypotheses (Gay 1987). Second, ethnography is iterative, or cyclical (Byrne 2001). As ethnographers collect data, they analyze them, revising their working hypotheses and creating new working hypotheses. Therefore, ethnographers work in a cycle beginning with working hypotheses, collecting data, revising hypotheses and creating new working hypotheses, and then collecting more data about those hypotheses. This cyclical process contrasts with the linear processes of other research methods discussed in this chapter.

In order to understand cultures, ethnographers amass great volumes of detailed data while on studies in the field. Therefore, another characteristic of ethnography is that the researchers live or work with the population they are studying. For example, Hill and Tyson (1997) investigated the culture of clinical teaching conferences. They attended fifty-two sessions of morning report with the faculty physicians, house officers, and medical students and timed the length of people's comments, the commentator's status, and comment's content. In addition to the sessions of morning report, the researchers conducted thirty-four interviews lasting between thirty and sixty minutes with people from the three groups. The quantitative aspect of this study is that the researchers tabulated the minutes and averaged the time that members of each group spoke. The qualitative aspect of this study is that the researchers analyzed the comments for themes.

Ethnography has other unique characteristics, such as the attention that ethnographers pay to the environment (furniture, instruments, space, lighting, schedules, brochures, and clothing). For example, Hill and Tyson (1997) recorded data on X-ray equipment and the placement of a table and a sign-in sheet. In general, ethnographers also record details about members of the population, including jargon, feelings, points of view, beliefs, practices, and goals. In conclusion, the strength of ethnography is that researchers obtain insights not discoverable in other methods. Its weaknesses include volumes of data that are difficult to analyze, large investments of money and time, and the lack of generalizability and replicability.

Experimental Research

Experiments are another major category of research methods. These methods classify into two subcategories: quasi-experimental studies and experimental studies. Both subcategories involve *treatments* using the broad meaning of the term as some sort of intervention. The level of control that researchers establish differentiates experiments between quasi-experimental studies and experimental studies.

Campbell and Stanley (1963) wrote the classic text on experiments. They defined and described six major types of experiments, with three in the subcategory of quasi-experimental and three in the subcategory of experimental. Quasi-experimental studies include the one-shot case study, the one-group pretest-posttest method, and static group comparison. Experimental studies include the pretest-posttest control group method, the Solomon four-group method, and the posttest-only control group method. The key elements in the descriptions of these experiments are randomization, observation (pretest or posttest), control group, and treatment.

Quasi-Experimental Studies

In the *one-shot case study,* researchers study one group only once following the treatment. For example, researchers could provide a two-hour training session on utilization of voice recognition software to all the first-year medical students and then measure the students' level of utilization at the end of the academic year. The researchers can make no credible statement about the effect of the training session on the utilization of voice recognition software because they (1) have not established with an observation (pretest) the level of utilization prior to the training (treatment) to use as a comparison and (2) have no other group of medical students (control group) to use as a comparison.

The *one-group pretest-posttest method* corrects one flaw of the one-shot case study with the addition of the pretest. Pretests and posttests are observations. Similar to the word *treatment,* researchers use the words *pretest, posttest,* and *observation* broadly. They simply mean that they have measured the variable in some way. Therefore, the researchers investigating utilization of voice recognition software could improve their experiment by adding some measurement, or pretest, that establishes the medical students' level of utilization prior to the training session. However, adding the pretest only minimally improves their investigation. Statements made by the researchers about the utilization of voice recognition software still would be highly suspect because they have no control group. Therefore, readers of this research could reasonably wonder whether other factors in the hospital or in society "caused" the level of utilization.

The *static group comparison* corrects the other flaw of the one-shot case study with the addition of a second group, the control group, for comparison. In the research on utilization of voice recognition software, the researchers could allow half the students to choose to attend the training session. This group would be the experimental group, and the half who chose not to receive the training would be the control group. Unfortunately, there is no random assignment. Perhaps all the technophiles joined the experimental group and all the technophobes joined the control group. Then, the increased level of utilization of the experimental group could just be an effect of the group's inherent love of computers and not of the training session.

It should be clear from this example that experiments in an experimental study are very difficult to conduct. Nevertheless, they are extremely powerful research methods. The following three methods are true experimental studies.

Experimental Studies

The *pretest-posttest control group method* corrects both flaws of the one-shot case study. The researchers randomly assigned the first-year medical students to experimental and control groups. By some measure, the researchers established both groups' levels of utilization of voice recognition software. The researchers conducted the two-hour training session and measured both groups' utilization of voice recognition software at the end of the academic year. These researchers could reasonably attribute differences in utilization to their "treatment."

The *Solomon four-group method* is a complex variation of the pretest-posttest control group method. In some instances, taking a pretest affects performance on a posttest. For example, in the study of utilization of voice recognition software, how much of the utilization is due to mere familiarity with the software related to the original exposure? The Solomon four-group method provides a way to control for this possibility. Using this method, researchers would create two experimental groups and two control groups. They then would only administer the pretest to one of the experimental groups and to one of the control groups but would administer the posttest to all four groups. The difference in level of utilization between the two experimental groups would be the effect of the familiarity from pretesting. Therefore, the Solomon four-group method provides a valuable additional control. However, this additional control comes at a very high price: everything is doubled.

The *posttest-only control group method* is very similar to the static group comparison except for one very important element. The posttest-only control group method corrects for the lack of randomization in the static group comparison. In the posttest-only control group method, researchers randomly assign persons to either the experimental group or the control group. Therefore, in the research on utilization of voice recognition software, the researchers would randomly assign half the first-year medical students to the experimental group and half to the control group. The experimental group would receive the treatment of the training session, and the control group would not. This fairly simple method eliminates the potential bias introduced by pretesting.

HIM professionals also encounter this method in clinical trials. For example, parasitologists used this method to observe the effects of drug regimens on multidrug-resistant malaria (Vugt et al. 1999). Patients with malaria presenting at the clinical trial sites were randomly and blindly assigned to study groups or control groups. Two study groups were given the experimental drug regimen, and the control group was given the currently recommended regimen. Laboratory results demonstrated the effects of various drug regimens on the disease.

Experiments are important because they allow researchers to investigate cause and effect. The types classified as quasi-experimental studies begin to determine that a causal relationship could exist. Some experts state that very large quasi-experimental studies *weakly* determine a causal relationship. However, to truly establish causal relationships, researchers must use one of the types classified as an experimental study.

Secondary analysis is the analysis of the original work of another person or organization. Researchers make the distinction between primary analysis and secondary analysis. **Primary analysis** refers to analysis of original research data by the researchers who collected them. There are three types of secondary analysis:

- Secondary analysis of data sets
- Meta-analysis
- Content analysis

In *secondary analysis of data sets,* researchers reanalyze original data by combining data sets to answer new questions or by using more sophisticated statistical techniques (Cohen 1992). In the field of health information management, Osborn (1999, 2001) reanalyzed data sets to evaluate data quality. For example, Osborn reanalyzed clinical databases to identify problems in specific diagnosis-related groups in order to reveal variations in charges and lengths of stay and to detect trends (2001). Reanalysis of secondary data is a powerful tool for health information managers because it allows them to compare their data with local, regional, state, and national benchmarks.

Meta-analysis is the integrative analysis of findings from many studies that examined the same question. Studies that are included in a meta-analysis have common underlying characteristics (Cohen 1992). Glass (1976) coined the term *meta-analysis,* defining it as "the statistical analysis of a large collection of results from individual studies for the purpose of integrating findings" (1976, p. 3). Meta-analysis began as a sophisticated way to present a literature review but has become a research method in its own right.

The advantage of meta-analysis is that it weighs findings from many studies, some of which are contradictory. Researchers who use meta-analysis must specify their inclusion criteria; explain how they searched and found articles; code the studies' designs, methods, and outcomes; and analyze the coded data (Cohen 1992).

For example, Lan, Colford, and Colford (2000) conducted a meta-analysis that analyzed studies of antibiotic treatment for streptococcal tonsillopharyngitis. First, they specified their inclusion criteria. To be included, the study must possess the following four characteristics: (1) it had to be a randomized clinical trial that compared the efficacy of different dosing frequencies of ten-day oral penicillin or amoxicillin in the treatment of acute streptococcal tonsillopharyngitis; (2) diagnosis had to be based on both symptoms and positive clinical findings; (3) antibiotic treatment had to be initiated upon diagnosis; and (4) it had to be the most recent publication, if multiple publications arose from the same study. Second, the researchers explained their strategies to find all the studies. They searched Medline, dissertation abstracts, and abstracts of the annual Interscience Conference on Antimicrobial Agents and Chemotherapy. They used combinations of key words, such as *tonsillopharyngitis, pharyngitis, penicillin, amoxicillin, clinical trial, streptococcus,* and *streptococcal.* These search strategies yielded thirty potential documents. After review, only six met the inclusion criteria. The researchers then coded the studies' designs, methods, and outcomes. Finally, they conducted the meta-analysis statistical procedure called effect size analysis. "Effect size" is the strength of the impact of one factor on another (Shi 1997). Integrating the results of these studies revealed that two doses of penicillin per day are as efficacious as more frequent doses per day. Thus, using meta-analysis, the researchers synthesized the results from multiple studies in order to make an overall conclusion.

Content analysis is the systematic and objective analysis of communication. Most often, researchers analyze written documentation. However, they may analyze other modes of communication, such as speech, body language, music, television shows, commercials, and movies. The purpose of content analysis is to study and predict behaviors.

For example, consumer groups who notify the public about the "most violent" or the "most sexually graphic" shows on television have used content analysis to compile their reports. Healthcare personnel also use content analysis. For example, Wilson et al. (2000) evaluated the readability and cultural sensitivity of information on the National Cancer Institute's Web site. They used standardized tools to conduct this evaluation. From their analysis of forty-nine documents, they established that the reading level was the twelfth grade. Because most newspapers are written at the fourth-grade level, this level would be too advanced for many patients. Thus, content analysis was valuable to oncology nurses who use various means to educate their patients about cancer.

Several key points are important to remember about research design and methods. Research is the systematic, orderly set of procedures that individuals choose to expand their knowledge or to answer their question. They can investigate the same broad question or problem using several of the research designs. (See table 16.6.) Preliminary, exploratory

Table 16.6. Research Designs in a Progression of Studies within One Topic

Design	Example of Progression of Studies
Historical	The factors leading to the creation and expansion of The Medical Record (TMR) and the Regenstrief Medical Record System (RMRS) between 1970 and 1990
Descriptive	A survey of physicians to determine how and to what degree they use the computer-based patient record
Correlational	A study to determine the relationship among physicians' attributes, the setting, and use of the computer-based patient record
Evaluation	A study to evaluate the efficacy of the implementation of the computer-based patient record in an academic health center
Causal-Comparative (Quasi-Experimental)	A study to compare the use of the computer-based patient record of a group of physicians in a setting classified as low barrier and a group of physicians in a setting classified as high barrier
Experimental	A study to compare use of the computer-based patient record of two matched physician groups; one group trained in a low-barrier experimental computer laboratory and one group trained in a high-barrier experimental computer laboratory

investigations are often descriptive or correlational. As researchers refine these investigations, they conduct causal-comparative and experimental studies. The research design chosen depends on the purpose of the research. Certain methods, such as surveys and laboratory experiments, are associated with particular designs. However, methods can be associated with more than one design and overlap occurs. The key point is that how the problem or question is defined indicates the appropriate research design and method.

Check Your Understanding 16.4

Instructions: Answer the following questions on a separate piece of paper.

1. Which research method uses self-report data?
2. What type of question is question 1?
3. Why would researchers choose to conduct a structured interview using an interview guide?
4. If researchers wanted to investigate the impact of the Hill-Burton Act on a region's healthcare, which method would they choose?
5. Why would researchers choose to conduct a questionnaire survey?
6. If researchers wanted to establish that a new drug caused a reduction in blood pressure, which research method would they choose?
7. When would researchers choose to conduct a meta-analysis?
8. In questions 3 through 7, what common characteristic determined the researchers' choice of method?

Statement of Hypothesis

Formulation of precise and accurate hypotheses is a difficult task. In the statement of **hypothesis,** the researcher states the research question in measurable terms. Therefore, the statement of the hypothesis is more specific than the research question. Some experts explain that the statement of the hypothesis operationalizes the research question. Moreover, the statement of the hypothesis becomes the basis of the statistical tests. Therefore, there are two errors to avoid in the statement of the hypothesis: writing an ambiguous hypothesis and writing an untestable hypothesis. Finally, researchers should take care that the hypothesis actually reflects the intent of the research.

Researchers write null hypotheses and alternative hypotheses. The **null hypothesis** states that there is no association between the independent and dependent variables. (The word *null* means none.) The **alternative hypothesis** states that there is an association between the independent and dependent variables. Alternative hypotheses are one-tailed or two-tailed. If the researcher states that the association is more or less, the alternative hypothesis is a **one-tailed hypothesis.** If the researcher makes no prediction about the direction of the results (more or less), the alternative hypothesis is a **two-tailed hypothesis.** These hypotheses are matched pairs. For example:

- *Null hypothesis:* There is no difference in the levels of utilization of voice recognition software between the group of physicians receiving the training and the group not receiving it.
- *Alternative hypothesis (one-tailed):* The level of utilization of the group receiving the training is 10 percent higher than the level of the group not receiving it.
- *Alternative hypothesis (two-tailed):* There is a 10 percent difference in the levels of utilization of voice recognition software between the group of physicians receiving the training and the group not receiving it.

Researchers state what they believe in alternative hypotheses. Unfortunately, the properties of statistical techniques do not allow them to directly test the accuracy of the alternative hypotheses. Instead, statistical techniques test null hypotheses. Therefore, researchers also must write null hypotheses in order to conduct statistical analysis. If the null hypothesis is rejected, the alternative hypothesis is accepted.

Associated with the statement of the hypothesis is establishing the appropriate level of significance known as the alpha (α) level. The **level of significance** is the criterion used for rejecting the null hypothesis. Common alpha levels are 0.05 and 0.01. Researchers set the lower alpha level when they want to minimize the chance that they might erroneously reject the null hypothesis when it is actually true.

Researchers can make two types of errors associated with rejecting or failing to reject null hypotheses. A **type I error** occurs when the researcher erroneously rejects the null hypothesis when it is true; in actuality, there is no difference. A **type II error** occurs when the researcher erroneously fails to reject the null hypothesis when it is false; in actuality, there is a difference. For example:

- *Null hypothesis:* There is no difference in blood pressure levels between the group of patients receiving the new drug and the group receiving the placebo.

- *Alternative hypothesis (one-tailed):* The blood pressure of the group of patients receiving the new drug is 15 percent lower than the blood pressure of the group receiving the placebo.

A researcher committing a type I error would reject the null hypothesis. Continuing in the error, he or she would report the efficacy of the new drug. Unfortunately, the fact is that there is no difference between the blood pressures of the two groups of patients; the new drug does not work as predicted. Researchers who set the alpha level at 0.05 have a five percent chance of making this error whereas those who set the alpha level at 0.01 have a one percent chance of making the error. Thus, an alpha level of 0.01 is stricter than an alpha level of 0.05.

Beta (β) designates the probability of making a type II error. In the previous example, the researcher would make a type II error if he or she failed to reject the null hypothesis and it was indeed false. The researcher would erroneously state that there was no difference between the blood pressure of the group taking the new drug and the blood pressure of the group taking the placebo. In fact, there was a difference and the new drug was working as predicted.

The level of significance is established prior to conducting statistical techniques. Statistical tests for significance result in a ρ value. A ρ value indicates the probability of obtaining the result by chance if the null hypothesis is true. Therefore, if the ρ value is 0.05, the probability that the difference occurred by pure chance is five percent. If the ρ value obtained from the statistical test is less than or equal to the level of predetermined alpha value, the study's results are considered unlikely to be mere chance and the null hypothesis is rejected.

The statement of the hypothesis is a crucial step in the development of the research plan. The statement of the hypothesis leads to the establishment of the appropriate statistical techniques and the determination of the level of significance. These two actions, in turn, affect the interpretation of the consequences of the treatment.

Selection of a Research Method

In selecting a research method, researchers first and foremost should consider their purpose as reflected in their research question. If they want to establish a causal relationship, they should conduct one of the experimental studies. If they are breaking new ground in a poorly understood area of practice, they may want to consider an exploratory study in a qualitative design.

Other factors are associated with the researchers' expertise and resources. Researchers should establish a match between the method and the following factors:

- *Expertise:* Can the researcher conduct, interpret, and explain sophisticated statistical techniques, or are more basic statistical techniques within the researcher's comfort zone?

- *Skills:* Can the researcher conduct the laboratory experiments necessary for research? For example, to investigate physicians' utilization of clinical guidelines, is the researcher able to insert code into a computer-based patient record? Is the researcher able to insert a time clock into the software and design a query mechanism?
- *Personal attributes:* If the researcher is considering interviewing people, is he or she able to easily establish rapport with people? Or, do conversations with strangers make the researcher feel awkward?
- *Time:* Does the researcher have the time to devote to conduct the research plan well? For example, investigating the change in attitude of students in HIM programs from the freshman year through graduation is a meritorious idea. However, graduate programs have time frames within which students must complete their studies. A four-year research study may not fit the time frame.
- *Money:* Can the researcher afford the postage for a census survey of all 40,000 AHIMA members?
- *Potential subjects:* The Solomon four-group method is excellent and beautifully controlled; however, it requires double the number of subjects. If subjects are in short supply, would this method be feasible?

Finally, researchers should strive for parsimony or elegance. *Parsimony* means that the researcher has eliminated extraneous, unnecessary complications. Just as the best theory is the simplest, so too is the best method.

Validity and Reliability

There are three types of validity. Internal validity and external validity involve the integrity of the research plan. Validity without a modifier refers to an attribute of measurement instruments. Reliability involves the consistency of measurements.

Validity

Internal validity and external validity are key issues when implementing a research plan. Campbell and Stanley (1963) identified eight threats to internal validity (figure 16.4, p. 386). **Internal validity** is an attribute of a study's design that contributes to the accuracy of its findings. Threats to internal validity are potential sources of error that contaminate the study's results. These sources of error come from factors outside the study (confounding variables). Therefore, if internal validity is breached, researchers cannot state for certain that the independent variable caused the effect. **External validity** refers to the extent to which the findings can be generalized to other people or groups. **Generalizability** is the term that researchers use to mean the ability to apply the results to other groups, such as hospitals, patients, and states. Are the findings representative of many people or groups? Internal validity represents the bare minimum; internal validity combined with external validity is the ideal.

Figure 16.4.   Threats to Internal Validity

History:	Unplanned events occur during the research and affect the results
Maturation:	Subjects grow or mature during the period of the study
Testing:	Taking the first test affects subsequent tests; "practice effect"
Instrumentation:	Lack of consistency in data collection
Statistical Regression:	Subjects selected because of their extreme scores
Differential Selection:	Control group and experimental group differ and the difference could affect the study's findings
Experimental Mortality:	Loss of subjects during the study
Diffusion of Treatment:	Members of the control group learn about the treatment of the experimental group

For example, researchers within the Department of Veterans Affairs (VA) evaluated the use of automated encoders in the VA system (Lloyd and Layman 1997). Eight VA medical centers tested encoding software programs from three vendors. During the course of the study, an earthquake badly damaged one of the VA medical centers, which never reopened. Therefore, no final data on the software program were available from that center. This event represents the threat to internal validity of **mortality (attrition),** meaning the loss of subjects. In addition, the VA centers were not covered by Medicare's inpatient prospective payment system (PPS) at the time. This uniqueness represents a threat to external validity because most hospitals are covered by the PPS. Thus, the findings lacked generalizability. Therefore, both internal validity and external validity are important considerations for researchers.

Validity in terms of an instrument means the extent to which the instrument measures what it is intended to measure. Multiple aspects of an instrument's validity are assessed. Two important aspects are content validity and construct validity. **Content validity** concerns whether the instrument's items relate to the topic (content). For example, an ICD-9-CM coding test with content validity would have items related to key aspects of coding, such as the definition of principle diagnosis, 5th digits, complications and comorbidities, V codes, E codes, and the neoplasm table. **Construct validity** is the instrument's ability to measure hypothetical, nonobservable traits called constructs. Classic examples of constructs are psychological concepts, such as intelligence, motivation, and anxiety. Although intelligence itself is not visible, its effects are. Therefore, if an instrument is intended to measure patient satisfaction, it should include issues associated with patient satisfaction. Researchers will state in their journal articles the validity of the instruments they used. References about instruments also provide the validity of instruments.

Reliability

Reliability represents consistency. Instruments that have reliability are stable. Repeated administrations will result in reasonably similar findings. **Intrarater reliability** means that the same person repeating the test will have reasonably similar findings. **Interrater reliability** means that different persons taking the test will have reasonably similar findings. Thus, **reliability** means that, over time, a test or observation dependably measures whatever it was intended to measure.

Check Your Understanding 16.5

Instructions: Answer the following questions on a separate piece of paper.

1. In which hypothesis does the researcher state what he or she believes?
2. If the researcher believes that the treatment increases output, would he or she write a one-tailed or a two-tailed hypothesis?
3. What is the difference between a type I error and a type II error?
4. What does the ρ value represent?
5. What issues are involved in internal validity?
6. Why is reliability important in tests?

Selecting an Instrument

An **instrument** is a standardized, uniform way to collect data. Common examples of instruments are interview guides and questionnaires, although many other types exist (figure 16.5). Researchers can find standardized instruments in several reference books (figure 16.6) and in electronic databases. Of particular interest to HIM professionals are three electronic databases: Health and Psychosocial Instruments (HAPI), Buros Institute of Mental Measurements, and ERIC/AE Test Locator. These databases provide descriptions and critiques of instruments.

Researchers should select instruments that other researchers have already developed and refined. The reliability and validity of these instruments are established. Construction of a reliable and valid measure is a research project in and of itself. Osborn (1998) explained that the construction of a questionnaire includes deciding on the content, considering the audience, determining the level of measurement, pilot testing, analyzing the validity and reliability, and confirming the scales. Researchers should undertake the difficult task of developing an instrument only after they have investigated and verified that one does not already exist.

Factors that determine the selection of an instrument include:

- Purpose
- Satisfactory ratings for reliability and validity
- Clarity of language
- Brevity and attractiveness
- Match between the theories underpinning the instrument and the researcher's investigation
- Match between the level of measurement (nominal, ordinal, interval, or ratio scales) and the proposed statistical analyses
- Public domain or proprietary
- Cost

Figure 16.5.   Types of Measurement Instruments

Checklists	Projective techniques
Clinical screenings and assessments	Psychological tests
Coding schemes and manuals	Questionnaires
Educational tests	Rating Scales
Index measures	Scenarios
Interview guides (schedules)	Vignettes
Personality tests	

Figure 16.6.   Print Sources of Measurement Instruments

Buros Institute. 1938–1995. *The Mental Measurements Yearbook: The Yearbook 1938-1995.* Highland Park, N.J.: Buros Institute.

Chun, Ki-Taek, Sidney Cobb, and John R. P. French Jr. 1975. *Measures for Psychological Assessment: A Guide to 3,000 Original Sources and Their Applications.* Ann Arbor, Mich.: Survey Research Center, Institute for Social Research.

Herndon, Robert M., editor. 1997. *Handbook of Neurologic Rating Scales.* New York City: Demos Vermande.

Keyser, Daniel J., and Richard C. Sweetland, editors. 1991. *Test Critiques.* Kansas City, Mo.: Test Corporation of America.

McDowell, Ian, and Claire Newell. 1996. *Measuring Health: A Guide to Rating Scales and Questionnaires,* second edition. New York City: Oxford University Press.

Redman, Barbara K., editor. 1998. *Measurement Tools in Patient Education.* New York City: Springer.

Spreen, Otfried, and Esther Strauss. 1997. *A Compendium of Neuropsychological Tests: Administration, Norms, and Commentary,* second edition. New York City: Oxford University Press.

Sweetland, Richard C., and Daniel J. Keyser, editors. 1991. *Tests: A Comprehensive Reference for Assessments in Psychology, Education, and Business,* third edition. Austin, Tex.: Pro-Ed.

Of these factors, purpose is the most important. Researchers should match their purpose and the instrument's purpose. They should obtain the instrument and then read it in its entirety to be sure that it is collecting what they want to collect and that the terms in it match their meaning for the terms. For example, if the instrument is measuring social support, does it mean social support in the workplace or social support in the family and home? A researcher studying the effect of social support from colleagues and coworkers in the workplace should select an instrument about social support in the workplace. Selecting an instrument about social support in the family would be a grave error with negative consequences for the validity of the research. Thus, merely reading the description and critique in the reference database is insufficient.

Instruments in the public domain can be copied and used freely; instruments that are proprietary must be purchased and cannot be copied. However, researchers can often obtain samples of instruments for review at little or no cost. In addition, researchers must consider the quality of the research. Of what use is an instrument that collects inaccurate data only tangentially related to the researcher's topic? The instrument must match the purpose and contribute to the collection of accurate data that build knowledge.

Obtaining or developing the proper instrument is a key step. Researchers should carefully consider the various factors as they review and select instruments. Carelessness or haste during this step can lead to unusable, unanalyzable data. Purpose should drive the decision.

Gathering the Data

All too often, researchers fail to plan how they will gather data. Researchers who make mistakes during this phase of the research violate one of the factors of internal validity—instrumentation. They have contaminated data and may have compromised their ability to analyze their data. Researchers must write a step-by-step, day-by-day plan for gathering data prior to implementation.

Data Sampling Methods

A **sample** is a set of units selected for study. It is a subset of a **target population,** which is the large group that is the focus of the study. For example, researchers cannot poll all U.S. citizens for their opinions on storing their health data on the Internet. Researchers can identify a sample, meaning a group of citizens representative of the entire population. Individuals are one set of units. In other studies, the sets of units could be bacteria, mice, families, schools, television shows, historical documents, and Web sites. There are two major types of samples: random and nonrandom.

Random Samples

Random sampling underpins many statistical techniques that HIM professionals encounter. To generate random samples, researchers can use either a feature of spreadsheet applications called the random number generator, an option of statistical packages called select cases, or a table of random numbers from a basic statistics textbook. The four types of random sampling are **simple random sampling, stratified random sampling, systematic sampling,** and **cluster sampling.** (See table 16.7, p. 388.) Researchers using these methods attempt to make the sample as representative of the population as possible.

Nonrandom Samples

Two common types of **nonrandom sampling** are convenience sampling and purposive sampling. Convenience samples cast doubt on the generalizability and usefulness of the research. Purposive sampling, on the other hand, serves a valuable function in qualitative research.

Researchers use convenience samples when they "conveniently" use any unit that is at hand. For example, HIM professionals investigating physician satisfaction with departmental services could interview physicians who came to the department. Unfortunately, this convenience sample ignores the opinions of all the physicians who did not come to the department and these physicians may find services substandard. Therefore, use of a convenience sample diminishes the credibility of the research.

Table 16.7.   Types of Random Sampling

Type of Sampling	Description
Simple	The selection of units from a population so that every unit has exactly the same chance of being included in the sample. When a unit has been selected, it is returned to the population so that the other units' chances remain identical.
Stratified	Some populations have characteristics that divide them. For example, the human population is male and female. The male and female subgroups are called strata (singular, stratum). The percentage of the stratum in the population should equal the percentage of the stratum in the sample. Therefore, the sample should be 50% male and 50% female. Other percentages would cast doubt on the results.
Systematic	Units of the sample are selected from a list by drawing every nth unit. For example, health information professionals could choose every fourth surgery on the surgical schedule for surgical case review.
Cluster	The sample is clusters of units. The population is first divided into clusters of units, such as family, school, or community.

Purposive sampling is a strategy of qualitative research. In purposive sampling, researchers use their expertise to select both representative units and unrepresentative units. This strategy reflects the qualitative view that there are many truths. For example, Freud's work is purposive sampling because it focuses on unusual cases. Psychiatrists investigating the psychopathology of mass murderers would use purposive sampling becauses mass murder is not generalizable (Chadwick, Bahr, and Albrecht 1984). Thus, purposive sampling has very specific applications.

Adequacy of the Sample Size

Sample size is the number of subjects the researcher determines should be included in the study in order to represent the population. The adequacy of the sample's size is a common concern. The size of the sample depends on the purpose of the study, the nature of the population, and the researchers' resources (Chadwick, Bahr, and Albrecht 1984). Some experts state that the general rule is to use the largest sample possible (Borg and Gall 1989; Gay 1987). However, Kish (1965) factored in utility to arrive at economic samples. An economic sample provides the level of detail needed to answer the question. Overall, although no absolute rule dictates the size of the sample, researchers should strive for a level of accuracy that makes the study worth conducting.

If a researcher's purpose was to explore areas of inconsistency between paper and electronic records, ninety randomly selected records at one academic health center may be sufficient (Mikkelsen and Aasly 2001). However, a study comparing the efficacy of various treatment protocols for breast cancer warrants a sample size in the thousands. If the researcher's purpose includes many variables, the sample size needs to be larger. Thus, purpose is a critical concern.

The nature of the population includes heterogeneity and typical response and attrition rates. **Heterogeneity** means variation or diversity. The more heterogeneous a population, the larger the sample. The sample needs to be larger in order to ensure that the sample includes all the diverse units in the population. Typical response rate is a factor for surveys. In the literature, other researchers report their response rates. The response rate is the number of people who returned the questionnaire or were reached for interview. If the typical response rate is 50 percent, the researcher will need to distribute twice as many surveys to achieve an adequate response. Attrition (mortality) rates are the numbers of subjects lost during the course of the study. Attrition is a threat to internal validity. High attrition rates also require a larger sample. Understanding the nature of the population contributes to the accuracy of the research.

Resources, namely time and money, also can affect sample size. Sometimes researchers must provide answers in a short time frame. For example, to respond in a timely fashion to a legislative initiative regarding photocopy charges, HIM professionals may conduct a quick survey of a small sample. Individual researchers often face financial constraints. These constraints sometimes result in smaller samples than purists would prefer.

Sample size calculation refers to the qualitative and quantitative procedures used to determine the appropriate sample size. Some experts have offered rules of thumb to calculate sample size (table 16.8). These rules of thumb try to account for frequency of the behavior, numbers of variables, and statistical technique. Other experts (Khan 1997; Osborn 2000b) offer statistical formulae to calculate adequate sample sizes. Formulae depend upon the sampling method used, such as simple random sampling or stratified random sample, and on the amount of information the researcher has about the population. For health information managers, Osborn's text offers excellent examples and step-by-step procedures. Finally, however, specific considerations should override reliance on these rules of thumb and formulae.

The following example outlines the procedure for arriving at an optimal sample size (figure 16.7). Suppose the HIS director at a large academic health center wanted to determine the sample size for a study on the medical staff's opinion of electronic medical records. One commonly used formula for determining sample size requires the researcher to know or decide on the size of the population, the proportion of subjects needed, and an acceptable amount of error. In this instance, the director knows that the number of attending physicians on the medical staff is 800 but has little other information. Therefore, $p = .5$ and $B = .05$. Using the basic formula, the director calculates that, in this situation, a sample of 267 is needed if he or she is willing to accept five percent error due to variability in the sampling.

Table 16.8.   Rules of Thumb for Sample Size

Rule	Source
General: Minimum of 30 cases or responses	Bailey 1994
Descriptive study: Minimum 10 percent of population	Gay 1987
Descriptive study: Minimum 20 percent of small population	Gay 1987
Correlational study: Minimum of 30 cases or responses	Borg and Gall 1989
Causal-comparative and experimental research: 15 to 30 cases per comparison group	Borg and Gall 1989; Gay 1987
Major subgroup: 100 each Minor subgroups: 20 to 50 each per subgroup	Sudman 1976
General: 200 cases or responses	Chadwick, Bahr, and Albrecht 1984

Figure 16.7.   Basic Example of Sample Size Calculation

Sample size = n
Size of the population = N
Proportion of subjects needed = p
Acceptable amount of error = B

Formula

$$n = \frac{Np(1 - p)}{(N - 1)\frac{(B^2)}{4} + (p)(1 - p)}$$

Data from the Case

$N = 800$
$p = .5$
$B = .05$

Calculations

$$n = \frac{(800)(.5)(1 - .5)}{(800 - 1)\frac{(.05^2)}{4} + (.5)(1 - .5)}$$

$$n = \frac{200}{(799)(.000625) + .25}$$

$$n = \frac{200}{.75}$$

$$n = 267$$

Data Collection Procedures

The research plan should consider every logistical detail of the collection of the data from start to finish. Lack of attention to detail at this point will breach factors of internal validity. Some issues related to data collection affect many of the methods; other issues are unique to the method. Data collection issues include:

- Obtaining approvals of oversight committees
- Listing each data element required to perform the appropriate statistical techniques
- Training for data collection procedures
- Performing a pilot study
- Considering the response rate
- Conducting the treatment
- Collecting the data
- Assembling the data for analysis

Federal regulations govern research on human subjects (Penslar 2001). Their purpose is to protect humans from researchers' abuses, such as those that occurred in the Tuskegee Syphilis Study (figure 16.8). To comply with federal regulations, organizations have **Institutional Review Boards** (IRBs). IRBs (sometimes called human subjects committees) are administrative bodies established to protect the rights and welfare of human research subjects recruited to participate in research activities associated with institutions. They approve, require modifications in, or disapprove of all research activities within their jurisdictions as specified by both federal regulations and institutional policies. As human health and life are at stake, the federal government imposes severe penalties on institutions and individuals who fail to comply.

Prior to conducting studies, researchers must obtain written approvals from the IRB and other oversight entities of their organizations. To obtain approvals, researchers complete the organization's documentation, providing descriptions of their research plan and copies of their informed consent forms. Sufficient time must be allowed in their plan for the board to review the research, meet, and respond.

Researchers should compile a list of each data element required for each statistical analysis they plan to conduct. Prior to beginning data collection, researchers should ensure that their data collection strategies will obtain all the data. Therefore, it is advisable to conduct mock statistical analyses on fabricated data and to create tables and figures for the manuscript early in the planning of the research. For example, suppose researchers were investigating whether the time from heart transplant to the first rejection episode differed by ABO blood type and Rh factor. The blood types and Rh factors are not evenly distributed in the general population nor are they evenly distributed by national origin. Running mock statistical analyses would reveal that the researchers need a large sample size. Too often, graduate students have had to write in their theses or dissertations, "I did not have sufficient cases to run the statistical analysis." Planning can avoid this embarrassment.

Researchers and those they employ to assist them may require special training. For example, publishers of some psychological tests require verification of training to administer

Figure 16.8.   Tuskegee Syphilis Study

The Tuskegee Syphilis Study is a notorious chapter in medical research in the United States. From 1932 to 1972, the U.S. Public Health Service conducted research that had the stated purpose of obtaining more information about the clinical course of syphilis. The medical researchers from the U.S. Public Health Service experimented on 399 African American males in Macon County, Alabama. The medical researchers told the men that they were being treated for "bad blood." In fact, the researchers were deceiving the men and were denying them treatment for syphilis. Many of the men's wives were infected, and their children were subsequently born with congenital syphilis. The U.S. Public Health Service continued the study despite the advent of penicillin in 1947. The Tuskegee Syphilis Study is a symbol of unethical research.

the tests. The researchers must obtain this verification (or select another instrument). To effectively conduct interviews or to observe vignettes, researchers and their assistants also need training.

Performing a pilot study enhances the likelihood of the study's successful completion. When researchers conduct pilot studies, they work out the details of their research plan. The maxim, "The devil is in the details," is only too true. Pilot studies can reveal the following information:

- Biases in sample selection
- Volumes required
- Associated costs
- Performance features of equipment
- Defects, such as poorly worded cover letters, unclear questionnaire items, and leading questions in interviews
- Possible log jams (gridlock) in the mailing method
- Errors in the scoring key
- Discrepancies between the order of items on the data collection instrument and the order on the computer screen

Pilot studies demonstrate that the research study is logistically feasible. Even researchers conducting naturalistic studies perform simulations that test their instruments prior to the event. Pilot studies are as necessary as disaster drills.

Ensuring an adequate response rate is of particular concern for surveys. Low response rates jeopardize study accuracy and generalizability. Therefore, researchers strive to increase their response rates. To increase response rates, researchers can use the findings of Berdie and Anderson (1974). These researchers conducted the classic research study on the process of questionnaire surveys. Their research revealed many strategies to increase the response rate (figure 16.9). Their primary recommendation was that researchers know their topic and their target population. This knowledge underpins decisions about the strategies and techniques to increase response rates.

Strategies to increase the response rate for questionnaire research include using a brief cover letter and multiple mailings. The cover letter should explain the purpose of the study and its benefits for the participants. Obtaining the sponsorship of a professional association or officials is desirable. Moreover, the letter should thank the responder, provide a deadline, and offer the study results. In the field of health information management, ensuring the confidentiality of the response also is particularly important. Key characteristics of effective cover letters are shown in figure 16.10. Multiple mailings in a timed sequence can significantly improve the response rate. For example, the total design method routinely achieves response rates of 74 percent (Dillman 1978; Salant and Dillman 1994).

Researchers also must be on guard for bias in response. For example, do persons who volunteer to participate in the research differ from those who do not volunteer? Do the persons who responded to the survey (responders) differ from

Figure 16.9.   Summary of Berdie and Anderson's Strategies to Increase the Response Rate in Questionnaire Surveys

General
1. Physical attractiveness of cover letter, postcard, and questionnaire
2. Quality of printing and paper
3. Pleasingly colored paper
4. Error-free documents
5. Incentives, such as an offer of the study's results or money ($0.25 maximum)

Cover Letter
1. Salutation's formality is tailored to the target population.
2. Prestigious sponsor
3. Time frame for response is exact (10 days) or "as soon as possible," depending on the population.
4. Tone of sincerity and honesty
5. Assurance of confidentiality

Questionnaire
1. Title
2. Easy to complete
3. Clear instructions included in the body of the questionnaire
4. Reasonable length
5. Contact information and return mailing address at the bottom

Mailing
1. Initial contact (postcard) that is an appeal for participation
2. Self-addressed, stamped return envelope
3. Properly timed follow-up

those who did not (nonresponders)? Finally, how similar are the participants, nonparticipants, responders, and nonresponders to the population?

In conducting the study, researchers must be careful to follow the plan they have written. Deviations from the protocol result in potential bias and inaccurate data. For example, in questionnaire research, the Dillman (1978) method depends on a strictly timed series of mailings. Does the researcher have staff to track the responses and to physically assemble the mailings?

Researchers must include a mechanism in the plan for compiling their data. If videotapes are involved, where will they be stored? Because sensitive data may be on personality tests, how will confidentiality be maintained? If the research includes measurement instruments, who will score them?

After researchers have collected the data, they must organize them in a way that allows analysis. In this step, the researchers must decide how they will enter the data into a software package. Who will enter the data? How will they ensure accuracy of data entry? Who will transcribe the contents of videotapes or audiotapes?

Data collection is a systematic, planned procedure that results in internal validity. Conducting a pilot study is a key step in assuring a thorough and carefully conceived plan. The methods section of the study report documents the plan's execution. The methods section is also a recipe that other researchers can use to replicate the study. Therefore, careful attention to documentation and vigilant adherence to procedures are demanded.

Instructions: Answer the following questions on a separate piece of paper.

1. Why would a researcher choose to use an instrument that someone else has created?

2. What is an adequate sample?

3. Would directors of departments of health information services be considered a heterogeneous population or a homogenous population?

4. Why are IRBs important?

5. What is a pilot study?

6. Why are survey researchers concerned about their response rates?

7. What common mistake do researchers make in data collection?

Analyzing the Data

In this phase of the research process, researchers try to determine what they have found or what the data reveal. Many researchers fall into the common error of allowing too little time for analysis. Researchers should be sure to allocate sufficient time in their research plan to analyze and interpret the data.

Before conducting their study, researchers should determine which statistical techniques they will use. These techniques are specified in the methods section of the manuscript. The description of the statistical techniques should be clear so that other researchers can duplicate them.

Techniques for Data Analysis

Three broad categories of statistical analysis exist: descriptive statistics, inferential statistics, and test statistics. **Descriptive** (summary) **statistics** describe the data. **Inferential statistics** allow the researchers to make inferences about the population characteristics (parameters) from the sample's characteristics. Finally, **test statistics** examine the psychometric properties of measurement instruments.

Figure 16.10.   Sample Cover Letter

Letterhead	ZHIMA 1800 Carriage Oxford, ZB 31002 October 1, 2002 Dear Colleague:
Purpose	The healthcare system and our field are rapidly changing. These changes place increasing demands on health information practitioners. Little research exists that explores stress and the buffers in directors of hospital health information management departments.
Study's Importance Participant's Importance	Therefore, you have been randomly selected to participate in a national survey on stress in the workplace. Please take the time to complete and return the survey. The accuracy of the results and the possible benefits for the profession depend on your participation.
Sponsor Time to Complete	This research is being sponsored by the AHIMA. The entire survey should take 15 to 20 minutes of your time. A detailed, personalized report on your coping resources is available. Should you wish to receive it, please write your name and address at the bottom of the pink Demographic Form. — Offer of Results
Time Frame	Please return the survey within 10 days in the postage-paid envelope. — SASE
	A vital concern of the health information management profession is confidentiality in research. The code number on your questionnaire is for mailing and follow-up purposes only. Only aggregate data will be reported, and at no time will the questionnaires be identified by respondent. — Confidentiality
Appreciation Contact Instruction	I truly appreciate your participation, and I think the findings of the survey will benefit many members of our profession in these stressful times. If you have any questions about the survey, please write or call me.
	Sincerely Jane Edwards, PhD 123 Anyplace Street Anytown, IL 12345 (123) 456-7890 Enclosures

Generally, researchers should begin with descriptive techniques to verify the accuracy of their data entry and to provide an overview of their respondents. Descriptive techniques include means, frequency distributions, and standard deviations. These statistical techniques are also called **univariate** because they involve one variable.

Researchers investigating the differences between groups would use a paired *t* test or analysis of variance (ANOVA). These are examples of inferential statistics.

Test statistics describe and explore the validity and reliability of tests. Researchers conducting test statistics calculate the validity coefficient (correlation coefficient) and each item's validity. They also could perform factor analysis. Examples of approaches to verify reliability include test-retest and Kuder-Richardson formulae. Finally, test statistics include an index of difficulty, which is the percentage of persons correctly answering each item.

Most research data can be subjected to more than one statistical technique. Researchers should maximize the use of their data by using a variety of techniques to look at their data from multiple views. Multiple views of the data shed light on different aspects of the issue and expand the body of knowledge.

Appropriate statistical techniques vary by the purpose of the research (research design), the number of variables, the type of data, and the nature of the target population. This discussion briefly describes a few common techniques. (For a detailed discussion, see chapter 15.)

Purpose of the Research

Researchers should match their purpose and their statistical technique. For example, researchers using a correlational design are investigating relationships. How do the variables relate to one another? Therefore, these researchers would use correlational statistics. One correlational technique is the **bivariate** correlational coefficient. The bivariate correlational coefficient allows the researcher to describe the strength of the relationship between two variables in mathematical terms.

Number of Variables

The number of variables also affects the choice of statistical technique. **Multivariate** correlational methods involve many variables. For example, multiple linear regression examines the strength of relationship between several independent variables and one dependent variable. Other more complex forms of regression exist.

Type of Data

Another factor in the choice of statistical technique is the type of data. There are five types of data:

- **Discrete data** are separate and distinct values or observations. Patients in the hospital represent discrete data because each patient can be counted.
- **Categorical data** are values or observations that can be sorted into a category, for example, gender.

- **Nominal data** are values or observations that can be labeled or named (*nom* = name). Therefore, the data can be coded, for example, Married = Y and Single = N or Male = 0 and Female = 1. Nominal data cannot be ranked or measured.
- **Ordinal data** represent values or observations that can be ranked (ordered). Ranking scales are common examples of ordinal data. For example, physicians often ask patients to evaluate the severity of their pain on a scale from 1 to 10. HIM professionals could use ordinal data when investigating customer satisfaction. For example, a health information manager could ask physicians how satisfied they were with the department's service on a scale from 1 to 5. However, because these rankings are subjective, the difference in satisfaction between 2 and 3 may be much less than the difference between 4 and 5.
- **Metric data** can be measured on some scale. Two subtypes are interval and ratio. The scale for **interval data** does not begin with a true zero. Time, as humans measure it, does not begin with a true zero. Interval data represent values or observations that occur on an evenly distributed scale. Time in years is an evenly distributed scale. The interval between 1985 and 1990 is the same as the interval between 1991 and 1996. On the other hand, the scale for **ratio data** does begin at a true zero. Height, weight, and temperature are examples of ratio data.

Metric data are **continuous data.** They represent values or observations that have an indefinite number of points along a continuum. For example, measurements made with a ruler can be a foot, an inch, a half-inch, a quarter, an eighth, to infinity. Continuous data also exhibit characteristics of the other types of data; they can be counted (discrete) and ordered (ordinal) and can be grouped.

The type of data depends on the way the variable is measured, not some inherent attribute of the variable. For example, height can be measured in inches or categorized as short or tall. Therefore, researchers should be careful to collect data in the form that matches their intended statistical technique.

Nature of the Target Population

The nature of the target population also affects the choice of statistical technique. For example, some statistical techniques are based on the assumption that the variable is normally distributed in the population. **Parametric techniques,** such as Student's *t* test, ANOVA, and Pearson *r*, are used in these cases. However, this assumption is not always true. In some cases, researchers use **nonparametric** or **distribution-free techniques,** for example, chi square and Spearman rho. Nonparametric techniques also are used for nominal and ordinal data.

Statistical Software Packages

Many software packages are available to assist researchers in the analysis of data. For basic descriptive statistics, researchers can use spreadsheet software, such as Excel™. However, most researchers will choose to use dedicated statistical packages because these packages require less manipulation of the data than spreadsheet packages and because they perform many more statistical procedures. Other factors that influence the choice of software are type of data, planned analytical techniques, and cost.

Several software packages are commonly used in research projects. For example, Code-A-Text is used to code and analyze documents, transcripts, and sound files. Coding is labeling words or word groups (segments) with annotations or scales. These labels are characteristics of the segments. This software allows researchers to specify labels and easily insert them into the document or sound file. Once the researcher has coded what the subjects said, the researcher can analyze the content of the document or sound file also using this software. The software produces descriptive statistics and tables and charts that support analysis. The software also assists researchers to categorize the segments into themes, known as content analysis. Code-A-Text can be applied to field notes, open-ended questionnaires, and interviews. A multimedia version codes video and pictures.

Epi-Info is freeware from the Centers for Disease Control. This integrated package, which includes word processing, database, and statistics, is designed for public health. The software allows the handling of epidemiological data in questionnaire format, calculating the required sample size, analyzing data, and presenting results.

LISREL is a software package that conducts factor analysis. Factor analysis is used to evaluate the psychometric properties of measurement instruments. LISREL generates test statistics. For example, Aish and Wasserman (2001) used LISREL to evaluate the properties of a psychological test that predicts suicidal behavior.

Qualitative Solutions and Research Non-numerical Unstructured Data Indexing Searching and Theorizing (QSR NUD*IST) 4.0 is a software package used to analyze qualitative data. NUD*IST searches text to generate categories and indexes. This software assists qualitative researchers to generate themes and theory. Mechanic and Meyer (2000) used NUD*IST to analyze transcripts from audiotapes. The software broke responses down into individual phrases that expressed a single theme.

Statistical Analysis System (SAS) is a powerful software package that integrates data access, data management, data analysis, and data presentation. Researchers use SAS to enter data, retrieve and manage data, analyze data with statistical and mathematical techniques, write reports, and generate graphics.

Statistical Package for Social Sciences (SPSS) offers a broad array of analytical and graphic software. Its many components range from basic statistical techniques to advanced, specialized techniques. Basic statistics performs counts and cross-tabs. Advanced techniques include factor, regression, cluster analysis, binomial and multinomial logistic regression, and correspondence analysis.

Check Your Understanding 16.7

Instructions: Answer the following questions on a separate piece of paper.

1. How do descriptive and inferential statistics differ?
2. How many variables do bivariate statistical techniques involve?
3. What inferential statistical techniques emphasize differences in groups?
4. What are two types of continuous data?
5. Why must researchers know the type of data they are collecting?
6. Why might a researcher use Epi-Info as his or her statistical package?

Presenting Results

A common research pitfall is that researchers do not allow adequate time to write their results. As stated earlier, the purpose of research is to build knowledge. Knowledge confined to the researchers' heads is of little use to practitioners in the workplace.

Researchers follow a two-step process when presenting their results. In the first step, they report their research findings with no commentary, explanation, or interpretation. This section of a manuscript is called research findings. In the second step, the researchers comment on, explain, and interpret their findings. This section of the manuscript is called discussion. Also included in the discussion are conclusions and recommendations for future research.

Researchers describe their results in the past tense; general truths are stated in the present tense. The style of writing for scientific manuscripts is objective, precise, and factual. Researchers avoid subjective interjections and emotional hyperbole. In the research findings, researchers must be very careful to maintain a neutral tone. They are merely recording their findings in narrative form.

In research findings, researchers describe the results for each hypothesis. Restating the hypothesis aids the readers. Researchers state whether or not the results support the hypotheses. They also record characteristics about the sample and describe the results of the statistical analyses that investigate whether the sample is similar to or different from the population. Supplemental statistical analyses also are described.

For research findings, researchers generate tables and graphs to support the readers' understanding of their findings. (See chapter 15 for more detailed descriptions of some common tables and graphs.) Day's (1988) rule of thumb is that data should be presented in only one way or mode. Researchers should present the particular data element in narrative text, in a table, or in a figure, but not in multiple modes. Graphics should clarify the data, not confuse the readers. Figure 16.11 lists ten important points to remember

Figure 16.11.   Considerations for Effective Graphics

1. Tables, graphs, and figures have titles.
2. Tables have subheads, spanner heads, and column heads for clarification.
3. Sources are cited.
4. Time frames and dates are noted.
5. Multiple tables, charts, graphs, and figures are numbered.
6. Both axes of graphs are labeled (bar titles, legends, scale captions).
7. Keys show the meaning of shadings and colors.
8. Scales start at zero.
9. Wedges (slices) of a pie chart represent percentages, and the percentages convert to 360 degrees.
10. Graphics are for emphasis; do not dilute the effect with clutter.

when constructing graphics. Researchers must carefully consider which mode of communication is most effective for the particular data element. For example:

- *Tables* summarize data in a grid or matrix. The elements and numbers should be in the columns, not in the rows.
- *Pie charts* with their segments visually show the relationships among variables and the whole. They also can represent categorical data.
- *Bar charts* show comparisons between and among items. They often illustrate major characteristics in the distribution of data (male or female, age ranges). They can be used to represent categorical, nominal, or ordinal data.
- *Line charts* show comparisons over time.
- *Histograms* are similar to bar charts. They show major characteristics in the distribution of data and summarize data about variables whose values are numerical and measured on an interval scale. Histograms are used for large data sets.

Writing the discussion section requires energy and creativity. Too often, researchers short-change this section. The discussion section is not a superficial repetition of the findings section. Rather, it is where researchers create new knowledge.

In the discussion section, researchers should compare their findings to the findings in the literature, explaining similarities and discrepancies. More important, they should provide some rationale to explain why their findings were the same or different. In writing this section, researchers should return to why they conducted the study in the first place. They should answer the following questions:

- What theoretical significance or practical worth do their findings have?
- How do their findings explicitly link to the larger body of knowledge?
- How have their findings improved the field's research model?
- How have they expanded the body of knowledge?
- What new definitions have they added to the field's area of practice?

- How do their findings support practitioners in the workplace?
- What problems do their findings solve?
- What valid conclusions can the researchers and the readers draw?

Research always raises new questions. These new questions become the suggestions for further research.

The discussion section closes the presentation of the findings. To accurately represent the time and effort that went into the research study, the discussion section should be rich and insightful. Sufficient time for reflection and contemplation should be scheduled into the research plan. The researchers' goal should be to put usable information into the hands of practitioners in the workplace.

Publishing Research

Knowledge is disseminated and examined in professional journals. To be useful, this information must be available and accessible. Therefore, researchers have an ethical obligation to publish their research. To prepare their results for publication, researchers face two major tasks: selecting the appropriate journal and following its submission guidelines.

Selecting the Appropriate Journal

As mentioned earlier, in the field of health information management, research is published in three journals: *Educational Perspectives in Health Information Management (EPHIM)*, the *Journal of the American Health Information Management Association (JAHIMA)*, and *Topics in Health Information Management (THIM)*. However, depending on the topic, researchers should consider journals in other disciplines, such as informatics, public health, epidemiology, healthcare management, allied health, nursing, bioethics, health services, health policy, and health education. Researchers can obtain lists of journals from a library.

Selecting the appropriate journal requires thought and investigation, and researchers should take the time to skim through a number of journals. This investigation allows them to match their purpose, topic, research design, and style to the journal's scope, content, and audience.

First, researchers should determine their purpose. Is it altruism, service, or promotion and tenure? Certain journals are better suited to one purpose than another. For example, some journals have a practice orientation and others have a research orientation.

For altruism and service, researchers may send their manuscripts to journals oriented to practice, such as the *JAHIMA*. The researchers want to help their profession by putting effective techniques into the hands of practitioners. For example, if the researcher found that a particular graphical interface increased coder accuracy by 10 percent, he or she may decide to send that manuscript to the *JAHIMA* or to *THIM*.

In addition to altruism and service, some researchers must meet work standards for promotion and tenure and publish as a condition of employment. Sometimes the work standards for publication specify quantity and quality. Quantity is the number of articles. Quality is less easily evaluated than quantity. One indirect measure is the prestige of the journal as indicated by its status as refereed or nonrefereed and its rejection rate. Researchers publishing to meet work standards should consider the refereed journals that have high rejection rates.

Second, researchers should match the content of their manuscript with the focus of the journal. For example, researchers should send manuscripts about research on the management of health information services to journals in the field of health information management. If their results have an impact on reimbursement or health policy, the researchers should consider journals with a broader base.

Third, researchers must match the design and method of their research to the types of designs and methods in the journal. Some journals include mostly experimental and quasi-experimental research; others include ethnographies, case studies, and personal histories. Researchers who match the design and method of their study with the types of typical designs and methods in the journal increase the likelihood of their manuscripts being accepted.

Fourth, researchers should strive for a match between their writing style and the preferences of the journal's audience. Journals that are oriented toward practice prefer brief articles written in simple, direct sentences. On the other hand, journals oriented toward scholarly work prefer a more formal and pedantic tone.

Finally, understanding the journal's audience combines the issues of topic and design. Researchers should submit their manuscripts to journals with audiences that would be interested in the topic. If the intended audience includes a broad range of fields, researchers should write manuscripts that are of interest to all potential readers. Moreover, researchers should clearly state how their manuscript affects and benefits the journal's intended audience.

Following the Journal's Submission Guidelines

Journals have rules for the format of manuscripts. The rules are both explicit and implicit. Explicit rules are openly stated; implicit rules are unwritten, but important. Editors and peer reviewers assume that researchers will naturally know and follow them. Different fields tend to have their own unique sets of implicit rules.

Journal editors state their explicit requirements for manuscripts in their style manual and submission guidelines. There are four major style manuals (figure 16.12). Selection of style manual relates to the field. For example, journals in education generally require APA style whereas biomedical journals require AMA style. Journals in health information management use an adapted University of Chicago style. The variance in style manuals is illustrated in table 16.9.

The journal's submission guidelines include details such as the word-processing package, width of margins, length, and organizational structure (figure 16.13, p. 396). For instance, the editors of EPHIM prefer an organizational structure that generally includes the following elements:

- Introduction/background
- Literature review
- Objectives

Figure 16.12.   Common Style Manuals

American Psychological Association. 1994. *Publication Manual of the American Psychological Association,* fourth edition. Washington, D.C.: APA. [Referred to as **APA Style.**]

Gibaldi, Joseph. 1999. *MLA Handbook for Writers of Research Papers,* fifth edition. New York City: Modern Language Association of America. [Referred to as **MLA Style.**]

Iverson, Cheryl. 1998. *American Medical Association Manual of Style: A Guide for Authors and Editors,* ninth edition. Baltimore: Williams & Wilkins. [Referred to as **AMA Style.**]

University of Chicago Press. 1993. *Chicago Manual of Style,* fourteenth edition. Chicago: University of Chicago Press. {Referred to as **Chicago Style.**]

Table 16.9.   Variation in Style Manuals

Organization	Book	Journal
AMA	Jencks C, Riesman D. *The Academic Revolution.* Chicago: University of Chicago Press; 1977.	Lloyd SC, Layman E. The effects of automated encoders on coding accuracy and coding speed. *Top Health Inf Manage* February 1997;17(3):72–79.
APA	Jencks, C., & Riesman, D. (1977). *The academic revolution.* Chicago: University of Chicago Press.	Lloyd, S. C., & Layman, E. (1997, February). The effects of automated encoders on coding accuracy and coding speed. Topics in *Health Information Management,* 17(3), 72–79.
Chicago	Jencks, Christopher, and David Riesman. 1977. *The Academic Revolution.* Chicago: University of Chicago Press.	Lloyd, Susan C., and Elizabeth Layman. 1997 (February). The effects of automated encoders on coding accuracy and coding speed. *Topics in Health Information Management* 17(3):72–79.
MLA	Jencks, Christopher, and David Riesman. *The Academic Revolution.* Chicago: University of Chicago Press, 1977.	Lloyd, Susan C., and Elizabeth Layman. "The Effects of Automated Encoders on Coding Accuracy and Coding Speed." *Topics in Health Information Management* 17.3 (1997): 72–79.

Figure 16.13.   Content of Submission Guidelines

Information needed about the author and contact
Style manual
Length and representativeness of title
Length of abstract in words
Length of manuscript in maximum number of pages or number of words
Font and font size
Line spacing
Justification
Margins
Pagination
Inclusive (nonsexist) language
Blinding (names of authors on separate page)
Format of charts and tables
Format of citations in text
Format of references (sometimes vary slightly from style manual)
General organizational structure of manuscript
Word-processing software
Number of paper copies
Diskette or electronic submission

- Methodology
- Analysis
- Results
- Discussion
- Conclusions

However, most editors do state that the organizational structure is flexible and that researchers should adapt the structure to suit their research. Researchers can find guidelines in journals or at the publishers' Web sites.

A journal's implicit rules reflect the culture of its audience. Culture is reflected in the use of the first person, anthropomorphism, passive voice, and tone. For example, an audience of qualitative researchers would accept use of the first person whereas its use probably would cause an audience of experimental researchers to doubt the article's credibility. Purists reject anthropomorphism as giving human traits to inanimate objects. Audiences that reject first person and anthropomorphism also tend to prefer passive voice and a detached, neutral tone. Time spent skimming journals would provide insight into the implicit rules of the various journals.

Some editors and peer reviewers assume that sloppy writing indicates sloppy research. Moreover, some editors and peer reviewers believe that the inability to follow submission guidelines indicates the inability to follow research protocols. Therefore, attention to detail is important. Researchers seeking more information about writing and publishing manuscripts should read the style manuals and review samples of submission guidelines. For grammar and clarity, Strunk and White's book on writing is a classic (2000). First published in 1959 and periodically revised, its succinct discussions and precise examples provide clear guidance. Finally, researchers should carefully read Day's book (1988), which is dedicated to research writing and publishing.

Check Your Understanding 16.8

Instructions: Answer the following questions on a separate piece of paper.

1. How do the research findings and discussion sections differ?
2. What two factors should researchers consider when determining how to present a particular data element?
3. What three questions should a researcher answer when writing the discussion section?
4. What three factors should researchers consider when selecting a journal for manuscript submission?

Search Techniques

Conducting searches of databases, Web sites, and library holdings is particularly well suited to health information managers. Their ability to organize and manage information is put to good use. Search techniques are used in a wide variety of media and settings. This section describes various sources of data and corresponding search techniques.

Literature Review

A well-developed literature review begins with a systematic plan to categorize, obtain, and organize the literature. Categorizing includes listing all types of sources of information on the topic. Although traditional literature may constitute the major portion of the plan, other sources (such as videos, newscasts, and the Internet) can contribute and should be considered. Tables and lists are essential tools.

The following steps for literature searches focus on refereed journal articles. Researchers can use similar tactics in other media and for popular literature.

1. Generate a list of key terms and synonyms (in the databases of medical literature these are medical subject headings or MeSH headings).
2. Generate a list of target databases (such as Healthstar, MedLine, CINAHL).
3. Search each database with each term. Use an advanced "All Fields" search and document each search.
4. Use the "Limit" function to narrow the searches to refereed journals.
5. Print articles from on-line journals.
6. Copy articles from print journals (bring an adequate supply of change or purchase a copy card).
7. Read and analyze the literature obtained to date.
8. Identify key journal articles.
9. Obtain the references cited at the end of the key articles. Track their order and receipt.
10. Note the medical subject headings (MeSH headings) of the key articles. If the original list missed these terms, rerun the search of the databases on the new terms.
11. Identify key researchers in the topic. Run advanced searches on "author." Obtain all their articles and books on the topic.

12. Alphabetize all the copies of the articles by author. This strategy avoids duplication and allows prompt access.

To avoid rework during the manuscript's composition, researchers should capture all data about the source when they first obtain it. The various style manuals have different requirements. To meet all the requirements, researchers should be sure to note the following information about their sources:

- Full name of the author, including first name and middle initial or name
- Full title of the journal, book, video, or Internet site
- Complete information about dates of publication, including the year, month, and season
- Complete name and address of the publisher (for books and videos)
- Inclusive page numbers
- Volume number and issue number (sometimes these data are only on the front of the publication)
- Accurate URL and access date (for the Internet)

Bibliographic software packages are available to assist researchers. These packages allow researchers to create bibliographic databases. The contents of the database can be imported into word-processing software. The software packages contain algorithms that transform the bibliographic entry into the required style (styles editor). Some also include search engines and allow direct download of the bibliographic entry without rekeying. Commonly used bibliographic packages include Reference Manager, EndNote, and ProCite.

Library Research

The holdings of a library include all of its books, reference manuals, maps, videotapes, audiotapes, and literary and other databases. Many libraries list their holdings on the Internet. Book holdings can typically be accessed through the library's catalog. The databases and on-line journals usually can be found under electronic resources. Libraries purchase licenses that allow their users access to the various databases. Just as different libraries have purchased different books, different libraries have purchased different licenses.

Students have access to the holdings of their educational institutions' libraries. In addition, AHIMA members have access to the National Information Center for Health Services Administration (NICHSA), which has access to thousands of books and more than 300 healthcare-related databases. Public libraries offer access to many information resources. Finally, healthcare organizations have libraries or access to libraries, and working professionals have access to their organizations' libraries.

Although Web sites may have information that has not been peer reviewed, they may have valuable government reports and other documents. Some libraries have developed Web sites that explain the features of various Internet search engines. The Web sites of two libraries, the University of South Carolina Beaufort Library (http://www.sc.edu/beaufort/library) and the Kansas City Public Library (http://www.kclibrary.org/resources/search/chart.cfm), provide tutorials on search engines.

Other Sources of Data

Several other sources of data are available to researchers. For example, several states post Medicaid data on the Internet. Specific examples of available data include:

- Labor force, earnings, and prices (Bureau of Labor Statistics)
- Crime, demographics, education, and health (Social Statistics Briefing Room)
- Statistics and information from seventy federal agencies (FedStats)
- Health statistics (National Center for Health Statistics, FASTATS A–Z)
- Medicare data (Medicare Provider Analysis and Review [MEDPAR] of Short-Stay Hospitals)
- Demographic data on U.S. population (Population Reference Bureau)
- Business, economic, and trade data from the federal government (STAT-USA)
- Hundreds of files from various governments (Statistical Resources on the Web)
- U.S. census data (U.S. Census Bureau)

The problem is that in order to transform the data into information, researchers must understand the underlying structure of the data and how they were collected. Each data source has its own unique characteristics.

For example, one hospital database contained a field related to death, which is typically a discharge status. However, with its death field (Field 342), the hospital could track the number of intraoperative deaths, postoperative deaths, autopsied deaths, and medical examiner's cases. The death field was a multiple-entry field, with each category having a number (intra-operative deaths = 1; postoperative death = 2; autopsied death = 3; and medical examiner's case =4). A surgeon requested a report on the number of intra-operative deaths. The worker who usually ran reports was on vacation and another worker attempted to run the query. This worker wrote the query as Field 342 = "1." As a multiple-entry field, the query should have been written as Field 342 contains "1." The erroneously written query excluded all intra-operative deaths that were also postoperative deaths (2), autopsied deaths (3), and medical examiner's cases (4). Some cases are all four. The case of a multiple stabbing victim illustrates the point. From the emergency room, the patient is initially brought to the operating room (OR). His wounds are explored and sutured. Postoperatively, the patient is sent to the intensive care unit. While in the ICU, he begins to bleed internally again and is brought back to the OR. While in the OR the second time, the patient dies. This patient is both a post-operative death and an intra-operative death (2 and 1). In addition, the body was sent for autopsy, and as a crime victim, the patient is a medical examiner's case (3 and 4). Therefore, researchers must either learn the underlying structure of the database and query it directly or download the data into a database or spreadsheet with which they are familiar.

Similar to the approach to literary databases, researchers must take a systematic and orderly approach. HIM professionals, such as Osborn (2001), have queried Medicare's large databases to analyze reimbursement data. Secondary analysis is a productive research method for HIM professionals.

Data Access

Access to data depends on the type of data and their location. It can range from totally uncontrolled to highly secured. For example, data on the Internet are easily accessed whereas data in health records require approvals from Institutional Review Boards (IRBs).

Data can be public or proprietary. Public data are often accessible under the Freedom of Information Act; some have been posted on the Internet. State registry data also are often accessible. Proprietary data require permission of the owner of the database.

Data can be individual or aggregate. Data that identify one individual are less accessible than aggregate data. Protections exist for identifiable data. In research using patient records, Bell and Hudson (2001) obtained approvals from three different IRBs. One approval was from the IRB of the university where they worked and the other two were from the IRBs of the two hospitals in which they reviewed patient records. Some organizations may require informed consents to review data. In addition, access to personally identifiable data may become more complex as the regulations related to the Health Insurance Portability and Accountability Act of 1996 are implemented.

After approvals or permissions are obtained, the location of data also affects ease of access. For data in databases, researchers can transfer the files over the Internet. For paper records, they must physically go to the site of storage where they must abide by the hours of operation and rules for security. In addition, they must arrange in some way to collect their data, for example, entering them into a laptop.

Access to data becomes critical for researchers who conduct secondary analyses or combine their primary research with public databases. The key points for researchers who want to mine these rich resources are obtaining the approvals and allowing sufficient time.

Research's Relationship with the Professional Body of Knowledge

One of the defining characteristics of a profession is that it has a body of knowledge. By definition, a field of work without a body of knowledge becomes an occupation or a job. Therefore, as a means to build and expand knowledge, research is the foundation of a profession.

As an emerging profession, health information management is developing and articulating its body of knowledge. Leaders of the AHIMA recognize the importance of knowledge in advancing practice and professional learning (Kloss 2000). HIM professionals are conducting research in issues and topics related to health information. These topics and issues involve health information technology and systems, health data security and quality, management, benchmarks in practice and education, and informatics (figure 16.14). This research is defining, expanding, and refining the body of knowledge for the HIM profession.

Research results are made public in professional presentations, proceedings of meetings, and journals. The availability and accessibility of these results allow all HIM professionals to benefit. HIM professionals can put the results of the research into practice. For example, as a consequence of the medical sociologist's research on the chatter about patients in hospital elevators, orientation sessions specifically address the need to maintain confidentiality in all conversations and in all settings.

All HIM professionals can use the steps of research. Research provides a thorough, systematic approach. The problem-solving models of management and the decision-making models of decision sciences are based on the steps of research. Therefore, the logic of the approach allows HIM professionals to use it in their day-to-day activities. To find answers to common questions or solutions to everyday problems, research is a practical and effective tool. In the long term, the orderliness of the step-by-step approach saves time and results in the best decision.

Some HIM professionals have roles that are specifically related to research. These roles sort into three types: researcher, support staff to researchers in healthcare settings, and employee of a research company or agency.

Many HIM professionals are researchers. They conduct research for several reasons, including service to the profession, personal interest, and condition of employment. Many of the citations in this chapter represent HIM professionals in the role of researcher.

Figure 16.14.   Research Topics in Health Information Management

Compliance	Managed care
Use of computer applications in HIM education	HIM curriculum changes and their effectiveness
Information security	Best practices in HI services
Distance learning	Unique HIM instructional techniques
Vocabularies and terminologies	
Clinical education	Information technology
Management issues	Implementation of computer-based patient records
Graduate education	

The supervisor of research studies whose decisions were described at the beginning of this chapter is the second type. As previously noted, she evaluated and summarized research proposals that were related to data in the department's databases or to use of the hospital's paper patient records. In addition to these tasks, she assisted researchers in several ways. For example, she:

- Identified the location of the desired health data in databases, records, logs, reports, registers, or indexes
- Directed them to key persons
- Discussed the format of the data, such as paper records, microfilm, microfiche, and database
- Noted caveats, such as time frames and residual codes, related to the data
- Ran the computer queries to find the cases
- Arranged access to the computer databases
- Had the paper records related to their research pulled
- Managed the work area reserved for researchers
- Obtained signed confidentiality statements

The third role, employee of a research company or agency, represents one of the roles from AHIMA's Vision 2006. This role is the research and decision support analyst. In this role, HIM professionals collaborate "with product and policy organizations on high-level analysis projects such as clinical trials and outcomes research" (AHIMA 1999, p. 131).

Check Your Understanding 16.9

Instructions: Answer the following questions on a separate piece of paper.

1. How do researchers use key terms (MeSH headings)?
2. Why would a researcher limit the search of journal articles to refereed journals?
3. Why would a researcher use bibliographic software?
4. List five data sources, other than journal articles, that a researcher should consider when doing a comprehensive search.
5. What should researchers who use large databases for secondary analysis know about them?
6. How do public databases and proprietary databases differ?

Real-World Case

Recent articles in the *Journal of the American Medical Association* (Lee et al. 2000) and the *Journal of Quality Improvement* (Schneider et al. 2001) have discussed the use of databases and patient records in the collection of data for the Health Plan Employer Data and Information Set (HEDIS).

These articles interested several physicians in a large, urban physician group practice. The physicians wanted to evaluate the quality of care and services that their practice provided. Because its performance measures were easily accessible, the physicians decided to use the HEDIS. In addition, because the evaluation was purely voluntary, the physicians decided that, initially, they would address one HEDIS performance domain per month.

Many of the physicians in the practice were familiar with the HEDIS from either their readings or past involvement with managed care organizations. They knew that data from claims (administrative data) and patient records (clinical data) were required to calculate performance rates. Therefore, the physicians gave the HEDIS project to the practice's health information manager because of her expertise in these areas.

Upon receiving the project, the health information manager decided to implement the step-by-step approach of a research study. She made this decision for three reasons. First, the clearly defined steps in research would divide the large project into tasks of a manageable size. Second, the systematic approach would reduce the likelihood of overlooking important aspects of the project. Third, the physicians, her supervisors, would understand the scientific approach of a research study.

Based on her knowledge of research methods, she devised the following plan:

1. Identify a theoretical model.
2. Define the research problem (question).
3. Perform a literature review.
4. Determine a research design.
5. Select a research method.
6. Formulate a statement of the hypothesis.
7. Select an instrument to gather data.
8. Organize the collection of data, remembering to ensure a random sample and to pilot the study.
9. Analyze the data using appropriate statistical techniques.
10. Interpret the findings.
11. Present the data to physicians of the group practice.

Discussion Questions

1. Use of the HEDIS requires systematic data collection and reporting. Why is utilization of research methods in this process appropriate?
2. What other accrediting and regulatory requirements entail data collection and reporting?
3. Explain how AHIMA's Model of Data Quality could serve as a theoretical model for the health information manager's HEDIS project.
4. To assist the health information manager, identify at least three peer-reviewed journal articles on the topic. As she reads these articles and others in the literature, what should she take care to note?
5. In their article in the *Journal of Quality Improvement,* Schneider and colleagues collected data from claims and patient records and presented their findings using percentages. If the health information manager based her study on their study, what type of design and time frame could she use?
6. Rulon and Sica (1997) state that the HEDIS requires a random sample of at least 411 patients. How could the health information manager generate a random sample? What types of flaws could she detect during the pilot study?
7. In presenting the data, how should the health information manager structure the report? Explain what graphics would best convey the information from the study.

Summary

High-quality research depends on a carefully conceived plan and impeccable execution. Researchers' plans are similar to the blueprints that architects use to construct buildings. Researchers use their plans to conduct their studies and to build new knowledge. Research is systematic, and health information professionals can adapt its step-by-step approach to practical problems in the workplace.

Knowing the purpose of the research is a consistent theme in this chapter. Purpose drives decisions in each of the steps of research. These steps are defining the problem, reviewing the literature, determining the design and method, selecting the instrument, collecting and analyzing the data, presenting the results, and interpreting the findings.

The purpose of research determines the approach, whether qualitative or quantitative. Qualitative research is often exploratory and preliminary; quantitative research investigates numerically measurable observations or tests hypotheses.

Purpose also assists researchers in clarifying their research question. Considering their purposes helps researchers to concentrate or narrow the focus of the question to a researchable issue. Purpose also can ensure that researchers investigate meaningful problems that need solutions or significant questions that need answers.

The literature review is guided by purpose. In research, preference is given to articles in refereed journals. Purpose aids researchers in discriminating between relevant and irrelevant articles and between related and tangential articles. Finally, one purpose of the literature review is to identify gaps in the body of knowledge that researchers can fill with their studies.

There are six common designs of research: historical, descriptive, correlational, evaluation, causal-comparative, and experimental. The design a researcher chooses depends on the purpose of the research. Associated with each design are many methods of research, including survey, observation, case study, ethnography, experiments, secondary analysis, and meta-analysis. As with the choice of design, purpose is crucial in the choice of method.

Purpose also is crucial in selecting the research instrument. Instruments are standardized means to collect data. Although many factors should be considered in the selection of an instrument, the most important is the researchers' purpose.

The importance of purpose may be less obvious in the collection and analysis of data. However, the higher the stakes, the larger the sample. Moreover, research that involves many variables also needs larger sample sizes. Therefore, purpose is a critical concern in the collection of data. Purpose also is involved in the analysis of data because statistical approaches vary by research design.

Moreover, purpose underlies the presentation of results and interpretation of findings. Researchers provide other HIM professionals with knowledge and techniques to answer questions and to solve problems in the workplace. Without presentation and interpretation, the knowledge and techniques would be unavailable to practitioners. Thereby, research in the field of health information management improves health information practices in the continuum of care.

HIM professionals are well suited to the role of researcher. Typically, persons in the field recognize their abilities to plan and organize. Their abilities with analytical expertise create a powerful toolbox of skills that HIM professionals can use to increase the field's body of knowledge.

References

Abdelhak, Mervat. 1982. Hospital information systems applications and potential: a literature review. *Topics in Health Record Management* 3(1):8–18.

Abdelhak, Mervat, Patricia A. Firouzan, and Lynn Ullman. 1993. Hospital information systems applications and potential: a literature review revisited, 1982–1992. *Topics in Health Information Management* 13(4):1–14.

AHIMA Data Quality Management Task Force. 1998. Practice Brief: Data quality management model. *Journal of the American Health Information Management Association* 69(6).

Aish, Anne-Marie, and Danuta Wasserman. 2001. Does Beck's Hopelessness Scale really measure several components? *Psychological Medicine* 31(2):367–72.

Amatayakul, Margret K., and Makhdoom A. Shah. 1992. *Research Manual for the Health Information Profession.* Chicago: American Health Information Management Association.

American Health Information Management Association. 1999. *Evolving HIM Careers: Seven Roles for the Future.* Chicago: AHIMA.

American Health Information Management Association. 2001. Guidelines for submitting manuscripts. Accessed online from www.ahima.org/journal/index.html.

American Psychological Association. 1994. *Publication Manual of the American Psychological Association,* fourth edition. Washington, D.C.: APA.

Annual Reviews. 2001. Accessed online from www.annualreviews.org.

Association of Schools of Allied Health Professions. 2001. Guidelines for authors. Accessed online from www.asahp.org.

BBC Education. 2001. Medicine through time. Accessed online from www.bbc.co.uk/education/medicine.

Bailey, Kenneth D. 1994. *Methods of Social Research,* fourth edition. New York City: Free Press.

Becker, Howard S., Blanche Geer, Everett C. Hughes, and Anselm S. Strauss. 1961. *Boys in White: Student Culture in Medical School.* Chicago: University of Chicago Press.

Bell, Paul D. 1999. Evaluating the use of computer-assisted instruction in allied health professional education: a review of the literature. *Educational Perspectives in Health Information Management* 2(2):29–40.

Bell, Paul D., and Suzanne Hudson. 2001. Equity in the diagnosis of chest pain: race and gender. *American Journal of Health Behavior* 25(1):60–71.

Berdie, Douglas R., and John F. Anderson. 1974. *Questionnaires: Design and Use.* Metuchen, N.J.: Scarecrow Press.

Borg, Walter R., and Meredith D. Gall. 1989. *Educational Research,* fifth edition. White Plains, N.Y.: Longman.

Brodnik, Melanie S. 1993. Burnout and turnover potential among department leaders. *Journal of the American Health Information Management Association* 64(8):64–67.

Brown, Catana, William P. Moore, Darcee Hemman, and Amy Yunek. 1996. The influence of instrumental activities of daily living assessment method on judgments of independence. *American Journal of Occupational Therapy* 50(3):202–6.

Buros Institute. 1938-1995. *The Mental Measurements Yearbook: The Yearbook 1938–1995.* Highland Park, N.J.: Buros Institute.

Buros Institute of Mental Measurements. 2001. *The Fourteenth Mental Measurements Yearbook.* Accessed on-line from www.unl.edu/buros.

Byrne, Michelle. 2001. Ethnography as a qualitative research method. *Journal of the Association of Operating Room Nurses (AORN)* 74(1):82–84.

Campbell, Donald T., and Julian C. Stanley. 1963. *Experimental and Quasi-Experimental Designs for Research.* Chicago: Rand McNally.

Chadwick, Bruce A., Howard M. Bahr, and Stan L. Albrecht. 1984. *Social Science Research Methods.* Englewood Cliffs, N. J.: Prentice-Hall.

Chun, Ki-Taek, Sidney Cobb, and John R. P. French Jr. 1975. *Measures for Psychological Assessment: A Guide to 3,000 Original Sources and Their Applications.* Ann Arbor, Mich.: Survey Research Center, Institute for Social Research.

Clinicaltrials.gov. What is a clinical trial? Accessed on-line from www.clinicaltrials.gov.

Cohen, Peter A. 1991. Criteria for evaluating research reports. Handout, Educational Research Course, Fall 1991. Medical College of Georgia. Augusta, Ga.

Cohen, Peter A. 1992. Meta-analysis: application to clinical dentistry and dental education. *Journal of Dental Education* 56(3):172–75.

Day, Robert A. 1988. *How to Write and Publish a Scientific Paper,* third edition. Phoenix: Oryx Press.

Dillman, Don A. 1978. *Mail and Telephone Surveys: The Total Design Method.* New York City: John Wiley & Sons.

EBSCO Publishing. 2001. Database descriptions. Accessed on-line from www.epnet.com.

Ericae.net. 2001. ERIC/AE test locator. ERIC Clearinghouse on Assessment and Evaluation. Accessed on-line from www.ericae.net.

Flexner, Abraham. 1910. *Medical Education in the United States and Canada: A Report to the Carnegie Foundation for the Advancement of Teaching.* 1960 Reissue. Washington, D.C.: Health and Science Publications.

Garrard, Judith. 1999. *Health Sciences Literature Review Made Easy: The Matrix Method.* Gaithersburg, Md.: Aspen.

Garvin, Jennifer Hornung. 2001. Building on the vision: exploratory research in future skill areas of the clinical data specialist as described in evolving HIM careers. *Educational Perspectives in Health Information Management* 4(1):19–32.

Gay, L. R. 1987. *Educational Research: Competencies for Analysis and Application,* third edition. New York City: Macmillan Publishing.

Gibaldi, Joseph. 1999. *MLA Handbook for Writers of Research Papers,* fifth edition. New York City: Modern Language Association of America.

Giovannucci, Edward, Meir J. Stampfer, Graham A. Colditz, David J. Hunter, Charles Fuchs, Bernard A. Rosner, Frank E. Speizer, and Walter C. Willett. 1998. Multivitamin use, folate, and colon cancer in women in the Nurses' Health Study. *Annals of Internal Medicine* 129(7):517–24.

Glass, Gene V. 1976. Primary, secondary, and meta-analysis of research. *Educational Researcher* 5(10):3–8.

Grove, Cynthia. 1980. Foundation for the future of quality assurance: a literature review of the past. *Topics in Health Record Management* 1(2):13–23.

Health and Psychosocial Instruments (HAPI). Current ed. Pittsburgh: Behavioral Measurement Database Services.

Herndon, Robert M., editor. 1997. *Handbook of Neurologic Rating Scales.* New York City: Demos Vermande.

Hill, Robert F., and Edward P. Tyson. 1997. The culture of morning report: ethnography of a clinical teaching conference. *Southern Medical Journal* 90(6):594–600.

Iverson, Cheryl. 1998. *American Medical Association Manual of Style: A Guide for Authors and Editors,* ninth edition. Baltimore: Williams & Wilkins.

Jencks, Christopher, and David Riesman. 1977. *The Academic Revolution.* Chicago: University of Chicago Press.

Johnson, Martin. 1992. A silent conspiracy? Some ethical issues of participant observation in nursing research. *International Journal of Nursing Studies* 29(2):213–23.

Kansas City Public Library. 2002. Accessed on-line from www.kclibrary.org/resources/search/chart.cfm.

Kennedy, William C., and Ellen Jacobs. 1981. Literature review of legal aspects of medical records. *Topics in Health Record Management* 1(4):19–32.

Keyser, Daniel J., and Richard C. Sweetland, editors. 1991. *Test Critiques.* Kansas City, Mo.: Test Corporation of America.

Khan, Myrna. 1997. Basic components of a randomized clinical trial. *The Internet Journal of Anesthesiology* 1(1). Accessed on-line from www.icaap.org/iuicode?81.1.1.8.

Kish, Leslie. 1965. *Survey Sampling.* New York City: John Wiley & Sons.

Kloss, Linda. 2000. Growing the HIM body of knowledge. *Journal of the American Health Information Management Association* 71(10):27.

Lan, Andrew J., John M. Colford, and John M. Colford Jr. 2000. The impact of dosing frequency on the efficacy of 10-day penicillin or amoxicillin therapy for streptococcal tonsillopharyngitis: a meta-analysis. *Pediatrics* 105(2):e19.

Layman, Elizabeth J., and Janet A. Guyden. 1999. The relationships among psychological type, coping mechanisms, and burnout in directors of hospital health information management departments. *Educational Perspectives in Health Information Management* 1(2):29–41.

Lee, Frances W. 1996. Can computer-aided systems engineering tools enhance the development of health care information systems? *Topics in Health Information Management* 17(1):1–11.

Lee, Thomas H., James I. Cleeman, Scott M. Grundy, Clayton Gillett, Richard C. Pasternak, Joshua Seidman, and Cary Sennett. 2000. Clinical goals and performance measures for cholesterol management in secondary prevention of coronary heart disease. *Journal of the American Medical Association* 283(1):94–98.

Lewis, Carol A. 1980. Cost containment in medical records: a literature review. *Topics in Health Record Management* 1(1):21–30.

Lippin, Tobi M., Anne Eckman, Katherine R. Calkin, and Thomas H. McQuiston. 2000. Empowerment-based health and safety training: evidence of workplace change from four industrial sectors. *American Journal of Industrial Medicine* 38(6):697–706.

Lloyd, Susan C., and Elizabeth Layman. 1997. The effects of automated encoders on coding accuracy and coding speed. *Topics in Health Information Management* 17(3):72–79.

McDowell, Ian, and Claire Newell. 1996. *Measuring Health: A Guide to Rating Scales and Questionnaires,* second edition. New York City: Oxford University Press.

Mechanic, David, and Sharon Meyer. 2000. Concepts of trust among patients with serious illness. *Social Science & Medicine* 51(5):657–68.

Metz, Mary Haywood. 2001. Intellectual border crossing in graduate education: a report from the field. *Educational Researcher* 30(5):12–18.

Meyer, Gregg S., and David Blumenthal. 1996. TennCare and academic medical centers: the lessons from Tennessee. *Journal of the American Medical Association* 276(9):672–76.

Mikkelsen, Gustav, and Jan Aasly. 2001. Concordance of information in parallel electronic and paper-based patient records. *International Journal of Medical Informatics* 63:121–31.

Monsen, Rita Black. 1999. Mothers' experiences of living worried when parenting children with spina bifida. *Journal of Pediatric Nursing* 14(3):157–63.

National Institutes of Health. 2001. Accessed on-line from www.nih.gov/about/NIHoverview.html.

Osborn, Carol E. 1998. A methodology for construction of a survey questionnaire. *Educational Perspectives in Health Information Management* 1(1):3–13.

Osborn, Carol E. 1999. Benchmarking with national ICD-9-CM coded data. *Journal of the American Health Information Management Association* 70(3):59–69.

Osborn, Carol E. 2000a. Practices and productivity in acute care facilities. *Journal of the American Health Information Management Association* 71(2):61–66.

Osborn, Carole E. 2000b. *Statistical Applications for Health Information Management*. Gaithersburg, Md.: Aspen.

Osborn, Carol E. 2001. DRG analysis reveals potential problems, trends. *Journal of the American Health Information Management Association* 72(7):78–84.

Pamplona, M. Carmen, Antonio Ysunza, Mara Gonzalez, Elena Ramirez, and Carmelusa Patino. 2000. Linguistic development in cleft palate patients with and without compensatory articulation disorder. *International Journal of Pediatric Otorhinolaryngology* 54(2-3):81–91.

Penslar, Robin L. 2001. IRB Guidebook. Office for Human Research Protections. Accessed online from www.ohrp.osophs.dhhs.gov/irbguidebook.htm.

Redman, Barbara K., editor. 1998. *Measurement Tools in Patient Education.* New York City: Springer.

Rudolph, Frederick. 1990. *The American College and University: A History.* Athens, Ga.: University of Georgia Press.

Rulon, Vera, and JoAnn Sica. 1997. The evolution of HEDIS: 3.0 and beyond. *Journal of the American Health Information Management Association* 68(6):32–40.

Salant, Priscilla, and Don A. Dillman. 1994. *How to Conduct Your Own Survey.* New York City: John Wiley & Sons.

Schneider, Kathleen M., R. Todd Wiblin, Kimberley S. Downs, and Brian E. O'Donnell. 2001. Methods for evaluating the provision of well child care. *Journal of Quality Improvement* 27(12):673–82.

Shi, Leiyu. 1997. *Health Services Research Methods.* Albany, N.Y.: Delmar.

Siemon, James E. 1982. Case mix and data quality: a review of the literature. *Topics in Health Record Management* 2(4):13–22.

Singleton, Royce A., Jr., Bruce C. Straits, and Margaret Miller Straits. 1993. *Approaches to Social Research,* second edition. New York City: Oxford University Press.

Spreen, Otfried, and Esther Strauss. 1997. *A Compendium of Neuropsychological Tests: Administration, Norms, and Commentary*, second edition. New York City: Oxford University Press.

Strunk, William, Jr., and E. B. White. 2000. *The Elements of Style,* fourth edition. New York City: Longman.

Sudman, Seymour. 1976. *Applied Sampling.* New York City: Academic Press.

Sweetland, Richard C., and Daniel J. Keyser, editors. 1991. *Tests: A Comprehensive Reference for Assessments in Psychology, Education, and Business,* third edition. Austin, Tex.: Pro-Ed.

University of Chicago Press. 1993. *The Chicago Manual of Style,* fourteenth edition. Chicago: University of Chicago Press.

University of South Carolina Beaufort Library. 2001. Accessed on-line from www.sc.edu/beaufort/library.

Van de Mortel, Thea, and Louise Heyman. 1995. Performance feedback increases the incidence of handwashing by staff following patient contact in intensive care. *Australian Critical Care* 8(2):8–13.

Vugt, M. Van, P. Wilairatana, B. Gemperli, I. Gathmann, L. Phaipun, A. Brockman, C. Luxemburger, N. J. White, F. Nosten, and S. Looareesuwan. 1999. Efficacy of six doses of artemether-lumefantrine (benflumetol) in multidrug-resistant Plasmodium falciparum malaria. *American Journal of Tropical Medicine & Hygiene* 60(6):936–42.

Wilson, Feleta L., Lynda M. Baker, Christopher Brown-Syed, and Claudia Gollop. 2000. An analysis of the readability and cultural sensitivity of information on the National Cancer Institute's Web site, CancerNet. *Oncology Nursing Forum* 27(9):1403–9.

Application Exercises

1. Investigate the clinical trials at the Web site of the National Institutes of Health (http://clinicaltrials.gov). The Web site allows users to search by disease. Students should select a disease such as stroke, myocardial infarct, or diabetes. Compare and contrast three medical research studies (clinical trials) by completing table 16.10.

2. Read the following article: Carol E. Osborn, 2000. Practices and productivity in acute care facilities. *Journal of the American Health Information Management Association* 71(2):61–66.

   a. Write a cover letter that could have accompanied the survey.

   b. The response rate was 20 percent. Suggest strategies the researchers could use to increase the response rate.

3. Use the library to obtain one of the literature reviews cited in this chapter and write a research question based on it.

4. Using the on-line databases for instruments (Health and Psychosocial Instruments [HAPI] or Buros Mental Measurements Yearbooks), find three instruments in an area of interest, such as organizational culture, organizational climate, or leadership. Complete table 16.11.

5. Critically review an article in a refereed journal. Use the following set of questions (Cohen 1991) to guide your review:

   a. Is the problem clearly stated? Are terms defined as needed? Has the problem been appropriately delimited?

   b. Is the hypothesis stated? Does it relate to the problem? Is the way the researcher intends to test the hypothesis clear?

   c. Is the literature review thorough, complete, and pertinent? Is it clear and organized? Is the problem important? Does the literature review synthesize rather than merely summarize?

   d. Does the study's design relate to the problem? Is the population clearly defined? Is the method of creating the sample clearly explained? Is bias reduced in sampling? Is the sample representative of the population?

   e. Is the instrument specified? Is it related to the problem? Does the researcher state the instrument's reliability and validity?

   f. Does the researcher explain the method clearly enough and with sufficient detail that another person could replicate the study? Are confidential data protected?

   g. Does the researcher use the best mode to present the results? Do tables, figures, and graphs have clear titles? Do the numbers add up?

   h. Do the conclusions relate to the findings? Does the researcher provide alternative explanations? Does the researcher relate the findings back to the larger body of knowledge or theory?

   i. Do all the citations in the body of the article appear in the reference list? Is jargon kept to a minimum?

Table 16.10.   Comparison of Clinical Trials

Characteristic	Trial 1	Trial 2	Trial 3
Title			
Purpose			
Problem statement			
Research design			
Method			
Time frame			
Sample			
Study and control groups; randomization			
Intervention			
Data in health record			

Table 16.11.   Comparison of Instruments

	Instrument 1	Instrument 2	Instrument 3
Title			
Acronym			
Author			
Brief description			
Number of items (questions)			
Type of scale			
Reliability			
Validity			

Review Quiz

Instructions: Select the most appropriate answers for the following questions.

1. ___ The supervisor of research studies receives a request from a researcher to review the department's twenty-five patient records related to a randomized clinical trial. What type of research study does this request represent?
   a. Phase I clinical trial
   b. Descriptive study using a convenience sample
   c. Epidemiological study
   d. Correlational study

2. ___ What is the set of rules that controls research in each clinical trial called?
   a. Protocol
   b. Study
   c. Interview guide
   d. Bylaws

3. ___ On his first day of work, the new clerk in release of information processed three requests for information. He observed that all three requests were from law firms. He concluded that all requests for information come from law firms. What type of reasoning is the clerk using?
   a. Inductive
   b. Clinical
   c. Deductive
   d. General

4. ___ The Institutional Review Board of an academic health center received a researcher's request to conduct a retrospective review of 3,000 of the center's health records. In the documentation, the researcher stated that the purpose of the study was to prove, beyond a shadow of a doubt, that smoking caused a 10 percent higher death rate in patients with bleeding esophageal varices. What will be the board's decision?
   a. Disapprove based on the research's poor design
   b. Refer the request to the director of the department of health information services
   c. Approve with modifications
   d. Table until the finance office can provide cost estimates

5. ___ The hypothesis states that there is no difference in the levels of utilization of voice recognition software between group A, the students receiving the training, and group B, the students not receiving the training. What is the independent variable in this hypothesis?
   a. Training
   b. Voice recognition software
   c. Level of utilization
   d. Group A

6. ___ The administration of an academic health center sent a survey to all 800 members of its medical staff. What type of survey did the administration conduct?
   a. Census
   b. Sample
   c. Clinical trial
   d. Medical research

7. ___ A researcher is conducting correlational research. She wants to write a one-tailed alternative hypothesis about the relationship between organizational culture and staff turnover rate. How should she state the hypothesis?
   a. A positive organizational culture is associated with a 10 percent lower staff turnover rate.
   b. There is no relationship between organizational culture and staff turnover.
   c. A positive organizational culture is associated with a 10 percent difference in staff turnover rate.
   d. A positive organizational culture causes a 10 percent lower staff turnover rate.

8. ___ An educator in health information was conducting a longitudinal study of student persistence. The study tracked students from freshman orientation through graduation. During the study's time period, a hurricane and a flood shut down the university for two weeks. What threat to internal validity does this represent?
   a. History
   b. Maturation
   c. Testing
   d. Statistical regression

9. ___ From a review of the literature, the researcher knows that the variable she is investigating is not normally distributed in the population. Which statistical analysis should she consider?
   a. Chi square
   b. Student's t test
   c. ANOVA
   d. Pearson r

10. ___ Researchers Allen, Bates, and Camden conducted a study. The sample consisted of 107 nurses in one community hospital. Self-report instruments were distributed at a meeting and mailed back to the researchers. Forty-four nurses returned the survey. What is the response rate?
    a. 41 percent
    b. 107
    c. 44 percent
    d. Cannot be calculated for one hospital

Chapter 17
Clinical Quality Management

Vicki L. Zeman, MA, RHIA

Learning Objectives

- To define *quality* within the context of clinical healthcare services and to explain who has ultimate responsibility for the quality of services provided by a healthcare organization
- To differentiate among the three types of performance measures used in clinical quality improvement: structure, process, and outcome
- To explain the benefits of having a quality improvement program and how each clinical department selects areas for review
- To describe the reason for an annual appraisal of a quality improvement plan/program
- To explain the significance of outcomes management, case management, clinical practice guidelines, and benchmarking in quality management
- To understand the concept of sentinel event
- To recognize when root-cause analysis is required
- To understand the impact of the concepts of medical staff appointment/reappointment, credentialing, and clinical privileges on the quality of care
- To explain the functions of the executive committee and to discuss the relevance of medical staff bylaws/rules and regulations in quality improvement
- To describe the medical staff quality applications required by JCAHO standards and to summarize the medical staff's patient care review functions
- To understand the utilization review process and its impact on the quality of care
- To understand the importance of integrating risk management into any quality improvement program
- To recognize the role of severity indexing in a quality improvement program
- To explain the importance of keeping quality improvement data confidential and secure

Key Terms

Agency for Health Care Policy and Research
Agenda for Change
Aggregate data
Benchmarking
Bylaws/rules and regulations
Clinical privileges
Commission on Accreditation of Rehabilitation Facilities
Core measures
Credentialing
Health Plan Employer Data and Information Set (HEDIS®)
Incident report review
Indicators
Indicator measurement system
Loss prevention
Loss reduction
Medical care evaluation studies (medical audits)
National Association of Healthcare Quality (NAHQ)
National Committee for Quality Assurance (NCQA)
National Practitioner Data Bank
Occurrence/generic screening

Orion Project
ORYX
Outcome
Outcomes management
Peer review organization (PRO)
Performance improvement (PI)
Performance measure
Potentially compensable events (PCE)
Practice guidelines
Process
Quality
Quality assurance (QA)
Quality improvement (QI)
Quality improvement organization (QIO)
Report cards
Risk prevention
Root-cause analysis
Scope of work
Sentinel event
Severity indexing
Structure
Tax Equity and Fiscal Responsibility Act (TEFRA)
Temporary privileges
Ten-step monitoring and evaluation process
Utilization management
Utilization review (UR)
Verification service

Introduction

In healthcare, the term quality means one thing to the patient and another to the healthcare provider. But to both, the objective of quality is to arrive at a desired outcome. Providing the best care in the most effective manner and for the least cost is something every healthcare organization strives to do. Improving healthcare quality is a fundamental consideration of the U.S. healthcare system today.

The world is constantly evolving and change is a sure thing. Whether making a change is chaotic or measured and controlled often speaks to the success of those involved in the change process. The more measured and controlled the change process, the greater the chance of success. People in healthcare are survivors of phenomenal change, both measured and chaotic, over the past two decades. Health information management (HIM) professionals have been a distinct part of the change process.

The gurus of managing the change process—Deming, Juran, and Crosby, for example—have developed methods to measure and monitor systems and processes in organizations. Their theories give managers methods to use in bringing about measured, focused change before crisis occurs. With encouragement from accrediting bodies and government agencies, healthcare organizations are trying to achieve continued, measured, and focused change with the purpose of improving healthcare.

Healthcare professionals are struggling to use the quality improvement methods offered in the business sector. Healthcare is a highly complex environment involving many specially trained individuals with a strong commitment to their way of providing care. Finding ways to help such individuals to work together effectively is a challenge.

This chapter discusses the history of quality management as well as how quality management is organized and evaluated in modern-day healthcare organizations. It then describes the clinical applications of quality improvement efforts, focusing on the medical staff, nursing, and ancillary services. Finally, the chapter looks at using comparative data in the process of managing clinical quality.

Theory into Practice

Dr. Jeffreys, chief of orthopedics, has been collecting information on the outcomes of joint replacement surgery (hip and knee) for the past six months and is interested in following up on this information using performance improvement as the approach. She contacts Dorothy Davis, manager of the quality improvement department, to set up a meeting to get some action.

In their meeting, Dr. Jeffreys mentions that her review of the outcomes data has raised several concerns. Significant variations include the cost to the hospital of performing joint replacement procedures, length of stay, and the types of ther-

apy following surgery. In addition, more and more patients appear to be returning postoperatively because of problems. She believes that everyone in orthopedics needs to start thinking about "how we can do things to get better results."

Dorothy explains that the hospital uses a definite quality improvement (QI) methodology. It is a basic problem-solving model developed by the Joint Commission on Accreditation of Healthcare Organizations (JCAHO) that looks like this:

Assess → Measure → Analyze →
Recommend Improvements/Changes → Measure → Analyze

She feels confident that she and Dr. Jeffreys can make general decisions, build a team of care providers to evaluate the current situation, and develop an action plan.

Dr. Jeffreys and Dorothy arrange a meeting with everyone who affects the care of patients undergoing joint replacement. They first will need to develop assessment information that is understandable to everyone involved. Dorothy asks the librarian do a literature search of the orthopedic literature so they can benchmark their results. On her part, Dr. Jeffreys contacts the American Academy of Orthopedic Surgeons to see whether it has any best practices available. Dorothy suggests that clinical practice guidelines, such as the ones adopted in the obstetrics department, be considered.

Dr. Jeffreys and Dorothy also decide to obtain information on the "change" process. Determined to "make a difference," Dr. Jeffreys is going to talk to all the orthopedic surgeons and the hospital's administration to ensure that everyone understands what she has found and how she plans to address the situation. Her goal is to improve the way the facility handles hip and knee joint replacement. However, improvement means change and change must be understood, encouraged, managed, and sustained if the healthcare environment is to improve.

QI is not an isolated event; it involves many people. Everyone from the physician to the housekeeping staff has an impact on the quality of care delivered. Understanding the QI process is a way to make a difference to the patients cared for at the hospital. QI is a problem-solving process used in a complex medical setting. Things will change only when everyone works together to achieve the common goal of improving patient care.

Overview of Clinical Quality Management

Clinical quality management involves the evaluation of direct patient care. Clinical performance is often measured around diagnosis, medical condition, or care processes along with outcomes. The relationship between the way care is provided and the outcomes or results of the medical intervention is the focus of clinical quality management. Clinical quality management includes the process of **quality improvement** as it is applied in healthcare organizations. Although both the administrative and clinical aspects of healthcare systems may be the subjects of QI processes, the focus is on the clinical applications of QI in healthcare systems today.

Quality Improvement and the Use of Aggregate Data

Quality is assumed to give an enhanced worth or value to a product or service. Each person brings his or her unique perspective to the quality of a product or service he or she receives. If a person sees a service as having quality, it follows that the service was perceived as being good. Further, cost affects the perceived quality of a product or service. Consumers believe that the greater the quality of a product or service and the lower the cost, the greater the value of that product or service. Americans demand high-quality products or services for the lowest possible cost. W. Edwards Deming stated that "Quality has meaning only in terms of the customer, his needs, what he is going to use it for" (Walton 1986, p. 28).

Individuals involved in quality improvement (QI) processes in healthcare organizations must determine who the customers are, what they want, and what must be done to meet their expectations. Expectations must translate into performance requirements so that healthcare professionals can evaluate whether customers' needs are being met. This leads to developing statements of expectation or performance called indicators. **Aggregate data** is analyzed to determine whether expectations are being met. The data are frequently analyzed and compared against other internal and/or external data in a process called **benchmarking.** This allows the organization an opportunity to determine whether it is providing the highest-quality care.

History of Quality Management in Healthcare

The evaluation of healthcare quality has been evolving for many years. Hippocrates said, "Do no harm," thereby making the physician responsible for a patient's care. In 1854, Florence Nightingale introduced new protocols for her nurses during the Crimean War. Changes were made in the ventilation and sanitation systems and in how the nurses related to their patients. These changes dramatically reduced mortality rates. In 1917, the American College of Surgeons (ACS) established minimum standards of care. In following years, the ACS began an accreditation program.

These first steps led to the creation of the JCAHO and standards for hospitals in 1952. The JCAHO published its first set of standards for hospitals in 1953. In 1965, Congress passed the Social Security Amendment, which initiated utilization review and medical care evaluation studies (audits). Evaluating clinical care was legislated in 1965 as part of Medicare/Medicaid. Medical care evaluation audits were mandated, and similar efforts were recommended by the JCAHO by the late 1960s. The JCAHO used the term **quality assurance** (QA) to identify its patient care improvement

efforts with the introduction of accreditation standards in 1980. QA focused on hospitalwide problem solving focusing on the administrative or business operations of the organization. The QA standards allowed flexibility in the approach used by the organization. Problem lists were created, and many problems were solved. Mainly administrative in nature, the problems focused on the environment and personnel working in the organization. As problem lists became more legally challenging and the numbers of problems were reduced, the JCAHO revised its standards in the mid-1980s.

The 1985 QA standards were revised as a process of monitoring and evaluating. The emphasis was still on an organizationwide effort, but the revised standards specified a ten-step monitoring and evaluation process to focus on the "important aspects of patient care and service" (JCAHO 1988, p.12)." The new standards emphasized actions taken to improve care and the evaluation of those actions to ensure the effectiveness of the QA efforts.

In 1986, the JCAHO launched a research and development project called the **Agenda for Change.** The Agenda for Change sought to develop better methods of evaluating healthcare effectiveness with regard to how the organization was governed and managed and how it provided clinical services. It included three initiatives that looked at the survey and accreditation process, education, and communication.

Developing valid and reliable quality indicators that could be used as screens to identify potential problems became a major part of the survey and accreditation initiative. Another goal of this initiative was to have accreditation decisions more accurately reflect the quality of care rendered by the organization.

By 1990, the monitoring and evaluation process had been expanded to include medical staff review activities. In 1992, the accreditation manual began to transition from quality assurance to the quality improvement (QI) processes used today. The monitoring and evaluation process was expanded to include a commitment to continuous improvement. In the mid-1990s, the JCAHO introduced the chapter on improving organizational performance and reorganized the accreditation manual. The revised standards were organized around functions common to all hospitals and healthcare organizations.

The indicator measurement system (IMS) was introduced for hospital use beginning in the mid-1990s. An organization could use approved indicators to screen their clinical performance to improve the quality of care. In addition, the JCAHO's **Orion Project** was launched in 1994. The Orion project was an initiative to test accreditation models. JCAHO regional representatives worked with healthcare organizations; introduced indicator-driven performance improvement measurement systems; and attempted to coordinate accreditation with other external review bodies.

In 1997, the **ORYX** initiative began. Its purpose was to establish a continuous, data-driven accreditation process by using performance measurement data focused on core measures. With the help of advisory panels, the JCAHO identified measures that give an overall picture of an organization's healthcare services. Data collection is scheduled to begin in 2002. In an effort to coordinate accreditation with other external review bodies, data collected on several of the measures also are being required by **quality improvement organizations** (QIOs). At the heart of the ORYX project is the development of continuous improvement processes that focus on clinical areas. This is a work in progress, with data collection using five core measure sets phased in over a period of years. Clinical QI efforts are more sophisticated and more clinically oriented today than at any other time in history.

Healthcare as an industry must strive to continually improve. Healthcare was slow to discover the link between improved processes and outcomes and increased effectiveness, efficiency, and cost savings. Some healthcare professionals still have a hard time recognizing the need to devote dollars to something that does not give an immediate payback.

The number of errors at any one hospital is likely to look insignificant but the issue is compounded when data regarding errors is aggregated. In 2000, the Institute of Medicine (IOM) published information that brought attention to the issue of patient safety. *To Err is Human: Building a Safer Health System* asserted that 44,000 to 98,000 Americans die each year as a result of preventable errors. Shine (2002) states that, in actuality, these figures may be low because they do not include nursing home deaths or ambulatory care deaths. Moreover, many errors were never recorded in patient records. Shine further points out that all the evidence gathered needs to do more than point to individual doctors. Information must be used to develop safer systems and processes less likely to fail. The numbers of adverse events and costs to society go far beyond anyone's expectation. Error reports show a gap between average care and best care. Additionally, there is evidence that physicians will change their performance if outcomes are measured. Much work needs to be done in the area of healthcare quality improvement.

Check Your Understanding 17.1

Instructions: Answer the following questions on a separate piece of paper.

1. What is quality? Why is it important to meet customers' expectations?

2. What role has the JCAHO initiatives played in the evolution of measuring healthcare quality?

3. What agencies have been important in the development of modern quality improvement processes?

Organization of Quality Management in Healthcare Facilities

Quality management in healthcare facilities is organized to meet the needs of the organization. Today, most organizations have a program of continuous improvement in all functional areas. Data collection and analysis and resulting improvements have become an accepted way of doing business. An organization must address how it is going to achieve a successful QI program.

Organization, Accountability, and Ownership

The success of any QI program begins with a strong commitment from the executive level of the organization. This means that the governing body and the administration show, by example, their commitment to improving the quality of patient care. As an organization develops or revises a QI program, it must consider certain key elements. The elements of a QI program include:

- A clear statement of mission
- A supportive environment
- Available resources
- Leaders with adequate qualifications
- Adequate personnel
- An attitude of improvement
- Coordinated and integrated efforts
- Comprehensive and continuous care processes

Responsibility for QI activities must be clearly designated so that the program functions effectively. In addition, the methods of reporting are made clear to all people involved in the QI program. (See figure 17.1.)

The governing body is ultimately responsible for the quality of care provided in any organization. Today, governing bodies are more involved in QI efforts than ever before. Board members are seeking training, asking questions, and insisting on seeing data confirming that care is improving within their organization. When a board expresses interest and concern about the quality of care being provided, it sets the bar for medical staff and administrative involvement.

Figure 17.1.   Organizational Communication and Reporting

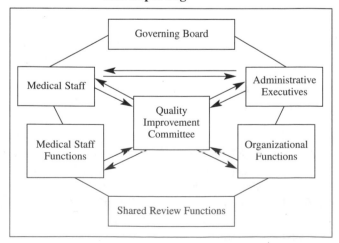

The Role of HIM Professionals

Many different types of professionals work in quality improvement. From a historical perspective, HIM professionals have been involved in QI from the time of medical evaluation audits. HIM professionals are a natural fit because they know the health record (still the primary data source) and understand the documentation process. The HIM professional can be involved in several ways, including:

- Collecting data/information
- Interpreting data in a meaningful way
- Knowing data sources
- Understanding clinical processes

Other professionals, such as registered nurses, are currently involved in QI in many facilities.

Quality Improvement and Management Program

Every healthcare organization needs to find QI methods that work for it. Organizationwide QI may be completed as part of health information service responsibilities, part of risk management, or a separate department in its own right. QI efforts must meet the needs of the facility.

The JCAHO requires that the approach, processes, and structures be described in writing (See figure 17.2.). The plan can be a separate document or incorporated into another

Figure 17.2.   Organizational Options for Quality Management Programs

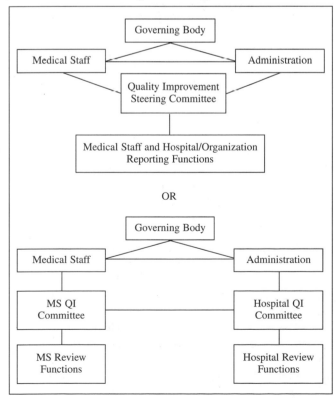

planning document. The Centers for Medicare and Medicaid Services (CMS) (formerly, the Health Care Financing Administration, or HCFA) also requires a plan in writing. Items commonly found in a plan include, but are not limited to:

- Statement of mission/vision
- Objectives
- Values
- Leadership
- Organizational structure
- Methodologies
- Performance measures
- Communication
- Annual plan appraisal

Plans need to be evaluated on a regular basis to determine their effectiveness. An annual appraisal should include a review of measurement and assessment activities and of documented improvements. The annual appraisal also should include a plan for the future direction of the program.

Definition of Quality Parameters

External regulators also are important factors in the quality puzzle. It is vital to understand who they are and what influence they have. The most influential external regulators in healthcare are voluntary accrediting agencies and the federal and state governments. There are also key judicial decisions that have had a profound impact on quality improvement processes.

Judicial Decisions

Three landmark court decisions help explain the direction of quality improvement: *Darling v. Charleston Community Memorial Hospital, Gonzales v. Nork and Mercy Hospital,* and *Johnson v. Misericordia Community Hospital.*

Darling v. Charleston Community Memorial Hospital (1965) is a landmark case that established a hospital's responsibility for patient care. Touching directly on quality are the issues of the facility's responsibility to have effective methods of credentialing in place and to have effective mechanisms for continuing medical evaluation. The facility is responsible for knowing whether the care it provides meets acceptable standards of care. The evaluation of medical care involves all professionals and must be done regularly so that both hospital and medical staff understand the results of patient care. The hospital must provide more than a place to practice and tools for physicians and other healthcare providers.

Gonzales v. Nork and Mercy Hospital (1973) supports a facility's responsibility for patient care. The hospital must establish a system to monitor the work and abilities of its physicians and other healthcare providers. In essence, the hospital owes its patients a duty to care.

Johnson v. Misericordia Community Hospital (1981) further supports the duty of the healthcare facility to select its medical staff and grant privileges using carefully defined criteria. In addition, the bylaws/rules and regulations adopted by the medical staff must be followed. Further, the hospital has a legal duty to ensure that the guidelines are followed. It must appoint and supervise qualified medical staff, and the medical staff has direct responsibility for the quality of care.

Federal Legislation

The federal government has had a profound impact on the development of quality improvement over the past thirty-five years. (See table 17.1.) The Social Security Amendments of 1965 and the Medicare Conditions of Participation, which followed in 1967, laid the groundwork for medical evaluation audits and utilization review if a facility was going to accept Medicare/Medicaid patients. In 1972, professional standard review organizations (PSROs) were legislated. The PSROs began to monitor the quality and appropriateness of Medicare/Medicaid patient care.

TEFRA not only introduced DRGs but also **peer review organizations** (PROs) to replace PSROs. In 1985, legislation was passed to deny Medicare payment for substandard care. In addition, the Conditions of Participation were revised to require a written QA plan in any facility accepting federal funds for Medicare/Medicaid patients.

In 1986, the Omnibus Budget Reconciliation Act (OBRA) required PROs to report adverse findings about healthcare providers to licensing and certifying agencies. That same year,

Table 17.1.   Major Legislation Relevant to Clinical Quality Management

Date	Act	Description
1965	PL 89-97	Health coverage for citizens 65 years of age and older (effective July 1, 1966)
1972	PL 92-603	Professional standards review organizations created
1982	Tax Equity and Fiscal Responsibility Act	Peer review organizations and the prospective payment system (PPS) created
1983	PL 98-21	PPS for Medicare established
1985	Consolidated Omnibus Reconciliation Act	Denial of Medicare payments for substandard care authorized
1986	PL- 99-509	PROs required to report substandard care to licensing and certifying boards
1986	PL 99-660	Health Care Quality Improvement Act
1989	PL 101-239	Agency for Health Care Policy and Research created Outcome measures research
1990	PL 101-508	PROs required to inform licensing boards of physician sanctions
1996	PL 104-191	Health Insurance Portability and Accountability Act

the Health Care Quality Improvement Act (HCQIA) was passed to help protect peer review activities from liability and laid the foundation for the **National Practitioner Data Bank.**

The Agency for Health Care Policy and Research (AHCPR) was legislated in 1989. This agency began to develop outcome measures and continues to be a resource in outcomes assessment.

In the 1990s, further federal efforts were undertaken to support quality improvement in healthcare. In 1990, legislation was passed requiring PROs to report physician sanctions to licensing and medical boards. In addition, the National Practitioner Data Bank legislated in 1986 was activated.

In 2002, peer review organizations were officially renamed quality improvement organizations (QIOs) to reflect changes in healthcare practice in recent years.

Legislative initiatives with the goal of improving the quality of care in the United States will most certain continue. The federal government finances healthcare for a number of designated populations and has an interest in ensuring that the services provided are effective and appropriate within an increasingly integrated delivery system.

Accrediting Standards

As mentioned earlier, the idea of using standards to bring healthcare practice to a minimum level was initiated by the American College of Surgeons (ACS). Standards were used and refined over the years until the Joint Commission on Accreditation of Hospitals assumed responsibility for them. Today, the commission is known as the Joint Commission on Accreditation of Healthcare Organizations (JCAHO).

The mission of the JCAHO is to improve the quality of healthcare. Since 1953, it has worked to develop standards that help healthcare organizations measure and evaluate the care they provide. The use of clinical indicators and continuous data-driven accreditation processes are currently being phased in.

However, the JCAHO is not the only organization developing and using standards to encourage high-quality care. Quality improvement (QI) efforts also are being supported by organizations such as the National Committee for Quality Assurance (NCQA) mentioned earlier. The Health Plan Employer Data and Information Set (HEDIS) is used to collect data on managed care plans. The **Commission on Accreditation of Rehabilitation Facilities** (CARF) has promoted high-quality healthcare in organizations serving patients who need rehabilitative treatment. The Accreditation Association for Ambulatory Health Care (AAAHC) is another private, nonprofit organization helping ambulatory healthcare organizations to improve the quality of their services. The National Association of Healthcare Quality (NAHQ) promotes continuous QI efforts in healthcare organizations by certifying qualified professionals. This organization offers QI professionals educational opportunities regardless of the healthcare setting they work in.

Check Your Understanding 17.2

Instructions: Answer the following questions on a separate piece of paper.

1. What basic elements should be included in a quality improvement program?
2. Who is responsible for the overall quality of care in a healthcare organization?
3. Why are HIM professionals an appropriate choice to work in a quality improvement program?
4. How can HIM professionals fulfill their role in the QI environment?
5. How have judicial decisions influenced quality improvement?
6. What role have the federal government and the JCAHO played in the development of QI processes?

Quality Management Process

Each stage of the evolution of quality management has involved some aspect of data collection, data analysis, and a resulting change to improve areas that are problematic. The focus of data collection efforts has been driven by diagnosis/procedure, problem, and, currently, clinical indicators.

Indicator Development

Indicators are quantifiable measures used over time to determine whether structure, process, or outcome supports the quality performance. They usually represent important aspects of care provided by the organization, department, or unit of service. Indicator development has been a linchpin for clinical quality improvement. After important aspects of care are identified, it is then possible to identify criteria or data elements that will identify care patterns.

The most common source of data is the health record. Data are collected, and the professionals involved in the QI process analyze them. A determination is made as to whether the data provide the information that is needed. A decision then is made about how best to improve the care provided. Key indicators addressing best practice have been developed and addressed in various ways during the evolution of quality improvement.

JCAHO's Quality Monitoring and Evaluation Process

The development of quality management included the **ten-step monitoring and evaluation process** developed by the JCAHO. The idea behind monitoring and evaluation is to continuously collect and analyze data and to address findings. The JCAHO's ten-step process was developed to help healthcare organizations have a more prescribed methodology of quality assurance. The basic premise is still applicable today. (See figure 17.3.)

Donabedian's Quality Assessment Model

Avidas Donabedian's QA model has been used and accepted for many years. The model's approach to the assessment of healthcare is based on three measures:

- **Structure** measures examine the organization's ability to provide services. Examples of measures of structure include policies and procedures, qualifications of staff, numbers of staff, physical space, and equipment.
- **Process** measures look at how care or service is provided to patients. The activities or protocols of care have some impact on the patient's outcome. Examples of process measures include protocols or methods of how treatment is delivered. For example, the patient's blood pressure is monitored hourly, patient education is completed before discharge, or the patient's discharge is determined to be appropriate. A healthcare provider (physician, nurse, or other allied health professional) usually carries out these functions.
- **Outcome** measures assess the end results of the care or services provided. Examples of outcome measures include mortality reviews, complications, or any adverse events. Any of these could indicate an undesirable outcome and indicate the need for further investigation.

JCAHO's Indicator Measurement System

The JCAHO's evolution to core performance measures is a story unto itself. In the late 1980s and early 1990s, the JCAHO began to develop an **indicator measurement system** (IMS) that would focus on clinical applications. During this time, the JCAHO determined that a program of continuous improvement was needed if a genuine impact on the quality of care was to be achieved. Additionally, the JCAHO wanted to move from a process/structure orientation to one more focused on outcomes. The objective was to affect both administrative and clinical patient care. One goal of the Agenda for Change initiative (discussed earlier) was to research and identify quality clinical indicators. Identified indicators represent sound clinical practice measures and reflect whether a healthcare organization is providing high-quality care to patients. The intention is to improve the quality of healthcare by improving performance in a given area of practice (for example, myocardial infarctions).

Figure 17.3. JCAHO's Ten-Step Monitoring and Evaluation Process

Step	1.	Assign Responsibility
Step	2.	Delineate Scope of Care
Step	3.	Identify Important Aspects of Care
Step	4.	Identify Quality Indicators
Step	5.	Establish Thresholds for Evaluation
Step	6.	Collect and Organize Data
Step	7.	Evaluate Data—Trends and Patterns
Step	8.	Take Actions to Solve Problems
Step	9.	Assess the Actions and Document Improvement
Step	10.	Communicate Relevant Information to the Organizationwide Quality Improvement Program

The complexity of the IMS project led first to the Orion project and then to the current ORYX initiative. The ORYX initiative integrates outcomes with **performance measures** and makes them both a part of the accreditation process. The use of nationally standardized performance measures or indicators has been considered a part of this initiative from the beginning. The term *core measures* is used in the ORYX initiative instead of the term *indicators*. **Core measures** are considered tools that provide an indication of an organization's performance. They are commonly tied to a process or outcome. Five initial core measurement areas are currently identified, including:

- Myocardial infarction
- Heart failure
- Pneumonia
- Surgical procedures and complications
- Pregnancy and pregnancy-related conditions

With the introduction of these core measures, healthcare facilities will be expected to send data to the JCAHO on a routine basis. Data from comparable organizations will be compared, and areas for improvement can be recognized. If any undesirable patterns or trends are found, further monitoring and evaluation will follow. The JCAHO is striving to make the accreditation process continuous and data driven. Review of the core measures is intended to help support current QI activities within the healthcare organization. In addition, it is hoped that the accreditation process will be seen as more relevant and valuable.

Outcomes Management

Quality improvement during the late 1980s was strongly focused on outcomes as the best way to judge the quality of patient care. Many national organizations worked to develop databases that allowed the comparison of outcomes. The JCAHO's IMS, the Maryland Quality Indicator Project, the Cleveland Health Quality Choice Program, and others were involved in developing indicators, collecting data, and analyzing outcomes. The Agency for Health Care Policy and Research (AHCPR) was funded to research clinical outcomes. A physician, Dr. Paul Ellwood, introduced the concept of outcomes management as a method to improve the quality of care. **Outcomes management** is the systematic collection of healthcare results using outcomes measurement. A database of outcomes experience is used to compare treatment modalities.

As a method of improving the quality of care, outcomes management looks for the best treatment process. A treatment process is determined and used, and data are collected and entered into a database. The data are analyzed and the treatment process changed as necessary. The goal is to find the best practice possible to benefit patient care. These identified best practices then can be considered guidelines for the treatment of patients.

Historically, the diagnosis and treatment of patients by their physician or primary healthcare provider has been a very personal process. **Practice guidelines** are intended to use a best practice concept to detail the care and treatment of a patient for a specific diagnosis or procedure. Clinical practice guidelines are identified by the Agency for Healthcare Research and Quality (formerly the AHCPR) as "systematically developed statements to assist practitioner and patient decisions about appropriate health care for specific clinical circumstances" (Schanz 1999, p.3). Practice guidelines are taken from a combination of current literature and expert knowledge. Clinical practice guidelines (also known as, practice parameters, Care Maps"™, and clinical indicators) are intended as tools to help make sound clinical decisions; they are not intended to replace sound clinical judgment.

Practice guidelines are intended to help standardize the care and treatment processes used by physicians. Deciding to use practice guidelines is an issue that needs to be addressed by every medical staff. The Institute of Medicine has published criteria to evaluate practice guidelines. (See table 17.2.)

The decision to use practice guidelines must be made carefully, considering both the clinical and financial implications. If used appropriately, the best practices concept resulting from the use of practice guidelines can reduce cost and improve the quality of care.

Managed Care Quality Criteria

The 1990s brought a renewed interest in managed care and dramatic increases in the number of people who received healthcare services under its auspices. The **National Committee for Quality Assurance** (NCQA) supports the quality of care provided by health plans. This organization sponsors,

Table 17.2.   Institute of Medicine Criteria for Practice Guidelines

Criteria	Description
Validity	Leads to predictable health and cost outcome
Strength of evidence	Documented expert judgment and research
Estimated outcomes	Result of implementation projected with consideration given to patient preference and perceptions
Reliability and reproducibility	Same results if studied by another group
Clinical applicability	Populations defined for clarity of results
Clinical flexibility	Exceptions to clinical guidelines specified
Clarity	Written in clear direct manner
Multidisciplinary	Guidelines developed allowing collaboration with appropriately interested care providers
Scheduled review	Delineated time for assessment of accuracy and relevance
Documentation	Process of development well documented and includes personnel involved, data source, and procedures used

Source: Schanz, S. J. 1999. *Developing and Implementing Clinical Practice Guidelines*. Chicago: American Medical Association.

supports and maintains the **Health Plan Employer Data and Information Set** (HEDIS) used by many health plans. HEDIS was actually developed through a combined effort of representatives of a variety of health plans and employers. This data set allows a health plan to evaluate the quality of care provided by measuring its practice against other health plans.

The results from the data collection can be used by the health plan to report the quality of care provided. Some health plans develop **report cards** and use HEDIS information to inform employers about both the quality of care and the cost of their health plan. HEDIS measures include items such as:

- Adolescent immunizations
- Antidepressant medication management
- Breast cancer screening
- Cervical cancer screening
- Childhood immunizations
- Cholesterol screening (after heart attack)
- Diabetic eye exams
- First trimester prenatal care

More than sixty different standards fall into the following five major categories:

- Access and service
- Qualified providers
- Stay healthy (wellness and preventative services)
- Getting better
- Living with illness

These data can help employers make decisions that are truly best for their organizations. The decision can include both the cost and quality aspects of the health plan and can allow intelligent dialogue when making decisions about what health plan is best for an organization. The NCQA Web site (www.ncqa.org) has a wealth of information about HEDIS.

Severity Indexing

Severity indexing is the process of identifying the level of resource consumption based on factors of clinical evidence. The more complications and comorbid conditions present, the sicker the patient and the higher the resource consumption. This method of trying to judge the level of illness is useful for reimbursement, utilization, and quality of care programs. Reimbursement should be higher when more resources are consumed, length of stay (LOS) should be longer or shorter based on resources needed and degree of illness, and quality could be compromised when a patient requires more care because of complications or comorbid conditions but does not receive it.

An organization using some form of severity indexing can use the information for a variety of purposes. Databases are available that allow the organization to make accurate determinations about the care rendered, the appropriateness of care, and the level of reimbursement. Adopting severity indexing can also impact reimbursement by providing a more complete picture of the patient care provided. The severity indexing can be especially effective if an organization wants to determine reasons for longer or shorter LOS or to provide information supporting or refuting statistics regarding the quality of care rendered.

Check Your Understanding 17.3

Instructions: Answer the following questions on a separate piece of paper.

1. How are indicators used in QI processes?
2. How are the assessment approaches of structure, process, and outcome and indicator development tied together?
3. What are the similarities and differences of core measures, outcomes management, and clinical practice guidelines?
4. What contributions did managed care make to quality improvement?
5. How can severity indexing contribute to improved patient care?

Quality Management in Clinical Applications

The first QA efforts using the JCAHO model from 1980 focused on problems. The problems were most often administrative in nature. For example, the mechanics of moving patients through admitting to their rooms and placing safety devices in patient rooms and hallways were addressed in the first wave of QA efforts. Making changes in the clinical practice of physicians was approached more slowly. Clinical applications are the current focus of QI efforts.

Medical Staff Applications

The medical staff is a key player in the evaluation of clinical services and any clinical process improvement efforts. The medical staff organization (MSO) works closely with the healthcare organization's administration but is directly responsible and accountable to its governing body. The **bylaws/rules and regulations** guide the medical staff regarding the organization's structure, functions, and responsibilities. In addition, the MSO must be responsive to internal requests from the administration or the governing body as well as external entities such as accrediting bodies and state and federal regulators.

Organization of the Medical Staff

Like any organization, the medical staff, as a self-governing entity, needs to have structure. The JCAHO identifies key characteristics of the medical staff in its accreditation manual as:

- Being fully licensed independent practitioners as permitted by law and the facility
- Having delineated clinical privileges defining the scope of services
- Being subject to medical staff and departmental bylaws, rules and regulations, and policies
- Being subject to review as part of the performance improvement activities

These characteristics help explain the role of the medical staff within the healthcare organization.

Committees are used to help most MSOs to function. The executive committee is the only MSO committee required by the JCAHO. It is usually made up either elected or appointed medical staff officers, department directors, and an administrative representative. Actual membership (size, composition, functions) is defined in the medical staff's own bylaws/rules and regulations (discussed below). The majority of those serving on the executive committee must be fully licensed physicians. The members of the executive committee make decisions, determine policy, and act on behalf of the medical staff as a whole. In addition, this group provides leadership to the medical staff and works to support performance improvement efforts.

The executive committee makes recommendations directly to the governing board in matters such as:

- Structure of the medical staff
- Mechanisms used to review credentials
- Medical staff membership
- Clinical privileges
- Participation in organizational performance improvement activities
- Termination of medical staff membership
- Fair hearing procedures

Further, the executive committee receives and/or acts on reports from medical staff committees and/or departments/units and makes recommendations regarding those reports.

Many MSO structures today are departmentalized or divided into functioning units; only very small, uncomplicated MSOs are not. The JCAHO does not specify how a medical staff will organize. It is the responsibility of the medical staff to determine its method of self-governance with approval of the governing body. The bylaws/rules and regulations contain descriptions and definitions necessary to the operation of the MSO.

A departmentalized MSO must decide on the mechanism for acting and reporting. The JCAHO recommends defining the leadership of each medical staff department. It further states that the department director must be qualified with appropriate education and training. The medical staff bylaws/rules and regulations specify the responsibilities of the department director. These responsibilities include:

- Determining clinical activities of the department
- Determining administrative responsibilities of the department
- Establishing mechanisms for the surveillance of the clinical activities performed by all individuals in the department
- Establishing criteria for clinical privileges for care provided within the department

- Recommending clinical privileges for each department member
- Determining the competence and qualifications of department personnel
- Integrating department functions into the organization
- Determining mechanisms for assessing and improving the quality of services and care provided within the department

The bylaws/rules and regulations of the medical staff provide the guidelines and framework or structure needed for the medical staff to function. In addition, the bylaws/rules and regulations define:

- Medical staff membership
- Credentialing procedures
- Process of awarding clinical privileges
- Committee structure (including the executive committee)
- Departmentalization
- Categories of the medical staff
- All the other areas determined appropriate for the medical staff to function effectively

The bylaws/rules and regulations must be approved by the medical staff and by the governing body of the organization. Once approved, they are intended to provide an agreement between the medical staff and the organization's administration.

Credentialing of the Medical Staff

Since its inception, the JCAHO has supported healthcare organizations by developing processes to ensure that only the most qualified professionals practice in healthcare organizations. The JCAHO's standards guide healthcare organizations in the credentialing process. Each healthcare organization must have its own credentialing process; thus, each healthcare organization will have a different process. Using the JCAHO standards results in a credentialing process with a certain commonality among healthcare organizations. A sound credentialing process is the foundation of high-quality care.

Credentialing is the process of reviewing and validating qualifications, granting professional or medical staff membership, and awarding delineated privileges. Specific policies and procedures are used by healthcare organizations to accomplish this process. The credentialing process verifies the education, training, experience, current competence, and ability to perform the privileges requested or any other background information pertinent to an individual requesting membership on the medical staff. The medical staff bylaws/rules and regulations delineate what needs to be collected and reviewed and the process of approval or denial of medical staff membership and clinical privileges.

The credentialing process begins with a potential medical staff member submitting an application to the medical staff for membership and a request for clinical privileges. After the information on the application has been verified, the department chair reviews the request for clinical privileges and makes a recommendation. The application, the results of the verification process, and the department chair's recommendations are reviewed by a selected group of medical staff members. The credentials committee commonly performs this function. The recommendation goes from the credentials committee to the executive committee. The executive committee then reviews the recommendations and makes its recommendation to the governing board. The governing board reviews the information and makes the final decision to accept or reject the application. (See figure 17.4).

Figure 17.4.   Flowchart of the Credentialing Process

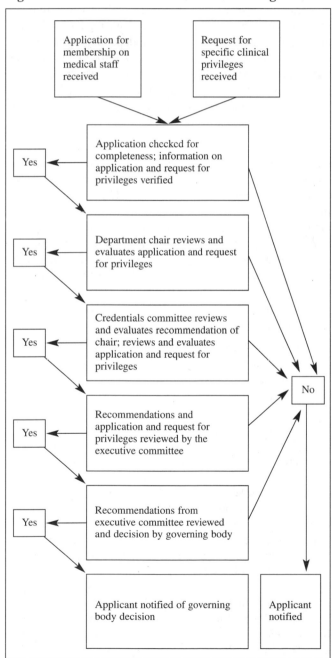

The application to the medical staff contains categories of information as specified by the NCQA. Some categories suggested by the NCQA include:

- Licensure
- Hospital privileges
- Drug enforcement agency registration
- Medical education, including specialty board certification
- Malpractice insurance
- Liability claims history
- NPDB queries (as required by law)
- Medical board sanctions
- Previous applications for medical staff membership/privileges

Items such as the above, plus additional items designated by the medical staff, are included on the application.

During the credentialing process, each applicant to the medical staff requests specific clinical privileges. According to the JCAHO, granting **clinical privileges** refers to the authorizing of a practitioner to provide specific patient care services within well-defined limits. The criteria for awarding clinical privileges must be detailed in the medical staff bylaws/rules and regulations. Criteria include, but are not limited to, preestablished definitions of minimum levels of education, training, experience, and competence (JCAHO 2002, p. 272).

Most healthcare organizations maintain lists of the procedures, services, and/or treatments that are most likely to be requested based on the services they offer. After the request for clinical privileges is made, the verification process begins. If the MSO is departmentalized, the department director uses the criteria to make recommendations regarding the appropriateness of the requested privileges. If the MSO is not departmentalized, the chief (president) of the medical staff or designee performs this function.

Clinical privileges may be categorized in a variety of ways. The JCAHO gives examples of ways to categorize clinical privileges, for example, by:

- Practitioner specialty
- Level of training or experience
- Patient risk categories
- Lists of procedures or treatments
- Any combination of the above

The delineation of privileges includes any limitations imposed on the individual provider, including the ability to admit, treat, or direct the course of treatment of patients admitted to the facility.

In today's healthcare environment, credentials are verified by either the healthcare organization (usually by a medical staff services professional) or a **verification service.** In either case, primary sources should be checked when possible. According to the Health Care Quality Improvement Act, the National Practitioner Data Bank must be queried when verifying applicants to the medical staff. All queries must be completed before any appointments are made or privileges awarded. In all cases, the verification process needs to be done in a timely manner, which is usually specified in the bylaws.

Initial appointment and awarding of privileges is done for no more than a two-year period. Typically, appointment and the designation of clinical privileges are done together. The credentialing process is ongoing. The reappointment and renewal or revision of clinical privileges is completed at least every two years. The reappointment/reappraisal process is continuous within the time line delineated in the medical staff bylaws.

The reappraisal process includes reviewing objective information collected on each individual who provides patient care services. Data are gathered and maintained on the practice patterns of all healthcare providers. Included in the data are the performance improvement activities completed within the defined time line. A credentials file is maintained on each member of the medical staff. This information is considered confidential and must be handled in accordance with established policies and procedures contained in the medical staff bylaws/rules and regulations. State and federal peer review and confidentiality legislation should be reviewed.

The initial granting of medical staff membership and privileges, along with any revisions or revocations of clinical privileges, must follow the medical staff bylaws/rules and regulations. All applicants have the right to appeal decisions and to a fair hearing before a panel of their peers.

Temporary privileges may be awarded when special circumstances arise. The medical staff bylaws/rules and regulations specify how temporary privileges are applied. The JCAHO requires that the chief executive officer or designee base the granting of temporary privileges on the recommendation of the department chair, when possible, or the president of the medical staff. Temporary privileges must fall under state and federal regulations. Examples of when temporary privileges are appropriate include pending verification of credentialing information and the need for a highly specialized individual to provide care in an emergency situation.

Medical staff bylaws/rules and regulations must specify the criteria used to appoint/reappoint or award clinical privileges. The medical staff and governing board approve the criteria. The bylaws must be applied to all applicants equitably. All individuals providing patient care services in the healthcare organization must be included in the credentialing process. It is imperative that the information provided as part of the application and request for privileges be reviewed and verified. Failure to verify information jeopardizes the healthcare organization from a liability standpoint. Courts consistently hold healthcare organizations liable for the failure to verify application/request for privileges information.

Independent Practitioners and Credentialing

Individuals who provide healthcare services without supervision or direction are considered to be independent practitioners. Independent practitioners can work as employees of the organization or may work privately or through a group of physicians. Physicians, dentists, podiatrists, and clinical psychologists most commonly practice as independent practitioners.

Licensed independent practitioners also must go through a credentialing process as described in the section on medical staff credentialing. Medical staff bylaws will delineate the process for credentialing independent practitioners. Independent practitioners go through an appointment/reappointment process and have specific privileges delineated within the scope of their license and the rules and regulations of the organization and medical staff. Independent practitioners must seek appointment and request specific clinical privileges and practice within that framework. The objective of this process is to ensure patient safety by assuring that only trained, competent, and qualified individuals provide healthcare services within the organization.

Other Medical Staff Quality Applications

Because the medical staff is responsible for ensuring the quality of care provided to patients treated in the healthcare facility, it is involved in collecting and analyzing data and improving both clinical and nonclinical functions in the organization. For the QI process to be successful, the medical staff must be engaged in QI activities. Data collection and analysis and recommendations are done on an ongoing basis, and changes are made to improve the patient care services offered in the organization. The medical staff and the healthcare organization can then judge whether the services provided are meeting standards of care.

Patient Care Review

Physician leadership is critical to the success of the continuous **performance improvement** (PI) program of any organization. Medical practice has changed remarkably over the last century. The practice of medicine has moved into the twenty-first century with the medical paradigm shifting from individuality to one of teamwork and collaboration. Physicians still work in an atmosphere of infallibility and have great difficulty acknowledging mistakes or lack of knowledge (Shine 2002). Yet, they persist in looking for ways to provide the best possible medical care for their patients. Physicians, the government, and accrediting agencies continue efforts to determine the best way to collect information about patient care that allows a consistent and objective patient care review process.

Currently, PI incorporates the evaluation of outcomes and processes. The medical staff must lead the way in improving clinical and nonclinical processes used in organizations. Involvement of the medical staff in patient care review is critical. This means the medical staff is involved in the measurement, assessment, and changes resulting from the review of patient care processes. The JCAHO provides guidelines to the medical staff.

No matter how the medical staff implements performance improvement, the process of evaluating peers needs to be clearly defined, have identified participants, have properly designed methods, time frames, and conditions for peer review functions. Characteristics of peer review are identified by the JCAHO as:

- Consistent
- Timely
- Defensible
- Balanced
- Useful
- Ongoing

Using these guidelines, the medical staff can provide leadership in evaluating of the clinical processes of peers.

Health Record Review

Health record review is necessary to ensure that the documentation captured is complete and accurate and reflects the care provided to the patient. At a minimum, the team involved in this improvement process consists of medical staff, nursing, health information management, and administrative services. The review includes health record documentation on both open and closed cases, with the total number of records being reviewed at approximately 5 percent of the overall discharges. Elements being evaluated are identified in the JCAHO standards. Findings must be shared with the healthcare organization's healthcare providers. Problems identified should be corrected, and the healthcare organization must be able to demonstrate how this is done.

Surgical Review

Data collection systems must be developed and used by healthcare organizations to evaluate all operative procedures. Both invasive and noninvasive procedures should be included in this improvement process. All procedures are a potential risk to the patient, and so the appropriateness of the procedure must be determined. The procedures established to have the greatest risk are reviewed closely. Procedural processes and outcomes need to be addressed. Again, the JCAHO helps guide the medical staff and healthcare organization in developing a system to measure the use of operative and other procedures. The procedural processes to be measured include:

- Selection of the appropriate procedure
- Patient preparation for the procedure
- Performance of the procedure and patient monitoring
- Postprocedure care
- Postprocedure patient education

Medication Usage Review

Medication use is an important method of treatment in healthcare. Because of the growing number of available medications

and the potential for adverse effects, such as short-term side effects, interactions of medications, and toxicity, it is essential that the healthcare organization measure the administration and use of medications. Moreover, the healthcare facility should evaluate medication use. Priority is based on:

- Number of patients receiving a medication
- Risk versus therapeutic value
- Known or suspected problem-prone drugs
- Therapeutic effectiveness

In addition, attention should be given to medication processes. Again, the JCAHO provides guidelines for data collection regarding:

- Ordering or prescribing
- Preparing and dispensing
- Administrating
- Monitoring the effects on patients

Blood and Blood Component Usage Review

Blood and blood components are used to treat patients. Treatment has the potential of offering patients risks as well as benefits. The JCAHO provides standards to guide the healthcare organization and the medical staff in the evaluation of use of blood and blood components. PI processes should examine the ordering, distribution, handling and dispensing, administration, and monitoring effects of blood and blood components. Other considerations include when blood and blood components are ordered, but not indicated; when they are indicated, but not given; or when they are administered incorrectly.

Mortality Review

Review of mortality (death) is an important outcome indicator. Establishing a meaningful evaluation of mortality is essential in the analysis of ongoing outcome and process improvement.

Infection Control

The medical staff and the healthcare organization should work together to provide an environment that reduces the risk of infections in both patients and healthcare providers. The healthcare organization should support activities that look for, prevent, and control infections. This is done with the involvement of the medical staff. Information is collected regularly on endemic and epidemic nosocomial infections. As appropriate, the healthcare organization must report significant information to both internal groups and public health agencies. The organization must also take the necessary steps to prevent and reduce the risk of infection in visitors to the facility. Monitoring should be ongoing, and the healthcare organization should support a process focused on reducing risks and lowering infection trends. In today's healthcare environment, processes must be in place to support the results of bioterrorism activities in preventing the transmission of disease.

Nursing Staff Applications

Nursing leadership and nurses providing patient care services are part of the organization's overall quality improvement program. Nursing works with the governing body, medical staff, administration, and other healthcare providers to collect and analyze data, implement changes where necessary, and improve services. Focus is placed on areas where the largest numbers of patients are provided services, where there is highest risk, or where there are known problems.

Nurses provide the majority of hands-on care. They not only provide direct nursing care but also work closely with other professionals in carrying out treatment plans. Their impact on the patient is all-embracing. Nursing professionals must provide care that is consistent with current literature and that meets nationally recognized standards.

Nursing executives and staff must provide the appropriate guidance for all nursing care. Policies and procedures, standards of nursing practice, nursing standards of patient care, and standards to measure, assess, and improve patient outcomes must be defined, documented, available, and used to improve patient care processes. Nurses must work in conjunction with management, the medical staff, and other healthcare providers as part of an organizationwide PI program.

Ancillary Services Applications

All patients should receive information about the care they are provided. Information about how data are collected, used, and evaluated can be incorporated into this message. A number of individuals are involved in the data collection and analysis and system/process redesign. Data may be collected from patients about their experiences by using patient satisfaction surveys. In addition, patients need to be informed of the healthcare organization's process improvement activities.

Utilization Management

Ensuring the appropriate and efficient use of a facility's or health plan's resources is the focus of **utilization management** (UM). Abdelhak et al. (2001) define utilization management as the systems and processes that ensure that the organization's resources, both human and nonhuman, are used most effectively to meet patient care needs. In addition to the appropriate use of the organization's resources, utilization management incorporates the process of utilization review. A utilization management program helps ensure that patients receive appropriate care in an efficient and cost-effective manner. Utilization management programs are required by the CMS (formerly, the HCFA), the Medicare/Medicaid Conditions of Participation, many state regulations, and the JCAHO. Data collected as part of this program offer insight into the quality of care provided.

Utilization review (UR) is a formal review of patient resource use. Data collected during this formal review help determine the appropriateness of the services provided. UR ensures the medical necessity of treatment provided and the cost-effective use of resources and identifies over- or underuse of available services. Both the federal government and many state regulations require the healthcare organization to have a written UR plan. Although the JCAHO does not require a written UR plan, it does require that UR incorporate a review of all patients, not just those who are federally funded.

History of Utilization Management

Utilization review was legislated as part of the 1965 amendments to the Social Security Act. The focus of this legislation was on LOS review using physician reviewers. It also initiated **medical care evaluation studies** or audits. UR affected only federally funded patients until the JCAHO published standards in the early 1970s. It then was expanded to include at least a sampling of patients with private payment sources.

As healthcare organizations try to improve their efficiency, utilization management becomes a resource for collecting information to help determine how best to treat patients. To coordinate utilization management activities, a utilization review coordinator collects the required information, uses screening criteria, and works with physicians and the administration to ensure that patients are being treated appropriately for medically necessary reasons.

Utilization Management Staffing

Utilization review coordinators have a variety of backgrounds. Registered nurses have moved into the field very successfully because of their clinical backgrounds and rapport with physicians. Health information managers also can be successful in the field because of their knowledge of documentation practices, their clinical backgrounds, and their understanding of reimbursement requirements. Utilization review coordinators must be able to work with physicians and employees of insurance companies and managed care organizations. In addition, they must also be able to work with various committee structures and to be active participants on the utilization management committee.

The utilization management committee consists of individuals who provide clinical services to patients and those involved in reimbursement. It will include representatives from administration, nursing, health information management, utilization management, physicians, and others who are thought to play a role in the care and treatment of patients. The composition of the committee should be detailed in the utilization review plan. The purpose of the committee is to review and evaluate the medical necessity of care provided and the appropriateness of treatment. In addition, the committee may be involved with the quality improvement studies initiated by the QIO.

Utilization Management Processes

In actuality, the utilization review process was implemented slowly. An organization must use screening criteria as a tool to make its determinations. Milliman and Robertson, a healthcare consulting organization, publishes the evidence-based guidelines used by many facilities today. These screening guidelines are a collection of best practices drawn from a variety of sources. Time frames for review are determined by the facility and are a part of the utilization review plan. Several types of review are common in healthcare organizations today.

Preadmission Review

Preadmission review is done prior to the patient's admission. It is required by most managed care plans. Its purpose is to determine if the admission and/or procedure are medically necessary and appropriate in an acute care setting. The preadmission review identifies patients who are unsuitable for admission or for a particular procedure and then directs them to the appropriate care setting to obtain healthcare services.

Admission Review

Admission review is done at the time the patient is admitted to the facility. This review is done to determine/verify the medical necessity and appropriateness of admission.

Continued-Stay or Concurrent Review

Continued-stay/concurrent review ensures that the patient is remaining in the facility because of medical necessity and is being treated appropriately. The review ensures that the patient is evaluated at preset intervals to determine the appropriateness of care rendered and that beds are utilized efficiently. The specific interval is commonly tied to the diagnosis and/or procedure.

Discharge Planning

Discharge planning ensures that a patient is ready for placement in a nonacute setting when he or she leaves the facility. This process often begins either at preadmission or upon admission to ensure that the patient is placed or receives services needed at the time of discharge. Client education is an important part of the discharge planning process. Readiness for discharge is determined by preestablished criteria.

Retrospective Review

Retrospective review is completed after patient discharge. Its purpose is to determine medical necessity and appropriateness of services rendered. When care is determined inappropriate or medically unnecessary, reimbursement is denied. The QIO is responsible for performing retrospective review on federally funded patients. Insurance companies and managed care organizations also do retrospective reviews. Reimbursement can be withdrawn when documentation does not support the medical necessity or appropriateness of care rendered. In addition, retrospective review can help determine problems with overutilization, underutilization, inefficient scheduling of services, and patterns of nonacute days.

Observation care is appropriate for patients with a condition that requires some time to determine whether admission is medically necessary. Different managed care plans have different criteria to determine the appropriate use of observation beds. In any case, care must be taken because the time spent in an observation bed is billed as an outpatient service and may not be covered under the patient's insurance.

Ancillary Services Review

Ancillary services review is tied to ordering, scheduling, and preparation for and performance of various tests and services. Data should be collected to determine whether ancillary services are being used in an efficient and effective manner. QI programs frequently address the appropriate use of ancillary services.

Medicare Review

Medicare review began with introduction of the professional standard review organizations (PSROs). PSROs were nonprofit agencies made up of physicians who examined the medical necessity of care. In addition, energy was put into ensuring that the most economical care was rendered to meet the needs of the patient. PSROs introduced the concept of denying payment for care determined to be unnecessary. In addition, quality objectives were introduced to healthcare through the PSROs. Their effectiveness was questioned until their demise in the early 1980s.

The 1982 Tax Equity and Fiscal Responsibility Act replaced the PSROs with the peer review organizations (PROs). The PRO program was established to ensure that Medicare beneficiaries were provided services that are medically necessary, appropriate, and recognized as meeting professional standards of care. The name PRO was changed to QIO (quality improvement organizations) in 2002.

QIOs review the appropriateness of admission, continued stays, and discharges. The QIO contracts with the CMS (formerly the HCFA) to provide specific initiatives during a designated period of time (currently three years). Their current **scope of work** is focused on quality-related issues, payment error prevention, and other areas. The most current scope of work involves a shift to a more national clinical QI focus. (See table 17.3, p. 420.)

Notices of noncoverage were required by both the PSROs and the PROs, and are still a part of the utilization review process. A notice of noncoverage is required for various situations, including:

- *Preadmission notice of noncoverage:* In this situation, the client is made aware, prior to admission, that care or services may not be covered or may be obtained at a lesser level of care. The client then is informed that if admission takes place, he or she will be responsible for all charges that result from the stay.

Table 17.3.   Quality Improvement Organizations' Current Scope of Work

Topic	Quality Indicators
Acute Myocardial Infarction	• Early administration of aspirin • Aspirin at discharge • Early administration of beta blockers • ACE inhibitor at discharge for low LVEF • Beta blocker at discharge • Timely reperfusion • Smoking cessation counseling
Heart Failure	Appropriate use and nonuse of ACE inhibitors
Pneumonia/ Immunization	• Time to initial antibiotic administration • Initial antibiotic administration • Assessment of bacteria involved • Statewide influenza immunization rate • Statewide pneumococcal (PPV) immunization rate • Blood cultures collected prior to antibiotic administration
Stroke Prevention	• Antithrombotics for stroke and TIA • Warfarin for atrial fibrillation • Avoidance of sublingual nifedipine, a short-acting calcium channel blocker for acute hypertension
Diabetes	• Biennial retinal eye exam • Annual HbA1c testing • Biennial lipid profile
Breast Cancer	Biennial screening mammography
Payment Error Prevention	Reduction in rate of Medicare Payment errors

Source: StratisHealth. 2000. *The Sixth Scope of Work—National Priorities and Indicators*. Bloomington, Minn.: StratisHealth.

- *Admission notice of noncoverage:* In this situation, the patient is informed that acute care is not required and that he or she will be responsible for charges resulting after a specific grace period (forty-eight hours).
- *Continued-stay notice of noncoverage:* In this situation, the patient is notified that acute care services are no longer required and that he or she will be responsible for charges after a specific grace period (forty-eight hours).

The content and wording of the notices is prescribed by the CMS through the PRO. A policy and procedure regarding these notices must follow the prescribed methodology. The QIO monitors each notice of noncoverage and closely reviews these cases.

External Agency Review

Third- and fourth-party reviewers complete external agency reviews. Reviewers include commercial health insurance companies, managed care plans, and auditors. The focus of the reviews includes resource utilization, quality of care, reimbursement issues, and cases meeting specific criteria such as readmission within seven days after discharge.

Medicaid Review

The Medicaid program was established by Title XIX of the Social Security Amendments of 1965. Federal money is distributed to each state under a block grant methodology, and each state administers disbursement based on federal guidelines. Medicaid reviews differ from state to state. Range of services, qualifying factors, methods of payment, and LOS limitations are handled differently. Utilization review plans also differ from state to state. However, most states do require a prior-approval process for inpatient care and selected outpatient procedures. Retrospective and prospective reviews may be a part of the process. Understanding each state's UR requirements is essential.

Managed Care Review

Managed care plans use utilization management to keep costs down and quality up. Each managed care plan will have a unique approach to doing utilization management. Managed care organizations frequently use preadmission certification. Continued-stay review is handled by the managed care organizations collecting information on the acuity and the timeliness of services. The managed care organization will request information both concurrently and retrospectively to determine medical necessity and appropriateness of care. Utilization review coordinators work closely with a variety of managed care organizations to ensure that payment is made for services rendered.

Risk Management

Risk management is a program designed to reduce/prevent injuries and accidents and to minimize or prevent financial loss to the organization. The concept of reducing injuries and accidents has been around for thousands of years. The Code of Hammarabi (400 B.C.) actually addressed the issue of physician liability. When a physician inflicted certain injuries on a patient, punishment for the injuries was prescribed in the code. During the 1970s, the dramatic increase in malpractice claims supported the need for more aggressive management of risk in healthcare organizations. Risk management systems today are sophisticated programs that function to identify, reduce, or eliminate **potentially compensable events,** thereby decreasing the financial liability of injuries or accidents to patients, staff, or visitors.

The JCAHO and other accrediting bodies recommend risk management programs, state and federal laws and regulations give guidance with regard to risk management, and a variety of professional organizations offer professional guidelines that address the importance of risk management. Even third-party payers expect organizations to have systems in place to keep patients, staff, and visitors as safe as possible. Liability insurance carriers require and support an organization's efforts to develop and sustain risk management programs. Policies and procedures addressing risk must be developed and used to control injuries and accidents and to reduce the organization's financial liability.

Healthcare organizations today are faced with ever-increasing costs for liability insurance. Internally, an organization must collect information on injuries and accidents. Incident/event reporting is frequently organized with the help of the insurance carrier. Along with these data, occurrence/generic screening tools can be used to collect data on the risk management of patients. In addition, patient satisfaction surveys, mortality and morbidity reviews, infection control data, patient complaints, hazard reports, claims management, as well as the development of appropriate policies and procedures to collect and analyze the data, all contribute to the well-being of the organization.

The healthcare organization must provide personnel to support the efforts of risk management. This can be accomplished by hiring a risk manager who has adequate authority to make changes as necessary, or these duties can be part of the quality and safety areas of the organization. In either case, it is essential that the organization recognize the need to collect and analyze data, make changes, and improve current facility systems and to do so in conjunction with current efforts to improve the quality of care.

Risk Management Processes

For a risk management program to be successful, it must include certain processes. **Loss prevention** is a risk control strategy that includes developing and revising policies and procedures that are both facilitywide and department specific. It also involves educating staff, including medical personnel, healthcare executives, volunteers, and employees. Credentialing activities must be thorough. Compliance must be assured with federal, state, and accrediting bodies standards, laws, and regulations. Complete and thorough patient education must be provided.

Another component of a successful risk management program is loss reduction. **Loss reduction** encompasses techniques used to manage events or claims that have already taken place. Ways to reduce losses incurred include:

- Investigating reported incidents or addressing occurrence reports promptly
- Reviewing claims made against the facility
- Managing workers' compensation programs
- Being knowledgeable about alternate dispute resolution processes
- Treating employee injuries on site
- Implementing back-to-work programs
- Assisting with depositions or other pretrial activities
- Working closely with defense counsel

Another component of a successful risk management program is **risk prevention.** Some of the ways that risk prevention can be attained include:

- Educating all employees and medical staff to recognize and properly report all potentially adverse occurrences
- Ensuring that all employees and medical staff are doing their jobs to the best of their ability.

- Developing early warning and reporting systems that identify areas of potential adverse effect
- Creating databases to track events and help point out areas where systems can be improved
- Making changes to systems requiring improvement and monitoring these areas to determine success
- Providing employees with appropriate safety training

Risk Management Reporting Tools

Several areas require special mention because they are basic tools in an effective risk management program.

Incident Report Review

Incident report review is a process in which incident reports are analyzed or descriptions of adverse events are evaluated. Common examples include needle sticks; patient, employee, or visitor falls; and medication errors. Reviewing incident reports and developing a database of incidents with report capability can help identify patterns or trends that signal potential adverse events.

Occurrence/Generic Screening

Occurrence/generic screening is a methodology where predefined criteria are used to review medical records to find cases that may indicate adverse patient outcomes. These criteria are not disease or procedure specific. Rather, they are generic in focus and include items regarding whether an informed consent was signed, whether the patient was returned to the operating room, whether hospital-acquired infections were noted, and whether there was a failure to respond to significant X-ray or laboratory results.

Safety Programs

Every organization must have a safety program in place to focus on the environmental concerns of patient care. Fire, radioactive materials, and air quality are examples of areas addressed in a safety program. Federal and state laws require safety programs and accrediting bodies have standards that address safety. Safety and risk are closely linked, and data should be shared.

Internal/External Disaster Preparedness Programs

An emergency preparedness program addresses disasters and emergency situations both inside and outside the healthcare organization. The September 11, 2001, tragedy involving the World Trade Center and the Pentagon created new challenges for this program. Management plans the response to crisis situations. The organization must have protocols on how patients will be treated, admitted, and discharged. The plan must be developed in cooperation with agencies and organizations within the community. All entities responding to emergency situations must be ready to work together to handle any type of disaster. Additionally, everyone working within the organization must be trained to respond to emergency and disaster situations.

The emergency preparedness plan must address certain areas, for example, how the organization will address the need for backup utilities, communication systems, and radioactive and chemical decontamination and isolation. Personnel must know their roles and responsibilities in a crisis situation. Practice sessions, also called disaster drills, should be held to help personnel react appropriately. Whether the emergency is internal or external to the organization, the appropriate policies and procedures need to be in place and well understood by the organization's personnel to ensure that the response is timely and meaningful.

Informed Consent Review

Healthcare organizations deal with many liability issues, including ensuring that clients understand and agree to treatment through the informed consent processes. Consent can be given either orally or in writing (expressed consent). It also may be implied through the actions or circumstances of the client's behavior.

Appropriate informed consent is one in which the client or patient acknowledges his or her understanding of the nature of the treatment or procedure to be performed. In addition, he or she must understand the risks, benefits, and alternatives to the treatment or procedure. The informed consent process involves an exchange of information between the healthcare provider and the patient or client, along with permission or assent. Failure to obtain informed consent can result in liability issues for both the healthcare organization and the healthcare provider.

Sentinel Event Review

The JCAHO's Sentinel Event Policy went into effect on April 1, 1998. Its purpose was to improve the quality of care. A **sentinel event** is an unexpected occurrence involving death or serious physical or psychological injury, or the risk thereof. *Serious injury* is defined as the loss of a limb or function. Events are deemed sentinel because they signal the need for immediate investigation and response. Examples of clinical events needing this kind of response are significant medication errors, significant adverse drug reactions, and confirmed transfusion reactions.

The organization may need to perform an intense analysis when:

- Patterns, trends, or variations of performance are significant or unexpected
- Performance differs significantly from performance in other, similar facilities
- Performance varies significantly from accepted standards
- A sentinel event occurs

Policies and procedures must be in place to respond to a sentinel event.

When a sentinel event occurs, organizational leadership must support the process of investigation, analysis, and improvement. The expectation is that the organization will respond to all sentinel events. **Root-cause analysis** is the process used to identify the cause of the event. The organization looks for ways to decrease the likelihood of such an event happening again. The focus should be on organiza-

tional and clinical systems and processes, not on the person or people involved in the sentinel event.

Root-cause analysis examines both the clinical and administrative reasons for the event. After data collection and analysis, the organization should develop an action plan and move to make improvements in order to make such future events as unlikely as possible. The focus of the JCAHO's survey process will be on how the organization has handled the sentinel event.

An organization is encouraged (but not required) to report sentinel events to the JCAHO. A root-cause analysis and an action plan must be completed regardless. Healthcare organizations reporting a sentinel event can benefit by having an outside, objective third-party review their action plan and obtaining consultation as needed. In addition, the organization should show the public a sincere effort to remedy problems and improve.

Check Your Understanding 17.5

Instructions: Answer the following questions on a separate piece of paper.

1. What do utilization review and utilization management contribute to quality of care?

2. How do the different types of review (for example, preadmission, admission, continued stay, and discharge planning) support medical necessity, appropriateness of services, and length of stay review?

3. How does the notice of noncoverage affect the denial of reimbursement?

4. How does risk management contribute to the overall quality improvement program?

5. How do sentinel event policy and root-cause analysis contribute to the quality of care provided to patients?

Integration of Comparative Data into Clinical Quality Management

The JCAHO and the QIOs have developed performance measures requiring regular data collection. In addition, the healthcare organization needs to develop its own performance measures. Performance measures frequently are built around the categories of efficiency, effectiveness, safety, timeliness, and quality. Determining what data collection techniques will meet the needs of the QI process, which data displays and reporting methods are most effective, what to consider when analyzing and interpreting data, and how to affect systems and processes with meaningful changes all need to be considered.

Chapter 21 addresses the tools and techniques of PI. Those tools can be applied to clinical quality improvement.

Data Collection and Reporting Techniques

To collect the required data, performance measures must be developed or identified that collect the correct data elements. Clinical measures need to be detailed, diagnosis/procedure specific (usually), focused on process or outcome (most commonly), and selected by high-volume, high-risk, or known problems. It is necessary to determine "what you want to know" and how you can say it in numbers. The data can be reported as either meeting the element (for example, 98 percent of patients were free of infection) or not meeting the element (for example, two percent of the patients experienced infection). Each data element collected must be clearly defined, clearly understood, and agreed on by everyone involved in the data collection process. This helps ensure that the data collected support what the organization wants to know.

The scope of performance measurement activities requires clarity. The important areas of service are usually based on volume, risk, or known problem. The population targeted must be clearly identified and defined, and the sample size must be representative and allow for valid and reliable statistical measurement. (See chapters 16 and 18.) Descriptions of the raw data and data sources must be identified precisely so that everyone understands what the data elements will tell them. The medical record remains as the main data source.

It also is important to identify who will be involved in collecting and assessing the data, determining improvements, and performing ongoing evaluation. Data gathering is frequently done using forms, check sheets, surveys, questionnaires, or computer screens using database or spreadsheet applications as the tool to maintain consistency and accuracy. Further, it is necessary to determine how often data will be collected (daily, weekly, or monthly) and whether they will be collected concurrently or retrospectively and for how long.

Data displays need to be functional and meet the needs of reviewers. It is important to remember that effective data displays are visual supports that allow reviewers to understand data at a glance. Data display tools include, but are not limited to, pie charts, histograms, scatter charts, line charts, and bar graphs. (See chapter 15). Narrative data also can be used effectively. Narrative information can address performance goals, data sources, and data collection procedures.

Data Analysis and Interpretation

The analysis and interpretation of data demonstrates whether a performance measure is being met. Changes plotted over time can answer questions about whether systems are doing what they are intended to do or whether they require change. Analysis and interpretation can help point out what change will have the most impact. The HIM professional and others involved in the QI activity can work together to use the displayed information to improve the care provided patients.

The QI activities follow a problem-solving process of access, measure, analyze, and improve. Determining the best way to effect change can be challenging. Langley et al. (1996) recommend a combination of a thorough understanding of the current system or process, creative thinking, and use of improved technology, when possible. Some ideas for developing creative thinking include:

- Know current boundaries before making changes
- Rearrange the steps of the process
- Looks for ways to level the current flow of tasks or activities
- Challenge why you are doing the QI activity
- Describe what would be ideal
- Do not allow the current way of doing to continue

Different techniques can be used to improve the patient care process. Traditional approaches include training or education of personnel, administrative changes such as decreasing wait times, more thorough credentialing, and working closely with risk management to decrease liability.

Results Reporting and Follow-up

Because QI is an organizationwide effort, reporting lines must be clear and direct. Reporting begins with a hospital and/or medical staff committee or some other organizational unit and follows a clear and defined route. It is essential that communication be thorough and complete. The QI plan must delineate how reporting will flow through the organization. All levels of the organization must know that results will be shared throughout the organization.

After changes are made to improve systems or processes, there must be a way to determine whether the change was meaningful. This involves determining what needs to be known and selecting a few data elements that will give that information. If the changes have been successful, it may be necessary to either reduce the frequency of review for this performance measure, or make an alternative change if no significant improvement can be identified.

For a quality management program to be effective, the risk management, safety, and disaster programs must work in conjunction with the quality improvement program. Data collected to meet the needs of the different programs designed to keep patients, staff, and visitors safe and to allow response to community needs must be shared to benefit the overall organization. Developing methods for reporting and evaluating the results of the different programs and systems is a complex, continuous challenge. Results from any of the above areas can give an indication of high-quality care or point out areas requiring improvement or change.

Data Security and Confidentiality

The confidentiality and security of QI data needs to be addressed through effective policies and procedures. QI information must move through the organization's communication systems and yet be protected. State statutes may be used to help develop policies that are supported by legislation. Peer review activities are addressed by legislation in every state. Data must be kept in a secure environment, and access to the data must be carefully delineated and supported by statute whenever possible. Release of QI information must be handled in accordance with statutes, policies and procedures, and medical staff bylaws/rules and regulations.

Use of Computer-Based Comparative Data

Computerized data must be kept in a secure environment. Passwords, fingerprints, retinal scans, and limited access are basic security features used to protect QI data. (The handling of computerized information is addressed thoroughly in chapters 2 and 5.) Adapting security and confidentiality practices for general computerized information is essential.

Check Your Understanding 17.6

Instructions: Answer the following questions on a separate piece of paper.

1. Why is it necessary to clearly define indicators, criteria, and/or data elements used in data collection?

2. What is the main source of data?

3. How does thinking creatively improve the quality of patient care?

4. Why must quality improvement data be kept confidential?

5. What impact could poor communication practices have on a quality improvement program?

Real-World Case

According to an Associated Press article published in the *News-Tribune,* March 25, 1995, an award-winning 39-year-old health columnist, who was being treated for breast cancer, died as a result of receiving the wrong dosage of cyclophosphamide (a cancer-fighting agent) and an overdose of another drug meant to keep her from suffering side effects. This happened at a reputable facility that specializes in the treatment of cancer.

At least a dozen doctors, nurses, and pharmacists missed the medication error for four days. Her husband reported that she suffered tremendously as the lining of her intestine was shed, resulting in her literally vomiting sheets of tissue. The doctors had reassured the patient and her husband that all was normal. Her heart failed after receiving four times the recommended amount of medication.

An autopsy revealed no visible signs of cancer in her body, which indicated that the treatment had worked. Another woman died of a similar mistake two days earlier. Human error was felt the only possible explanation, according to the treatment center. Incorrect doses of medication through either dispensing error, administration error, or prescription error can be deadly. Moreover, many adverse events go unreported. The Institute of Medicine released information on medical errors in November of 1999. Medical errors kill an estimated 44,000 to 98,000 Americans each year and affect every healthcare setting; medication errors are responsible for more than 7,000 deaths per year.

Discussion Questions

1. What type of event is this? Provide reasons to support your answer.

2. What is the process used to identify the cause of this death, who needs to be involved in the investigation, and what tools should be used to analyze the situation?

3. Discuss what kinds of changes are likely to result in an improved system of treating patients using toxic medications.

Summary

In the twentieth century, the American College of Surgeons paved the quality improvement (QI) road by establishing standards of care. In the last half of the twentieth century, the Joint Commission on Accreditation of Healthcare Organizations (JCAHO) and other accrediting bodies having clearly led the way in developing modern QI initiatives. The federal government, through the Medicare Conditions of Participation and quality improvement organizations, also has contributed to the development of high-quality patient care. In addition, judicial decisions have made—and will continue to make—significant progress toward improving healthcare.

Every healthcare organization has its own version of quality. In general, however, the attributes of quality must be both administrative and clinical in nature and involve both the medical and facility staff. The organization's focus should be on customer satisfaction, professional standards of care, and process and system performance. The organization must collect and analyze data and use the results to make improvements in its processes and systems and in the healthcare it provides. Instituting a methodology of performance improvement will bring ordered change and improve the quality of healthcare.

Numerous QI methodologies have been used over the years, beginning with the medical care evaluation audit. The JCAHO has introduced several methodologies and is currently moving toward a data-driven, continuous accreditation process. Other accrediting organizations have developed methodologies that require assessing, measuring, and improving the quality of healthcare. Outcomes management practice guidelines are examples of techniques frequently used in healthcare to help ensure that patients receive high-quality care.

The medical staff must be a part of the organization's QI efforts. The QI process begins with a well-functioning credentialing process to ensure that the medical staff is qualified to perform requested clinical privileges. The medical staff's bylaws/rules and regulations must support the QI processes. Medical staff leadership is critical when evaluating clinical processes as part of the performance improvement program. Moreover, the QI processes in any organization include a variety of programs.

The utilization management function contributes to high-quality healthcare by providing information on how effectively and efficiently the organization's resources are being used. Risk management contributes to patient safety by directly linking known risks to improving patient care. Use of generic criteria to monitor patient care helps to identify areas of risk, which enables the organization to be proactive in preventing or reducing injuries and accidents. The emergency preparedness program and safety programs also contribute to the quality of care.

Today, accrediting agencies, government agencies, and healthcare organizations use performance measures. Collecting information to evaluate an organization's processes is critical to improving the care the organization provides patients. Using effective data analysis and interpretation techniques helps determine whether the processes are effective.

Making meaningful changes is a constant challenge. Communicating performance measurement information to all parties who might benefit is difficult. Healthcare in the United States today is a highly technical, complex environment. All who practice in this environment must constantly be aware of the need to improve the processes and systems with which they work.

References

Agency for Healthcare Research and Quality. 2001. Reducing and preventing adverse drug events to decrease hospital costs. *Research in Action* 1(March). AHRQ Publication Number 010020.

Arrichiello, Lark. 2000. *HEDIS 101*. St. Paul, Minn.: Blue Cross/Blue Shield of Minnesota.

Brandt, M. 1994. Clinical practice guidelines and critical paths: roles of HIM professionals. *Journal of the American Health Information Management Association* 95(6).

Committee on Quality Healthcare in America, Institute of Medicine. 2001. *Crossing the Quality Chasm: A New Health System for the 21st Century.* Washington, D. C: National Academy Press.

Crosby, P. B. 1979. *Quality Is Free: The Art of Making Quality Certain.* New York City: Penguin Books.

Donabedian, A. 1980. *Exploration in Quality Assessment and Monitoring,* Vol. 1. The definition of quality and approaches to its assessment. Ann Arbor, Mich.: Health Administration Press.

Elliott, C., P. Shaw, P. Isaacson, and E. Murphy. 2000. *Performance Improvement in Healthcare: A Tool for Programmed Learning.* Chicago: American Health Information Management Association.

Governance Institute. 2000. *The Board's Role in Monitoring Quality.* Washington, D.C.: Governance Institute.

Graham, O. N., editor. 1995 *Quality in Health Care: Theory, Application and Evaluation.* Gaithersburg, Md.: Aspen Publishers.

Joint Commission on Accreditation of Healthcare Organizations. 1996. *Hospital Accreditation Standards.* Oakbrook Terrace, Ill.: JCAHO.

Joint Commission on Accreditation of Healthcare Organizations. 1996. *When Bad Things Happen to Good Health Care Organizations: Meeting the Joint Commission Sentinel Event Policy Requirements Leaders Guide,* Part 1. Oakbrook Terrace, Ill.: JCAHO.

Joint Commission on Accreditation of Healthcare Organizations. 2002. *Hospital Accreditation Standards.* Oakbrook Terrace, Ill.: JCAHO.

Langley, G. J., K. M. Nolan, T. W. Nolan, C. L. Norman, and L. P. Provost. 1996. *The Improvement Guide: A Practical Approach to Enhancing Organizational Performance.* San Francisco: Jossey-Bass Publishers.

Leape, L. 1990. Practice guidelines and standards: An overview. *Quality Review Bulletin* 16:42–43.

Lumsdum, K. and M. Haglund. 1993. Mapping care. *Hospitals and Health Networks.* October 20, 1993, p. 34–40.

Mellott, Susan, editor. 1996. *NAHQ Guide to Quality Management,* sixth edition. Glenview, Ill.: National Association for Healthcare Quality.

Milliman and Robertson. 2002. Milliman Care Guidelines. Seattle, Washington: Milliman, USA.

Prophet, Sue. 1997. Fraud and abuse implications for the HIM professional. *Journal of the American Health Information Management Association* 68(4):52–56.

Schaffer, W. A. 1991. Introducing data to medical staffs. In *Quantitative Methods in Quality Management: A Guide for Practitioners,* edited by D. R. Longo and D. Bohr. Chicago: American Hospital Publishing.

Schanz, S. J. 1999. *Developing and Implementing Clinical Practice Guidelines.* Chicago: American Medical Association.

Shine, K. I. 2002. Health care quality and how to achieve it. *Academic Medicine* 77(1):92.

Slee, V. N., and D. A. Slee. 1991. *Health Care Terms.* St. Paul, Minn.: Tringa Press.

Slovensky, D. J. 2001. Quality management and clinical outcomes. In *Health Information: Management of a Strategic Resource,* revised edition, edited by M. Abdelhak et al. Philadelphia: W. B. Saunders Company.

Spath, P. L. 2000. *Fundamentals of Health Care Quality Management.* Forest Grove, Ore.: Brown-Spath & Associates.

StratisHealth. 2000. *The Sixth Scope of Work: National Priorities and Indicators.* Bloomington, Minn.: StratisHealth.

Walton, M. 1986. *The Deming Management Method.* New York City: Putnam Publishing Group.

Youngberg, B. J. 1990. *Essentials of Hospital Risk Management.* Rockville, Md.: Aspen Publishers.

Application Exercises

1. Secure several sample quality improvement plans, accreditation standards, and the Conditions of Participation. Use these resources to identify the required components of a QI plan and then analyze the plans to determine whether they contain all the appropriate elements. Also identify any missing elements. Share your findings with the other students or develop presentations identifying how the QI plans might be improved.

2. Visit at least three separate Web sites of groups or agencies that are concerned about the quality of healthcare. Then submit a written critique of each Web site. The critique should include items you found most helpful and how the Web sites might be of value to you as an HIM professional.

3. Perform a literature search to find an example of a quality improvement activity. Use the data in the article to create an original data display of the data. Then display the data and include a written analysis of the display and submit a copy of the article.

4. Read the following scenario and answer the questions as completely as possible:

   The surgical floor has anecdotally noticed that patients who have received a spinal anesthetic are complaining more and more frequently of severe, persistent headache within four hours of surgery. The anesthesia department has decided that this needs further investigation. It is well established in the literature that spinal headaches can be avoided with proper education of staff and patients.

   • How can the anesthesia department establish whether a problem exists?

   • Develop a measurable statement that can be used to determine desired performance regarding spinal anesthetic and headache.

   • Using the information gathered in the previous activity, develop a formula that will give the rate of spinal headaches on the surgical unit.

   • Identify the most likely data sources used to gather the above information.

Review Quiz

Instructions: Choose the most appropriate answer to the following questions.

1. All of the following are characteristics of an organized medical staff as recognized by the JCAHO except ___.
   a. Peer review activities are optional.
   b. Fully licensed physicians are permitted by law to provide patient care services.
   c. Clinical privileges are delineated.
   d. The medical staff is subject to medical staff and departmental bylaws/rules and regulations, and policies.

2. A person who states that "our main job is to prevent injury and property loss" is primarily concerned with ___.
   a. Credentialing
   b. Utilization management
   c. Risk management
   d. Severity indexing

3. The medical staff committee that is most likely to be responsible for evaluating applicants to the organized medical staff is the ___.
   a. Credentials committee
   b. Infection control committee
   c. Joint conference committee
   d. Utilization management committee

4. The body that has final authority for appointing applicants to the medical staff and for awarding privileges is the ___.
   a. Credentials committee
   b. Governing body
   c. Administrative staff
   d. Executive committee

5. The database established to identify the level of resource consumption based on clinical evidence is best described as___.
   a. Utilization review
   b. Severity index
   c. Risk management
   d. Credentials review

6. Quality improvement focuses on the three performance measures of ___.
   a. Process, results, mortality
   b. Training, process, results
   c. Structure, process, outcome
   d. Surgery, outcomes, admission

7. The most commonly used data source during quality improvement activities is the ___.
   a. Medical record
   b. Pathology report
   c. Operative index
   d. Incident reports

8. Fundamental tasks that are part of the QI process include all of the following except ___ .
   a. Assessment
   b. Performance
   c. Improvement
   d. Measurement

9. The theme addressed in three judicial decisions on quality improvement was ___.
   a. Postoperative infection control
   b. Emergency care of patients
   c. Future care of patients
   d. Credentialing of the medical staff

10. The Health Care Quality Improvement Act (HCQIA) established the ___.
    a. National Practitioner Data Bank
    b. Peer Review Management Control Board
    c. Board of Medical Examiners
    d. Federal Licensing Bureau

Part V

Knowledge-Based Healthcare Data and Information

Chapter 18
Biomedical and Research Support

Carol E. Osborn, PhD, RHIA

Learning Objectives

- To understand the role of biomedical research in evaluating the safety and efficacy of diagnostic and therapeutic procedures in order to solve human problems
- To relate the measures outlined by the Nuremberg Code, the Declaration of Helsinki, and the Belmont Report for the protection of human subjects
- To outline the contents of informed consent for the protection of human subjects as required by federal regulation
- To discuss the Health Insurance Portability and Accountability Act (HIPPA) and its privacy provisions for the protection of human subjects
- To understand the various research designs for conducting biomedical research
- To understand the purpose of outcomes and effectiveness research
- To describe the various types of outcomes and effectiveness measures
- To relate the purpose of the Health Plan Employer Data and Information Set (HEDIS®) sponsored by the National Commission for Quality Assurance (NCQA)
- To explain the purpose and requirements of the ORYX measurement process

Key Terms

Attributable risk (AR)
Case-control study
Clinical trial
Cohort study
Controls
Core measures
Cross-sectional study
Double-blinded study
Epidemiological studies
Experimental study
Food and Drug Administration (FDA)
Health Plan Employer Data and Information Set (HEDIS®)
Healthcare Cost and Utilization Project (HCUP)
Human subjects
Informed consent
Observational study
Odds ratio
Outcomes and effectiveness research (OER)
Principal investigator
Prospective studies
Protocol
Relative risk (RR)
Retrospective study
Single-blinded study
Sponsor

Introduction

Biomedical research is a search for knowledge that often leads to advances in medicine. It uncovers what new drugs and other types of treatments, as well as new technology, are safe and effective for patients. When new treatments and/or technologies ultimately reach the consumers of healthcare, long-term studies of outcomes and effectiveness begin.

This chapter explores the various methods by which biomedical research is conducted. It also examines methods of assessing outcomes and effectiveness, including programs initiated by the Agency for Healthcare Research and Quality, the Joint Commission on Accreditation of Healthcare Organizations, and the National Commission for Quality Assurance.

Theory into Practice

A physician in a healthcare facility is conducting a retrospective study of pathological fractures in women age 65 and over. He asks the HIM professional to provide medical records of these patients for the past five years.

The facility's information warehouse is queried for the number of cases that fall into DRG 239, Pathological Fractures and Musculoskeletal and Connective Tissue Malignancy, for the years 1997 through 2001. The cases selected have a principal diagnosis code of 733.xx.

The HIM professional is also asked to review the informed consent for a clinical trial that compares a new drug with the traditional drug for treating peripheral neuropathy. In the consent, the HIM professional notices the following paragraph (the consent is written in the first person):

> I understand that all or part of my medical record will be sent to the Gynecology Oncology Group (GOG) administrative office in Philadelphia, PA, as well as to the GOG statistical data center in Buffalo, NY, to be reviewed and analyzed by physicians and other study personnel, along with the records of all other patients participating in this study from this and other institutions. I understand that hospital records; doctor's office records; and laboratory, operating room, and other records may be audited by representatives of the GOG and the National Cancer Institute.

The HIM professional has been asked to advise the principal investigator on whether this statement is in compliance with the privacy rule of the Health Insurance Portability and Accountability Act (HIPAA).

Clinical and Biomedical Research

Biomedical research studies are conducted to evaluate disease processes and interventions and the safety, effectiveness, and usefulness of drugs, diagnostic procedures, and preventive measures such as vaccines and diets. The broad objective of these studies is to establish reproducible facts and theory that help solve human problems.

Ethical Treatment of Human Subjects

Human subjects are used in biomedical research studies. Federal regulations state that **human subjects** are living individual(s) about whom an investigator conducting research obtains either (1) data through intervention or interaction with the individual or (2) identifiable private information.

In the United States, the Belmont Report: Ethical Principles and Guidelines for the Protection of Human Subjects of Research, prepared by the Commission for the Protection of Human Subjects of Biomedical and Behavioral Research, guides the conduct of biomedical research. The Belmont Report was issued in 1979 and is still followed today. The Office for Human Research Protections (OHRP) of the Department of Health and Human Services monitors compliance with the federal regulations that govern the conduct of biomedical research. The federal regulations can be found in the *Federal Register* (1991, volume 56, number 117).

International guidelines also govern the ethical conduct of human research: the Nuremberg Code and the Declaration of Helsinki. The Nuremberg Code outlines research ethics that were developed during the trials of Nazi war criminals following World War Two. The code was widely adopted as a standard for protecting human subjects in the 1950s and 1960s. The basic tenet of the Nuremberg Code is that "voluntary consent of the human subject is absolutely essential" (Nuremburg Code 1949, p. 181). Additionally, it is the duty and responsibility of the individual initiating, directing, or conducting the experiment to ensure the quality of the informed consent.

The Declaration of Helsinki is a code of ethics for clinical research approved by the World Medical Association in 1964. It is a statement of ethical principles that provide guidance to physicians and other participants in medical research involving human subjects, including research on identifiable human material or identifiable data. The document has been revised a number of times, most recently, at the Fifty-second World Medical Association Assembly held in Edinburgh, Scotland, in October 2000.

Informed Consent

In most cases, biomedical research requires that subjects be given informed consent. **Informed consent** is a person's voluntary agreement to participate in research or to undergo a diagnostic, therapeutic, or preventive procedure. It is based on adequate knowledge and an understanding of relevant information that is provided by the investigators. In giving informed consent, subjects do not waive any of their legal rights nor do they release the investigator, sponsor, or institution from liability for negligence. Federal regulations require that certain information be provided each human subject:

- A statement that the study involves research, the purpose of the research, the expected duration of subject participation, a description of the procedures to be followed, and the identification of procedures that are experimental
- A description of reasonably foreseeable risks or discomforts
- A description of the benefits to the subject or others who may reasonably benefit from the research

- A disclosure of the appropriate alternative procedures or courses of treatment, if any, that might be advantageous to the subject
- A statement describing the extent to which confidentiality of records identifying the subject will be maintained
- For research involving more than minimal risk, an explanation as to whether any compensation or medical treatments are available if injury occurs, and, if so, what they consist of, or where further information may be obtained
- An explanation of whom to contact for answers to pertinent questions about the research and research subjects' rights and whom to contact in the event of a research-related injury to the subject
- A statement that participation is voluntary, refusal to participate will involve no penalty or loss of benefits to which the subject is otherwise entitled, and the subject may discontinue participation at any time without penalty or loss of benefits to which the subject is otherwise entitled

The regulations further require that additional consent information be provided when appropriate [Federal Policy 45 CFR 46.116], including:

- A statement that the treatment or procedure may involve risks to the subject (or embryo or fetus if the subject is pregnant) that are unforeseeable
- Anticipated circumstances under which the subject's participation may be terminated by the investigator without regard to the subject's consent
- Any additional costs that a subject may incur as a result of participating in the research
- The consequences of a subject's decision to withdraw from the research and procedures for orderly termination of participation by the subject
- A statement that significant new findings developed during the course of the research that may relate to the subject's willingness to continue participation will be provided to the subject
- The approximate number of subjects involved in the study

A model consent form appears in figure 18.1.

In institutions where biomedical research is conducted, consent forms are usually maintained in storage facilities monitored by the principal investigator, not in the hospital medical record. Consent forms often contain sensitive information such as that related to genetic testing. Information regarding genetic testing is not to be provided to insurers or other parties, and sometimes not to the subject. To help ensure that this information is not released inadvertently in the regular course of business related to the release of information process, it is important to keep these files separately. Examples of documents that are kept in the study center files are listed in figure 18.2 (p. 432).

Figure 18.1.   Template for Informed Consent for Research Involving Human Subjects

---

Consent to Investigational Treatment or Procedure

I, _____ , hereby authorize or direct _____ or associates of his/her choosing to perform the following treatment or procedure (describe in general terms), upon _____ (myself).

The experimental (research) portion of the treatment or procedure is:

This is part of an investigation entitled:

1. Purpose of the procedure or treatment:

2. Possible appropriate alternative procedure or treatment (not to participate in the study is always an option):

3. Discomforts and risks reasonably to be expected:

4. Possible benefits for subjects/society:

5. Anticipated duration of subject's participation (including number of visits):

I hereby acknowledge that _____ has provided information about the procedure described above, about my rights as a subject, and he/she answered all questions to my satisfaction. I understand that I may contact him/her at phone no. _____ should I have additional questions. He/she has explained the risks described above, and I understand them; he/she has also offered to explain all possible risks or complications.

I understand that, where appropriate, the U.S. Food and Drug Administration may inspect records pertaining to this study. I understand further that records obtained during my participation in this study that may contain my name or other personal identifiers may be made available to the sponsor of this study. Beyond this, I understand that my participation will remain confidential.

I understand that I am free to withdraw my consent and participation in this project at any time after notifying the project director without prejudicing future care. No guarantee has been given to me concerning this treatment or procedure.

I understand that in signing this form that, beyond giving consent, I am not waiving any legal rights that I might have, and I am not releasing the investigator, the sponsor, the institution, or its agents from any legal liability for damages that they might otherwise have.

In the event of injury resulting from participation in this study, I also understand that immediate medical treatment is available at _____ and that the costs of such treatment will be at my expense; financial compensation beyond that required by law is not available. Questions about this should be directed to the Office of Research Risks at _____ .

I have read and fully understand the consent form. I sign it freely and voluntarily. A copy has been given to me.

Figure 18.2.   Study Center File Contents

Investigational brochure

Signed protocol

Revised protocol (if applicable)

Protocol amendments (if applicable)

Informed consent form (blank)

Copy of signed forms

Curriculum vitae (resumes) of investigators and subinvestigators

Documentation of Institutional Review Board (IRB) or Ethical
Review Board (ERB) Compliance

Documentation of IRB approval of consent form, any protocol
amendments, and any consent form revisions

All correspondence between the investigator, IRB, or ERB, and study
sponsor or contract research organization, relating to study conduct

Copies of safety reports sent to the FDA

Lab certifications

Normal laboratory value ranges for tests required by the protocol

FDA's Clinical Investigator Information Sheet

Clinical Research Associate monitoring log

Drug invoices

Study site signature log

Financial disclosure statement

Privacy Considerations in Clinical and Biomedical Research

The Health Insurance Portability and Accountability Act (HIPAA) of 1996 includes certain privacy provisions that apply to human subject research. The privacy rule protects medical records and other individually identifiable health information used or disclosed in any form. The rule became effective on April 14, 2001, and organizations covered by the rule have until April 2003 to comply.

The privacy rule defines the means by which human research subjects are informed of how their personal medical information will be used or disclosed. It also outlines their rights to access the information. The privacy rule protects the privacy of individually identifiable information while ensuring that researchers continue to have access to the medical information they need to conduct their research. Investigators are permitted to use and disclose protected health information for research with individual authorization or without individual authorization under limited circumstances.

It is believed that the privacy rule will promote participation in clinical trials. For example, in genetic studies at the National Institutes of Health (NIH), nearly 32 percent of eligible people offered a test for breast cancer risk declined to take it. The reason cited most often is concern about health insurance discrimination and loss of privacy should the information be released. The privacy rule provides human subjects with some assurance about the privacy of their health information.

Types of Biomedical Research

The more common types of designs for research involving human subjects include:

- Epidemiological studies
- Case-control studies
- Cohort studies
- Cross-sectional study
- Clinical trials

Epidemiological Studies

The purpose of **epidemiological studies** is to compare two groups of individuals: one group with the risk factor of interest and one without it. In such studies, the investigator is attempting to identify risk factors for diseases, conditions, or behaviors or risks that result from particular causes, such as environmental factors and/or industrial agents.

Epidemiological studies are concerned with finding the causes and effects of diseases/conditions and/or the whys and the hows. The goal is to quantify the association between exposures and outcomes and to test hypotheses about causal relationships. Epidemiological research has several objectives, including:

- To identify the cause of disease and its associated risk factors
- To determine the extent of disease in a given community
- To study the natural history and prognosis of disease
- To evaluate new preventive and therapeutic measures and new modes of healthcare delivery
- To provide the foundation for public policy and regulatory decisions relating to environmental problems

Epidemiologial studies may be observational or experimental. In an **observational study,** the exposure and outcome for each individual in the study is studied (observed). In an **experimental study,** the exposure status for each individual in the study is determined and the individuals are then followed forward to determine the effects of the exposure.

Observational studies are used to generate hypotheses for later experimental studies. They may consist of clinical observations at a patient's bedside. For example, Alton Ochsner observed that every patient that he operated on for lung cancer had a history of cigarette smoking (Gordis 1996). If he had wanted to explore the relationship further, he would have compared the smoking histories of a group of his lung cancer patients with a group of his patients without lung cancer. This would be a case-control study. Research designs that are considered observational are prospective cohort study, retrospective cohort study, case-control study, and cross-sectional studies.

In biomedical research, experimental studies consist primarily of randomized clinical trials. In randomized clinical trials, individuals are randomized to experimental and control groups in order to study the effect of an intervention, such as an experimental drug.

A major purpose of epidemiological studies is to determine risk. In prospective studies, a 2×2 table is a tool that is used to evaluate the association between exposure and disease. (See table 18.1.) The table is a cross-classification of exposure status and disease status. The total number of individuals with the disease is $a + c$, and the total number without disease is $b + d$. The total number exposed is $a + b,$ and the total number not exposed is $c + d.$

The number of individuals who had both exposure and the disease is recorded in cell *a*; the number who had exposure, but no disease, is recorded in cell *b*; the number who had the disease, but no exposure, is recorded in cell *c*; and the number who had neither the disease nor exposure is recorded in cell *d*.

Case-Control Study

Case-control studies are the mainstay of epidemiological research. In them, persons with a certain condition (cases) and persons without the condition (controls) are studied by looking back in time. The objective is to determine the frequency of the risk factor among the cases and the frequency of the risk factor among the controls in order to determine possible causes of the disease. In a case-control study, if there is an association between exposure and disease, the prevalence of history of exposure will be higher in persons with the disease (cases) than in those without it (controls). For a case-control study, the 2×2 table in table 18.1 is modified in table 18.2. The proportion of cases exposed is $a/a + c$, and the proportion of controls exposed is $b/b + d$.

The advantages of case-control studies are that they are easy to conduct and cost-effective, with minimal risk to the subjects. Also, existing records are used to conduct the studies. Case-control studies also allow the researcher to study multiple causes of disease. Because they usually involve small groups, case-control studies are easily repeatable to determine whether the results are consistent.

Although the use of existing medical records is advantageous, there are problems associated with using them for retrospective research. One major problem is that the cases are based on hospital admissions. Admissions are based on patient characteristics, severity of illness and associated conditions, and admission policies. All of these vary from hospital to hospital, making standardization of the study difficult. In addition, there are problems related to poor documentation, illegibility, and missing records. Lack of consistency in diagnostic and clinical services between hospitals also make comparability difficult. Further, validation of the information can be difficult. An important aspect of epidemiological studies is the identification of risk. In studies using medical records, the population at risk is generally not defined.

Cohort Study

A **cohort study** is a prospective study in which the investigator selects a group of exposed individuals and unexposed individuals who are followed for a period of time to compare the incidence of disease in the two groups. The length of time for follow-up varies from a few days for acute diseases to several decades for cancer and cardiac diseases. If there is an association between exposure and disease, the incidence of disease is greater in the exposed group ($a/a + b$) than in the unexposed group ($c/c + d$). New cases of the disease are identified as they occur so that it can be determined whether a time relationship exists between exposure to disease and development of disease. The time relationship must be established if the exposure is to be considered the cause of the disease. For a cohort study, the 2×2 table in table 18.1 is modified in table 18.3.

One of the most famous cohort studies is the Framingham Study that began in the 1950s. The research project was designed to monitor the incidence of coronary artery disease in more than 5,000 residents who were examined every two years for a period of twenty years. This study has provided important data demonstrating the relationship between the development of heart disease and risk factors such as smoking, obesity, diet, and high blood pressure.

Cohort studies offer several advantages. First, the researcher can control the data collection process throughout the study. Also, outcome events can be checked as they occur; many outcomes can be studied, including those that were not anticipated at the start of the study. The disadvantages of cohort studies are that they are costly and there is a long wait for the study results. Also, subjects may be lost to death, withdrawal, or follow-up.

One difference between case-control and cohort studies is that the former is a retrospective study and the latter is a prospective study. A **retrospective study** is conducted by reviewing records from the past; a **prospective study** is designed to observe events that occur after the subjects have been identified. The advantages and disadvantages of prospective and retrospective studies are outlined in tables 18.4 and 18.5 (p. 434).

Another difference is that in a cohort study the subjects are individuals with or without the disease and the focus is disease status; in the case-control study, the subjects are individuals who have been exposed or not exposed to the disease and the focus is exposure status.

Table 18.1. 2×2 Table for Classifying Disease Status and Exposure Status

		Disease Status		
		Yes	No	Total
Exposure Status	Yes	*a*	*b*	$a + b$
	No	*c*	*d*	$c + d$
		$a + c$	$b + d$	$a + b + c + d$

Table 18.2. 2×2 Table for Case-Control Studies

	Cases (with disease)	Controls (without disease)
Exposed	*a*	*b*
Not exposed	*c*	*d*
Total	$a + c$	$b + d$
Proportions exposed	$a/a + c$	$b/b + d$

Table 18.3. 2×2 Table for Cohort Studies

	Disease Develops	Disease Does Not Develop	Totals	Incidence Rates of Disease
Exposed	*a*	*b*	$a + b$	$a/a + b$
Not Exposed	*c*	*d*	$c + d$	$c/c + d$

Cross-Sectional Study

In a **cross-sectional study,** both the exposure and the disease outcome are determined at the same time in each subject. A cross-sectional study also may be referred to as a prevalence study because it describes characteristics and health outcomes at a particular point in time. It provides quantitative estimates of the magnitude of a problem. After the population has been defined, the presence or absence of exposure and of disease can be established for each individual in the study. Each subject is then categorized into one of four subgroups that correspond to the 2×2 table that appears in table 18.6.

The prevalence of disease in persons with the exposure, $a/a + b$, is compared with persons without exposure, $c/c + d$. Alternatively, the prevalence of exposure in persons with the disease, $a/a + c$, to the prevalence of exposure to persons without the disease, $b/b + d$.

A major advantage of the cross-sectional study is that it is relatively easy to conduct and may produce results in a short period of time. The disadvantage is that because exposure and disease are determined at the same time in each subject, the time relationship between exposure and onset of the disease cannot be established. It describes only what exists at the time of the study.

Clinical Trials

Epidemiological studies that are experimental are referred to as clinical trials. **Clinical trials** are used to assess the safety and efficacy of new drugs, devices, treatments, or preventive measures in humans by comparing two or more regimens or interventions. They are prospective in nature. Many clinical trials are multicentered; that is, a number of research institutions cooperate in conducting the study. In randomized clinical trials, participants are assigned to a treatment or a control group. They may be **single-** or **double-blinded studies,** in which case the investigator, the participants, or both do not know who is in the treatment or control group until the end of the study.

Most clinical trials consist of three phases. In a phase 1 drug trial, studies are performed on twenty to eighty healthy volunteers who are closely monitored. The objective of phase 1 drug trials is to determine the metabolic and pharmacological actions of the drug in humans, to determine the side effects associated with increasing dosages, and to gain early evidence of effectiveness. Historically, phase 1 trials are considered the safest and usually involve administering a single dose to healthy volunteers. But they also can pose a high level of unknown risk because this is the first administration of a drug to a human. When the drug is highly toxic, such as cancer chemotherapies, cancer patients are usually the subjects for phase 1 trials.

In the phase 2 drug trial, the number of participants is usually increased to between 100 and 200. The purpose of this trial is to evaluate the drug's effectiveness for a certain indication in patients with the condition under study and to determine the short-term side effects and risks associated with the drug. Subjects included in phase 2 studies are usually those with the condition the drug is intended to treat. Phase 2 studies are randomized, well controlled, and closely monitored. They may include randomization to treatment and control groups and be double-blinded. Treatment and control groups allow for comparison between subjects who received the drug and those who did not.

Table 18.4.   Advantages and Disadvantages of Retrospective Studies

Advantages	Disadvantages
Short study time	Control group subject to bias in selection
Relatively inexpensive	Biased recall possible
Suitable for rare diseases	Cannot determine incidence rate
Ethical problems minimal	Relative risk is approximate
Hospital medical record may be used	
Small number of subjects	
No attrition problems	

Table 18.5.   Advantages and Disadvantages of Prospective Studies

Advantages	Disadvantages
Control group less susceptible to bias	Requires more time
No recall necessary	Costly
Incidence rate can be determined	Relatively common diseases only
Relative risk is accurate	Ethical problems may be considerable and influence study design
	Volunteers needed
	Results may not be generalizable to a larger population
	Requires a large number of subjects
	Problems with attrition

Table 18.6. 2×2 Table for Cross-Sectional Studies

	Disease	No Disease	Totals	Prevalence of Disease for Exposed/Not Exposed
Exposed	a	b	$a + b$	$a/a + b$
Not Exposed	c	d	$c + d$	$c/c + d$
Totals	$a + c$	$b + d$	$a + b + c + d$	$a + b + c + d$
Prevalence of Exposure for Disease/No Disease	$a/a + c$	$b/b + d$		

Group a: Persons exposed with the disease
Group b: Persons exposed without the disease
Group c: Persons with the disease, but not exposed
Group d: Persons without disease and without exposure

Phase 3 drug trials involve the administration of a new drug to a larger number of patients in different clinical settings to determine its safety, effectiveness, and appropriate dosage. The number of subjects involved may range from several hundred to several thousand. Phase 3 trials are conducted only after evidence of effectiveness has been obtained. Phase 3 studies are designed to collect more information on drug effectiveness and safety for evaluating the drug's overall risk benefit.

The **Food and Drug Administration** (FDA), in collaboration with the sponsor, may decide to conduct a phase 4 postmarketing study. Phase 4 studies are designed to obtain more information about the drug's risks, benefits, and optimal use. They may include studying different doses or schedules of administration than what was used in phase 2 studies, the use of the drug in other patient populations or other stages of the disease, or the use of the drug over a longer period of time.

Risk Assessment

As stated earlier, one objective of epidemiological studies is to assess risk. Risk is the probability that an individual will develop a disease over a specified period of time, providing that he or she did not die as a result of some other disease process during the same time period. It is usually expressed as **relative risk** (RR). RR is calculated from cohort studies and compares the risk of some disease in two groups differentiated by some demographic variable such as sex or race. The group of interest is referred to as the exposed group and the comparison group is the unexposed group. The risk ratio is calculated as:

$$\text{Risk for exposed group} \div \text{Risk for unexposed group}$$

A relative risk of 1.0 indicates that there is identical risk in both groups. An RR that is greater than 1.0 indicates an increased risk for the exposed group, and an RR of less than 1.0 indicates a decreased risk for the exposed group.

Odds Ratio

In a case-control study, the objective is to identify differences in exposure frequency associated with one group having the disease under study and the other group not having it. The incidence of disease in the exposed and unexposed populations is not known because persons with the disease (cases) and without the disease (controls) are identified at the onset of the study. Thus, relative risk cannot be calculated directly. So the question becomes, What are the odds that an exposed person will develop the disease? or What are the odds that a nonexposed person will develop the disease?

In a case-control study, the **odds ratio** compares the odds that the cases exposed to the disease to the odds that the **controls** were exposed. Using the 2 × 2 table in table 18.1 as a reference, the odds ratio is calculated as:

$$\frac{a/b}{c/d} = \frac{a \times d}{b \times c}$$

The odds ratio measures the odds of exposure of a given disease. For example, an odds ratio of 1.0 indicates that the incidence of disease is equal in each group; thus, the expo-

sure may not be a risk factor for the disease of interest. An odds ratio of 2.0 indicates that the cases were twice as likely to be exposed as the controls. This implies that the exposure is associated with twice the risk of disease.

Attributable Risk

The **attributable risk** (AR) is a measure of the public health impact of a causative factor on a population. In this measure, the assumption is that the occurrence of a disease in an unexposed group is the baseline or expected risk for that disease. Any risk above that level in the exposed group is attributed to exposure to the risk factor. It is assumed that some individuals will acquire a disease, such as lung cancer, whether or not they were exposed to a risk factor such as smoking. The AR measures the additional risk of illness as a result of an individual's exposure to a risk factor. The AR is calculated as:

$$AR = \frac{(\text{Risk for exposed group}) - (\text{Risk for unexposed group})}{\text{Risk for exposed group}} \times 100\%$$

Check Your Understanding 18.1

Instructions: Answer the following questions on a separate piece of paper.

1. What is the origin of the Nuremberg Code? What is its basic tenet?
2. What are the basic elements that should be contained in an informed consent for human subjects?
3. Describe the relationship of the privacy rule to clinical research.
4. What are some of the common types of research designs used in studies of human subjects?
5. What are the objectives of epidemiological studies?
6. In what type(s) of studies are medical records used?
7. What are the characteristics of a case-control study?
8. What are the characteristics of randomized controlled clinical trials?
9. What is relative risk?
10. What is attributable risk?

Outcomes and Effectiveness Research in Healthcare

The major objective of **outcomes and effectiveness research** (OER) is to understand the end results (outcomes) of particular healthcare practices and interventions. Examples of outcomes include the ability of a patient to function, quality of life, patient satisfaction, and mortality. By linking the care that patients receive to the outcomes they experience, OER has become the key to developing better ways to monitor and improve the quality of care.

The history of outcomes research can be traced back to the 1860s when Florence Nightingale laid the foundation for collecting and evaluating hospital statistics. Hospital mortality rates were the basic measures used for evaluating patient outcomes. The major finding was that mortality rates varied significantly from hospital to hospital.

The Flexner Report (1910), the Codman studies (1914), the establishment of hospital standards by the American College of Surgeons (1913), and the founding of the Joint

Commission on Accreditation of Hospitals (1952) are landmarks in the development of outcomes research. More recently, the passage of Medicare (1965) and subsequent legislation accelerated interest in outcomes research.

Outcomes Movement

The current outcomes movement gained momentum in the 1980s when the prospective payment system (PPS) for Medicare inpatient care was implemented. The public and policy makers were concerned that Medicare patients were being forced out of hospitals because "their DRG had run out." The fear was that patients were being discharged based on their length of stay rather than when they were clinically ready for discharge. William Roper, who became HCFA (Health Care Financing Administration, now the Centers for Medicare and Medicaid Services [CMS]) administrator in 1986, promoted the use of Medicare databases to monitor the quality of care through measurement of mortality rates, readmission rates, and other adverse outcomes.

Simultaneously, others were advancing the outcomes movement, which contained elements of research, measurement, and management. John Wennberg, director of the Center for the Evaluative Clinical Sciences at the Dartmouth Medical School, and others developed methods for exploring the impact of healthcare services on patient outcomes. Other research efforts on geographic variations in medical practice, appropriateness of care, and the poor quality of medical evidence to support various interventions and treatments resulted in establishment of the Agency for Health Care Policy and Research (AHCPR) in 1989. The Healthcare Research and Quality Act of 1999 changed the agency's name to the Agency for Healthcare Research and Quality (AHRQ). The mission of the AHRQ is to support research designed to improve the outcomes and quality of healthcare, reduce its costs, address patient safety and medical errors, and broaden access to effective services. The research sponsored by the AHRQ provides information that helps people make better decisions about healthcare.

The goals and research priorities of the AHRQ include:

- Supporting improvement in health outcomes
- Strengthening quality measurement and improvement

- Identifying strategies to improve access, foster appropriate use, and reduce unnecessary expenditures

An analytical tool that the AHRP supports is the **Healthcare Cost and Utilization Project** (HCUP). The HCUP is a database system for research, policy analysis, and quality measurement and improvement. It contains some Web-based tools that can be used to identify, track, analyze, and compare trends in hospital care at the national, regional, and state levels.

A component of the HCUP is the HCUP Quality Indicators. This is a set of clinical performance measures developed as a quick and easy-to-use screening tool for use with administrative databases. The indicators span three dimensions of care:

- Potentially avoidable adverse hospital outcomes
- Potentially inappropriate utilization of hospital procedures
- Potentially avoidable hospital admissions

Examples of HCUP measures appear in table 18.7.

Outcomes and Effectiveness Research Strategies

OER may be conducted at the community level, system level, institutional level, or patient level. At the community level, outcomes research focuses on the population as a whole or on specific communities. For example, the *Dartmouth Atlas of Musculoskeletal Health Care* (Center for the Evaluative Clinical Sciences 2000) has found that the rate for leg amputations in the southern tip of Texas is more than two times higher than the national average. The amputation rate in the Corpus Christi region is 3.7 leg amputations per 1,000 Medicare patients, three times higher than in Amarillo.

OER at the system level refers to the healthcare system as a whole. It may include the entire country or a specific region. Examples of geographic variations in medical care at the national level cited by the *Dartmouth Atlas of Health Care* include:

- In Bend, Oregon, the rate for back surgeries is 7.3 for every 1,000 Medicare recipients, more than four times higher than in Syracuse, New York, where there are 1.5 surgeries for every 1,000 Medicare recipients.

Table 18.7.   Examples of HCUP Quality Indicators

Type of Measure	Indicator	Relationship to Quality	Population at Risk
Outcome	Pulmonary compromise after major surgery	Although patients who receive general anesthesia are at risk for subsequent pulmonary complications, meticulous postoperative care should prevent such occurrences.	Postoperative discharges with pulmonary congestion, lung edema, or respiratory insufficiency or failure in any secondary diagnosis
Utilization	Hysterectomy	Hysterectomy is performed for more indications than any other single procedure. Studies have shown that 41 percent of hysterectomies are performed for reasons that may be considered inappropriate.	All nonmaternal/nonneonatal discharges of females age 18–64 years
Access to primary care	Pediatric asthma discharges	Asthma that is under good medical control rarely requires hospitalization. A strong relationship has been found between hospitalization for asthma and low socioeconomic status, particularly among children and adolescents. It has been demonstrated that adequate ambulatory care can prevent hospitalization for asthma.	All nonmaternal/nonneonatal discharges age under 18 years

- Heart patients in Elyria, Ohio, receive angioplasties at a rate more than seven times higher than in York, Pennsylvania, 360 miles away.
- Men in Baton Rouge, Louisiana, undergo prostate removal surgery at a rate more than eight times higher than do men in Tuscaloosa, Alabama.

OER at the institutional level refers to the sites in which healthcare is delivered: hospitals, clinics, or health maintenance organizations. At the patient level, the interest is on the interaction between one provider and one patient. An example outcome study performed at the institutional level is a review of medical records and/or clinical data of patients with a principal diagnosis of acute myocardial infarction who expire during hospitalization. A second example is the ongoing assessment of patient satisfaction.

There is no standard method for conducting outcomes research at the institutional level or any level. Donabedian (1966) proposed the first model for evaluating patient outcomes. His model focused on measuring the structure, process, and outcomes of medical care. Structure is the setting in which the healthcare is provided and the resources available to provide it. Process is the extent to which professionals perform according to accepted standards. Process is a set of activities that take place between providers. Outcomes include changes in the patient's condition, quality of life, and level of satisfaction. Characteristics of structure, process, and outcome appear in table 18.8. Other models used for the study of outcomes include the disease model and the health and wellness model. Epidemiological approaches are often used to study outcomes. In the hospital setting, the medical record often serves as the data source for outcome studies.

Outcomes and Effectiveness Measures

Several types of measures are used in OER: clinical performance, patient perceptions of care, health status, and administrative/financial performance.

Clinical performance measures are designed to evaluate the processes or outcomes of care associated with the delivery of clinical services. Clinical measures allow for intraorganizational and interorganizational comparisons to be used to improve patient health outcomes. Clinical measures should be condition specific or procedure specific or should address important functions of patient care, such as medication use and infection control.

Patient perceptions of care and/or services focus on the delivery of clinical services from a patient's perspective. Aspects of care that may be addressed are patient education, wait times, medication use, pain management, practitioner's bedside manner, communication regarding current care and future plans for care, and improvement in health status.

Health status measures address the functional well-being of specific populations, both in general and in relation to specific conditions. They indicate changes that have occurred in physical functioning, bodily pain, social functioning, and mental health over time.

Table 18.8.   Characteristics of Structure, Process, and Outcome

Structure	Process	Outcome
System characteristics: Organization Specialty mix Workload Access/convenience	Technical: Visits Medications Referrals Test ordering Hospitalizations	Clinical endpoints: Symptoms and signs Laboratory values Death
Provider characteristics: Specialty training Preferences Job satisfaction	Interpersonal: Interpersonal manner Counseling Communication level	Health-related quality of life: Physical Mental Social Role
Patient characteristics: Diagnosis/condition Severity Comorbidity Health habits		Satisfaction with care: Access Convenience Quality General

Administrative/financial performance measures address the organizational structure for coordinating and integrating service, functions, or activities across organizational components. Examples of administrative/financial measures are those related to financial stability, utilization, length of stay, and credentialing.

Defining expected clinical outcomes is a major section of the **protocols** for clinical trials. The **principal investigator** or organization sponsoring the study must specifically state the expected outcomes of the clinical trial before the investigation can begin. Investigators also must state at what point the research study will stop if adverse events occur. Examples of study objectives and outcome variables are listed in figure 18.3 (p. 438).

Use of Comparative Data in Outcomes Research

Healthcare organizations such as the National Commission for Quality Assurance (NCQA) and the Joint Commission on Accreditation of Healthcare Organizations (JCAHO) have developed measures for evaluating the effectiveness of healthcare providers. The purpose of the measures developed by the NCQA is to provide purchasers of healthcare, primarily employers, with information about the cost and effectiveness of organizations with which they contract for services. The JCAHO measures also are designed primarily to encourage organizations to improve their own performance and to provide a comprehensive picture of the care provided within the organization.

National Commission for Quality Assurance

The National Commission for Quality Assurance (NCQA) is an accountability system for managed care organizations. The NCQA began accrediting managed care organizations in 1991. The goals of the NCQA include:

- Fostering the development and strengthening of internal systems for quality improvement
- Assessing the quality of medical management

- Developing more reliable and comparable measures of system performance

As part of these efforts, the NCQA developed a set of performance measures known as the **Health Plan Employer Data and Information Set,** more commonly known as HEDIS. These measures are designed to provide both purchasers and consumers of healthcare with information to compare the performance of managed care plans. The information can help purchasers select health plans that provide employees with high-quality, cost-effective healthcare. The NCQA supports, sponsors, and maintains HEDIS. The goals of HEDIS include:

- Providing employers with the information needed to assess the performance of managed care plans
- Obtaining agreement on a set of baseline measures
- Standardizing data reporting to employers
- Demonstrating accountability to the public
- Building consensus among networks regarding data system investment

Three methods are used in collecting HEDIS data: examining claims data, reviewing health records, or a combination of both. The health record can provide the most complete information, but it is the more time-consuming, costly, and difficult method. Health record review is time-consuming because a statistically valid sample of records must be reviewed. The stated minimum is 411 charts. It is costly because the reviewers must have technical skills that require higher salaries.

Figure 18.3.   Sample Objectives and Outcome Variables for Clinical Research

---

Objective: To determine whether the treatment drug is a safe and effective treatment in patients with advanced chronic heart failure and is effective in reducing the incidence of cardiovascular hospitalization and/or mortality due to all causes.

Primary Outcome Variable: The primary outcome variable is the time from entry into the study to mortality from all causes of cardiovascular hospitalization. A hospitalization is a nonelective admission for medical therapy that results in at least one overnight stay. A cardiovascular hospitalization is one that is due to heart failure, myocardial infarction, coronary insufficiency, stroke, atrial or ventricular dysrhythmias, or symptomatic heart block.

Secondary Outcome Variables:

Time from study entry to all-cause mortality or all-cause hospitalization

Time from study entry to all-cause mortality or worsening heart failure hospitalization

Patient global assessment at the six-month visit

Six-minute walk test at the six-month visit

Other Outcomes of Interest:

All hospitalizations, classified by cause (heart failure, cardiovascular, vascular, noncardiovascular) in regard to frequency, length of stay, and cost

Number of emergency department visits classified by cause (heart failure or nonheart failure)

Mortality classified by cause (heart failure, cardiovascular, vascular, noncardiovascular)

All-cause mortality, all-cause hospitalization, cardiac transplant, and left ventricular assist device insertion

Myocardial infarction and cardiac revascularization

The safety and tolerability of the drug as determined by the occurrence of adverse events, permanent treatment withdrawals, changes in laboratory tests, physical exam, and ECG

Moreover, health records must be reviewed from the offices of many physicians because there is usually more than one primary care provider in any health plan.

HEDIS performance measures cover a number of areas: effectiveness of care, access and availability of care, satisfaction with care, health plan stability, utilization of services, cost of care, healthcare choices, and health plan descriptive information. A list of specific HEDIS measures is provided in table 18.9.

Providers and consumers of care are often interested in different performance measures. Providers are usually more interested in process and outcome measures whereas consumers (patients) are more interested in measures that pertain directly to them. For patients, the most important reasons for choosing a healthcare plan are physician communication, respect toward patients, time spent with physicians, and location of the physician's office. (Detailed information about NCQA programs and HEDIS measures can be found online at www.ncqa.org.)

Joint Commission on Accreditation of Healthcare Organizations

In 1997, the Joint Commission on Accreditation of Healthcare Organizations (JCAHO) introduced a set of performance measures known as ORYX. ORYX is a performance measurement process that the JCAHO has integrated into the accreditation process. ORYX is a data-driven process that encourages healthcare organizations to examine their processes for providing care in order to improve the results of care. JCAHO-accredited hospitals, long-term care facilities, home care, and behavioral health organizations must participate in the program.

ORYX uses standardized performance measures, referred to as **core measures,** that are applied across accredited healthcare programs. The use of core measures allows for benchmarking based on processes and outcomes of patient care. Core measures are designed to provide a comprehensive picture of the care provided in a given area.

The data collected from the JCAHO's core measures will be used for the following functions:

- Monitoring the performance of healthcare organization on an ongoing basis
- Focusing triennial surveys on areas within the organization that offer the greatest potential for clinical improvement
- Helping organizations identify issues that require attention
- Establishing a national comparative database to support internal quality improvement activities, benchmarking, and health services research
- Identifying both exemplary performance and best practices to facilitate the provision of benchmarking services to healthcare organizations
- Providing the content for publicly available comparative reports on organizational performance
- Fostering standardization of performance measurement

Currently, five core measurement areas contain twenty-five measures for acute care facilities:

- Acute myocardial infarction (eight)
- Heart failure (five)
- Community-acquired infections (two)
- Pregnancy and related conditions (three)
- Surgical procedures and complications (seven)

Examples of core measures from each category appear in table 18.10. Accredited hospitals are required to collect core measure data. To reduce duplication of effort, the JCAHO has included seventeen measures contained in the CMS's (formerly, HCFA) PRO Sixth Scope of Work. The CMS measures

Table 18.9.   HEDIS Performance Measures

Effectiveness of Care	Access/Availability of Care	Use of Services
Childhood immunization status	Availability of primary care providers	Well-child visits in third, fourth, fifth, and sixth years of life
Adolescent immunization status	Availability of behavioral health providers	Adolescent well care visit
Advising smokers to quit	Availability of OB and prenatal care providers	Frequency of selected procedures
Flu shots for older adults	Initiation of prenatal care	Inpatient utilization—general hospital/acute care
Breast cancer screening	Low birth weight deliveries at facilities for high-risk deliveries and neonates	Ambulatory care
Treating children's ear infections	Availability of language interpretation services	Inpatient utilization—nonacute care
Beta blocker treatment after a heart attack		C-section and vaginal birth after cesarean section
Eye exam for individuals with diabetes		
Satisfaction with Care	**Health Plan Stability**	**Health Plan Descriptive Information**
Member satisfaction surveys	Disenrollment	Case management
	Provider turnover	Recredentialing
	Years in business/total membership	Utilization management
	Indicators of financial stability	Preventive care
		Risk management
Cost	**Informed Healthcare Choices**	
Rate trends	New member orientation and/or education	
High-occurrence/high-cost DRGs	Language translation services	

Table 18.10.   Example ORYX Core Measures

Core Measure	Type of Measure	Measure	Description	Rationale
Surgical Procedures and Complications	Outcome	Surgical site infection within 30 days (for selected surgical procedures)	Patients undergoing selected surgical procedures who develop a surgical site infection (SSI) within 30 days of the procedure	Surgical site infections affect 2 to 5% of the 16 million patients undergoing surgical procedures each year in acute care hospitals. These infections lead to a significant increase in morbidity and mortality, accounting for 24% of all nososcomial infections, second only to urinary tract infection in overall frequency.
Heart Failure	Process	Patients with atrial fibrillation receiving oral anticoagulation therapy (warfarin/Coumadin) unless a relative or absolute contraindication to warfarin/Coumadin exists	Use of warfarin in atrial fibrillation	In the United States, an estimated 4.7 million patients have diagnosed heart failure. Mortality rates are high, and as our population ages, the incidence and mortality rates are expected to increase. Arterial thromboemboli have been reported to occur with an incidence of 0.9 to 42.4 events per 100 patient years in patients with heart failure due to left ventricular systolic dysfunction. A number of studies have demonstrated the efficacy of oral anticoagulation therapy in reducing the risk of stroke and systemic embolism in patients with nonrheumatic atrial fribillation.
Community-Acquired Pneumonia	Process	Oxygenation assessment within 24 hours of hospital arrival	Increase awareness of oxygenation assessment which can improve outcomes in patients with community-acquired infections	Hypoxemia is a known risk factor for poor outcomes in patients with pneumonia, and supplemental oxygen has been shown to decrease mortality in patients with pneumonia.
Acute Myocardial Infarction	Outcome	Inpatient mortality	Patients with a principal diagnosis of AMI who expire during hospitalization	Mortality of patients with AMI represents a significant outcome potentially related to quality of care. High rates over time may warrant an investigation into the quality of care provided.
Pregnancy and Related Conditions	Outcome	Vaginal birth after cesarean section (VBAC)	Prenatal patient evaluation, management, and treatment selection concerning vaginal deliveries in patients who have a history of previous cesarean section	A trial of labor may be offered to women who have had a previous cesarean section. Although trial of labor is usually successful and is relatively safe, major maternal complications can occur.

are in the pneumonia, acute myocardial infarction, and heart failure measure sets.

Each facility selects its own core measures based on the services it provides. For example, if a hospital does not provide obstetrical services, it would not be required to select measures from the pregnancy and related conditions category. Hospitals that serve patient populations that have conditions that match two or more of the core measure sets will be required to choose two measure sets. Hospitals should select measures that correlate to the greatest degree of high-risk, high-volume, and problem-prone areas within the organization. Data are submitted quarterly to the JCAHO.

The ORYX requirements have been simplified for small hospitals. Small hospitals are designed as with an average daily census of less than ten and outpatient visits of less than 150 per month. Because the ORYX core measures may not be appropriate for small hospitals, small hospitals may select performance measures available from other sources. Measures contained in the healthcare-related literature, those developed by professional associations, and/or measures developed internally may be chosen.

How an organization uses its selected core measures will be evaluated during a JCAHO accreditation on-site survey. The organization will have to demonstrate the reliability of the data, conduct credible analysis of the data, and initiate system and process improvements. JCAHO review of submitted ORYX data may trigger a response outside the regular triennial survey. Failure to provide ORYX data for two consecutive quarters may result in a Type I recommendation. A Type I recommendation indicates that the organization is in compliance with most performance areas but has deficiencies that require resolution within a specified period of time. Continued failure to submit data could result in the organization receiving conditional accreditation. Conditional accreditation indicates that the organization has failed to comply with one or more specified accreditation policy requirements but is believed to be capable of achieving acceptable compliance within a stipulated time period.

Check Your Understanding 18.2

Instructions: Answer the following questions on a separate piece of paper.

1. What is the purpose of outcomes and effectiveness research?
2. What types of outcomes are studied?
3. What is the mission of the Agency for Healthcare Research and Quality (AHRQ)?
4. Who sponsors the Health Care Utilization Project (HCUP)? What is the purpose of the HCUP database?
5. What is the focus of the HCUP quality indicators?
6. What types of performance measures are used in outcomes and effectiveness research?
7. What is the purpose of the HEDIS measures developed by the National Commission on Quality Assurance?
8. How are HEDIS data collected?
9. What is the purpose of the ORYX core measures developed by the JCAHO?
10. What are the ORYX five core measurement areas?

Real-World Case

A managed care organization is about to be surveyed by the National Commission on Quality Assurance (NCQA). The surveyors have requested data on cervical cancer screening rates for the past four years (see table 18.11).

Discussion Questions

1. Analyze the above data. What problems do you see? What explanations would you give if NCQA questioned you about this data?
2. What would you propose as the goal for 2002? What information would you use to set the goal for 2002 and the years to follow?

Summary

Biomedical research conducted on human subjects should follow guidelines set forth in the Belmont Report, the Nuremberg Code, and the Declaration of Helsinki. Further, biomedical research on human subjects requires informed consent.

Many study designs are used to conduct biomedical research, including case-control studies, cohort studies, cross-sectional studies, and clinical trials. In a case-control study, the frequency of the exposure in the diseased cases is compared with the frequency of exposure in the controls. In a cohort study, a set of group characteristics by risk factor in a group of individuals is followed over time for outcome. In a cross-sectional study, the frequency of a risk factor and an outcome of interest in a geographically defined population is studied at one point in time. Clinical trials are controlled studies that involve human subjects. They are designed to evaluate prospectively the safety and effectiveness of new drugs, devices, or behavioral interventions.

A major objective of biomedical research is to quantify the risk of obtaining a particular disease as the result of exposure to a risk factor. Relative risk, odds ratio, and attributable risk are measures used to quantify or assess risk. Relative risk compares the incidence of disease in the exposed group to the incidence of disease in the control group. The odds ratio, the odds of exposure in a diseased group, is divided by the odds of exposure in the nondiseased group. And attributable risk is the proportion of total risk for a disease or outcome attributable to a particular exposure.

Lastly, various models for outcomes and effectiveness research are available. The Agency for Healthcare Research and Quality (AHRQ) serves as a resource for individuals engaged in outcomes research. The AHRQ sets a national agenda for the types of outcomes research that should be conducted. In addition, the Joint Commission on Accreditation of Healthcare Organizations conducts the ORYX program, which has a set of core measures for evaluation effectiveness of care in various types of healthcare organizations. And lastly, the NCQA administers HEDIS, a program for evaluating the quality of services provided by managed care organizations.

Table 18.11.   Data for Real World Case: Cervical Cancer Screening Rates

Year	Goal	Performance Rate
1998	Baseline performance rate	60%
1999	60%	65%
2000	60%	68%
2001	70%	72%

References

The Belmont Report: Ethical Principles and Guidelines for the Protection of Human Subjects of Research. 1978. Washington, D.C.: U.S. Government Printing Office. DHEW Publication No. (OS) 78-0012. Reprinted in *Federal Register* 44 (April 18, 1979): 23192.

Center for the Evaluative Clinical Sciences at Dartmouth Medical School. 2000. *Dartmouth Atlas of Healthcare.* Available online from www.dartmouthatlas.org.

Code of Federal Regulations Title 45 Part 46, Protection of Human Subjects. June 18, 1991. Department of HHS, NIH, Office for Protection from Research Risks.

Donabedian, A. 1966. Evaluating the quality of medical care. *Milbank Memorial Fund Quarterly: Health and Society* 44(3; pt. 2):166–203.

Federal Policy for the Protection of Human Subject (Basic DHHS Policy for Protection of Human Research Subjects). Source: 56 FR 28003, June 18, 1991.

Friis, R. H., and T. A. Sellers 1999. *Epidemiology for Public Health Practice.* Gaithersburg, Md.: Aspen Publishers.

Gordis, Leon. 1996. *Epidemiology.* Philadelphia: W. B. Saunders.

Jekel, J., J. G. Elmore, and D. L. Katz. 1996. *Epidemiology, Biostatistics and Preventive Medicine.* Philadelphia: W. B. Saunders.

Joint Commission on Accreditation of Healthcare Organizations. 2001. *Candidate Core Measures Profiles: Acute Myocardial Infarction.* Available online from www.jcaho.org.

Joint Commission on Accreditation of Healthcare Organizations. 2001. *Candidate Core Measures Profiles: Community-Acquired Pneumonia.* Available online from www.jcaho.org.

Joint Commission on Accreditation of Healthcare Organizations. 2001. *Candidate Core Measures Profiles: Heart Failure.* Available online from www.jcaho.org.

Joint Commission on Accreditation of Healthcare Organizations. 2001. *Candidate Core Measures Profiles: Pregnancy and Related Conditions.* Available online from www.jcaho.org.

Joint Commission on Accreditation of Healthcare Organizations. 2001. *Candidate Core Measures Profiles: Surgical Procedures and Complications.* Available online from www.jcaho.org.

Joint Commission on Accreditation of Healthcare Organizations. 2001. *Facts about Core Measures.* Available online from www.jcaho.org.

Joint Commission on Accreditation of Healthcare Organizations. 2001. *First Complement Hospital Core Measure Sets.* Available online from www.jcaho.org.

Joint Commission on Accreditation of Healthcare Organizations. 2001. *ORYX: The Next Evolution in Accreditation.* Available online from www.jcaho.org.

Joint Commission on Accreditation of Healthcare Organizations. 2001. *Plan for Introducing Joint Commission Hospital Core Measure Requirements.* Available online from www.jcaho.org.

Morton, R. F., J. R. Hebel, and R. J. McCarter. 1990. *A Study Guide to Epidemiology and Biostatistics.* Gaithersburg, Md.: Aspen Publishers.

Murphy, G. F., M. A. Hanken, and K. A. Waters. 1999. *Electronic Health Record: Changing the Vision.* Philadelphia: W. B. Saunders.

National Institutes of Health, Office of Extramural Research, Office for Protection from Research Risks. 1993. *Institutional Review Board Guidebook: Protecting Human Subjects.* Bethesda. Md.: National Institutes of Health.

The Nuremburg Code. 1949. Reprinted in *Trials of War Criminals before the Nuremburg Military Tribunals under Control Council Law No. 10,* Vol. 2, pp. 181-182, Washington, D.C.: U.S. Government Printing Office. Also reprinted in Levine, R. J. *Ethics and Regulation of Clinical Research,* 2nd Edition. Baltimore: Urban and Schwarzenberg, pp. 425–26.

U.S. Department of Health and Human Services. 2001. *HHS Fact Sheet: Protecting the Privacy of Patients' Health Information.* Accessed July 2001. Available online from www.hhs.gov/news/press.

U.S. Department of Health and Human Services. 2001. Standards for Privacy of Individually Identifiable Health Information. Administrative Simplification. Available online from aspe.os.dhhs.gov/admnsimp.

U.S. Government Printing Office. 1949. *Nuremberg Military Tribunals and Control Council Law* 2(10):181–82. Available online from ohsr.od.nih.gov/nuremberg.

Vergano, Dan. 2000. The geography of surgery. *USA Today,* September 18.

World Medical Association. 1964. Declaration of Helsinki. As amended by the 41st World Medical Assembly, Hong Kong, September 1989. Reprinted in *Law, Medicine and Health Care* 19(3–4):264–65 (1991).

Application Exercise

According to the AHRQ, hysterectomy is performed for more indications than any other single procedure. Studies have shown that 41 percent of hysterectomies are performed for reasons that may be considered inappropriate. The purpose of this exercise is to evaluate the medical necessity of hysterectomies performed at Community Hospital and to benchmark hospital performance with national data.

1. Define the population at risk.

2. Using ICD-9-CM codes, identify cases for review.

3. Are there cases that should be excluded from the study?

Review the Community Hospital data set table in table 18.12 (pp. 442–43) for this exercise and answer the questions that follow.

4. Rank-order the reasons for hysterectomy.

5. How many physicians performed hysterectomies? Categorize the reason for hysterectomy by physician. Can you detect a pattern on the need for hysterectomy by physician?

6. What is the average length of stay (LOS) and average age of patients receiving hysterectomy for each physician? Can you identify any trends?

7. How many hysterectomies were performed for the age groups listed in the National Comparison Data Table in table 18.13 (p. 444) for this exercise? Copy table 18.13 on a separate piece of paper and fill in all the empty boxes in the National Comparison Data Table. What is the LOS and average charges for each age group? How do hospital data compare with national data? Use HCUPnet to run your query (http://hcup.ahrq.gov/HCUPNet.asp).

8. If the hospital's data varies from national data, can you identify a reason?

9. After analyzing the data, identify what questions need further exploration. How will you answer these questions?

Table 18.12.   Data for Application Exercise #3: Community Hospital Data Set Table, Hysterectomies, January–March 2000*

MRN	DRG	RW	Disch Date	PDX	DX1	DX2	DX3	DX4	DX5	Pproc	LOS	Age	Age Group	Surgeon	Total Charges	Payor Class
924084380	358	1.1902	1/4/2000	626.2	218.9	620.2	622.7	424.0		68.51	1	51	2	3	$7,681.00	MNGD CARE
373305379	359	0.8165	1/22/2000	218.1	218.2	621.0	401.9			68.4	3	52	2	19	$10,623.00	MEDICARE
900257145	359	0.8165	1/27/2000	618.2	401.9	716.98				68.59	2	57	2	19	$9,761.00	MEDICAID
901328256	359	0.8165	1/11/2000	218.2	617.0	621.0	626.2	285.9		68.4	2	47	2	2	$7,270.00	MNGD CARE
903920624	358	1.1902	1/5/2000	218.1	788.20	620.2	625.3			68.29	3	33	1	12	$9,938.00	MNGD CARE
900144577	359	0.8165	1/11/2000	617.1	617.3	218.9	401.9	620.1		68.4	2	45	2	16	$9,647.00	MNGD CARE
908815122	359	0.8165	1/7/2000	626.2	617.0	218.2	620.2	278.01	780.57	68.4	2	47	2	18	$10,748.00	COMMERCIAL
900488642	359	0.8165	1/26/2000	626.9	218.9	620.2	617.0			68.4	2	53	2	5	$9,620.00	MNGD CARE
960490222	359	0.8165	1/31/2000	218.9	451.9	311	278.01			68.4	3	43	1	13	$8,217.00	SELF PAY
960901159	359	0.8165	1/18/2000	218.9	625.3	788.43				68.29	1	40	1	12	$5,806.00	MNGD CARE
960147125	359	0.8165	1/13/2000	218.9	626.2	625.3	620.2	614.8		68.4	3	37	1	13	$8,391.00	MNGD CARE
690147988	359	0.8165	1/3/2000	620.0	616.0	625.3	625.9		311	68.4	2	36	1	18	$7,018.00	MEDICARE
906941619	359	0.8165	1/30/2000	218.0	401.9	789.06				68.4	7	52	2	13	$11,520.00	MNGD CARE
970680716	359	0.8165	1/6/2000	617.0	788.33	626.2				68.4	3	36	1	10	$8,693.00	SELF PAY
907891047	358	1.1902	1/25/2000	218.2	280.0	617.1	620.2	626.2		68.51	1	44	1	3	$9,151.00	MNGD CARE
970942975	359	0.8165	1/7/2000	628.2	218.9	614.1				68.29	2	36	1	18	$7,515.00	MNGD CARE
907422455	359	0.8165	1/4/2000	218.0	626.2	625.6	285.9	244.9		68.4	3	52	2	18	$11,289.00	MNGD CARE
907564804	359	0.8165	1/4/2000	617.0	625.9					68.59	1	33	1	10	$7,081.00	MNGD CARE
970205482	359	0.8165	1/9/2000	v26.0	493.90					66.79	1	32	1	9	$6,615.00	MNGD CARE
907629693	359	0.8165	1/8/2000	625.3	617.3	218.9	620.1	788.1		68.4	3	41	1	18	$9,113.00	COMMERCIAL
907852967	358	1.1902	1/6/2000	623.8	218.9	280.0	623.8			68.29	1	48	2	13	$7,513.00	MNGD CARE
906209459	359	0.8165	1/5/2000	218.0	614.1	401.9				68.29	2	36	1	12	$9,176.00	MNGD CARE
960300551	358	1.1902	1/12/2001	220	616.0	135	493.90	564.1	426.4	68.4	3	55	2	11	$8,695.00	GOV MNGD CARE
942480388	358	1.1902	2/28/2000	218.2	285.1	599.0	401.9			68.4	3	52	2	16	$10,894.00	MNGD CARE
900122573	358	1.1902	2/17/2000	218.9	244.9	250.00	616.0	620.1	690.8	68.4	3	46	2	10	$8,535.00	MNGD CARE
900255145	359	0.8165	2/15/2000	218.0	626.8	401.9	617.0			68.3	1	47	2	10	$11,940.00	MNGD CARE
900862277	359	0.8165	2/2/2000	218.2	626.8	620.2	530.81	401.9	285.9	68.4	2	47	2	5	$8,066.00	MNGD CARE
900372967	358	1.1902	2/29/2000	218.0	620.1	626.2	625.9	280.0		68.4	3	43	1	11	$7,267.00	MNGD CARE
900333891	359	0.8165	2/16/2000	218.9	625.9	620.8				68.29	2	44	1	5	$7,190.00	GOV MNGD CARE
900773300	359	0.8165	2/19/2000	218.2	626.2	616.0	493.90			68.4	3	49	2	18	$7,769.00	COMMERCIAL
900462422	359	0.8165	2/2/2000	617.0	620.8					68.4	2	42	1	5	$8,095.00	MNGD CARE
900664382	358	1.1902	2/28/2000	617.0	621.0	625.3	530.81	424.0	311	68.4	2	45	2	5	$8,369.00	MNGD CARE
900105623	359	0.8165	2/21/2000	617.3	218.8	568.89	616.0			68.4	2	45	2	4	$7,908.00	MNGD CARE
900415253	359	0.8165	2/2/2000	218.1	625.3	617.0	616.0	614.1		68.4	3	49	2	14	$9,827.00	MNGD CARE
960310882	359	0.8165	2/28/2000	218.2	616.0	620.1	625.3	626.2	V10.3	68.4	3	42	1	4	$8,425.00	MNGD CARE
609208203	359	0.8165	2/27/2000	218.1	617.0	620.1	626.8	218.1		68.4	3	42	1	17	$7,217.00	MNGD CARE

609411828	359	0.8165	2/10/2000	218.2	615.1	620.2	526.2			68.4	3	50	2	6	$7,948.00	MNGD CARE
609721017	359	0.8165	2/23/2000	617.0	620.2	620.2			729.1	68.4	3	49	2	16	$8,098.00	MNGD CARE
960741867	358	1.1902	2/3/2000	218.1	625.3	620.2	710.0	564.1		68.4	3	42	1	13	$8,699.00	MNGD CARE
960522918	359	0.8165	2/7/2000	616.0	218.9	278.00	250.00		401.9	68.59	1	43	1	19	$9,140.00	MNGD CARE
960672299	359	0.8165	2/19/2000	620.2	618.4	617.0	788.30	530.81	401.9	68.4	3	66	3	18	$14,013.00	MEDICARE
960003138	359	0.8165	2/14/2000	218.9	220	617.0	625.9	618.2	616.0	68.51	1	54	2	2	$6,748.00	MNGD CARE
960233972	359	0.8165	2/1/2000	618.1	218.9	616.0	625.6	724.5	787.01	68.59	1	39	1	3	$5,663.00	MNGD CARE
709390003	359	0.8165	2/3/2000	218.9	285.9	285.9				68.29	2	37	1	17	$7,855.00	MNGD CARE
970893422	359	0.8165	2/2/2000	218.0	626.2	285.9				68.29	1	34	1	4	$7,145.00	MNGD CARE
970244885	359	0.8165	2/7/2000	625.3	626.2	618.0	244.9	555.9		68.59	1	34	1	16	$6,776.00	MNGD CARE
790664394	359	0.8165	2/19/2000	218.0	616.0	622.1	626.2	285.9	214.1	68.4	3	40	1	16	$10,523.00	MNGD CARE
970058342	359	0.8165	2/23/2000	617.0	621.0	616.0				68.4	2	38	1	13	$7,190.00	MNGD CARE
904084986	358	1.1902	2/1/2000	626.2	218.9	617.0	401.9	285.9	614.6	68.4	3	45	2	4	$8,955.00	MNGD CARE
940368973	359	0.8165	2/16/2000	218.9	626.2	616.0	617.0	620.2		68.59	1	46	2	19	$8,001.00	MEDICAID
906300974	358	1.1902	2/16/2000	616.0	218.9	625.9				68.4	2	55	2	8	$8,303.00	COMMERCIAL
970792206	359	0.8165	2/7/2000	218.0	218.2	285.9	614.6	626.2	628.2	68.29	2	31	1	10	$10,656.00	COMMERCIAL
960362409	358	1.1902	2/16/2000	220	553.1	303.93	560.9	998.3	571.3	68.4	9	40	1	10	$15,900.00	GOV MNGD CARE
195104599	359	0.8165	3/14/2000	617.1	626.2	616.0	280.9	218.9		68.4	2	54	2	5	$7,335.00	MNGD CARE
900011042	359	0.8165	3/7/2000	220	218.9	218.9				68.4	2	58	2	5	$9,445.00	MNGD CARE
900501239	359	0.8165	3/6/2000	617.0	218.1	620.1	625.3	626.2	787.02	68.51	2	45	2	16	$10,042.00	MNGD CARE
900462299	359	0.8165	3/15/2000	218.1	285.9	455.0	560.1	568.0	998.11	68.4	5	46	2	4	$14,193.00	MNGD CARE
900713217	359	0.8165	3/13/2000	218.0	285.9	218.2				68.4	2	40	1	5	$7,438.00	SELF PAY
900023586	359	0.8165	3/21/2000	218.2						68.4	2	40	1	5	$8,856.00	MNGD CARE
900923451	359	0.8165	3/17/2000	218.1	626.2	621.5	617.1	617.0	280.0	68.29	3	46	2	3	$8,771.00	MNGD CARE
900344443	358	1.1902	3/21/2000	626.2	424.0	625.0	625.3			68.51	2	30	1	4	$9,237.00	GOV MNGD CARE
900644348	359	0.8165	3/13/2000	617.0	616.0	218.9	626.2			68.59	1	41	1	2	$6,128.00	MNGD CARE
900415705	358	1.1902	3/13/2000	218.1	626.8	620.2	620.0	617.0	280.0	68.4	2	52	2	5	$9,323.00	MNGD CARE
900387033	358	1.1902	3/1/2000	218.0	625.6	626.2	280.0	401.9		68.59	4	38	1	16	$9,933.00	MNGD CARE
960540073	358	1.1902	3/23/2000	218.2	621.0	614.6	593.9	428.0	414.01	68.4	3	57	2	19	$12,728.00	MEDICAID
960511566	359	0.8165	3/13/2000	218.1	625.3	626.2	626.2			68.29	2	33	1	12	$6,248.00	COMMERCIAL
960420355	359	0.8165	3/14/2000	626.2	626.6	626.6	218.9	285.9	401.9	68.4	2	48	2	10	$12,931.00	SELF PAY
970920422	359	0.8165	3/2/2000	218.1	616.0	553.21	311	216.5	788.33	68.4	4	41	1	10	$16,038.00	MNGD CARE
970581979	359	0.8165	3/24/2000	218.9	625.9	617.0	617.0			68.4	3	57	2	1	$9,051.00	MNGD CARE
970338402	359	0.8165	3/23/2000	620.5	620.1	220	220			65.49	1	25	1	10	$8,610.00	MNGD CARE
970664982	359	0.8165	3/31/2000	626.2	618.0	218.9	218.9	250.00	625.6	68.59	3	45	2	18	$10,716.00	MNGD CARE
970308784	359	0.8165	3/19/2000	218.9						68.29	1	40	1	9	$7,905.00	MNGD CARE
908257695	359	0.8165	3/21/2000	218.2	617.1	617.0	617.0	250.00		68.4	2	49	2	13	$7,922.00	MNGD CARE

*Column headings are explained on p. 444.

Column heading key for Table 18.12:

MRN = Medical record number of the patient
DRG = Diagnosis related group that is assigned to the patient after the patient has been discharged and the record is coded
RW = Relative weight of the DRG assigned; hospital payment is based on the relative weight of the DRG
Disch Date = Date the patient is discharged from the hospital
PDX = Principal diagnosis—the main reason for the patient's admission to the hospital
DX 1 = Secondary diagnosis number one
DX 2 = Secondary diagnosis number two
DX 3 = Secondary diagnosis number three
DX 4 = Secondary diagnosis number four

DX 5 = Secondary diagnosis number five
Pproc = Principal procedure—the procedure performed for definitive treatment; the procedure most closely related to the principal diagnosis
LOS = Length of stay—total number of days the patient was hospitalized
Age = Age of patient upon admission
Age groups: 1 = 25–44; 2 = 45–64; 3 = 65–84
Surgeon = Identifying number of the surgeon who performed principal procedure
Total Charges = Total amount of money charged to the payor for the patient's hospital stay
Payor Class = Type of third party payer who is responsible for payment

Table 18.13.   Data for Application Exercise #7: National Comparison Data Table for Hysterectomies

Age Group	Hospital Discharges	Hospital ALOS	Hospital Average Charges	National Discharges	National ALOS	National Average Charges
18–44						
45–64						
65–84						
85+						
Total						

Review Exercise

Instructions: Choose the most appropriate answer for the following questions.

1. ____ In the United States, biomedical research is guided by which of the following?
   a. The Belmont Report
   b. The Nuremberg Code
   c. The Declaration of Helsinki
   d. All of the above

2. ____ Which of the following elements is not required in an informed consent for research on human subjects?
   a. Social Security number
   b. Description of foreseeable risks
   c. A disclosure of alternate treatments
   d. A statement that the study involves research

3. ____ In which type of research study does neither the researcher nor the subject know the treatment group assignments of individual subjects?
   a. Single-blinded study
   b. Double-blinded study
   c. Experimental study
   d. Cross-sectional study

4. ____ What is attributable risk?
   a. The measure of an occurrence of an illness
   b. The measure of the impact of a disease on a population
   c. A measure that compares the risk of disease between two groups
   d. A measure that provides the odds that an individual will acquire a certain illness

5. ____ Which of the following statements is true of the HIPAA privacy rule?
   a. It compels patients to participate in human subject research.
   b. It requires release of hospital medical records upon request of the principal investigator in a research study.
   c. It protects identifiable health information from disclosure.
   d. It allows principal investigators in research studies to release subject information without consent.

6. ____ Which of the following is an objective of epidemiological research?
   a. To identify the cause of disease and its associated risk factors
   b. To track down individuals within a community who have been identified as having infectious disease
   c. To advise the public of health issues
   d. To approve new technology before it is made available to the healthcare community

7. ____ Which of the following is an advantage of a retrospective epidemiological study?
   a. Ethical problems
   b. Relatively inexpensive
   c. Research bias possible
   d. Large number of subjects required

8. ____ What is "low-birth-weight deliveries at facilities for high-risk deliveries" a measure of?
   a. Access/availability
   b. Utilization of services
   c. Effectiveness of care
   d. Cost

9. ____ You have completed a study of the number of hysterectomies performed at Community Hospital for the year 2000. For hospital discharges, what is the population at risk?
   a. All hospital inpatient discharges for the year 2000
   b. All female inpatient discharges for the year 2000
   c. All nonmaternal, nonneonatal female inpatient discharges for the year 2000
   d. All nonmaternal, nonneonatal female inpatient discharges, age 18–64 for the year 2000

10. ____ What type of measure is "surgical site infection within 30 days?"
   a. Outcome
   b. Process
   c. Utilization
   d. Satisfaction with care

Chapter 19
Expert Systems and Decision Support

J. Michael Hardin, PhD

Learning Objectives

- To understand the concept of decision support and the process of decision making
- To recognize the valuable assets contained within the organization's current data systems and how to better use the data
- To understand the background and history of decision support systems in general
- To identify the different structures used to develop decision support systems
- To differentiate between decision support systems and other information systems
- To understand the general types of decision support systems and to recognize the key architectural differences
- To understand the concept of data warehousing and how it is applicable to decision support
- To understand the process and tools of data mining and how they are used in decision support systems
- To recognize the different classes of decision support systems found in healthcare
- To understand some of the basic models of artificial intelligence used in developing decision support systems
- To recognize some of the career opportunities available to health information management professionals

Key Terms

Applied artificial intelligence
Artificial neural network (ANN)
Association rule analysis
Clinical decision support systems (CDSS)
Clinical repository
Data miners
Data mining
Data warehouse
Decision support system (DSS)
Decision tree
Expert system
Graphical user interface (GUI)
Graphics-based DSS
Health management information system (HMIS)
Hospital information system (HIS)
Hybrid on-line analytical processing (HOLAP)
Inference engine
Intellectual capital
Linkage analysis
Machine learning
Multidimensional data structure
Multidimensional database management system (MDDBMS)
Multidimensional on-line analytical processing (MOLAP)
Normalization
On-line analytical processing (OLAP)
Operations research (OR)
Relational database management system (RDMS)
Relational on-line analytical processing (ROLAP)
Return on investment (ROI)
Satisficing
Simon's decision-making model
Snowflake schema
Star schema
Structured query language (SQL)
Supervised learning
Unsupervised learning

Introduction

In *Future Health: Computers and Medicine in the Twenty-First Century*, Kaufman and Paterson (1995) identified seven goals that must be addressed in order to meet the future computing needs of physicians. Of critical importance, they observed, was the continued development and research of decision support systems (Pickover 1995).

But what are expert and decision support systems? For many people in healthcare, the mention of these systems evokes notions of a computer application that assists the clinician in caring for patients. Based on symptoms and other data from a patient, the computer system formulates possible diagnoses for the patient's condition and presents these suggestions to the clinician. In difficult cases, possibly involving rare conditions, these suggestions may greatly assist the clinician in formulating a decision regarding the best course of treatment for the patient.

Computer systems that provide such aid and recommendations to clinicians in making clinical decisions for individual patients are an important group of expert and decision support systems used in healthcare. This group of systems typically is called **clinical decision support systems** (CDSS).

This chapter examines the many types of expert and decision support systems that are found in today's healthcare environment. It also describes the infrastructure requirements for decision support systems. Finally, the chapter looks at how artificial intelligence is applied in healthcare and discusses the roles of health information management professionals in decision support.

Theory into Practice

Jewish Hospital HealthCare Services (JHHS) is a regional network providing healthcare services at thirty-five locations throughout Kentucky and southern Indiana. The JHHS network owns two acute care hospitals, one rehab hospital, a home health agency, and a hotel; manages six hospitals; and operates two primary care centers, nine outpatient rehabilitation centers, and three healthy lifestyle centers. In total, JHHS services more than 300,000 patients annually.

JHHS's corporate planning department is responsible for developing strategies and making recommendations on a variety of business issues with costs ranging from $5 to $50 million. Some of these business decisions include:

- Ambulatory care development
- Community needs assessments
- Optimal placement of physicians to maximize patient access and service
- Competitor analysis (physicians and facilities)
- Market analysis (customer location, market share by type of service)
- Employer analysis (where they are and how they use JHHS)
- Drive time and access studies
- Healthcare site selection

As an example, in planning a new healthcare facility, the group must advise corporate officers on the ranking of several sites using identified variables, determine which site is most optimal, and recommend what services each site should incorporate.

To accomplish its healthcare site selection model, the team uses a decision support system, in particular, a geographical information system, that incorporates healthcare statistics and business data in various planning and allocation models. The system is called ArcView Business Analyst from ESRI. (See www.esri.com/software/businessanalyst/index.html.) Using DSS, the corporate planning team has been very successful in helping the corporation to make good, strategic decisions and helping the JHHS to remain competitive.

Decision Support Systems

As business in general and healthcare in particular have entered into the twenty-first century, a new economic reality has emerged. Known by many different names, this new reality often is called "a knowledge economy" (Hardin et al. 1999). Businesses in a knowledge economy are more reliant on information, and this information resides in their employees and in their corporate data systems. The sum of all this knowledge represents a new form of business asset: **intellectual capital** (Stewart 1997). To be competitive and provide high-quality products and services in a knowledge economy, a business must learn to make right decisions quicker than their competitors do (Senge 1990).

The key point here is decision making. Decision making is a critical task for managers and clinicians. There is no shortage of computers and information technologies. What is important is not simply having information technology to collect data (although in healthcare this is very important as has been seen in the earlier chapters), but how a healthcare organization uses its information to make decisions. Stewart notes that "a corporation becomes a true knowledge company when it becomes aware of and involved in the 'deeper level,' where information is pursued for its own intrinsic value and not simply to automate or report on other activities" (1997, p. 6).

Expert and decision support systems enable business (healthcare) to move beyond automation of activities and begin to use computers to gain knowledge about its customers and its operations. Decision support systems include the establishment of repositories and data warehouses to efficiently store the organization's data in such a way as to make them accessible to managers as they make decisions. It also includes activities associated with **data mining,** which is the process of sorting through the organization's data to identify unusual patterns or to apply analytical models that will assist in predicting future events. Current applications of data-mining activities in healthcare include models to support fraud detection, utilization review, and clinical pathways.

Decision support systems (DSSs) also assist hospital chief financial officers (CFOs) in allocating financial resources (Friend 1992) and assist health plan administrators in managing the medical care market and formulating appropriate payment plans (Forgionne 1991). Additionally, DSSs assist hospital administrators in evaluating resource utilization (Cunningham and McKenna 1986) and improving the distribution of pharmaceuticals for inpatient patients (Zaki 1989). DSSs are being used and evaluated as tools to prevent medical errors and adverse events (Berner et al. 1999) in response to the serious issues noted in *To Err Is Human: Building a Safer Health System* (Kohn, Corrigan, and Donaldson 2000). The study described in this book shocked many people when it reported that as many as 98,000 people die as a result of medical errors such as:

- *Adverse events,* which are injuries to patients caused by medical mismanagement instead of the patient's underlying disease or medical condition
- *Medication-related errors,* such as accidental drug poisoning
- *Medication adverse events,* which are injuries resulting when, for example, an antibiotic drug is prescribed for patient with a history of allergic reactions to the antibiotic

The recent Institute of Medicine report entitled *Crossing the Quality Chasm: A New Health System for the 21st Century* (2001) recommends that greater use of DSSs by healthcare providers and organizations will improve the quality of care for patients and help minimize the likelihood of the occurrence of these serious problems.

Definition and Types of Decision Support Systems

Although computers are integral to the implementation of decision support and expert systems, these systems are really about people—how they solve problems, how they think, how they use information and decide which information to use. In essence, these systems indicate how people make decisions. Hence, a study of decision support and expert systems also must incorporate some discussion of people issues.

A **decision support system** is a computer-based system that gathers data from a variety of sources and assists in providing structure to the data using various analytical models and visual tools in order to facilitate and improve the ultimate outcome in decision-making tasks associated with nonroutine and nonrepetitive problems. However, this is but one of many definitions of a DSS. Because the goals involved in these systems have such breadth, no universally agreed-upon definition exists (Turban 1995). Nevertheless, this is a good working definition and captures the important characteristics commonly identified for DSSs. Table 19.1 provides a list of some of these characteristics.

Table 19.1.   Common Characteristics of a Decision Support System

- Is used in semistructured or unstructured decision contexts
- Is intended to support decision makers rather to replace them
- Supports all phases of the decision-making process
- Focuses on the effectiveness of the decision-making process rather than its efficiency
- Is under the control of the DSS user
- Uses underlying data and models
- Facilitates learning on the part of the decision maker
- Is interactive and user-friendly
- Is generally developed using an evolutionary, iterative process
- Provides support for all levels of management from top executives to line managers
- Can provide support for multiple independent or interdependent decisions
- Provides support for individual, group-based, and team-based decision-making contexts

Source: Marakas 1999, p. 3.

Notice that the words "expert system" do not appear in the definition above. Was this an oversight? Well, yes and no! Most commonly, an **expert system** is a computer-based system that can perform problem-solving tasks equal to the performance of human experts and, in some cases, can actually exceed the abilities of human experts. Expert systems were developed as part of a branch of computer science known as **applied artificial intelligence,** and the vision of some of these efforts has been to replace human experts with computers.

Some people argue that although they have some unique features in their architecture, expert systems also satisfy the concepts contained in the definition of DSS. Hence, an expert system is simply one type of DSS. However, if the notion in the definition relating to the facilitation role of the DSS is seen as one in which the system suggests possible actions, but the final decision rests with the human decision maker, expert systems may go beyond DSSs. Artificial intelligence and this view of expert systems is discussed later in this chapter, but for now it suffices to include the expert system as a type of DSS.

History and Background of Decision Support Systems

The roots of DSS emanate from two works that appeared in the early 1970s: *Models and Managers: The Concept of a Decision Calculus* by J. D. Little (1970) and *A Framework for Management Information Systems* by G. A. Gorry and M. S. Scott-Morton (1971). Using ideas from the research of Simon (1957, 1960) on how people, in particular, managers, make decisions, these two works proposed computer-based systems to assist in unstructured decision making.

Simon argued that decisions were arrayed on a spectrum from highly structured to unstructured. *Structured decisions* arise from very established, repetitive kinds of problems, ones for which standard solutions are available. Examples of areas that provide such decisions are accounts receivable, patient entry, and so on. Structured decisions depend on the context that produced the need for the decision to provide a framework for the solution.

During the Second World War, a new branch of applied mathematics, **operations research** (OR), was developed to analyze situations arising out the war and to propose mathematical models for their solutions. OR proved very effective in providing solutions to structured problems arising in this context. After the war, this new discipline was applied to business problems and a new business discipline, management science, was launched. During the 1950s and 1960s, these new disciplines assumed that decision makers could follow logical and systematic processes for arriving at business decisions by applying the scientific method to business problems. Thus, business problems were analyzed and classified into various general groups, for example, inventory control and scheduling. The key features of each of these general problems were analyzed, and elegant mathematical

models and solutions were developed for them. Computer programs then were developed to perform the computations in a quick and efficient manner. Thus, by the late 1960s, the use of computers to provide assistance and support in the solution of structured decisions had become an important tool for business decision makers.

However, more research was still needed for unstructured decisions. According to Simon, *unstructured decisions* arose from those contexts in which there were no clear-cut solutions and for which the particular problem or decision at hand may never have been encountered previously and may never be encountered again. The set of possible alternatives as well as the relevant data may not be available to the decision maker in these complex decisions.

Decision-Making Process

When faced with decisions, Simon (1960) observed that people use a three-phase approach. A schematic of **Simon's decision-making process** is shown in figure 19.1.

Figure 19.1.   Simon's Decision-Making Process

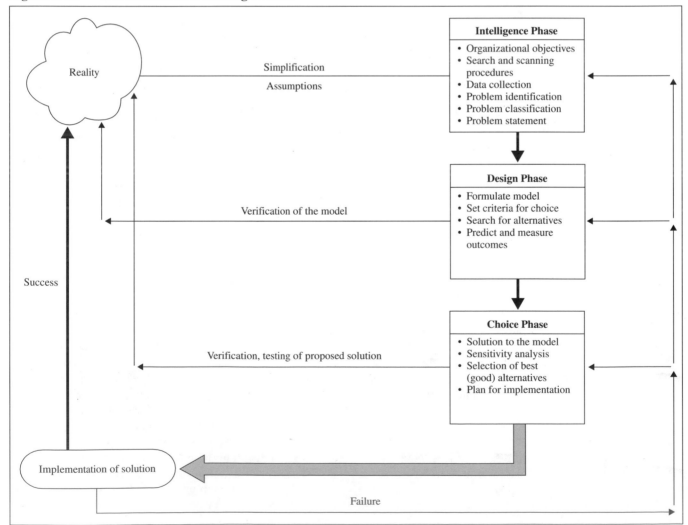

The Intelligence Phase

The first phase of Simon's decision-making model is the intelligence phase. In this phase, the decision maker is attentive to the organization's goals and is on alert for issues that run counter to those goals. The key activities of this phase are problem identification and organizational objective formulation, for example, defining the objectives of the problem and what needs to be accomplished. Other activities during this phase may include breaking the problem down into smaller subproblems, problem classification, and data collection. However, the final outcome of this phase should be a careful statement of the problem to be solved or decision to be made.

The Design Phase

In the design phase of the decision-making process, the decision maker identifies possible courses of action and the varieties of decision alternatives, locates the various knowledge sources of relevance to the problem, formulates a basic model for the problem, and determines the criteria to be used to evaluate possible alternatives. Also in this phase, the decision maker may seek to gather various data pertinent to the problem. In developing a model, the decision maker identifies various sets of variables to be included.

The sets of variables used in the modeling aspect of this phase include:

- The outcome, or dependent or target variable(s)
- The variables that can be manipulated or controlled
- The variables that cannot be controlled but are simply part of the context of the problem

The relationships among these variables also must be specified.

Often the decision maker has available standard decision-making models. For example, models developed in management science (such as linear and nonlinear programming, goal programming, integer programming) are helpful in this process; the decision maker simply identifies and gathers the appropriate data and information from within the organization to apply these models accurately to a given situation. Illustrative of this phase, one main aim of a data warehouse is to provide a convenient location from which to obtain any data needed in formulating and then solving such models.

The Choice Phase

In the choice phase, the decision maker applies the criteria decided on in the second phase and searches for the appropriate decision alternative. When the decision has been chosen, it must be evaluated and then a recommendation made as to the final solution to the given problem. Certainly, there is overlap between phases two and three with respect to enumerating the possible alternatives and in evaluating and selecting a decision alternative. This concept of postulating various decision alternatives and then selecting from among them is the classic view of decision making and is illustrated in figure 19.2.

Figure 19.2.   Classic View of Decision Making

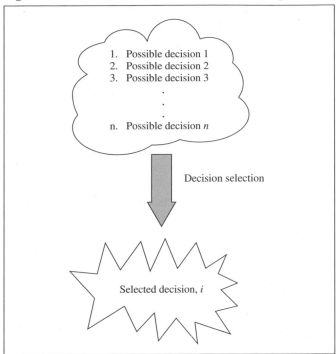

A number of interesting questions can be posed about this process, including:

- How are the alternative decisions postulated?
- How many alternatives should be identified?
- What if there are too many alternatives (as is possible in complex problems)?
- What are possible strategies for selecting among the alternative decisions?

The answer to how the alternatives are postulated lies to a large degree in the creativity of the decision maker; however, having as many sources of data and information available will enhance this activity. In choosing a possible criterion for selecting among alternatives, various options are available depending on the situation. For example, a problem involving the expenditure of capital may involve a large number of alternatives. Hence, the decision maker might select the criterion of maximizing the **return on investment** (ROI) and seek the alternative that gives the greatest ROI.

Because it can be difficult to determine exactly what the ROI will be for various investments, one might elect to use the criterion that the solution should make a "good" ROI possible. Because the definition of "good" in this case is fuzzy, some minimum ROI might be set and the first alternative accepted that exceeds this minimum. The general idea here is that the decision maker will accept any solution that meets the minimum requirements for a solution; it does not have to be the very best solution or even the optimal solution. Simply providing a solution to the problem that meets the requirements renders it a "good" solution. Such an approach is sometimes called a "good enough" solution or a **satisficing** solution (Simon 1976, 1977).

The examples above go through phase two of the decision-making process. The next question concerns how to go about searching through all the alternatives to identify one that fulfills the criterion. This search is part of phase three activities and has various options. One option is to use a "try-one-and-see" approach. The idea is simply to begin evaluating the criterion on a given alternative and see if it works. If it does, we are done; if not, we move on. Selection of alternatives is by chance, and so this option may be called a blind search.

Another option would be to use the mathematical optimization tools developed in operations research and management science and to attempt to select the analytically optimal alternative, one that either maximizes some objective such as ROI or minimizes something like loss. Both blind search and optimal searches, however, may take an exceedingly long time, even on a computer, so other options may need to be considered.

In some situations, other information might be incorporated into the search process. This additional information can be in the form of rules of thumb, hunches, or experience but is nevertheless felt to be accurate. When this type of information is used to help in the search, it is called a "heuristic" search. In cases where the criterion of satisficing is employed, search techniques such as genetic algorithms (a new area in artificial intelligence and machine learning) can be used.

Structure of Decision Support Systems versus Information Systems

Based on the account above of how people make decisions, it is easy to see various types of support that would be helpful to a decision maker. For example, having a data warehouse would facilitate the generation of solutions to ad hoc problems concerning patient case mix, patient payer mix, typical patient flow, length of stay, and so on. Another type of support is assistance in performing any of the searches mentioned. For any realistic problem, such searches would exceed the cognitive limits of most people. Computer-based DSSs were developed to meet these needs.

Functionality of a DSS will be much different from that of an information system. Information systems developed as managers began to recognize the need for periodic reports from the transactional or operational systems within the organization. Transactional systems are the systems that perform electronic data processing and storage. They were among the first implementations of computer technology to business during the 1950s and 1960s and are still a primary application today. Such systems include payroll systems, patient billing systems, patient registration systems, accounting systems, and so on.

Tan (1998, 2001) applies the term **hospital information system** (HIS) to the transactional systems found in health-care and uses the term **health management information system** (HMIS) for those systems whose purpose is to provide reports on routine operations and processing. Examples of HIMSs are pharmacy inventory systems, radiological systems, and patient tracking systems. Many of these systems have been discussed in earlier chapters of this book. Neither the HIS nor the HMIS has decision support as its explicit purpose.

As stated earlier, DSS is about people and making decisions, not about data processing. Thus, the structure or architecture of the DSS will reflect this emphasis. Figures 19.3, 19.4, and 19.5 may be used to compare the differences between an HIS, an HMIS, and a DSS. Figure 19.3 presents a conceptual model of a typical HIS (or data-processing system). The key elements of the system relate to data acquisition and entry, storage, retrieval, record keeping, and so on. Typical outputs would include a patient bill, a listing of patient charges, and a list of patients admitted on a given day.

The HMIS presented in figure 19.4 (p. 452) includes some of the same elements as the HIS, in particular, data entry and storage. The key difference is that a standard reports element is added to the system. Thus, the outputs from the system will assist managers in monitoring the operations of the organization. For example, the system may generate a standard report on the number of admissions per week for the past six months. In addition, it could generate a report on the average cost per patient over a given period of time.

Figure 19.5 (p. 453) focuses on the role of the system as a decision tool. First, there is the user interface element. This element provides a friendly and interactive environment for the user interaction with system. Ideally, this will be through a **graphical user interface** (GUI), allowing the user to point, click, drag, and drop icon objects on the computer screen to accomplish desired tasks. Input devices include the standard keyboard and the computer mouse.

The second element of the model identifies the sources of data that populate the DSS. These sources are those that a decision maker would turn to in order to obtain more information and knowledge about the problem's background and setting. Such sources would include data from the organization's operational/transactional systems (HIS, HMIS) and could include other sources of external data such as state, regional, or national comparative data.

The DSS must contain some element or subsystem to manage all of this information. This element may be divided into a database management subsystem and a model or knowledge-based management subsystem, depending on the sophistication of the DSS.

Perhaps the key element in the DSS is the one that assists in reasoning from the data and knowledge. This element enables the DSS to recognize and solve the problem. In expert systems, this element is often called the inference engine. Overall, it is where the DSS integrates the data and knowledge provided from the various sources, uses the structure of the problem as presented to it by the user, and applies its models/reasoning to suggest a feasible decision.

Figure 19.3.   Conceptual Model of a Health Information System

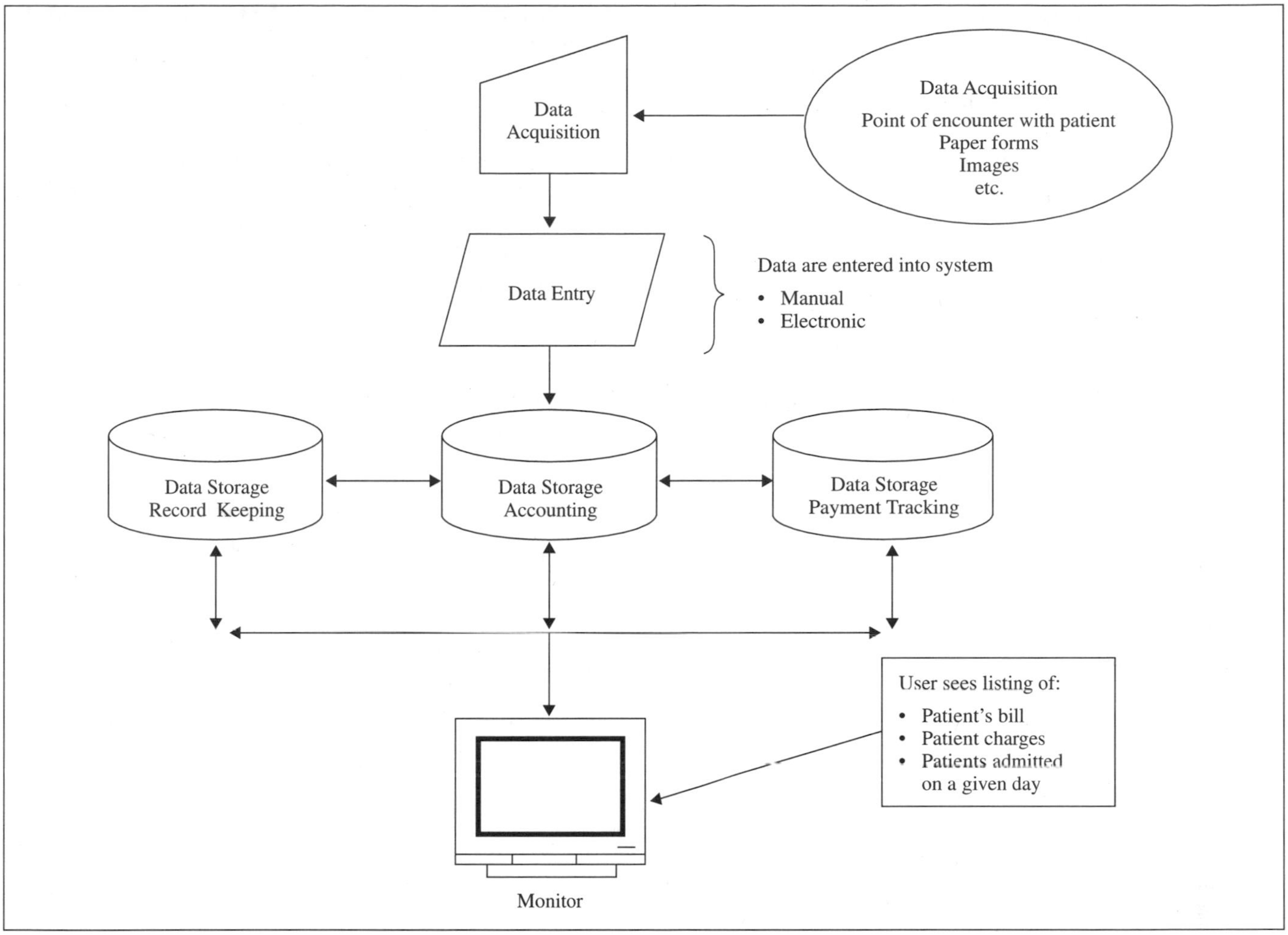

Finally, the DSS must communicate proposed decision options to the user/decision maker. Most often, this communication is accomplished through the same user interface that was used to specify the problem to the system, although it could use a separate system.

DSSs can be classified according to the exact nature of the various elements represented in its model as:

- Data-based decision support systems
- Model-based decision support systems
- Knowledge-based decision support systems
- Graphics-based decision support systems

Data-Based Decision Support Systems

A data-based DSS uses a database management approach for its overall organization. Its central focus is on providing access to the various data sources within the organization through one system. In essence, all the data and knowledge management is performed through the database subsystem. The input user interface generally allows the user to specify many forms of ad hoc queries through a graphical interface. The system uses its knowledge system to translate the user's

requests into a query format acceptable to the database component. A typical implementation of this system allows the user to specify queries in a pick-and-click or drop-down manner via the GUI. The system then translates those requests into the database language SQL (**structured query language**). The SQL is submitted to the database system containing the various data sources, and a report is sent back to the user. In healthcare, the STARS® system from ViPS, Inc., is an example of a data-based DSS. Most data warehouse systems also fall into this category of DSS.

Model-Based Decision Support Systems

The famous statistician George Box once quipped, "All models are wrong, but some are useful" (Box 1979, p. 202). A model is a generalized, abstract representation of the world in which the decision or problem is located. In fact, all individuals depend on models to help interpret and organize everyday experiences. Experiences and decisions are interpreted and formed in terms of these mental models. These models are constructed from our experiences and education and those of the society in which we live.

A good model-based DSS will attempt to include as many different models as can be accommodated to provide the user the greatest flexibility in framing the decision situation. For example, the SAS® Enterprise Miner™ tool for data mining provides a large collection of models that the user can select and combine into an overall description of the problem. Other systems may provide specific models such as financial risk analysis or forecasting, depending on the area for which the DSS was developed.

In the model-based DSS, the key element is the subsystem that manages the system's models. The models make up the system's knowledge. The user describes the decision situation to the system in terms of the models available in the system or by using a modeling language. Internal and external data relevant to the needs of the model are accessed and supplied to the model. The reasoning element in this system consists primarily of the modules needed to perform the computations or searches as required by the model. Results are provided via the user interface or output system.

Many examples of model-based DSS exist in healthcare. For example, the Episode Treatment Groups system from Symmetry Health Data Systems, Inc., can assist both buyers and providers of healthcare services with case-mix analysis of patients, provider profiling, and severity-of-illness adjustments when making quality of care and financial decisions.

Figure 19.4.   Conceptual Model for a Health Information Management System

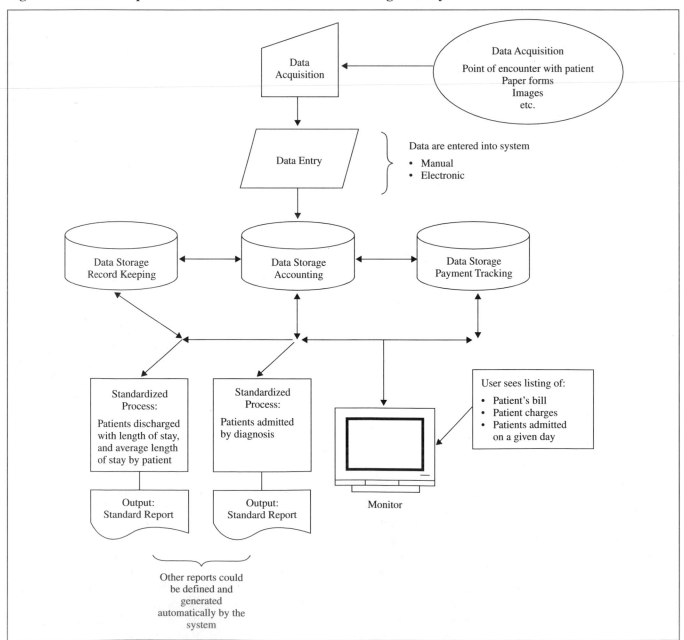

Knowledge-Based Decision Support Systems

A knowledge-based DSS is one in which the key element is the knowledge base. Knowledge-based DSSs are often referred to as "rule-based" systems because the knowledge is stored in the form of rules. For example, a simple rule system is the familiar IF, THEN, ELSE format—if a certain condition is true, then this is an indication of a certain other condition, else the condition is not indicated. By applying general rules of this form to a given situation, a decision is suggested to the user. The form of the rules can be generalized to allow them to have a probabilistic nature. For example, a rule might state that if a given condition is present, there is some probability that another condition is present.

In a knowledge-based DSS, the reasoning element is usually referred to as the inference engine. The **inference engine** is a module that can apply and link the appropriate rules together based on the inputs provided by the user. Often the user in a dialog format supplies the input in these systems. The user interface asks the user a question and the user responds. Through the inference engine, the DSS applies the appropriate rule or rules and determines whether more input is needed. This iterative process between user and DSS continues until the DSS either is able to make a suggestion or determines that its knowledge base is not sufficient to make a determination.

Because many of the ideas of the knowledge-based DSS arose from the early work in artificial intelligence in computer

Figure 19.5.   Conceptual Model of a Decision Support System

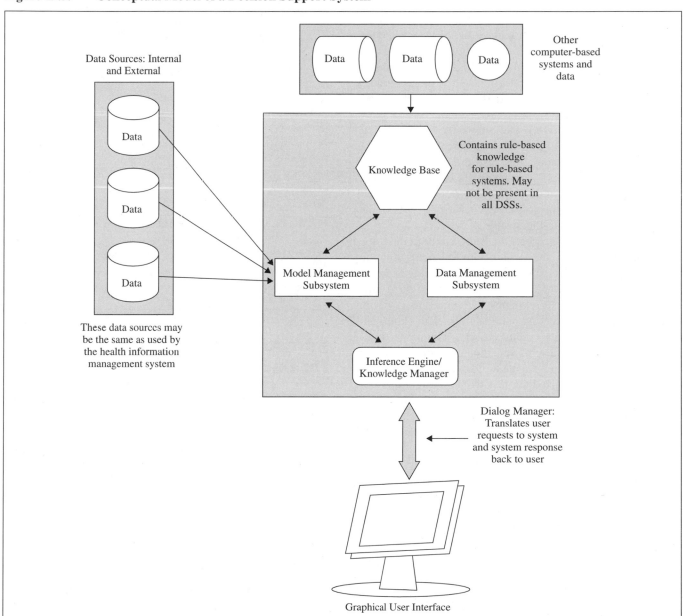

Adapted from Turban 1995, p. 88.

science, it is often considered under the framework of expert systems. Examples of knowledge-based systems in healthcare include the early work of Shortliffe (1976) on his MYCIN system. The MYCIN system provided assistance in diagnosis and therapy selection for patients with blood-borne bacterial infections. Other systems that developed later along these lines are QMR (Quick Medical Reference) by Miller et al. (1986) and DXplain by Barnett et al. (1987). Artificial intelligence and these types of systems are discussed in later sections of this chapter.

Graphics-Based Decision Support Systems

Graphical tools are becoming more and more important in helping people make decisions. Perhaps the old adage that a picture is worth a thousand words is really true. **Graphics-based DSSs** exploit the human ability to glean patterns and insight from visual presentations of data. Thus, the key element in the architecture of a graphics-based DSS is the user interface. This interface must be carefully constructed and include both hardware and software. The hardware must be able to present detailed visualizations in a timely manner. Further, the type of graphic itself is of fundamental importance.

In a graphics-based DSS, the knowledge base is the collection of graphics that the system is capable of displaying. Common graphics include maps, histograms, and bar charts. However, many systems today involve a complex combination of various graphical displays for both output and input. Depending on the purpose of the DSS, various types of data also must be available to the system.

Many types of graphics-based DSSs have been developed for healthcare. In 1995, the Health Care Financing Administration (HFCA), now renamed the Centers for Medicare and Medicaid Services (CMS), contracted with Los Alamos National Laboratory to develop new techniques for reviewing Medicare claims to detect potentially fraudulent claims and/or providers (http://www.c3.lanl.gov/ccs3web/index2.html). Los Alamos used a variety of new mathematical models and algorithms from the emerging area of **machine learning** and data mining to accomplish their tasks. One result of this work was development of a visualization system that gave the user the ability to spot potential patterns of fraud and abuse. In this case, the data/knowledge element of the system is the claims data, the reasoning element consists of the models and algorithms, and the user interface is the graphical display.

Similar graphical techniques have been developed by other people to detect fraud. These methods use a data-mining technique called linkage analysis. **Linkage analysis** portrays relationships discovered within data sets by a linked network graph. The graph shows interactions among items in the data set and has been applied to fraud investigations in money laundering (for example, Davis 1981; Davidson 1993). Netmap from Alta Europe (www.altaeurope.com), Daisy (www.daisy2000.com), and SAS®'s Enterprise Miner™ are examples of general software programs that implement this approach. Today, many healthcare organizations as well as government agencies are investigating linkage analysis as a DSS tool for containing the increasing cost of healthcare due to fraud and abuse.

Another important graphics-based DSS is the geographical information system (GIS). The example cited at the beginning of this chapter illustrates just one use of these types of graphics-based DSSs within healthcare. Other areas of application are also interesting. For example, Begur, Miller, and Weaver (1997) reported on their use of the package MAPINFO (www.mapinfo.com) for the development of a graphics-based GIS system to assist in the routing of home healthcare nurses during their daily visits to ensure the shortest commuting distances and thereby minimize travel expenses.

Check Your Understanding 19.1

Instructions: Answer the following questions on a separate piece of paper.

1. Why is decision support important for modern healthcare?
2. What are some of the challenges facing healthcare that decision support can assist in addressing?
3. What is a decision support system?
4. What is the key difference between a decision support system and an expert system?
5. Out of what discipline from World War Two did the study and development of decision support systems come?
6. What are the three phases in Simon's model of the decision-making process?
7. Describe the class view of decision making.
8. What is the key element in the architecture of a decision support system, and what does it do?
9. Name the four classes of decision support systems.
10. Name at least one important medical decision support system that can be classified as a knowledge-based decision support system. Explain why it falls into this classification.

Infrastructure Requirements for Decision Support Systems

What types of organizational and technical infrastructure are required to enable the effective use of decision support systems? To implement effective DSSs, an organization first must have developed at least four key components: (1) a data warehouse or operational data store, (2) a set of data-mining or data-querying tools, (3) a trained group of data analysts or data miners, and (4) a trained group of data users. A definition and brief overview of these elements follows. Chapter 20 thoroughly explores data warehousing and data-mining concepts and tools.

Data Warehouses

Data warehouse is a popular concept in information technology (IT) circles today. Almost any conference on IT contains a presentation on some aspect of the corporate data warehouse. The term was coined primarily by William Inmon

(1992). Basically, a **data warehouse** is a database that has the following functions:

- It serves as a neutral storage area for data extracted from an organization's transactional systems.
- It serves as a storage area organized around specific business functions or requirements.
- It provides easy access to business data for analysis or data mining (that is, decision support).

Although various people have proposed different definitions of the data warehouse, all agree that one of its critical aspects is that it is a database. Its content is organized in a subject-specific, integrated, time-invariant, nonvolatile manner using one of several possible data models.

Because its architecture is so important, some people simply define data warehouse as an architecture and not as an application or thing. Its architecture refers to how the system is put together or constructed; it is the system's blueprint. Thus, a data warehouse could be thought of as a collection of software systems that includes:

- A database engine allowing access, manipulation, and storage of transactional data
- An application software that allows business analysts to conduct complex business tasks, such as decision support
- A connectivity system that allows the system to communicate with the data sources as well as the end users (that is, client and server[s])

A simplified model of a data warehouse is shown in figure 19.6.

A comparison of the database components of a data warehouse and a transactional system shows that their underlying goals are very different. In a transactional system, the database has been constructed according to well-established principles of relational database design, in particular, normalization. **Normalization** seeks to eliminate redundancy in data storage. The design goal of a transactional system is to eliminate potential errors arising from updating, deleting, or inserting new records into the system, as well as minimizing data redundancy. Thus, a data model for these systems includes many tables, each containing nonredundant data. A data warehouse, on the other hand, is designed to assist the user in querying corporate data. Thus, the underlying design sacrifices data redundancy for query speed and ease of access and use. The data warehouse is not highly normalized.

Two well-known data models are used in designing data warehouses:

- The **star schema** seeks to represent the data within the business context by key business dimensions (time, location, and so on) and by the quantities of interest that are characterized by these dimensions (units sold, dollars spent, length of stay, and so on). For example, suppose the data of interest pertain to patient costs and lengths of stay over time. The star schema organizes the data around a central fact table containing these key

Figure 19.6.   Simplified Model of a Data Warehouse

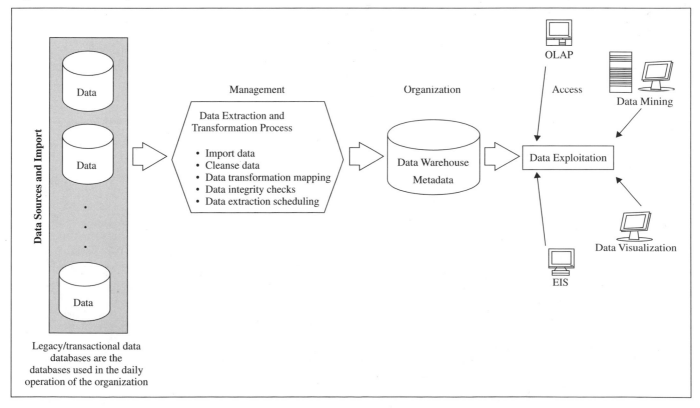

business data items, and relates the other dimensions of these data items (for example, physician, patient information, procedures, hospital service, time, and so on) through tables linked to the central fact table. The links are accomplished through variables called keys (for example, patient_ID). Figure 19.7 illustrates the star schema.

- The **snowflake schema** allows the dimensions in the star schema to be normalized. Figure 19.8 illustrates the general notion of the snowflake schema.

In healthcare, a closely associated idea is the clinical repository. The **clinical repository** likewise is a database that has been developed using a consistent clinical data model and clinical vocabulary and provides accurate clinical data from the various patient care systems. The clinical repository requires that the other health information and patient care systems be integrated with it to allow data to flow between it and the other systems. Thus, the clinical repository is like the data warehouse in that is serves as a database for storing data from transactional systems.

However, the data warehouse and the clinical repository differ in architecture. Because the clinical repository is integrated into the overall information system, its architecture is best described by the systems with which it interacts. The star and snowflake schemas are typically not utilized in its design. Further, although nonclinical data warehouses are static in nature (their data do not change except as specified on a periodic basis), the clinical repository is constantly changing as new clinical data are available for patient care. And finally, the nonclinical data warehouse is focused on retrospective analyses of business data; the business analyst wishes to tap the corporate data to assist with future decisions. However, the clinical repository is focused on assisting with patient care in a near real-time environment.

Figure 19.7.   Example Star Schema for a Data Warehouse

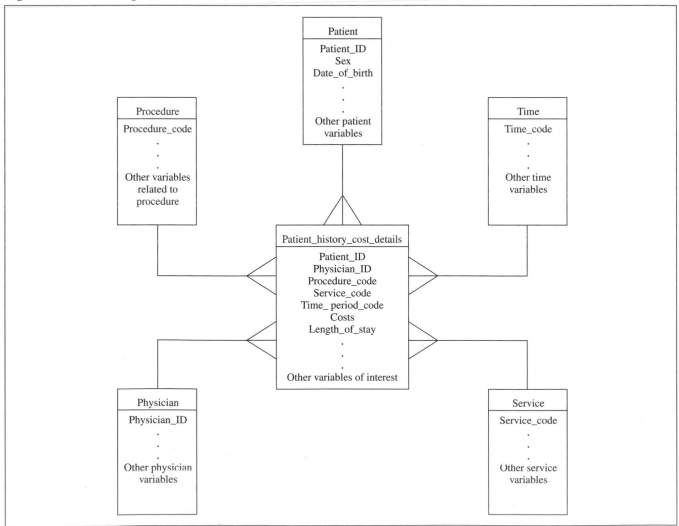

The symbol ————< indicates a one-to-many relationship.

Data-Mining Tools

Data-mining tools exploit the resources of the data warehouse. They enable the end user to query the warehouse, to drill down into the details of the information, to develop models for prediction, and to allow discovery algorithms to highlight new patterns of potential interest.

On-Line Analytical Processing

One set of tools is **on-line analytical processing** (OLAP). In discussing the data warehouse, it was mentioned that a key design feature is to recognize that complex business problems are multidimensional in nature. Thus, the data warehouse attempts to identify the key business dimensions of the data and organize the data around those dimensions.

OLAP is an application architecture that was developed to explore the multidimensional aspects of such business data. OLAP stores the data in a **multidimensional data structure** (multidimensional database, or MDDB) and enables the user to examine and view the data along dimensions that may be specific to the context and will be defined by the business rules of the organization. For example, total cost of stay in a hospital has dimensions of time, type of charges involved, and so on. Often this data structure is conceptualized as a data cube, where its dimensions represent the dimensions of the data and the data item of focus, such as cost or length of stay, is viewed as being located in one of the cells of the cube. This process is often referred to as slicing and dicing or drilling down into the data.

The MDDB is often stored in memory, which results in a very fast response to the user. The data in the MDDB are usually aggregated, and many statistics are calculated prior to loading them into the system.

The OLAP database does not have to be part of the data warehouse, but it does extract data from it. The data ware-

Figure 19.8.   General Snowflake Schema

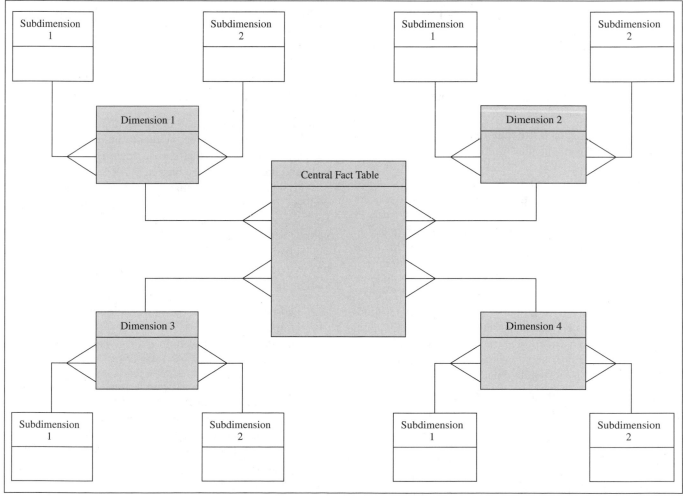

Notes:

1. All dimensions have been shown with exactly two subdimensions for illustrative purposes only. A dimension can have as many subdimensions as necessary.

2. Only generic table names are shown, for example, Dimension 1. In practice, the corresponding variables would appear in the table.

house database model, though, is often designed with OLAP in mind.

Although OLAP is based on the concepts of multidimensional databases, its implementation by different vendors has resulted in specialized data structures. Thus, OLAP tools have been categorized into several different groups, including:

- **Multidimensional on-line analytical processing** (MOLAP): MOLAP vendors developed specialized multidimensional data structures, that is, **multidimensional database management systems** (MDDBMSs). A typical business context in which this has worked well is decision support for business problems involving applications of trend or time series analyses.
- **Relational on-line analytical processing** (ROLAP): ROLAP vendors have sought to develop systems that can access the two-dimensional tables found in a typical **relational database management system** (RDBMS). Using these tables, the user can create a multidimensional view of the data without having to create the multidimensional data structure. ROLAP has been evolving rapidly among vendors, and various implementations are available.
- **Hybrid on-line analytical processing** (HOLAP): HOLAP is actually a catchall group. With the rapidly changing landscape of technologies, vendors are adopting system architectures that blur the lines of distinction among these various groups.

As mentioned, the data structure on which OLAP is based can provide a convenient platform from which to perform other data mining. However, one important distinction must be noted: data mining and OLAP are different. As noted above, OLAP gives the user the ability to view and query the data in a multidimensional manner, but it is up to the user to determine which query to submit or what view is required to support a given decision problem. Data mining, on the other hand, seeks to learn from the data or to discover patterns not previously recognized by the user. Additionally, data mining seeks to search for new solutions to problems whereas OLAP must remain passive. Not all people agree with this distinction. Many vendors currently market systems as data-mining systems when, in essence, their true nature is OLAP. They simply provide the user an environment from which to provide drill downs into corporate data.

Machine Learning Techniques

Artificial neural networks (ANNs) and **decision trees** are examples of data-mining tools that use machine learning techniques called **supervised learning.** Both ANNs and decision trees are discussed in chapter 20. In supervised learning, the algorithm learns the inherent patterns hidden in the data that predict a specified outcome or target variable. In supervised learning algorithms, this outcome or target variable must be present in the supplied data set in order for the algorithm to proceed.

Another class of machine learning techniques is **unsupervised learning.** Unsupervised learning techniques seek to group cases or data records together that are similar or alike in certain respects. The goal of the analysis is to discover previously unknown groupings that exist in the data. A common unsupervised learning algorithm is k-nearest neighbor clustering.

One last machine learning technique that has received a lot of attention for data mining is rule induction, or **association rule analysis.** Association rule analysis does not fit neatly into either of the previous categories of learning techniques. Rule induction seeks to uncover the co-occurrences of items within the database. For example, the classic illustration of association rule analysis is the "market basket" analysis. In this case, the analyst wished to determine customer-purchasing behaviors by examining associations among the various items customers place in their shopping baskets.

For instance, if the customer has placed milk in the basket, how likely is he or she to also place bread in the basket? If the customer has placed bread and cheese in the basket, how likely is he or she to also purchase soup? Thus, association rule analysis examines the co-occurrence of items in customers' baskets and produces sets of rules or associations that describe customer-buying behavior. A typical rule produced by an association rule analysis is as follows:

Milk & bread → cheese [support = 2%, confidence = 80%]

Support is the percentage of times that all three items occurred together in all the baskets examined; confidence is the percentage of time that cheese occurred given that both milk and bread were in the basket.

Although this type of analysis may seem of great use to retailers, how can it be used in healthcare? Suppose the "basket" was a person's tenure with a particular company. The various activities, projects, buildings, and jobs that the individual had or was involved in while with the company might be the items in the basket. Interesting questions that an association rule analysis could reveal include:

- Did people who worked in a specific building develop lung cancer?
- Did individuals in certain management positions also experience certain stress-related diseases?

Another example in healthcare is fraud detection. In this case, a "basket" would be a suspected provider or group of providers and the items in the basket would be the codes they billed. An association rule analysis then would suggest interesting co-occurrences of codes billed together. For example,

{short office visit and patient age > 65} → {CBC ordered}
[support = 20%, confidence = 98%]

A payer integrity officer may find this association unusual and investigative whether the provider has some financial interest in the lab to which the patients are being referred.

Data Miners

Data miners are those individuals who use the data warehouse and the various analytical tools and software applications to support the decision-making activities of the organization. In this sense, they are decision support analysts. Moreover, data miners understand and can effectively use various data-mining algorithms such as those mentioned above.

In healthcare organizations, data miners may hold degrees in either a clinical or business area. Such an educational background is, in fact, very helpful because it enables the data miner to better understand the context of the decision support problem. However, data miners will need to have other skills as well, including the ability to use relational databases, advanced statistics, and computer programming.

Data Users

Data users include a range of individuals within the organization. At one end of the spectrum is senior management. A senior manager uses reports prepared from the data, often extracting data from the data warehouse, in managing and making decisions for the business. In some cases, a senior manager might use a decision support system called an executive information system (EIS). An EIS can provide easy access to a variety of corporate data without the need for programming or making requests to other information technologists. Such systems provide predefined queries and reports specifically tailored to address issues of continuing concern to management. For example, the CEO of a health system would be interested in always knowing the past week's number of patients admitted, average length of stay, and total dollars billed and collected. Using available data, an EIS would allow the CEO to generate such reports in her or his office.

Other data users include clinical staff and business staff. Clinical staff use patient data in the routine care of their patients; business staff use data in determining bills, sending out invoices, and crediting accounts.

Thus, many individuals in an enterprise use data. Data miners use data to develop answers for specific issues currently facing the organization, and others use data in their day-to-day jobs.

Check Your Understanding 19.2

Instructions: Answer the following questions on a separate piece of paper.

1. What are the three functions of a data warehouse?

2. What does normalization seek to do in a database?

3. What are two well-known data models used in constructing a data warehouse?

4. How is a data warehouse different from a clinical repository?

5. What do the acronyms OLAP, MOLAP, ROLAP, and HOLAP stand for?

6. What is supervised learning? Unsupervised learning?

7. Name two important data-mining tools.

Uses of Decision Support Systems in Healthcare

Decision support systems are used in a variety of contexts in contemporary healthcare organizations.

Healthcare Decision Support

The term *healthcare decision support* is used here to cover a variety of decision support systems used in healthcare, other than clinical decision support, executive decision support, or nursing decision support. In general, these systems all seek to provide the same assistance as a decision support system in general, namely, to assist the user in the decision-making process within the domain of the system.

Examples of these systems include medication management and pharmacy order-entry DSSs. These systems assist in warning of possible drug interactions and prescribing errors (Poikonen and Leventhal 1999). Other examples of a healthcare DSS are alert and monitoring tools built into patient information systems.

During the last several years, healthcare has given a lot of attention to quality of care and has used the tools of TQM to measure progress in this arena. Various systems have been proposed and developed that assist in combining data from financial units within a hospital as well as from the clinical areas to allow both administrators and clinicians to examine quality improvement and cost efficiency of services provided to patients. Several recent articles discussing these systems can be found in Howe et al. (1999), Hohmann et al. (1998), and Dexter et al. (2001). These systems all fall within the definition of healthcare decision support.

Clinical/Medical Decision Support

Clinical decision support systems (CDSS) were mentioned at the beginning of this chapter. As noted earlier, for many people, the whole notion of the use of computers in medicine conjures an image of the physician interacting with a computer system to reach a decision regarding a diagnosis for a patient. However, in the broadest sense, a **clinical decision support system** is any computer system that assists a health professional in making clinical decisions. Some CDSSs include reminder and other alert systems as part of the integration with a general clinical information system.

CDSSs were one of the earliest applications of computers in healthcare. The research on CDSSs dates back to the late 1950s with papers by Ledley and Lusted (1959) and Warner et al. (1964). Particularly illustrative of the early work in CDSSs is Shortliffe's (1976) seminal work on the MYCIN system. MYCIN was developed to assist physicians in the selection of appropriate antibiotic therapy and was evaluated for patients with blood-borne bacterial infections (Yu et al. 1979). The system was designed using ideas that emerged out of the computer science field of artificial intelligence.

Research in artificial intelligence provided new models for developing computer systems that could process and reason from "rules" provided to the system. Most software systems process numbers as input. "Knowledge" of the context of the numbers resides within the program and is "hard-coded" into the system.

Work in artificial intelligence and the resulting area of expert systems provides a means for a computer system to be supplied with a collection of rules that the system can then reason with or chain together to draw new inferences or make new decisions. A typical rule from the MYCIN is given in figure 19.9 (p. 467). Basically, a rule is a conditional statement, expressed in an if-then format. Given a condition such that the "if" part of the statement is true, the "then" part of the rule indicates what conclusions are indicated. These rules may be referred to as production rules, condition–action rules, situation–action rules, or if–then rules.

MYCIN used a collection of about 450 rules that were elicited from in-depth interviews with medical experts in the area of antibiotics. The rules then were stored in the system's knowledge base. A knowledge base is the collection of all rules from which an expert system can draw in reaching a decision. The component of the system that chains the rules together or reasons from the rules is called the inference engine. Two common methodologies for performing this chaining process are forward chaining and backward chaining (Russell and Norvig 1995).

During these early years of research in CDSSs, several other systems also were developed. Gorry and Barnett (1968) developed a model for diagnosis using a sequential Bayesian reasoning system. Using this work, F. T. de Dombal and his colleagues developed a CDSS for diagnosing abdominal pain (de Dombal 1969). In 1975, R. A. Miller and his associates presented the INTERNIST-I system (Pople, Myers, and Miller 1975; Miller et al. 1982). This system, initially called DIALOG, has undergone much development and research over the years and is now best known as QMR (Miller et al. 1986). In the late 1980s, Otto Barnett and his colleagues proposed the DXplain system (Barnett et al. 1987).

Today, there are many CDSSs, each attempting to address various areas in clinical care. Currently, many researchers are examining how best to integrate these systems into overall medical work flow, in particular, linking these systems to a patient's computer-based health record (Berner et al. 1999). Several examples of recent work in this include Durieux et al. (2000), Gerbert et al. (2000), and Dayton et al. (2000). A recent commercial implementation of a CDSS is found at www.dynasty.com/goSolutions/triage. Two Web-based systems for patients are http://easydiagnosis.com and http://askred.dynasty.com/drd.

Executive Decision Support

Executive decision support systems, often called executive information systems (EISs), are special types of DSSs specifically designed to facilitate and support the decision-making needs of the organization's top executives. They provide easy access to both internal and external data sources relevant to monitoring critical success factors and making strategic decisions. EISs provide overall views of the organization's operations and offer a wide range of views of the data, including drill-down tools and various summarization tools. Table 19.2 lists some common characteristics of a typical EIS.

The term EIS was coined at the Massachusetts Institute of Technology (MIT) in the late 1970s and early 1980s (Marakas 1999). Originally, the EIS consisted of a mainframe computer program that pulled together various corporate data and packaged them in an easily readable and accessible format for decision makers. The intent was to assist corporate officers who were either unfamiliar or uncomfortable with working with computers.

Since the early days of EISs, however, the demand for such data and decision support has grown. Today, EISs support not only top-level executives, but also mid- and lower-level managers who require such support. With the advent of the PC and local area networks, such support can easily be offered to an organization's various levels of management.

Although EISs are types of decision support systems, it is important to note a few key differences. First, the EIS generally will not provide the sophisticated modeling and database capabilities that a DSS does. The EIS targets the top-level view and is not intended for the more in-depth analyses provided by a DSS. Second, the EIS is intended to allow executives to gain a quick view or "snapshot" of the organization as a whole whereas a DSS often provides more detailed support in a particular area of the organization's operation. Third, generally speaking, EISs incorporate external data into the information given to the user whereas DSSs typically use internal data.

Table 19.2.   Characteristics of Typical Executive Information Systems

Characteristic	Description
Degree of use	High, consistent, without need of technical assistance
Computer skills required	Very low, must be easy to learn and use
Flexibility	High, must fit executive decision-making style
Principal use	Tracking, control
Decisions supported	Upper-level management, unstructured
Data supported	Company internal and external
Output capabilities	Text, tabular, graphical, trend toward audio/video in future
Graphic concentration	High, presentation style
Data access speed	Must be high, fast response

Source: Dobrzeniecki 1994.

The use of EISs in healthcare has grown over the years. Dobrzeniecki (1994) listed four examples of EIS use in healthcare settings:

- Baylor University Medical Center uses an EIS system called Performance Advisor to assist in creating flexible budgets that allow for different levels of customer activity. The program is a mainframe, general-ledger system.
- Meriter Hospital, in Madison, Wisconsin, adopted a product called Alternative View from Gerber Alley. This product provides an EIS for the hospital's clinical applications and has been part of its TQM effort.
- Samaritan Health Services, in Phoenix, Arizona, adopted the IBM product, Destiny, as its EIS system. The system provides a "briefing book" feature, which organizes information into several folders on key areas of interest. Users can monitor the various areas by selecting the appropriate folder. The system provides summary and trend information in graphical formats.
- The Florida Acute-Care and Teaching Hospitals Healthcare Cost Containment Board adopted MAXPAR, which allows executives to monitor financial, productivity, and physician-related data in all 220 acute care and teaching hospitals in the state of Florida. MAXPAR is an EIS product specifically designed for healthcare. A variety of summary information is available (for example, comparisons of practice patterns and average length of hospital stays for particular procedures).

Nursing Decision Support

The role of nursing in the care and treatment of patients is best thought of as complementary to the role of the physician. Physicians diagnose diseases, obtain medical histories, identify disease risks, and prescribe treatments. Nurses, on the other hand, contribute to the cure of patients through their special role of patient care. Nurses assess how patients respond to treatment and therapy and how patients are coping with their conditions and treatments. Nurses develop patient care plans and seek ways to assess patients and alleviate suffering.

Nursing decision support systems assist nursing staff in their delivery of patient care. Clearly, the decisions faced by nurses are broad and complex, making the development of such systems difficult. For this reason, to date, there are few nursing decision support systems as such, although some systems have been developed that are similar to the clinical diagnostic DSSs mentioned above. For example, Lagina (1971) developed a system for assessing the anxiety of patients awaiting surgery. A recent interesting study by Ruland (1999) examined the use of decision support to elicit patient preferences and include them in the nursing care plan.

In a broad sense, however, decision support is built into current nursing information systems, especially those that are a part of emerging comprehensive patient information systems. These systems provide nurses with important, timely data on the patient and include alerting and monitoring mechanisms.

Artificial Intelligence Applications in Healthcare

Throughout this chapter, applications in healthcare and decision support have been mentioned from a branch of computer science called artificial intelligence (AI). AI is actually a fairly new branch that originated formally in 1956 when the term was coined (Russell and Norvig 1995). Although AI is generally thought of as being the development of programs for playing games such as chess, making robots, or creating computer systems that talk and interact with people, it is concerned primarily with understanding and building intelligent entities or agents in addition to studying intelligence. Thus, all the things mentioned are part of AI, plus more.

Four areas of AI are discussed in the following subsections.

Natural Language Processing

In 1950, Turning proposed his now-famous test for defining computer or machine intelligence. He proposed a test in which a human integrator would ask questions and interact via teletype with a computer presumably in another location out of the integrator's sight. A computer passed the test when the integrator could tell whether he or she was interacting with a human or a computer at the other end.

For a computer system to pass this test, it must possess at least the capability of natural language processing. Natural language processing is the ability of a computer to understand the full range of meaning contained in languages such as English. The system must be able to process the commands, instructions, or other input when provided by sentences as spoken in normal human discourse. Computer systems have excellent capabilities to process structured or constrained input where the user is limited to certain phrases or when a very specific manner in which to provide input to the system is prescribed. However, natural language has proved to be a very difficult capability for a computer system to acquire.

Recently, some systems have come to market with the ability to learn spoken language. Dictation programs that type as the user speaks have become widely available, and Microsoft Windows XP comes with speech recognition as a standard module. Nevertheless, the user must train these programs by providing as much as thirty minutes of spoken language to the system. Typically, these programs ask the user to read a predefined passage into the system. After the selection is read, training algorithms in the system process the recorded speech and train the system to recognize the user's unique speech patterns. Often such systems require additional training and adjustments. Once trained, however, the user can give verbal commands to the system and have them be performed.

In healthcare, natural language processing would be a tremendous tool for capturing physician notes and other bits of clinical communication that occur among healthcare workers. Such information could be directly entered into the patient's computer-based health record, thus enhancing other decision support tools. However, such systems are still some distance in the future. Although natural language processing is an active area of research within both the computer science and informatics communities, many challenges still must be overcome. Issues such as a consistent or standard medical vocabulary must be addressed in addition to other technical issues in the speech recognition process.

Expert Systems

Earlier in this chapter, a distinction was made between decision support systems and expert systems. Discussion of both the knowledge-based DSS and the CDSS, particularly the MYCIN system, has introduced many of the features that characterize an expert system.

An expert system (ES) is a system that attempts to replicate a human expert's ability to solve complex problems in a particular domain. In solving a particular problem, the system employs a set of rules obtained through a knowledge-gathering or engineering process by the developers of the ES. Reasoning is accomplished via an inference algorithm (as mentioned previously) from AI. As mentioned previously, the reasoning component is the inference engine.

ES users are not experts in the particular problem domain. Rather, the ES is developed (ideally) as a surrogate for the expert. Thus, the user is typically inexperienced in the problem domain. In a sense, the goal of an ES is to capture an expert in the computer system.

One of the most difficult tasks in developing an ES is the capture of expert knowledge. This task is exceedingly difficult for several reasons. First, experts do not always know exactly how they arrive at their decisions. Often they have many years of experience and have developed an intuition about the problems and their solutions within the domain. Asking experts to state their knowledge in if–then rules becomes impossible. Second, even when if–then rules can be elicited from an expert(s), ensuring that the rules are consistent is a major challenge. Consistency of the rules means that when the rules are applied, the consequence will not contradict other rules in the collection or simply be circular.

Over the years, ESs have received mixed reactions from researchers and practitioners alike. The early work on MYCIN and other similar systems was groundbreaking. Many ES researchers and developers took as their goals the replacement of the expert with the computer. However, this goal was never fully accomplished. By the mid- to late 1980s, many clinicians questioned the idea of a system that treated the physician as a passive user, unable to solve a given diagnostic problem. Miller (1994) termed this early model of diagnostic support the "Greek oracle" model and noted its weaknesses. He observed that more recent systems have attempted to allow the user more control. The goal is no longer to allow the computer system to be the expert but, rather, to enhance the performance of user.

In general, people are wary of giving a computer "expert status," especially in healthcare. In a few cases, ESs have been able to meet the goal of practically replacing the expert. An example is the XCON system developed in the 1980s by Digital Equipment Corporation (DEC) to be used by sales and service people for configuring DEC computer systems for customers. XCON was able to mimic the performance of computer engineers in configuring systems and was used by DEC for several years.

In healthcare, a variety of CDSSs have been developed using ES methodologies. Some of these systems have undergone rigorous evaluation (Berner et al. 1994). Yet, the reactions to these systems remain mixed. Carter (1999) observed the activity in this area as being one of "impressive creativity coupled with limited successes, small gains, [and] cynical resignation" (p. 194). He concluded: "Do physicians really want help with the diagnostic process? This is a question of social and cognitive processes for which the answer to-date appears to be a very cool 'perhaps'" (p. 194).

Artificial Neural Networks

Artificial neural networks (ANNs) are another important area in artificial intelligence. ANNs seek to provide mathematical models and computer algorithms that operate in a similar manner to the nervous system, in particular, the brain. The basis for ANNs consists of simple units called perceptrons (similar to the biological unit, neuron). These perceptrons are connected together and work in parallel. As data are presented to the ANNs, learning takes place through the adjustment and modification of weights embedded in the construction of the perceptron.

Research in ANNs began in the late 1940s and 1950s as an attempt to create programs that could reason similarly to human reasoning ability. Although the initial goal of the early researchers was never realized, over the years various ANN models have been developed that are very useful in pattern recognition, clustering, and predictive modeling. Many examples of ANN applications can be found in recent medical literature. Examples include applications involving the use of ANNs to assist radiologists in reading (classifying images), predicting patient outcomes, and developing clinical pathways.

Virtual Reality

Virtual reality (VR) is a very recent area of artificial intelligence. Jaron Lanier, founder of VPL research, coined the term in 1989 (Beier 2001). Since then, the term has been associated with a variety of closely related topics such as artificial reality, artificial life, virtual worlds, virtual environments, and cyberspace. VR is not purely an area of artificial intelligence but, rather, combines elements from computer simulation and computer graphics and visualization to provide an interactive, computer-mediated experience for the user. In the typical application, the user actually perceives him- or herself as an active participant in the "virtual" world constructed by the computer. To achieve this highly interactive, "virtual" experience, VR applications often require the user to wear some type of sensory device to achieve the immersive experience. Such devices range from a sensory glove or a head-mounted vision display, or both, to recent devices in which the user wears a complete sensory suit. These devices register the user's reactions to various actions occurring in the virtual environment and provide visual feedback and, in some cases, even physical sensations.

The application of VR to medical and healthcare issues has been rapidly occurring. Many other examples are available on the Web as well as in numerous articles and reference materials (for example, Isdale 1993).

The application of VR to decision support, however, is still in its infancy. Some promising directions are in the application of VR to assist in simulating emergencies and training and in monitoring different healthcare workers' reactions. More business-oriented VR applications include examining the location of new facilities, studying traffic flow patterns, and modeling local residents' reactions to real estate development.

Check Your Understanding 19.3

Instructions: Answer the following questions on a separate piece of paper.

1. Name four types of decision support systems found in healthcare.

2. What are the main characteristics of a clinical decision support system?

3. What was the name of one of the earliest CDSSs?

4. What type of inference engine did the system given above use?

5. What are some of the difficulties in maintaining a CDSS?

6. What is a key characteristic of an EIS?

7. What makes the task of decision support for nursing so complex?

Future Roles for HIM Professionals

In 1996, the American Health Information Management Association (AHIMA) initiated its Vision 2006 (AHIMA 1999). Working through Delphi Groups, this initiative charted new roles for HIM professionals in response to identified needs within healthcare organizations today. Two new roles outlined by the Delphi Group examining the area of decision support were the research specialist and the decision support specialist.

Research Specialist

Data and vocabulary managers will perform many of the tasks of the research specialist (RS). As outlined by Johns et al. (2001), the RS works to create and support decision- and knowledge-based activities within an organization by gathering and analyzing data. Typical job descriptions for RSs will include skills such as proficiency in Microsoft Access and/or SQL server, Visual Basic or Cold Fusion, and a statistical package such as SPSS or SAS.

In addition, the RS will need excellent communication skills and the ability to manage data (verification, examination, and collection). The AHIMA sample position for the RS is shown in table 19.3.

Table 19.3.   AHIMA Sample Position Description: Research Specialist

Position Title: Research Data Analyst

Immediate Supervisor: Department Director

General Purpose: The Research Data Analyst ensures the quality of data collection, coordination, and analysis for clinical research projects.

Responsibilities:

- Verifies, examines, and collects data

- Ensures that clinical data are quality assured, consistent, and relevant to projects and the organization's goals

- Ensures the integrity of the data and safe and proper management of study parameters

- Maintains expert knowledge of relevant FDA guidelines and other regulatory procedures

- Monitors protocol at study sites

- Retrieves data from numerous clinical databases within the organization as well as from proprietary and nonproprietary databases available through outside sources

- Uses structured query language and downloads data into the organization's custom databases for review and analysis

- Manipulates and analyzes data by using statistical software, such as SPSS and SAS, and identifies and determines significant variances and trends for quality control

- Reviews proposed research design to ensure that the data collected are adequate to meet the project's goals

- Prepares periodic progress and monitoring reports on study recruitment, data collection, and data quality

- Participates in team meetings

- Prepares and provides overviews, demonstrations, and presentations to wide variety of audiences

Qualifications:

- Master's degree in health science or related field

- Baccalaureate degree in health information management, business, or closely related area

- Experience in health science and administration

- Certification as RHIA preferable

Decision Support Specialist

The second new role developed by the AHIMA Delphi Group was that of the decision support specialist (DSSp). The DSSp's job is to support strategic planning and operational improvement activities in support of management and the overall organization. (The AHIMA sample position for the DSSp is shown in table 19.4). Both DSSps and RSs must have the same abilities for managing, manipulating, and analyzing data. Moreover, both must be able to use statistical software packages such as SAS and SPSS.

Data Miner/Data Analyst

The skills for a data miner/data analyst are best described as a combination of the skills required for both the DSSp and the RS roles. In most cases, a data miner also should have at least a master's degree in an area such as health informatics, biostatistics (or applied statistics), epidemiology, or some quantitative health science field.

One difference between the data manager and the data miner, however, is that the data miner will not necessarily be involved directly in the collection and management of data

Table 19.4.   AHIMA Sample Position Description: Decision Support Specialist

---

Position Title: Decision Support Specialist

Immediate Supervisor: Director, Decision Support

General Purpose: The Decision Support Analyst coordinates data and research for senior managers at the corporate level of the integrated system.

Responsibilities:

- Participating and assisting in the design of a comprehensive program to lend support and analysis to management

- Performing scientific and technical planning, direction, and analysis of selected surveillance systems used by management

- Investigating existing national data and performing descriptive and analytic studies using statistical techniques

- Providing ongoing data analysis to entity decision makers that is relevant to the healthcare market and assisting in problem solving, solution development, decision making, and strategic planning

- Recommending focus and direction of resources toward management goals

- Preparing and providing decision support overviews, demonstrations, and presentations to a wide variety of audiences

- Serving as technical expert advisor and consultant to collaborating organizations in the area of management goals

Qualifications:

- Bachelor's degree in health information management, business, healthcare, or information systems technology

- Certification as RHIA or RHIT

- Understanding of healthcare delivery systems and health science administration

---

from the clinical or other setting. Instead, he or she will use the tools of data mining to better utilize the organization's data resources in making strategic and other business decisions.

Future Development of Decision Support Systems

Many directions are possible for future development of decision support systems. The incorporation of natural language processing into patient information systems may enable quick capture of physicians' clinical observations. Another avenue of development is to help consumers of healthcare services make more informed decisions. Examples of this direction of development include the APACHE system mentioned in the real-world case and systems such as one that assists low-literacy women in making decisions about options of care and treatment for breast cancer. Jimison and Sher (1999) have written a helpful review that summarizes much of the activity in this area. Future directions also may include the development of systems that can guide nonexpert individuals to provide care for critical individuals during catastrophic events such as natural disasters when trained medical personnel are taxed to their limits and unable to meet the needs of all the people who need care.

Real-World Case

According to a recent article published in the *Naples Daily News* on January 22, 2001 (www.naplesnews.com), Naples Community Hospital in Naples, Florida, recently completed the installation of a computerized decision support system for the hospital's intensive care unit (ICU). The software program assists both physicians and families in making decisions regarding treatment options for seriously ill or injured patients. Using the information available through the hospital's information systems, the new system is able to predict the mortality of the sickest patients cared for by the hospital. The system is called APACHE, which stands for Acute Physiology, Age, Chronic Health Evaluation, from APACHE Medical Systems, Inc. (www.apache-msi.com).

The physician, Dr. William Knaus, developed the APACHE manual (or paper-based) scoring system for critically ill patients in 1991. He wanted a way of tracking his patients to monitor their outcomes. According to Vi Shaffer, president of APACHE Medical Systems, Inc., in McLean, Virginia, since 1991, data collected by physicians using APACHE scoring has been obtained on over 700,000 patients in critical care environments. This data has been used to develop the current APACHE computerized decision support system.

The predictive model that lies at the heart of the system is based on a set of twenty-nine variables. These variables are a mix of various physiological and demographic information on the patient. A second set of data provides information on where the patient was before he or she was admitted to the intensive care unit.

The APACHE system can assist hospital administrators in assessing and monitoring the quality of care within the intensive care area and in monitoring the care received by critically ill patients. Second, it assists physicians in planning the most appropriate course of treatment and care for the patient. Other hospitals that have implemented the system have realized millions of dollars in savings in variable costs because physicians were able to make improved decisions on treatment options for patients.

Naples Community Hospital has 34 ICU beds and is owned by the nonprofit NCH Healthcare System. Two other hospitals in Florida also have implemented the APACHE system: Sarasota Memorial Hospital in Sarasota and Baptist Memorial Hospital in Miami.

Discussion Questions

1. One of the features of the APACHE system is that it assists family members in making decisions with regard to treatment options for critically ill patients. This type of decision support has not been previously discussed. What are the pros and cons of providing such assistance?

2. According to the article, the APACHE system was developed using data from 700,000 patients in critical care environments across the country. Twenty-nine variables relating to patient body functioning and demographics were measured and included in the data, along with mortality, the outcome variable of interest. The data then were used to develop a model that could predict mortality for new patients. Measurements of the variables for each new patient are obtained and supplied to the model, which, in turn, computes a prediction of his or her mortality. Identify the type of learning algorithm that was used to construct this model. What types of predictive modeling tools could be used to build it?

3. In addition to helping physicians make decisions regarding patient care, the APACHE system helps hospital administrators monitor resource use and quality of care. Does this system fit within the classification scheme discussed in this chapter? If so, in which group of decision support systems would you classify it, and why? If not, what name would you give to the class of decision support systems such as this one?

Summary

Decision support systems will play an important role in the future of healthcare. Clinical decision support systems, which have received much attention in the past, will continue to play a key role—and perhaps an even more important role than before. As computer-based patient record and patient information systems emerge and develop, the incorporation of clinical decision support in the form of clinical reminders, clinical alerts, and medication alerts and drug interaction monitoring offers great potential for improving the quality of patient care and for eliminating many of the medical errors cited in recent reports. With strong mandates from both consumers and the government, the opportunities for advances in clinical decision support are numerous.

Other areas of decision support also offer great promise for the future. The development of data warehouses, and the use of data-mining tools to exploit this vast mountain of data, will be an important competitive advantage for healthcare organizations. Many already are employing and studying the use of data-mining tools to identify medical errors and adverse events. In other examples, applications of this technology are proving beneficial in developing predictive models to assist in patient care and diagnosis, new facility location, clinical pathway development, identification of inappropriate utilization of healthcare resources, emergency vehicle scheduling in times of crisis, and improved quality of care for patients.

References

American Health Information Management Association. 1999. *Evolving HIM Careers: Seven Roles for the Future.* Chicago: AHIMA.

Barnett, G. O., J. J. Cimino, J. A. Hupp, and E. P. Hoffer. 1987. DXplain—an evolving diagnostic decision-support system. *Journal of the American Medical Association* 258(1):67–74

Beier, K. P. 2001. Accessed online from www-vrl.umich.edu/intro/.

Begur, S. V., D. M. Miller, and J. Weaver. 1997. An integrated spatial DSS for scheduling and routing home-health-care nurses. *Interfaces* 27(4):35–48.

Berner, E. S., et al. 1994. Performance of four computer-based diagnostic decision support systems. *New England Journal of Medicine* 330(25):1792–96.

Berner, Eta S., Richard S. Maisiak, C. Glenn Cobbs, and O. D. Taunton. 1999. A computer alert system to prevent injury from adverse drug events development and evaluation in a community teaching hospital. *Journal of the American Medical Informatics Association* 6(5):420–27.

Berson, Alex, and Stephen J. Smith. 1997. *Data Warehousing, Data Mining, & OLAP.* New York City: McGraw-Hill.

Box, G. E. P. 1979. Robustness in the strategy of scientific model building. In *Robustness in Statistics,* R. L. Launer and G. N. Wilkinson, editors. New York City: Academic Press.

Carter, Jerome H. 1999. Design and implementation issues. In *Clinical Decision Support Systems: Theory and Practice,* Eta S. Berner, editor. New York City: Springer.

Classen, D. 1998. Clinical decision support systems to improve clinical practice and quality of care. *Journal of American Medical Association* 280(15):1360–61.

Cunningham, M., and O. McKenna. 1993. Market model addresses hospitals' need for decision support. *Journal of Medical Systems* 10:65–71.

Davidson, C. 1993. What your database hides away. *New Scientist* 137(1855):28–31.

Davis, R. H. 1981. Social network analysis: an aid in conspiracy investigations. *FBI Law Enforcement Bulletin* 50(12):11–19.

Dayton, C. S., J. S. Ferguson, D. B. Hornick, and M. W. Peterson. 2000. Evaluation of an Internet-based decision-support system for applying the ATS/CDC guidelines for tuberculosis preventive therapy. *Medical Decision Making* 20(1):1–6.

de Dombal, F. T., J. R. Hartley, and D. H. Sleeman. 1969. A computer-assisted system for learning clinical diagnosis. *Lancet* 1:145–148.

Dexter, P., S. Perkins, J. M. Overhage, K. Maharry, R. Kohler, and C. J. McDonald. 2001. A computerized reminder system to increase the use of preventive care for hospitalized patients. *New England Journal of Medicine* 345(13):965–70.

Dhar, Vasant, and Roger Stein. 1997. *Seven Methods for Transforming Corporate Data into Business Intelligence.* Upper Saddle River, N.J.: Prentice-Hall.

Dobrzeniecki, A. 1994. *Executive Information Systems.* Chicago: ITT Research Institute.

Durieux, P., R. Nizard, P. Ravaud, N. Mounier, and E. Lepage. 2000. A clinical decision support system for the prevention of venous thrombo-embolism effect on physician behavior. *Journal of the American Medical Association* 283(21):2816–21.

Dutta, A., and S. Heda. 2000. Information systems architecture to support managed care business processes. *Decision Support Systems* 30:217–25.

Elson, R., J. Faughnan, and D. Connelly. 1997. An industrial process view of information delivery to support clinical decision making: implication for systems design and process measures. *Journal of the American Medical Informatics Association* 4(4):266–78.

Forgionne, G. 1991. Effectively marketing prepaid medical care with decision support systems. *Health Marketing Quarterly* 8(3/4):107–18.

Forgionne, G., A. Gangopadhyay, J. Klein, and R. Eckhardt. 1999. A decision technology system for health care electronic commerce. *Topics in Health Information Management* 20(1):31–41.

Friend, D. 1992. Building an EIS your CFO will really use. *Chief Information Officer Journal* 5(1):32–36.

Gerbert, B., A. Bronstone, T. Maurer, R. Hofmann, and T. Berger. 2000. Decision support software to help primary care physicians triage skin cancer: a pilot study. *Archives of Dermatology* 136(2):187–92.

Gorry, G. A., and G. O. Barnett. 1968. Experience with a model of sequential diagnosis. *Computers and Biomedical Research* 1:490–507.

Gorry, G. A., and M. S. Scott-Morton. 1971. A framework for management information systems. *Sloan Management Review* 13:55–70.

Hardin, J. M., P. Miller, A. Whelton, and S. Bellile. 1999. A new role for HIM in the knowledge economy. *Journal of American Health Information Management Association* 70(7):56–59.

Hohmann, S., E. L. Buff, and G. Wietecha. 1998. Monitoring performance improvement using decision support systems. *Journal of American Health Information Management Association* 69(10):36–39.

Holsapple, Clyde W., and Andrew B. Whinston. 1996. *Decision Support Systems: A Knowledge-Based Approach.* St. Paul, Minn.: West Publishing.

Howe, R. S., M. B. Terpening, and S. Wadhwa. 1999. Disease management and clinical decision support. *Journal of Healthcare Information Management* 13(2):53–66.

Inmon, William H. 1992. *Building the Data Warehouse.* New York City: John Wiley.

Institute of Medicine, Committee on Quality of Health Care in America. 2001. *Crossing the Quality Chasm: A New Health System for the 21st Century.* Washington, D.C.: National Academy Press.

Isdale, J. 1993. Available from www.isdale.com/jerry/VR/index.html.

Jimison, H. B., and P. R. Sher. 1999. Decision support for patients. In *Clinical Decision Support Systems,* E. Berner, editor. New York City: Springer.

Johns, Merida L., J. M. Hardin, and Karel M. Weigel. 2001. Research and decision support. In *Ethical Challenges in the Management of Health Information,* L. B. Harman, editor. Gaithersburg, Md.: Aspen Publishers.

Kaufman, David M., and Grace I. Paterson. 1995. Preparing future physicians: how will medical schools meet the challenge? In *Future Health: Computers and Medicine in the Twenty-first Century,* Clifford A. Pickover, editor. New York City: St. Martin's Press.

Kohn, Linda T., Janet M. Corrigan, and Molla S. Donaldson, editors. 2000. *To Err Is Human: Building a Safer Health System.* Washington, D.C.: National Academy Press.

Kvedar, J. 2000. Decision support is changing health care. *Archives of Dermatology* 136(2):249–50.

Lagina, S. 1971. A computer program to diagnose anxiety levels. *Nursing Research* 20(6):484–92.

Ledley, R., and L. Lusted. 1959. Reasoning foundations of medical diagnosis. *Science* 130:9–21.

Little, J. D. 1970. Models and managers: the concept of a decision calculus. *Management Science* 16(8):B466–85.

Los Alamos National Library. 2002. Modeling, algorithms and informatics group. Accessed online from www.c3.lanl.gov/ccs3web.

Marakas, George M. 1999. *Decision Support Systems in the 21st Century.* Upper Saddle River, N.J.: Prentice-Hall.

Miller, R. A. 1994. Medical diagnostic decision support systems—past, present, and future: a threaded bibliography and commentary. *Journal of the American Medical Informatics Association* 1(1):8–27.

Miller, R. A., F. E. Masarie, and J. Myers. 1986. Quick Medical Reference (QMR) for diagnostic assistance. *MD Computing* 3(5):34–48.

Miller, R.A., H. E. Pople, Jr., and J. Myers. 1982. Internist-I, an experimental computer-based diagnostic consultant for general internal medicine. *The New England Journal of Medicine* 307(8):468–76.

Musen, M. A., Y. Shahar, and E. H. Shortliffe. 2001. Clinical decision support systems. In *Medical Informatics: Computer Applications in Health Care and Biomedicine,* E. H. Shortliffe, L. E. Perreault, G. Wiederhold, and L. M. Fagan, editors. New York City: Springer.

Payne, T. 2000. Computer decision support systems. *Cardiopulmonary and Critical Care Journal* 118(2):47S–52S.

Pickover, C. A., editor. 1995. *Future Health.* New York City: St Martins.

Poikonen, J., and J. M. Leventhal. 1999. Medication-management issues at the point of care. *Journal of Healthcare Information Management* 13(2):43–52.

Pople, H. E., J. D. Myers, and R. A. Miller. 1975. DIALOG: a model of diagnostic logic for internal medicine. In *Proceedings of the Fourth International Joint Conference on Artificial Intelligence.* Cambridge, Mass.: MIT Artificial Intelligence Laboratory Publications.

Ruland, C. M. 1999. Decision support for patient preference-based care planning: effects on nursing care and patient outcomes. *Journal of American Medical Informatics Association* 6(4):304–12.

Russell, S., and P. Norvig. 1995. *Artificial Intelligence: A Modern Approach.* Upper Saddle River, N.J.: Prentice-Hall.

Sanders, G. D., C. G. Hagerty, F. A. Sonnenberg, M. A. Hlatky, and D. K. Owens. 1999. Distributed decision support using a Web-based interface. *Medical Decision Making* 19(2):157–66.

Sauter, Vicki. 1997. *Decision Support Systems: An Applied Managerial Approach.* New York City: John Wiley.

Senge, P. 1990. *The Fifth Discipline: The Art and Practice of the Learning Organization.* New York City: Doubleday.

Shams, K., and M. Farishta. 2001. Data warehousing: toward knowledge management. *Topics in Health Information Management* 21(3):24–32.

Shortliffe, E. H. 1976. *Computer-Based Medical Consultations: MYCIN.* New York City: Elsevier.

Sim, I., P. Gorman, R. Greenes, et al. 2001. Clinical decision support systems for the practice of evidence-based medicine. *Journal of the American Medical Informatics Association* 8(6):527–34.

Simon, Herbert A. 1957. *Models of Man.* New York City: John Wiley.

Simon, Herbert A. 1960. *The New Science of Management Decision.* New York City: Harper & Row.

Stewart, T. A. 1997. *Intellectual Captial.* New York City: Doubleday/Currency.

Tan, Joseph K. 2001. *Health Management Information Systems: Methods and Practical Applications,* second edition. Gaithersburg, Md.: Aspen Publishers.

Tan, Joseph K., and Samuel Sheps, editors. 1998. *Health Decision Support Systems.* Gaithersburg, Md.: Aspen Publishers.

Teich, J., and M. Wrinn. 2000. Clinical decision support systems come of age. *MD Computing* 17(1):43–46.

Turban, Efraim. 1995. *Decision Support and Expert Systems: Management Support Systems,* fourth edition. Englewood Cliffs, N.J.: Prentice-Hall.

Turning, A. 1950. Computing machinery and intelligence. *Mind* 59:433–60.

Warner, H. R., R. M. Garner, and A. F. Toronto. 1964. Experience with Bayes' theorem for computer diagnosis of congenital heart disease. *Annals of the New York Academy of Science* 115:2–16.

Wyatt, J. 2000. Decision support systems. *Royal Society of Medicine* 93(12):629–33.

Yu, V. L., et al. 1979. Antimicrobial selection by a computer: a blinded evaluation by infectious disease experts. *Journal of the American Medical Association* 242(12):1279–82.

Zaki, A. 1989. Developing a DSS for a distribution facility: an application in the healthcare industry. *Journal of Medical Systems* 13:331–46.

Application Exercises

1. Suppose you want to develop a decision support system to support a quality of care improvement initiative within your hospital. Using Simon's decision-making model, develop a list of activities for each phase.

2. When patients arrive at the emergency department complaining of chest pains, they must be triaged as quickly as possible so that appropriate care and treatment can be initiated. In the mid-1980s, researchers developed several systems to help clinicians with this task. Find three articles on this work in the library and write a one-page summary of each. Hint: One of the first articles in this area was written in 1982 by L. Goldman, et al. and titled A computer protocol to predict myocardial infarction in emergency department patients with chest pain (*New England Journal of Medicine* 307:588–97). The authors have since written other articles on this topic, and several other teams of investigators have developed and evaluated decision support techniques in this area.

3. An important part of DSS development is evaluation. Read the following two papers related to the evaluation of clinical DSSs and identify key elements involved in conducting an evaluation: Performance of four computer-based diagnostic decision support systems, written by E. S. Berner, G. D. Webster, A. A. Shugerman, et al. in 1994 (*New England Journal of Medicine* 330:1792–96); and Relationships among the performance scores of four diagnostic decision support systems, written by E. S. Berner, J. R. Jackson, and J. Algina in 1996 (*Journal of the American Medical Informatics Association* 3:208–15).

4. Developing and maintaining the rules in a rule-based decision support architecture is difficult. Pick an area of interest in healthcare and make a plan for developing rules for your rule base. Using your plan as a guide, interview an expert in your chosen area to try to gather rules. Your rule base should be in the form of IF *condition* THEN *result (action).* The *condition* should be in the form of test results = 2.0 or blood pressure is greater than 120/70. You may use AND in the *condition.* The rules you develop should have the same form as that illustrated in figure 19.9. Try to develop a set of rules (knowledge base) consisting of at least ten rules. These rules could form the basis of a DSS for the area chosen. Write a short diary describing your experiences. If possible, work in teams of three or four people.

5. Find an article on a successful DSS implementation in healthcare. Try to determine the factors that drove the need for the system, who the chief advocate for the system was in the organization, who the users are, and how long implementation took to accomplish. Finally, develop of a list of factors that you consider critical to the successful implementation of a DSS within a healthcare organization.

Figure 19.9.   A Typical Rule from the MYCIN System

	Rule 507
IF:	(1) The infection which requires therapy is meningitis
	(2) Organisms were not seen on the stain of the culture
	(3) The type of infection is bacterial
	(4) The patient does not have a head injury defect, and
	(5) The age of the patient is between 15 years and 55 years
THEN:	The organisms that might be causing the infection are *Diplococcus pneumoniae* and *Neisseria meningitidis*

Source: Musen, Shahar, and Shortliffe 2001, chapter 16.

Review Quiz

Instructions: Choose the best answer for the following questions.

1. ____ Which of the following terms refers to the sum of all the knowledge and information that resides in an organization's employees and information systems?
   a. TQM
   b. Corporate data
   c. Organization infrastructure
   d. Intellectual capital

2. ____ What is the computer-based system called that gathers data from a variety of sources and assists in providing structure to the data using various analytical models and visual tools in order to facilitate and improve the ultimate outcome in decision-making tasks associated with nonroutine and nonrepetitive problems?
   a. Decision support system
   b. Health information system
   c. A six-sigma system
   d. An electronic patient record system

3. ____ The intelligence phase, the design phase, and the choice phase are the three phases of which of the following processes?
   a. The relaxation response
   b. The six-sigma process
   c. Simon's decision-making process
   d. The renewal process

4. ____ HIMS is an acronym for which of the following terms?
   a. Health information manipulation system
   b. Hardin's intelligence mapping system
   c. Health information management system
   d. Health intelligence management system

5. ____ What is the reasoning element usually referred to in a knowledge-based DSS?
   a. A database
   b. A gathering place
   c. A GUI
   d. An inference engine

6. ____ Which of the following is not a class of decision support system?
   a. Linux-based system
   b. Model-based system
   c. Knowledge-based system
   d. Graphics-based system

7. ____ Which of the following is not a function of a data warehouse?
   a. It provides the most recent transaction data available within the organization.
   b. It serves as a neutral storage area for data extracted from an organization's transactional systems.
   c. It is organized around specific business functions or requirements.
   d. It provides easy access to business data for analysis or data mining (that is, decision support).

8. ____ What is a star schema?
   a. A map to the homes of movie stars
   b. A data model used to construct data warehouses
   c. An outline of the constellations
   d. A method of statistical analysis

9. ____ Machine learning is a branch of which scientific discipline?
   a. Physics
   b. Chemistry
   c. Computer science
   d. Biology

10. ____ MYCIN was an example of which type of decision support system?
   a. Nursing decision support system
   b. Executive decision support system
   c. Healthcare decision support system
   d. Clinical decision support system

Chapter 20
Knowledge Management

Kam Shams, MA, and Mehnaz Farishta, MS

Learning Objectives

- To understand knowledge management as a business discipline
- To recognize the importance of knowledge assets
- To discern the components of a knowledge management initiative/program
- To explore key knowledge management applications in healthcare, such as data warehousing, data mining, and customer relationship management
- To apply knowledge management to decision making
- To describe the role of a chief knowledge officer in a healthcare organization

Key Terms

Analysis session
Branding communications
Business intelligence
Core communications
Customer relationship management (CRM)
Data mine/data mining
Decision tree
Explicit knowledge
Fuzzy logic
Genetic algorithms
Information assets
K-nearest neighbor (K-NN)
Knowledge
Knowledge assets
Knowledge management
Knowledge workers
Learning organization
Neural networks
On-line analytical processing (OLAP) engine
Operations support systems (OSS)
Predictive modeling
Relational database management system (RDMS)
Rule induction
Strategic communications
Structured analysis
Tacit knowledge
Unstructured analysis
Wisdom

Introduction

Hidden deep within the minds of individuals and embedded in business processes are nuggets of information and knowledge regarding the data, processes, and organizational components that can lead to effective strategic and tactical decisions. Leveraging this knowledge at the right time by the right people is necessary to add value to the healthcare organization's daily decision-making process.

The process of knowledge management, with its various components and applications, can enhance clinical and financial decision making and transform data into business intelligence and wisdom. By applying the knowledge management discipline, healthcare organizations can allow their knowledge base to be updated and maintained by knowledge workers, closing the gap between the knowledge worker and the organization. Reducing turnaround time for meeting business objectives results in a progressive organization that can maximize the use of its knowledge assets for tangible benefits.

This chapter discusses how healthcare organizations can transform data into information and then into wisdom through the process of knowledge management. In addition to defining knowledge management, the chapter presents a five-step framework for a knowledge management initiative and explains how the process can be applied in healthcare organizations using different performance improvement tools.

Theory into Practice

Hospital A began as a small community hospital in Texas. Over the past ten years, it has become the largest medical center between Austin and Dallas. Founded in 1956 by a charity organization, the hospital has grown in response to growth in the area population. Today, hospital A has four campuses and is part of the ABC Regional Health Network. The health system provides a network of services, including a cancer center, home care health management, women's health centers, rural clinics, and family, emergency, cardiac, and psychiatric services. As part of the ABC Health Network, hospital A is operating as a private for-profit institution. For the past four years, it has been generating modest revenues for the network although the other hospitals within the network have been operating at break-even levels.

Hospital A has undertaken an initiative to increase revenues for the entire network by improving current processes in the areas of data management and customer relationship management. The hospital has a valuable leader in its chief information officer (CIO), who is known for his leadership skills and innovation. The CIO has been promised that in the next fiscal year, he will be allocated a budget of $2 to $3 million to purchase information technology tools to help in the areas his initiative intends to address.

The CIO created a think tank composed of members from various hospital departments, including finance, scheduling/ admissions, human resources, medical records, management information systems, accounting, nursing, and medical staff. The team identified the following areas that need data/ information and reports:

- The insurance contracts that are currently making money for the hospital
- How to lower the cost for the largest employer in town and whether the hospital should consider direct contracting
- Accounts the collectors should go after when they come to work every morning
- Volume, cost, and profitability by service and location
- Trends in drug use and costs for pharmacy contract negotiations

The team decided to embark on a knowledge management initiative and identified the following tasks:

- Deciding which information technology tools or applications should be used to fulfill the hospital's data/ reporting needs
- Cataloging the knowledge assets of the organization and sharing the findings, especially to determine what has already been achieved in those areas
- Identifying gaps that exist in the current system and explaining the underlying reasons
- Selecting the knowledge management application(s) to address the information needs identified
- Developing recommendations for creating a culture of knowledge management in the organization
- Deciding whether to recommend the creation of a chief knowledge officer role in the organization

From Knowledge to Wisdom

The healthcare industry has long cited the uniqueness of its business as the reason for being slow to adopt innovations in information technology (IT). However, increased regulation and competitive market forces have required the industry to become more efficient, effective, and customer oriented. Thus, decision support systems and knowledge management applications have assumed an increasingly important role in enabling the industry to adjust to change. These applications are being applied in several healthcare areas in an effort to:

- Determine the cost-effectiveness of treatment protocols
- Understand cost structures of services
- Find patterns in data that are of significance
- Forecast trends to make sense of the monumental amount of healthcare data
- Implement process redesign initiatives to enhance customer service

The creation, communication, and absorption of information within a system pose enormous challenges for healthcare management, especially when dealing with legacy healthcare information systems (HIS). Most legacy information applications still operate in a linear fashion, creating information in isolated stages in the same way that cars are manufactured (Loshin 2001). Legacy systems focus primarily on providing operational applications to meet day-to-day hospital clerical and tactical needs. They are transaction based, with single platforms and hierarchical databases that provide fragmented decision support. Although this continues to be essential in running many aspects of today's healthcare environment, it poses quite an interesting challenge in the rapidly changing world of healthcare in which the acute care service component has shifted toward ambulatory care, and there is renewed emphasis on chronic and long-term care management. Thus, in the new paradigm, the emphasis is on knowledge management applications rather than traditional HIS systems. Knowledge management applications are end-user centric, with graphical user interface (GUI) and Web-based applications, and use the power of relational database technology to provide holistic decision support. (See figure 20.1 for a comparison of the paradigm shift in healthcare organizations.) Moreover, there is a tremendous need to integrate all components of the local healthcare delivery system, which is reflected in the new healthcare economy. Traditional HIS vendors have struggled to handle this evolving healthcare model. They also have struggled with the adaptation of emerging technology to meet the changing needs of the new marketplace.

Information growth is accelerating beyond the scope of most healthcare information systems. In 2000, for example, the International Data Corporation predicted that the information distributed through corporate systems would undergo a phenomenal growth of more than thirty-seven times by the year 2002. Regardless of the actual growth percent, this is a lot of information to deal with, and most healthcare IT systems and organizations will struggle with its effective management and utilization (Grammer 2000).

Thus, it is not surprising that most organizations are seeking new IT tools that are based on open systems and have the capabilities to perform knowledge management–related functions. In stride, the IT marketplace is exploding with options and software that allow organizations to add on to their current HIS systems in order to make them more useful, more productive, and less costly and, at the same time, to leverage their current investment.

In *Post Capitalist Society,* Peter Drucker wrote: "The basic economic resource is no longer capital, nor natural resources, nor labor. It is and will be knowledge. Value is now created by 'productivity' and 'innovation,' both applications of knowledge to work" (Penny 2000). The organizations that can leverage technology to exploit their data through the use of data warehousing, customer relationship management (CRM), and data mining not only have business intelligence as a corollary but also create a competitive advantage for themselves. By identifying trends, unusual patterns, and hidden relationships that a competitor may not realize, these organizations can create new opportunities for growth and will thrive in the changing healthcare marketplace. The extent of use of information technology in the organization is directly related to the adoption of knowledge management.

Knowledge Management Defined

Knowledge, or the awareness and understanding gained through experience, is not held within an organization itself but, rather, by the various individuals who make up the organization. An organization's viability directly depends on how the organization captures and harnesses knowledge to help it identify the best business practices and to refine and improve them during changing times.

As described in a white paper by Gallagher Financial Systems, Inc. (1999), **knowledge management** is a process that attempts to identify and capture knowledge to enable individuals to share it, to leverage existing knowledge in the creation of new knowledge, and to use it to define and improve business practices. Additionally, knowledge management may be defined as the practice of treating knowledge like any other business asset, in other words, as something to be used, maintained, and expanded to the benefit of the organization.

It is only when healthcare leadership realizes the potential power of information as a critical corporate asset that the foundation of a knowledge-centric organization can be laid. This signals the migration from an industrial age view of data to a knowledge age view, where many data sets are aggregated, fused, enhanced, and broadcast to share an enterprisewide knowledge base (Loshin 2001). Thus, knowledge management accelerates learning and decision making and leverages expertise and technology to enable smart organizations to achieve peak performance. It is a process, not an end product.

Most corporate knowledge resides in the heads of employees digesting vast amounts of information. Although information is captured, knowledge is not. Bits of it leave at the end of every employee's tenure (Grammer 2000). Thus, knowledge management must be acknowledged as a business

Figure 20.1.   Comparison of Information Management Paradigms in Healthcare Organizations

Old Healthcare Paradigm	New Healthcare Paradigm
Health information system	Enterprisewide knowledge management system
Operation oriented	Analysis oriented
Hierarchical database	Relational database
Programmer centric	End-user centric
Silo based	Process based
Character based	GUI/WEB based
Fragmented decision support	Holistic decision support

discipline that depends on various **knowledge assets,** or sources of knowledge for an organization, and not merely as a software application. The Gartner Group captures this concept in its definition of knowledge management. According to its definition, knowledge management is a discipline that promotes an integrated and collaborative approach to the process of information asset creation, capture, organization, access, and use. **Information assets** include databases, documents and, most important, the tacit expertise and experience resident in the organization's employees.

The key to this definition is identifying knowledge management as a discipline rather than a technology. Healthcare management must recognize that, as a discipline, knowledge management requires cultural and process changes in order for the organization to have a return on investment (ROI). Technology is certainly the enabler to ascertain business/ corporate intelligence, but without cultural change, organizations cannot reap the full benefits of adopting a knowledge management initiative. Knowledge management puts forth the goal of achieving competitive advantage by leveraging the vast knowledge of collective corporate memory.

Knowledge Management Process

Knowledge management also transforms data to information and then to knowledge, which eventually creates wisdom or business intelligence for the organization. (See figure 20.2.) Several sources define the various building blocks of the knowledge transformation process with slight variations. This section describes the constituents of **business intelligence,** or rather, the end product of knowledge management, which improves an enterprise's ability to make good decisions and makes information available to everyone in the enterprise.

Figure 20.2.   Transformation of Data to Information to Knowledge to Wisdom

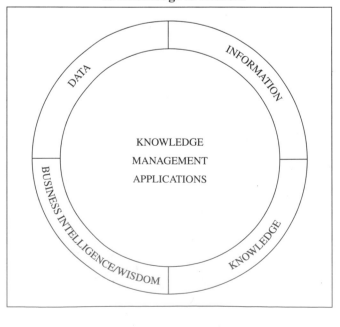

As explained in earlier chapters, data can be broadly defined as a collection of facts—facts about specific events, objects, and about an industry in general—that can be analyzed. The facts originate from a variety of sources and include raw statistics such as demographic, billing, nursing, pharmacy, laboratory, and marketing information. Thus, data can form the basis of knowledge as they are gathered, analyzed, and synthesized by individuals within the organization. Healthcare heavily relies on transaction processing systems because they are capable of collecting and processing large amounts of data, which is crucial for knowledge management solutions.

Sometimes referred to as explicit knowledge, information results from the collection and communication of ideas and experiences. The process involves combining and/or summarizing data from different sources to create information that affects decisions because it influences the way people interpret their environment and the underlying trends in their day-to-day operations (Allison 2000).

Knowledge management or business intelligence applications that have ad hoc query and reporting capabilities enable users to extract data from a database. By placing data in a context that produces meaning, these applications give users the ability to create information. The creation of information is an extensive process that involves constantly separating and regrouping data to extend its value. Applications that have **on-line analytical processing** (OLAP) **engines** allow users to analyze data and determine relationships, patterns, trends, and exceptions. An OLAP engine is an optimized query generator that can retrieve the right information from the warehouse to accommodate "what if" business queries. This process further paves the way for the ultimate transition of information into knowledge and business intelligence.

Knowledge involves much more than storing information and recalling it when the time is appropriate. Translating information into knowledge requires robust IT tools, experience, and reflection. Combining information with experience, knowledge helps provide a context in which new information can be created and interpreted when compared to previously acquired information. Because knowledge comprises ideas, experiences, and insights, true knowledge is often referred to as tacit knowledge. It is important to note that knowledge in itself means nothing if appropriate action does not follow. This leads to the end goal of the knowledge management process—creating business intelligence for the organization. For this reason, intelligence, or **wisdom,** is defined as the *empowerment* and *courage* to act (English 1999).

Knowledge represents the intelligence that individuals apply to data and information in order to make decisions and draw conclusions. Without intelligence, information cannot become knowledge. Thus, the possession of knowledge, along with intelligence and the ability to create new knowledge, determines an organization's success in accelerating business processes and reducing and eliminating non-value-added activities, which is one of the major goals for a knowledge management initiative.

Return on Knowledge Assets

The implementation of knowledge assets in the organization's IT infrastructure maximizes its ROI. Data warehousing, data mining, CRM, and OLAP are all tools and applications that bring knowledge management to the forefront of the organization. Data stored in the organization's databases and other data sources are retrieved and used to perform various functions and to make important decisions. When data are inaccurate, missing, or used ineffectively, the processes performed and decisions made by the organization will be impaired. Therefore, it is important that the organization adopts the discipline of knowledge management to become a learning organization. A learning organization focuses on acquiring and sharing knowledge and making information available to all.

Knowledge management initiatives play a key role in the organization's overall health in numerous ways, including by:

- Reducing costs of information gathering and decision support that add no value to the business
- Improving customer support processes so that questions are answered faster and more accurately
- Identifying new market opportunities
- Reducing the knowledge gap that exists when key personnel leave an organization

When all identified knowledge assets are documented and communicated, it is possible to capture and retain information as well as tacit knowledge. Finally, if a sound knowledge management mechanism is in place, the knowledge acquired can be shared among users, which raises the strategic acumen of the organization in general. As workers share knowledge, they improve their performance, are able to make better decisions, and are transformed into **knowledge workers.** Thus, the organization is able to respond in a timely manner to changes in the marketplace. Moreover, as knowledge is documented and shared, it becomes easier to retain tacit knowledge for new employees and to reduce errors.

Knowledge management or business intelligence applications that have data-mining capabilities enable users to identify hidden trends and unusual patterns within the data. Without the use of a data-mining application, this effort would be extremely time-consuming. Similarly, data warehousing is a knowledge management application that aids knowledge acquisition and knowledge transfer. Using a variety of data sources, business processes, and organizational departments, data warehousing puts information into context. In addition, it extracts strategic knowledge from the raw data, enabling organizations to deliver the knowledge to the right people for timely and powerful responses to changing healthcare needs. This is how the adoption of knowledge management takes advantage of intellectual assets and increases business performance.

Knowledge Management Programs and Initiatives

Before embarking on a knowledge management initiative, it is important to identify the sources of knowledge, or knowl-edge assets, of an organization. (See figure 20.3.) This includes printed documents, unwritten rules, work flows, customer knowledge, databases/spreadsheets, and human expertise and know-how. Knowledge as information in a context that supports proper decisions and actions exists as both explicit and tacit knowledge. **Explicit knowledge** refers to knowledge that is fully and clearly expressed and defined, and it includes documents, databases, and other types of recorded and documented information. On the other hand, **tacit knowledge** is implied by or inferred from actions or statements. Hence, the actions, experiences, ideals, values, and emotions of an individual constitute tacit knowledge. Tacit knowledge tends to be highly personal and difficult to communicate. Corporate culture, organizational politics, and professional experience are common examples of tacit knowledge.

It also is crucial to develop an organized framework to capture knowledge and transform it into business intelligence. The basic framework of a knowledge management initiative consists of five steps. Underlying these steps are two general principles that help chart the course toward knowledge management. The first principle is to realize the challenges faced by the organization; the second is to develop principles for success (figure 20.4). Principles for success include an emphasis on learning, integrating, and sharing data/information/knowledge across an enterprise, regardless of individual departments; on identifying the ROI; and finally, on selecting robust solutions,

Figure 20.3.   Knowledge Assets in a Healthcare Organization

Explicit Knowledge
Documents
Spreadsheets
Databases
Recorded and documented information
Health information systems
Inventory of all applications and tools to leverage information

Tacit Knowledge
Human expertise and know-how
Actions, ideals, values, and emotions of individuals
Corporate culture
Work flow
Professional experience
Corporate memory
Intellectual assets

Figure 20.4.   The Course of Knowledge Management

Individual Challenge	Available
Admit that knowledge is inaccessible	Data warehousing
Identify business problems	OLAP tools
Identify target audience	Smart EMR
	DSS EIS
Principles for Success	Document warehousing
Analyze return on investment	
Integrate sharing of culture between HIS and HIM	
Learn! Learn! Learn!	
Keep WWW in mind	
Aim for robust solutions	

such as data warehousing, OLAP, data marts, data mining, and so on, that create business intelligence.

The following five steps of a knowledge management initiative guarantee the transformation of an ordinary organization into a learning organization.

Step 1. Categorize the Organization's Knowledge Assets

As mentioned earlier, the organization's knowledge assets include both explicit physical assets (spreadsheets, documents, databases, and so on) and tacit intellectual assets (the collective knowledge, human expertise, and know-how of the organization's employees and staff). They also include an inventory of all applications and tools that are in place to leverage information, such as data warehousing applications, data marts, transaction processing systems, and so on. While categorizing explicit knowledge assets (even though this knowledge is documented), it is not always clear where to find the desired information because it exists in many locations and forms. Additionally, it can be difficult to determine correlations among different information components to form useful knowledge and to separate out-of-date information from current information. Similarly, grouping tacit knowledge assets is a challenge. Tacit knowledge is shared via word of mouth and shared experiences, but at some point, it becomes impractical to rely on word of mouth to convey appropriate tacit knowledge throughout an organization.

It is important to realize that data and information can exist in the absence of people. However, knowledge can exist only as a characteristic in people when they apply their experience and reason to recognize the significance of information. Wisdom requires actions that lead to the accomplishment of good results. It also requires empowered and motivated people to act on knowledge. Therefore, the first step in categorizing knowledge assets is to recognize that merely doing an audit is not sufficient. It is equally important to consider whether the knowledge assets can be shared with others in the organization. It is in this process of sharing lessons learned that knowledge can be leveraged, and it is this leveraging of knowledge and information that multiplies the value of the organization's knowledge assets (English 1999).

Steps 2 and 3. Analyze the Cost and Value of Current Knowledge Assets and Identify Problems That Current Assets Cannot Solve

Completion of the first step, creating an inventory of systems and information within an organization, makes it easier to determine the value of the information and its associated update and maintenance costs. Outdated information often makes it difficult to retrieve important information in a timely manner. Other times, new information is created that may or may not add to the overall picture. Thus, it is important to take stock of information that is of value to the organization.

In addition, a detailed analysis is prudent at this stage to ensure that the existing applications and systems, such as the HIS, on-line transaction systems, and others, are producing results that are in line with the organization's objectives. Key questions to consider include:

- Is the organization able to use the information effectively?
- Is the information readily available?
- Is the information accessible to all decision makers in a timely manner?
- Is the information creating a strategic advantage for the organization?

In addition, costs are associated with these systems and applications in terms of hardware, software, and manpower. When there is no ROI in terms of leveraging information and using these systems to their optimum potential, it is even more crucial to embark on a knowledge management initiative that can support these applications and add innovation where it is lacking to ensure an affirmative response to the preceding key questions.

Thus, analyzing the cost and value of current assets and identifying problems that current assets cannot solve are crucial steps in identifying gaps in the current system and seeking appropriate solutions that will bridge them and strategically maneuver the organization to survive in today's competitive healthcare environment.

Step 4. Build a Culture That Encourages the Capture of Knowledge Targeted to Achieve the Organization's Objectives and Goals

The emphasis on knowledge retrieval is a key component of this step to make explicit knowledge readily available to users and to have tacit knowledge documented. Additionally, this step requires organizations to use communication technologies and virtual teams to break down the cultural and geographic barriers to knowledge sharing (Penny 2000).

Another important part of this step is to create a process that will motivate employees to share knowledge. Employees sometimes hesitate to share their knowledge because of a perception that their job or role in the organization could become obsolete. Technology can enable the organization to overcome some of these cultural barriers (Penny 2000). Creating a culture of knowledge also requires that steps be taken to encourage the use of information by all users. For this purpose, information/knowledge must be easily available to knowledge workers across the organization.

Step 5. Deploy and Implement Knowledge Management and Business Intelligence Applications

After a culture of knowledge management is adopted, the final step of a knowledge management initiative is to deploy and implement knowledge management and business intelligence applications. The combination of data warehouses and analytical tool sets has given organizations the ability to drill down into integrated data to reveal cost savings and competitively differentiating findings. Organizations can rely on business intelligence analysis to provide hard facts that will help them make better, more informed decisions and reap unforeseen rewards (Goldman 2001).

The term *data warehousing* is often used synonymously for the term *business intelligence*. Whatever the name, data warehousing is by far one of the most important knowledge management applications. It promises to eliminate the barriers between data and the business analysts who need them, improve data quality, and integrate internal and external data. All of these promises make knowledge discovery more efficient, improve knowledge transfer, or provide information that, as a byproduct, points the organization to areas in which it needs to gain more knowledge (Allison 2000).

Although data warehousing is vital to the data-intensive healthcare industry, it cannot be a panacea. A well-designed business intelligence system also exploits technologies such as on-line analytical processing, client/server computing, the Internet and intranets, new **relational database management systems** (RDMS), parallel processing, and advanced microprocessors. Success in adopting any of these business intelligence applications lies in proper planning and implementation and in management support and leadership, which are necessary to remove barriers to change that may exist in the organization.

Check Your Understanding 20.1

Instructions: Answer the following questions on a separate piece of paper.

1. In what ways does knowledge management apply to healthcare services?

2. Where is knowledge found in healthcare organizations?

3. List and describe the five steps or components of a knowledge management program.

4. What is the difference between information and knowledge?

5. What is the difference between knowledge and wisdom?

6. What is the difference between explicit knowledge and tacit knowledge?

Knowledge Management Applications in Healthcare Organizations

Bill Gates, CEO of Microsoft, described the qualities of leadership in a magazine interview (*Industry Week,* November 20, 1995) as "vision, innovation, long-term thinking, and risk-taking." Maximizing the return on data warehousing requires these qualities. If healthcare leadership is ready to become a knowledge management organization, the sky is the limit.

As IBM chairman and CEO Louis V. Gerstner Jr. stated at the Securities Industry Association's annual convention in Boca Raton, Florida, in October 1997, "Today and in the future, companies that succeed will be those that know how to manage knowledge faster than competitors. It isn't a question of getting new information. It's the ability to extract information from your existing business, to see trends and insights faster than your competition." If knowledge is

indeed power, the importance of knowledge management systems and applications for tapping into this power cannot be ignored. The healthcare industry is in a constant state of flux. It is only through the transition of data into knowledge that healthcare organizations can compete strategically in this evolving industry. Although most organizations have transitioned from data to analysis, only those that understand the value of data and technology have advanced to knowledge and wisdom, which has led to the competitive advantage these organizations currently enjoy. Business intelligence and/or knowledge management applications, such as data warehousing, data mining, and customer relationship management, are the cornerstones of the healthcare landscape. These applications transform knowledge into wisdom, which gives organizations the ability to make decisions in a timely manner, improve their performance and operations, and respond to their most important customers—the patients.

In today's healthcare marketplace, fast and easy access to information about the key factors driving the business is paramount. To meet this need, most organizations are consolidating data from operational systems into central data warehouses or data marts that are structured to support decision making. A recent survey conducted by a knowledge management company in December 2000 elucidates this trend. According to the survey, in 2001–2002, the amount that most healthcare organizations budgeted for acquiring strategic knowledge management applications was growing at a healthy pace. Specifically, 58 percent of the facilities surveyed believed that spending would increase, 29 percent stated that spending would remain the same, and 13 percent planned to spend less on new intelligence software. (See figure 20.5.) Of those planning to increase software purchases in the next twelve months, the main reason given was their emphasis on improving decision making in a managed care environment. Many IT organizations also understand that these robust and powerful business intelligence tools are more expensive than the traditional character-based HIS

Figure 20.5.   Results of a Healthcare Industry Survey on Future Growth in the Acquisition of Strategic Information Technology Applications

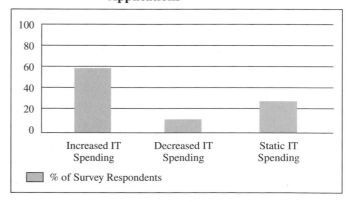

applications. However, when traditional HIS applications do not meet the organization's needs and when the cost is greater in the long run because of inefficiency and difficulty of use, the organization's eventual success will more than compensate for the initial investment.

As reported in the keynote address at the TDWI World Conference, fall 2001, in Orlando, Florida, by William McKnight, president of McKnight Associates, business intelligence (knowledge management) technology revenues will increase at a compound annual growth rate of 27 percent from $3.6 billion in 2000 to $11.9 billion in 2005 (Brohan 2001). These applications are designed to improve a healthcare organization's ability to make good business decisions by making necessary information available at all levels of the enterprise, from senior management to the knowledge worker. The healthcare industry is faced with making more complex decisions in shorter time frames and managing colossal amounts of data under tighter budgets and cost constraints in the delivery of high-quality services. It is more important than ever to empower more people within an organization to become knowledge workers. When knowledge workers use smart business intelligence or knowledge management applications, they can address these challenges in a consistent and effective manner and become the champions of a learning organization.

In a learning organization, the focus is on delivering information quickly, clearly, and visually to everyone within the organization, with a strong emphasis on data integrity and the ability to see every aspect of the business relationship in a true perspective. Therefore, data are given prime importance for developing trends, aggregates, and summarizations over time and for discerning valuable information.

The tools, often referred to as business intelligence or knowledge management applications, that help accomplish this also share great importance and reverence in a learning organization. Howard Dresner of the Gartner Group coined the term *business intelligence* in the early 1990s to encapsulate the end-user query and reporting (EUQR) tools, decision support tools, and the on-line analytical processing (OLAP) tools market. Since the term was coined, business intelligence has been driven by activities in data warehousing and data mart technology, including extraction, transformation, and loading (ETL); data cleansing; databases; information portals; data mining; and business modeling. Of these various knowledge management/business intelligence applications, data warehousing, data mining, and customer relationship management (CRM) applications play a key role in a healthcare setting.

Data Warehousing

Industry and market research indicates that knowledge management and strategic decision making powered by data warehouses have dominated IT industry attention since the 1990s (Boar 1993). Numerous companies in multiple industries, including healthcare, are achieving tremendous benefits from data warehousing, including faster and better decision making, employee empowerment, and leveraging of operational data and scenario analysis.

A data warehouse is a platform that contains all of an organization's data in a centralized and normalized form and in one place for deployment to users in order to fulfill simple reporting of data to complicated data analysis, decision support, and executive-level reporting/archiving needs. Typically, a data warehouse consists of a set of programs that extract data from the operational environment, a database that maintains data warehouse data, and systems that provide data to users (Lambert 1996). Physically, a data warehouse is a repository of information that businesses need to thrive in the information age. Analytically, a data warehouse is a modern reporting environment that provides users direct access to data.

Data Warehousing Applications

Data warehousing applications include information retrieval, analysis, and reporting. The data sources for these types of applications are often triggered extracts from on-line transaction processing (OLTP) systems or **operations support systems.** Figure 20.6 lists the attributes of data warehouses.

Benefits of Data Warehousing

Data warehousing offers healthcare organizations a number of benefits, including:

- *Immediate information delivery:* Data warehouses shrink the length of time between the business event and the delivery of relevant event information for decision support.
- *Data integration from across and outside the organization:* Data warehouses combine data from multiple sources, such as billing systems and clinical management systems.

Figure 20.6.   Attributes of a Data Warehouse

DATA
INFORMATION
KNOWLEDGE
INTELLIGENCE

Periodic or real-time refreshment of the database from the source OLTP or OSS applications

Extended-time accumulation of data

Simple restore/recovery

Ability to "can" repetitive user requests

Flexible import/export facilities

Information sharing

Analyst workbench that may include graphics tools, report writers, statistical modeling tools, spreadsheets, simulators, query languages, word processors, desktop publishing, project management software, artificial intelligence tools, data-mining tools, information discovery/exchange tools, and development tools (Boar 1993)

- *Ability to perform trend and outcome analysis:* Data warehouses contain multiple years of cross-departmental data for effective business analysis.
- *Unlimited query and reporting capability:* Data warehouses allow users to run any type of queries/reports to answer any strategic questions that arise during day-to-day operations.
- *Ability to analyze and present data to create business intelligence:* Data warehouses give users tools to look at data differently, for example, tables and graphs that make information available quickly and in easy-to-read formats.
- *Freedom from information systems department resource limitations:* With a data warehouse, users can create most of their reports themselves, thus saving considerable time.

Compared to the costs associated with implementing data warehouses (including hardware/software, development personnel/consultants, and operational costs), the benefits are infinite, including added revenue and reduced costs generated by process redesign. The success of data warehousing is most evident when data warehouses are conceptualized, implemented, and managed as a decision support tool for strategic decision making.

Data Warehousing as a Decision Support Tool

Data warehousing as a decision support tool is invaluable for an organization to incorporate business intelligence. For healthcare organizations, using clinical, financial, and operational information in an integrated decision support database to provide immediate access to healthcare practitioners and management is becoming crucial. Many healthcare organizations struggle with the utilization of data collected throughout their OLTP systems, which is not integrated for management, decision making, and clinical care processes.

Managed care pressures are on the rise, and the marketplace is observing government efforts to better manage Medicare/Medicaid. Expense control, cost avoidance, utilization management of resources, direct provider-to-employer contracting, utilization of data for competitive advantage, and adoption of information technology/automation for increased productivity are no longer mere buzzwords but, instead, are paramount strategic areas of the managed care marketplace. Hence, most healthcare facilities are giving precedence to case management, continuum management, and disease state management initiatives to manage cost, integrate care across the continuum, and align clinical pathways with clinical best practices for optimum patient care at lower costs. Unquestionably, a decision support strategy with data warehousing as its application is critical to meet these challenges.

With its powerful set of tools, data warehousing maximizes a user's ability to leverage and exploit the captured operational data and creates a strategic advantage for organizations. Time is the key factor. A data warehousing strategy allows organizations to compete across time by enabling employees to strategically learn from the past, adapt in the present, and position themselves for the future with the help of the powerful tools supported by this technology (Boar 1993). During the course of business, employees perform many tasks, control processes, share information, and make many decisions. When better information is made available in a timely manner and at the point of need, employees become more empowered, which creates leverage for the organization. Through data warehousing, potent information is made available to all employees so that they can solve problems and make good decisions. This is why data warehousing is considered a rising-tide strategy. When the tide comes in, it raises all the ships in the harbor; similarly, data warehousing raises the strategic acumen of all employees (Boar 1993). In the information age, data warehousing is a key strategic weapon for organizations.

Data Warehousing as a Performance Improvement Tool

As financial and marketplace pressures force healthcare organizations to better integrate all the components of the local healthcare delivery system, many forward-looking organizations have recognized the fact that they cannot improve what they cannot measure. More and more enlightened organizations are empowering their staff, including managers and key stakeholders, with data warehouse–based critical thinking and knowledge management tools to completely transform the way they do business. Instead of running the organization from stacks of paper reports received thirty to forty days after the fact, managers can proactively identify opportunities for performance improvement, cost savings, and revenue enhancements by using point-and-click data-mining tools. The backlog of reports that once existed in information systems is diminishing, and IS departments are shifting from being the total provider of reports to all users to being a conduit and facilitator of knowledge management.

With the power of data warehousing, management can make more complex decisions and manage more data in a shorter time frame with tighter budgets and cost constraints. And, as mentioned earlier, employees are empowered with the right tools so that they can make better and more timely decisions for the benefit of the organization. Data warehousing and disease and case management are crucial for healthcare institutions if they are to integrate all critical service lines to create a healthcare delivery system that offers customers the best experience in a high-quality and cost-effective manner.

For healthcare organizations facing growing pressures to cut costs and maintain high-quality patient care, adopting a data warehouse strategy is a key decision to make. For this strategy to be successful, management must perform an analysis of current systems/processes to identify areas for improvement and target areas that can benefit from the powerful tool of data warehousing. By analyzing the organization's goals, objectives, and vision and comparing them to the decision support systems already in place, management will be able to determine how best to implement a data ware-housing strategy. For the healthcare facility without the abil-ity to provide the right data to the right decision makers at the right time and in the right manner for the areas of patient care, budgeting, planning, research, process improvement initiatives, external reporting, benchmarking, trend analysis, and marketing, data warehousing is the right answer. Imme-diate access to accurate information is the driving force behind the adoption of a data warehouse strategy.

Planning and Implementation of a Data Warehouse

After management has decided to adopt a decision support strategy that involves the establishment of a data warehouse, steps must be taken to properly plan and implement the data warehouse application. These steps include:

1. The business objectives and goals of the healthcare organization must be identified, followed by gap analy-sis for data needs and finalization of the hardware and software requirements.

2. The source systems used to collect data within the healthcare organization must be identified, along with the resources required to establish the data warehouse and data marts for each of the service lines. This includes selection of an implementation team. It is recommended that a decision support core team be designated as the primary repository for financial and clinical data. This core team must collaborate efforts with the IS team, including representation from clinical departments, health information management, information services, and administration. Additionally, it should work with the owners of the source systems to identify the core data elements to feed into the data warehouse.

3. The data to be fed into the data warehouse must be edited and cleansed. Also, time lines for downloading data from the source system to the data warehouse must be defined, along with audits within the ware-house to ensure data integrity.

4. Following the business objectives, data marts should be built and rolled out for identified service lines. The first data mart built should be the executive informa-tion system (EIS), with the data needed by administra-tion to answer the questions that keep them up at night. What follows is the identification, validation, and transfer of needed data from the data warehouse to the EIS. Other service line data marts can be built and cus-tomized as appropriate.

5. Finally, an education program should be implemented to enhance the transition of end users toward knowl-edge management.

To ensure successful implementation of a data warehouse decision support strategy, it is crucial to elicit organizational resources, including management support. Furthermore, meas-ures of success should be delineated to evaluate the strategy's viability and durability. These measures could include the achievement of business goals and objectives such as in-creased revenue/market share, increased patient volume, improved patient outcomes, increased volume of activity on the data warehouse/data marts, increased number of requests for the development of new data marts, and the ability to respond quickly to changes in healthcare. In addition, imple-mentation of a successful data warehouse decision support strategy can produce significant cost savings by eliminating the costly report-writing maintenance of legacy applications, reducing support costs by simplifying operations, and elimi-nating nonessential reports (Evans 1997).

A recent study by a group called IDC, which used infor-mation gathered from more than sixty organizations that had implemented data warehouses, found that data warehousing generated an average ROI of 401 percent over a three-year period. In addition to cost savings and increased revenues, there are other benefits that magnify the ROI for this decision support strategy. These benefits include (Evans 1997):

- More timely information access for decision makers
- Customized information delivery for end users
- Ability of the system to handle large amounts of data while providing fast response time
- State-of-the-art analysis tools that require minimal training time
- Improved management ability to identify trends and change a course of action through increased access to data
- Integrated information from multiple systems in a process that organizes information to allow comparison of multiple time periods from multiple sources

Data Mining

Successful healthcare organizations empower their manage-ment and staff with data warehousing–based critical thinking and knowledge management tools for strategic decision mak-ing. Many healthcare organizations struggle with the utiliza-tion of data collected through their OLTP system, which is not integrated for decision making and pattern analysis.

Healthcare data can be classified into four categories:

- Patient-centric data, which are directly related to patients
- Aggregate data, which are based on performance and utilization/resource management data
- Transformed base data for planning, clinical, and management decision support, which consist of data elements from various sources that are combined, sum-marized, and thus made more relevant and meaningful to decision makers
- Comparative data for healthcare services research and outcomes measurement

The data source is usually the enterprise's OLTP system or operations support system. Thanks to years of accumu-lated disparate data, these systems are data rich, but information poor (Shams and Farishta 2001). With the adoption of data warehousing and data analysis/OLAP tools, an organization can make strides toward leveraging data for better decision making.

Data mining, also known as database exploration and information discovery, brings the practice of information processing closer to providing the answers that organizations want from their data (Ferguson 1997). Healthcare involves massive amounts of data that have no organizational value until they are converted into information and knowledge. Data mining provides automated pattern recognition and attempts to uncover patterns in data that are difficult to detect with traditional statistical methods. Without data mining, it is difficult to realize the full potential of the data collected within an organization because the data under analysis are copious, highly dimensional, widely distributed, and uncertain (Ferguson 1997). For healthcare organizations to succeed, they must be able to capture, store, and analyze their data (Shams and Farishta 2001).

In the early days of data warehousing, data mining was viewed as a subset of the activities associated with the warehouse. Today, data mining is recognized as an independent activity that is paramount for success with data warehouse–based DSSs. It enables users to discover hidden patterns without a predetermined idea or hypothesis about what the patterns may be.

Data-Mining Process

The data-mining process can be divided into two categories: (1) discovering patterns and associations and (2) using the patterns to predict future trends and behaviors (Ferguson 1997). As mentioned earlier, the power of data mining is that it can reveal patterns that the user has not considered in his or her search, producing answers to questions that were never asked. This is especially helpful when dealing with a large database with an infinite number of patterns to identify. Interesting to note is the fact that "the more data in the warehouse, the more patterns there are, and the more data we analyze, the fewer patterns we find" (Parsaye 1996). What this means is that in a large database, it may be best to data-mine different data segments separately so that the influence of one pattern does not dilute the effect of another. At this junction, the user should not fear the loss of certain indicators or patterns in a smaller segment. When a trend or pattern is applicable in an entire database, it also is evident in a smaller segment. Thus, depending on the circumstances and the nature of data in a warehouse, data mining generally can be performed on a segment of data that fits a business objective rather than on the whole warehouse (Parsaye 1996).

Data-mining technology and techniques are invaluable to healthcare management in analyzing clinical and financial data for strategic decision making. Such techniques can help organizations to meet their business objectives for cost control and revenue generation, while maintaining high-quality care for the patients. Moreover, data-mining tools and techniques can ease the burden for management and staff faced with the growing pressures of lower payer reimbursements, increased labor costs, and a highly competitive healthcare marketplace. These tools can work as strategic weapons to convert data into information, creating business intelligence in the process.

In a data mine, analysis for pattern identification is done on a data segment and the process of mining this segment is called an **analysis session.** For example, management may want to predict the response to a flu vaccination initiative for the elderly in the community by analyzing previous initiatives or to know the patient sample over various geographic regions. When a user begins the analysis with a specific task, for instance, analyzing reimbursement by DRGs, the analysis is called a **structured analysis.** Structured analysis is generally done on a routine basis (for example, analysis of quarterly costs, revenues, expenses, and so on) to identify and forecast trends. When the user wanders through a database without a specific goal, he or she may discover interesting patterns or randomly hidden facts. In this case, the analysis is called an **unstructured analysis** (Parsaye 1996). For example, a supermarket may mine their customer data and find that 65 percent of the people who buy tuna fish in a can also buy orange juice at the same time.

The following types of techniques are used in data mining:

- Decision trees
- Genetic algorithms
- Neural networks
- Predictive modeling
- Rule induction (associated rule analysis)
- Fuzzy logic
- K-nearest neighbor

Decision Trees

A **decision tree** is a tree-shaped structure that visually describes a set of rules that caused a decision to be made. For example, it can help determine the factors that affect kidney transplant survival rates.

Decision trees also are techniques that learn and discover patterns from data that have been presented to them. One nice feature of a decision tree is ease of interpretation. Decision tree algorithms operate by searching through the data for the best possible variables on which to divide the data so that new groups resulting from the split will be more alike than the original overall group. The process continues again with each new group. That is, for each new group, the algorithm searches for the best variable on which to split so that the new groups that result from the split will be more alike. The process continues until the algorithm reaches a stopping point using criteria supplied by the user. A classic example of decision tree methodology is the DRG algorithm process used in Medicare reimbursement.

Genetic Algorithms

Genetic algorithms are optimization techniques that can be used to improve other data-mining algorithms so that they derive the best model for a given set of data. For example, algorithms can help determine the optimal treatment plan for a particular diagnosis.

Neural Networks

Neural networks are nonlinear predictive models that learn how to detect a pattern to match a particular profile through a training process that involves interactive learning, using a set of data that describes what the organization wants to find. For example, they can help determine what disease a susceptible patient is likely to contract. Neural networks are good for clustering, sequencing, and predicting patterns. Their drawback is that they do not explain why they have reached a particular conclusion.

Predictive Modeling

Predictive modeling can be used to identify patterns. The patterns then can be used to predict the odds of a particular outcome based on the observed data.

Rule Induction

Rule induction, also referred to as association rule analysis, is the process of extracting useful if–then rules from data based on statistical significance.

Fuzzy Logic

Fuzzy logic handles imprecise concepts. It is more flexible than other techniques. For example, it can help identify patients who are likely to respond to hospital/community initiatives to raise awareness of the cause of AIDS prevention.

K-Nearest Neighbor

K-nearest neighbor (K-NN) is a classic technique for discovering associations and sequences when the data attributes are numeric (Ferguson 1997).

Forms of Data Mining

In the early days, organizations generally followed the "build a warehouse first, mine later" paradigm. Classified by Parsaye as the "sandwich paradigm," this "build first, think later" approach can be considered a "data dump paradigm" because in many cases it leads to the construction of a toxic data dump whose contents are not easily salvageable. A much better way is to "sandwich" the warehousing effort between two layers of mining. The first, preliminary round of mining is considered "premining." Thus, one understands the data before warehousing it. Then the warehouse is built based upon information uncovered during premining. This approach ensures that data mining complements the data warehouse (Parsaye 1995, 1996).

Data mining can exist in the following basic forms:

- *Above the warehouse:* This form of data mining provides a minimal architecture for analysis and pattern identification and is prescribed only when data mining is not a key objective for the warehouse.
- *Beside the warehouse:* This form of data mining allows data mining to be done in specific data segments with specific business objectives, and the exploratory nature of the data-mining exercise does not interfere with the warehouse's routine processes of query and reporting. Data are moved from the warehouse to the mine, restructured during the transformation, and then analyzed.
- *Within the warehouse:* This form of data mining works like a "republic within a republic" and is independent of the warehouse structures. However, it usually leads to loss of flexibility, most often due to the centralization within the warehouse. This form limits significant benefits because problems with mining within the warehouse, once begun, multiply quite rapidly.

In most cases, the beside the warehouse approach is prescribed. Stand-alone data mines also can exist in situations where it takes too long for an organization to build its corporate warehouse. In fact, the stand-alone data mine can be used later as a guide to design the warehouse architecture following the sandwich paradigm mentioned above (Parsaye 1995, 1996).

Selection of Data-Mining Tools

When selecting a data-mining tool or product, it is important to consider how well it integrates with other components of the data warehouse. A two-way exchange interface with an OLAP tool should be done. This allows the OLAP tool to pass selected subsets of the data warehouse to the data-mining tool to be mined for patterns that the OLAP tool has difficulty observing. The data-mining tool then can forward its findings to the OLAP tool to verify them in a larger database.

Additionally, it is important for a data-mining tool to support rule conversion. Converting mined rules into SQL queries allows OLAP and other analysis tools to use the mined rules immediately for data segmentation purposes and makes them available for reuse by other OLAP applications (Ferguson 1997). It is equally important for a data-mining tool to have visualization capabilities. The success of data mining relies on how well the user can view, evaluate, and act on discovered patterns through the user interface tool. The user must have a natural way to view the results of a data-mining activity, and the user interface must integrate seamlessly into the user's current environment for ease of use. The power of automatic pattern discovery is enhanced when patterns can be viewed via charts and tables using color, position, and size differentiators (Ferguson 1997).

Other requirements need to be considered to have success with a data-mining product. The data-mining product architecture must account for scalability and run-time performance in its design and must use multiprocessors to take full advantage of performance-enhancing technology. The product must support a full range of data-mining activities and techniques to enable users to see the same problem from many different angles. In addition, it must support various possible data sources, both internal and external. Finally, the data-mining tool should support data preparation activities, such as data cleansing, data description, data transformation, data sampling, and data pruning (Ferguson 1997).

Customer Relationship Management

Customer relationship management (CRM) is another key knowledge management/business intelligence application. Today, the healthcare industry has to react to empowered customers almost as much as any other industry. The number of people who have searched the Internet for healthcare information doubled in two years to 98 million, with IntelliQuest predicting that the number would grow to 100 million by the end of 2001. Moreover, healthcare consumers are willing to spend their own money to get the kind of care they want. According to the federal Health Care Financing Administration (now renamed the Centers for Medicare and Medicaid Services), private spending on healthcare moved beyond $1.1 trillion in 1998. That number is expected to more than double by 2008, and support for defined contribution plans is rising. Finally, consumers are dissatisfied with the current healthcare picture in which physicians spend less and less time with patients. Increasingly, patients want more personalized care and information. According to a study of patients and physicians conducted by Harris Interactive and AriA Marketing's research group, U.S. consumers want to manage their healthcare through a combination of on-line, phone, and nurse triage services. These findings are echoed by PriceWaterhouseCoopers Healthcast 2010, which found that "speed and service will be the keys to consumer satisfaction" (Paddison 2001a, 2001b).

In this environment, healthcare must take the patient perspective and communicate with patients based on their needs, not solely on the healthcare organization's need to promote its strategic vision. This is not to discount the provider's responsibility to create and maintain organizational awareness and loyalty through more traditional marketing approaches, but it does call for a new model. This paradigm leads to event-driven, one-to-one marketing, which is enabled by CRM solutions (Paddison 2001a, 2001b).

CRM is all about providing products and services to meet customer need when and where the customer wants them. Therefore, CRM requires a focus on business strategy, organizational structure, and organizational culture, as well as technology. CRM aligns these elements with customer information and technology so that all customer interactions can be conducted to the long-term satisfaction of the customer and to the benefit and profit of the organization (Imhoff, Loftis, and Geiger 2001). Thus, the redefined CRM solution for healthcare is built on understanding customer needs and health histories and allowing practitioners to effectively implement and track health promotion and disease prevention programs targeted for specific patients and prospects. This is how CRM enables healthcare to build and maintain individual relationships to increase the lifetime value for each customer (Paddison 2001a, 2001b).

Core Communications Programs

In healthcare, the CRM philosophy is based on communications that include **core communications** at the center, supported and surrounded by branding and strategic communications. (See figure 20.7). The term *core communications* refers to the basic communications that inform customers and others in the community about how they can maintain and improve their health. Core communications are a series of triggered, event-specific communications based on need and data such as age, sex, and health profile that give providers an appropriate time and personalized reason to communicate with the recipients. They include events such as recommended immunizations (tetanus, for example) and screenings (mammography and prostate cancer exams) as well as classes, newcomer programs, physician referral programs, satisfaction and outcome surveys, and customized newsletters.

Branding communications include messages sent to increase awareness and enhance image in the marketplace. A branding program should differentiate the organization from its competitors and persuade consumers that it is the best place to receive such care. Because most traditional tools used in branding (such as media advertising) are not necessarily launched from a CRM system, it is helpful to show how branding fits with and benefits from the CRM structure.

Finally, **strategic communications** are programs created to advance specific organizational goals such as promoting a new center or service, establishing a new program, or positioning the organization as a center of excellence in a specific discipline (for example, cardiology or oncology). Even though strategic goals differ from organization to organization, the CRM system can be used to identify the most attractive candidates for those strategies and to develop messages and offers that promote the organization to customers and track campaign results. These three layers form a complete CRM marketing approach, with core communications and strategic communications largely event driven (Paddison 2001a, 2001b).

Benefits of Core Communications Programs
The core communications program offers the organization several key benefits. Most healthcare organizations want to improve and maintain the health and wellness of their

Figure 20.7.   Application of CRM Philosophy in Healthcare Organizations

CORE COMMUNICATIONS
Triggered and event-driven communications based on need and data (for example, age, gender, and health profile)

BRANDING COMMUNICATIONS
Messages sent to increase awareness and enhance image in the marketplace

STRATEGIC COMMUNICATIONS
Programs created to advance specific organizational goals

communities. The essence of a core communications program is to inform people of events designed to improve their health, thus making it an important and effective tool in achieving a wellness mission. Customer retention also will increase as organizations engage customers in activities that are of interest and importance to them. This, in turn, will increase loyalty and foster long-term relationships and greater customer lifetime value.

In addition, because these communications are targeted only to the individuals for whom they are most relevant, organizations can lower marketing costs significantly and either retain the savings or apply them to other marketing programs. The core communications program also is a great way to begin leveraging the several hundreds of thousands of dollars required to develop and implement the CRM solution. Finally, after an organization has identified the events to include in its core communications and has created the messages for various channels, the program runs itself. An automated program sends out the event-triggered communications and notifies the appropriate individuals of the action (Paddison 2001a, 2001b).

Implementation of Core Communications Programs

Putting a core communications program into action involves the following steps:

1. Identify the need. Different individuals have different healthcare needs at different times in their lives. Identifying those needs and matching them to events the organization wants to promote is extremely crucial.
2. Identify the events to promote. These might include immunizations, screenings, wellness classes, and so on.
3. Define selection criteria. These criteria are used to determine who should receive each communication based on information in the CRM database. This information will minimally include age and sex but also could include information such as payer type, health status, and so on.
4. Determine the timing for the campaign.
5. Determine the message to communicate. The message should go to the selected audiences with an offer that will prompt a response.
6. Determine how to communicate on a customer-by-customer basis, for instance via the Internet, direct mail, or calls from the call center (Paddison 2001a, 2001b).

Adoption of a Customer Relationship Management Philosophy

Adoption of the true CRM philosophy will change the order of things within the organization. CRM implementation requires careful planning, an understanding of its critical success factors, and the ability to manage its success factors while continuing to facilitate change. A sustainable CRM-friendly culture must be established in an organization. Several factors can be monitored to ensure that the culture will enable a customer focus. Service staff must understand the positive impacts that can result from satisfied customers. They must be generally accepting and enthusiastic about the customer satisfaction aspects of their positions. Finally, their job skills must be assessed and be adequate for implementing a CRM strategy (Imhoff, Loftis, and Geiger 2001).

The presence of an information management structure is very important in the adoption of a CRM philosophy. The information management infrastructure needs to be in place on both the IT and business sides. Building a CRM strategy without excellent customer information is similar to building a house without a foundation. Managing customers depends on being able to manage large amounts of information about them. And like every other asset, information should be controlled, maintained, and enhanced. However, unlike other assets, information is used by everyone in the organization. Controlling and maintaining information is a very complex task. As a supporting block of a CRM initiative, the information must be accurate and up-to-date. Therefore, customer information management is critical to CRM success (Meza 1998).

Many organizations today have legacy systems, and every line of business has its own customer database. The reality is that the information in these disparate databases is rarely shared effectively across business lines. This so-called silo approach creates an environment that breeds poor data quality and leads to a poor understanding of the organization's customers. Organizations must encourage enterprisewide understanding of their customer relationships and ensure that all distribution channels and customer touch points share consistent information regarding customer relationships (Meza 1998).

In addition to the emphasis on a customer-based culture and the importance of a solid information management structure, technology plays a key role in the adoption of a CRM philosophy. The ability to develop the CRM program requires the creation of a marketing database powered by the Web. The unique blueprint or data model must be industry focused, market driven, and technology enabled (Paddison 2001a, 2001b). The components of a mature healthcare data repository that provides a near-complete view of individual patient and prospect activities are necessary. The correct tools must be applied to make the database fulfill the tasks for which it was designed, which include analyzing and mining the data for information opportunities. This software, based on algorithms and statistics, can be grouped into three categories: information delivery and data analysis, data mining, and campaign management. All information should be accessible to the user on the desktop through standard word-processing and spreadsheet software (Paddison 2001a, 2001b).

After the data warehouse is built, the organization must develop a strategic plan to take full advantage of the CRM program's capabilities. Key questions to consider include:

- What do I want to accomplish with my CRM program?
- Where are my opportunities?

- Who are my individual customers?
- What is the makeup of their household?
- What do they need? What is their health status?
- Are they insured?
- What message do I need to communicate to them?

A CRM market plan might include an overall evaluation of services and products for value and efficiency, an overall market evaluation for revenue opportunities and growth areas, identification of the size of the market by total number of customers and analysis of the current market share compared with the competitors' share, the development/marketing of programs that can improve wellness and quality of life, and the tracking and evaluation of communications efforts and annual refinement (Paddison 2001a, 2001b).

The CRM strategy must be flexible and remain relevant to changing times (Meza 1998). Understanding the customer base as an asset, with a strategy of differentiation through customer service, provides the foundation for a successful CRM solution (Byrne 2001). When implemented correctly, a CRM program can give organizations the ability to fully understand their customers' needs and expectations across the lines of business and at every point of interaction. Moreover, it can integrate sales, marketing, and customer service initiatives in a manner that optimizes the customer relationship and the customer experience (Meza 1998).

The degree to which an organization is able to change depends on its ability to strengthen customer relationships through improvements in the availability, access, and accuracy of customer information and to eliminate non-value-added activities to streamline business processes across the organization. It also is important to develop a learning organization that addresses the issues of training and change because information and processes alone are not sufficient when the right people to service the customer are unavailable.

A training program must include all levels of the organization and stress the importance of customer information management and data quality and how they relate to the successful implementation of a CRM strategy (Meza 1998). In conclusion, healthcare organizations must not forsake the ultimate goal of providing high-quality and consistent service to each customer during each interaction, regardless of the channel. CRM is the cornerstone for accomplishing this goal.

Check Your Understanding 20.2

Instructions: Answer the following questions on a separate piece of paper.

1. What is a learning organization?

2. What are the four categories of healthcare data?

3. What is a data warehouse? What purpose does it fulfill in knowledge management?

4. What function(s) does data mining play in knowledge management?

5. Name the three basic forms of data mining.

6. What is customer relationship management?

7. Explain the differences among core communications, branding communications, and strategic communications.

Application of Knowledge Management to Decision Making

The preceding sections of this chapter focused on providing an overview of key knowledge management applications in healthcare—data warehousing, data mining, and customer relationship management. These applications play a key role in a learning or knowledge management organization in which data act as the primary source of manipulation to navigate through the decision-making process. Data can be used in several areas, including patient care, process reengineering, quality improvement, clinical and management decision making, basic and applied research, health services research, external reporting, strategic planning, market trend analysis, and more. Various sources of the healthcare data include operational information systems and on-line transaction processing systems, legacy systems, departmental databases, primary research data, and secondary research data sources.

As mentioned previously, there is immense data chaos in healthcare because of disparate data sources and extensive amounts of data. Hence, business intelligence inquiry can rarely begin with a precisely framed question. Often knowledge workers need to navigate through the data and ask questions based on what they see at the time in order to discover valuable information in the form of trends and patterns. For this reason, data from different sources need to be analyzed and summarized to get meaningful insight, which needs to be presented to other users in the system for effective and timely decision making.

Thus, the decision-making process can be divided into the following three phases:

1. The *discovery phase* involves looking at comparisons and exceptions and examining data from many different dimensions to identify trends and patterns. Discovery tools include OLAP, data mining, and other query tools.
2. The *analysis phase* focuses on proving that the identified trends do exist, understanding them, forecasting them over time, and making solid predictions about their consequences. Analysis tools include modeling, market research, what-if analysis, and so on.
3. The *presentation phase* involves the creation of the reports that are most appropriate for the organization's goals and objectives. Presentation tools include data visualization, geographical analysis, bubble charts, and multimedia viewers. These tools must be easy to use and data driven, with drag-and-drop functionality and summarization logic.

It is important here to further explore on-line analytical processing (OLAP) as one of the discovery tools besides data mining. OLAP is a software configuration that provides a fast way to view and analyze data from any perspective without having to specify the perspective and the exact level of detail required in advance. In other words, OLAP offers fast access to multidimensional information for exploitation in a wider business intelligence context. To leverage an organization's operational data to create strategic acumen, OLAP supports data warehousing as a decision support tool. Using OLAP, enterprises can drive decision support, do trend analysis, compare business units, and monitor strategic business decisions.

An OLAP engine is an optimized query generator that can retrieve the right information from the warehouse to accommodate what-if business queries. OLAP data are presented in a way that reflects multiple business dimensions: patients admitted per quarter by disease category, costs per service line by region, medical supplies shipped on time per department per hospital, and so on. This type of information allows managers to conduct effective comparison and trend analysis. OLAP makes it possible to analyze potentially large amounts of data with very fast response times. It also enables users to slice and dice through the data and drill down or roll up through various dimensions as defined by the data structure (Hettler 1997).

A knowledge worker may want to move progressively into more detail or drill down into summarized data. This capability is extremely valuable in investigating what exists at different levels of detail. By enabling multidimensional analysis, business performance reporting, and business modeling, OLAP data sources play a pivotal role in a data warehousing initiative. In addition, OLAP is ideal for meeting business users' requirements because with it, information is stored in an intuitive business structure, is easy to use, and can be delivered to many users within the enterprise. Users can ask questions of the data naturally—in the way they think—without worrying about how the database will interpret their queries. OLAP is also faster, which means users obtain answers more quickly and are likely to use it more often (Hettler 1997).

An organization's success depends on its ability to make timely and efficient decisions. Most HCOs have the data but do not have the ability to turn the data into information and knowledge. This ability to provide complete and high-quality information and knowledge for better decision making will determine not only who survives, but also who thrives in today's constantly changing and competitive healthcare marketplace.

For healthcare organizations to survive under current market pressures, they must react quickly to seize growth- and quality-enhancing opportunities as they arise. Moreover, they must give their customers the ability to interact effortlessly with the organization. This requires that all departments and functions of the organization be integrated with coherent data and information flow among all users. Organizations must work collectively with all their departments to understand how to access the information to improve business and clinical decision making.

In addition, organizations must track progress toward goals and targets across the various departments to provide an integrated picture of where the hospital stands. Finally, they must provide a balanced view of the organization that transcends both financial and clinical data to create direct cause-and-effect relationships between operational and strategic directives.

Data warehousing, data mining, CRM, and other knowledge management applications help organizations address these essential needs. They also help organizations meet their objectives for smart organizational planning and operations; process and outcomes improvement; disease, case, and care management; risk management; cash flow improvement; outcome measurement; cost and clinical effectiveness assessment; and so on.

These applications help transform data into business intelligence so that an organization can make strategic decisions and act on the knowledge it has acquired to improve overall performance.

Without question, an organizational culture that cultivates knowledge sharing is critical to the successful implementation of knowledge management applications. As economist Lester C. Thurow discusses in *Building Wealth: The New Rules for Individuals, Companies, and Nations in a Knowledge-Based Economy,* people tend to resist sharing their knowledge when they believe that doing so will undermine their value to the organization (Allison 2000). If the organization aims to successfully integrate knowledge management at its core, management must eliminate this barrier by creating an environment of trust. This is a distinguishing characteristic of a learning organization, which focuses on efficiently acquiring knowledge from different sources, both within and outside the organization. A learning organization uses technology such as data warehousing to ensure that information is available to all employees at the right time and in the right way in order to raise the organization's strategic acumen.

Chief Knowledge Officer

With the importance of a knowledge-sharing culture in mind, a healthcare organization can successfully implement knowledge management applications through the creation of a chief knowledge officer (CKO) position. The individual in this position would oversee the entire knowledge acquisition, storage, and dissemination process and identify subject matter experts to help capture and organize the organization's knowledge assets. Management should give the CKO authority to research and obtain enabling technologies that would capture and leverage information from the various knowledge assets. To organize this process, the CKO creates a knowledge map to ensure that relevant information sources within the organization are identified and obsolete and/or incorrect information sources are discarded. The CKO also can ensure that an incentive system is in place to encourage knowledge workers to share their knowledge with others in the system. A useful technique might be to reward workers for reusing knowledge and contributing to the corporate knowledge base. This position also might create a "one-stop shop" where knowledge would be accessible to all. Finally, the CKO position can take the leadership in advocating constant change and innovation to capture and improve the use of knowledge.

Check Your Understanding 20.3

Instructions: Answer the following questions on a separate piece of paper.

1. What role(s) do knowledge workers play in organizational decision making?

2. Describe the roles of discovery, analysis, and presentation in the decision-making process.

3. What is OLAP, and what role does it play in decision support systems?

4. What role does the CKO play in a healthcare organization?

Real-World Case

Begun in 1935 as the 47-bed Gregg Memorial Hospital, Good Shepherd Medical Center (GSMC) has since grown to a 349-bed regional referral center for specialized care with the largest trauma center in Longview, Tex. A nonprofit medical center, GSMC is funded solely from patient revenue and community support and receives no public support from any taxing authority. In 1996, the center provided $28 million of uncompensated care to the residents of eastern Texas, largely through the ongoing support of the Good Shepherd Foundation, the Good Shepherd Guild, and the Good Shepherd Prospectors. In 1999, it was named one of the 100 top hospitals nationally for case management and its orthopedic departments and intensive care units.

Wiley Thomas, CIO at GSMC, was faced with the challenges of effective knowledge management that many hospitals face today. The hospital had embarked on a case management program, and data/administrative automation was critical to its success. As Thomas explained, "Appropriate clinical utilization is the name of the game. It is vital that we have technology that meets our very special needs of disease and case management, and also has the capability to empower our clinical decision makers, which includes physicians, to feel comfortable with the data to make clinically appropriate changes in practice patterns."

Thomas responded to these challenges by making data warehouse technology GSMC's computer-based patient record (CPR) foundation using a data warehousing/data repository solution. To date, the hospital has saved more than $3 million in case management and been recognized in *Modern Healthcare* for its success.

Before case management was implemented at Good Shepherd, the average length of stay (ALOS) for a coronary artery bypass patient also having a cardiac catheterization during his stay was 14.7 days. At that time, the HCFA ALOS for that patient type was 12.1 days. Two years after GSMC implemented its case management initiative, the ALOS for these patients plummeted to 10.3 days, less than the HCFA average of 10.8 days.

The case management software used by GSMC pinpoints areas where costs are excessive, allowing doctors and case managers to work together to find an equally effective and less costly treatment option. Quarterly reports consisting of charts and graphs show precisely which physicians are using effective, cost-efficient treatment options. The reports are seen by physicians and reviewed by administration and the executive board. One of the reports includes a top ten DRG section that lists the physicians with the highest dollar charges. Another report shows the top five physicians with the highest expenditures.

Case managers are assigned to specific areas to determine the average cost of patient treatment and to compare it with Medicare. Case management software not only organizes and calculates the information but also allows each case manager to track individual patients and to tie them back to the physicians who treated them.

Financial outcome is another aspect that is affected by the case management software, which reduces the time required to track treatments and ALOS. Case management has grown tremendously since the software's implementation. Initially, one nurse was the liaison to cardiovascular patients, but because of the tremendous savings, twelve case managers now handle the steadily growing workload. The case management software helped give GSMC the means to cut costs without sacrificing patient care.

Discussion Questions

1. Aside from the challenges mentioned in the case study, what are some other issues that the CIO would need to consider? Could these issues be solved with the alternative that was chosen for the hospital? If not, can you think of any other alternative that would solve these issues?

2. It was stated by the CIO that when choosing a solution, he would have to make sure that the physicians "feel comfortable with the data to make clinically appropriate changes in practice patterns." To what extent will these changes affect the hospital?

3. Take the five steps of the knowledge management process and apply them to this case study. If you were the CIO of the hospital, would you add, skip, or change any steps? Which ones and why?

4. Would any other knowledge management application mentioned in this chapter help in the data management problem of the hospital? Keeping in mind the cost (both in time and money) to implement an application, how much would it benefit the hospital?

5. After reviewing this case study, discuss how important you believe data warehousing is to the success of a healthcare organization. Keep the section entitled *Data Warehousing as a Performance Improvement Tool* in mind as you answer this question.

Summary

Knowledge management is the process of collecting and processing information, using it, sharing it, and enhancing it to improve the business practice of healthcare organizations. The maintenance of knowledge is crucial to an organization's viability and ability to reach its peak performance level. Knowledge management involves the transformation of data into information, then into knowledge. The process of knowledge management, with its various components and applications, can enhance clinical and financial decision making.

Before embarking on a knowledge management initiative, it is important to identify the sources of knowledge, or knowledge assets, of an organization. It is also crucial to develop an organized framework to capture knowledge and transform it into business intelligence. There are five steps in a knowledge management initiative that guarantee the transformation of an ordinary organization into a learning organization. The final step involves the deployment and implementation of knowledge management and business intelligence applications. These applications play a key role in a learning or knowledge management organization in which data act as the primary source of manipulation to navigate through a decision-making process.

This chapter addressed three of these applications in detail, including data warehousing, data mining, and customer relationship management, which are the cornerstones of the healthcare landscape. These applications transform knowledge into wisdom, which gives organizations the ability to make decisions in a timely manner, improve their performance and operations, and respond to their most important customers—the patients.

It is also important to understand the decision-making process and its phases and to have an organizational culture that cultivates knowledge sharing when the organization aims to successfully integrate knowledge management at its core.

References

Allison, Bryan. 2000. Catching the next wave. *DM Direct,* July.

Boar, B. 1993. *The Art of Strategic Planning for Information Technology: Crafting Strategy for the 90s.* New York City: John Wiley & Sons.

Brackett, M. 1995. *The Data Warehouse Challenge: Taming Data Chaos.* New York City: John Wiley & Sons.

Brohan, M. 2001. The changing face of business intelligence applications. *DM Review,* November.

Byrne, Rory. 2001. Unified customer interaction: bridging the physical/virtual world gap. *DM Direct,* May.

English, Larry P. 1999. Information quality in the knowledge age. *DM Review,* October.

Evans, Jim. 1997. Need for analysis drives data warehouse appeal. *Health Management Technology* 18(11): 28–31.

Farishta, Mehnaz. 2001. Mining your data for decision-making success. *Journal of the American Health Information Management Association* 72(10): 29–32.

Ferguson, Mike. 1997. Evaluating and selecting data mining tools. *InfoDB,* November.

Gallagher Financial System, Inc. 1999. Knowledge management and knowledge automation systems. White paper.

Goldman, Lawrence. 2001. Customer relationship management: refine, not rebuild your data warehouse. *DM Review Online,* November.

Grammer, Jeff. 2000. The enterprise knowledge portal. *DM Review,* March.

Hettler, Mark. 1997. Data mining goes multidimensional. *Healthcare Informatics,* March.

Imhoff, Claudia, Lisa Loftis, and Jonathan Geiger. 2001. *Building the Customer-Centric Enterprise.* New York City: John Wiley & Sons.

Kimball, R., et al. 1998. *The Data Warehouse Lifecycle Toolkit: Expert Methods for Designing, Developing, and Deploying Data Warehouses.* New York City: John Wiley & Sons.

Lambert, Bob. 1996. Data warehousing fundamentals: what you need to know to succeed. *Data Management Review,* March.

Loshin, David. 2001. Intelligent information processing. *DM Review,* July.

Meza, Juan. 1998. Customer information management: the critical foundation to a CRM strategy. *DM Direct,* September.

Paddison, Nancy. 2001a. Benefits of event-driven CRM in healthcare, part 1. *DM Direct,* January.

Paddison, Nancy. 2001b. Benefits of event-driven CRM in healthcare, part 2. *DM Direct,* February.

Parsaye, K. 1995. The sandwich paradigm for data warehousing and mining. *Database Programming and Design,* April.

Parsaye, K. 1996. Data mines for data warehouses. White paper. Information Discovery Inc.

Penny, Paul. 2000. Knowledge management: maximizing the return on your intellectual assets. *DM Direct,* September.

Shams, K., and M. Farishta. 2001. Data warehousing: toward knowledge management. *Topics in Health Information Management* 21:(3): 24-32.

Wu, Jonathan. 2000. Business intelligence: the transition of data into wisdom. *DM Review Online,* November.

Application Exercises

1. Define the role of decision support systems in the healthcare industry.

2. Define knowledge management as a business discipline and explain why knowledge management might be defined as a discipline rather than a technology.

3. Compare and contrast the old and new healthcare paradigms and discuss the role of knowledge management in the new paradigm. Identify which paradigm your healthcare organization falls under and explain your choice.

4. Discuss some of the challenges that healthcare organizations face with regard to data management and how knowledge management can play a positive role in addressing these challenges.

5. Explain how knowledge management helps in transforming data into knowledge and wisdom.

6. Explain the framework of a knowledge management initiative and how you might apply it to your healthcare organization.

7. Name and briefly describe some knowledge management applications in the healthcare industry and discuss whether they are being used in your organization.

8. Discuss why healthcare management and staff should be empowered with data warehousing skills and explain why data warehousing is a rising-tide strategy.

9. You are charged with implementing a data warehouse at a 256-bed acute care facility in a rural area. How will you begin this project, and what steps will you follow during its implementation?

10. As a knowledge worker in a health network, you have been assigned the task of determining which patients from your healthcare database are likely to respond to hospital/community initiatives to raise awareness of AIDS prevention. How will you begin this assignment, and what knowledge management application(s) will you use?

11. As vice president of operations in a large community hospital, you have been asked to present a report on the importance of a CRM solution to your board of directors. What will you include in your preliminary report?

12. You have recently been promoted from your current position to the newly created position of a chief knowledge officer (CKO) as part of the knowledge management initiative undertaken at your hospital. Discuss how you will position yourself as CKO, and discuss your roles and responsibilities.

Review Quiz

Instructions: Choose the best answer to the following questions.

1. ___ What is knowledge management?
   a. The process of managing knowledge
   b. The process of collecting data and manipulating it to make an organization look intelligent
   c. The process of transforming data into information, then into knowledge that can be shared within an organization
   d. The process of ensuring that the managers of an organization are well-informed

2. ___ What do information assets include?
   a. Databases, documents, tacit knowledge, and so on
   b. Documents only
   c. Information not shared among workers
   d. Confidential information about patients

3. ___ What are the building blocks of knowledge management?
   a. Workers
   b. Data
   c. Computers
   d. CIOs

4. ___ What is the difference between information and knowledge?
   a. Knowledge is derived from information
   b. Information is mundane and knowledge is not
   c. Information cannot be shared but knowledge can be shared
   d. Information is more important to an organization than knowledge

5. ___ What is the difference between explicit knowledge and tacit knowledge?
   a. Tacit knowledge is documented while explicit is not
   b. Certain workers cannot know about explicit knowledge
   c. Certain workers cannot know about tacit knowledge
   d. Explicit knowledge is documented while tacit knowledge is implied

6. ___ What is one benefit of knowledge management implementation in a healthcare setting?
   a. Users can make intelligent decisions
   b. Workers can get their work done faster and more efficiently
   c. Hospital users can extract all patient data from a central database
   d. All of the above

7. ___ What is a data warehouse?
   a. The metaphorical term for a computer lab in a large organization
   b. A location in an organization where workers meet to share knowledge
   c. A centralized location that contains all of an organization's data
   d. Pattern recognition

8. ___ What are the attributes of a data warehouse?
   a. Periodic or real-time refresh of the database from the source OLTP application
   b. Extended time accumulation of data
   c. Information sharing
   d. All of the above

9. ___ What are the business/financial benefits of a data warehouse?
   a. Immediate information delivery
   b. Data integration from across and outside the organization
   c. Ability to perform trend and outcomes analysis
   d. Unlimited query and reporting capability
   e. All of the above

10. ___ What challenges does the healthcare industry face in the area of data management?
   a. The healthcare industry does not have enough resources to implement information technology tools
   b. The healthcare industry is data rich and information poor
   c. Hospitals have too many patients and not enough beds
   d. Doctors feel that hospitals are not well managed

11. ___ What are the prerequisites for a successful implementation of a data warehouse?
   a. Ensure that management support is elicited
   b. Ensure that the right resources are allocated
   c. Ensure that the measures of success are delineated to evaluate the viability of the data warehousing strategy
   d. All of the above

12. ___ How are healthcare data categorized?
   a. Patient-centric data, aggregate data, transformed base data, comparative data
   b. Patient data, family history data, disease data, personal data
   c. Policy data, registration data, operation data, case management data
   d. Big data, small data, important data, irrelevant data

13. ___ What is data mining?
   a. Automatic search of incorrect data in patient records
   b. Random data generation to replace missing data in patient records
   c. Uncovering of hidden patterns in data
   d. None of the above

14. ___ What does OLAP do?
   a. Shows multiple amounts of data on one page
   b. Offers fast access to multidimensional information from any different perspective
   c. Analyzes data to predict future trends
   d. All of the above

15. ___ What are the various techniques of data mining?
   a. Decision trees and genetic algorithms
   b. Neural networks and predictive modeling
   c. Rule induction, k-nearest neighbor, and fuzzy logic
   d. All of the above

16. ___ What is an analysis session?
   a. Supervisors meet to detect flaws in the system
   b. Analysis for pattern identification on a data segment
   c. Patient records are broken apart to create categorical data
   d. None of the above

17. ___ What is a prerequisite for selecting a data mining tool?
   a. Consider whether integration will be successful
   b. Make sure there are no visualization capabilities
   c. Ensure that doctors do not feel comfortable using the selected tool
   d. None of the above

18. ___ What is customer relationship management?
   a. Providing products and services to meet customer needs
   b. Management of patients' personal needs
   c. Ensuring that the customer does not violate hospital codes
   d. Both a and c

19. ___ How can healthcare organizations benefit from a CRM philosophy?
   a. They can ensure patient satisfaction
   b. The hospital can focus on making more money
   c. Healthcare organizations will thrive when no one is in need of care
   d. None of the above

20. ___ What is the goal of a core communications program?
   a. Make sure that patients are clearly aware of hospital rules
   b. Create a clear communication path among patients and doctors
   c. Create a clear communication path between doctors and administration
   d. Inform patients of events designed to improve their health

21. ___ What are the three phases of the decision-making process using business intelligence or knowledge management applications?
   a. Review, discuss, decide
   b. Discuss, decide, approve
   c. Discovery, analysis, presentation
   d. Research, analyze, resolve

22. ___ What is the role of a chief knowledge officer (CKO) in a learning organization?
   a. A CKO is in charge of managing the healthcare organization's administrative operations
   b. A CKO ensures that patient information does not fall into the wrong hands
   c. A CKO encourages workers to share knowledge and ensures that knowledge is accessible to all
   d. A CKO is responsible for data security and the management of workers in the organization

Part VI

Management of Health Information Services

Chapter 21
Principles of Management and Leadership

David X. Swenson, PhD

Learning Objectives

- To introduce the management discipline, the evolution of management thought, and the key functions and skills of management
- To identify significant trends in managerial models
- To understand that management approaches emerge in response to change drivers of a particular period
- To identify key theorists in the development of management practices
- To describe the four functions of management
- To describe the ten roles of a manager
- To describe the relationship between management functions and skills, and levels of management

- To explain the differences between managers and leaders
- To recognize the traits related to leadership effectiveness
- To understand that leadership style needs to adjust to various situations
- To describe the steps in effective problem solving and decision making
- To explain the importance of effective communication
- To recognize the stages of organizational change
- To recognize ways of facilitating transition in order to minimize stress to people and production

Key Terms

Acceptance theory of authority
Active listening
Administrative management
Appreciative inquiry
Balanced scorecard (BSC)
Baldridge Award
Benchmarking
Bounded rationality
Break-even analysis
Bureaucracy
Business process reengineering (BPR)
Champion
Change agent
Change drivers
Charisma
Conceptual skills
Consideration
Contingency model of leadership
Control
Critic
Critical path method
Decentralization
Delegation
Diffusion S curve
Discipline
Downsizing

Early adopters
Early majority
Effectiveness
Efficiency
85/15 rule
Ending
Evidence-based management
Executive dashboard
Expectancy theory
Forecasting
Fourteen principles of management
Gantt chart
Great person theory
Hawthorne effect
Hierarchy of needs
Human relations movement
Initiating structure
Innovators
Interpersonal skills
Intuition
Inventor
ISO 9000
Laggards
Late majority
Leader-member relations
Leadership grid
Leading

Least Preferred CoWorker Scale (LPC)
Line authority
Linear programming
Management by objectives (MBO)
Management functions
Mission statement
Neutral zone
New beginnings
Nonprogrammed decision
Normative Decision Model
Operational plan
Operations management
Organization development (OD)
Organizing
Paradigm
Path-goal theory
Piece-rate incentive
Planning
Position power
Program evaluation and review technique (PERT)
Programmed decisions
Queuing theory
Reflective learning cycle
Refreezing
Satisficing

Scalar chain
Self-monitoring
Simulation and inventory modeling
Span of control
Sponsor
Staff authority
Stages of grief
Strategic plan
Survey feedback
Synergy
System
Systems theory
Tactical plan
Task structure
Team building
Technical skills
Theory X and Y
Time and motion studies
Total quality management (TQM)
Trait approach
Transactional leadership
Transformational leadership
Unfreezing
Vertical structure
Worker Immaturity–Maturity

Introduction

"Permanent whitewater" is the phrase often used to describe the turbulent nature of the emerging business environment, the world that managers must understand and in which they operate daily (Vaill 1996). Models for management originally were based on traditional ways of organizing people to accomplish tasks. For thousands of years, these involved small family cottage industries, military organizations, or church-directed structures. With the advent of the industrial revolution, migration to cities, and specialization of labor, the former methods of management no longer worked effectively. Workers did not necessarily carry on family traditions, could not be commanded to comply with orders, and did not serve out of dedication to some larger corporate value. New ways of thinking about management were needed.

In 1962, Thomas Kuhn published *The Structure of Scientific Revolutions.* Translated into twenty languages and cited by scholars in numerous fields, it has been a reference point for new management thinkers. Kuhn introduced the concept of a **paradigm,** a mental model or structure for perceiving, understanding, and responding to the world. Paradigms make thinking more efficient by drawing attention to certain things, but they also filter out exceptions to the rules where innovations may lie. He argued that scientific progress, rather than growing slowly and incrementally, more often occurs when complexity increases to a high degree and cannot be adequately dealt with by the current paradigm. A paradigm shift then occurs, and the old one is replaced with a new one.

A key idea in management is the recognition that management theories and practices grow out of the unique constellation of forces or change drivers that operate at the time. These large-scale forces consist of demographic, social, political, economic, technical, and, more recently, global and informational factors. In a competitive environment, each organization seeks to position itself to succeed against other organizations and does so by the effective and efficient allocation of its resources to respond to these demands. Leadership is a key component of organizations, and the role of leadership throughout the organization is expanding.

This chapter describes some of the historical landmarks in management theory that have led to the present thinking about management. It also describes the role of the organizational leader, the process of organization development, and how such transition can be facilitated. Finally, it identifies some of the trends that may help us understand the future directions of organizational behavior that must be managed and the skills for doing so.

Theory into Practice

Three years ago, Northern General Hospital merged with St. Vincent Hospital. The merger was intended to take advantage of the complementary specialized services each hospital provided, and both had equally talented staff and strong reputations in the region. Although the organizations had blended rather well, unforeseen problems emerged.

After the merger, duplicate positions were eliminated, a single vision statement had been formulated, and the organizational hierarchy was flattened. Yet, morale was low and turnover continued to be higher than expected, even among staff who were secure in their positions. Conflict between employees, and between managers and employees, became a constant concern.

As management began to examine the problem areas, it became clear that the two hospitals were financially, operationally, and organizationally compatible; however, much less attention and preparation had been given to the human aspects of organizational change. Although executed fairly, the downsizing disrupted long-standing relationships, job security, and management–employee trust. Knowing that merged organizations often experience two to three subsequent downsizings, employees were waiting for the next round of layoffs. The flatter structure and lower staff sizes required remaining staff to take on multiple roles and heavier workloads. High performers were encouraged to take on more leadership roles in addition to their regular work; many such ad hoc managers were talented in their fields but had little managerial or leadership experience.

Moreover, the cultures of the two facilities were markedly different, both a strength and a source of conflict. Before the merger, Northern General provided a wide range of health services including abortion and contraception; St. Vincent traditionally limited such services. Several groups of physicians left the merged facility to avoid ethical conflicts.

The health information management (HIM) department was at the heart of the organization in many ways. HIM staff were integrating two different information systems, taking on key roles in developing the new balanced scorecard, and trying to orient staff to the new forms of documentation—all the while dealing with their own uncertainties. They were discovering how essential it was to have a clear understanding of successful management styles and theories that could become the blueprint for the emerging organization.

Landmarks in Management as a Discipline

A **discipline** is a field of study characterized by a knowledge base and perspective that is distinctive from other fields of study. The knowledge base and perspective form a foundation for the discipline's practices, guide research for continuing refinement, and create its literature base. As the study of management found its way into academic settings, theories and practices of management began to emerge. Changing social conditions and growing technological innovations often contributed to the way that management theories were framed.

Scientific Management

The late nineteenth and early twentieth centuries marked the emergence of many elements of modern management theory. German sociologist, lawyer, and political economist Max Weber (1864–1920) was formulating his ideas of the ideal or prototypic organization. Recognizing the inefficiency that was occurring with high variability in standards, he proposed that organizations become **bureaucracies.** He believed that variability could be reduced by having a formally structured hierarchy of relationships, by formulating rules and regulations to standardize behavior, and by using trained specialists for jobs. As a result, efficiency could be promoted, subjective judgment and favoritism could be eliminated, and planning could be based on the position rather than the person. At a time when organizational procedures were highly variable, bureaucratic theory offered the structure necessary to improve performance. In the modern marketplace where competitive advantage is maintained through innovation, bureaucracy has come more often to refer to slow decision making, unresponsiveness, ignoring the uniqueness of individuals, and rules without reasons.

About the same time that Weber was forming his ideas about bureaucracy, Frederick W. Taylor (1856–1915) was a young engineer working at the Midvale Steel Company. He discovered that his company and most others had tremendous unused potential. Pay and working conditions were poor, waste and inefficiency were prevalent, and management decision making was unsystematic and not based on research of any sort. Taylor introduced new practices whose success led to his being recognized as the Father of Scientific Management. Although many of his ideas are commonly accepted today, they were revolutionary at the time.

Taylor defined the main objective of managers to be that of securing maximum prosperity for employer and employee. He viewed management and the workforce as interdependent and promoted the idea that people were inherently capable of hard work. The problem, he argued, was that the old management stifled workers and could be remedied by his four principles:

1. Management should develop a scientific approach to work, involving precise, measurable guidelines for output; pay could be linked to performance.
2. Management should scientifically select, train, and develop workers to be first class so that the right person has the right job.
3. Management and workers should collaborate to ensure that the job matches plans.
4. Management should provide equal division of work and responsibility between workers and management.

To implement his ideas, Taylor and his followers developed new techniques. **Time and motion studies,** for example, were conducted in which tasks were subdivided into their most basic movements. Detailed motions were timed to determine the most efficient way of carrying them out. After the one best way was found, the best worker match for the job was hired, tools and procedures were standardized, instruction cards were written to guide workers, and breaks were instituted to reduce fatigue. From implementing new practices, one mining company increased production from 12.5 to 47 tons of loaded pig iron per day and reduced the number of yard laborers from 600 to 140 with no reduction in output. A **piece-rate incentive** system also was developed in which workers received additional pay when they exceeded the standard output level for their task.

Taylor's principles were quickly embraced and later refined by Frank and Lillian Gilbreth, Henry Gantt, and others. The Gilbreths were a husband and wife team who developed many of the early ideas of ergonomics and work efficiency. Their original studies focused on bricklaying, part of Frank's background, in which they noticed that workers developed their own ways of working and that no two workers used the same method. The Gilbreths divided the process into detailed individual motions they called "therbligs" (Gilbreth nearly spelled backwards) to identify unnecessary or inefficient motions. Seeking the single best way to perform the tasks, they reduced the number of motions for bricklaying from 18 to 4.5, which resulted in much higher productivity, less fatigue, and better planning. Lillian (1878–1972) was known for her studies on finding innovative ways to design efficient kitchen and home living areas for patients with cardiac-limited conditions.

Frank Gilbreth (1868–1924) embraced time saving with a passion and gained notoriety with his experiments. For example, he would experiment to see whether it would be faster to button his vest from top to bottom or the reverse. He tried to shave with two razors, but the time saving was reduced by having to patch his several cuts. Two of his children wrote the popular book Cheaper by the Dozen in which they detailed the family's preoccupation with innovations.

Henry Gantt (1861–1919) worked for Taylor and was known for his promotion of favorable psychological work conditions. He may be best remembered for his development of the **Gantt chart,** which is still used for project management to show how the components of a task are scheduled over time. His chart contributed to development, in the late 1950s, of the **program evaluation and review technique (PERT)** developed by the U.S. Navy and the **critical path method** developed by Dupont. He also contributed his Task and Bonus Plan to management, which provided bonus payment for workers who exceeded their production standards for the day.

Many of these developments were rapidly applied to the growing market demand for popular products in the United States. Sears and Roebuck probably designed the first manufacturing assembly line for meeting mail-order delivery. In the automobile industry, Henry Ford (who employed Taylor) became intrigued by the moving conveyer belt of carcasses in a Chicago slaughterhouse. He quickly developed this idea into his assembly line for automobile manufacturing, streamlining production from a one-person assembly time of 12.5 hours to about 93 minutes per car. The idea was taken to its extreme in healthcare in the early 1970s when Russian ophthalmologists attempted to introduce assembly-line radial keratotomy, a surgery for correcting eye lens problems. The idea did not catch on widely, although there have been attempts in other countries to promote this idea to cut medical costs.

The legacy of scientific management is pervasive and persists in many areas of modern management. At a time when most businesses were growing in size and complexity, but lacked sound organization, Taylorism provided principles for increasing standardization and consistency. It emphasized the role of research in understanding how tasks were done, in selecting and training people, and in providing consistency in rules and procedures to promote efficiency. However, Taylorism was not without critics. Although scientific management helped managers routinize the internal workings of the business, it essentially ignored the external environment. In addition, critics complained that it was based on simplistic economic motivation, that workers were viewed as mechanistic parts of an organizational machine, and that senior management tasks were excluded from analysis.

Administrative Management

Attempting to compensate for scientific management's exclusion of senior management, **administrative management** argued that management was a profession and could be learned. Henry Fayol (1841–1925), a French engineer and director of mining, published a book summarizing his executive experiences in 1916. Fayol's major contribution includes both a description of five functions of management and fourteen principles for organizational design and administration.

Fayol's five **management functions** have persisted with some variation into modern organizations and identify key functions that define the manager's role. These managerial functions were:

- **Planning** consists of examining the future and preparing plans of action to attain goals.
- **Organizing** includes the ways in which the managed **system** is designed and operated to attain the desired goals. It involves the way that tasks are grouped into departments and resources are distributed to them.
- **Leading** (sometimes also called directing) is the process of influencing the behavior of others. It involves motivating, creating shared culture and values, and communicating with all levels of the organization.
- **Controlling** refers to the monitoring of performance and use of feedback to ensure that efforts are on target toward prescribed goals, making course corrections as necessary.

Fayol's fifth function, coordination or unifying and harmonizing activity and effort, has been absorbed by the other functions (primarily controlling) in modern versions.

Fayol formulated **fourteen principles of management** to guide managerial activities within the total organization. (See figure 21.1.) Like his managerial functions, most have been incorporated into modern organizations and are widely accepted today. For example, authority was proposed as the right of an executive to give orders and expect obedience. *Unity of command* meant that each employee reports to only one boss. The **scalar chain,** or line of authority, ensured that everyone in the organization appears in the chain of command and reports to someone. *Esprit de corps* emphasized the work climate in which harmony and cohesion promoted good work.

Chester Barnard (1886–1961), a former president of the New Jersey Telephone Company and the Rockefeller Foundation, published *The Functions of the Executive* in 1938. In this book, he elaborated the role of top executives. He proposed that the leader needed information from those below, that the communication system is designed and implemented by the executive, and that the role of middle management is to implement plans and solve problems. Barnard developed the **acceptance theory of authority,** which proposes that people have free will to choose whether they follow work orders. In addition, he emphasized that the measure of organizational cooperation is effectiveness and efficiency. **Effectiveness** refers to the degree to which the organization achieves its intended outcomes; **efficiency** refers to how well a minimum of resources is allocated to achieve the outcomes.

Another major contributor to the administrative approach was Mary Parker Follett (1868–1933). In contrast to what was often considered a mechanistic view by Taylor, she was

Figure 21.1.   Fayol's Fourteen Principles

1. *Specialization of labor:* Work allocation and specialization allow concentrated activities, deeper understanding, and better efficiency.
2. *Authority:* The person to whom responsibilities are given has the right to give direction and expect obedience.
3. *Discipline:* The smooth operation of a business requires standards, rules, and values for consistency of action.
4. *Unity of command:* Every employee receives direction and instructions from only one boss
5. *Unity of direction:* All workers are aligned in their efforts toward a single outcome.
6. *Subordination of individual interests:* Accomplishing shared values and organizational goals take priority over individual agendas.
7. *Remuneration:* Employees should receive fair pay for work.
8. *Centralization:* Decisions are made at the top.
9. *Scalar chain:* Everyone is clearly included in the chain of command and line of authority from top to bottom of the organization.
10. *Order:* People should clearly understand where they fit in the organization, and all people and material have a place.
11. *Equity:* People are treated fairly and a sense of justice should pervade the organization.
12. *Tenure:* Turnover is undesirable and loyalty to the organization is sought.
13. *Initiative:* Personal initiative should be encouraged.
14. *Esprit de corps:* Harmony, cohesion, teamwork, and good interpersonal relationships should be encouraged.

interested in broader social ideas and championed the role of relationships in organizations. Although she drew mixed attention in the late 1920s, she foresaw the development of a systems view of business, the role of empowered employees in organizational development, and the use of workgroups to implement solutions. Her ideas have enjoyed a revival in recent years, acknowledged by such management gurus as Peter Drucker and Henry Mintzberg. Follett promoted using teamwork and creative group effort, involving people in organizational development, and integrating the organization, which contained many elements of **systems theory.**

Humanistic Management

Although the United States has always touted itself as the home of democracy, the equity of power in the workplace has not always existed between workers and management. By the early 1900s, there were growing social pressures to treat workers in a more enlightened manner. Building on Barnard's and Follett's ideas that people should be treated fairly and that effective controls come from individual workers, the stage was set for a shift in management thought stimulated by an experiment at an electric power plant.

At the turn of the century, gas and electricity companies were intensely competitive about their respective products, and it appeared that electricity had edged out gas. To firm up its advantage, Thomas Edison and the Committee on Industrial Lighting proposed a study that would confirm the advantage of electric lighting. The Hawthorne plant of the Western Electric Company was elected to serve as the laboratory for examining the effects of illumination. From 1924 to 1932, Harvard professors Elton Mayo and Fritz Roethlisberger conducted the series of experiments. In some cases, the lighting in the plant was changed to see how it affected productivity. Although performance initially increased when illumination was improved, it paradoxically also improved when lighting was lowered to about the level of moonlight. The study concluded that although light was not the motivator they intended, positive attention and human relations improved performance—the so-called **Hawthorne effect.**

This revolutionized thinking about how to treat workers to improve productivity and initiated the **human relations movement.** Sometimes referred to as the contented cow approach (they give more milk), the belief was that satisfied workers are more productive. Interestingly, reexamination of the original research design and data suggests that financial incentives had a good deal to do with motivating people, and yet the impact of the human relations emphasis continues (Parson 1974). This movement reached its peak during the 1960s and 1970s.

Human Resources Management

In the 1950s, the field of psychology in the United States was just coming into its own prominence, as were theories of motivation. Observing that many problems derived from an inability to meet needs, Abraham Maslow (1908–1970) suggested that a **hierarchy of needs** might help to explain behavior and provide guidance for managers on how to better motivate workers. His now-famous hierarchy began with physiological existence needs and progressed through safety, social belongingness, self-esteem, and finally self-actualization or creativity needs. This developmental view of needs meant that to motivate people, lower-order needs should be satisfied before higher-order needs could serve as motivators. Although these were useful generalizations, in the emerging global economy with diverse populations, motivators can vary considerably by culture. What works as a management approach in American organizations may not work as well in other countries or cultures.

Douglas McGregor (1906–1964) recognized the shift in conceptual models from assumptions that workers were incapable of independent action to beliefs in their potential and high performance. He formulated the contrasting views as **theory X and Y** (1960). Theory X presumed that workers inherently disliked work and would avoid it, had little ambition, and mostly wanted security; therefore, managerial direction and control was necessary. Theory Y took a more enlightened view and assumed that work was as natural as play, that motivation could be both internally and externally driven, and that under the right conditions people would seek responsibility and be creative. Although Theory Y is most favored at present, theory X may still be appropriate in some military, corrections, and immature workforce settings. In contrast, the innovative Saturn Corporation has based nearly all its auto manufacturing practices on Theory Y.

Despite its simplicity, the human relations view brought management to focus on the human side of enterprise (to use McGregor's term). Managers and researchers began to consider the possible role of social and psychological factors on performance. This gave balance to a view of workers that was too heavily laden with mechanistic and economic explanations.

Operations Management

The innovations resulting from wars, the space race, and other international crises have often been the impetus for innovation. With the Second World War came the problems of planning, organizing, distributing, and monitoring huge collections of troops and materiel on a global basis. Advances in the fields of statistics, mathematics, and quantitative methods were brought to bear on decision making and strategy in an approach called operations research. **Operations management** later emerged as an application of these techniques in the business setting to better understand how products and services could be manufactured and delivered.

A variety of techniques is now commonly found in many organizations, including:

- **Forecasting** is regularly used for planning in which previous conditions (such as sales and inventory) are projected into the future. Increasingly sophisticated software can provide projections of changes in technology, demographics, and human resources needs. However, in a rapidly changing environment, predictions based on past performance can be uncertain.

- **Linear programming** is used to identify an optimal decision given a set of planned constraints or limited resources.
- **Break-even analysis** helps planners determine when a project "breaks even," that is, the level of sales at which total revenues equal the total costs. Revenues beyond that are profits.
- **Queuing theory** is a mathematical technique for determining the flow of customers or for designing optimal wait times for services.
- **Simulation and Inventory modeling** is a recent development in management science based on computerization and systems concepts. The key components and processes of a system are represented in a computer model so that planners can experiment with different operating strategies and designs to get the best results before committing to their actual implementation.
- PERT was originally developed by the Navy in 1958 to coordinate the building of submarines. Now facilitated by powerful computer packages, PERT allows large, long-term, and complex projects to be shown graphically in order to clarify critical task sequences, potential bottlenecks, and the time required for them. For complex situations such as healthcare systems, computer decision support can help explore and optimize decisions.

Although many of these programs and techniques are challenging to learn, their ability to deal with vast amounts of data provides considerable advantage to the managers who can fully use them.

Contemporary Management

Often referred to as the guru of management gurus, Peter Drucker (1909–) more clearly formulated the practice of strategy by integrating formulation, tactical planning, and budgeting into a single system of management (Kerker 2001). He revolutionized the role of strategy by wresting it from the hands of top management and making it everyone's job, helping workers understand how mission, strategy, goals, and performance were related. Because strategy was action oriented, starting in the 1950s, Drucker elaborated on the technique of **management by objectives** (MBO), in which clear target objectives could be stated and measured and could direct behavior. The four elements of an MBO system include (Drucker 1986):

- Top management's planning and setting of goals
- Managers with subordinates setting individual objectives related to organizational goals
- Autonomy in the means of achieving objectives
- Regular review of performance in obtaining objectives

From the late 1970s to the mid-1980s, the United States was beset with a series of economic setbacks. Serious recessions, a growing trade deficit, government deregulation, and huge operating losses led to the downsizing of hundreds of thousands of workers. Quality became the focus as a means of increasing competitive position, and much of the idea was derived from W. Edwards Deming (1900–1993), an American statistician. Deming had initially developed his ideas in the 1950s, but the American economy was booming at the time and seemed to believe it had found the "one best way" to do things. Consequently, American industry was inattentive to Deming's ideas about improvement and his statistical control procedures for monitoring quality. However, the Japanese were suffering from an all-but-destroyed economy and were eager to hear new ideas about production. They quickly adopted the concept of **total quality management** (TQM).

TQM purported to overcome the limitations of MBO, criticizing the use of quotas because workers too often spent too much time trying to look good or protect themselves by seeking short-term objectives and ignoring long-term and critical outcomes. TQM offered a way to build in high performance by maximizing employee potential and continuous improvement of process. The **85/15 rule** of TQM proposes that 85 percent of problems encountered are the result of faulty systems rather than unproductive employees. The manager's job then becomes one of anticipating and removing barriers to employee high performance. Deming proposed his fourteen principles for TQM implementation. (See figure 21.2.)

Figure 21.2.   Deming's Fourteen Principles

1. Create a constancy of purpose toward continual improvement of products and services, with the objectives to stay in business, be competitive, and provide jobs.
2. Adopt the new philosophy for a new economic age by correcting superstitious learning, calling for a major change, and looking at the customer rather than competition.
3. Cease dependence on inspection to achieve quality by eliminating emphasis on mass inspection and building quality in from the beginning.
4. Don't award business based on price tag alone, and minimize total costs by developing trusting and loyal long-term relationships with single suppliers.
5. Constantly and continually improve production and service systems and thereby improve quality and decrease costs.
6. Institute training on the job, where barriers to good work are removed and managers provide a setting that promotes worker success.
7. Institute leadership with the aim of revising supervision to better help people, machines, and processes do a better job.
8. Drive out fear so everyone can work effectively toward company goals.
9. Break down barriers between departments so that various departments can work as a team and anticipate problems of production or use of a product or service.
10. Avoid asking for new levels of productivity and zero defects through slogans and targets because most problems of low productivity lie with the system rather than the worker.
11. Replace work standards such as quotas, numerical goals, and MBO with good leadership.
12. Remove barriers that rob people at all levels of their pride of workmanship; shift from numbers to quality.
13. Institute a program of education and self-improvement by emphasizing lifelong learning and employment.
14. Transformation of the workplace occurs through everyone's action.

Variations of TQM also were promoted by Juran and Crosby, and many of the ideas now find expression in a variation called **business process reengineering** (BPR). In the 1990s, when recognition of the high level of business competition was reaching a peak, Hammer and Champy (1993) published *Reengineering the Corporation*. They proposed that a radical redesign of the organization might be necessary to reduce costs, streamline operations, and improve quality of service. By the mid-1990s, the idea was often used to justify **downsizing,** or the reduction of labor costs by laying off portions of the workforce, often without achieving the improvements desired.

The popularity of these approaches has demonstrated the growing importance of customer satisfaction, **benchmarking,** employee involvement, and teamwork. Quality has become a national goal. In 1987, Congress established a national award to recognize excellence in the manufacturing and service industries, small business, and, in 1999, healthcare and education. The **Baldridge Award,** named after the Secretary of Commerce, is based on meeting several criteria: leadership, strategic planning, customer focus, information and analysis, human resources and process focus, and business results. ISO 9000 is another example of the drive toward quality improvement. **ISO 9000** is an internationally agreed-upon set of standards for quality management established in 1987. Adopted by more than 90 countries, the generic standards can be applied to organizations of any size. It involves defining, executing, and auditing best practices in production or service delivery (ISO Online 2002).

Although elements of most major theories can be found within the practices of successful managers, new developments and refinements in thinking continue to thrive. In 1982, Peters and Waterman published *In Search of Excellence*. Based on a sample of highly successful business firms, they described the management practices that led to their success. Eight characteristics were described that became the rage in management circles for a time, with managers hoping to reproduce in their own organizations what top firms had done. (See figure 21.3.) Although the eight practices are very important, a follow-up of the same organizations four years later showed disappointing results. In that short time, 66 percent had fallen from a top position and 19 percent were in a troubled position (Pascale 1990).

Although researchers continue to search for the essential ingredients that will make firms most successful, the lesson from the excellence studies highlights some important principles, including:

- When you succeed or fail, try to understand what brought that about.
- When you succeed, recognize that the success factors are not static, but continually changing.
- Do not let past success strategies keep you from discovering new ones for the future.
- What may contribute to the success of one type of organization or competitive setting may not be as useful to other types and settings or at other stages of organizational development.

Figure 21.3.   Characteristics of Highly Successful Firms

1. *A bias for action:* They establish a value for action and implementation rather than overanalyzing and delaying with endless committees.
2. *Close to the customer:* They listen and respond to customers to satisfy their needs.
3. *Autonomy and entrepreneurship:* They empower people and encourage innovation and risk taking.
4. *Productivity through people:* They increase employees' awareness that everyone's contributions lead to shared success.
5. *Hands on, value driven:* Their managers should be visible, involved, and know what is going on.
6. *Stick to the knitting:* They stay with the core business, what they do well, and avoid wide diversification.
7. *Simple form, lean staff:* They have fewer administrative layers and keep the structure simple.
8. *Simultaneous loose–tight properties:* They maintain dedication to core principles but encourage flexibility and experimentation in reaching goals.

Check Your Understanding 21.1

Instructions: Answer the following questions on a separate piece of paper.

1. What are some of the important management concepts that have persisted over the decades? Why have they persisted?

2. Why have some management ideas been rapidly accepted, and others have required years to become popular?

3. Using the example of the Gilbreth time-motion study, identify some complex activity you engage in (such as packing for a trip, dressing in the morning, and so on) and see how you can streamline the sequence to become more efficient.

4. Explore reasons why the top companies identified in Peters and Waterman's *In Search of Excellence* dropped from their top position within a few short years. How might that have been prevented?

Functions and Principles of Management

As mentioned earlier, Fayol identified four functions of management. Related to these functions are certain categories of skills that are needed to carry them out.

Managerial Functions

As theories of management began to be refined, so too did the formal nature of the manager's role. As organizations increased in diversity, complexity, and size, managers often shifted their expertise from expert knowledge in doing a task to expert knowledge in managing other people. As Mary Parker Follett is reputed to have said, "Management is the art of getting things done through people" (Stoner and Freeman 1989). Specific functions of management came to be defined, as did a range of skills and subroles that contribute to successful problem solving.

Fayol's management functions of planning, organizing, leading, and controlling continue to be useful categories for examining the work of the manager. After the enterprise is begun, these four stages become a cycle for continuous improvement in which the last function of control is fed back into planning for plan revision.

Planning

Planning is the first step in management and involves determining what should be accomplished and how. Although planning occurs at all levels, top-level or strategic planning is most critical in formulating the mission and providing direction for change. When these strategies are defined, they can be implemented at the lower levels of the organization. Planning provides competitive advantage over those who minimize the importance of planning, as reflected in higher levels of performance such as profits (Shrader, Taylor, and Dalton 1984).

Plans are usually organized hierarchically, with a **mission statement** driving the enterprise by defining exactly what business the organization is in and what is valued. The **strategic plan** follows from the mission. It is formulated by top management, sets the priorities and positioning of the organization for a time period, and is based on the constellation of internal strengths and weaknesses and external opportunities and threats. These are translated through the lower levels of the organization by middle management, which formulates **tactical plans** for the organization's major divisions. At the lower departmental levels, these finally become **operational plans** that are implemented as daily activities.

Plans are usually expressed in terms of goals. Goals are statements of intended outcomes that provide a source of direction and motivation as well as a guideline for performance, decision making, and evaluation. Good goals cover key result areas of the strategy; have the characteristics of being specific, measurable, and challenging, but achievable; and are set for a given period of time.

Organizing

After the goals have been specified, the task changes to deciding how resources can be allocated to achieve them. Traditionally, division of labor has been used to divide work into separate jobs. This specialization allows for development of greater expertise and standardization of tasks and for clear selection and training criteria. However, too narrow or specialized a task, as in assembly-line work, may produce more boredom than productivity. As Bridges notes (1994), the emerging economy with downsized and flatter organizations may require workers to take on multiple roles and, consequently, to have portfolios of skills rather than highly defined job descriptions.

Jobs are most often organized by positions, and the positions are arranged hierarchically in the business by an organizational chart. (An example of a typical hospital organizational chart is shown in figure 21.4.) The organizational

Figure 21.4.   Sample Hospital Organizational Chart

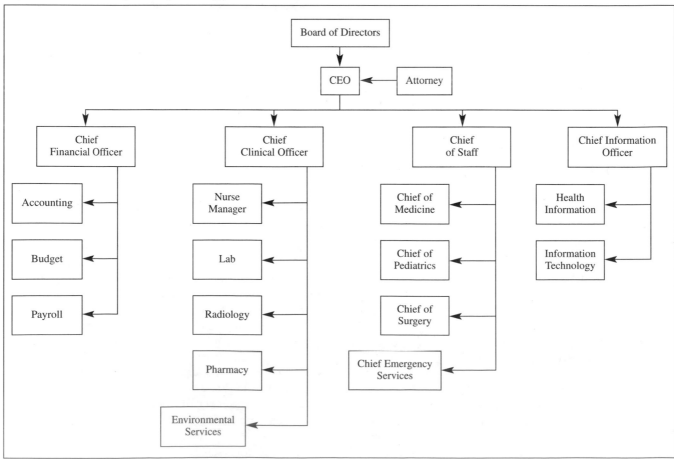

chart often includes departmental subdivisions and follows the scalar principle and unity of command discussed earlier. The **vertical structure** of the organization refers to the formal design of positions within departments and divisions, the lines of authority and responsibility, and the allocation of resources to them. Two kinds of authority are found in organizations. **Line authority** is the right of managers to direct the activities of subordinates under their immediate control; **staff authority** is related to the expert knowledge of specialists and involves their advising and recommending courses of action.

Each supervisor has a certain number of people who report to him or her, which is referred to as the span of management or the **span of control.** Although the span of control is determined more often by tradition or accident, there are several factors to consider in optimally balancing it. In general, the span is larger when work is routine and homogeneous, workers have similar tasks, rules and guidelines are available, people are well trained and motivated, workers are located together, and task times are short (Jacques 1996). Deciding how a combination of factors leads to a particular span has been facilitated by technology. For example, the Healthcare Management Council (HMC) provides a comprehensive measurement of organizational factors leading to a span of management recommendation. The HMC Span of Control Analysis considers organizational flatness, departmental fragmentation, and layers of management using organizational charts. The HMC report can be used by managers to optimize organizational structure, set staffing and financial targets, and determine needs (Healthcare Management Council 2001).

Related to span is **delegation,** in which managers transfer authority to subordinates to carry out a responsibility. With an increasing focus on customers and rapid response, frontline workers are now trained to make decisions that once were made levels above them. When authority and responsibility move from the organization's top levels to its lower levels where they can be competently exercised, centralized decision making becomes decentralized. Although this **decentralization** enables top managers to take on new responsibilities or spend time with other priorities, it places an additional burden on workers.

Leading

The third managerial function accomplishes goals by influencing behavior and by motivating and inspiring people to high performance. At the turn of the century, an autocratic view of leadership was considered to be appropriate, but as humanistic views have prevailed over the decades, leadership has become decentralized and distributed throughout the organization.

Leading is most often accomplished by communicating, directing, and motivating, all intended to influence behavior to perform well. Power, the ability to influence, is central to leadership and derives from several sources, including:

- *Authority or legitimate power* comes from the right of the position in the organization to direct the activities of subordinates.

- *Reward power* is based on the leader's ability to withhold or provide rewards for performance.
- *Coercive power* maintains control over punishments.
- *Referent power* exists when the leader possesses personal characteristics that are appealing to the constituency, and the constituency follows out of admiration, charismatic impact, or the desire to be like the leader.
- *Expert power* occurs when the leader has knowledge or expertise that is of value (French and Raven 1959).
- *Information power* is based on the persuasive content of the person's message, apart from personal characteristics (Raven 1983).

Leadership behaviors and most models of leadership fall into two categories: task-oriented behaviors, and social or group-oriented behaviors. *Task-oriented behaviors* are directed toward defining tasks, creating structure and rules, ensuring production, and placing emphasis on quality and speed of output. *Social orientation* focuses on interpersonal behaviors that develop and maintain harmonious work relationships, encourage morale, reduce stress and conflict, and build worker satisfaction. Several models of leadership, such as the Blake-Mouton Managerial Grid, use these two dimensions and are discussed in a later section of this chapter.

Controlling

The final managerial function refers to the monitoring of performance, determining whether it is on or off course in achieving the goals and making course corrections as needed. Managers are obligated to ensure that progress is made toward achieving goals, although recent trends indicate that employees are empowered to monitor themselves and each other, rather than being monitored from the top. This obviously requires selecting employees who have the maturity and integrity to accept this responsibility, but it corrects for the distortion and delay that can occur in a very hierarchical organization.

Significant breakthroughs have occurred in control with the development of the executive dashboard and **balanced scorecard** (BSC) introduced in 1992 (Kaplan and Norton 1996). The **executive dashboard** is often characterized as a manager's version of a pilot's cockpit dashboard; it contains all the critical information for leading the organization. The dashboard typically contains regularly updated information on key strategic measures such as forecasts, customer satisfaction, billings, profit, and so on. The BSC is an extension of strategic planning in which key performance indicators are measured at all levels of the organization and progress with workers and management receiving ongoing feedback. Categories of feedback usually include financial, customer satisfaction, internal processes (for example, quality, response time), and learning and growth. The customer satisfaction component was highlighted in a report by the Ontario Hospital Association, which sent surveys to 55,000 former acute care patients of their 89 Canadian hospitals. The study focused on clinical utilization and outcomes, financial performance, patient satisfaction, and future directions for the hospitals. The information obtained has been used for revisions in strategic planning, improvement of services, and public information (Leahy 2000).

The four functions of management vary in emphasis according to the level of management involved. (See figure 21.5.) In general, as one moves from first-line to middle management to top managers, planning increases, organizing increases, leading decreases, and controlling stays about the same (Mahoney, Jerdee, and Carroll 1965).

Managerial Skills

The categories of skills required to perform the four management functions are conceptual, interpersonal, and technical skills (Katz 1974). As management has become increasingly complex, the requisite skills for carrying out the four managerial functions also vary by level in the organization. (See figure 21.6.)

The need for **conceptual skills** has increased significantly over the decades. Where it once was important only to have good technical skills, now a successful manager must be able to understand diverse fields and deal with complex situations. According to Tenner (1996), the lack of sufficient conceptual and planning skills has led to revenge effects. Revenge effects are unexpected and usually undesired outcomes that emerge from good intentions, but failure to understand the long-term and ripple effects of an action in an interconnected organization or system.

For example, Medical insurance companies are always searching for ways to contain the costs of medical care. Traditional gallbladder surgery was costly, risky, uncomfortable, and required an inpatient stay. Newer laparoscopic surgery involved only a small abdominal incision, caused less discomfort, required fewer days of care, and enabled people to return to work more quickly. It was so attractive and embraced by HMOs that the rate of gallbladder surgery increased by 50 percent in one HMO, unexpectedly raising the total costs on gallbladder care by 11 percent (Legorreta et al. 1993). In addition, the number of errors increased because of poor resolution on TV's guiding miniaturized instruments (Swenson 2001).

Interpersonal skills involve the ability to work with and through others to accomplish goals. Depending on the nature of the work and the level of interaction needed among individuals, interpersonal skills may or may not be a critical skill for employee success. However, managers, in their interactions with employees and with each other, need to cultivate impeccable interpersonal skills.

That the interpersonal domain is important is shown in a review of top management texts in which this was the only category that they all shared in common (Bigelow 1993). However, as the Institute for Employment Studies reports, managers too often have a skill gap between what is required and the actual level of interpersonal effectiveness (Kettley and Strebler 1997).

Interpersonal competency is based on self-awareness and understanding, and the best managers are those who can articulate both their strengths and weaknesses (Goleman 1998). Yet self-awareness is not enough, and consistently high performers also demonstrate self-monitoring (Church, 1997). **Self-monitoring** refers to the ability to observe the reactions that one's behavior elicits in others and then adjusting one's behavior to improve the relationship. Other important interpersonal skills include communicating, motivating and influencing, managing conflict, credibility, and learning how to complement different ways of interacting (Page, Wilson, and Meyer, 1999).

Understanding and mastering the technical information, methods, and equipment involved in a discipline constitute the **technical skills.** Although most important at the employee level of the organization, they are still required for upper management so that there is a comprehensive understanding of the workings of the organization. However, the conceptual and interpersonal skills are probably more useful in obtaining promotion in most organizations. This is true because, at higher levels in organizations, interpersonal and conceptual skills are used more often and are more important than technical skills. Conceptual skills are more useful for the leading and planning function because they involve understanding the systems view of the total organization.

Effective managers are different from *successful* managers (Luthans, Hodges, and Rosenkranz 1988). Effective managers are identified as those who have satisfied and committed subordinates and produce results; successful managers are those that have been promoted rapidly. Such promotions are often related to interpersonal effectiveness.

Figure 21.5.   Management Functions by Level in the Organization

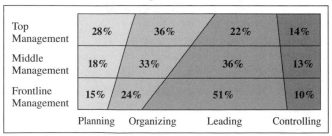

	Planning	Organizing	Leading	Controlling
Top Management	28%	36%	22%	14%
Middle Management	18%	33%	36%	13%
Frontline Management	15%	24%	51%	10%

Figure 21.6.   Functional Skills by Level in the Organization

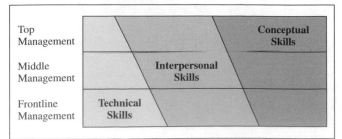

Managerial Roles

Henry Mintzberg (1939–), Cleghorn Professor of Management at McGill University, completed his dissertation at MIT in which he examined the roles of managers. Suspecting that what managers did might be difficult to classify in the categories covered in this chapter, he shadowed managers and recorded their actual activities. His findings defied many common assumptions about the work that managers do. It is widely believed that managers are systematic, reflective thinkers who carefully analyze situations before making decisions and acting. In practice, Mintzberg (1992) found that most chief executives spent less than ten minutes on any activity and that supervising foremen in industry averaged one activity every forty-eight seconds! Managers opened thirty-six pieces of mail, attended eight meetings, and toured a building. Whatever was planned, something unexpected usually emerged. Another study of British middle and top-level managers showed that they were able to secure a half hour for concentrated work without interruption only once every two days. Mintzberg summarized his findings by saying that managers completed a great deal of work at an unrelenting pace, but the activities were characterized by variety, fragmentation, and brevity.

Mintzberg's subsequent research with managers showed that their activities could usually be described by ten roles organized into three categories. The categories include informational, interpersonal, and decisional management (table 21.1).

Interpersonal activity arises from the manager's formal authority in the organization and is supportive of the informational and decisional activities. It includes the roles of figurehead for ceremonial and formal occasions, leadership for motivating and using power, and liaison to link and network for information and support. The *informational* activity includes the roles of monitor of performance information, disseminator of values and information, and spokesperson for the organization with outside groups. Finally, the decisional activity includes the roles of entrepreneur to promote improvement and change, disturbance handler to deal with disruptions, resource allocator for overseeing resources and setting priorities, and negotiator for arrangements with other organizations.

These roles are intricately intertwined and not easily separated by a particular problem when it comes to team management, where responsibilities are often distributed among team members. However, they provide a realistic portrayal of the wide range of skilled behaviors required of effective managers.

When Peter Senge published *The Fifth Discipline: The Art and Practice of the Learning Organization* (1990), it was likely that not many people expected his ideas to influence management thinking as much as they have. As with Taylor's theory, the marketplace was ready for, and receptive to, new ways of thinking about increasingly complex organizations and how they could adapt to equally complex competitive environments. When introduced in the 1940s by von Bertalanffy and others, **systems theory** was a reaction against reductionism in which complex processes were reduced to their constituent elements and analyzed. Proponents of systems theory believe that important information is lost by too specific a focus and, in turn, emphasize the interconnections and organization of these constituents rather than their inspection in isolation. In management, systems decisions implemented in good faith and with planning may have an adverse ripple effect in other parts of the organization or in relationship to the external environment.

The learning organization was an idea with a good fit for the questions managers were asking: How do we adjust to all the changes in the marketplace? Senge's answer: learning. All systems (individual, team, organizational) adapt to a changing environment by learning. The more rapidly they learn, the faster they can take a stronger competitive position. This has led Robert Weiler, CEO of GIGA Information Group, to paraphrase the Darwinian principle: "It's not the strongest that survive, it's those most responsive and adaptive to change" (Pratt 2000).

Comparing the workings of organizations during the twentieth century with those emerging in the twenty-first century, there is a clear need for a new way of thinking on the part of managers. Although the managerial skills used in conceptualization, relationships, and technology will persist, they will have to be applied in a different manner. The **change drivers** of globalization, demographic and marketplace diversity, information and technological changes, and others will mean that managers will seldom be able to focus

Table 21.1.   Mintzberg's Managerial Roles

Managerial Activities	Related Roles
Interpersonal	• *Figurehead:* The manager represents the organization and is a symbol for ceremonial, social, legal, and inspirational duties. • *Liaison:* The manager maintains networks of relationships outside his or her organizational unit to gather information and favors. • *Leader:* The manager directs, guides, motivates, and develops subordinates.
Informational	• *Monitor:* The manager oversees internal and external information sources. • *Disseminator:* The manager communicates facts and values to others in the organization. • *Spokesperson:* The manager communicates with others outside the organization.
Decisional	• *Entrepreneur:* The manager promotes development and planned change in the organization. • *Disturbance handler:* The manager resolves crises and unexpected problems. • *Resource allocator:* The manager uses authority to allocate budget, personnel, equipment, services, and facilities. • *Negotiator:* The manager resolves dilemmas and disputes and determines the use of resources.

on the status quo as they have in the past. The new status quo is one of change and how people can be helped through transitions.

•Again coming full circle, Taylor and other proponents of scientific management emphasized an important criterion for managerial success—It should be based on research whenever possible. As Stacy demonstrated in his diagram of the managerial fads from the 1960s to 1990s, many ideas were without empirical foundation, were short-lived, had limited application, and in some cases caused more problems than they solved. In healthcare, as well as other fields of management, decisions are based more on political and value considerations than on empirical sources. With the increased interest in alternative approaches to healthcare (for example, acupuncture, nutrition), determining which methods are legitimate and produce the best outcomes can reduce liability and enhance sound program promotion. An emphasis on **evidence-based management,** or information-based management, is emerging in which more informed decisions are made based on the best clinical and research evidence that proposed practices will work. For example, Australia-based CSIRO works with healthcare organizations to determine factors that influence the use of health information by at-risk segments of a population and also develop performance measures for staff. Their procedures have increased the use of data and information by senior managers in strategic and daily planning. Increasingly, all levels of managers are having information available on performance evaluation and the outcomes of the decisions they make.

Check Your Understanding 21.2

Instructions: Answer the following questions on a separate piece of paper.

1. Discuss reasons for the four management functions changing in emphasis over the three levels of management. For example, why would there be less emphasis on the leadership function for top-level managers compared with the strong emphasis for first-line managers?

2. Examine a job description for a position in your field. What is the distribution of conceptual, interpersonal, and technical skills required?

3. Make a list of daily activities engaged in by observing or asking a manager what he or she does. Then, categorize the activities into Mintzberg's ten managerial roles.

4. Draw an organizational chart of your college, a hospital, or some other organization with which you are familiar. Be sure to designate both line and staff positions.

5. What does *quality* mean in your work? Identify several tasks you perform, define *quality* for each task, and consider how you would measure it.

Trends in Management Theory

What we have seen in the several management theories presented in this chapter is that as change drivers have an impact on the marketplace and organizations, organizations must adapt in order to survive and thrive. Management theories become a template for thinking about the structure and processes by which business is conducted. As the marketplace changes, old theories may lose their explanatory power and be replaced with more accurate theories and principles for managing the organization. (See table 21.2.) At the same time, as managers become accustomed to, and develop expertise with, a certain viewpoint, they may become biased in its use and fail to see exceptions to it. A requisite skill for managers is to know when to use a particular framework and when to change it.

Although Taylor and others at the turn of the twentieth century faced a host of changes, the unrelenting pace of change is an even more constant companion to managers today. The successful manager must be able to see patterns of change and prepare others to respond to them.

Problem Solving and Decision Making

Problems are defined as impediments to the attainment of goals. While some managers view problems as negative and something to be avoided, problem solving can also be viewed as an opportunity for managers and organizations to build experience and resilience. Solving problems requires that they be framed or defined in useful and understandable ways, that creative approaches are applied to them, and that efficient methods are applied to recurrent problems. Problem solving involves understanding and resolving the barriers to goal attainment, while decision making refers to making the best choices from among available alternatives.

Table 21.2.   Paradigm Shift in Management

Traditional Management Paradigm	The New Management Paradigm
Multilevel hierarchical organizations	Flatter organizations
Centralized decision making	Decentralized decision making
Status measured by the amount of turf controlled	Status reflected in success in achieving outcomes
Quantity	Quality
Individual leadership	Teamwork
Think local	Think global and systems
Maintain stability	Change and adapt
Job security	Job flexibility
Focus on profit	Focus on customers
Short-term view	Long-term view
Homogeneous workforce and market	Diverse workforce and market
Competition	Collaboration
Work at office	Telecommuting and home office
Capital	Information
Physical labor	Knowledge workers
Terminal education	Continuous learning

Two primary responsibilities of managers are solving problems and making decisions. In the early years of management practice, these activities were often based on personal preferences and limited experience, with little regard for long-term consequences. Since then, however, formal models of dealing with issues have been developed and managers are encouraged to proceed systematically through several stages, including:

1. Defining the problem and the desired outcome
2. Analyzing and understanding the nature of the problem
3. Generating alternatives
4. Selecting desired alternatives (decision making)
5. Planning and implementing the alternative
6. Evaluating and gathering feedback about the attained outcome

At each step in the problem solving model, decisions need to be made that lead to the final choice of how to implement a means for solving the problem. Given the changing circumstances of the modern healthcare marketplace, it is unlikely that all the information managers desire will be available. They will need to decide using less than perfect or less than complete information, and under ambiguous or risky circumstances.

In recent years the importance of rational decision making has become essential in management, and a variety of models have been developed. The Vroom-Yetton (1971) normative decision tree, which is discussed in detail in a later section of this chapter, is an example of a system for responding to key questions, branching to alternatives, and arriving at a conclusion. For more complex decision making where there are several choices and criteria for selection, but the criteria cannot be ordered sequentially as in the Vroom-Yetton model, a decision matrix can be constructed for evaluating and comparing alternatives (see figure 21.7). Using this method, the decision maker lists the criteria for a good outcome and then rates each possible alternative for the solution to the problem. Each alternative is identified, and each is rated on the extent to which it fulfills the desired outcome criteria. Finally, the criteria weightings are multiplied by the choice ratings and totaled. The alternative with the highest total is considered to provide the best combination of characteristics that meet the most important criteria. This can be a tedious process with very complex problems, and various computer programs and expert systems have been developed to systematically walk the user through the decision process and perform the calculations. An example is StatCon or "statistical consultant," a simple expert system that prompts the user to answer questions about research data, and then recommends which statistical procedure to use to analyze it (Andrews, et al., 1981).

Although this classical model of problem solving illustrates what managers *should* do, the most accurate assessment of a manager's effectiveness is determined by what he or she *actually* does.

Bounded Rationality

Most, if not all, problem solvers and decision makers operate within the limits of bounded rationality. **Bounded rationality** recognizes that problem situations can be overwhelmingly complex and in states of constant change, that not every fact about a situation can be known, and that people are not always rational. As a result, bounded rationality accounts for the limits of time and information, and encourages action despite uncertainty.

Intuition and Satisficing

Because of bounded rationality, managers often tend to rely on intuition and satisficing. **Intuition,** unconscious decision

Figure 21.7.   Decision Matrix

Example—Choosing the Job Offer That Best Meets Your Career Criteria				
		Rating of extent to which this job meets each criterion (1 = high, 5 = low)		
Key decision criteria for a good job	Rating of the Importance (1 = high)	Job Choice 1 Rating : Product	Job Choice 2 Rating : Product	Job Choice 3 Rating : Product
Criterion 1: Good pay	5	3 : 15	4 : 20	2 : 10
Criterion 2: Preferred region of country	2	2 : 4	3 : 6	4 : 8
Criterion 3: Interesting work	4	3 : 12	5 : 20	4 : 16
Additional criteria		↓	↓	↓
Total ratings for each choice		31	46	34

Step 1: Identify and rate (1–5, 5 high) the importance of the criteria for your desired job.

Step 2: Rate the extent to which each of the job choices meet your criteria (1–5, 5 high).

Step 3: Multiply each rating by the criteria rating.

Step 4: Total the products for all ratings and compare across the choices.

Decision: The higher product total of job choice 2 (e.g., 46) offers greater fit with the applicants preferred criteria than do choices 1 and 3.

making based on similar conditions, can be useful as a quick way for highly experienced persons to make decisions when the current problem is similar to prior experiences. This kind of decision making is neither impulsive nor arbitrary but is based on decision pathways that have become so automatic as to become unconscious.

Satisficing is a less precise method than intuition and refers to a manager adopting the first alternative that is sufficient to meet the minimum requirement for a solution to the problem. Although this method is efficient and saves time and effort, it may have unexpected long-term effects that have not been considered. For example, the first apparent solution is not necessarily the most efficient in terms of time and money or the most appropriate. Without further analysis, the first solution is simply the first idea that appeared.

Programmed and Nonprogrammed Decisions

Decisions can be programmed or nonprogrammed. **Programmed decisions** are those in which a problem is so predicatable, uniform, and recurring that rules have been developed to standardize or automate the procedure. Such rules enable managers to delegate authority to others to make decisions using predetermined criteria or to develop expert systems in which computers can make decisions. An example of such automation is an inventory system that automatically requests an order for restocking by a supplier when stock reaches a certain level.

Nonprogrammed decisions involve situations that are unpredictable, extremely complex, or ill defined. These situations defy simple decision criteria and usually require careful deliberation, often in consultation with others. Examples of nonprogrammed decisions include those found in market development, strategic management, and new product or service development.

Managerial Communication

As noted earlier in this chapter, Follett observed that managers get things done through people, and this in turn is accomplished by communicating with them. Communication is the interpersonal process by which information is transferred from one person to another. Nearly everything we do can potentially communicate something to someone, or more economically stated, "you cannot, not communicate" (Watzlawick, Beavin, and Jackson, 1968). About 75 percent of the working time people spend in organizations is used for interpersonal interactions. Still, ineffective communication remains a significant problem in most organizations. For example, a survey of workers who voluntarily quit their organizations found that about 25 percent of their reasons were because they perceived their managers to be poor communicators (American Quality Institute 2002). Executives tend to agree, citing as much as 14 percent of a 40 hour work week is wasted due to poor staff–manager communication (Mills 1998).

Communication can take place through formal or informal channels. Formal communication consists of those intentional messages that are directed to people through their role relationships in the organization, and usually through established channels such as e-mail, phone, face-to-face interaction, memo, letter, or other forms of announcement. This kind of communication usually focuses on task accomplishment and related matters. In contrast, informal communication may occur across role or department boundaries or organizational levels. It tends to employ face-to-face interactions, and focuses on the interpersonal aspects of work—rumors, and topics outside the immediate scope of the workplace. It is through informal communication that most relationships develop between employees and influence is exercised.

Complex organizations also have a variety of barriers to the richness or completeness of communication, both structural and interpersonal. Structural barriers include the distortion that can occur when a message is passed through several people, each adding or deleting information based on their own perceptions and needs. The increasing use of e-mail in organizations also eliminates the nonverbal cues of voice tone, volume and inflection, as well as facial and gestural cues that add so much to face-to-face communication. Interpersonal barriers include distraction and partial listening, tendency to judge, assuming we know what others mean, and fear in asking questions. In general, low richness channels are one-way communication tools such as reports, bulletins, memos and e-mail; high richness channels include telephone and face-to-face interactions.

As the workforce continues to become more diverse, there will be greater challenges to managerial communication. A Los Angeles multinational firm, for example, provides new employee orientation in 17 different languages. In many Asian countries where courtesy and "saving face" is very important, a person might say "maybe" when they really mean "no" in order to avoid hurting feelings. While most task-oriented Americans prefer to get right down to business, many South Americans prefer to spend time getting to know who they are doing business with, and Arabs may have conversations where they shift from business to personal and other interests and then loop back several times. In addition to verbal language differences, nonverbal communication also differs culturally; what may be a benign gesture in one place may be very offensive in another (Axtell, 1991). For example, while many Americans feel quite comfortable crossing their legs and leaning back in a chair, showing the sole of the foot in such a manner is very offensive to most Arabs and most Japanese would consider a slouched posture a sign of poor character. Beckoning by curling the index finger back is a common way for Americans to say "come here," but in Indonesia and Australia, such a gesture is used only for calling animals. Appreciating communication differences and customs is an important part of being an effective communicator, cosmopolitan traveler, and respected manager.

To communicate effectively, managers must pay just as much attention to how the other person receives and interprets the message as to the informational content of the message. The following practices can enhance the accuracy and acceptance of communication (Okum, 1985; Morgan and Baker, 1985):

- Minimize "noise" that can distort the message. Make sure all parties have minimal distractions, undivided attention, and sufficient time to get their message across.
- Know what outcome you want in communicating the message—then check to see if you get that outcome.
- Monitor others' nonverbal behaviors for cues that they are following or are confused.
- Consider the effect that different interpersonal styles, cultural backgrounds, and experiences may have on interpretation of the message or how it is delivered.
- Use **active listening** in which you (or the other person) restate in your own words what you have heard the other person saying.
- Respond to the feelings, attitudes, and values in the message as well as the content. Show empathy, concern, and compassion as appropriate.
- Use examples or visual aids to make the message clearer.
- Ask for feedback and listen to it without being judgmental.
- In writing, be clear and concise.
- Remember that how well you model communication skills sets the norm for others.

Functions and Principles of Leadership

Leadership is the art of setting a direction and influencing people to move in that direction. Given the changing nature of the workplace and marketplace, leaders are in a unique position to influence the shaping of vision and mission in order to inspire people to make their best effort. Leaders also are the ones that others rely on to help make organizational change meaningful and to enable the transition. Yet, clarifying exactly who leaders are and what they do is not an easy task. Several specialists in the field have lamented that in spite of so much research on the subject of leadership, there is little to show for it in the way of real insight and practical results (Bennis 1959; Burns 1978; Yukl 1998). Even in an inspiring study by the Gallup Organization in which 80,000 managers from 400 companies were examined, the managers were found not to share a great deal in common other than "breaking rules" (Buckingham and Coffman 1999).

Functions of Leadership

Leadership is a central strategic concern for most organizations because it makes a difference. Each year, *Fortune* magazine and the Hay Group conduct a survey of the world's most-admired companies (Hay Group 1999). Hay interviewed the top companies in twenty-one industrial groupings and found that they were differentiated from the other companies by their exceptionally strong focus on several leadership areas. They put a great deal of effort into identifying and selecting people with leadership potential. In addition, they matched people whose needs fit the company culture and strategic goals. Moreover, they had organizational cultures that emphasized the importance and value of people. Finally, they intentionally developed leadership competencies, such as orientation to achievement, self-confidence, self-management, empathy, and teamwork. Asked about their level of satisfaction with leadership, 91 percent expressed satisfaction with the quality and breadth of their leadership, compared to a group of global 500 companies that only showed a 72 percent satisfaction.

In addition, the top companies reported that leadership success was related to emotional intelligence and social skills, and technical skills were considered only half as important. Supporting this was another Hay study in which CEO failure was most related not to flawed strategy or vision but, rather, to poor execution and problems in interpersonal relations (Charan and Colvin 1999). There is still some controversy about the extent to which leadership affects an organization. However, a growing body of evidence suggests it can make a strategic difference. Effective leadership has been found to improve financial performance of the organization, with fiscal improvements ranging from 7 to 15 percent (Salancik and Pfeffer 1977), to a high of 44 percent (Weiner and Mahoney 1981). The essential role of the leader during organizational change has also been explored (Burke, Richley, and DeAngelis, 1985). Nonetheless, leadership is one of several important factors influencing the health of an organization.

In modern organizations, leadership does not just reside at the top but, instead, is perfused throughout the organization. In a CIO survey of 300 information management executives, 78 percent identified "inculcating leadership in their staff" as their most important job (Blodgett 1999). Every few years, a Human Resource Development National Executive Survey is conducted to assess organizational trends in training. The findings from a 1998 survey show that the importance of leadership development is increasing. About 84 percent of organizations reported that they promote some form of leadership training and employee development. Although it is still reserved primarily for managerial positions, leadership development is gradually finding its way throughout all levels of organizations (National HRD 1998). The most commonly mentioned skills of effective leaders included communication (57 percent), vision (53 percent), interpersonal skills

(50 percent), strategic planning (40 percent), and change management (37 percent). Regardless of what the desired characteristics include, they appear deficient, as reflected in the topics the organizations preferred to see in training: change management (74 percent), leadership styles (73 percent), and performance management (65 percent).

The trend in leadership in modern organizations is to develop the leadership potential of employees to their full capacity. This allows the employees to exercise the empowerment they are given, demonstrate their value to the organization, and perhaps participate in leadership succession in the organization.

Leadership versus Management

As seen in several chapters of this text, the workplace and the marketplace are beset with continuous adaptations to large-scale change drivers over which there is little control. Management must provide stability and consistency for workers and at the same time prepare them for the transition to new structures and processes. Managers and leaders must collaborate closely to ensure clear understanding and smooth transitions in ways that minimize disruption to people and production. Although the activities of leaders and managers can be distinguished, there is considerable overlap between the roles, and effective leaders and managers usually carry out both functions to some degree.

The terms *leader* and *manager* are often used interchangeably, and although they overlap, they are technically—and in some aspects, practically—different. In general, the responsibility of managers is to ensure that current operations run smoothly whereas leaders strive to help the organization adapt to changing conditions. Managers tend to focus more on structured and analytical modes of thinking whereas leaders tend to use more flexible and creative modes. Managers are often more attentive to danger and uncertainty whereas leaders seek opportunities in undefined and unknown risk areas. Managers are said to determine the scope of problems whereas leaders search for alternative solutions. Managers seek methods and ask how something can be done whereas leaders seek motives and wonder why things are as they are and how they can be different. In general, then, managers work to create efficiency with the status quo whereas leaders move the organization into its unfolding future. (See table 21.3.)

These differences have been attributed to the influence of different developmental experiences in these individuals' lives. When asked about their early family and personal experiences, managers often describe uneventful early childhoods and see life as a steady normative progression of positive events and security. Being involved in social and organized activities from an early age, they tend to gain a strong sense of belonging, identity, and self-esteem from others. In contrast, leaders more often describe disruptive experiences in early family and childhood in which they were confronted by conflicts and stresses. These crises required reflection and mastery through which self-efficacy was

Table 21.3.   Differences between Managers and Leaders

Managers	Leaders
Administer, replicate, and maintain	Innovate, originate, and develop
Emphasis on structure	Emphasis on people
Short-range view	Long-range view
Focus on bottom line	Focus on the horizon
Relies on control and rules	Relies on trust and inspiration
Avoids risks as problems	Takes risks as opportunities
Does things right	Does the right thing
Uneventful early childhood	Developmental conflicts requiring reflection and mastery
Life seen as steady progression of positive events and security	Life punctuated with series of disruptions and challenges
Feel strong sense of belonging	Feel separateness; create rather than inherit identity
Transactional	Transformational

developed. Because confidence grows out of problem solving rather than relationships, leaders may be more attached to a vision that drives their achievement and inspires others than to an immediate situation (Hickman 1990; Kotter 1990; Zaleznik 1977).

Attesting to the relevance of developmental experiences, biographical data have been found to be predictive of good leadership. At a time when human resources directors use caution about the types of questions they can ask in employment interviews, inquiring about the kinds of experiences that have led managers and leaders to be the kind of people they are can be insightful. It is important to remember that both roles are required in organizations, and it is in collaboration that leaders and managers provide balance for organizations in transition.

Trends in Leadership Theory

Recently, several leadership theories have emerged to focus more attention on the interpersonal role of managers. In addition, as opposed to focusing on roles at the top leadership levels, recent theories encourage and explore a flatter distribution of leadership roles and responsibilities within an organization.

Early theories were more basic views of leadership, consisting primarily of traits that leaders were expected to possess. As the limitations of these simple conceptualizations became evident, and the workplace and the marketplace became increasingly complex, the definitions and characteristics of effective leadership necessarily broadened to account for different circumstances. These situational or contingency views emphasize a leader's skills in assessing a situation and adjusting behavior accordingly. Although leadership theories have attempted to account for more complex behavior over time, nearly all of them continue to include task-oriented and people-oriented aspects.

Classical Approaches to Leadership Theory

The classical approaches to leadership refer to those early theories that formed the foundation for thinking about leadership and provided a basis for advancing research and new practices. Based on hierarchically structured organizations of the time, classical leadership theories tended to focus on the principled and effective use of authority. This emphasis began to change with the many social changes that were emerging in the early to mid 1900s. Inventions and innovations in manufacturing increased competition, which made managers more open to new ideas. Workers became increasingly better educated and skilled, thereby requiring managers with authoritative styles to adopt more democratic approaches. The workforce also became increasingly diverse, much like today, and this required a broader understanding of different cultures and motivational approaches.

Great Person Theory

The course of human history is marked with the contributions of great people. Such outstanding individuals originally led to the conception of leadership as an inborn ability, sometimes passed down through family, position, or social tradition, as in the cases of royal families in many parts of the world. The problem with the **great person theory** is that some of those who took positions of such greatness were terribly lacking, as in the case of such notables as Caligula in Rome, Idi Amin in Uganda, and Pol Pot in Cambodia. In the United States, there have been people who were leaders in one sphere, but who failed in others. General Ulysses S. Grant excelled as a general, which largely got him elected president, a role that he performed miserably. Braniff Airlines struggled with the leadership of Harding Lawrence who, despite his strategic brilliance, *demotivated* employees. On flights, his tantrums were notorious and he resorted to screaming and throwing food, violent behaviors that would be considered arrestable offenses today (Harris 1982).

Trait Approach

The **trait approach** gradually replaced the great person model and proposed that leaders possessed a collection of traits or personal qualities that distinguished them from nonleaders; in other words, they had "the right stuff." During the 1930s and 1940s, hundreds of studies on the trait approach to leadership were conducted, and as many as 18,000 traits were identified (Allport and Odbert 1936). Traits were often grouped into categories related to physical needs, values, intellect, personality, and skill characteristics. Some researchers have organized traits on the three leadership requirements of conceptual, interpersonal, and technical skills. Others add a fourth category, administrative skills, that includes the four managerial functions of planning, organizing, directing, and controlling (Yukl 1998).

Unfortunately, in much of the early research, only a weak relationship was discovered between traits and individuals who would emerge as leaders, and many leaders did not share all the traits in common. During later studies in which traits and skills were correlated with leader effectiveness rather than leader emergence, stronger connections appeared. Some of the more important traits included adaptability, social alertness, ambition, assertiveness, cooperativeness, decisiveness, dominance, energy, stress tolerance, and confidence. Skills included intelligence and conceptual abilities, creativity, tact, verbal fluency, work knowledge, organization, and persuasion (Stogdill 1974). Despite this extensive work, it appears that no single traits are absolutely required for leadership. Having certain traits and skills leads to a greater likelihood that such attributes may be more helpful in a situation and to leader effectiveness.

Autocratic versus Democratic Leadership

As Douglas McGregor noted in his formulation of Theory X and Y, two types of environments and leaders corresponded to autocratic and democratic behaviors. In the late 1950s, stimulated by the cold war between political democracies and communism, researchers at Iowa State University conducted studies on democratic and autocratic leaders (White and Lippitt 1960). They found that groups under the direction of autocratic leaders performed well as long as they were closely supervised, although levels of member satisfaction were low. In contrast, democratic leadership led members to perform well whether the leader was present or absent, and members were more satisfied. This kind of research led to the emphasis on participative management in many organizations, although the studies have been strongly criticized for studying groups of young boys at a summer camp and then generalizing the findings to corporate behavior (Lee 1982).

However, the autocratic-democratic dimension was useful for understanding a range of managerial behavior. Tannenbaum and Schmidt (1973) designed a continuum that described seven degrees of managerial involvement in a decision (figure 21.8, p. 508). At one end of the continuum, the manager makes a decision alone and announces it; at the other, the manager encourages his or her subordinates to make their own decisions within prescribed limits. This model reflected a shift away from looking at the leader in isolation or in terms of a rigid or permanent style and suggested that a person had available a range of behaviors depending on the situation. But what were the behaviors that made leaders successful?

Check Your Understanding 21.3

Instructions: Complete the following activities and answer the questions on a separate piece of paper.

1. Make two lists of effective and ineffective leaders. What makes them different from each other? Consider their personalities, limitations in skills or adaptability, and changes in the situation and what it required of them.

2. Make a list of your traits and skills. Rank them in order of how effective they make you as a leader in a given situation. Change the leadership situation and see which traits and skills might also change to give you advantage or which ones might unexpectedly become a disadvantage. How could you develop these skills further?

3. Imagine you have been asked to be a consultant to an aspiring political or managerial figure. You are asked to recommend how this person should appear in order to increase his or her chances for election or promotion. What behaviors would you advise for and against? What are the ethical issues involved in this type of image building?

Figure 21.8.   Tannenbaum and Schmidt's Leadership Continuum

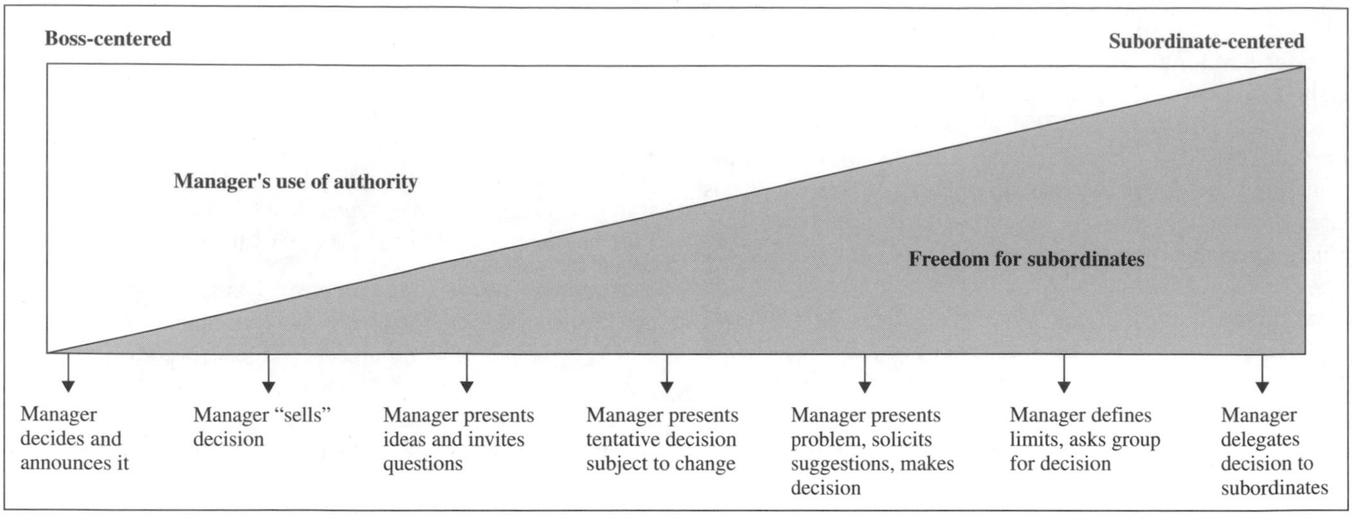

Behavioral Theories of Leadership

Earlier theories focused on what leaders *should* do and what was expected of them. In contrast, the emerging behavioral theories described what managers actually do. These emerging theories clearly emphasized a leader's orientation toward both tasks and people and enabled leaders to describe a variety of styles rather than just the "right" one.

Normative Decision Tree

Victor Vroom and Philip Yetton (1971) developed the **Normative Decision Model** in the early 1970s. Using a continuum similar to Tannenbaum and Schmidt's, they identified a series of intermediate questions and decisions, which could be answered yes or no, that would lead to each outcome (figure 21.9): crucial aspects of the situation related to the quality of the decision required, the degree of subordinate support for the decision, the amount of information available to leaders and followers, and how well structured or defined the problem was. A decision made exclusively by the leader without member input could create problems in acceptance, just as delegating a decision to a group could be costly in time and effort, if unnecessary. The Vroom-Yetton model enables a manager to decide on the level of decision-making involvement: autonomous, consultative, or delegative. A more recent revision of the model by Vroom and Jago (1988) replaced the limiting features of the yes–no response options with five choices. It also incorporated consideration for subordinate development, decision time, and the manager's rating of the criteria as new decision rules. The resulting formula is complex and most easily applied with a software program.

Another way to view both autocratic-democratic and leadership continuum models is by describing them along a task-social dimension. For example, both the linear models of Tannenbaum and Schmidt and of Vroom and Jago allowed behavior to be described from a task to a social orientation. However, these linear models only allowed leaders to be placed along a single point on the continuum, and did not allow them to favor both aspects at the same time. By "bending" the linear continuum into orthogonal axes (figure 21.10, p. 510), it is possible to create a grid or a two-by-two table that has a greater area for describing more varieties of leadership behavior. Using this matrix format, a person could be described as having both task and social orientations, not just one or the other.

Ohio and Michigan Studies

During the 1950s and 1960s, researchers at The Ohio State University examined the behavior of leaders in several hundred studies and reduced them to two categories: consideration and initiating structure (Shartle 1979). **Consideration** referred to attention to the interpersonal aspects of work, including respect for subordinates' ideas and feelings, maintaining harmonious work relationships, collaborating in teamwork, and showing concern with the subordinates' welfare. **Initiating structure** was more task focused and centered on giving direction, setting goals and limits, planning, and scheduling activities. During the same period, researchers at the University of Michigan developed a similar model. Comparing effective and ineffective managers, they found that a key difference was that the former employee-centered managers focused more on the human needs of their subordinates whereas their less effective job-centered managers emphasized only goal attainment (Likert 1979).

Leadership Grid

Building on the Ohio and Michigan studies, Blake and Mouton (1976) at the University of Texas identified the same two dimensions: concern for people and concern for production. Their **leadership grid** marked off degrees of emphasis toward orientation using a nine-point scale and finally separated the grid into five styles of management based on the combined people and production emphasis. For example, a

Figure 21.9.   **Normative Decision Tree**

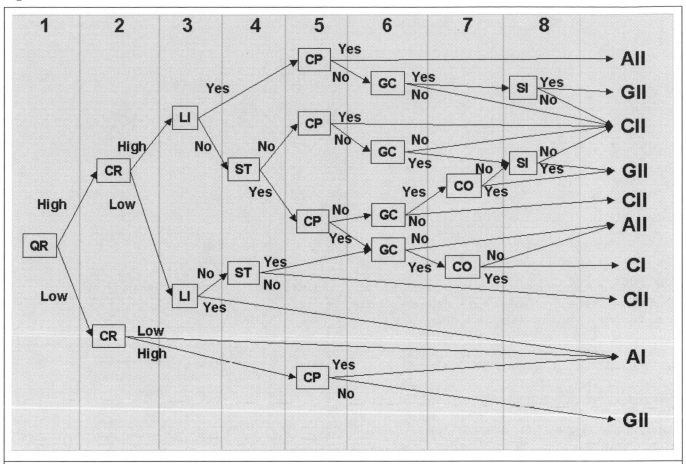

At each step in the process, a question is asked and the response determines the next branch and question. Each node of the tree has a critical criterion for determining the outcome, including:

- *Quality requirement (QR):* How important is the technical quality of the decision?

- *Commitment requirement (CR):* How important is subordinate commitment to the decision?

- *Leader's information (LI):* Do you (the leader) have sufficient information to make a high-quality decision on your own?

- *Problem structure (ST):* Is the problem well structured (e.g., defined, clear, organized, lends itself to solution, time limited, etc.)?

- *Commitment probability (CP):* If you were to make the decision by yourself, is it reasonably certain that your subordinates would be committed to it?

- *Goal congruence (GC):* Do subordinates share the organizational goals to be attained in solving the problem?

- *Subordinate conflict (CO):* Is conflict among subordinates over preferred solutions likely?

- *Subordinate information (SI):* Do subordinates have sufficient information to make a high-quality decision?

Decision Outcome	Description
Autocratic I (AI)	Leader solves the problem alone using information that is readily available.
Autocratic II (AII)	Leader obtains additional information from group members, then makes decision alone. Group members may or may not be informed.
Consultative I (CI)	Leader shares problem with group members individually and asks for information and evaluation. Group members do not meet collectively, and leader makes decision alone.
Consultative II (CII)	Leader shares problem with group members collectively but makes decision alone.
Group II (GII)	Leader meets with group to discuss situation. Leader focuses and directs discussion but does not impose will. Group makes final decision.

Figure 21.10.   The Shift from Leadership Continuum to Matrix Leadership Model

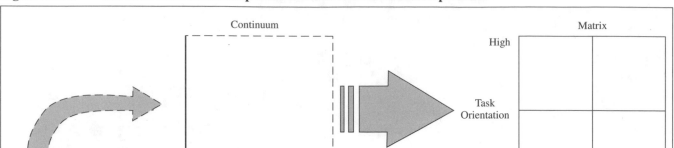

---

score of 9,9 (emphasizing both people and production) was called "Team Management." Blake and Mouton considered it the best orientation because it emphasized harmonious cooperation in production to achieve goals. A score of 9,1, an "Authority-Compliance" orientation with an emphasis on production and operational efficiency, afforded little attention to human needs. The 1,9 "Country Club" orientation emphasized group harmony, esprit de corps, and cooperation over production. The 1,1, "Impoverished" orientation reflected inattention toward both relationships and work production. A mix of both dimensions, but less than a team orientation, is the 5,5 "Middle-of-the-Road" approach, which tries to balance the two. (See figure 21.11.)

Later Models of Leadership

To this point, most theories have emphasized identifying a cluster of traits or a single style or orientation for leadership. As research in leadership has continued, it has become apparent that successful leadership does not depend on style or skills alone but, rather, on matching a leader's style with the demands of a specific situation.

Fiedler's Contingency Model

Fred Fiedler at the University of Illinois designed his **contingency model of leadership** to compensate for the limitations of the classical and behavioral theories of leadership (Fiedler 1967). Fiedler kept the social-task orientation as the cornerstone of his theory and designed an innovative test to determine the leader's preferred style. **The Least Preferred CoWorker (LPC)** scale presented a series of sixteen to twenty-two bipolar adjectives along an eight-point rating scale. Sample items included unfriendly to friendly, uncooperative to cooperative, and hostile to supportive. When the leader described a least-preferred coworker with positive terms, he or she was considered to have a relationship orientation. That is, although the leader might not want to work

Figure 21.11.   Leadership Matrix Models

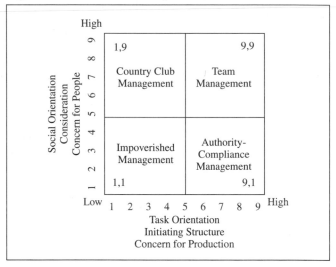

with the coworker, the leader's interpersonal orientation allows him or her to still perceive the coworker in a positive light. In contrast, a task-oriented leader would be one who described the LPC in negative terms; if he or she cannot work with the coworker, this biases the leader's view of the person on other behaviors.

The second aspect of Fiedler's model was the favorability of the situation in which the leader would operate. Because contingency means "depends on," the favorability or fit of a leader depends on the following three situational factors:

- **Leader-member relations** or "group atmosphere" is much like social orientation and includes the subordinates' acceptance of, and confidence in, the leader and the loyalty and commitment they show toward the leader.
- **Task structure** is obviously related to task dimension described by other theories above and refers to how

clearly and how well defined the task goal, procedures, and possible solutions are.

- **Position power** refers to the authority the leader has to direct others and to use reward and coercive power.

In general, the greater the favorability to the leader, the more the subordinates can be relied on to carry out the task and the fewer challenges to leadership. Situations more favorable to leadership are those in which leader-member relations are positive, task structure is high, and position power is high. Situations in which these factors are reversed are considered unfavorable to leaders because they have less leverage to influence their followers. Task-oriented leaders tend to perform better in situations that are either high or low in favorability; relationship-oriented leaders do better under moderately favorable conditions.

Although the idea of a contingency or leadership style varying in effectiveness depending on circumstances has gained in popularity, research has not shown extensive support for certain aspects of Fiedler's model and its utility remains in dispute. The LPC, for example, does not appear to be exclusively related to task and relationship styles, and may measure other, unrelated features. Fiedler originally believed that personality was "fixed" and that one should engineer or change a situation to be more compatible with a leader's style. Although Fiedler introduced a variety of useful strategies for changing the three contingencies, it is now clear that leaders have much more flexibility in applying their style than was once thought. Finally, several studies have shown that leaders in high or low favorability situations are about equally effective in goal attainment. Nonetheless, Fiedler's important contribution was his promotion of the idea of contingency.

Hersey and Blanchard's Situational Model

One of the more popular leadership models used for training, and one that has attempted to integrate other ideas from management, is Hersey and Blanchard's situational model of leadership (Hersey, Blanchard, and Johnson 1996). As Dubrin (2001) points out, this is more a model than a theory because it does not explain why things happen but, rather, offers recommendations for behaving differently under various conditions. To the already widely used task and social dimensions, Hersey and Blanchard added a third: the maturity of the followers. **Worker immaturity–maturity** is a concept borrowed from Chris Argyris, who suggested job and psychological maturity also influence leadership style. *Job maturity* refers to how much work-related ability, knowledge, experience, and skill a person has; *psychological maturity* refers to willingness, confidence, commitment, and motivation related to work. Behaviors associated with maturity include initiative, dependability, perseverance, receptiveness to feedback, goal orientation, and minimal need for supervision. Argyris (1957) has suggested that to apply a directive approach with mature workers can result in stifling their maturity and even in forcing them back to lower levels of maturity. Hence, adjusting

leadership style to worker maturity is an important consideration. (See figure 21.12.)

Hersey and Blanchard also adapted the grid format of their predecessors and structured it in a developmental sequence. Borrowing the idea that teams and organizations progress through developmental stages of a life cycle (Miller and Friesen 1984; Tuckman 1965), they suggested that leadership style should be adjusted to the stage of team development. For example, their Situation-1 (S1) involves high-task, but low-social, emphasis, thereby indicating that the leader should focus on task duties such as goal setting, identifying resources and constraints, and so on. As the team moves to Situation-2 (S2), task and social functions of the leader are both involved as members attempt to influence each other and to explore how their styles may conflict with or complement each other. In Situation-3 (S3), members clearly know the task and need little direction, but social interaction around team norms may require intervention and guidance. Finally, Situation-4 (S4) is the stage of high team performance in which both task and relationships require little intervention by the leader. Worker maturity is high, and the leader may be active only in encouraging higher performance and removing barriers to performance. Hersey and Blanchard also incorporated Tannenbaum and Schmidt's autocratic-democratic continuum, which they distributed across the developed stages and labeled telling, selling, participating, and delegating. (See figure 21.13.)

Figure 21.12.   Argyris's Worker Immaturity–Maturity Continuum

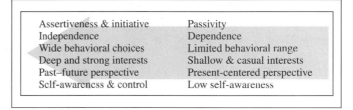

Assertiveness & initiative	Passivity
Independence	Dependence
Wide behavioral choices	Limited behavioral range
Deep and strong interests	Shallow & casual interests
Past–future perspective	Present-centered perspective
Self-awareness & control	Low self-awareness

Figure 21.13.   Situational Leadership Model

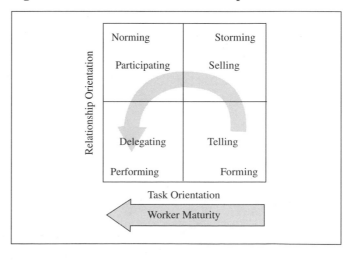

Path-Goal Theory

A more recent model of leadership, initially introduced by House (1971), is **path–goal theory.** This theory was based on the **expectancy theory** of motivation that proposes that one's effort will result in the attainment of desired performance goals. Path-goal theory states that a person's ability to perform certain tasks is related to the direction and clarity available that lead to organizational goals. For example, if a worker is unclear about what a task involves and what should be done, performance will be improved when clear instructions are given. The role of leaders, then, is to facilitate the path toward the goal by removing barriers to performance.

Path-goal theory identifies four different situations, each requiring a different facilitative response from leadership (figure 21.14). When workers lack self-confidence, leaders provide support by being friendly, approachable, concerned about needs, and equitable. This increases the worker's confidence to achieve the work outcome. When the worker has an ambiguous job, the leader is more directive in providing the worker with direction, schedules, rules, and regulations that clarify the path. When workers do not have sufficient job challenge, the leader uses an achievement approach, combining demanding and supporting by setting challenging goals, continually seeking improvement, and expecting high performance, for example. Finally, when the reward is mismatched with worker needs, the leader takes a more consultative or participative role in which workers share work problems, make suggestions, and are included in decision making to ensure more appropriate rewards. All four strategies result in improved task performance and satisfaction—again, the task and social dimensions.

Theories of Transactional and Transformational Leadership

This discussion goes back to the difference between managers and leaders discussed earlier. In 1978, when James MacGregor Burns published his Pulitzer prize-winning *Leadership,* he emphasized this distinction among political leaders, calling them transactional and transformational styles. **Transactional leadership** refers to the role of the manager who strives to create an efficient workplace by balancing task accomplishment with interpersonal satisfaction. In contrast, **transformational leadership** is considered more complex and powerful. In this leadership style, leaders promote innovation and organizational change. In the mid-1980s, Bernard Bass extended the model into the business world (1985).

An important aspect of transformational leadership is **charisma,** or the ability to inspire and motivate people beyond what is expected with exceptionally high levels of commitment (Bass and Avolio 1993; Klein and House 1995). Charisma refers to influence by force of personality in which the leader inspires commitment, loyalty, and faith in a vision. Examples of people who have wielded such power include Martin Luther King, Normal Schwarzkopf, Winston Churchill, Adolph Hitler, and David Koresh. Although the rhetoric and imagery can be stimulating to followers, there is a risk that with the leader's passing, leadership succession may fail and progress may falter.

In a five-year study, Bennis and Nanus (1985) conducted extensive interviews with ninety top leaders. Their study reinforced differences between transformational (leaders) and

Figure 21.14.   Path–Goal Theory

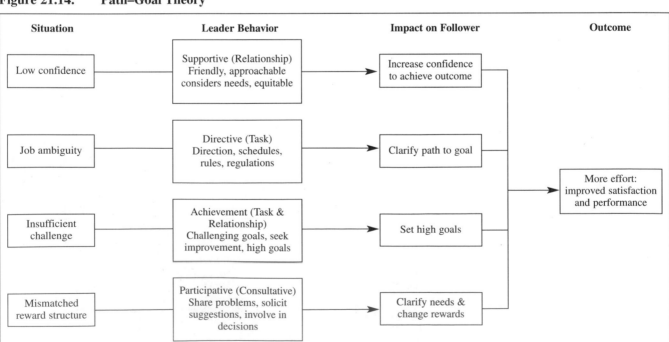

transactional (managers) roles, finding that transformational leaders were distinguished by their "four Is": idealized influence (leader as role model), inspirational motivation (team spirit and meaningfulness), intellectual stimulation (innovation and creativity), and individual consideration (mentoring).

Attempting to define the leadership practices of transformational leaders, Kouzes and Posner (1989) surveyed 550 middle and senior managers in private and public sectors. They used a series of questions that identified how leaders performed during their personal best leadership achievements. They reduced the results into five leadership practices and ten behavioral commitments:

- *Challenging the process* included the search for opportunities and taking risks.
- *Inspiring a shared vision* involved envisioning the future and enlisting others.
- *Enabling others to act* was based on fostering collaboration and strengthening others.
- *Modeling the way* included setting an example and planning small wins.
- *Encouraging the heart* referred to recognizing and celebrating accomplishments.

Kouzes and Posner stressed that the relationship between leaders and followers has a **synergy,** in which the combination of their efforts produces more than either acting alone. This enthusiasm for change is essential in dealing more effectively with the innovations and changes that face modern organizations.

Check Your Understanding 21.4

Instructions: Complete the following activities on a separate piece of paper.

1. Think of a decision you might be confronted with as a supervisor at work. Use the Vroom-Yetton decision tree to trace how you might arrive at the choice of either making the decision yourself, consulting with others, or delegating the decision to someone else.

2. Describe how your approach to leading people should change as they move through the stages of worker maturity. Explain what might happen if your style mismatches what they need at these stages.

Diffusion of Innovations

Innovations have occurred throughout history, but little attention was given to exactly how they were adopted until Rogers and Shoemaker (1971) clarified the process in their book, *Communication of Innovations*. Although Rogers and Shoemaker were not the first to develop ideas about diffusion, their presentation of the adopter categories or stakeholders and diffusion S-curve came at a time that businesses were eager to understand consumers

Viewing the organization in much the same way that marketers view market segments, Rogers and Shoemaker identified five categories of adopters of an innovation that generally fits the normal curve (figure 21.15):

- **Innovators:** This venturesome group comprises about 2.5 percent of the organization and individuals who are eager to try new ideas. They tend to be more cosmopolitan, to seek out new information in broad networks, and to be willing to take risks.
- **Early adopters:** This respectable group accounts for about 13.5 percent of the organization. The individuals in this group have a high degree of opinion leadership. They are more localized than cosmopolitan and often look to the innovators for advice and information. These are the leaders and respected role models in the organization, and their adoption of an idea or practice does much to initiate change in the organization.
- **Early majority:** This deliberate group comprises about 34 percent of the organization. Although usually not leaders, the individuals in this group represent the backbone of the organization, are deliberate in thinking and acceptance of an idea, and serve as a natural bridge between early and late adopters.

Late majority: This skeptical group comprises another 34 percent of the organization. The individuals in this group usually adopt innovations only after social or financial pressure to do so.

Laggards: The traditional members of this group are usually the last ones to respond to innovation and make up as much as 16 percent of the organization.

Figure 21.15.   Characteristics of Innovation Stakeholders

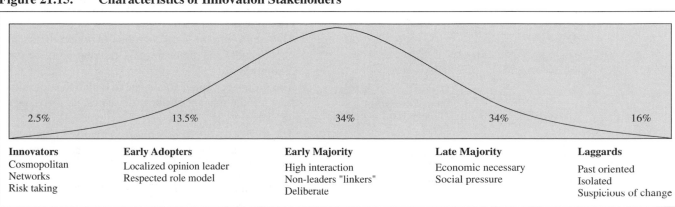

Innovators	Early Adopters	Early Majority	Late Majority	Laggards
Cosmopolitan	Localized opinion leader	High interaction	Economic necessary	Past oriented
Networks	Respected role model	Non-leaders "linkers"	Social pressure	Isolated
Risk taking		Deliberate		Suspicious of change

2.5%   13.5%   34%   34%   16%

The laggards are often characterized as isolated, uninformed, and mistrustful of change and change agents, but they may serve a function by keeping the organization from changing too quickly.

When planning a change, each of these groups should be considered as a market segment whose needs must be responded to by leaders. In general, people who are more receptive to innovation have more education, are more literate, and have stronger aspirations for achievement. In addition, they have higher socioeconomic status, occupational prestige, higher income, and social mobility. Moreover, they are better socially networked, cosmopolitan, diverse in interests, and well integrated into the organization and the community (Rogers 1995).

Each of the adopter categories engages innovation at a different time and a different acceptance rate, as shown by the diffusion S curve (figure 21.16). Note that during the early stages of diffusion, there is a shorter period between becoming aware of an innovation and its adoption. Over time, each of the adopter categories becomes aware of the innovation but increasingly takes longer periods to adopt it, which can affect how well an innovation is introduced into the marketplace or how fully it is practiced in the organization. In addition, how quickly an innovation is accepted is based on a number of factors, including whether it offers an advantage relative to its alternative, its compatibility with the potential adopters' values and lifestyles, how easy it is to understand and use, the degree to which it can be experimented with, and the degree to which the results are visible to others (Rogers 1995)

In the late 1960s and early 1970s, the literature reflected a new interest in the roles of innovators within organizations who become gatekeepers or nodes for the flow of information (Allen and Cohen, 1969). Four roles have been identified for the successful implementation of an innovation (Daft and Marcic 1998):

- The **inventor** (innovator) is the individual who develops a new idea or practice in the organization. However, it is not sufficient to merely originate and understand the new

idea. Rather, the idea must be facilitated by several other roles in the organization before it is adopted or brought to market (Daft 2000).

- The **champion** is someone in the organization who believes in the idea, acknowledges the practical problems of financing and political support, and assists in overcoming barriers.
- The **sponsor** is usually a high-level manager who approves and protects the idea, expedites testing and approval, and removes barriers within the organization.
- The **critic** is a crucial, but sometimes overlooked, role. This role is essential in challenging the innovation for shortcomings, presenting strong criteria, and, in essence, providing a reality test for the new idea.

In an innovative environment, all these roles are important and good examples of how role responsibilities are distributed in an organization.

Change Management

A more global role for practitioners of organizational change is often referred to as the change agent. The **change agent** is a specialist in organizational development and facilitates the change brought about by the innovation. He or she may be internal or external to the organization, as in the case of a consultant specifically hired to assist with the change. **Organization development** (OD) is the process of an organization reflecting on its own processes and consequently revising them for improved performance. Beckhard has provided a widely accepted definition of OD: "Organization Development is an effort planned, organizationwide, and managed from the top, to increase organization effectiveness and health through planned interventions in the organization's processes, using behavioral-science knowledge" (1969, p. 9).

Blake and Mouton (1976) suggested that OD consultants might perform a range of five functions with management:

- The *acceptant function* uses counseling skills to help the manager sort out emotions to gain a more objective perspective of the organization.
- The *catalytic function* helps collect and interpret data about the organization.
- The *confrontation function* is one in which the change agent challenges the manager's thinking processes and assumptions.
- The *prescriptive function* is one in which the consultant may tell the manager what to do to correct a given situation.
- The *theory and principle function* involves helping the client system internalize alternate explanations of what is occurring in the organization.

The work of change agents is captured in the seven stages of OD (Kolb and Frohman 1970):

Figure 21.16.   The Diffusion S-Curve

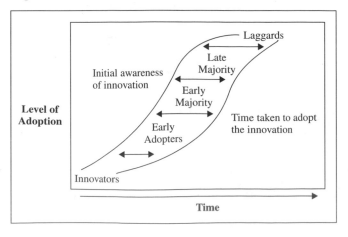

1. *Scouting stage:* The change agent inquires and observes to determine how receptive the organization is, where the leverage points for change are located, and what the fit is between his or her skills and the system's requirements.

2. *Entry and contracting stage:* The working relationship between the change agent and key organizational members is built, expectations are set, roles are clarified, credibility is established, and resources and constraints are identified.

3. *Diagnosis, or data-gathering and feedback, stage:* This stage is one of the central features of OD. Rather than using the so-called medical model in which an expert makes the diagnosis and delivers it to the patient, the OD practitioner obtains data from the organization and involves the organization in interpreting the data and considering their implications.

4. *Planning stage:* The system moves toward a conclusion about the information. Responsibility is shifted from the change agent to the organization, which commits to the change and often formulates policy regarding it.

5. *Implementation stage:* The plan is carried out as designed and agreed to, with the change agent available for further consultation as needed.

6. *Evaluation stage:* This stage involves selecting appropriate measurements, monitoring the change process and its outcomes, and keeping people informed.

7. *Termination stage:* The change agent meets with key organizational members to review the change process, to determine what and how they have learned from the experience, and to end the consulting relationship.

OD methods are quite varied and have grown out of extensive research and innovation in the behavioral sciences. Cummings and Huse (1989) identified more than twenty different techniques that practitioners use to promote change, and new ones are emerging regularly. Popular examples include:

- **Survey feedback** is widely used, especially during the diagnostic stage when questionnaires are used to identify attitudes and values about aspects of the change process. The results of the survey are given to decision makers as feedback, with the intention that any discrepancies between what they believe and what is actually occurring in the organization will prompt corrective action.

- **Team building** involves identifying performance goals and then building cohesion by involving members in activities that enhance acquaintance, resolve conflicts, build healthy group norms, and build skills in reflecting on team processes to continue performance improvement.

- **Appreciative inquiry** is based on the belief that whatever is needed in organizational renewal already exists somewhere in the organization. It seeks to identify where the change already works and how it can be amplified and transferred elsewhere in the organization.

Stages of Change

People and organizations move through stages of change; and as they do, they have different needs and require different skills from the leader. One of the first models of change was proposed by Kurt Lewin, one of the early behavioral scientists who contributed to the knowledge base of information on group work, leadership, and organization development. Lewin's model identified the initial stage of change to be one of **unfreezing** the status quo, often by presenting the discrepancies between the status quo and the desired goals. Unfreezing often creates a state of cognitive dissonance, which is an uncomfortable awareness of two incompatible perceptions or beliefs—in this case, the discrepancy. This motivates the person to resolve the dissonance, usually by changing the situation to make the perceptions congruent. This marks the second stage of change or moving to the new desired state for the organization. In the final stage of **refreezing,** the new behaviors are reinforced to become as stable and institutionalized as the previous status quo was. Lewin originally conceptualized this three-stage process as one in which the organization would plateau and stabilize for a time before the next change was required. More recent beliefs about organizational change characterize the change process as continuous with little respite for workers, managers, or leaders. The status quo has become one of dealing with continual change, which can be stressful.

Elizabeth Kubler-Ross (1969) examined the stress of change in her classic study of the **stages of grief** experienced by terminally ill patients and their families. Change in the healthcare system often involves mergers, acquisitions, downsizing, and other transitions that usually involve losses and grief. Her five-stage model has become useful in anticipating and working with people in a dramatic transition (Rogers 2000). The five stages of her model are (figure 21.17):

1. In the *shock and denial* stage, workers have difficulty believing the proposed transition. They may deny that change is imminent and go about business as usual rather than prepare for the adjustment. News of the change also may stun workers to the extent that they

Figure 21.17.   Kubler-Ross's Stages of Grief

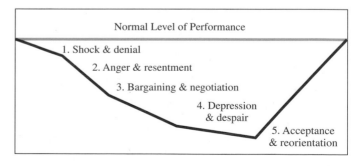

Normal Level of Performance
1. Shock & denial
2. Anger & resentment
3. Bargaining & negotiation
4. Depression & despair
5. Acceptance & reorientation

cannot concentrate or work efficiently, and they may isolate themselves.

2. In the *anger* stage, workers begin to understand the inevitability of the change. They may direct their resentment at the organization or the managers for allowing it to happen. In addition, they may engage in unproductive complaining, organize resistance, or even sabotage operations in attempts to reduce the threat.

3. In the *bargaining* stage, workers make a final attempt to avoid the change. They may actually try to bargain with managers to delay the change or work intensively to prove their value and reduce the risk of loss.

4. In the *depression* stage, workers may lose their self-esteem and be unresponsive to encouragement.

5. In the *acceptance* stage, workers begin to redirect their energy toward the new organization.

Resistance to Change

Kurt Lewin is credited with saying, "If you wish to understand something, try changing it." What he was referring to was the observation that when one attempts to change a system, the mechanisms that maintain it spring to its defense. Change does not come easily to most people, and in organizations, "resistance to change is experienced at almost every step" (DeWine 1994, p. 281). The first step for leaders who are trying to reduce resistance to change is to understand its source.

Resistance to change occurs for a number of reasons, including self-interests and anxiety about the unknown, different perceptions, suspiciousness, and conservatism. When confronted with change, the first thing most workers want to know is how it will affect them and their jobs. Because the turbulence of the marketplace makes many changes uncertain, the workers may not receive satisfactory answers to their questions. Those who have attained expertise and status from their positions now may face new job descriptions or expanded or new duties. For example, many managers in downsized organizations have been reassigned as coaches to newly formed teams. This new role raises questions about their authority, status, and responsibility.

Other workers may resist change simply because they perceive the situation differently and believe the proposed change is unjustified. The result of ongoing change is to make many people uneasy about, and even mistrustful of, any innovation. Some people view all change as just another fad based on the whim of management rather than a survival strategy for the organization. And finally, some people are very conservative in their beliefs, are isolated in their social networks and information, and dislike the inconvenience of change.

Resistance can distract workers from their tasks, preoccupy them with gossiping, and contribute to stress and workplace violence. To confident change leaders, indications of resistance can be viewed as useful information about what stakeholders need before the transition can continue.

Facilitation of Change

In recognition of the stresses that change imposes on the organization's employees, Bridges (1980) extended Lewin's three-stage model with recommendations for transition management to ease the struggle. The transition process starts with the recognition that the old way of doing things is **ending.** Workers begin to anticipate and experience losses with resulting grief, blame, shock, and fear. They need help to let go of the way things were. The transition can be facilitated by providing reasons for the ending and by indicating what will not change. It is usually best to overcommunicate to ensure that everyone has sufficient information about ongoing developments in the change process. Acknowledging losses and accepting grieving also can assist people in the ending stage.

The second stage, the **neutral zone,** begins when the old system has been left behind, but the new one has not yet been fully accepted. This stage fosters anxiety, uncertainty, and confusion. However, the organization can facilitate the transition by providing support, encouragement, protection, reassurance, and protection. The employees need to know where they are and the direction in which they are going. Creativity can be stimulated by having people generate innovative ideas about how they can move toward the new organization.

In the third stage, **new beginnings,** people accept, orient themselves, and engage in the new organization. New goals are created to provide direction, and the workers' relationships with the organization and their jobs are reinvented and integrated. Attitudes and behaviors that support the new beginning are supported by workers and role-modeled by leaders. Retraining, performance feedback, and recognition of new behavior serve to reinforce it.

Importance of Reflection

Reflection is the process of examining one's experience. It is an essential skill for developing leadership skills and an important component of team and organization development. However, reflection alone is not sufficient for changing behavior. Reflection involves awareness. Reflective learning, on the other hand, uses awareness to formulate an interpretation of what has been observed, considers what difference can be made by applying what has been learned, and executes the efforts toward change through deliberate action. Several remarkably similar models of the **reflective learning cycle** have been developed over the years, including those by John Dewey (1938), David Kolb (1970), W. Edwards Deming (1986), and Donald Schon (1983). These models share the following four stages in common (figure 21.18):

- *Doing:* At this stage, people are concentrating and working directly on a task. Although most people reflect on a task after it is accomplished, this is often too late to make midcourse or more frequent changes. The reflective process should be used often, although too much reflection sometimes is used to avoid task completion.

Figure 21.18.   Reflective Learning Process

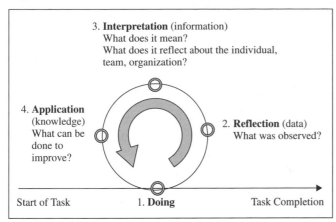

As the marketplace continues to change, organizations will have to adapt in order to maintain their competitive advantage. Organizational leaders play a key role in helping employees to reduce their resistance to change and to inspire and motivate them to accept change. By understanding leadership theories and the stages and techniques of planned change, and by using the reflective learning cycle, managers will be better prepared to meet the challenge.

Check Your Understanding 21.5

Instructions: Answer the following questions on a separate piece of paper.

1. If you were an OD consultant, what would you tell an executive team about a pending reorganization? What should they expect?

2. If you were informed that your job was being eliminated due to reorganization but that you could reapply for new positions, how would you react? What would you need to cope with the stress?

3. Use the reflecting learning process to examine a group meeting. What did you notice? What do you think that your observations reflected about the group processes? What could you do differently to improve the next meeting?

Real-World Case

The corporate director of health information services consulted an organization development specialist about recurrent problems she had been having with one of two departments under her direction. The two medical information depart-

ments were similar in size and structure and were located in branch clinics only a few miles apart, but that is where the similarity ended. Although one department had only four union grievances over a four-year period, the other generated as many phone calls to the corporate director on a weekly basis.

The consultant visited the troubled department to meet with the manager and determine the problem. The manager had been promoted to the position that year based on her exceptional technical knowledge. She told the consultant that when she arrived, she found the department terribly disorganized. She took on the burden of raising the standards, requiring compliance, monitoring performance, and pushing people to perform at their best. The consultant was impressed with her dedication and eager to speak with members of her department. However, when he suggested doing so, he was surprised by her response: "What do you mean you want to talk to my staff! Do you think I'm lying? Do you think I don't know what I'm talking about?"

The intensity of her reaction puzzled the consultant, but he persisted, emphasizing that any change effort necessarily involves understanding the perspectives of all the organization's stakeholders. When he finally scheduled meetings with the employees, he was met with silence, even though he had assured them of confidentiality. With the encouragement of the corporate director, a few relented and expressed how fearful they were of the manager. They explained that under her dominating style, the job had become a "survival game." Curious, the consultant asked them to explain the game. They replied that they despised the manager, but that the job and benefits were too good to leave. Therefore, they had devised a way to work around her by rating her moods from one to six. One through three required them to avoid her at all cost, four to five required them to carefully evaluate whether they really needed to speak with her, and a six indicated that something nice had happened in her life that day and she could be approached.

Incredulous, the consultant asked if this was a joke. The employees suggested that he come early some morning and he would see the game in action. A few weeks later, he arrived at 8 a.m., just as the first employee entered the manager's office. When the employee emerged ten minutes later, heads poked up from all of the cubicles in the office area to see the employee holding three fingers aloft, indicating that it was best to avoid the manager that day.

Confronted by the consultant and the corporate director, the manager refused to acknowledge that her employees were afraid of her. She said that neither the consultant nor the corporate director understood what she was trying to do and that she could teach them a thing or two about effective management. She simply was unaware of how ineffective her style was; nor was she receptive to feedback. After a short probationary period during which she showed no response to further coaching, she resigned. The consultant found out later that the staff had celebrated by having a "funeral" in which they dug a hole and threw in reminders of their most memorable interactions with her, using the occasion to debrief the reign of intimidation.

The next manager had a better combination of technical and interpersonal skills, but it took nearly two years to establish trust.

Discussion Questions

1. How could this problem situation have gotten so far without intervention?

2. What could the corporate director have done to resolve the situation sooner?

3. What difference might a 360-degree performance evaluation, an organizational culture assessment, or a management feedback system have made?

4. If the manager had been more receptive to intervention, how might you have used coaching or some other support to help her change?

Summary

As the marketplace has expanded to a global perspective and workplace settings have become more diverse and complex, the discipline of management has likewise evolved. Classical management theories focused on formal authority, hierarchical avenues of communication and accountability, and operational efficiency. Weber's concept of bureaucracy, Taylor's scientific management, and Gilbreth's and Gantt's operational innovations provided such structure.

As management became professionalized, effective practices and responsibilities became more formal and were incorporated into the administrative model of management. In addition to describing the functions of planning, organizing, leading, and controlling, Fayol formulated fourteen principles for management. Prior to emergence of the humanistic approach to management, Bernard proposed the acceptance view of authority and emphasized the balance of effectiveness and efficiency. The Hawthorne effect marked the shift from operations and authority to the human relations movement and attention to worker motivation. Maslow described a hierarchy of needs that provided managers with a model for targeting efforts to motivate workers. And McGregor recognized the shift from authoritarian to humanistic orientation in his Theory X and Y.

As technology and strategy were emphasized in response to international conflicts and competition, management science developed a variety of new tools. Operations management, statistical forecasting, break-even analysis, queuing, modeling, and PERT were used to reemphasize production to balance the renewed emphasis on people.

More contemporary approaches to management have emphasized improved quality of products and services through greater efficiency and increased focus on people. TQM, the Baldridge Award, and the search for best practices have fine-tuned many management and business processes.

Effective management involves not only understanding Fayol's four functions, but also understanding and developing conceptual skills for strategy, interpersonal skills for working effectively with people, and technical skills for dealing with the specific business field. Moreover, managers must learn to perform multiple roles while working at an unrelenting pace.

More recent theories have emphasized the complexity of modern organizations. Senge's emphasis on systems theory, for example, helps managers understand how the organization's components are connected much as a living system, and that change in one component can affect other components.

Change management requires strong leadership. Managers traditionally maintain a highly efficient workplace and establish procedures; leaders look to the future and promote change. Both solve problems and make decisions. Recurrent problems lend themselves to clear rules for programmed decisions that can be used routinely; unique, complex, or changing situations require careful thought when nonprogrammed decisions are made. Formal decision making progresses through several stages, including problem definition, problem analysis, generation of alternatives, selection of alternatives, plan implementation, and evaluation and feedback. In practice, managers more often use intuition or satisficing.

Leadership theories provide a way to examine what is required in a situation to facilitate change through people. Classical approaches to leadership emphasized collections of traits that became unwieldy in practice. However, as society embraced democratic ideals, management began to reflect greater worker participation and involvement in decision making. Vroom and Yetton's normative model of decision making enables managers to decide when to make a decision alone and when to delegate. Studies from Ohio State University, Michigan State University, and Blake and Mouton have enabled leadership styles to be described along a continuum of task and social dimensions. Building on the need for leaders to adjust their styles to meet the unique characteristics of each situation, more recent models have emerged, including Fiedler's leadership contingency model, work done by Hersey and Blanchard, and the path-goal theory.

Change goes through different stages in an organization, and each stage has its own group of stakeholders. Plotting actual change results in an S-shaped curve with a slow start, rapid development, and a plateau of saturation and adoption. Within the organization, innovations require the key roles of inventor, champion, sponsor, and critic. The change agent spearheads the organization's change efforts.

A variety of tools and techniques for helping organizations change has been developed. Surveys, team-building activities, and appreciative inquiry are examples of structured approaches to helping organizations examine how they deal with change. Understanding the stages of change also can relieve resistance to change. The stages of change often parallel the stages of grief identified by Kubler-Ross in her classic study. Similarly, the stages of organizational change can be thought of as an end to the old ways, a neutral time of transition, and new beginnings.

References

Allen, T. J., and S. I. Cohen. 1969. Information flow in two R&D laboratories. *Administrative Science Quarterly* 14(1):12–19.

Allport, G. W., and H. S. Odbert. 1936. Trait-names: a psycho-lexical study. *Psychological Monographs* (47):171–220.

American Quality Institute. 2002. Employees cite poor managers as primary reason for quitting, according to new national survey by the Supplee Group. Accessed online at www.americanquality.com.

Andrews, F., et al. 1981. *A Guide for Selecting Statistical Techniques for Analyzing Social Science Data.* Ann Arbor, Mich.: University of Michigan Institute for Social Research.

Argyris, C. 1957. *Personality and Organization.* New York City: Harper & Row.

Artell, R. E. 1991. *Gestures: The Do's and Taboos of Body Language around the World.* New York City: John Wiley & Sons.

Bass, B. M. 1985. *Leadership and Performance beyond Expectations.* New York City: Free Press.

Bass, B. M., and B. J. Avolio. 1993. Transformational leadership: a response to critics. In *Leadership Theory and Research: Perspectives and Directions,* edited by M. M. Chemers and R. Ayman. San Diego, Calif.: Academic Press.

Beckhard, R. 1969. *Organization Development: Strategies and Models.* Reading, Mass.: Addison Wesley.

Bennis, W. 1959. Leadership theory and administrative behavior: the problem of authority. *Administrative Science Quarterly* 4:259–301.

Bennis, W. 1989. *Why Leaders Can't Lead.* San Francisco: Jossey-Bass Publishers.

Bennis, W. 1997. Champions of change. Leadership Symposium 1997, GNP, Ltd., UK.

Bennis, W., and B. Nanus. 1985. *Leaders: The Strategy for Taking Charge.* New York City: Harper & Row.

Bigelow, J. 1991. Managerial skills texts: how do they stack up? Organizational Behavior Teaching Conference, Bellingham, Wash., June 26–29, 1991.

Blake, R. R., and J. S. Mouton. 1976. *Consultation.* Reading, Mass.: Addison Wesley.

Blodgett, M. 1999. Teaching Johnny to lead. *CIO Magazine.* Accessed online from www.cio.com.

Bridges, W. 1980. *Transitions: Making Sense of Life's Changes.* Reading, Mass.: Addison Wesley.

Bridges, W. 1994. *Jobshift: How to Prosper in a Workplace without Jobs.* Reading, Mass.: Addison Wesley.

Buckingham, M., and C. Coffman. 1999. *First, Break All the Rules: What the World's Greatest Managers Do Differently.* New York City: Simon & Schuster.

Burke, W., et al. 1985. Changing leadership and planning processes at the Lewis Research Center, National Aeronautics and Space Administration. *Human Resources Management* 24(1):81–90.

Burns, J. M. 1978. *Leadership.* New York City: Free Press.

Charan, R., and G. Colvin. 1999. Why CEOs fail. *Fortune,* June 21, p. 69.

Church, A. H. 1997. Managerial self-awareness in high performing individuals in organizations. *Journal of Applied Psychology* 82(2):281–92.

Cummings, T. G., and E. F. Huse. 1989. *Organization Development and Change.* New York City: West.

Daft, R. L. 2000. *Management.* Fort Worth, Tex.: Dryden.

Daft, R. L., and D. Marcic. 1998. *Understanding Management.* Fort Worth, Tex.: Dryden.

DeJanasz, S., K. Dowd, and B. Schneider. 2002. *Interpersonal Skills in Organizations.* New York City: McGraw-Hill.

Deming, W. E. 1986. *Out of the Crisis.* Cambridge, Mass.: Massachusetts Institute of Technology, Center for Advanced Engineering Study.

Dewey, J. 1938. *Experience and Education.* New York City: Collier.

DeWine, S. 1994. *The Consultant's Craft: Improving Organizational Communication.* New York City: St. Martin's Press.

Drucker, P. 1986. The appraisal of managerial performance. *Management Decision* 24(4):67–78.

Dubrin, A. J. 2001. *Leadership: Research Findings, Practice, and Skills.* Boston: Houghton Mifflin.

Fiedler, F. E. 1967. *A Theory of Leadership Effectiveness.* New York City: McGraw-Hill.

French, J. R. P., and B. Raven. 1959. The bases of social power. In *Studies in Social Power,* edited by D. Cartwright. Ann Arbor, Mich.: Institute for Social Research.

Gilbreth, F. B., Jr., and E. G. Carey. 1945. *Cheaper by the Dozen.* New York City: Thomas Y. Crowell Company.

Goleman, D. 1998. What makes a leader? *Harvard Business Review,* Nov-Dec.

Hale, B. 2002. Kenneth Lay: a fallen hero. BBC News. Accessed online on January 24, 2002, at www.news.bbc.co.uk.

Hammer, M., and J. Champy. 1993. *Reengineering the Corporation.* New York City: Harper.

Harris, B. 1982. The man who killed Braniff. *Texas Monthly,* July, pp. 116–20, 183–89.

Hay Group. 1999. New Fortune/Hay Group ranking of "the world's most admired companies." Press release. Accessed online from www.haygroup.com.

Healthcare Management Council. 2001. Web site address: www.hmc—benchmarks.com.

Hersey, P., K. H. Blanchard, and D. E. Johnson. 1996. *Management of Organizational Behavior: Utilizing Human Resources,* seventh edition. Upper Saddle River, N.J.: Prentice-Hall.

Hickman, C. R. 1990. *Mind of a Manager, Soul of a Leader.* New York City: John Wiley & Sons.

House, R. J. 1971. A path-goal theory of leader effectiveness. *Administrative Science Leadership Review Quarterly* 16:321–39.

ISO Online. www.iso.ch.

Jacques, E. 1996. *Requisite Organization.* Arlington, Va.: Cason Hall.

Kaplan, R. S., and D. P. Norton. 1996. *The Balanced Scorecard.* Boston: Harvard Business School Press.

Katz, R. L. 1974. Skills of an effective administrator. *Harvard Business Review* 52:90–102.

Kerker, S. 2001. Kerker reflects: Drucker's development of the strategy-focused organization. *The New Corporate University Review* 9(1). Accessed online from http://www.traininguniversity.com/magazine/jan_feb01/index.html.

Kettley, P., and M. Strebler. 1997. Changing roles for senior managers. Institute for Employment Studies, EIS Report 327.

Klein, K. J., and R. J. House. 1995. On fire: charismatic leadership and levels of analysis. *Leadership Quarterly* 6(2):183–98.

Kolb, D. A., and A. L. Frohman. 1970. An organization development approach to consulting. *Sloan Management Review* 12(1):51–65.

Kotter, J. P. 1990a. *A Force for Change: How Leadership Differs from Management.* New York City: Free Press.

Kotter, J. P. 1990b. What leaders really do. *Harvard Business Review,* May-June, pp. 103–11.

Kouzes, J., and Posner, B. 1989. *The Leadership Challenge: How to Get Extraordinary Things Done in Organizations.* San Francisco: Jossey-Bass Publishers.

Kubler-Ross, E. 1969. *On Death and Dying.* New York City: Simon & Schuster/Touchstone.

Kuhn, T. S. 1962. *The Structure of Scientific Revolutions.* Chicago: University of Chicago Press.

Leadership Symposium. 1997. Survey tracks views of the leaders and the led. GNP, Ltd., Encouraging Excellence Series. Accessed online from www.gnp.co.uk.

Leahy, T. 2000. Tailoring the balanced scorecard. *Business Finance,* August, p. 53. Accessed online from www.businessfinancemag.com.

Lee, James. 1982. *The Gold and Garbage in Management Theories and Prescriptions.* Athens, Ohio: Ohio University Press.

Legorreta, A. P., et al. 1993. Increased cholecystectomy rate after the introduction of laparoscopic cholecystectomy. *Journal of the American Medical Association* 270(12):1429–32.

Likert, R. 1979. From production- and employee-centeredness to systems 1-4. *Journal of Management* (5):628–41.

Luthans, F., R. Hodgetts, and S. Rosenkrantz. 1988. *Real Managers.* Cambridge, Mass.: Ballinger.

Mahoney, T. A., T. H. Jerdee, and S. J. Carroll. 1965. The job(s) of management. *Industrial Relations* 4(2):97–110.

McGregor, D. 1960. *The Human Side of Enterprise.* New York City: McGraw-Hill.

Miller, D., and P. H. Friesen. 1984. A longitudinal study of the corporate life cycle. *Management Science,* pp. 1161–83.

Mills, K. 1998. Failure to communicate costly for companies. *NARTE News* 16(3). Accessed online at www.narte.org.

Mintzberg, H. 1992. The manager's job: folklore and fact. In *Managing People and Organizations,* edited by John J. Gabarro. Boston: Harvard Business School Publications.

Morgan, P., and K. Baker. 1985. Building a professional image: improving listening behavior. *Supervisory Management,* November, pp. 34–38.

National HRD Executive Survey: Leadership development, first quarter survey report. 1998. American Society for Training and Development. Accessed online from www.astd.org.

Page, C., M. Wilson, and D. Meyer. 1999. A three domain, two dimensional model of managerial effectiveness. Paper presented at the Academy of Business and Administrative Sciences Conference, Barcelona, Spain.

Parson, H. M. 1974. What happened at Hawthorne? *Science* 183:922–32.

Pascale, R. T. 1990. *Managing on the Edge.* New York City: Simon & Schuster.

Peters, T. J., and R. H. Waterman. 1982. *In Search of Excellence: Lessons from America's Best-Run Companies.* New York City: Harper & Row.

Pratt, D. 2000. Adaptation is key in the digital economy. Barnstable Patriot, Hyannis, Mass. Accessed online from www.barnstable—patriot.com.

Raven, B. H. 1983. Interpersonal influence and social power. In B. H. Raven and J. Z. Rubin, *Social Psychology,* pp. 399–444. New York City: John Wiley & Sons.

Rogers, E. 1995. *Diffusion of Innovations,* fourth edition. New York City: Free Press.

Rogers, E., and F. F. Shoemaker. 1971. *Communication of Innovations: A Cross Cultural Approach.* New York City: Free Press.

Rogers, K. A. 2000. Transition management as an intervention for survivor syndrome. *Canadian Journal of Leadership Nursing* 13(4). Accessed online at www.acen—cjonl.org.

Salancik, G. R., and J. Pfeffer. 1977. Constraints on administrator discretion: the limited influence of mayors in city budgets. *Organizational Dynamics* 12(4):475–96.

Schön, D. A. 1983. *The Reflective Practitioner.* New York City: Basic Books.

Senge, Peter. 1990. *The Fifth Discipline: The Art and Practice of the Learning Organization.* New York City: Currency/Doubleday.

Shartle, C. L. 1979. Early years of the Ohio State University leadership studies. *Journal of Management* 5:126–34.

Shrader, C. B., L. Taylor, and D. R. Dalton. 1984. Strategic planning and organizational performance: a critical appraisal. *Journal of Management* 10(2):149–71.

Stogdill, R. M. 1974. *Handbook of Leadership: A Guide to Understanding Managerial Work.* Englewood Cliffs, N.J.: Prentice-Hall.

Stoner, J. A. F., and R. E. Freeman. 1989. *Management.* Englewood Cliffs, N.J.: Prentice-Hall.

Swenson, D. X. 2001. The Ouroboros Effect: the revenge effects of unintended consequences. Accessed online from http://www.css.edu/users/dswenson/web/revenge.htm.

Tannenbaum, T., and W. Schmidt. 1973. How to choose a leadership pattern. *Harvard Business Review,* May-June.

Tenner, E. 1996. *Why Things Bite Back: Technology and the Revenge of Unintended Consequences.* New York City: Alfred A. Knopf.

Tuckman, B. W. 1965. Developmental sequence in small groups. *Psychological Bulletin* 63:384–99.

Vaill, P. B. 1996. *Learning as a Way of Being.* San Francisco: Jossey-Bass Publishers.

Vroom, V., and P. Jago. 1988. *The New Leadership? Managing Participation in Organizations.* Englewood Cliffs, N.J.: Prentice-Hall.

Vroom, V., and P. Yetton. 1971. *Leadership and Decision Making.* Pittsburgh, Pa.: University of Pittsburgh Press.

Watzlawick, P., J. H. Beavin, and D. D. Jackson. 1968. *The Pragmatics of Human Communication.* New York City: Norton.

Weiner, N., and T. A. Mahoney. 1981. A model of corporate performance as a function of environment, organization, and leadership influences. *Academy of Management Journal* 24:453–70.

White, R. K., and R. Lippitt. 1960. *Autocracy and Democracy: An Experimental Inquiry.* New York City: Harper.

Yukl, G. 1998. *Leadership in Organizations.* Upper Saddle River, N.J.: Prentice-Hall.

Zaleznik, A. 1977. Managers and leaders: are they different? *Harvard Business Review,* May/June, 68–78.

Application Exercises

1. Follow and observe a manager during his or her daily activities. Make a list of the activities engaged in and determine the proportion that can be classified in terms of the four management functions, three manager's skills, and Mintzberg's management roles.

2. Assume you are applying for a managerial position in a healthcare facility. How would you describe your managerial style during the interview? Which management theory best explains the managerial style you described?

3. Rapid changes are occurring in most areas of healthcare. Identify a change that is occurring presently in a facility or department you are familiar with. Interview people to learn how they are reacting to the changes. If you were a manager, what could you do to facilitate the employees' transition?

Review Quiz

Instructions: Choose the answer that best completes the sentence or answers the question.

1. ___ Which of the following is not one of the traditional four managerial functions?
   a. Leading
   b. Controlling
   c. Negotiating
   d. Planning

2. ___ In a management sense, controlling means ___.
   a. Directing people to carry out tasks
   b. Monitoring performance
   c. Providing little choice in job descriptions
   d. Making people do what a manager wants

3. ___ The scalar chain is one in which ___.
   a. Everyone is included in the organizational chart.
   b. Decisions are made only by top management.
   c. Each person on an assembly line has a different job.
   d. Quality is rated on a five-point scale.

4. ___ Which is more accurate regarding the relationship between levels of management and managerial skills?
   a. Interpersonal skills increase as one goes from lower to upper management.
   b. The highest level of technological skills is at the top of the organization.
   c. Conceptual skills are greatest at the top level of management.
   d. Interpersonal, technical, and conceptual skills are required in equal amounts at all levels of the organization.

5. ___ Staff authority refers to ___.
   a. Advising and making recommendations
   b. Directing actions
   c. Allocating resources
   d. Setting budgets

6. ___ The practice of quality is most focused on ___.
   a. Top management
   b. Successful product lines
   c. The customer
   d. Frontline workers

7. ___ Systems theory is based on the idea that ___.
   a. Organizations should be broken into their constituent components for study.
   b. A system was popular in early management but is no longer popular or useful.
   c. Parts of an organization will fare better in isolation from other parts.
   d. Parts of an organization are interconnected and can affect each other.

8. ___ A learning organization has as its central purpose ___.
   a. Profit
   b. Standards
   c. Adaptability
   d. Structure

9. ___ The span of management refers to ___.
   a. The number of roles a manager performs
   b. The number of subordinates a manager supervises
   c. The ratio of managers to workers in an organization
   d. How diverse the range of products or services is

10. ___ Which of the following is the best reason for team building?
    a. To quickly move from acquaintance to strong task effort
    b. To identify a leader
    c. To help members build skills to work more effectively at each developmental stage of the team
    d. To ensure that the leader situation is favorable

11. ___ The person in the organization who believes in an idea and obtains financial and political support is in the organizational change role of ___.
    a. Facilitator
    b. Inventor
    c. Critic
    d. Champion

12. ___ One of the differences between leaders and managers is that leaders more often ___.
    a. Have more turbulence in their early lives
    b. Are strongly dependent on others for their security
    c. Pay attention to present efficiency
    d. Use structured and analytical thinking

13. ___ The term executive dashboard refers to ___.
    a. The short amount of time in which top level managers have to complete tasks
    b. The summary page for project management computer programs
    c. An information system maintaining current information on key strategic variables
    d. A brief version of an executive's resume regarding change efforts

14. ___ The advantage of self-monitoring is that it enables the person using it to ___.
    a. Maintain better inventory control using information systems
    b. Adjust one's behavior depending on reactions from others
    c. Pay much less attention to the behavior of others
    d. Decide whether to make a decision alone or to delegate the decision

15. ___ ISO 9000 refers to ___.
    a. The financial standards of accounting that all organizations must conform to
    b. A European company that has set the standard for excellence in strategic planning
    c. The newest information management system allowing decision makers to monitor all organizational databases
    d. A set of international standards for quality management

Chapter 22
Work Design and Performance Improvement

Madonna LeBlanc, MA, RHIA, and Andrea Weatherby White, PhD, RHIA

Learning Objectives

- To explain how standards can be applied to each of the resources of management and to identify alternative ways in which they can be communicated
- To identify the criteria for effective standard setting
- To explain the purpose and function of work measurement and work measurement techniques and to assess the strengths and weaknesses of each as a management tool
- To express production (quantitative) standards in terms of time/unit and units/time and to calculate quantitative standards using data obtained via various methodologies
- To identify the steps involved in a work sampling effort and the tools that can be used with certain steps
- To determine sample size for a work sampling effort by using precision interval method and by formula involving various scenarios of desired certainty factor and acceptable error in the study results
- To identify potential areas for improvement in the health information services (HIS) functions given data obtained through work measurement activities and appropriate benchmarks
- To develop production standards for HIS functions

- To forecast staffing requirements for HIS functions on the basis of predicted work volume increases/decreases
- To distinguish between quantitative and qualitative standards and to identify examples of each for HIS functions
- To write effective, well-written quantitative and qualitative performance standards
- To identify common symptoms of process problems, generally and specific to HIM services
- To differentiate among the terms *effectiveness, efficiency,* and *adaptability* as goals of process improvement
- To describe the components of a system and how they are related
- To summarize the steps of the systems analysis and design process
- To describe the tools that can be used to assist managers in determining the efficiency of work flow and the distribution of work responsibilities in a work unit
- To discuss the principles incorporated in the philosophy of continuous quality improvement (CQI)
- To explain the purposes of the various CQI tools and techniques
- To discuss the similarities and differences among systems analysis and design, CQI, and reengineering

Key Terms

Affinity grouping	Flow process chart	Performance measurement	System
Benchmarking	Flowchart	Precision factor	Systems analysis and
Brainstorming	Force-field analysis	Productivity	design
Check sheet	Goal	Qualitative standards	Systems thinking
Common cause variation	Histogram	Quantitative standards	Telecommuting
Certainty factor	Job procedure	Reengineering	Time ladder
Closed systems	Job sharing	Run chart	Unit work division
Compressed workweek	Movement diagram	Scatter diagram	Volume logs
Continuous data	Multivoting technique	Serial work division	Work distribution analysis
Continuous quality	Nominal group technique	Service	Work distribution chart
improvement (CQI)	Objective	Shift rotation	Work division
Cybernetic systems	Open systems	Special cause variation	Work flow
Ergonomics	Parallel work division	Standard	Work measurement
Fishbone diagram	Pareto chart	Statistical process control	Work sampling
Flextime	PDSA cycle	chart	

Introduction

Management has been defined as getting work done through and with people. It may be thought of as both a science and an art. Management is a science because it is based on theory and principles that have been—and continue to be—tested and explored. It is an art because effective management depends on the use of sound judgment, intuition, and communication and interpersonal skills. Management uses specific functions including planning, organizing, directing, and controlling. These functions enable work processes to flow smoothly. It is the manager's responsibility to create and facilitate effective work processes so that the desired outcome can be achieved in a cost-efficient manner.

Management of human resources is one of the most challenging and critical functions in healthcare organizations. Whether as a lead staffperson, a supervisor, an assistant director, or a health information management (HIM) department director, the key to success lies in the practitioner's people and performance management skills. Performance management does not occur by accident or by osmosis. Careful consideration of the resources available and their organization is key to the effectiveness and efficiency of HIM services, as is a well-designed set of tools and strategies to facilitate staff management.

Budgets need to be met, and variances in those budgets need to be addressed intelligently and swiftly. In order to respond to fiscal demands, it is essential to have a plan of action, which includes staffing, work division, job procedures, ergonomic considerations, and performance or work measurement.

This chapter introduces key concepts, tools, and techniques associated with designing/redesigning and implementing effective and efficient work processes within an organization. It also discusses components of work processes and the development and use of performance standards and various methodologies in performance improvement.

Theory into Practice

Health information services (HIS) in any healthcare setting is a complex array of task-oriented functions. HIS is a strongly customer service–driven department and needs to be in constant communication with its different customers.

Following is a pointed example of one department's ready response to customer concerns taken from "Changes for the Better: Implementing Four Best Practices" by Cynthia Doyon, Kim Thompson, and Lori Meottel in the May 1999 issue of *Journal of the American Health Information Management Association:*

> Valley Presbyterian Hospital is a 347-bed, nonprofit acute care facility in Van Nuys, CA. The hospital houses specialty care units including skilled nursing, acute rehabilitation, pediatric intensive care, and newborn intensive care. The facility has a cardiac surgery and reha-
> bilitation program and one of the largest and busiest birthing centers in the San Fernando Valley. Today, the medical record services department (MR Services) has 29 full-time equivalents, including 5.5 transcriptionists. 4.23 FTEs are involved with the discharges, patient record retrieval, and assembly/analysis processes discussed in this article. When these functions were reengineered in 1991–92, Monica Pappas, RHIA, was director of the department.
>
> MR Services had been receiving complaints from both administration and physicians, so the department's management team knew that changes had to be made to improve overall practices within the department. The department was not meeting the needs of its customers—administrators, physicians, or patients. Days in accounts receivable due to outstanding coding were high; physicians were not completing their records in a timely manner; record control was virtually nonexistent; delinquent chart count was high; and the Joint Commission on Accreditation of Healthcare Organizations was coming in several months. To fix the problems, the managers realized process reengineering was necessary.
>
> The group conducted an analysis of the areas receiving the most complaints. Part of this analysis included a survey of the medical staff's satisfaction with the department. Guided by the analysis results and survey recommendations, the management team conducted a literature search and drew on previous experience at other facilities. Using the results of the review and the research, the management team was able to identify priority areas to be addressed.

Health information managers can successfully address customer issues and performance variances by fully understanding the components of work processes and the application of performance/work measurements.

Methods of Work Division

Staffing involves the determination of which types of employees are needed, how many of each type are needed, and what kind of work schedule is needed. Employee selection depends on the skills, experience, and education required by the work. The number of employees needed depends on the volume of work and the pattern of work division that has been selected. Work scheduling is based on when employees are needed and/or what services are required.

Work Division Patterns

Any of a number of basic **work division** patterns can be followed in process-oriented departments. The type pattern depends in large part on the type of work to be performed and the number of employees available to perform it. Three types of work division patterns are:

- **Serial work division:** This refers to the consecutive handling of tasks or products by individuals who perform a specific function in sequence. Often referred to as a production line–type of work division, serial work division tends to create task specialists. For example, three transcriptionists might be used to transcribe medical reports. A transcription clerk would support their work by performing functions such as sorting copies, answering telephones, and duplicating and disseminating the completed transcriptions. In this staffing model, the transcription clerk cannot perform his or her duties until the transcriptionists have completed their work.

- **Parallel work division:** This pattern is the concurrent handling of tasks. Multiple employees do identical types of tasks and basically see the process through from beginning to end. In parallel work division, the transcription function might include four transcriptionists, each responsible for transcribing medical reports, sorting copies, answering telephones, and duplicating and disseminating the transcribed reports. Thus, all four transcriptionists would be expected to perform the same duties independent of the others.

- **Unit work division:** This type of work division enlists simultaneous assembly in which everyone performs a different specialized task at the same time. The tasks are all related to the same end product but are not dependent on each other. The work is specialized, but the sequence of tasks is not fixed. Unit assembly is rarely referred to in HIM departments but is typical of manufacturing. Examples of unit assembly in an HIM department might include discharge record analysis and registry data abstracting. Both functions are vital to the completed medical record and may be performed by several individuals simultaneously, but independently.

Work Distribution Analysis

Work distribution analysis is a function of effective work process management and is one element of organizational analysis. It is used to determine whether a department's current work assignments and job content are appropriate. Making time to perform this analysis can lead to one or more of the following observations:

- Large amounts of time are being dedicated to functions of minor importance.
- Small amounts of time are being dedicated to functions of key importance.

- There is too much or too little job function specialization.
- There is duplication of efforts or functions.
- Some employees are overloaded with work assignments.
- Some employees do not have enough work to keep busy.
- Staff are performing tasks inappropriate to their positions.

Basic distribution data can be collected via a **work distribution chart,** which is filled out by each employee and includes all responsible task content. (See table 22.1.) Task content should come directly from the employee's current job description. In addition to task content, each employee tracks each task's start time, end time, and volume or productivity within a typical unit of a workweek.

Work Scheduling

After management has determined the equity of work distribution within a department and made adjustments accordingly, it is ready to consider a work-scheduling system. Determining the work schedule for departmental staff involves more than simply assigning hours. Effective scheduling results in the following:

- A core of employees on duty at all times when services must be provided
- A pattern of hours (shifts) to be worked and days off that employees can be reasonably sure will not be changed except in extreme emergencies
- Fair and just treatment of all employees with regard to hours assigned

Several staffing issues should be considered when devising an effective staff schedule. Answers to the following questions will help determine the department's course of action:

- *How is the workweek defined by policy?* The workweek is generally established to begin on Sunday, but organizational policy may dictate otherwise.

Table 22.1.   Work Distribution Chart

Position/ Employee	Supervisor/J. Johnson		Admissions Clerk/A. Jones		Discharge Clerk/B. Olson		File Clerk/R. Smith	
Activity	*Task*	*# of Hours*	*Task*	*# of Hours*	*Task*	*# of Hours*	*Task*	*# of Hours*
Release of information	Post requests; give depositions	2 10	Photocopy	8	Certify content	15	Retrieve records	10
Analysis	Chart IRS	2	File in MD box	3	Tag for incomplete	15	Collect charts	9
Filing	Audit file room	2	—	—	Pull for MDs	4	File and pull records	20
Administrative overhead	Attend meetings; supervise employees	12 10	Receive visitors; typing	14 14	Generate MD letters	5	—	—
Training	Read literature, etc.	2	Attend software training	1	Attend computer training	1	Attend computer training	1
Totals	40 hours/40 hours		40 hours/40 hours		40 hours/40 hours		40 hours/40 hours	

- *What days of the week is the department open? How many and what hours/days are covered?* When the coverage policy has been set, the number of personnel can be set.
- *What functions must be performed each day and within what timeframe?*
- *How many full-time equivalents (FTEs) are needed on the basis of the organization's definition of full-time?* The Fair Labor Standard Act Wage and Hour Law defines the full-time standard as forty hours per week, eighty hours per two-week period, or eight hours per day. The act also defines the difference between *exempt* (management) and *nonexempt* (nonmanagement or hourly) employees.

HIM departments often are on a standard Monday through Friday, eight-hour-day pattern but also may need evening/weekend coverage to handle specific functions that must be provided twenty-four hours per day, seven days a week. Uninterrupted work stretches should be no less than two days and no more than seven days.

Shift Rotation and Shift Differential

Employee schedules may involve shift rotations and shift differentials when the department has more than the standard Monday through Friday, eight-to-five staffing needs. Rotation among morning, afternoon, and evening shifts is not the ideal scheduling situation but is often necessary when coverage is needed and personnel have not been specifically hired to work afternoons or evenings on a regular basis. Specific start and end times should be determined for every shift, and at least twelve hours should elapse between the time an individual ends one shift and begins another. Time spent on the more undesirable shifts should not exceed time spent on the preferred shift. For example, a schedule of two weeks of days, one week of afternoons, and one week of evenings is acceptable, but a schedule of one week of days, one week of afternoons, and one week of evenings can create problems. In situations where weekend coverage is an issue, employees should have at least alternate weekends off. Many employers pay a slightly higher hourly wage to employees who work less desirable shifts (evening, night, weekend). This is referred to as a *shift differential.*

Mandatory activities and the minimal staff needed to cover them should be defined when determining weekend or holiday coverage. All employees should participate in holiday/weekend rotation. Holiday rotations should be posted one year in advance and weekend rotations at least three months in advance. Employees should be required to provide their own holiday or weekend replacements but should not be responsible for providing replacements when their absence is due to illness.

Vacation and Absentee Coverage

To keep productivity optimal, the HIM department manager must plan appropriately for vacation staffing and absentee coverage. Temporary FTEs hired to cover for vacationing employees are most desirable, but not always feasible financially. Moreover, some positions are too complex to be filled with FTEs. For example, it is unlikely that a temporary assistant director could be hired to fill in for an assistant director on a two-week vacation.

When additional employees are unavailable, the department must determine which of the absent employees' tasks must be done and distribute the work among the available employees. A week or more of absent staff can add undue stress on the remaining employees and adversely affect department service levels; thus, it would be advisable to hire temporary help when more than one week of absence is expected.

Alternate Work Schedules

Another aspect of determining work schedules is that of considering alternatives to the regular workweek. Following are some examples:

- *Compressed workweek:* A **compressed workweek** is a week in which more hours are combined within fewer days, for example, four ten-hour days, three twelve-hour days, seven ten-hour days with seven days off (seven on/seven off), and so on. This type of scheduling has advantages but may present child care issues and psychological/physical fatigue that could reduce efficiency and productivity.
- *Flextime (also called gliding time or bandwidth flextime):* With **flextime,** employees choose their arrival and departure times within a fixed core. For example, if management feels full coverage is essential between 10 a.m. and 2 p.m., employees could start as early as 5:30 a.m. or end as late as 6:30 p.m. and still provide the department with core coverage.
- *Job sharing:* **Job sharing** divides one job between two part-time employees, each with partial benefits (as they apply). In some organizations, the two employees split full-time benefits, for example, one takes insurance coverage and one takes vacation time. Job sharing can be problematic because it requires two like-minded individuals. Should one terminate employment, finding a compatible partner could present a challenge.
- *Telecommuting:* In this scenario, employees work full- or part-time in their own homes. The first employees in the HIM department to take advantage of **telecommuting** were transcriptionists; they were soon followed by at-home coders. These telecommuters use computers (often provided by the facility) at home to transcribe or code information and then send it over telephone lines to the HIS department. The advantages to this type of work scheduling are that it saves space in the department, reduces long commutes to the workplace, retains parents who prefer to be home, and offers opportunities to the physically challenged.

The benefits of alternative work schedules to employers include easier staff recruitment and better retention, increased morale, decreased absence and tardiness, and some productivity improvements. For employees, the benefits can include less home stress, reduced commuting time, and a perception of greater autonomy in the workplace.

On the other hand, employers may feel a loss of control when employees telecommute. And some employees in alternative work situations, such as telecommuters, need core time contact hours with other employees to avoid feeling disconnected from the department. There is further discussion about managing telecommuters in chapter 24.

Management of Work Procedures

A **job procedure** is a structured, action-oriented list of sequential steps involved in carrying out a specific job or solving a problem.

Rules of Procedure Writing

To be effective, the writing of procedures requires considerable attention to detail. Meeting the following criteria can facilitate pertinent procedure development:

- Display the title accurately and clearly.
- Number each step of the procedure for ready reference.
- Begin each activity with an action verb.
- Keep sentences short and concise.
- Include only procedures, not policies, in procedure manuals. Policy manuals should be maintained as separate documents.
- Identify logical beginning and end points to simplify directions.
- Consider the audience and construct the procedure to be of most help. For example, new staff, temporary staff, or cross-trained staff who perform these procedures only occasionally need a basic, simplified version to ensure completion of a new or seldom-performed task.

In addition, the written procedure should provide completed ("filled in") samples of forms used during the procedure being documented.

It is considered best practice to have the individual who does the job write the procedure because he or she knows it best. Supervisory personnel should collect all the written procedures and determine whether they are complete and follow a consistent format.

Procedure Formats

When determining the appropriate format for a procedure, the HIM manager needs to consider the audience as well as the complexity of the task. Several formats can be followed in documenting procedural documentation, including:

- *Narratives:* Narrative formats are the most common for procedure writing. The author details the processes of the procedure in a step-by-step description method.

- *Playscript:* This format describes each player, the action, and the player's responsibility regarding the process from start to completion of a specific task, function, or procedure.
- *Flowcharts:* Flowcharts use standard flowcharting symbols provided in software programs such as PowerPoint® and VISIO® to depict the steps associated with a procedure. Figure 22.1 (p. 528) shows an example of flowcharting applied in the HIS setting.

Sometimes a combination of narrative and flowchart formats is used. However, whatever format is chosen, all procedures should be available to employees at any time.

Procedure Manuals

A procedure manual is a compilation of all of the procedures used in a specific unit, department, or organization. Procedure manuals may be kept as hard copies that have been printed out and bound together in a book or binder, or they may be maintained on an organization's secure Web site or intranet. The functions of procedure manuals include:

- Promoting teamwork
- Promoting conformity
- Reducing training time
- Establishing guidance on standards
- Explaining what is expected of employees
- Answering employee questions

The manual's content and format are relatively straightforward. Procedure manuals should include the following elements:

- *Title page:* Name of the facility, name of the manual, name of the department, and date
- *Foreword:* Paragraph form, purpose of manual, suggestion for use by employees
- *Table of contents:* List of all procedures in the manual referenced to page number
- *Job instruction and execution:* Step-by-step procedures to be followed, including forms used in each procedure, preferably completed ones together with explanations
- *General rules and regulations:* Information that includes department- or unit-specific details often influenced by state or federal law and/or regulatory agencies
- *Index:* Alphabetical list of topics covered in the manual (optional)

Work Environment

Considering the fact that the average FTE spends more waking hours in the work environment than in the home, it would be prudent for management to create a workplace ambiance that evokes comfort and productivity. Whether creating new space or evaluating current space, development of the work environment involves certain fundamental principles that address space and equipment, aesthetics, and ergonomics.

Figure 22.1.   Loose Chart Filing Flowchart

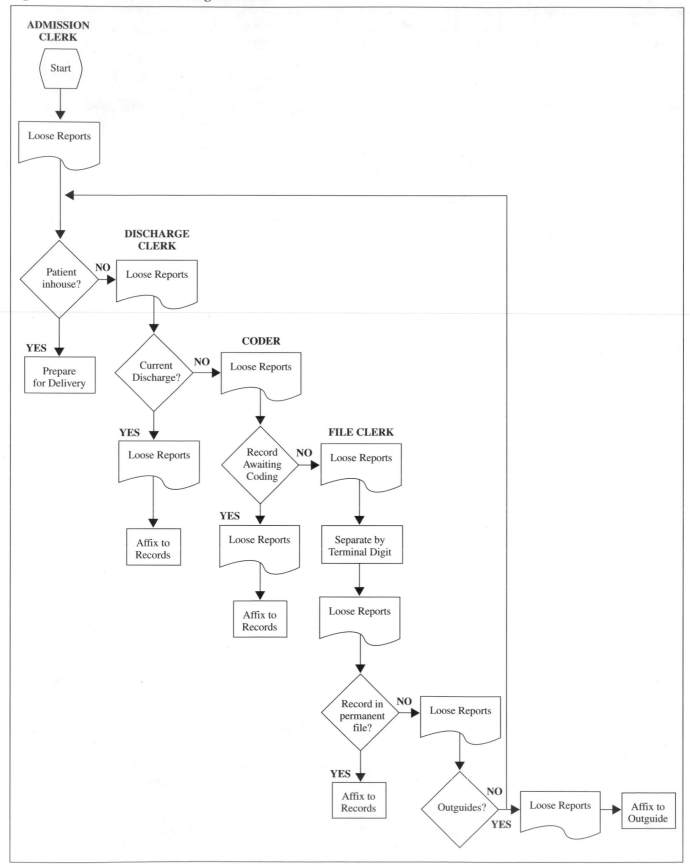

Work Flow

The **work flow** in a departmental setting is the established path along which tasks are sequentially completed by any number of staff to accomplish a function. According to Keister (2001), "Workflow has been defined as the automation of a business process, in whole or in part, during which documents, information, or tasks are passed from one participant to another for action in a way that is governed by a set of procedural rules."

Well-designed work flow is critical to achieving optimal efficiency and productivity when a function requires the coordinated activity of a group of employees. In a manual process environment, spatial relationships among people who perform tasks and the equipment required to perform them are critical factors in planning efficient work flow.

Creating a layout diagram, sometimes called a movement diagram or layout flowchart, helps the manager to visualize the functions and related tasks performed in a defined work area and how they are related. (See figure 22.2, p. 530.)

Space and Equipment

Workspace design can influence morale, productivity, and job satisfaction. The design of efficient office space involves a number of considerations, the first of which is typically location. If the department is located on any floor other than ground level, it is important to determine how much weight the suspended floor can support. This is especially critical when planning for additional shelving to store paper medical records. The combined weight of the records and shelving can be extreme, and the floor must be designed to support weights of potential proportion.

The amount of space designated for the department is the determining factor in considering office design and equipment specifications. Space is considered a precious and costly commodity in healthcare facilities and must be used efficiently. Designing efficient office space is a highly specialized and intricate process.

Department managers should understand basic facility planning techniques. They also must consider the facility's master plan in developing a plan for the department. This ensures maximum efficiency, consistency, and flexibility. The department plan also should address:

- The department's physical environment
- Office space utilization
- Space planning techniques, guidelines, and standards
- Office furniture and equipment

In an ideal situation, a move into a new space is the reason for engaging in space planning. Reorganization of a department because of changes in workforce numbers resulting from downsizing or from taking on new functions constitutes a space planning process. Departmental reorganization in response to changes in methods or functions, such as a move to home-based transcription or development of a CPR, can trigger a call for revised space planning. Sometimes the basic need to improve work flow and/or the appearance of a department can be a pivotal reason for space planning.

Remodeling existing space, as opposed to designing new space, presents special challenges. There may be space problems that cannot be changed, such as walls and pillars that cannot be moved and inadequate wiring. In addition, employees may resist changes and find it difficult to think creatively. In such instances, managers need to be inventive and creative in their space utilization.

Another consideration in designing efficient and effective space utilization is hard space versus soft space. *Hard space* is space that cannot be converted easily to service another function. For example, a file area could have certain structural needs or radiology may require lead walls. *Soft space* is space that is readily expandable or contractible to adjust to changing needs.

Determining how soft and hard space will be utilized is a major component of office space planning. Effective space planning has the following characteristics:

- Keeping costs to a minimum
- Contributing to the quality of the work
- Contributing to employee satisfaction
- Contributing to services provided by the department

Space needs change in the course of time and should be reevaluated periodically to determine whether principles of good space planning are being followed.

Four separate, self-explanatory types of office space are needed:

- Private office space
- General office space
- Service area
- Storage area

Another space consideration is personal space or the area of privacy surrounding an employee. Territoriality is a natural development because employees instinctively control the physical areas where they work.

Aesthetics

The physical environment factors, or aesthetics, of the workplace have the most physiological as well as psychological effects on employees. Aesthetic elements include the lighting of both the office and the workspace, the colors of the walls and furniture, auditory impacts, and atmospheric condition and temperature.

Light should be of sufficient brightness and diffusion for the work situation. Exposures (north, south, east, and west in order of preference) to natural light must be considered when creating new space because natural light is best and easiest on the eyes. Luminance is the quality of light, and lux is a unit of measure. (Candlelight equals 10 lux. A well-lit office equals 500 to 700 lux whereas the noonday sun produces 160,000 lux.) Desk or task lighting is more physically supportive than overhead florescent lighting alone. Many HIS

Figure 22.2.   Movement Diagram: Inefficient (top) and Efficient (bottom)

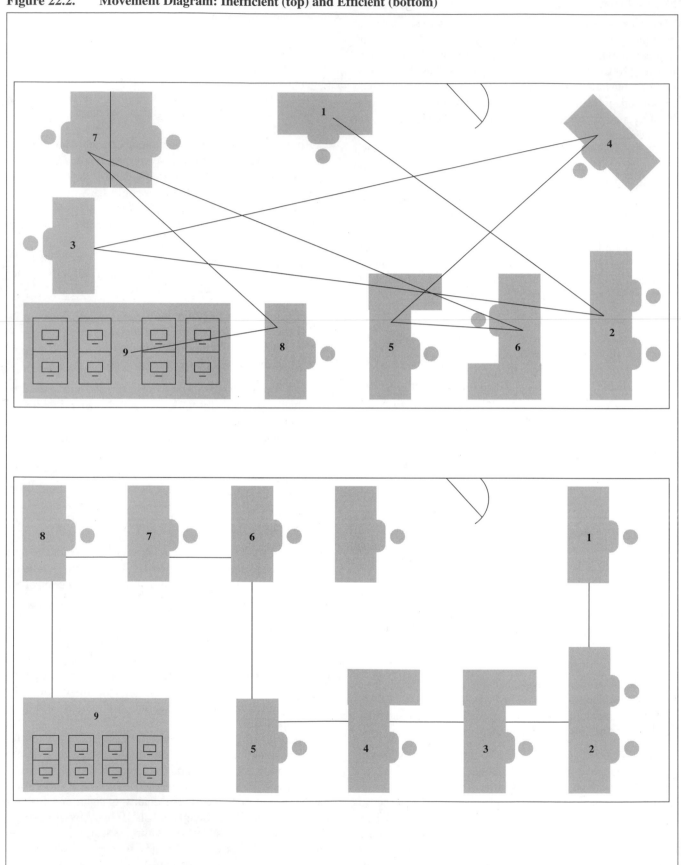

functions include PC monitors, and the contrast between the print and the background can influence the employee's comfort level. Typically, a light background with dark print is least taxing on the eyes. Glare from light sources or PC screens can cause discomfort. Display screen fixtures can be used to help reduce glare. In addition, it is important to factor in the age of the staff; people over forty have an increased level of discomfort from glare. For additional information on office light, visit IBM at www.pc.ibm.com/ww/healthy computing/vdt19c.html.

Color influences how people feel. For example, dark areas feel brighter and/or lighter when painted with light colors. Moreover, certain colors evoke a variety of sensations and feelings. Blues are cool, reds are warm, greens evoke luxury, and so on. When choosing color schemes, it is important to consider the area and who will occupy it. Neutral colors can have a calming effect and help avoid the subliminal friction that some prism colors trigger. Also, the finish of the paint should be taken in consideration. Matte surfaces absorb more light and reduce glare but are typically not cleanable. On the other hand, gloss surfaces are cleanable, but reflective, and can exacerbate glare.

Music and sound can be incorporated to improve working conditions and relieve both mental and visual fatigue. Certain kinds of music can reduce tension and make employees generally feel better. Sound conditioning and soundproofing are important considerations because a noisy office is seldom efficient. A certain level of routine office background noise is expected and usually is not irritating. However, loud or abrupt sounds can be alarming, distracting, and disruptive. Planning separate space for noisy work processes, such as copying and printing, is effective because it addresses the source of the noise. Carpeting, drapes, and partitioning can offer noise control because they absorb significant amounts of sound.

Air-conditioning regulates temperature, circulation, and moisture content and determines cleanliness. When considering normal ventilation for the space, at least 2000 cubic feet per person per hour should be configured to maintain a healthy respiratory atmosphere. Air that is too warm or too cold is equally distracting and a balance can be difficult to maintain. A range of 68 to 72 degrees Fahrenheit is generally acceptable to most people.

Ergonomics

The word *ergonomics* is derived from the Greek word *ergon,* which means "work," and *nomos,* which means "natural laws of." Developed in the 1950s by a group of scientists and engineers, the discipline of **ergonomics** has helped redefine the employee workspace with consideration for comfort and safety.

Questions to consider in office layout and design include:

- Do staff members assume fixed working postures that remain static for the majority of the workday? For example, do they sit at a keyboard all day?

- Do staff members perform repetitive motions such as filing, stamping, hole punching, and so on?
- Has the psychological stress caused by uncomfortable workstations been taken into consideration?

In effective ergonomic planning, the designer must know the work requirements of the job and the tasks involved. The physical traits of the worker assigned to each workstation also influence ergonomic considerations. For example, height or leg length or back waist length will determine specific needs. Another consideration is whether a single person or multiple persons share one workstation throughout the workweek. Finally, one must consider what equipment is currently available at the workstation and what equipment must be purchased to create an ergonomically correct work environment?

When the work environment is not ergonomically sound, common cumulative trauma disorders and repetitive strain injuries associated with office personnel can occur, including:

- *Carpal tunnel syndrome* is considered an occupational illness rather than an injury because it takes a long time to develop to the point of debilitation. The syndrome causes flexion, with ulnar deviation. Symptoms include tingling, numbness, and pain in the wrist and lower arm.
- *Upper back and neck strain* is caused by poor posture. Symptoms include tension headaches and muscle pain.
- *Eyestrain* is caused by incorrect viewing distances and poor illumination. Symptoms include burning, watery eyes, and headaches.

Good preventative, proactive ergonomic management includes educating staff on how to care for themselves to reduce potential ergonomic injuries or discomfort. A few simple principles help raise employees' awareness of their physical relationship with the work environment. Managers should encourage, if not insist, that staff working at a PC for the majority (more than two-thirds) of a shift take hourly neck, shoulder, and wrist roll breaks, along with stretch routines. In addition, employees should be aware of, and assessed on their use of, the ten basic principles of good sitting posture:

- Feet should rest flat on the floor or footrest.
- A fist-width space should be measurable between the back of the knees and the edge of the seat pan of the chair.
- The hips should be at a 90-degree angle (or slightly greater) in relation to the body. To help ensure this angle, the knees should be at or below hip height.
- The lower back (lumbar region) should be supported.
- Shoulders should be relaxed, not shrugged, slouched, or rolled forward.
- Elbows should rest comfortably at the side or on armrests. When typing, elbows should be at 90-degree angles and preferably supported by an adjustable armrest at an appropriate height.

- Wrists should be maintained in a neutral (straight) position while typing or using any variety of keyboard.
- Head and neck should be in an upright position. To confirm this, the ears should be directly over the shoulders, which are directly over the hips.
- Computer monitors should be positioned so that they are directly in front of the worker. The top line of print should be horizontal with the eyes when looking directly forward.
- Ergonomic aids should be used to help maintain comfortable posture. Examples include footrests, wrist rests for keyboard and mouse, antiglare screens for computer monitors, copy stands, and adjustable chair height for those working at a multitask station.

These basic activities can help employees to stop the tension cycle and reduce potential long-term discomfort.

Careful consideration and professional assessment of individual needs will help reduce or eliminate physical barriers to employee comfort and productivity. Preemptive, ergonomically correct practices markedly reduce employee absence and worker's compensation usage due to workplace injury.

Check Your Understanding 22.1

Instructions: Answer the following questions on a separate piece of paper.

1. Looking at the sample vacation schedule in table 22.2, for which weeks would the department be well advised to secure temporary help?
2. List the potential problem areas a work distribution analysis can reveal.
3. Who should write a job description? Who should collect the necessary information?
4. What is the best way to plan an efficient work flow?
5. Name the elements of good work environment planning.

Performance and Work Measurement Standards

Work is the task to be performed; performance is the execution of the task. Effective management involves discerning what work is to be done, what performance standards are achievable and appropriate, how performance can be meas-

ured in terms of efficiency and efficacy, and how performance can be monitored for variances from the standards set. Most employees simply want to know what tasks they are responsible for, what is expected of them, and how they are performing with regard to that expectation. Through performance standard setting and measurement processes, managers can determine success or opportunities for improvement.

A **standard** may be defined as a performance criterion established by custom or authority with the purpose of assessing factors such as quality, productivity, and performance. Managers are responsible for controlling the resources available to them, including men (staff), materials, machines, methods, and money. Thus, managers are expected to set standards for each of these resources and then use them as ways to judge (assess, evaluate) the quality, productivity, and/or performance of those resources.

Criteria for Setting Effective Standards

To create viable, significant standards, it is important to identify the criteria for effective standard setting. Effective standards are:

- *Understandable:* The persons affected by the standard know what it means, and it makes sense to them.
- *Attainable:* It is reasonable to expect that the person(s) affected by the standard can actually achieve it.
- *Equitable:* If more than one person is affected by the standard, all are held accountable for it.
- *Significant:* Meeting the standard is important to the goals of the work unit or organization; the effort it takes to meet the standard is worth it.
- *Legitimate:* The standard has been formally accepted within the organization and is documented in appropriate places and ways.
- *Economical:* The standard can be met and monitored without incurring costs that are beyond the value of that which is gained by having it. In other words, is the standard worth the expense?

Keeping the definition of effective standards in mind, it is possible to set about writing new standards for the staff or

Table 22.2.   Sample Vacation Schedule

Employee	Title	Hire Date	Week #	7/1	7/8	7/15	7/22	7/29	8/5	8/12	8/19
Brown	Transcriptionist	2001	1					x			
Dorsey	Transcriptionist	2000	2	x							x
Grunch	Transcriptionist	1999	3		x				x	x	
Glass	Clerk	2000	2			x	x				

Diewell Community Hospital Vacation Policy	
General Employees	**Department Managers/Administrators**
3 years or less = 1 week	3 years or less = 2 weeks
4 to 7 years = 2 weeks	4 to 7 years = 3 weeks
8 to 10 years = 3 weeks	8 years and over = 4 weeks
11 years and over = 4 weeks	

reviewing and revising current standards. Several examples of effective resource management standards include:

- Standards related to human resources *(staff)*
  - *Quality:* Coders code inpatient services with 98 percent accuracy.
  - *Productivity:* Coders code twenty-five to thirty inpatient discharges per eight-hour workday.
  - *Performance:* Employees maintain an acceptable or better rating on peer evaluations of effectiveness as team members.
- Standards related to supplies *(materials)*
  - *Quality:* Paper-based health record forms must be printed on twenty-pound paper stock, or pens used for health record documentation must contain waterproof ink.
  - *Performance:* Paper-based health record forms must be two-hole punched on the top margin and three-hole punched on the left-hand margin to accommodate both the chart binder used on the care unit and the permanent file folder.
- Standards related to budgetary resources *(money)*
  - *Performance:* Major budget expense categories (salaries, supplies, postage, telephone, travel, and maintenance) must remain within plus or minus three percent of the budgeted amount monthly.
  - *Standard states:* Paid dollars per key statistic (P$PKS) must be less than $2 plus or minus the target P$PKS indicator established for the department.
- Standards related to *methods*
  - *Quality:* Health record forms must be assembled (organized) in accordance with the organization's standard chart order guidelines, or the health record of a discharged patient must be logged into health information services for processing by 7:00 a.m. the day following discharge.
  - *Performance:* The health record of a discharged patient must follow this work flow pattern in the department's assembly, analysis, coding, chart completion (when appropriate), and permanent file.
- Standards related to equipment *(machines)*
  - *Quality:* Each file shelf unit must support up to 100 pounds of file weight.
  - *Productivity:* The copier must be able to collate and staple up to ten fifty-page packets at a time.
  - *Performance:* The printer must be able to produce prints (hard-copy paper and transparencies) from PowerPoint™ software using at least four different types of design templates.

Methods of Communicating Standards

After the standards have been created, they must be communicated to staff. All of the above types of standards can be provided to staff in a number of ways, including through:

- *Written specifications,* as used in job descriptions, equipment specification sheets, and forms design guidelines
- *Documented rules, regulations, or policies,* as used in policy manuals, procedure manuals, regulations manuals, and employee handbooks
- *Demonstration models,* as in sample health records
- *Verbal confirmations,* as in the reinforcement of a standard whenever possible and appropriate

Standards are worded differently at various levels within the organization depending on whether they reflect a goal or an objective. A **goal** is a generalized statement of a unit, departmental, or organizational standard, typically without measurable content. An **objective** is a statement of end result in measurable terms with time and cost limits, as applicable. For example, the HIM department might have a general standard (most commonly called a goal) for its transcription function, such as "to support patient care through accurate and timely transcription of medical reports." The transcription function then might state an **objective**-level standard in more specific language to make it more understandable and more measurable, for example, "to report routine history and physical, operative, and consultation dictation within twelve hours of dictation." This objective is related directly to the timeliness aspect of the preceding goal.

Qualitative and Quantitative Standards

Standards are also characterized in two other ways: as quantitative standards and as qualitative standards.

Qualitative standards specify the level of service quality expected from a function, such as:

- Accuracy rate (For example, assignment of diagnostic and procedure codes for inpatient records is at least 98 percent accurate.)
- Error rate (For example, mistakes in the assignment of diagnostic and procedure codes occur in no more than two percent of inpatient records coded.)

Quantitative standards specify the level of measurable work, or productivity, expected for a specific function, such as:

- Number of units of work per specified period of time or amount of time allotted per unit of work (For example, seventy records per FTE per day or no more than fifteen minutes are allotted to coding an inpatient record.)
- Turnaround time (TAT) (For example, dictation must be transcribed within twenty-four hours.)
- Response time (For example, requests are responded to within seven working days of receipt.)

Quantity (also called productivity) and quality (also known as **service**) standards are generally used by managers to monitor individual employee performance and/or the performance of a functional unit or the department as a whole. To properly communicate performance standards, managers need to make the distinction between quantitative and qualitative standards and identify examples of each for HIS functions.

Key Indicators

Key indicators are live (versus retrospective) measurement thresholds that alert a department or work unit to its level of competent customer service. After the department's standards have been determined, the focus is on compliance. Managers must watch the key indicators to determine whether the department is on course. Two red flags that indicate that targets are being missed are:

- *The number and severity of complaints increase.* When the number or severity of complaints increases, the circumstances surrounding the complaints need to be assessed immediately so that corrections to the process or personnel involved can be made.
- *Surveys to assess performance on accreditation, legal, or regulatory standards indicate that the organization has failed to comply in one or more areas.* When the organization fails to comply with one or more external standards during a survey, the organization needs to correct the variance(s) and return to compliance.

Methods of Developing Standards

Any of a number of methods can be used to develop standards for **productivity** (the creation of products using an organization's financial and human resources) in a work unit. Two approaches are commonly used: (1) benchmarking comparable performance, and (2) measuring actual performance.

Benchmarking Comparable Performance

Benchmarking is based on research into the performance of similar organizations and programs or on standards established by national or local sources, such as professional associations and standard-setting organizations. It has become a more prevalent management approach in HIM in the past few years because this type of information is now being published more regularly.

To engage in a benchmarking effort, the manager should first select key functions of the department that will be benchmarked (coding service, transcription service, release of information service, and so on). Relating benchmarks to the specific process is critical. Thought must be given to the types of performance measure(s) desired as indicators (for coding, for example, payments remaining in accounts receivable due to uncoded records and payments remaining in accounts receivable due to coding disputes; for transcription, for example, TAT [dictation to charting] for consultations, operative reports, history, and physicals).

Once the key functional areas have been selected and the types of indicators identified, the research of benchmarks through published sources (preferably) may begin. Investigation of benchmark standards involves assessment of their relevance to the department's specific situation. Then the idea can be sold to the rest of the organization. Benchmarking involves the following steps:

1. Identifying peer organizations/departments that have achieved outstanding performance based on some key indicator (for example, 98 percent of health records coded within two days postdischarge)
2. Studying the best practices within that organization that make it possible to achieve that performance level

3. Acting to implement those best practices in one's own organization to achieve a similar performance

Routinely gathering performance data enables a manager to monitor actual performance against the benchmark and then evaluate factors in department processes that must be changed to move actual performance into the benchmark range.

Measurement of Actual Performance

Work measurement is the process of studying the amount of work accomplished and the amount of time it takes to accomplish it. It involves the collection of data relevant to the work, such as the amount of work accomplished per unit of time. Its purpose is to define and monitor productivity.

Work measurement can support a manager in many activities, including:

- Setting production standards
- Determining staffing requirements
- Establishing incentive pay systems
- Determining direct costs by function
- Comparing performance to standards
- Identifying activities for process/methods improvement

Gathering the information available through work measurement efforts will be invaluable to the manager in making administrative decisions. But how does a manager know which work measurement will serve them best?

When selecting the work measurement technique that would best suit the manager's department, the following factors should be considered:

- The amount of financial resources available
- The availability of qualified personnel to take part in the study
- The amount of time available to devote to study
- The attitudes of employees toward participation in a study

Work measurement can be accomplished through a variety of techniques, including:

- *Analysis of historical (past performance) data:* The analysis of historical data generally uses work volume (direct or estimated) and hours paid from past records to establish the standard. When using historical data, managers are cautioned to keep in mind that volume figures are not adjusted for the level of quality and the number of hours paid is different from the number of hours actually worked.
- *Employee self-logging:* Employee self-logging is a form of self-reporting in which the employees simply track their tasks, volume, and hours worked. Employee logging incorporates a **time ladder,** which is a form used by the employee to document the amount of time spent (worked) on various tasks. It can be modified to include the number of units produced per task throughout the day. **Volume logs** are sometimes used in conjunction with a time ladder to obtain information about

the volume of work units received and processed in a day by simply keeping track of the number of products produced or activities done (table 22.3).

- *Scientific methods:* The scientific methods of work measurement include time studies and the use of preestablished time/unit standards. For example, time studies use a stopwatch to record and document the time required to accomplish a specified task.
- *Work sampling:* Work sampling is a technique of work measurement that involves using statistical probability (determined through random sample observations) to characterize the performance of the department and its work (functional) units.

Each one of the varieties of work measurement techniques offers calculations of employee productivity in either unit/time or time/unit. For example, with the completion of a Daily Time Ladder Summary (table 22.4), a manager can determine simple unit/time productivity statistics by dividing the number of units produced by the number of hours worked. The following illustrates calculating a coder and a clerk's weekly employee self-logging activities:

Work sampling is an especially valuable technique in the development of performance standards. Work-sampling data can help the manager to:

- Catalog the activities being performed
- Determine the time devoted to each activity

- Identify inefficiencies
- Set employee performance standards

Work-sampling projects follow an established sequence of steps and use specific tools:

1. Decide which work activities to monitor during the study.
2. Design the form that will be used to record the observations collected during the study. The sample observation record form shown in table 22.5 (p. 536) captures activities by individuals and by units of function (supervisory, transcription, clerical, and coder).
3. Determine the best size of the study sample by using the precision interval method, a standard formula used to determine sample size. The formula allows for various scenarios of desired certainty factor (confidence factor) and precision factor (acceptable error) in the study results. The **certainty factor** is a numerical representation of the confidence the manager has that the results will show the level of acceptable error. The **precision factor** is the level of tolerable error in the sampling process.

$$\text{Sample size} = 0.25 \times \left[\frac{\text{certainty factor \%}^2}{\text{precision factor \%}} \right]$$

*Note that the 0.25 is a fixed (not variable) part of the formula.

If the precision factor is 5 percent, the confidence factor needed is 95 percent. (Note that the precision factor plus the confidence factor equal 100 percent). For example:

$$25 \times (0.95 \div 0.025)^2 = 0.25 \times (38 \times 38) = 361$$

4. Determine the length of the study and establish appropriate observation times. When the sample size (total number of observations required) has been determined, the number of observations per day can be determined on the basis of the number of days, weeks, or months available to complete the study. The actual

Table 22.3.   Sample Volume Log

Task	Number of Worked Hours	Number of Units
Coding	40 worked hours	120 records
Loose filing	36 worked hours	48 inches

The coding standard calculates at three records per worked hour for this employee (120 records/40 hours) and a filing standard of 1.3 inches per worked hour (48 inches/36 hours). It does not capture any interruptions or unworked time in the eight-hour day but is a simple way to arrive at a ballpark figure.

Table 22.4.   Sample Daily Time Ladder Summary

Unit: <u>Reception</u>   Date: <u>07-04-02</u>

Note: 7.5 worked hours (two 15-minute breaks)

Employee	Code/Task	Total Time/%	Work Units
Jane	A. Answer phones	3hr/40%	64
	B. Write requisitions	1.75 hr/23%	92
	C. Personal/set up, etc.	.5 hr/7%	NA
	D. Mail handling	2.25 hr/30%	Incoming 80 **Outgoing 100**
Betty	A. Answer phones	5 hr/66%	100
	B. Write requisitions	.5 hr/7%	15
	C. Personal/set up, etc.	.5/7%	NA
	D. Mail handling	0	NA
	E. Stat chart delivery	1.5/20%	10

Table 22.5.   Sample Observation Record Form

Activity	Mason	Davis	Perry	Kent	Martin	Carter	Roth	Evans	Larson	Owens .5 FTE	
	Supervisor	Transcriptionists			Clerical				Coders		Total
Supervision											
Coding											
Transcription											
Record A & A											
Record retrieval/filing/transport											
Release of Information											
Assisting physicians											
Other clerical											
Idle: Gone, rest											
Total observations											

Observation Times:

1.   6.
2.   7.
3.   8.   Recorded by: _____
4.   9.
5.   10.   Date: _____

Figure 22.3.   Observation Generator

Time Block Number	Clock Time	Time Block Number	Clock Time
0	8:00 a.m.	25	12:10 p.m.
1	10	26	20
2	20	27	30
3	30	28	40
4	40	29	50
5	50	30	1:00 p.m.
6	9:00 a.m.	31	10
7	10	32	20
8	20	33	30
9	30	34	40
10	40	35	50
11	50	36	2:00 p.m.
12	10.00 a.m.	37	10
13	10	38	20
14	20	39	30
15	30	40	40
16	40	41	50
17	50	42	3:00 p.m.
18	11:00 a.m.	43	10
19	10	44	20
20	20	45	30
21	30	46	40
22	40	47	50
23	50	48	4:00 p.m.
24	12:00 p.m.	etc.	

time of each observation each day must be determined by using a random observation generator (figure 22.3) and a random numbers table (figure 22.4). To create the observation generator, list the period of time the study will take place in a workday (in figure 22.3, from 8 a.m. until 4 p.m., with 10-minute increments) and number each predetermined time increment. Then using a random numbers table (figure 22.4 is a partial table of tables found in any statistics book), randomly select the first number and then a direction to read the numbers (horizontally, vertically, or diagonally). Looking at the first number, refer to the observation generator to find the time of day assigned that corresponding number. If it does not exist, proceed to the next number until the optimal number to complete the study has been selected. For example, if 500 observations were needed and fifty workdays were allotted to complete the study, 10 observations would need to be made each day of the fifty-day study. (See figure 22.5.)

5. Explain the purpose of the study and how it is conducted to observers and staff. Orientation of observers and personnel is very important because it encourages consistency in data collection among observers and ensures that unbiased and reliable observations are collected on the basis of the observation schedule. At this point in the study, those who will be observed also must be informed of its purpose. It is important that workers perform normally throughout the process. They also should understand that the outcome of the study will be shared with them at the conclusion of the study period.

6. Collect and record observation data at random points. (See table 22.6.)

7. Report the results of the study. (See tables 22.7 and 22.8 on p. 538 and table 22.9 on p. 539.)

Performance Measurement

Performance measurement is the process of comparing the outcomes of an organization, work unit, or employee to preestablished performance plans and standards. The results of the performance measurement process are expressed as percentages, rates, ratios, averages, and other quantitative assessments. Performance measurement is used both in assessments of quality of clinical care and for management applications. Examples of performance measures maintained by acute care hospitals include the rate of nosocomial infection, the percentage of surgical complications, the average length of stay, and the ratio of live births to stillbirths. Examples of performance measures maintained by an HIS department include transcription lines transcribed and turnaround times per report type, turnaround times for release of information and chart retrieval, and loose filing inches filed and existing.

Performance measurement is a fundamental managerial activity that supports two of the basic functions of management: controlling and planning. The control function is concerned with ensuring that the work unit or organization is doing what it should be doing in the right way. The function of planning is to define the expectations of performance (or standards), the processes required for achieving those expectations (or objectives), and the desired outcomes of performance (or goals). The goals, objectives, and standards established during the planning process become the criteria that are used in the control process to evaluate actual performance.

Performance Controls

In the control process, specific monitors (controls) are established and outcomes data are collected. The outcomes data are then analyzed to determine the extent to which actual performance corresponds to the performance expectations established during the planning process.

The characteristics of effective controls include:

- *Flexibility* refers to the fact that controls must be adaptable to real changes in the requirements of a process. For example, a budget is a control on the use of money. Money budgeted in one category (equipment) may need to be spent in another category (travel) because of a change in a program, a new law/regulation, and so on.
- *Simplicity* refers to the fact that those involved in the process must find the controls understandable and reasonable.

Figure 22.4.   Random Numbers Table (Partial)

69	18	82	00	97		32	82	53	05	27
90	04	58	54	97		51	98	15	06	54
73	18	95	02	07		47	67	72	62	59
54	01	64	90	04		66	28	13	10	03
75	75	87	64	90		20	97	18	17	49
08	35	86	99	10		78	53	24	27	85
28	30	30	32	64		81	33	31	05	91
53	84	08	62	33		31	59	41	36	28
etc.										

Note: Entry may be made at any point, proceeding horizontally or vertically.

Figure 22.5.   Example of a First Day's Observation Times

Observation Times	
1. 8:50 a.m.	6. 1:00 p.m.
2. 9:40 a.m.	7. 1:10 p.m.
3. 10:20 a.m.	8. 1:20 p.m. Recorded by: _____
4. 12:00 noon	9. 2:20 p.m. Department: _____
5. 12:40 p.m.	10. 2:30 p.m. Date: _____

Table 22.6.   First Day's Observations, Cure-All Hospital's HIM Department

	Mason	Davis	Perry	Kent	Martin	Carter	Roth	Evans	Larson	Owens .5 FTE	
Activity	**Supervisor**	**Transcriptionists**			**Clerical**				**Coders**		**Total**
Supervision											2
Coding											0
Transcription											24
Record A & A											10
Record retrieval/filing/transport											16
Release of information											8
Assisting physicians											8
Other clerical											15
Idle: Gone, rest											10
Total observations	10	10	10	10	10	10	10	10	10	3	93

- *Economy* implies that controls should not cost more than they are worth. The time and money spent to implement a control should be in line with the level of risk (loss) involved if the process fails to meet performance expectations. For example, loss of a life calls for a significant investment in controls; criminal liability calls for significant investment in controls; a day of overtime to correct clerical errors calls for a minimal investment in controls.

- *Timeliness* suggests that controls should be implemented so as to detect potential variances within a time frame that allows for corrective action before any adverse effect has occurred. For example, the accuracy of a record number assignment should be confirmed at the time of registration or the coding checked before a bill is mailed or transmitted to avoid the adverse effects associated with errors that are transmitted to other areas of the organization or to the insurance carrier.

- A *focus on exceptions* demands that controls be targeted at those aspects of a process that are most likely to vary significantly from expectation. For example, a new transcriptionist who is likely to make more errors that could do damage to customer service ratings is generally monitored more closely and more often than one who is experienced and has performed well for the past year.

There are two general types of controls: preventive (self-correcting) and feedback (non-self-correcting). Preventive controls are front-end processes that guide work in such a way that input and/or process variations are minimized. Simple things such as standard operating procedures, edits on data entered into computer-based systems, and training processes are ways to reduce the potential for error by using preventive controls.

Feedback controls are back-end processes that monitor and measure output, and then compare it to expectations and identify variations that then must be analyzed so correction action plans can be developed and implemented. Processes with feedback controls in place are also called cybernetic processes or systems. Some may be self-regulating (such as thermostatic systems), but most are non-self-regulating, meaning that they require intervention by an oversight agent (a supervisor, manager, or auditor) to identify the variance and take action to correct it.

Table 22.7.   Observation Summary, Cure-All Hospital HIM Department

Activity	Previous Observation Days	3/10/00	Study Total	% Total
Supervision	—	2	90	2.2
Coding	—	0	18	0.4
Transcription	—	24	1,053	25.9
Record A & A	—	10	540	13.3
Filing/retrieval/transport	—	16	618	15.2
Release of information	—	8	381	9.4
Assisting physicians	—	8	273	6.7
Other clerical	—	15	711	17.5
Idle: Gone, rest	—	10	378	9.4
Total observations	—	93	4,062	100.0

Note: This particular work sampling effort involved a total work sampling of 500 planned observations (10 observations per workday for 50 days). This number of observations gives a ±2.75% precision interval for = >10% activities, a 5.5% accuracy rate, and 94.5% confidence level.

Variance Analysis

When variations are identified (when actual performance does not meet or significantly exceeds expectations), further analysis is called for. Analysis of the performance factors involved in the work (people, supplies, equipment, and money) is conducted to help determine what, if any, changes should be made. Changes may involve activities such as additional staff training; modifications in procedures, work flow, or policies; purchases of updated equipment; or improvements in maintenance procedures. The analysis may lead to changes in performance criteria and expectations.

Table 22.8.   Work Sampling Results, Cure-All Hospital's HIM Department: Actual Activity versus Expectations

Activity	Normal Range of Expectations	Department Expectations	Department Actual	Estimated Variation
Supervision	NA	15%	2.2%	−13%
Coding	2–4.5%	3%	0.4%	−2%
Transcription	30–40%	30%	25.9%	−4%
Record A & A	10–13%	12%	13.3%	+1%
Record retrieval/filing	2–5%	3%	15.2%	+12%
Release of information	6–9%	7%	9.4%	+2%
Assisting physicians	6–10%	8%	6.7%	−1%
Other clerical	8–13%	10%	17.5%	+7%
Idle: Gone, rest	7–14%	12%	9.4%	−3%
Total	NA	100%	100%	NA

Table 22.9.   Work Sampling Results, Cure-All Hospital's HIM Department

Activity Area/Expected %	% of Time	Minutes*	Hours*	Work Volume for Period	Work Units
Supervision/15%	2%	4,560	76	NA	NA
Coding/3%	1%	0.01 × 228,000 or 2,280	0.01 × 3,800 or 38 hours	775	Dx coded
Transcription/30%	26%	0.26 × 228,000 or 59,280	0.26 × 3,800 or 988	150,000	Lines transcribed
Record assembly and analysis/12%	13%	29,640	494	2,964	Records analyzed
Record filing, retrieval, etc./3%	15%	34,200	570	11,400	Records pulled/filed
Release of information/7%	9%	20,520	342	1,050	Requests handled
Assisting physician/8%	7%	15,960	266	NA	NA
Other clerical/10%	18%	41,040	684	NA	NA
Idle: Gone, rest/12%	9%	20,520	342	NA	NA
Total	100%	—	—	—	—

Notes:

Working days in the period: 50 days

Current workforce: 9.5 FTE, including the supervisor

Work minutes/day per FTE: 480 minutes (8 hr × 60)

Total study work hours: 3,800 hours (9.5 FTE × 8 × 50)

Total study work minutes: 228,000 minutes (9.5 FTE × 480 × 50) or (3,800 × 60)

*Minutes and hours are calculated based on the percentage of total time represented by each activity area. For example, 2% of 228,000 minutes – 4,560 minutes; 2% of 3,800 hours = 76 hours.

Assessment of Employee Performance

When establishing an employee performance assessment program, the steps in the control (evaluation) process include:

1. Monitoring and measuring outcomes performance
2. Comparing performance to established goals and standards
3. Evaluating variance and developing action plans
4. Taking appropriate action

Monitoring and Measuring Outcomes Performance

Monitoring and measuring performance involves taking an aggregate look at performance over a period of time. Options include operating on a self-reporting method such as self-logging, using computerized monitoring to audit productivity, manually auditing work samples, or relying on customer feedback to measure departmental performance.

Outcomes performance monitoring depends on employee productivity and management execution. Focus is on indicators such as turnaround time, cost/revenue reports, and customer feedback. The indicators highlight collective performance as a department and at the same time presents discrepancies in goals and standards.

Consider this practical application of performance monitoring. Assume that one established expectation of the transcription function in your department is that the routine release of information in response to a consent for use or a disclosure of health information request occurs within five working days of receipt in the department.

The first step in controlling a function would be to set up a data collection and reporting activity to obtain information that can be used to monitor the time it takes the department to respond to a routine request for information. (See table 22.10.)

Next, the department should determine the kinds of controls it wants to establish. The department wants to monitor routine requests, but how are "routine requests" defined? They may be any requests that are not stat or emergency or do not have to be handled within minutes, hours, or some stipulated amount of time under five working days. For example, a subpoena for a record that must be handled within three days or a request for a record needed for an appointment in a clinic the next morning would not be considered routine requests.

Table 22.10.   ROI Requests

On June 6, 2000, Total Routine ROI Requests in Processing: 130					
Days Since Receipt	6–10 Days	11–15 Days	16–20 Days	>20 Days	Summary
Number of total	12 9%	15 12%	2 2%	1 1%	30 24%
Unable to locate record	0	2	0	1	3 10%
Incomplete record	12	12	2	0	26 87%
Issue with authorization	0	0	0	0	0
Unavailable record	0	1	0	0	1 3%
Other	0	0	0	0	0

The line related to release of information requests in the middle of the performance report shown in table 22.11 indicates the average number of days it took the HIS department to respond to all of the routine ROI requests in January (3), February (3), March (6), and April (5). However, the numbers tell nothing about the routine ROI requests the department has received but not yet responded to.

The average TAT number is calculated by dividing the total response days attributed to the volume of routine requests responded to within the reporting period by the volume of routine requests responded to. For example, if the department responded to 300 routine requests in the month of May and 100 were responded to in six days, 100 in two days, and 100 in four days, the average TAT in May would be four days:

$$\frac{600 \text{ days} + 200 \text{ days} + 400 \text{ days}}{300 \text{ requests}} = 4 \text{ days (TAT average)}$$

The data used to arrive at the average TAT for the report are also quite useful because they allow the department to see what really makes up the four-day average and to focus on aspects of a process that might need some attention in order to prevent a crisis later on. Having the information on a monthly basis to include as part of the regular performance reporting within the organization allows the manager to review monthly trends and identify potential focus areas for future process improvement activities.

In addition, the underlying data indicates that a considerable number of requests do not get responded to within the five-working-days expectation (for example, 33 percent were responded to in six working days). A direct supervisor of the ROI activity would likely want access to information of this nature more often than once a month. For example, a weekly report showing the number of routine requests in the system for five days or more that have not yet been answered would allow the supervisor or ROI clerk to identify problem requests and take corrective actions over the course of the following week.

Comparing Performance to Established Goals and Standards

The next step in monitoring and measuring outcome performance is to compare current performance against established goals (standards). Continuing with the example in the preceding section, when comparing performance against the standard performance indicator of responding to routine requests for information within five days, the data in table 22.11 show an upward trend in March and April. The trend was appropriately reversed in May, which indicates that the function appears to be under control but obviously needs to be monitored.

Evaluating Variance and Developing Action Plans

When comparisons are done, the manager should evaluate any variances and develop an action plan specific to each. The routine response to consent for use or disclosure of health information performance information does not indicate the need for significant action. Other variances in department functions may take priority, such as Transcription TAT for H & Ps, Days in Assembly/Analysis, Coding: Days in Accounts Receivable, etc.

Table 22.11.   Sample Health Information Services Performance Report

Indicator	January 2000	February 2000	March 2000	April 2000
DCEs	5,000	5,400	5,360	5,500
Labor cost per DCE: <$10.00	$10.00	9.25	9.33	9.90
FTE budgeted at 50	50	50	50	48
Days in assembly/analysis at end of month <2days	1	2	2	3
Delinquency rate <50%	35%	40%	43%	45%
Coding: Days in AR due to uncoded records <5 days	3	5	4	5
Lines transcribed	120,000	130,000	128,000	132,000
Transcription: TAT for H&Ps <24 hours	12	16	18	26
ROI requests received	200	245	300	260
Release of Info: TAT <5 days	3	3	6	5
File pull requests	2,000	2,200	2,300	2,500
Retrieval rate: >95%	%94	%96	%93	%91%
Loose filing inches received	100 average 25/week	120 average 30/week	80 average 20/week	130 average 32/week
Loose filing inches at end of month: <16	15	20	12	15
Filing: Misfiles <1%	.05%	.08%	.06%	.08%
Resignations: <1%	0	0	0	2/50 = 4%
Education hours	4	16	2	8
Unproductive hours (sick, vacation): <15%	10%	12%	20%	10%

In an evaluation of variances, it is important to routinely collect data that would provide the following types of information to disclose the triggers of the variances:

- Are any open ROI requests in the department with a date of receipt of more than five working days? (This is the focus on exceptions rule in action.)
- If so, what is the total number and what is the percentage of the total open ROI requests? How many are six to ten working days, ten to fifteen working days, sixteen to twenty working days, or more than twenty days?
- If so, what are the reasons the requests are still open?
- If so, on what date(s) has the requesting party been notified of the reason for the delay?

After the variances have been evaluated, action plans can be formulated to address them as follows:

- Establish a procedure to ensure weekly contact with the requestor to determine continuing need for the information and update on the status of the request.
- Flag the incomplete record with a ROI REQUEST PENDING to ensure that it is routed to ROI immediately when required documentation is complete.
- Track the missing record.
- Check the status of the unavailable record and contact user to obtain it so that ROI can occur and then (if necessary) the record can be returned to the user.

Taking Appropriate Action

Continuing with the consent for disclosure requests, appropriate actions are taken to put the plan in place and to monitor its effectiveness. Action plans should be revisited often to ensure that they are the appropriate approach to the problems originally identified by the data collecting and analysis.

Identification of Improvement Opportunities

When defining processes and identifying common symptoms of process problems, generally and specific to HIM services, how do we know whether we have process problems? We need only be observant to:

- Inaccuracies and errors in work
- Complaints from customers
- Delays in getting things done or lots of interruptions
- Low employee morale or high rates of absenteeism/turnover
- Poor safety records and on-the-job injuries

Efforts to measure employee performance will alert management to the inaccuracies and errors in the work processes. The accuracy rate can be realized in a performance measurement plan. Any and all variances of quality must be addressed with expedient performance data collection and analysis.

Customer complaints indicate that a system or performance is not meeting expectations. Managers need to consider each complaint and determine whether it is circumstantial or a signal of something bigger. When chart delivery is delayed, customer expectations and patient needs should be examined and adjusted accordingly.

Delays in getting things done or continuous interruptions to a process can warn of roadblocks to success. Delays give time to revisit the current work flow and analyze what might be improved. If transcribed operative reports are not on the patients' charts within the prescribed time, how can the reason for the delay be identified and how can the improvement activity be planned to eliminate the delay?

Low employee morale and a high rate of absenteeism or turnover are serious indicators that procedures need to be improved. A lack of job satisfaction is typically caused by a lack of or incomplete training. High turnover and absenteeism are budget draining and call for a defined plan of action to avert a continued pattern. High turnover in positions that are especially difficult to fill can be exceptionally taxing to the budget and department alike because of the retraining and redistribution of workloads caused by reduced FTE levels.

Poor safety records or injuries are indicative of urgent process improvement opportunities. Work-related injuries and accidents are management markers regarding a poorly designed process, failing equipment, or poor training. Again, work injuries are a costly burden for the department and the goals and standards it has labored to establish. Are the charts too tightly packed on the shelves, creating extraordinary resistance to storing and retrieving records? Are personnel consistent in checking that aisles are clear before operating an automated movable filing system?

Being alert, collecting meaningful data, and observing and listening to customers and key staff are all ways to identify improvement opportunities. It is a continuous process that has no tolerance for complacency. Excellence is not an accident but, rather, a carefully planned outcome.

Principles of Performance Improvement

The general principles of work improvement, process improvement, and methods improvement are essentially synonymous. They all relate to a management philosophy that is systems oriented; that is, a management philosophy that views the work processes in an organization as being systematic in nature, and seeks to constantly improve them by adjusting various components of the system.

A **system** is set of related elements (components) that are linked together according to a plan in order to meet a specific objective. Systems come in both manual and automated forms. The basic systems model demonstrates that a system is made up of the following components (figure 22.6, p. 542):

- *Input* refers to human resources (attitudes, abilities), money, procedures (documents that describe how the department does things), equipment, supplies, and data.

Figure 22.6.   Basic Systems Model

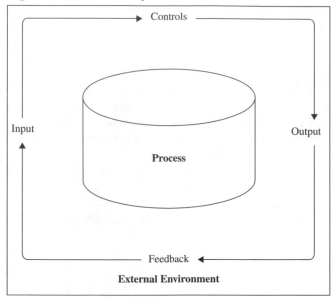

• *Process* refers to the transformation of the inputs. What is done to or with the inputs results in something being accomplished. For example, assembling a medical record and coding the medical record are processes.

• *Output* is the finished product or the result of the process, such as an educated student, a transcribed report, a coded record, and so on.

• *Controls/standards* are the expectations of what the output should be and the mechanisms in place to monitor, track, and observe how well actual performance measures up to expectations. Examples of controls/standards are quality and production standards, such as twenty-four-hour TAT, ROI requests responded to within five working days from receipt, and records coded within three days postdischarge. Also, laws, policies, and established procedures are standards that must be incorporated into the systems the facility manages.

• *Feedback* refers to the fact that when monitoring efforts indicate that expectations have been exceeded, it is time to compliment the folks involved and celebrate. Conversely, when expectations have not been met, it is time to sit down to discuss what can or should be done differently the next time. Feedback includes receiving complaints as well as indicators that something is not meeting customer expectations.

• *External environment* refers to anything outside the system that affects how it functions, for example, laws or regulations set by the local, state, or federal government. External factors that affect how the system functions include:
—The HIPAA regulations related to patient information security
—Medicare's Conditions of Participation requirements for what must be kept in a patient's medical record

—The ICD-9 (soon to be ICD-10) coding systems, which drive the reimbursement systems in hospitals
—A tight labor market, which makes it difficult to find well-educated employees

Systems such as those described here also are called **open systems** because they are affected by what is going on around them and must adjust as the environment changes and **cybernetic systems** because they have standards, controls, and feedback mechanisms built into them. Diametrically occurring is the closed system. A **closed system** operates in a self-contained environment; that is, it is not affected by outside factors. A mechanical system (engines, motors, and so on) is the best example of a closed system.

Thus, work improvement, process improvement, and methods improvement are simply three different phrases that are very closely related as concepts. They all relate to systematic approaches that managers take to determine what needs to be changed in the systems they manage in order to get the systems to meet expectations.

The aim, then, of all performance/method/process improvement efforts is to determine why actual output varies from expected output and then to take actions to increase the effect.

• *Effectiveness* indicates how closely the output from a process matches what is expected of the process. If a department is effective, it is getting done what it is supposed to get done.

• *Efficiency,* on the other hand, indicates how well the department is using its resources. Is it getting the most bang for its buck, or is it wasting time, money, energy, and other resources?

• *Adaptability* refers to the ease with which the system can adjust when circumstances require it to change to meet new demands or expectations. Adaptable systems respond appropriately to changing needs.

Customer Service

Customers are the people, external and internal, who receive and are affected by the work the healthcare facility does. They have names and needs, and are the reason(s) for the collective work of the organization.

Internal customers are located within the organization. They may be anyone within the work unit who is affected by the HIS function. Physicians and clinical staff need high-quality, expedient patient health information in order to deliver high-quality patient care. Administrative staff members are customers of the information harvested from collective databases for use in planning facilities and services. And not the least of internal customers are the HIM associates who rely on HIS to provide access to timely, reliable data to assist in clinical decision making.

External customers reside outside the organization. Physicians seen by patients who originated at the facility for care are considered external customers, as are purchasers and payers who need information so they can reimburse their enrollees in a timely manner. Regulatory agencies look to HIS for data on conditions of accreditation or participation. Vendors assist HIS, with the department's direct input, in making optimal selections of products. Communities look to HIS for information and data on their state of collective health and to earmark services the population needs to maintain a healthy existence.

All process improvement environments today focus on the customer and work to create a true customer orientation within the work environment by listening and responding to customers, thinking about their needs, and using that information to modify and improve the way our systems work for them.

In the process of customer orientation, management and staff must:

- Identify who the customers are
- Define quality from a customer perspective
- Determine how to judge service
- Obtain regular feedback

The Joint Commission on Accreditation of Healthcare Organizations (JCAHO) has standards that specifically require accredited organizations to have performance improvement efforts as an integral aspect of their day-to-day operations, as follows:

PI.1. The leaders establish a planned, systematic, organization-wide approach to process design, performance measurement, analysis, and improvement.

PI.2. New or modified processes are well designed.

PI.3. Data are collected to monitor the stability of existing processes, identify opportunities for improvement, identify changes that will lead to improvement, and sustain improvement.

PI.4. Data are systematically aggregated and analyzed on an ongoing basis.

PI.5. Improved performance is achieved and sustained.

Performance Improvement Methodologies

Three principal methodologies are available to healthcare facilities interested in performance improvement: systems analysis and design, continuous quality improvement, and reengineering. All three approaches have the same goal and use many of the same tools. However, they differ in focus and breadth of improvement effort.

Systems Analysis and Design

Systems analysis and design can be applied to any type of system. For example, it can be applied to the selection of a new information system or it can be applied to the redesign of a work process. Included in this section are discussions of the concept of systems thinking, steps of the systems analysis and design process, and tools frequently used in systems analysis and design.

Systems Thinking

When considering performance improvement, a fundamental concept to understand is systems thinking. **Systems thinking** has been defined as "a conceptual framework, a body of knowledge and tools that have been developed over the past fifty years, to make patterns clearer and to help us see how to make changes effectively in the system" (Senge 1990, p. 7). It enables us to recognize and better view a process in its entirety, rather than just focusing on its individual parts.

It is impossible to appropriately examine systems, detect potential problems, and offer constructive suggestions without understanding what systems are and how they work. All organizations, departments, and work units can be viewed as systems. Johns (1997, p. 310) defines a system as "a group of components that have the ability to self-adapt and that interact through defined relationships working to accomplish a goal or objective." (From this definition, it is clear that a variety of entities that have complex, interrelated elements working together toward a common purpose are systems.)

Systems may be classified as:

- *Mechanical:* A heating and air-conditioning system is an example of a mechanical system.
- *Human:* A human system would be a family unit or employees working in a particular department.
- *Man-machine:* A man–machine system relies on either human–human interactions or human–technology interactions, for example, a monitoring system for patient care or a unit in HIM that uses the organizations' health information system.

Most complex systems have numerous subsystems, and these subsystems frequently have still smaller subsystems.

All systems and subsystems are affected by resource constraints and subject to certain controls. Controls may originate from within the entity or from outside. *Internal controls* include organizational policies and procedures or the prevailing organizational culture that helps shape and influence the organizational norms and values of the employees operating in the system. *External controls* include laws, regulations, or societal values. Both internal and external controls shape and constrain the system to function in a particular manner.

As mentioned earlier, all systems and subsystems have four components: inputs, conversion processes, outputs, and a feedback loop. Inputs may include the knowledge, abilities, skills, and attitudes of employees, as well as supplies and equipment. They are processed in some manner and transformed into an output. The actual output is then compared to the anticipated output to determine whether it complies with what was expected. This information is the feedback. In most cases, good inputs and good processes produce desirable outputs. The feedback loop is critical for determining whether changes should be made with either the input component or the process component to produce an actual output that is in line with the expected output.

Outputs of subsystems frequently become inputs of other subsystems. Consider a new patient being seen in a physician's office. This encounter initiates a number of systems. Looking at the system from a macro level, the inputs would be the patient, the physician, the physician's staff, and the computer and instruments the physician used. The conversion processes could include registration, examination, assessment, treatment, and reimbursement. The outputs for the patient might be prescriptions and a bill or receipt.

However, a closer examination of the patient–physician encounter reveals activation of multiple subsystems, each with its own inputs, conversion processes, outputs, and feedback. For example, the registration process is a subsystem consisting of several smaller subsystems. The patient first completes the information form. The pencil, the patient's knowledge, and the patient's insurance card are all inputs into this subsystem. As the patient completes the form, he is engaging in the process. The completed form is the output.

The output of the registration subsystem becomes the input for the next subsystem initiated. The receptionist takes the completed form and, using the computer and her knowledge of the process (inputs), enters the patient's data into the practice information system (process). At this point, the output is the start of the encounter form. The physician uses the registration information as input, along with interview information, and then begins to examine the patient (process). After completing the examination, the physician may make notes in the patient's chart, write some prescriptions, and complete a form noting what was done so that the clerk can generate a form for billing.

The Systems Analysis and Design Process

The systems analysis and design process includes six distinct steps:

1. *Determine the need for the system and the system requirements.* The need for the system is often expressed as objectives established by management. Information must be obtained on the purpose of the system. Interviewing the people who participate and interact with the system is one way to determine the system requirements.
2. *Analyze the system requirements.* System analysis involves gathering, organizing, and evaluating facts about the current system. Data may be gathered by interviewing employees who participate in or interact with the system, conducting a focus group, administering a survey, reading organizational documents, and so on. The facts then must be organized in some systematic, meaningful way, for example, according to problems or steps in the process. The information then can be evaluated to determine whether the system's goal or purpose is being achieved currently in the most effi-

cient and effective manner or whether it could be better achieved through a redesign.
3. *Propose a system design or redesign.* Actually designing the new system requires input from many personnel. Both managers and employees must buy in to the potential benefits of the new or redesigned system and be committed to working out the "bugs" that always accompany the implementation of something new. A number of systems or redesigns should be considered. From these alternatives, the design that seems to have the best potential for producing the desired outcome should be selected.
4. *Evaluate the proposed system.* Evaluation of the proposed system must take into consideration its impact on all of the system components. Does the proposed system appear capable of meeting organizational goals and satisfying employee needs? Critical success factors should be developed that permit comparison of what is wanted with what is actually produced. At this point, it may be helpful to pilot-test the proposed system on a small scale to see how well it meets its objectives. Data should be collected and compared to the critical success factors identified earlier. Conducting a small test of change can provide valuable information and perhaps spare the organization the expense of implementing a system that may have unanticipated and negative consequences. If the proposed system appears to meet the criteria for success, it is ready to be implemented.
5. *Implement the system.* The implementation phase takes a great deal of time and planning. For example, the people involved in the system change must be given adequate training. Documentation of the changes, accompanied by flowcharts and revised policies and procedures, also can contribute to a smooth transition. Information obtained during the pilot test mentioned above may be used to facilitate the implementation organizationwide.
6. *Conduct ongoing evaluation and maintenance of the system.* Systems, particularly new and newly revised systems, will always need monitoring and maintenance to ensure that they are providing the desired results. Again, it may be helpful to think about the feedback loop. A method should be included in the design that would indicate whether the system is performing as expected.

Basic Tools of Systems Analysis

Tools are frequently used to gather the facts used in systems analysis. Three tools that provide valuable information on work flow and employee work activities are the work distribution chart, the movement diagram, and the flow process chart.

Work Distribution Chart

A work distribution chart can be very helpful in determining the nature of the work being performed in the unit, which employees are performing the activities, and the amount of time spent on each activity. As mentioned earlier, a work distribution chart shows job activities, time spent on them, and the names or titles of the employees who perform them. It can be very helpful in determining whether adequate time is available and appropriate for each task and whether employees are overburdened or have time for additional responsibilities. In addition, it can help the manager assess whether the work is organized and distributed appropriately.

Work distribution charts can be formulated in a variety of ways but frequently are tables with work tasks forming the row headings and a double column of employee names and hours spent on tasks forming the column headings. (See table 22.1, p. 525.) Data for the work distribution chart come from self-reported activities and hours or parts of hours spent on tasks gathered by employees over a designated period of time. Actual data collection time varies depending on what is needed to get a representative sample of activities and times. When adequate data have been collected, the manager compiles them, clusters similar job tasks together, and completes the chart.

Movement Diagram

A **movement diagram** is a visual graph of the layout of the workspace with all of the furniture, equipment, doorways, and so on sketched in. Superimposed on the layout are the movements of either individuals or paper. (See figure 22.2,

p. 530.) Ideally, individuals or paper move in a relatively straight line; the movement diagram can indicate whether the work is flowing smoothly or whether there is bottlenecking or backtracking. The manager then can use the movement diagram to redesign the flow of work and improve its efficiency (Abdelhak et al. 1996).

Flow Process Chart

A flow process chart is useful in operations analysis. (See figure 22.7.) It charts the flow of work of a material or a task but is limited to the flow of only one unit at a time. Each step of a particular process is shown in chronological order and in great detail (for example, the distance a material moves in each step, the time needed, the quantity moved, and specific notes about the process). Standard symbols are used on the chart to indicate specific processes. An operation is symbolized with a circle, transportation with an arrow, storage with a triangle, inspection with a rectangle, and a delay with a figure resembling an uppercase D. When the symbols are connected with a line, the manager can see the actual flow of work.

The flow process chart is an excellent method for indicating time problems with work flow. It can show duplication and inefficiency and also can be very useful in verifying procedures or planning a workstation redesign (Liebler, Levine, and Rothman 1992). Some flow process charts include two charts in one, a chart showing the current flow of work and a second chart proposing a redesigned work flow.

Figure 22.7.   Flow Process Chart

	PRESENT		PROPOSED		DIFFERENCE		
	NO.	TIME	NO.	TIME	NO.	TIME	
○ OPERATIONS							Job _____
⇨ TRANSPORTATIONS							Date _____
□ INSPECTIONS							
D DELAYS							Man □ Material □
▽ STORAGES							Chartered by _____
DISTANCE TRAVELED		FT.		FT.		FT.	

DETAILS OF (PRESENT/PROPOSED) METHOD	OPERATION	TRANSPORT.	INSPECTION	DELAY	STORAGE	DISTANCE IN FEET	QUANTITY	TIME	ANALYSIS		ACTION
									WHY	NOTES	CHANGE
1	○	⇨	□	D	▽						
2	○	⇨	□	D	▽						
3	○	⇨	□	D	▽						
4	○	⇨	□	D	▽						
5	○	⇨	□	D	▽						
6	○	⇨	□	D	▽						

Continuous Quality Improvement

Continuous quality improvement (CQI), frequently referred to as total quality management (TQM) or service excellence, is a management philosophy that seeks to "involve healthcare personnel in planning and executing a continuous flow of improvements to provide quality health care that meets or exceeds expectations" (McLaughlin and Kaluzny 1999, p. 3). Its focus is on improving the quality of services provided to customers, whether internal (employees) or external (patients, physicians, payers). The approach is to make efforts to meet or exceed customer expectations by conducting small tests of change aimed at improving the quality of services. Of course, not all customer expectations can be met at the same time. In fact, some customers have expectations that conflict with the expectations of other customers. However, the goal is worth pursuing, even when only partly achievable.

CQI casts off the notion of ignoring problems until they become too big to ignore. Rather, it subscribes to the theory of seeking ways to improve the system through the testing of small, incremental changes with the expectation that, over time, the changes will continually improve the quality of care that health facilities provide to their patients (Berwick 1989). To achieve this, CQI relies on the gathering and analysis of data that can be used to make informed decisions.

More than the latest buzzword in healthcare, CQI is a way of thinking, a way of being, a way of managing, a way of conducting business. It can be applied to individuals as well as organizations. The expression "If it ain't broke, don't fix it" is alien to the CQI philosophy. Moreover, CQI does not seek to blame problems on individuals but, instead, suggests that systems or processes may have inherent flaws that contribute to problems.

CQI attempts to involve people in the examination and improvement of existing systems. Several principles are incorporated into the CQI philosophy, including:

- *Constancy of variation:* Systems will always produce some normal variation in their output; the manager's job is to reduce the amount of variation as much as possible so that the process can become more stable and produce a more reliable output. Managers should not assume that any variation is a defect but should monitor and measure data over time to ensure that any variation is, in fact, caused inherently by the system. This type of variation is **common cause variation.** A greater-than-expected variation is a **special cause variation.** Sometimes a change is initiated with the express purpose of producing an improvement effort, in which case it should be encouraged. Other times, changes result in negative outputs and these must be eliminated.

  An example of variation in HIS departments might be found in the coding and processing of records. A coder may complete twenty records one day, but only eighteen the next. The variation is not due to the clerk's lack of productivity, but perhaps to the size of the records that day. In other words, the change is attributed to common cause variation. A significant drop in coding might indicate that a special cause is in effect. Perhaps the coder was assigned duties that day in addition to coding.

- *Importance of data:* Far too often, decisions for improvement are based on faulty assumptions. CQI recognizes the importance of collecting sufficient data so that informed decisions can be made. Omachonu (1999, p. 71) states "that the ability to collect, analyze, and use data is a vital component of a successful performance improvement process. Healthcare organizations that do not devote sufficient attention to data collection may be able to speak of only marginal success in their process improvement journey." Individuals planning a CQI effort must take time to develop appropriate data collection methods and instruments (written surveys, direct observation, focus group interviews, reviews of medical records with criteria forms). Appropriate analysis must follow data collection to provide the knowledge on which improvement efforts can be built (White 2002).

- *Vision and support of executive leadership:* CQI gurus such as W. Edwards Deming and Brian Joiner stress that acceptance of the CQI philosophy must funnel down from the top to truly permeate the organization's culture. Executive leadership must communicate a clear vision and mission statement that every employee can understand and share.

- *Focus on customers:* To be successful, the organization must know and understand what its customers need and want. One way to obtain customer feedback is to administer satisfaction surveys on a regular basis. Any needs that are identified should be addressed.

- *Investment in people:* The CQI philosophy assumes that people want to do their jobs well. However, because this philosophy is relatively new, some employees may need training on how they can more adequately serve their customers. Management can empower employees by giving them opportunities to learn and grow and feel more competent in performing their jobs.

- *Importance of teams:* Because CQI seeks to improve processes that may extend beyond the boundaries of individual departments, the people directly involved with the processes must work together. Teams should include individuals with different expertise and from different levels of the organization. Team members should be knowledgeable about portions of the process and able to contribute to the improvement effort. Having members from different areas on the team brings fresh perspectives and opens communication. A good team also is able to communicate its purpose and activities to other parts of the organization.

Improvement Models

Several models exist for structuring performance improvement. One that is frequently used in hospitals is Hospital Corporation of America's FOCUS-PDCA model. This model includes five steps before initiating its PDCA (**P**lan, **D**o, **C**heck, **A**ct) cycle (described below in the Foundation for Improvement Model as the PDSA Cycle). The five initial steps of the FOCUS-PDCA include:

1. **F**ind a process to improve
2. **O**rganize a team that knows the process
3. **C**larify the current knowledge of the process
4. **U**nderstand causes of special variation
5. **S**elect the process improvement

A different, but highly effective, model that can be used for any process targeted for improvement is the Langley, Nolan, and Nolan Foundation for Improvement Model (1994). It is presented here because of its simplicity. The model has two parts. The first part requires an individual or team to answer three fundamental questions; the second part requires initiation of the PDSA cycle.

The three fundamental questions that must be answered for any improvement project are:

- *What is my aim?* This question forces the responder to determine his or her overall goal.
- *How will I know a change is an improvement?* This question requires the responder to define measures (preferably quantitative, but also some qualitative) that will indicate progress made toward his or her goal. These measures will enable the individual or team to collect data.
- *What changes have the potential to result in improvement?* This question requires the responder to brainstorm a number of changes that might lead to improvement. He or she must recognize that not all changes do result in improvement.

After changes have been brainstormed, one change deemed to have significant potential for effecting improvement should be tried. This is a small test of change made with one change strategy. If it is successful, other changes may be added. The change strategy is tested using the **PDSA cycle.**

PDSA stands for **P**lan, **D**o, **S**tudy, and **A**ct. It is actually a trial and learning cycle. (See figure 22.8.) The phases of the cycle break down as follows:

1. During the *plan phase,* preparations are made for implementing the selected change. This is the time to consider who, what, where, when, and how. In addition, this is the time to plan how to collect data that will be used in determining the progress of the implementation. It may be necessary to develop a data collection instrument. Having already determined what the measurements will be, it also may be necessary to collect baseline data before implementing the change. Finally, this phase is the time to decide how often and how long to collect data before the results are analyzed.

2. During the *do phase,* the change strategy is implemented and data are collected. Perhaps the change strategy and the data collection will go on for two weeks before the analysis. The length of time depends on how frequently data were collected and how long the PDSA cycle is intended to last.

3. During the *study phase,* the data are analyzed. Is progress being made toward the defined aim? Are there any unanticipated problems? This phase indicates whether a change is an improvement. If it appears to be, the decision will likely be to continue the change strategy. If it is not showing as much improvement as expected, it may be necessary to adjust the change strategy. If it shows no improvement, it may be time to abandon the change strategy and test another one.

4. During the *act phase,* the knowledge obtained from the PDSA trial and learning cycle is applied, which leads to three possible actions: continue with the current change strategy, adjust it, or try a new one. At this point, a second PDSA cycle is implemented to continue the quest for knowledge about what affects the process and what permits progress. The more knowledge, the greater the likelihood of a successful improvement effort.

Figure 22.8.   PDSA Cycles Expedite Improvement

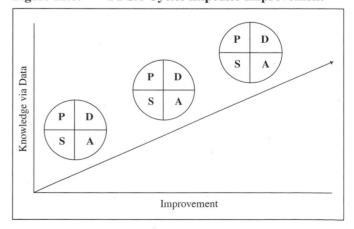

Basic CQI Techniques and Tools

A number of tools and techniques are frequently used with performance improvement initiatives (Brassard and Ritter 1993; Johnson and McLaughlin 1999; Cofer and Greeley 1993). Some of them are used to facilitate communication among employees; others are used to assist people in determining the root causes of problems. Some tools show areas of agreement or consensus among team members; others permit the display of data for easier analysis. The following section presents a brief description and discussion of the purpose of tools and techniques commonly used by improvement teams (White 2002).

Brainstorming

Brainstorming is a technique used to generate a large number of creative ideas. It encourages team members to think "out of the box" and offer ideas. There are some variations in using the technique—one can use an unstructured method for brainstorming or a structured method. The unstructured method involves having a free flow of ideas about a situation. The team leader writes each idea down as it is offered so all can see. There should be no evaluative discussion about the worthiness of the idea because we want to do nothing that will inhibit the flow of ideas. Each idea is captured and written for the team to consider at a later point.

Structured brainstorming uses a more formal approach. The team leader asks each person to generate a list of ideas for themselves and then, one by one, the team leader proceeds around the room eliciting a new idea from each member. The process may take several rounds. As team members run out of new ideas, they pass, and the next person offers an idea until no one can produce any fresh ideas.

Brainstorming is highly effective for identifying a number of potential processes that may benefit from improvement efforts and for generating solutions to particular problems. It helps people to begin thinking in new ways and gets them involved in the process. It is an excellent method for facilitating open communication.

Affinity Grouping

Affinity grouping allows the team to organize and group similar ideas together. Ideas that are generated in a brainstorming session may be written on Post-it notes and arranged on a table or posted on a board. Without talking to each other, each team member is asked to walk around the table or board, look at the ideas, and place them in groupings that seem related or connected to each other. Each member is empowered to move the ideas in a way that makes the most sense. As a team member moves the ideas back or places them in other groupings, the other team members consider the merits of the placement and decide if further action is needed. The goal is to have the team eventually feel comfortable with the arrangement. The natural groupings that emerge are then labeled with a category. This tool brings focus to the many ideas generated. (See figure 22.9.)

Figure 22.9.   Affinity Grouping

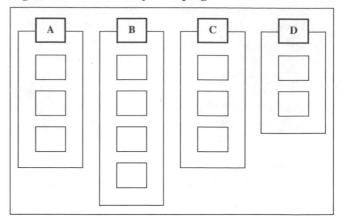

Nominal Group Technique

Nominal group technique (NGT) is a process designed to bring agreement about an issue or an idea that the team considers most important. It produces and permits visualization of team consensus. In NGT, each team member ranks each idea according to its importance. For example, if there were six ideas, the idea that is most important would be given the number 6. The second most important idea would be given the number 5. The least important idea would have the number 1. After each team member has individually ranked the list of ideas, the numbers are totaled. The ideas that are deemed most important are clearly visible to all. Those ideas that people did not think were as important are also made known with their low scores. NGT demonstrates where the team's priorities lie.

Multivoting Technique

The **multivoting technique** is a variation of NGT and has the same purpose. Rather than ranking each issue or idea, team members are asked to rate the issue using a distribution of points or colorful dots. Weighted multivoting is a variation of this process. For example, a team member may be asked to distribute 25 points among 10 total issues. Thus, one issue of particular importance to him may receive 12 points, four others may receive some variation of the remaining 12 points, and five others may receive no points. After the voting, the numbers are added and the team is able to see which issue has emerged as particularly important to the team.

This process can also be done with colored dots. For example, if there are eight items, on a chart, each team member may be given four dots to distribute on the four items that are most important to him or her. This method particularly enables team members to see where consensus lies and what issue has been deemed most important by the team as a whole.

Flowchart

Whenever a team examines a process with the intention of making improvement, it must first thoroughly understand the process. Each team member comes to the team with a unique perspective and significant insight about how a portion of the process works. To help all members understand the process, a team will undertake development of a **flowchart.** (See figure 22.1, p. 528.) This work allows the team to thoroughly understand every step in the process and the sequence of steps. It provides a picture of each decision point and each event that must be completed. It readily points out places where there is redundancy and complex and problematic areas.

Root-Cause Analysis (Fishbone Diagram)

When a team first identifies a problem, it may use a **fishbone diagram,** also known as a cause-and-effect diagram, to help it determine the root causes of the problem. (See figure 22.10.) The problem is placed in a box on the right side of the paper. A horizontal line is drawn, somewhat like a backbone, with diagonal bones, like ribs, pointing to the boxes above and below the backbone. Each box contains a category. The categories may be names that represent broad classifications of problem areas, for example, people, methods, equipment, materials, policies/procedures, environment, measurement, and so on. The team determines how many categories it needs to classify all of the sources of problems. Usually there are about four. After constructing the diagram, the team brainstorms possible sources of the problem. These are then placed on horizontal lines extending from the diagonal category line. The brainstorming of root causes continues among team members until all ideas are exhausted. The purpose of this tool is to permit a team to explore, identify and graphically display all of the root causes of a problem.

After identifying a number of causes of a problem, a team may decide to begin working to remove one of the causes of the problem. CQI involves continually making efforts to improve processes; certainly removing one cause, and then working to remove another cause, will eventually improve the process. The question may arise, however, about which cause to remove first. Techniques such as multivoting or nominal group technique, discussed above, can help bring consensus among the team about what to work on first.

Pareto Chart

When a team decides to use multivoting or nominal group technique to determine consensus among the members about the most important problem to tackle first, each team member places a number or mark next to an item indicating that individual's opinion about the item's importance. When the numbers are tallied, the items can be ranked according to importance. This ranking can then be visually displayed in a **Pareto chart.** (See figure 22.11, p. 550.) A Pareto chart looks very much like a bar chart except that the highest-ranking item is listed first, followed by the second highest, down to the lowest-ranked item. Thus, the Pareto chart is a descending bar chart. This visualization of how the problems were ranked allows team members to focus on those few that have the greatest potential for improving the process. The Pareto chart is based on the Pareto principle, which states that 20 percent of the sources of the problem are responsible for 80 percent of the actual problems. By concentrating on the vital few sources, a large number of actual problems can be eliminated.

Force-Field Analysis

A **force-field analysis** also visually displays data generated through brainstorming. The team leader draws a large T formation on a board. (See figure 22.12, p. 550.) Above the crossbar and on the left side of the T is written the word drivers, and above the bar and written on the right side of the T is written the word barriers. Team members are then asked to brainstorm and list on the chart under the crossbar the reasons or factors that would contribute to a change for improvement and those reasons or factors that can create barriers. Thus, the force field enables team members to identify factors that support or work against a proposed solution. Often the next step in this activity is to work on ways that would either eliminate barriers or reinforce drivers.

Check Sheet

A **check sheet** is a data collection tool permitting the recording and compiling of observations or occurrences. It consists of a simple listing of categories, issues, or observations on the left side of the chart and a place on the right for individuals to record checkmarks next to the item when it is observed or counted. (See figure 22.13, p. 550.) After a period of time, the checkmarks are counted, and patterns or trends can be revealed. A check sheet is a simple tool that allows a clear picture of the facts to emerge. It enables data to be collected. After data are collected, several tools can be used to display the data and help the team more easily analyze them.

Figure 22.10.   Fishbone Diagram

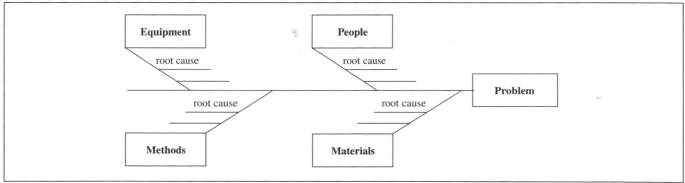

Figure 22.11.   Pareto Chart

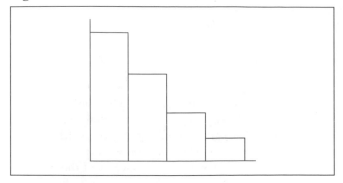

Figure 22.12.   Force-Field Analysis

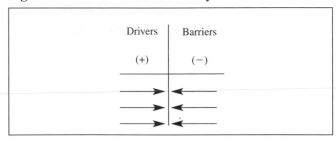

Figure 22.13.   Check Sheet

	1	2	Total
A	⊬⊬⊬⊤	/ / /	8
B	/ / / /	/ / / /	8
C	/ /	/	3

Scatter Diagram

A **scatter diagram** is data analysis tool used to plot points of two variables suspected of being related to each other in some way. For example, to see whether age and blood pressure are related, one variable, age, would be plotted on one line of the graph, and the other variable, blood pressure, would be plotted on the other line. After several people's blood pressures are plotted along with their ages, a pattern might emerge. If the diagram indicates that blood pressure increases with age, the data could be interpreted as revealing a positive relationship between age and blood pressure. (See figure 22.14.)

In some cases, a negative relationship might exist, such as with the variables "age" and "flexibility" or with the number of hours of training and number of mistakes made. Whenever a scatter diagram indicates that the points are moving together in one direction or another, conclusions can be drawn about the variables' relationship, either positive or

Figure 22.14.   Scatter Diagram

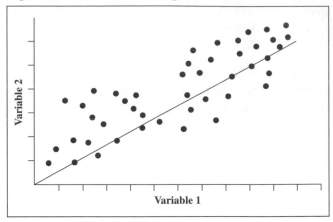

negative. In other cases, however, the scatter diagram may indicate no linear relationship between the variables because the points are scattered haphazardly and no pattern emerges. In this case, the conclusion would have to be that the two variables have no apparent relationship.

Histogram

A **histogram** (figure 22.15) is a data analysis tool used to display frequencies of response. (See also chapter 11.) It offers a much easier way to summarize and analyze data than having them displayed in a table of numbers. A histogram displays **continuous data** values that have been grouped into categories. The bars on the histogram reveal how the data are distributed. For example, an HIM administrator may want to show the number of minutes it takes to respond to patient requests for information. Minutes may be categorized into four groupings, for example, 1–30 minutes, 31–60 minutes, 61–90 minutes, and more than 90 minutes. Checkmarks may be recorded indicating the category of minutes taken to respond to the request. After a period of time, the checkmarks are added and the histogram is plotted with the frequencies shown on the vertical, or *y* axis, and the minute intervals shown on the horizontal, or *x* axis.

This graph indicates the different intervals patients had to wait for their requests to be filled. A histogram can give an excellent idea of how well a process is performing. Thus, it can show how frequently data values occur among the various intervals, how centered or skewed the distribution of data is, and what the likelihood of future occurrences is.

Run Chart

A **run chart** displays data points over a period of time to provide information about performance. (See figure 22.16.) Measured points of a process are plotted on a graph at regular time intervals to help team members see whether there are substantial changes in the numbers over time. For example, suppose an HIM administrator wanted to reduce the number of incomplete records in the HIS department. He might first plot on a graph the number of incomplete records each month for the past six months and then enact a change in the processing of records designed to improve the process. Following the improvement effort, data would continue to be collected on the number of incomplete records and would continue to be plotted on the graph. If the run chart shows that the number of incomplete charts has actually decreased, the HIM administrator could attribute the decrease to the improvement effort. A run chart is an excellent tool for providing visual verification of how a process is performing and whether an improvement effort appears to have worked.

Statistical Process Control Chart

A **statistical process control** (SPC) **chart** looks very much like a run chart except that it has a line displayed at the top, called an upper control limit (UCL), and a line displayed at the bottom, called a lower control limit (LCL). (See figure 22.17.) These lines have been statistically calculated from the data generated in the process and represent three units of dispersion above and below the midline (three standard deviations) (Omachonu 1999).

Like the run chart, the SPC chart plots points over time to demonstrate how a process is performing. However, the two control limit lines enable the interpreter to determine whether the process is stable, or predictable, or whether it is out of control. CQI statisticians Walter Shewhart and W. Edwards Deming first presented the idea of variation that routinely occurs in systems. Remembering the constancy of variation principle, it is easy to see the purpose of the SPC chart. The SPC chart indicates whether the variation occurring within the process is a common cause variation or a special cause variation. It indicates whether it is necessary to try and reduce the ordinary variation occurring through common cause or seek out a special cause of the variation and try to eliminate it.

Business Process Reengineering

Unlike CQI, which focuses on conducting small tests of change to achieve continuous, but incremental, improvement over time, business process **reengineering** focuses on the potential revamping of the entire process from head to toe to achieve improvement. (See table 22.12 for a comparison of reengineering and quality management.) Reengineering implies making massive changes to the way a facility delivers healthcare services. In *Reengineering the Corporation: A Manifesto for Business Revolution,* Hammer and Champy (1993) defined reengineering as "the fundamental rethinking and radical redesign of business processes to achieve dramatic improvements in critical contemporary measures of performance such as cost, quality, service, and speed" (McBrierty 1995, p. 46).

Philosophy of Reengineering

Reengineering, or business process reengineering, entered the healthcare sector after first being used in the business community. It is a radical approach that seeks to reevaluate and redesign organizational processes in order to achieve dramatic performance improvement (Abdelhak et al. 1996).

Figure 22.15.   Histogram

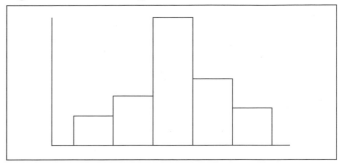

Figure 22.16.   Run Chart

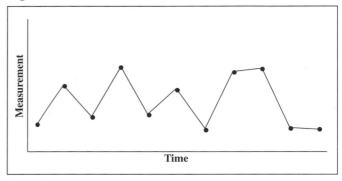

Figure 22.17.   Statistical Process Control Chart

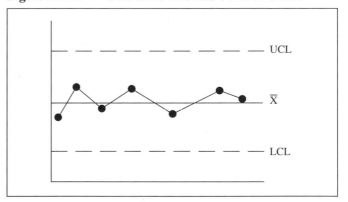

Table 22.12.   Reengineering Compared to Quality Management

Reengineering		Quality Management	
Rethinking and Radical Redesign	Focus	Incremental Improvements	Focus
Rethink	Think out of the box	Quality planning	Focus on the customer
Redesign	Think both process and outcome	Quality control	Measure and monitor performance
Retool	Use technology to control and define work processes	Quality improvement	Use data, eliminate boundaries, and empower work

It may be applied to the entire organization or to processes recognized as needing increased efficiency.

In reengineering, the entire manner and purpose of a process is questioned. The purpose is to achieve the process goal in the most effective and efficient manner possible. Thus, the expectations for reengineering include:

- Increased productivity
- Decreased costs
- Improved quality
- Maximized revenue
- More satisfied customers

However, it should be clearly understood that the main focus is on reducing costs (Palmer 1995).

Used extensively in the mid-1980s and early 1990s, reengineering has met with significant criticism in the healthcare sector because of the fear it has invoked among healthcare workers. As would be expected, reengineering frequently results in the loss of jobs. Because salaries and benefits comprise 50 to 60 percent of a healthcare facility's total expenses, a drop in personnel can have a significant impact on reducing expenditures and is often used as an effective strategy in reengineering.

Process of Reengineering

When an organization decides to use reengineering as an improvement strategy, it commits itself to looking at selected processes within the organization in fine detail. Processes are selected for reengineering based on a number of criteria, including:

- Frequency and severity of problems created by the process, such as slow turnaround time or excessive waiting time
- Impact on customer satisfaction
- Complex processes involving multiple departments, procedures, and employees
- The feasibility of actually creating improvement (Umiker 1998)

Selecting a process for reengineering raises several questions, including:

- What is the intended purpose of the process? Is that purpose being accomplished efficiently?
- Is the process absolutely necessary? Are there redundancies or non-value-added activities that could be eliminated?
- Which employees are involved in the process, and which ones are actually needed? In other words, what are the minimum qualifications and minimum number of employees needed to do the job?
- Is the process as efficient as it could be, or are there more efficient means for accomplishing the goal?
- Is the process contributing to the efficiency of other processes that may be affected by its results?

- Is there an opportunity for processes to be combined and for employees to be trained or utilized to perform more functions than they currently perform?
- Can any steps of the process be eliminated?
- Is outsourcing a feasible and more cost-effective alternative?
- Would new equipment or new technologies improve the process?

Many of the tools and techniques used in systems analysis and CQI also are used in reengineering. In reengineering, it is essential to thoroughly understand how the process contributes to how the organization functions and to determine whether a better method exists. Therefore, observation of processes, customer input, interviews with employees, and the use of cross-functional teams to discuss the current steps of the process are frequently used methods for obtaining data. Data must be collected for a sufficient period of time to actually reflect the effectiveness of the process.

In addition, the data must be analyzed appropriately, and the analysis should include the input of individuals qualified to interpret the findings. Thus, a team composed of individuals involved in various aspects of the process should be permitted access to the data and should give input about alternative strategies. Moreover, the team can investigate the acceptability of new technologies that might allow for greater efficiency. Before new technologies are adopted, however, the team should thoroughly analyze the potential benefits, costs, and feasibility of using them in the organization.

After a reengineered process has emerged, new policies and procedures must be written and distributed to the people involved in the process. In addition, employees should be thoroughly trained in the redesigned process. However, it is very important that they be given adequate time to master the process. Managers play an important role in reengineering through their support, encouragement, and commitment to the process.

Factors for Success in Reengineering Efforts

One critical factor for the success of the reengineering effort is the visible and persistent commitment of senior administration. A second critical factor is management's commitment to excellence. Managers must demonstrate a "can-do" attitude in working through the change. In addition, the fact that change is needed to address an unacceptable problem must be effectively communicated throughout the organization. Having everyone, or almost everyone, acknowledge that a problem exists creates a great deal of buy-in. Employees, including physicians, should be encouraged to overcome any reluctance to participate in the change process due to fears about restructuring. Many healthcare organizations make the mistake of not including their physicians in critical decision making. The likelihood of a successful reengineering effort will increase when every stakeholder is involved in the process.

Reengineering takes anywhere from one to three years to achieve. The organization should realize that change cannot be achieved overnight and should avoid trying to change too many processes at once. Instead, it should focus its efforts on a few processes at a time. A great deal of planning, information gathering, and analysis must occur before an actual redesign can be implemented. When the planning phase has been completed, the organization should revise or develop policies and procedures accordingly and distribute them throughout the organization.

Finally, implementation of the redesigned processes requires patience. Glitches may occur with any new system, but with careful monitoring and persistent adjusting, reengineering can produce significant performance improvement.

Check Your Understanding 22.3

Instructions: Indicate whether the following sentences are true or false and, on a separate piece of paper, correct any false statement to make it true or explain why it is false.

1. ___ The goal of CQI—to meet and/or exceed the expectations of all the organization's customers—is generally attainable and achievable.

2. ___ A manager's job with regard to performance improvement is to seek ways to reduce the amount of normal variation that occurs within systems and processes.

3. ___ Obtaining and using actual data to inform managers who need to make decisions is a critically important element of the CQI philosophy.

4. ___ Reengineering is particularly focused on efficiency.

Real-World Case

On January 4, 2001, the *New York Times* published an article about an innovative redesign of the appointment system at the Kaiser Permanente Medical Center in Roseville, California. The physician office practice appeared very successful: the waiting rooms were usually filled with patients, and the appointment books showed several weeks of nonemergency patient appointments. Of course, problems would routinely occur when patients needed to be seen immediately and worked into the schedule. This situation usually backed up everything and created long waits. Patients, who already were feeling ill and irritated, became more irritated and physicians and staff had to apologize and find something or someone else to blame. In addition to creating an uncomfortable situation for everyone, the physicians often had to work longer hours than expected to see all of their patients.

Dr. Mark Murray, a family practice physician, questioned whether there might not be a better way to manage the situation. However, his colleagues assured him that the situation was typical of successful physician office practices. "After all," they said, "economically, it was better to have too many patients than too few patients, and as long as everyone eventually got seen, what really is the harm?" Nevertheless Dr. Murray wondered if there might not be another way.

Dr. Murray was aware of the work being done by the Institute of Healthcare Improvement, a Boston-based, nonprofit organization committed to the principles of continuous quality improvement. The proponents of this organization were physicians who had used many CQI methods, appreciated their benefits, and reported the improvements they had noted in the management of their own practices. Dr. Murray was eager to see if he could improve services for his patients, cut down on their wait time, and perhaps even create more consistency in working hours for his colleagues. He began to use several of the methods discussed in this chapter.

Realizing that neither he nor the staff really understood how the current system was working, he determined that it was essential to begin collecting data to learn what the process was like for their patients. The results were both surprising and validating. One surprising finding was that patients had to wait an average of fifty-five days to get nonemergency appointments. Not surprising was that there were more calls for appointments in the fall and winter than in the spring and summer. Generally, there were from sixteen to twenty-five calls for appointments each day for each physician, with each physician generally seeing about twenty-one patients per day. Data also revealed and supported the supposition that more patients came to the office on Mondays than on any other day. As a result, Monday appointments were generally backed up, which contributed to patient irritation and physician and staff exhaustion. This information equipped Dr. Murray to make appropriate recommendations about supply and demand.

He presented his findings to his colleagues and proposed several changes to improve patient service. His goal was to significantly reduce wait time for both patients trying to make appointments and those in the waiting room. He suggested that practice physicians plan to work longer hours on Mondays, particularly during the winter. They were working longer hours anyway, so why not just set their expectations at that level? He further suggested that physicians work longer hours temporarily to reduce the practice's current backlog of patients. Dr. Murray's ultimate goal was very ambitious: he wanted patients to be able to make appointments with their own physicians on the very day they called.

Although his colleagues agreed that his goal would be very satisfying to patients, if it were achieved, they were very concerned about not having the comfort of seeing several weeks of appointments listed in the appointment book. Could this new system actually work? When the goal was communicated to patients, they seemed pleased, but skeptical. No one had ever heard of such a thing. They were used to long wait times and could not imagine quick response times. Enlisting the support of his colleagues was quite a challenge, but eventually they agreed to implement the changes. Success was not immediate; it took about a year for the goal to be realized. Now, however, patients can get an appointment with their own physician generally on the same day they call. Everyone is much happier.

Summary

Competencies pivotal to excellence in management include being knowledgeable of the components of work processes and how to define, execute, and monitor performance/work measurements. The elements that are part and parcel to strategically managing staff productivity include employing appropriate numbers of FTEs to operate the functions of an HIS department and creating an effective environment in which to do just that.

Performance improvement involves three major approaches: systems analysis and design, continuous quality improvement, and reengineering. These approaches share many similarities: all are focused on bettering the system to provide quality service in a cost-effective manner. They also use similar data-gathering and analysis tools. The differences in the approaches may reflect the breadth of change, the duration of the change effort, and the specific area of interest. Systems analysis and design often occurs with the design of a new system. CQI is a test of small changes with the intention of improving services to customers over time. Reengineering is a massive reexamination and redesign of processes with the main purpose of reducing costs. All of these approaches have their place in improving healthcare service delivery.

References

Abdelhak, M., S. Grostick, M. A. Hanken, and E. Jacobs. 1996. *Health Information: Management of a Strategic Resource.* Philadelphia: W. B. Saunders Company.

Berwick, D. M. 1989. Continuous improvement as an ideal in health care. *New England Journal of Medicine* 320(1): 53–56.

Brassard, M., and D. Ritter. 1993. *The Memory Jogger™ II.* Methuen, Mass.: GOAL/QPC.

Cofer, J. I., and H. P. Greele. 1993. *Quality Improvement Techniques for Medical Records.* Marblehead, Mass.: Opus Communications.

Doyan, C., K. Thompson, and L. Meottel. 1999. Changes for the better: implementing four best practices. *Journal of American Health Information Management* 70(5): 40–43.

Hammer, M., and J. Champy. 1993. *Reengineering the Corporation: A Manifesto for Business Revolution.* New York City: Harper Business.

Johns, M. L. 1997. *Information Management for Health Professionals.* Albany, N.Y.: Delmar Publishers.

Johnson, S. P., and C. P. McLaughlin. 1999. Measurement and statistical approaches in CQI. In *Continuous Quality Improvement in Health Care,* edited by C. P. McLaughlin and A. D. Kaluzny, pp. 70–101. Gaithersburg, Md.: Aspen Publishers.

Keister, J. 2001. Workflow automation: streamlining the way things get done. *For the Record* 13(16): 16–20.

Langley, G. J., K. M. Nolan, and T. W. Nolan. 1994. The foundation of improvement. *Quality Progress* (June): 81–86.

Liebler, J. G., R. E. Levine, and J. Rothman. 1992. *Management Principles for Health Professionals,* second edition. Gaithersburg, Md.: Aspen Publishers.

McBrierty, L. 1995. Reengineering: a step beyond CPR. *Journal of American Health Information Management Association* 66(2): 46–48.

McLaughlin, C. P., and A. D. Kaluzny. 1999. *Continuous Quality Improvement in Health Care: Theory, Implementation and Applications,* second edition. Gaithersburg: Md.: Aspen Publishers.

Omachonu, V. K. 1999. *Healthcare Performance Improvement.* Norcross, Ga.: Engineering and Management Press.

Palmer, L. 1995. Reengineering healthcare: the future awaits us all. *Journal of American Health Information Management Association* 66(2):32–35.

Senge, P. M. 1990. *The Fifth Discipline: The Art and Practice of the Learning Organization.* New York City: Currency/Doubleday.

Umiker, W. 1998. *Management Skills for the New Health Care Supervisor,* third edition. Gaithersburg, Md.: Aspen Publishers.

White, A. 2002. Performance improvement. In *Health Information Management Technology: An Applied Approach,* edited by Merida L. Johns. Chicago: American Health Information Management Association.

Application Exercises

1. Use the model for improvement described in this chapter to design your own personal improvement project. Select some area in your life that you want to improve and then follow the steps of the model:

   • Determine and write your aim(s).

   • Identify measures (data you can collect) that will allow you to know if a change is an improvement.

   • Determine a change strategy to initiate that will help you make progress toward your aim.

   • Implement a PDSA Cycle

      —Plan how you will do the change; plan how you will collect data, plan when you will analyze the data.

      —Do the change, collect the data.

      —Study the data and determine whether the change is beneficial.

      —Act on your knowledge. Do you need to plan a new change, modify your change strategy, or maintain the change?

   • Frequently, it is beneficial to run another PDSA cycle.

2. On a piece of paper, write a procedure for frying an egg using the criteria for writing effective procedures. Have another person review your finished product for comprehensibility and ease of execution.

Review Quiz

Instructions: Select the correct answer for each of the following exercises.

Scenario for questions 1–3: By reviewing the records kept on filing unit performance over the past year, the filing unit has filed an average of 1,000 records per day. You have three FTE record filers in the department who are productive 88% of each workday (that is, 12% unproductive or 12% PFD). Based on this information, answer the following questions and show the formula you used to reach your answer. Round your answer to a whole number.

1. ___ The average number of records filed per productive hour in the file unit as a whole is ___.
   a. 143 charts/hour
   b. 110 charts/hour
   c. 48 charts/hour
   d. 42 charts/hour

2. ___ The average number of records filed per productive hour per FTE is ___.
   a. 48 charts/hour
   b. 37 charts/hour
   c. 16 charts/hour
   d. 14 charts/hour

3. ___ In the following list, label each standard that is stated in *measurable* terms with S (standard) and each that is stated in unmeasurable terms with UM.
   a. ___ To respond to a written ROI in a timely way
   b. ___ To complete timecards for payroll by 6:00 p.m. on the last day of the payroll period
   c. ___ To drop file one inch of loose documents per hour
   d. ___ To maintain an accurate master patient index
   e. ___ To transcribe reports with 98% accuracy in spelling and word usage

4. ___ Identify each standard below as a quality standard (L) or a quantity standard (N).
   a. ___ To deliver the record to the requester of a STAT request within 10 minutes of receiving the request
   b. ___ To respond to requests in two working days 95% of the time
   c. ___ To assign the correct MR# to a returning patient with 99% accuracy
   d. ___ To transcribe 1,500 lines per day
   e. ___ To file 50 to 60 records per hour
   f. ___ To complete five birth certificates per hour

5. ___ Which of the following system components allows one to determine whether the results that were actually achieved are the ones that were expected?
   a. Inputs
   b. Process
   c. Outputs
   d. Feedback
   e. Controls

6. ___ Indicate the logical order of the systems analysis and design process.
   a. Propose a system design or redesign, determine need for system and system requirements, analyze system requirement, evaluate proposed system, conduct ongoing evaluation and maintenance, implement system.
   b. Determine need for system and system requirements, analyze the requirements, propose a system design or redesign, evaluate proposed system, implement system, conduct ongoing evaluation and maintenance.
   c. Analyze system requirements, determine need for system and system requirements, evaluate proposed system, implement system, propose a system design or redesign, conduct ongoing evaluation and maintenance.
   d. Propose a system design or redesign, evaluate proposed system, implement system, conduct ongoing evaluation and maintenance, determine need for system and system requirements, analyze system requirements.
   e. Determine need for system and system requirements, propose a system design or redesign, evaluate proposed system, analyze system requirements, implement system, conduct ongoing evaluation and maintenance of system.

7. ___ All of the following tools are typically used in systems analysis and design except ___.
   a. Work distribution chart
   b. Movement diagram
   c. Flow process chart
   d. Multivoting technique

8. ___ CQI tools are intended to facilitate all of the following outcomes except ___.
   a. Group communication
   b. Problem identification
   c. Adherence to hierarchical roles
   d. Group consensus
   e. Data analysis

9. ___ A CQI tool frequently used to display data is ___.
   a. Scatter diagram
   b. Brainstorming
   c. Nominal group technique
   d. Multivoting
   e. Movement diagram

10. ___ Which of the following is not a true statement about reengineering?
    a. It is intended to make small incremental changes to improve a process.
    b. It seeks to reevaluate and redesign organizational processes to make dramatic performance improvements.
    c. It implies making massive changes to achieve significant improvements in cost, quality, service, and speed.
    d. Its main focus is to reduce costs.
    e. It frequently results in the loss of jobs.

Chapter 23
Human Resources Management

Shirley Eichenwald Maki, MBA, RHIA, CPHIMS

Learning Objectives

- To understand and differentiate among the concepts of chain of command, scope of command, and unity of command
- To differentiate among the hierarchical, bureaucratic, and team-based approaches to organization and management
- To develop organizational charts that accurately represent an organization's formal structure
- To construct mission, vision, and values statements
- To understand the unique responsibilities associated with each level of management in the organization: supervisor, middle manager, executive manager, and board director
- To identify the activities associated with the human resources management function in an organization
- To associate key federal legislation with each of the human resources management activities
- To develop position descriptions, performance standards, and staff schedules used as tools in human resource management
- To explain how job descriptions are used in recruitment and hiring
- To identify effective steps in conducting an interview
- To discuss the roles employee orientation and communication plans play in developing and retaining staff
- To articulate the benefits of teamwork in an organization and identify the steps in creating an effective team
- To identify and differentiate among the four methods of job evaluation
- To describe the relationship among performance standards, performance review, and performance counseling
- To identify the key steps a manager should take in performance counseling and/or disciplinary action
- To select the appropriate conflict management technique to use in each specific conflict situation
- To explain the process for handling employee complaints and grievances
- To identify the obligations an organization has to maintain the security of employee information and records
- To anticipate the impact of current workforce trends on the organization's human resources management activities

Key Terms

Ability (performance) tests
Age Discrimination in Employment Act
Americans with Disabilities Act (ADA)
Aptitude tests
Behavioral description interview
Board of governors (board of trustees, board of directors)
Bureaucracy
Chain of command
Civil Rights Act, Title VII (1964)
Civil Rights Act (1991)
Communications plan
Compensable factor
Effort
Equal Pay Act of 1963 (EPA)
Executive managers
Exempt employees
Factor comparison method
Fair Labor Standards Act of 1938 (FLSA)
Family and Medical Leave Act of 1993
Grievance
Grievance procedures
Hay method
Hierarchy
Job classification
Job evaluation
Job ranking
Labor relations

Mental ability tests
Middle managers
Mission statement
Nonexempt employees
Occupational Safety and Health Act of 1970 (OSHA)
Organization
Organizational chart
Panel interview
Performance standards
Point method
Policy
Position (job) description
Pregnancy Discrimination Act
Procedure
Progressive discipline
Recruitment
Reliability
Responsibility
Resume
Retention
Scope of command
Skill
Structured interview
Supervisory managers
Systems thinking
360-degree evaluation
Union
Unity of command
Validity
Values statement
Vision statement
Working conditions

Introduction

The process of management cannot be practiced or examined meaningfully outside the social, cultural, and ethical contexts in which human organizations of all kinds operate. In modern industrial societies, human resources represent every organization's most valuable asset.

Healthcare organizations are extremely complex. They must be operated as effective and efficient businesses in a very tight financial environment. They also must employ a variety of well-educated technical specialists and professional employees to provide or support increasingly sophisticated healthcare services. Contemporary healthcare managers work in a unique environment that is characterized by the need to control costs and at the same time meet the needs of healthcare workers and healthcare consumers.

Managers work at many levels within healthcare organizations: as supervisors of functional units, as middle managers of departmental units or service lines, and as executive managers of multiple departmental units or service lines. At each level of management, the practice of managing the human resources within the prescribed scope of authority and responsibility is critical to the manager's success and the success of the entire organization.

Managing human resources is both an art and a science. Managers can learn much in this arena by partnering with human resources management (HRM) specialists, observing experienced colleagues, reflecting regularly on their own experiences, and continuing to develop their competencies throughout their careers.

This chapter is not meant to provide the comprehensive background in human resources management that health information management (HIM) students will ultimately need. The purpose of this chapter is to present a general introduction to the subject of managing human resources in the context of health information management operations. This chapter begins with a brief overview of the principles and nature of organizations and a discussion of the roles of the various levels of management. The chapter's primary focus is the interrelationship of HIM managers and human resources professionals and the roles of the supervisor and middle manager as frontline implementers of the human resources policies and practices of healthcare organizations.

Theory into Practice

In 2000, healthcare organizations were challenged by the introduction of the ambulatory payment classification (APC) system and the outpatient prospective payment system for Medicare beneficiaries. The leadership of one hospital's HIM department needed to develop a plan to ensure compliance with the new reimbursement system. First, the department collected information about the regulations and APCs. Then, the department manager and coding supervisor met to discuss the staffing changes and workload issues involved in implementing the new system.

It was decided that all emergency room visits, nuclear medicine and invasive radiology procedures, and cardiac diagnostic tests would be individually coded. That is, coders would no longer rely on a charge master. However, all of the outpatient charge masters would need to be updated, and a regular review schedule established.

The number of cases was projected on the basis of estimated Medicare patient volumes for the next budget cycle and current patient volumes. Time studies were then undertaken to identify how much time it would take to code each case. It was determined that this new coding function would require 0.75 full-time equivalent (FTE) positions. In addition, a 0.25 FTE would be needed to accommodate the increased effort associated with the updating and continuous review of the hospital's charge masters as well as the quality control of all outpatient coding and documentation. As a result of the workload analysis, a new 1.00 FTE position was added to the next year's budget. In addition, the organization decided to contract with an appropriately experienced HIM professional to update all existing charge master documents on a preimplementation timeline. This plan gave the HIM department and the HR department several months before implementation to finalize the position description, recruit and select a qualified candidate, and establish policies and procedures for the new system.

Principles of Organization

Organization is the planned coordination of the activities of more than one person for the achievement of a common purpose or goal. Organization is accomplished through the division of labor, and it is based on a hierarchy of authority and responsibility (Schein 1980). Jobs and the people who perform them are arranged in a way that accomplishes the goals of the organization. Various organizational tools are used to communicate the structure, the purpose, and the methods for accomplishing the shared work of the organization's members.

Organizations are somewhat like sports teams in that they have specific positions, a predefined set of rules, and a shared goal (in the case of sports teams, the goal is winning). Organizations also use communications tools that are similar to a player's roster (position descriptions), a rule or play book (policies and procedures), and a record of wins and losses (a budget and financial records).

Like other types of businesses, healthcare institutions are a type of formal organization. That is, they have established goals and a specific purpose for existing. Although the purpose, structure, and methods vary widely, all healthcare organizations use common systems and tools to achieve their goals.

Nature of Organizations

By nature, humans are social creatures. They are biologically designed to live within groups of their own kind. Moreover, they continuously form and reform informal and formal groups of various sizes (two members to billions of members) and longevity (a few seconds to a few centuries). No two groups have identical purposes, membership, or rules. Therefore, every human group is unique.

There is an endless variety of groups. Groups range from relatively informal friendships, families, and social clubs to extremely formal businesses, educational institutions, and national governments. They can be loose, unstructured, and temporary. An example of an extremely loose, short-term group might be that of a dozen people who rode on a bus together on a given morning. But even the most informal groups have a purpose and a set of more or less well-communicated rules. In this example, the group's purpose was to get from point A to point B. The rules required that the bus driver follow a preestablished route and that the riders pay a preestablished fare.

Although every group of humans is unique, interactions among humans follow predictable patterns. Human behavior has been studied for centuries. Theories on organizational behavior have been offered ever since humans learned how to communicate with each other. Although few principles of organizational behavior go unchallenged, centuries of observation have produced some basic rules. For example, one unchanging principle of organizational behavior seems to be that the group's structure affects the way its members interact with each other. And the structural effects can have both positive and negative consequences for the group as a whole as well as for its individual members.

Organizational Structures

At least until recent decades, formal organizations such as healthcare and manufacturing institutions have tended to be structured as relatively inflexible hierarchies. In a **hierarchy,** every member of the organization is assigned a specific rank. Each rank, in turn, carries a specific level of decision-making authority as well as specific responsibilities within the institution. Hierarchies are authoritarian in nature. In other words, they are strictly controlled by a powerful elite working "at the top" of the organization. These few individuals make almost every significant decision on behalf of the entire organization.

Historically, large governmental institutions have tended to be organized as rigid bureaucratic structures. In a **bureaucracy,** as in a hierarchy, positions within the formal organization are assigned specific ranks. Hierarchical ranks are based on levels of decision-making authority. In contrast, bureaucratic ranks are based on levels of technical expertise.

The purpose of bureaucratic organizations is to conduct highly complex and regulated processes. The structure of the bureaucratic organization reflects the processes it was designed to carry out. Therefore, bureaucracies operate according to well-established and often-inflexible rules. Each individual within the bureaucracy is responsible for carrying out only a small, well-defined element of the larger process. The Social

Security Administration is a good example of a government bureaucracy. It was created in 1935 with the sole purpose of implementing the Social Security Act.

Both hierarchies and bureaucracies depend on authoritarian **chains of command. Scope of command** (that is, one manager oversees the work of many employees) and **unity of command** (that is, each employee is accountable to only one boss) are principles that are inherent in a traditional chain-of-command structure. The structures of military organizations, for example, are organized around extremely rigid chains of command.

In modern times, organizational structure has been studied systematically since the early twentieth century. In the subsequent decades, a number of new management theories were suggested, and each theory seems to have required innovations in organizational structure. The period of economic rebuilding after the Second World War ushered in the current era of business thinking. Business and management theorists W. Edwards Deming and Joseph M. Juran began developing modern management systems during the early 1950s.

Today's management systems are modern in that they are moving away from the traditional authoritarian models that have prevailed since the Industrial Revolution. Most of all, they are modern in that they recognize the potential value of change and treat it as an opportunity rather than as a threat.

Modern management systems are based on the objective statistical analysis of data and information. They emphasize the benefits of sharing authority among employees and managers. They also favor interdisciplinary and cross-functional cooperation and teamwork over bureaucratic regulation and authoritarian control. Modern management systems value continual learning and demand systems thinking (Senge 1990, pp. 6–8). **Systems thinking** is simply an objective way of looking at work-related ideas and processes with the goal of allowing people to uncover ineffective patterns of behavior and thinking and then find ways to make lasting improvements.

In large part, modern management systems represent a rejection of the traditional authoritarian, hierarchical, and bureaucratic approaches to organization and management. However, because traditional management systems have been the accepted norm since the Industrial Revolution began in the early eighteenth century, they have proved difficult to displace. They continue to be the core organizational structures in place in most businesses today. Management theorists continue to lead the movement to establish information-based management systems and team-based organizational structures in all types of business endeavors, including the business of healthcare delivery. (See chapter 21 for a fuller discussion of the evolution of management theory.)

Organizational Charts

An **organizational chart** is a graphic representation of an organization's formal structure. It shows the organization's various activities and the specific members or categories of members assigned to carry out its activities. The chart for a very small organization might list the actual names of employees or individual position titles. The chart for a very large organization might list the various functional groups or departments responsible for each area of operations.

Traditionally, the reporting relationships among individuals and groups also are indicated according to accepted labeling conventions. For example, a solid line between two elements on a chart indicates a direct reporting relationship, and a broken line indicates an indirect reporting relationship. (See figures 23.1, 23.2, and 23.3 for examples of organizational charts developed for different types of healthcare organizations.)

Today's healthcare organizations are somewhat less concerned with official lines of authority. Instead, they are concerned with the interrelationships of work groups and functions. Individual departments and interdepartmental

workgroups sometimes develop detailed organizational charts as a first step in redesigning work processes. The charts then can be used as the basis for creating workflow diagrams and flowcharts. The purpose of these graphic tools is to help work teams visualize current and proposed processes and then suggest and implement improvements.

Some organizations also include organizational charts in their official position (job) descriptions. In this context, the charts put the work of a specific position or employee into the larger context of how the whole organization works as a system of interdependent processes.

Mission, Vision, and Values Statements

Modern organizations use a variety of communication devices to communicate their purpose and goals to their members and

Figure 23.1.   Sample Organizational Chart for an Acute Care Hospital

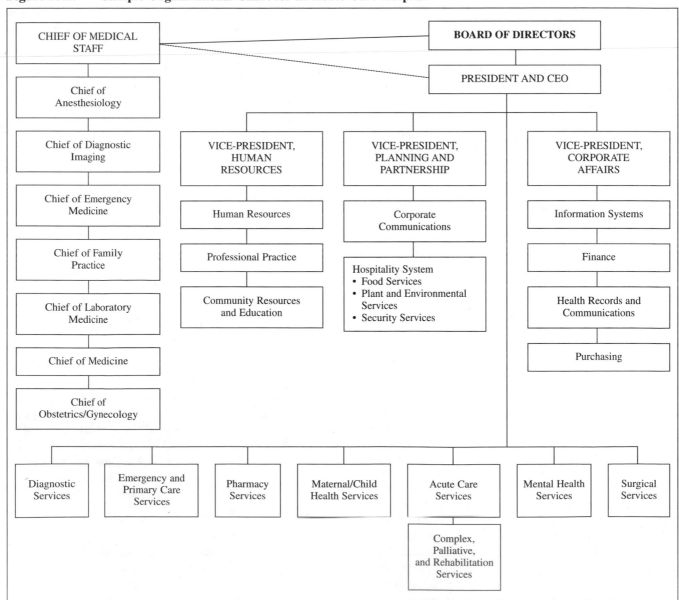

Figure 23.2.   Sample Organizational Chart for an Ambulatory Care Clinic

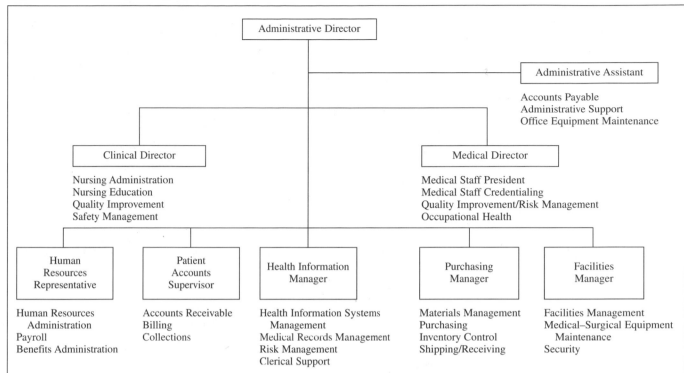

Figure 23.3.   Sample Organizational Chart for a Managed Care Organization

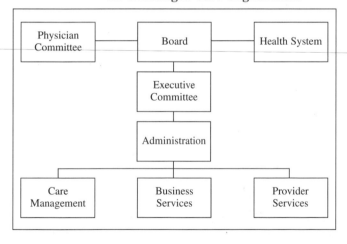

the communities they serve. A **mission statement** is a short description of the general purpose of an organization or group. For healthcare organizations, the mission statement usually includes a broad definition of the services the organization provides and the communities/customers it serves. Similarly, a **vision statement** is a short description of the organization's ideal future state. One way to make the distinction between an organization's mission and its vision is to think of the concepts in the following way:

- The mission is a *realistic* expression of what the organization actually does at the current time.

- The vision is an *idealistic* portrayal of what the organization would like to become sometime in the future.

Most healthcare organizations update their mission and vision statements regularly as part of the strategic planning process. The organization shares its mission and vision statements internally with its employees and medical staff and externally with its customers and the community it serves. The statements are meant to inform, guide, and inspire.

Healthcare organizations use mission and vision statements at many different levels. An individual organization usually develops statements for the enterprise as a whole. A multifacility healthcare system usually develops statements for the system as a whole as well as for each individual facility within it. Departments, work teams, and even temporary task forces often develop vision and mission statements. These groups use the statements to express and communicate their specific purpose and goals. Figure 23.4 (p. 562) provides examples of vision and mission statements from healthcare organizations. (See chapter 27 for a broader discussion of strategic planning.)

Many healthcare organizations also develop **values statements** that communicate their social and cultural belief system. The organization's values statement provides a way to support the type of behavior the organization wishes to encourage among its members. For example, the Benedictine Health System based in Duluth, Minnesota, clearly identifies "hospitality, stewardship, respect and justice" as its organizational core values (Benedictine Health System 2002, p. 1).

Figure 23.4.   Sample Mission and Vision Statements

General Hospital Affiliated with a Larger Healthcare System

Lutheran Hospital's **mission** is to improve the health of the communities we serve by providing high-quality services in a responsible and caring way.

Our **vision** is to become the leader in promoting healthy life-styles in an atmosphere of spiritual support, dignity, compassion, and mutual respect for all.

Community General Hospital

Anytown General Hospital's **mission** is to provide quality health services and technology to meet the changing healthcare needs of the people of southwestern Minnesota.

Anytown General Hospital's **vision** is to become the hospital of choice for residents of Polk, Sunny Isle, and Spring counties, a position we strive to strengthen by our long-term commitment to:

- Teamwork
- Service excellence
- Compassionate care
- Cost consciousness
- Continuous improvement

Academic Medical Center

Prairie University Hospital's **mission** is to provide the most up-to-date medical and surgical services available in the three-state area and to train medical students and graduate physicians to meet current and future challenges in healthcare.

Our **vision** is the achievement of healthy communities and progress toward the future of healthcare for Montana, western North Dakota, and northwestern South Dakota.

Specialty Hospital

The **mission** of Women's Hospital of Somewhereville is to meet the healthcare needs of our patients and to exceed their service expectations.

Our **vision** is of a hospital:

- Providing services with compassion and kindness
- Striving for performance improvement
- Fostering pride and integrity
- Aiming for increased cost-effectiveness and productivity

Specialty Clinic within an Academic Medical Center

The **mission** of the Midwest Asthma Center is to:

- Provide optimal medical care for persons with asthma and related illnesses
- Develop new knowledge about asthma and its management through medical research
- Promote improved understanding about asthma and related illnesses through providing educational programs and materials for our patients, for other healthcare providers, and for the community

The **vision** of the Midwest Asthma Center is to provide the highest quality of integrated comprehensive care for persons with asthma and related illnesses and to be one of the centers of excellence in the world for asthma treatment, research, and education.

Primary Care Physicians' Practice

The **mission** of Coastal Shores Primary Care Associates is to serve the unique needs of individuals and families by providing high-quality, coordinated, primary care medical services through an efficient, accessible, and responsive network of caring providers.

Our **vision** is to be the primary care medical group of choice in the Atlantic County area by delivering high-quality, individualized, and efficient patient care.

Check Your Understanding 23.1

Instructions: Indicate whether the following statements are true or false (T or F).

1. ___ Continuous performance improvement and total quality management are examples of industrial management theories.

2. ___ Systems thinking is a subjective way to look at work-related ideas and processes.

3. ___ Bureaucratic ranks are based on levels of technical expertise.

4. ___ Today's healthcare organizations are increasingly concerned with official lines of authority.

5. ___ Healthcare organizations develop mission statements to communicate their social and cultural belief systems.

Levels of Management

As noted earlier in this chapter, the various levels of management in organizations have different levels of responsibility and decision-making authority.

Supervisory Management

Supervisory managers (supervisors) oversee the organization's efforts at the staff level and monitor the effectiveness of everyday operations and individual performance against preestablished standards. Further, supervisory managers are responsible for ensuring that the organization's human assets are used effectively and that its policies and procedures are carried out consistently.

Supervisory managers work in small (two- to ten-person) functional work groups or teams. They often perform hands-on functions in addition to supervisory functions. They play an important role in staff training and recruitment/retention efforts. Supervisory managers direct daily work, create work schedules, and monitor the quality of the work and the productivity of the staff. They are important resources in revising procedures and conducting performance reviews because they are familiar with the work of the unit and the performance of individual staff members.

Supervisory managers usually have advanced technical skills that allow them to perform the most complex functions of the work team. However, most supervisors have limited financial authority and must seek the approval of higher-level managers before spending money or hiring staff. Depending on the size and structure of the organization, HIM supervisors report to another supervisory-level manager or to a department-level manager or assistant manager.

Effective supervisory managers are extremely important in healthcare organizations, because the greatest part of the healthcare organization's resources is expended at the operational level. Labor costs represent the greatest investment the organization makes. Staff and supervisory healthcare workers include nurses, clinical therapists, diagnostic technicians, dietary workers, laboratory workers, environmental support staff, and administrative support staff.

In healthcare organizations, health information technicians (HITs) often fill roles as supervisory managers. They provide vital administrative services and support patient care by protecting the accuracy and confidentiality of clinical databases and health records. They also ensure the financial health and future of their organizations by providing high-quality clinical coding services.

Middle Management

Middle management is concerned primarily with facilitating the work performed by supervisory- and staff-level personnel as well as by executive leaders. The responsibilities of **middle managers** include the following:

- Developing, implementing, and revising the organization's policies and procedures under the direction of executive managers
- Executing the organizational plans developed at the board and executive levels
- Providing the operational information that executives need to develop meaningful plans for the organization's future

Middle managers oversee operations of a broader scope in their work as managers or assistant managers of departments or disciplinary functions. For example, they direct health information management, nursing, risk management, and facilities management functions.

Middle managers can change department-level policies and procedures when necessary. For example, when a department manager finds that an employee is not following a specific procedure, he or she investigates and analyzes the department's systems and processes to determine whether the problem is with the employee's performance or shortcomings in the processes themselves. In contrast, supervisory managers enforce the policies and procedures that relate directly to the activities of their own work group or team. For example, when a supervisor finds that an employee is not following a specific procedure, he or she takes action to correct that individual's performance.

Typically, middle managers are responsible for performing a limited number of hands-on analytical and/or decision-making functions related directly to the departments they manage. In an HIM department, for example, a health information administrator (HIA) in an assistant director position might be responsible for tracking the quality of clinical databases and overseeing coding compliance programs. HIM department managers participate on a number of permanent

and temporary interdisciplinary committees within the organization and serve as resources to the committees on subjects that relate to the organization's information resources. They also initiate interdepartmental efforts to address issues that go beyond department-level operations. In small healthcare organizations, the HIM director may play additional managerial roles in risk management, quality management, and/or utilization management.

Depending on the size and structure of the organization, middle managers in HIM report to a department-level director or an executive-level manager (vice-president) on the organization's senior management team. In a multifacility healthcare delivery network, the director of HIM services might report to the vice-president of operations (sometimes referred to as the chief operating officer, or COO) or the vice-president of information services (sometimes called the chief information officer, or CIO). In a small community hospital, the HIM director might report to the CEO (chief executive officer), the CFO (chief financial officer), or the COO.

Executive Management and Governance

The third managerial level in healthcare organizations can be divided into executive management and governance, the realm of the **board of governors** (often called the board of directors or the board of trustees). (The word *governance* means government.)

Role of Executive Management

Executive managers are directly employed by the organization. They are hired either by the board or by the organization's chief executive officer with the board's approval. In publicly owned organizations, the stockholders elect board members. In privately owned organizations, the board members are appointed.

Executive managers are primarily responsible for working with the board to set the organization's future direction and establish its strategic plan. To that end, executive managers work to ensure that the organization uses its assets wisely, fulfills its current mission, and works toward achieving a meaningful vision for the future. Executive managers oversee broad functions, departments, or groups of departments. Executive managers are also responsible for establishing the policies of healthcare organizations and leading their quality improvement and compliance initiatives. In addition, executive managers work with community leaders to make sure that the healthcare organization contributes to the well-being of the community it serves.

Depending on the complexity of the organization, the titles of executive managers vary. The different titles include chief executive officer, president, executive vice-president, senior vice-president, vice-president, and director. Executive managers may report to other executive managers, to higher-level vice-presidents, or to the chief executive officer.

In most organizations, the chief executive officer is the highest-ranking executive manager. CEOs sometimes hold more than one title. For example, the head of an organization might have the title president and CEO. The CEO and/or president reports directly to the organization's board of directors.

Role of the Governing Board

Healthcare organizations such as hospitals, healthcare businesses, and multifacility healthcare delivery networks are organized as legal entities, or corporations. Every state has laws that dictate how corporations are to be structured and run within its jurisdiction. However, all state incorporation laws are consistent in one area: Responsibility for the operation of each healthcare organization ultimately lies with its board of governors. Thus, the board is the final authority in setting the organization's strategic direction, mission and vision, and general philosophy and ethical base. The name and structure of the board depend on the profit-making status of the organization, among other factors.

Typically, the board consists of a chairperson and ten to twenty board members. It represents the interests of the organization's owners. Any number of different entities may own large healthcare organizations, including federal, state, and local governments; investment groups; educational institutions; and religious organizations. Moreover, healthcare organizations may be owned privately or publicly. In publicly owned for-profit entities, investors purchase stock on national and international stock exchanges and receive a share of the profits in the form of dividends. Many private healthcare organizations operate as not-for-profit charitable organizations. In not-for-profit organizations, any excess income is reinvested in the organization rather than being paid out in profits or dividends.

Check Your Understanding 23.2

Instructions: Indicate whether the following statements are true or false (T or F).

1. ____ Supervisory managers set the organization's future direction and establish its goals.
2. ____ In general, middle managers perform the daily work of the organization.
3. ____ Vice-presidents are representatives of the executive level of management.
4. ____ The ultimate responsibility for the organization's operation lies with its chief executive officer.
5. ____ In publicly owned healthcare entities, investors buy stock and receive dividends.

Role of the Human Resources Department

In most healthcare organizations, payroll and benefits consume the majority of the organizations' financial resources. Therefore, adequate time and attention must be paid to the management of human resources. Effective HR management is also important for reasons beyond financial impact. HR management factors affect the attitudes and morale of health-care workers and other employees and so their ability to perform their work effectively. Obviously, employee moral becomes extremely important when the work involves caring for patients directly or indirectly supporting those who provide hands-on care.

Entities such as hospitals, large physician groups, and managed care organizations commonly have a dedicated human resources department that acts as a reference and support for managers at all levels. However, every manager must have an understanding of the principles of human resources management in order to implement them effectively within the scope of their authority and responsibility. Every manager must also know how to appropriately and effectively work with the organization's human resources department.

The HR department is responsible for several types of interrelated activities. Mathis and Jackson (2002) describe HR management as a set of closely related activities focused on contributing to an organization's success by enhancing its productivity, quality, and service. Each of these interrelated activities is shown in figure 23.5. Mathis and Jackson also emphasize the importance of performing HR activities with the organization's unique mission, culture, size, and structure in mind as well as the greater social, political, legal, economic, technological, and cultural environment in which it operates.

Human Resources Planning and Analysis

Human resources planning and analysis ensure the long-term health of the organization's human assets. Internal trends such as the aging of the organization's workforce or the changing nature of the skill mix required to handle the organization's evolving product lines must be addressed. The impact of external trends such as workforce shortages and evolving workforce expectations must also be assessed.

Equal Employment Opportunity Practices

The HR department takes the lead in ensuring that the various laws and regulations associated with equal employment opportunity (EEO) laws are scrupulously applied in the organization's hiring and promotion practices. Federally enacted EEO legislation includes the **Age Discrimination in Employment Act,** the **Americans with Disabilities Act (ADA),** the **Civil Rights Acts of 1964 and 1991,** and the **Pregnancy Discrimination Act** (Anthony, Perrewe, and Kacmar 1996).

Staffing

The HR department also helps managers to define staffing needs; develop job descriptions; and recruit, screen, and select staff. After an employee is brought into the organization, the HR department plays a significant role, in partnership with the employee's direct supervisor, by spearheading the employee's immediate orientation to the organization's policies, practices, and procedures. The HR department is also active in addressing the employee's ongoing training and development requirements.

Figure 23.5.   Human Resources Management Activities

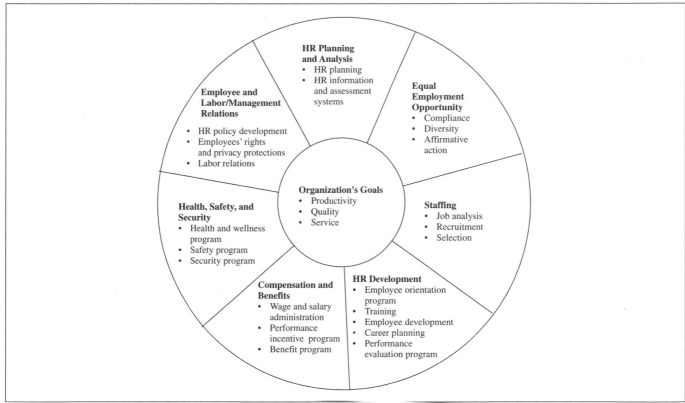

Adapted from Mathis and Johnson 2002, p. 4.

Compensation and Benefits Program

The management of the organization's compensation and benefits program is probably the most prominent activity associated with HR management because it is so directly connected to the employees' pocketbook. This activity involves the establishment of basic definitions of employment and compensation status for the organization (for example, full-time versus part-time, temporary versus permanent, independent contractor versus employee, wage versus salary). The **Fair Labor Standards Act of 1938** (FLSA) and the **Equal Pay Act of 1963** (EPA) serve as fundamental legislative mandates in this area.

The HR department also leads the development and administration of the organization's fringe benefits program, job evaluation and classification systems, wage and salary systems, and incentive pay systems. The **Family and Medical Leave Act of 1993** (FMLA) is an example of one legislative initiative that has a major impact on fringe benefit programs, as well as on staffing activities (Anthony, Perrewe, and Kacmar 1996).

Health and Safety Program

The HR department is also involved in activities designed to protect the health, safety, and security of the workforce. Healthcare organizations have given substantial attention to safety management since the enactment of the **Occupational**

Safety and Health Act of 1970 (OSHA). It's intended purpose is "to assure so far as possible every working man or woman in the Nation safe and healthful working conditions and to preserve our human resources." This act established a national reporting system for accidents and injuries on the job and led to the development of specific safety management programs in most businesses. More recently, health-related hazards associated with the use of technology or chemical substances in the workplace, injuries due to workplace violence and employee security concerns have begun to receive special attention by HR professionals (Anthony, Perrewe, and Kacmar 1996).

Labor Relations

Employee and labor/management relations are established through the day-to-day interactions between employees and their managers. However, the organization's managers and employees often seek leadership and support from the HR department. The HR department sets the stage for developing and sustaining the quality of these critical relationships by establishing and communicating to both managers and employees the contracts, policies, practices, and rules that constitute the organization's expectations of its employees.

HR management activities associated with **unions** and collective bargaining are referred to as **labor relations.** Labor organizations (unions) enter into negotiations with employers on behalf of groups of employees who have elected to join a union. The negotiations relate to compensation and safety and health concerns. In a unionized environment, three laws that came into existence over a period twenty-five years (1935–1960) constitute a code of practice for unions and management. HR departments pay strict attention to these three acts (Mathis and Jackson 2002; Anthony, Perrewe, and Kacmar 1996):

- Wagner Act (National Labor Relations Act)
- Taft-Hartley Act (Labor-Management Relations Act)
- Landrum-Griffin Act (Labor-Management Reporting and Disclosure Act)

For the manager who oversees a group of employees covered by a union contract, the contract provisions of these laws represent the basic rules for their interactions with employees in the areas of pay, benefits, safety, health, and performance evaluation.

Check Your Understanding 23.3

Instructions: Indicate whether the following statements are true or false (T or F).

1. ____ Internal and external environmental trends are significant factors in HR planning and analysis.

2. ____ The Fair Labor Standards Act is one piece of the EEO legislation package passed in the early 1960s.

3. ____ A national system for reporting workplace accidents and injuries was mandated by the Americans with Disabilities Act.

4. ____ Orientation for new employees and the ongoing training of employees are solely the responsibility of the HR department.

5. ____ The Fair Labor Standards Act, the Wagner Act, and the Equal Pay Act provide key guidelines for managing union relationships.

Role of the HIM Manager in Human Resources

Because the day-to-day management of the organization's human resources is the responsibility of supervisory, middle, and executive managers, every manager is responsible for the same HR activities as the HR professionals. In an HIM department, for example, the supervisor of coding services would be responsible for the day-to-day management of clinical coding specialists. Luckily, managers can use any of a variety of HR tools and processes to handle these responsibilities efficiently and effectively.

Tools for Human Resources Planning

Several tools may be used to plan and manage staff resources. **Position descriptions,** for example, outline the work and qualifications needed to perform a job. **Performance standards** establish the organization's expectations of how well a job must be done and how much work must be accomplished. Routine staff meetings and regular written communications (via departmental Web sites, bulletin boards, and newsletters, for example) establish a routine process for up-to-date information flow for employees.

Staffing Structures and Work Scheduling

In addition to these basic tools, managers establish staffing structures and use work schedules to ensure that there is adequate coverage and staff to complete the required work. Schedules are developed first to provide adequate coverage during the hours the organization or department is open for business.

In hospitals, it is not uncommon to find some part of the HIM department open twenty-four hours a day, seven days a week. This schedule ensures that HIM staff will be available to provide information for admissions to the hospital and emergency department, support patient discharges and transfers, and handle other HIM functions. In some healthcare organizations, the demand for HIM services outside of regular business hours is limited. In such cases, HIM functions can be provided by business office staff, nursing staff, and/or emergency department staff who have been cross-trained to perform basic HIM tasks.

Another scheduling consideration is space. Space limitations on the number of workstations in the department or the number of employees who can work in the file room may require that employees work in shifts or on weekends. In addition, staff preferences need to be considered in creating the work schedule. Balancing the demands of the organization with individual requests for flexible start times makes scheduling an important part of the manager's responsibility.

Written **policies and procedures** that explain the department's staffing requirements and scheduling procedures help the manager to remain fair and objective and help the staff to understand the rules. The amount of personal time off, as sick leave or vacation, also factors into the development of a staff schedule and the overall assessment of the number of staff positions required.

In addition, most healthcare organizations establish some type of job classification system that combines jobs with similar levels of responsibility and qualifications into job grades that determine salary ranges and benefit packages. For instance, all supervisory-level managers might be classified into one salary and benefit category, but each would have a unique job description. Job classifications also may determine whether an employee belongs to a union or is a candidate for unionization.

Position Descriptions

Position or job descriptions outline the work to be performed by a specific employee or group of employees with the same responsibilities. Position descriptions generally consist of three parts: a summary of the position's requirements and purpose, its functions, and the qualifications needed to perform the job. Position descriptions also include the official title of the job.

Position descriptions are used during the recruitment process to explain the work to prospective candidates. They also enable managers and human resources staff to set appropriate salaries and wages for the various positions. Moreover, they may be used to resolve performance problems. The manager can use the position description to clarify the tasks the employee is expected to perform.

Generally, job descriptions are needed in the following circumstances:

- When an entirely new kind of work is required
- When a job changes and the old description no longer reflects the work
- When a change in technology or processes dramatically affects the work to be accomplished

Sometimes top performers outgrow their job descriptions. They may find more efficient ways of doing part of their assigned tasks and/or want more interesting or meaningful work. Some employees request updated job descriptions to support an increase in salary and benefits or a change in title.

When writing new position descriptions, managers may use existing descriptions of other, related jobs or interview staff who are currently performing some of the tasks intended for the new job. They also might ask staff members to keep a record of how they spend their time for a period that reflects a comprehensive cycle of their work. Staff with more repetitive daily activities may only need to record their activities for a week. In contrast, staff with more diverse tasks may need a month to document the scope of their duties.

Performance Standards

In addition to a position description, **performance standards** are often developed for the key functions of the job. These standards indicate each function's level of acceptable execution. Performance standards are usually set for both quantity and quality and should be as objective and measurable as possible.

Some organizations establish measures that reflect various levels of performance. For example, one measure of a coder's performance might be coding a specified number of charts per day, perhaps no fewer than twenty charts per day. Other organizations might establish several levels of expected performance, for example:

30–35 charts per day	Outstanding
25–29 charts per day	Exceeds expectations
20–24 charts per day	Meets expectations
15–19 charts per day	Needs improvement
Fewer than 14 charts per day	Unsatisfactory

The following example shows how a quality standard might be used as a performance indicator of coding accuracy. For example:

96%–100% accuracy	Outstanding
92%–95% accuracy	Exceeds expectations
89%–94% accuracy	Meets expectations
84%–88% accuracy	Needs improvement
Less than 84%	Unsatisfactory

In the preceding example, a definition for coding accuracy might be helpful. For example, accurate coding includes cap-

turing accurate codes and sequencing them appropriately for all diagnoses and procedures that affect reimbursement.

Standards that are measurable and relevant to an employee's overall performance are helpful in setting clear expectations. They also are useful in providing useful feedback. (See chapter 22 for a full discussion of performance standards and measurement.)

Policies and Procedures

Policies and procedures are critical tools that may be used to ensure consistent quality performance. A **policy** is a statement about what an organization or department does. For example, a policy might state that patients are allowed to review their health records under certain conditions such as when a clinical professional is present or in the HIM department. Policies should be clearly stated and comprehensive. They must be developed in accordance with applicable laws, and they must reflect actual practice. And because they may be used as documentation of intended practice in a lawsuit, policies should be developed very carefully.

A **procedure** describes how work is to be done and how policies are to be carried out. Procedures are instructions that ensure high-quality, consistent outcomes for tasks done, especially when more than one person is involved.

One of the benefits of developing a procedure is that time is taken to analyze the best possible method for completing a process. This analysis may begin by developing a flowchart to document workflow, decision points, and the flow required to complete a procedure. (Flowcharting is discussed in detail in chapter 22.)

After a flowchart is completed, the steps in the process are written down in the order in which they are to be performed. When more than one person is involved in completing a procedure, each person who performs a task is documented. Anyone generally competent to perform a task should be able to complete it after reading a well-written procedure. This usually takes several drafts that have been reviewed by people who actually perform the work. Moreover, it might be useful to ask someone unfamiliar with the job to try to complete the task according to the written procedure.

Writing a procedure also offers a great opportunity to identify ways to streamline the process. Are supplies available and organized in a way that makes work efficient? Would it be faster to complete one type of task for all of the work, or should each job be completed before the next task is begun?

For example, a procedure for the process of logging in information requests might include the following steps:

1. The receptionist opens all incoming mail daily before 10 a.m. He or she then confirms that the date on the date stamp is accurate and stamps all mail in the upper right-hand corner.
2. The receptionist sorts requests for medical information into three categories: legal, medical, or insurance. He or she then counts the requests in each category, clips

or binds the requests for each category together, writes the count on a Post-it™ note, and places the note on the top request of each bundle. The bundles are then delivered to the release of information (ROI) inbox. (The inbox is located on the ROI coordinator's desk.)

3. The ROI coordinator picks up medical requests for information from the ROI inbox each morning after 10 a.m. He or she enters the number of requests on a daily work log (an Excel™ spreadsheet stored on G:roi/requests/medical).

Obviously, it would be inefficient for the receptionist to open, date-stamp, and deliver each piece of mail individually. This procedure would continue through the logging process. However, this example shows how a detailed procedure would be useful in training a new receptionist or ROI coordinator or in providing instructions to anyone needed to perform this task in the regular employee's absence. It also highlights the fact that the receptionist would need to be trained to identify different types of information requests.

Several tools may be used to effectively communicate the purpose, scope, and details of the work done by employees in the organization. The manager is responsible for developing and maintaining these tools. However, the manager's role does not end here. Given the tools described so far, he or she is ready to hire, train, and interact with employees.

Tools for Recruitment and Retention

Recruitment is the process of finding, soliciting, and attracting new employees. **Retention** is the ability to keep valuable employees from seeking employment elsewhere.

Staff Recruitment, Selection, and Hiring

Armed with a position description, the manager is ready to begin recruiting candidates for a new or open position. However, the manager should be sure to understand the organization's recruitment and hiring policies and seek the assistance of the HR department before the vacancy is publicized. This preparation ensures that the organization's legal obligations and policies and procedures are followed throughout the recruitment, selection, and hiring process.

Recruitment

The first thing to consider in recruiting candidates to fill a staff opening is whether to promote someone from inside the organization or to look for candidates outside the organization. The advantage of promoting from within is that the practice often motivates employees to perform well, learn new skills, and work toward advancement. To advertise a vacancy internally, the organization might post it on facility bulletin boards or list it in the organization's newsletter or Web site. The department manager may announce an opening at a routine staff meeting or use any other communication channels available. Management must communicate an opportunity for promotion to all staff rather than to just the employee who is the most likely candidate. Because employ-

ees see widespread posting as a fair practice, it communicates the underlying message that internal candidates are considered first whenever possible.

When the position cannot be filled from within, however, there are several ways to advertise it externally. For example, the organization might run an ad in a newspaper, post the job on Internet recruitment sites, announce the opportunity at professional meetings, contact people who have previously applied or expressed interest in working at the organization, or work through a professional recruiter.

In most cases, the approach used depends on the nature of the open position. For example, the facility might run an ad in a local newspaper for a file room position, but not in a professional journal. On the other hand, the facility might turn to a professional recruiter when trying to fill a department director or experienced coding position.

As in every industry, job seekers looking for professional-level healthcare positions submit detailed resumes. A **resume** describes the candidate's educational background and work experience and usually includes information on personal and professional achievements. Candidates often submit a cover letter describing the type of position in which they are interested along with the resume. Today, it is common for candidates and organizations to conduct the preliminary screening process through electronic mail.

Most organizations ask every candidate to complete a formal job application. People seeking entry-level positions may be asked to complete an application rather than to submit a resume.

Selection

Once a sufficient pool of applicants has been recruited, the selection process can begin. The goal of the selection process is identify the candidate most qualified to fill the position.

Testing with reliable and valid instruments designed to objectively assess the applicants' fit for the position and interviews are the two basic tools employed in the selection process. Testing is commonly conducted during the applicant's first visit to the facility. **Reliability** refers to the consistency with which a test measures an attribute. **Validity** refers to a test's ability to accurately and consistently measure what it purports to measure. HR professionals are generally familiar with a variety of **ability (performance) tests, aptitude tests, mental ability tests,** psychological/personality tests, and honesty tests that are suitable for use in the organization (Anthony, Perrewe, and Kacmar 1996). Many healthcare organizations also perform routine drug testing on candidates for employment.

Mathis and Jackson (2002) agree that the selection interview is generally considered the most important phase of the selection process. They also describe three effective interview formats:

- The **structured interview** uses a set of standardized questions that are asked of all applicants.

- The **behavioral description interview** requires applicants to give specific examples of how they have performed a specific procedure or handled a specific problem in the past.
- The **panel interview** includes a team of people who interview applicants at one time.

Interviewing is one of the most important skills that managers need for selecting new staff. Many managers, unfortunately, receive little formal training in interviewing techniques and/or have little practical experience. Even supervisors and managers with many years of experience sometimes dread the interviewing process. This shortcoming can be overcome through self-education, mentoring by more experienced managers, or instructional sessions with HR professionals in the organization.

Failure to adequately prepare for conducting the interview has consequences that are very serious for the organization and the applicant. Reviewing the position description, reading the applicant's resume and/or application form, and preparing appropriate and relevant questions are important steps to take before beginning an interview.

The interview itself has four basic purposes:

- To obtain information from the applicant about his or her past work history and future goals
- To give information to the applicant about the organization's mission and goals and the nature of the employment opportunity
- To evaluate the applicant's work experience, attitudes, and personality as a potential fit for the organization
- To give the applicant an opportunity to evaluate the organization as a potential fit for his or her current and future employment goals

Equal employment opportunity regulations dictate the types of questions that may be asked during interviews and on job applications. For example, questions pertaining to age, religious affiliation, and marital status should be avoided in most cases. These regulations apply during all activities associated with the interview, including the formal interview sessions, as well as the less formal lunches or dinners, hallway/elevator small talk when it is very easy to inadvertently lapse into discussions on these topics. Managers should always seek the advice of HR professionals when they are uncertain about which questions they may or may not ask.

Healthcare organizations, like other employers, must be certain to conduct careful background checks of potential employees. Managers or HR professionals also check the references of candidates and communicate with the past employers of candidates via telephone or correspondence. Checking references involves confirming the information provided by applicants on resumes and applications. Reference checks and/or a background investigation should also be conducted specifically to assess the applicants' fit with the position and to validate the accuracy of information the applicants provide on their applications and during their interviews. According to Mathis and Jackson (2002, p. 73), a recent survey of employers revealed that the false information furnished most commonly by candidates for employment dealt with the candidates' past lengths of employment, salary history, criminal record, and job titles.

Hiring

After all the internal and external interviews, tests, and reference/background checks are complete, the hiring manager usually has enough information to make a hiring decision. In some organizations, the manager shares the hiring decision with key staff, HR staff, and/or executive staff, depending on the level of the position.

Once the details of the job offer have been approved by the HR department, a formal job offer should be made. The HR department should prepare a letter that describes the duties and responsibilities of the position, states the employment start date, and explains the salary and benefits package. In addition, the hiring manager may choose to communicate the offer to the candidate through a personal telephone contact, which is subsequently confirmed by an official letter to the candidate (Anthony, Perrewe, and Kacmar 1996).

Staff Retention

It is normal to have a certain level of staff turnover. Employees move, retire, or seek other careers. A manager can do little to prevent turnover resulting from changes in the personal live of employees. However, the actions of managers and the policies of the organization can have an impact, either positive or negative, on staff retention. The following questions should be considered:

- Does the organization support continued education either financially or through flexible work schedules?
- Do employees have opportunities to advance their careers within the organization?
- Are salaries and benefits competitive with similar organizations?
- Do working conditions provide a comfortable and safe environment?

Although individual managers may have limited influence on some of these factors, they must always be aware of the impact that broader organizational HR policies and practices have on employees. Gone unnoticed or left unaddressed, employees' concerns in these areas are often what make employees look for other jobs. For example, employees can become dissatisfied when they feel that they are being treated unfairly or that HR practices are needlessly rigid. In some cases, employees become dissatisfied simply because they do not know the rationale for a particular HR policy or because a concern they have voiced about an unsafe condition in their work area is not acted on by the manager. The challenge to the manager is to anticipate or, at the very least, to find ways to be informed as soon as possible when employees express an HR-related concern.

Staff turnover is expensive in terms of both lost productivity and recruitment and training costs. To ensure effective management, turnover should be monitored across time and benchmarked with the rest of the organization and/or other organizations in the community or geographic area. Routine employee satisfaction surveys can help provide information about how employees feel about their jobs and insights into how the facility might improve working conditions. Conducting routine exit interviews with employees who leave the organization is another way to obtain information on how employees feel about their jobs and what issues cause them to leave.

New Employee Orientation and Training

One of the key ingredients in employee satisfaction is the feeling of being knowledgeable and competent. This feeling begins with an effective orientation and training program for new employees. Just as the manager prepared for the interview and selection of the new employee, he or she must plan how the new employee will learn about the organization, the department, and the job.

Most large organizations have a formal new employee orientation process. This process may involve a one-on-one session with human resources, group training with new employees from all over the organization, and/or some form of computer-based training.

In general, orientation programs in healthcare organizations address the organization's mission and vision, goals, and structure; general employment policies; employee conduct standards; communication processes; and confidentiality policies. Orientation also may include a tour of the facility and cover computer access and responsibilities. When the organization provides this type of orientation, the manager must understand the material covered and feel comfortable answering any questions or directing the new employee to the appropriate resource for follow-up.

The manager must be very patient during the employee's first days and schedule adequate time to spend with the new hire. Everyone learns in different ways and at a different pace. The first days not only establish how the employee will do the job, but also contribute to the employee's ongoing relationships with the manager and other staff. (A full discussion of the development of new employee orientation programs is presented in chapter 24.)

Tools for Effective Communication

Maintaining regular and effective communication with staff is one of the ongoing challenges in managing human resources. Communication is, however, very important because it contributes significantly to the morale of the staff and their ability to contribute to the department's operations as a whole. To address this challenge, a manager should establish a **communications plan** that includes routine and timely opportunities for both verbal and written information sharing within the department or work group. The plan should include, at minimum, the following types of communications:

- Daily personal contact with every employee to maintain a sense of connectedness and, as necessary, create opportunities for casual discussions of emerging work-related changes or issues
- Web-based or traditional bulletin boards located in an area convenient to staff to publicize official announcements, permissible personal news, written status updates, and written highlights from departmental meetings
- Weekly status update meetings with the staff for each functional unit in the department in larger organizations or the entire department in smaller organizations
- Monthly departmental meetings with highlights recorded for posting
- Quarterly performance discussions with individual employees
- Ad hoc verbal or electronic (e-mail) status updates, as appropriate, to alert staff to information of interest from organizational meetings

On a day-to-day basis, when problems emerge that require resolution within the department or when decisions are made that affect the employees in the department, the management team is responsible for establishing a unique communication plan that conforms to the situation. Such a plan identifies the full range of employees affected by the problem or the decision and defines the specific approach that managers will take to engage or inform each person appropriately.

In general, keeping staff well informed is a key factor in developing and sustaining a healthy level of trust in the relationship between employees and managers. Communication plans are simple tools that managers can use to ensure that this very critical aspect of their responsibilities is handled with the level of routine and regular attentiveness it requires.

Tools for the Empowerment of Staff

Creating an environment that encourages and allows employees to use and develop their problem-solving and decision-making competencies is an established HR management practice that has many benefits. For example, it increases the manager's capacity and productivity, improves the quality and timeliness of decision-making, enhances employee morale, and contributes to improved employee retention.

Team Building

Most people today want to work in a team. The team may consist of people who perform the same function within the same department, for example, a coding team. The team may bring together people who perform different functions within the same department to solve a problem they share. The team may bring together people from across the organization with different expertise to implement a new computer system or to study an issue that would affect the overall organization, for example, improvements in the employee evaluation system.

At their best, teams increase the creativity and improve the quality of problem solving. Often, team-based decisions are more widely accepted than managerial decisions because team members enlist support for the decisions from their peers and coworkers. In addition, teams can use their collective energy to produce more work than individuals can. Moreover, teamwork establishes strong relationships among employees. Teamwork also can enrich jobs and provide variety in work assignments. Finally, teams can develop new leaders and expose employees to issues that would not be within the usual scope of their jobs.

One thing that binds team members together is having a common purpose. The purpose for an ongoing work team, for example, might be to ensure cross-training, improve procedures, and monitor quality and/or productivity. In other cases, teams are created for a specific purpose. Some teams exist for long periods of time because they have an ongoing reason to exist. Other teams function for limited periods of time and disband after their purpose has been fulfilled.

However, having a common purpose is only one element of an effective team. The team also must have an effective leader. This individual must be able to create agendas and organize meetings, lead discussions, and ensure that the work moves forward. The team may either appoint or elect its leader, depending on its purpose and the experience and expertise of its members.

In addition, effective teams set ground rules. For instance, team members might decide that all meetings will start on time, minutes will be recorded, decisions will be reached by consensus, and everyone will participate in discussions. The early establishment of rules can reduce conflict as the team moves forward. Teams work through the same type of decision-making process described earlier in this chapter. However, their strength lies in engaging the collective brainpower of all of their members, and so the team leader should use techniques that effectively engage every member of the team.

Not all teams are effective, and the causes for problems vary. For example, a team without a clear purpose could create a product that does not accomplish the work it was designed to accomplish. A leader who dominates the team could reduce its effectiveness and frustrate its members. Members who do not participate, have insufficient expertise, or are unconcerned with the team's success could cause the team to fail. And members who work outside the team or do not support its decisions can create dissension and reduce support for the outcome.

Managing staff teams is an important aspect of every managers' responsibilities. Careful consideration should be given to developing the team's purpose and composition. Team members need to feel that their work is important and that their contributions make a difference. A well-run team can be an effective and productive force. A poorly run team can waste time and frustrate and demoralize its members.

Delegation of Authority

Managers have specific responsibilities and the authority to act within the scope of those responsibilities. A manager's responsibilities can never be delegated to another person; that is, the manager always remains the one accountable for outcomes in areas within his or her designated scope. However, with appropriate preparation and decision-making guidelines in place, managers can and should delegate the authority to make and act on decisions to employees as individuals or teams. Delegation of authority expands the manager's capacity, improves the timeliness of decisions, and develops the competencies of other staff members.

When delegating authority, managers make it possible for staff to succeed by preparing them in advance:

- By explaining exactly what needs to be done
- By describing clear expectations
- By setting clear deadlines
- By granting the authority to make relevant decisions
- By ensuring appropriate communication and outcomes reporting
- By providing the resources needed to complete the assigned task

(See chapter 24 for an expanded discussion of empowerment and delegation as workforce retention strategies.)

Check Your Understanding 23.4

Instructions: Indicate whether the following statements are true or false (T or F).

1. ___ To lead effectively, every manager should have an understanding of human resources management principles.
2. ___ Position descriptions outline the work that employees are expected to perform.
3. ___ Performance standards are developed to indicate the time frame in which each function of a job must be executed.
4. ___ Procedures are written explanations of how to perform tasks.
5. ___ In healthcare organizations, individuals applying for entry-level positions must submit a resume and a cover letter.
6. ___ Staff turnover is expensive in terms of lost productivity and recruitment and training costs.
7. ___ A manager's responsibilities include new employee orientation and training.
8. ___ One thing that teams have in common is that their members are usually from the same department.
9. ___ Managers can delegate responsibilities but not authority.
10. ___ The interview process is intended to give the applicant an opportunity to evaluate the organization as a potential fit for his or her current and future employment goals.
11. ___ To be effective communications with employees should be expressed in written form.
12. ___ Trust between managers and employees is enhanced by keeping employees well informed.

Compensation Systems

Employee compensation systems basically serve to reward employees equitably for their service to the organization. Organizations also use compensation systems to enhance employee loyalty and encourage greater productivity.

The Fair Labor Standards Act (FLSA), the Equal Pay Act (EPA), and several of the EEO laws (for example, Title VII of the Civil Rights Act, Age Discrimination in Employment Act, and the Americans with Disabilities Act) all have provisions that affect compensation systems. Provisions of the FLSA, for example, cover minimum wage, overtime pay, child labor restrictions, and equal pay for equal work regardless of sex. Federal regulations specify exemptions from some or all of the FLSA provisions for a number of groups of employees (Myers 1998). These groups are referred to as **exempt** employees. Covered groups are referred to as **nonexempt** employees.

Managers who control employee work schedules and process employee timecards at the close of each pay period become quite familiar with the provisions of the FLSA that relate to overtime pay. In general, the FLSA requires that employers pay time and a half for all hours that covered (nonexempt) employees work in excess of forty per week. Some organizations institute overtime pay for all worked hours in excess of eight hours per day. In calculations of worked hours, the FLSA specifies that rest periods of up to twenty minutes each be counted as worked time, but meal periods of thirty minutes or more are not counted as worked time. Time spent in mandated job-related training is considered worked time, and significant travel time (beyond the usual time required to commute to and from work) associated with a work-related event is counted as worked time. Compensatory time, taken in lieu of overtime pay, may be used when it is part of the organization's compensation plan (Myers 1998).

Because of the complexities and sensitivities associated with compensation issues, HR professionals are a manager's best advisor when questions related to compensation regulations and practices arise.

Compensation Surveys

The HR department routinely consults compensation surveys published by government agencies and professional and trade associations. In some cases, an HR department may choose to conduct an independent survey to obtain data more specific to the organization's needs. Often, consultants experienced with survey design and data analysis are employed by the organization to either assist in or to do the survey project to ensure a successful outcome from this costly activity. Compensation surveys provide benchmark data that the organization can use to evaluate or establish its compensation system for unique jobs within the organization or for the jobs throughout the organization (Myers 1998).

Job Evaluations

Job evaluation projects are undertaken by an organization to determine the relative worth of jobs as a first step toward establishing an equitable internal compensation system. Job evaluation is the process of applying predefined compensable factors to jobs to determine their relative worth (Myers 1998,

p. 630). Myers defines a **compensable factor** as "a characteristic used to compare the worth of jobs" (p. 631) and adds that "the EPA requires employers to consider [several] compensable factors in setting pay for similar work performed by both females and males." These factors include **skill, effort, responsibility,** and **working conditions.**

Four job evaluation methods are commonly used:

- **Job ranking** is the simplist and the most subjective method of job evaluation. It involves placing jobs in order from highest to lowest in value to the organization.
- **Job classification** method involves matching a job's written position description with a description of a classification grade. Jobs in the federal government are graded on the basis of this method of job evaluation.
- The **point method** is a commonly used system that places weight (points) on each of the compensable factors in a job. The total points associated with a job establish its relative worth. Jobs that fall within a specific range of points fall into a grade associated with a specific wage or salary.
- The **factor comparison method** is a complex quantitative method that combines elements of both the ranking and point methods. Factor comparison results indicate the degree to which different compensable factors vary by job, making it possible to translate each factor value more easily into a monetary wage (Mathis and Jackson 2002).

In recent years, the **Hay method** of job evaluation, officially known as the Hay Guide Chart-Profile Method of Job Evaluation, is being used extensively. It is adaptable to many types of jobs and organizations and easy for individuals within organizations to learn to use. The method is essentially a modification of the point method that numerically measures the levels of three major compensable factors: the know-how, problem-solving, and accountability requirements of each job (Myers 1998; Mathis and Jackson 2002).

Performance Management

Most organizations use some form of performance review system to evaluate the performance of individual employees. Although performance reviews should be a part of regular communications between managers and employees, formal performance review discussions are routinely held on an annual or biannual basis. The functions of performance reviews include the following:

- Assessment of the employee's performance compared to performance standards or previously set performance goals
- Development of performance goals for the future year
- Development of a plan for professional development

Reviews also may include employee self-assessments. In some organizations, other employees may contribute information to the reviews of colleagues and coworkers. In the case of a supervisory manager, his or her staff may participate in the evaluation. This form of evaluation to which managers, peers, and staff contribute is called a **360-degree evaluation.**

Many organizations base pay increases on the results of annual performance reviews. Whether or not the evaluation affects salary, the annual review is an opportunity to formally discuss past accomplishments, career development, and expectations for future performance.

Periodic Performance Reviews

Performance management is an ongoing challenge. Information about performance should be collected regularly and shared with employees, whether their jobs involve coding clinical records or directing a department. Good performance results should be shared to encourage and reward ongoing success.

Performance issues are rarely resolved by ignoring them. Understanding the causes of problems and working with employees to resolve them are important management tasks. Actions that can be taken to improve performance include retraining, streamlining responsibilities, reestablishing expectations, and monitoring progress.

Performance Counseling and Disciplinary Action

When actions taken to improve performance are unsuccessful, more formal counseling and even disciplinary action may be required. Most organizations have formal processes in place to ensure that all staff are treated fairly and that employment laws are followed. Managers should consult with the human resources department to ensure that any disciplinary actions comply with approved procedures.

The steps described in establishing performance standards, hiring and training employees, and conducting routine performance reviews are all necessary before doing performance counseling or taking disciplinary action. Moreover, steps to improve performance should be taken in all cases.

Performance counseling usually begins with informal counseling or a verbal warning. No record of these actions is maintained in the employee's file.

The **progressive discipline process** begins with a verbal warning. When a second offense occurs, the process progresses to a written reprimand with formal documentation of the problem and delineation of the steps needed to correct it. Employees may be required to submit a step-by-step action plan to resolve issues and improve their performance. A third offense results in suspension, and a fourth offense generally results in dismissal.

In some environments, disciplinary actions include suspension from employment without pay or demotion to a job with lower expectations and less pay. In some cases, more than one of these actions may be taken. Generally, however, suspension and demotion are less popular than the use of binding performance improvement plans because suspension and demotion create a punitive atmosphere. Such punitive actions also affect the morale of other employees and staff. Empowering employees to create a plan of action places the responsibility for performance improvement in their own hands.

Regardless of the counseling and disciplinary actions mandated by the organization, managers should take some key steps of their own:

- They should discuss performance problems and consequences for poor performance with the employee in a clear and direct manner.
- They should support the employee's efforts to improve performance or resolve performance issues.
- They should document the steps taken to improve performance.
- They should be careful to follow the organization's HR policies.
- They should consult human resources professionals before taking action.
- They should keep performance issues confidential.
- They should follow the same process for all employees.

Conflict Management

Sometimes problems arise because of conflicts among employees. It is not unusual for people to disagree. Indeed, sometimes a difference of opinion can increase creativity. However, conflict can also waste time, reduce productivity, and decrease morale. When taken to the extreme, it can threaten the safety of employees and cause damage to property.

Conflict management focuses on working with the individuals involved to find a mutually acceptable solution. There are three ways to address conflict:

- *Compromise:* In this method, both parties must be willing to lose or give up a piece of their position.
- *Control:* In this method, interaction may be prohibited until the employees' emotions are under control. The manager also may structure their interactions. For example, the manager can set ground rules for communicating or dealing with specific issues. Another form of control is personal counseling. Personal counseling focuses on how people deal with conflict rather than on the cause of specific disagreements.
- *Constructive confrontation:* In this method, both parties meet with an objective third party to explore their perceptions and feelings. The desired outcome is to produce a mutual understanding of the issues and to create a win–win situation.

Grievance Management

Employees have the right to disagree with management and can express their opinions or complaints in a variety of ways.

They should be encouraged to bring problems and concerns directly to their manager. When they do not achieve satisfaction at that level, the manager should explain other options to the employee. For example, dissatisfied employees should understand that they can either take their issues to the next management level or discuss them with human resources staff.

Organizations establish **grievance procedures** that define the steps an employee can follow to seek resolution of a disagreement they have with management on a job-related issue. A complaint becomes a **grievance** when it has been documented in writing. At that point, the formal grievance procedure is set in motion.

Employees who belong to a union should follow the grievance procedures set by their union. Union contracts usually specify the types of actions employees can take and the time frames for filing grievances. The contracts usually specify time frames for responses and define the formal process for elevating the consideration or resolution of a grievance. Grievances taken to the highest levels will likely have to be resolved through mediation or arbitration.

Each of these steps takes time and can cost money. Therefore, managers should try to avoid grievances by maintaining open and effective communication with their staff.

Maintenance of Employee Records

Official employee records must be maintained under the control of the HR department. Any personnel records maintained under the control of the manager must be kept secure at all times.

Federal legislation such as Title VII of the Civil Rights Act of 1964, the Age Discrimination in Employment Act, the Immigration Reform and Control Act, and the FLSA place numerous record-keeping and reporting requirements on the HR department. The Environmental Protection Agency (EPA) and the Occupational Safety and Health Administration (OSHA) also have record-keeping requirements. Myers (1998, pp. 125–26) outlines several additional record-keeping obligations:

- Employers must protect the confidentiality of personnel records and files.
- Employers must protect the health records of employees.
- Employers must avoid intruding into the personal lives of employees, such as their other associations, alcohol use, spending habits, and financial obligations unless there are valid job-related reasons for making such intrusions.
- Employers must prevent the public disclosure of personal information that maybe embarrassing to an employee.

- Employers must protect the results of employment-related tests, including written tests used in making selection decisions and the results of both preemployment and random drug testing.

Current Human Resources Trends

According to the U.S. Department of Labor (2001), the following trends in employment are likely to affect the labor market in the United States during the first decade of the twenty-first century:

- Total workforce growth will be slower between 2000 and 2006 than in previous decades.
- Only one-third of the entrants to the workforce between 2000 and 2006 will be white males.
- Women will constitute a greater proportion of the labor force than in the past, and 63 percent of all U.S. women will be in the workforce by 2005.
- Minority racial and ethnic groups will account for a growing percentage of the overall labor force. Immigrants will expand this growth.
- The average age of the U.S. population will increase, and more workers who retire from full-time jobs will work part-time.
- As a result of these and other shifts, employers in a variety of industries will face shortages of qualified workers.

From this information, it is obvious that employers must be prepared to function with an increasingly diverse workforce in terms of gender, age, health status, race, and ethnicity. In general, the management of an increasingly diverse workforce is receiving considerable attention in the human resources literature, and some organizations are initiating diversity-training programs. Mathis and Jackson (2002, p. 39) identify three content areas that are often included in diversity training programs:

- *Legal awareness:* federal and state laws and regulations on equal employment opportunity and the consequences of violating these laws and regulations
- *Cultural awareness:* attempts to deal with stereotypes, typically through discussions and exercises
- *Sensitivity training:* attempts to sensitize people to the differences among them and how their words and behaviors are perceived by others

According to Flynn Gillian (1998), mixed reviews regarding the effectiveness of the diversity training received from both public- and private-sector organizations suggest that either the programs or their implementation are ineffective. There seems to be considerable work still to be done within healthcare organizations and health information management departments to prepare for the anticipated growth in the multicultural profile of human resources assets over the coming decade.

The Department of Labor data also indicate that employees will increasingly seek ways to gain more control over their time. The time pressure associated with trying to balance work and personal lives (especially when both parents are working outside the family home) coupled with the time pressure associated with increasingly long commutes appear to be driving this concern to the surface in HR management. Flextime, job sharing, and home-based (telecommuting) staffing options are emerging as viable solutions to the workforce retention issue. Within transcription and coding work units in health information management services, flextime and home-based staffing options are being implemented to address the labor shortages that are already affecting departmental operations. (See chapter 22 for a full discussion of these staffing alternatives.)

Check Your Understanding 23.5

Instructions: Indicate whether the following statements are true or false (T or F).

1. ____ Employee compensation systems are used to enhance employee loyalty.

2. ____ Minimum wage and overtime policies are impacted by the Taft-Hartley Act.

3. ____ All employees are subject to the provisions of the Fair Labor Standards Act.

4. ____ Trade associations and government agencies are routine sources for compensation benchmark data.

5. ____ The Equal Pay Act requires employers to consider compensable factors when setting pay for similar work performed by both females and males.

6. ____ Job ranking is the most commonly used method for conducting job evaluations.

7. ____ The Hays method is a popular, specialized point method for conducting job evaluations.

8. ____ Formal performance review sessions are routinely done on an annual basis.

9. ____ A 180-degree evaluation involves evaluation feedback from supervisors, peers, as well as self-assessment.

10. ____ The first step in a progressive disciplinary process is a verbal, undocumented warning.

11. ____ Compromise is a method of conflict resolution with a goal to arrive at a win–win outcome.

12. ____ Grievances taken to the highest levels for resolution will likely be resolved through mediation or arbitration.

13. ____ Organizations are obliged to avoid intrusions into an employee's personal life unless there is a valid job-related reason for doing so.

14. ____ U.S. Department of Labor statistics indicate that a surplus of qualified labor will be available in most industries over the next decade (2000-2006).

15. ____ Flextime and home-based staffing alternatives are being employed in health information services to address labor shortage issues.

Real-World Case

Figure 23.6 (p. 576) shows the resume of one of the numerous candidates applying for a coding specialist position. The staff position is being added to the HIM department of a large metropolitan medical center. The purpose of the new position is to help the current staff to handle its increased workload since the implementation of the outpatient prospective payment system for Medicare patients earlier in the year. A registered health information administrator was hired six months ago to supervise the department's five-person outpatient services team.

The director of the HIM department has already developed a detailed job description for the new position. (See figure 23.7, p. 577.) The new manager is a bit nervous about taking on this part of her new job.

Discussion Questions

1. Look at the resume and think about the steps that will need to be taken before the new manager can decide which of the candidates she would like to interview first. What does the format and presentation of the resume say about the candidate?

2. Does he appear to have the qualifications described in the job description?

3. Should the manager add this candidate to the list of candidates to be interviewed? Why or why not?

4. If the manager decided to interview this candidate, what should the first question be? The second?

5. If the manager decided that she might want to hire this person, what questions would she want to ask the candidate's former employer?

Summary

Management is key in setting the direction of the organization, establishing policies, and maximizing the organization's assets. Included among those assets are the people who carry out the organization's mission as staff: the organization's human resources. Managers are diffused throughout the organization with different responsibilities assigned at different levels, and yet all have important roles to play in creating and maintaining an environment that is prudent in handling its financial resources, focused on providing quality services to its customers, and attentive to the basic human needs of the organization's workforce.

Effective management of human resources begins with attention given to the adoption of appropriate policies, procedures, and practices in each of the seven HR activity areas: HR planning and analysis; equal employment opportunity; staffing; HR development; compensation and benefits; health, safety, and security; and employee and labor/management relations. HR professionals working in close partnership with the organization's managers hire and retain qualified employees by following these guidelines and fostering

Figure 23.6.   Sample Resume

RESUME

Stephen Jeremy Johnsen
222 Brickpath Way   Born 1/23/1971
Chicago, ILL 60622   Height 5 ft 9 in
773/222-2222   Weight 180 lbs

Goal: Looking for a job that lets me use my education and my knowledge of hospital
   coding and billing

Salary: $30,000+, opportunitie for advancement

2001 Code Lincoln Valley Community Hospital
    I left to move to Chicago to be with my girlfried

2001 Billing specialist University Medical Center, Chapaigne,Illinois
    Was here for almost a year; disliked manager; needed more money

1999 School Oakwood Community College

    Worked as a orderly to earn money for classes, majored in health information
    technology and computer programming

1995 Army Stationed in South Carolina, Germany, trained as medical corpsman

1989 School, majored in business but dropped out to join Army and earn money for
    school

1989 Graduated Glenview high school, Computer club, Music Camp, Varsity
    football, worked in father's landscape business during summers

*References available

---

good working relationships between employees and management.

Effective recruitment, selection, and hiring practices involve the consistent use of the tools designed to identify the best-qualified candidates for each position. Once hired, ensuring that employees are well oriented and trained is the critical first step toward a successful long-term outcome. Subsequently, maintaining open and meaningful communications with employees, setting realistic performance expectations for employees, engaging employees in ways that give them appropriate control of their work schedule and environment, delegating appropriate levels of decision-making authority, and providing them with opportunities for ongoing staff development all serve to enhance their morale and increase job satisfaction.

Managing human resources is both a science and an art. As such, it is learned through a combination of study and observation. Published HR management resources are readily available to provide the knowledge foundation associated with this field. In the workplace, HR professionals are available to serve as advisors to managers who want to handle this complex aspect of their management responsibilities knowledgably and artfully.

References

Anthony, William P., Pamela L. Perrewe, and K. Michele Kacmar. 1996. *Strategic Human Resource Management.* Orlando, Fla.: Harcourt Brace & Company.

Armstrong, Michael. 1999. *How to Be an Even Better Manager,* fifth edition. London: Kogan Page Ltd.

Benedictine Health System. 2002. Advancing the BHS ministry through a renewed commitment to mission, values. *BHS System Spirit & Life* 6(3):1.

Daley, Dennis M. 2002. *Strategic Human Resource Management.* Upper Saddle River, N.J.: Prentice-Hall.

Figure 23.7.   Sample Job Description for the Real-World Case

Position Description

Position Title:	APC Coordinator
Immediate Supervisor:	Director of Health Information Management
General Purpose:	The purpose of this position is to create consistency and efficiency in outpatient claims processing and data collection to optimize APC reimbursement and facilitate data quality in outpatient services.

Responsibilities:

- Performs data quality reviews on outpatient encounters to validate the ICD-9-CM, CPT, and HCPCS Level II code and modifier assignments, APC group appropriateness, missed secondary diagnoses and/or procedures, and compliance with all APC mandates and outpatient reporting requirements.
- Monitors medical visit code selection by departments against facility-specific criteria for appropriateness. Assists in the development of such criteria as needed.
- Monitors outpatient service mix reports and the leading medical visit, surgical service, significant procedure, and ancillary APCs assigned in the facility to identify patterns, trends, and variations in the facility's frequently assigned APC groups. Once identified, evaluates the causes of the change, and takes appropriate steps in collaboration with the right department to effect resolution or explanation of the variance.
- Continuously evaluates the quality of clinical documentation to spot incomplete or inconsistent documentation for outpatient encounters that impact the code selection and resulting APC groups and payment. Brings identified concerns to medical staff committee or department managers for resolution.
- Provides and/or arranges for training to facility healthcare professionals on the use of coding guidelines and practices, proper documentation techniques, medical terminology, and disease processes appropriate to the job description and function as it relates to the APC and other outpatient data quality management factors.
- Maintains knowledge of current professional coding certification requirements and promotes recruitment and retention of certified staff in coding positions when possible.
- Reports to the facility Compliance Committee each quarter.
- Abides by the Standards of Ethical Coding as set forth by the American Health Information Management Association and monitors coding staff for violations and reports to the HIM Director when areas of concern are identified. Concerns involving compliance issues are forwarded to the Compliance Committee for action.
- Develops reports and collects and prepares data for studies involving outpatient encounter data for clinical evaluation purposes and/or financial impact and profitability.
- Serves as the facility representative for APCs by attending outpatient coding and reimbursement workshops and bringing back information to the appropriate departments. Communicates any APC updates published in third-party payer newsletters/bulletins and provider manuals to all facility staff that need this information.
- Keeps abreast of new technology in coding and abstracting software and other forms of automation and stays informed about transaction code sets, HIPAA requirements, and other future issues impacting the coding function.
- Demonstrates competency in the use of computer applications and APC Grouper Software, OCE edits and all coding, software and hardware currently in use in the HIM department.
- Performs periodic claim form reviews to check code transfer accuracy from the abstracting system and the chargemaster.
- Evaluates, records, and responds to the Peer Review Organization APC change and/or denial notices. Provides appropriate documentation from required source to the PRO when appealing a PRO decision.
- Monitors outpatient unbilled accounts report for outstanding and/or uncoded outpatient encounters to reduce Accounts Receivable days for outpatients.
- Serves on the Chargemaster maintenance committee.

Qualifications:

- Minimum of associate's degree in a health services discipline. Formal HIM education with national certification, RHIA or RHIT preferred.
- Coding certification required from the American Health Information Management Association or the American Academy of Professional Coders.
- Minimum of five years progressive coding or coding review experience in ICD-9-CM, CPT, and HCPCS with claims processing and/or data management responsibilities a plus.
- Good oral and written communication skills and comprehensive knowledge of the APC structure and regulatory requirements.
- Prefer someone with past auditing experience or strong training background in coding and reimbursement.

Duncan, W. Jack, and Peter M. Ginter. 2000. Principles of management. In *Health Information: Management of a Strategic Resource,* second edition, edited by M. Abdelhak et al. Philadelphia: W. B. Saunders Company.

Gift, Robert G., and Catherine F. Kinney, editors. 1996. *Today's Management Methods: A Guide for the Health Care Executive.* Chicago: American Hospital Publishing.

Gillian, Flynn. 1998. The harsh reality of diversity programs. *Workforce* 12:26-35.

Haiman, Theo. 1984. *Supervisory Management for Health Care Organizations,* third edition. St. Louis: Catholic Health Association of the United States.

Kouzes, James M., and Barry Z. Posner. 1995. *The Leadership Challenge.* San Francisco: Jossey-Bass Publishers.

Mathis, Robert L., and John H. Jackson. 2002. *Human Resource Management: Essential Perspectives,* second edition. Cincinnati: South-Western Publishers.

Myers, Donald W. 1998. *1999 U.S. Master Human Resources Guide.* Chicago: CCH Incorporated.

Peters, Tom. 1987. *Thriving on Chaos.* New York City: Alfred A. Knopf.

Rosner, Bob, Allan Halcrow, and Alan Levins. 2001. *The Boss's Survival Guide.* New York City: McGraw-Hill.

Senge, Peter M. 1990. *The Fifth Discipline.* New York City: Doubleday/Currency.

Schein, Edgar H. 1980. *Organizational Psychology,* third edition. Englewood Cliffs, N.J.: Prentice-Hall.

Application Exercises

1. Prepare your resume and complete a job application for a position that is advertised in the newspaper or on the Web. Consider how the resume and application reflect your qualifications for that unique position.

2. In groups of three, practice role-playing an interview. As a team, prepare the interview questions. One person plays the part of interviewer, one plays the role of the candidate, and one observes the interview and takes notes. End the practice session with a group discussion of what went well and what could be improved.

3. In groups of three, practice a conflict resolution session or a performance review session. As a team, prepare the conflict scenario or the performance evaluation scenario, as appropriate. One person plays the part of the manager/supervisor, one person plays the part of the employee, and one observes the interaction and takes notes. End the practice session with a group discussion of what went well and what could be improved.

4. Write an essay about a previous manager with whom you have worked. What human resources tools did the supervisor use in his or her position? How effective was your training and orientation? How did this person handle performance evaluation and reviews? How did this person handle conflict? How did this person coach and mentor his or her staff? What lessons did you learn from this experience?

5. In groups of five, develop a presentation for the class on one of the following labor relations laws: (1) National Labor Relations Act of 1935, (2) Labor Management Relations Act, and (3) Labor-Management Reporting and Disclosure Act of 1959.

6. Conduct a class discussion on the human resources challenges that managers face today. Are there local issues that affect any of these challenges? Discuss how would a manager prepare for these challenges.

Review Quiz

Instructions: Choose the best word or phrase to complete the following statements.

1. ___ The organization's mission ___.
   a. Is rarely referred to once developed
   b. Is a realistic expression of what the organization does
   c. Expresses the beliefs held by the organization
   d. Is an idealistic portrayal of the desired future

2. ___ A graphic representation of the organization's formal structure is called ___.
   a. The budget
   b. The mission statement
   c. An organizational chart
   d. Organizational values

3. ___ Supervisory managers are primarily responsible for ___.
   a. Developing the organization's policies and procedures
   b. Setting the organization's future direction
   c. Establishing the strategic plan
   d. Monitoring everyday performance

4. ___ A summary of the responsibilities of a position, a list of duties, and a list qualifications required to perform the job are all elements of a ___.
   a. Orientation plan
   b. Performance review
   c. Position description
   d. Schedule

5. ___ Performance standards are used to ___.
   a. Communicate performance expectations
   b. Assign daily work
   c. Describe the elements of a job
   d. Prepare a job advertisement

6. ___ Position descriptions, policies and procedures, training checklists, and performance standards are all examples of ___.
   a. Human resources tools
   b. Organizational policies
   c. Strategic plans
   d. Items on a training checklist

7. ___ The department's orientation checklist should not include a ___.
   a. Review of communication policies
   b. Discussion of problem employees
   c. Description of how to request time off
   d. Review of departmental goals

8. ___ Periodic performance reviews ___.
   a. Encourage good performance
   b. Take the place of annual reviews
   c. Are the only opportunity to discuss performance
   d. Are only important when there are problems

9. ___ The usual first step in performance counseling is ___.
   a. Suspension without pay
   b. A demotion
   c. A verbal warning
   d. Conflict resolution

10. ___ The focus of conflict management is ___.
    a. Getting personal counseling for the parties involved
    b. Separating the parties involved so that they do not have to work together
    c. Working with the parties involved to find a mutually acceptable solution
    d. Bringing disciplinary action against one party or the other

Chapter 24
Training and Development

Karen R. Patena, MBA, RHIA

Learning Objectives

- To understand the continuum of employee training and development
- To appreciate the role of staff development in retaining a competent workforce
- To understand how to respond to the needs of adult learners
- To understand how to respond to the needs of a culturally diverse workforce or the needs of employees with disabilities
- To understand how to apply appropriate delivery methods to various training needs
- To learn how to develop an orientation program for new employees
- To learn how to prepare and conduct appropriate in-service education programs for various healthcare employees
- To identify alternative staffing trends and discuss their role in workforce retention
- To understand how to apply appropriate methods for developing employee potential
- To learn how to assess the needs of current employees for continuing education
- To be able to prepare a training and development plan for a health information management department

Key Terms

Accountability
Asynchronous
Authority
Career development
Coaching
Competencies
Compressed workweek
Computer-based training
Continuing education
Cross-training
Delegation
Development
Distance learning
Diversity training
Employment contract
Empowerment
Flex years
Flextime
Habit
Incentive
In-service education
Intranet
Job description
Job rotation

Job sharing
Job specification
Learning curve
Lecture
Massed training
Mentoring
Motivation
Needs assessment
On-the-job training
Orientation
Outsourcing
Productivity
Reinforcement
Self-directed learning
Socialization
Spaced training
Strategic plan
Synchronous
Task analysis
Telecommuting
Trainee
Trainer
Training
Train the trainer

Introduction

As a service industry, healthcare relies on the availability of competent workers. The growth of new technologies, the application of new vocabulary and processes, and the decreasing numbers of employees with adequate skills to respond to the new environment mean that healthcare organizations must frequently assume responsibility for preparing and developing their own labor pool. However, providing the necessary training is costly in terms of both money and time. Moreover, after the organization has made the investment, it must do what it can to protect its investment by retaining its workforce.

Human resources are the healthcare institution's most valuable asset. Managing employees requires recognizing and meeting the needs of the employees as well as those of the organization. Healthcare organizations must provide employees with the tools for career success and personal achievement if they are to win their employees' long-term commitment.

This chapter focuses on training and retaining employees in the healthcare organization. It describes the orientation process and different methods for training new employees as well as current employees taking on new job responsibilities. It also discusses adult learning strategies, techniques for delivering employee training, and methods for enhancing job satisfaction. Finally, the chapter describes how to implement a departmental employee training and development plan.

Theory into Practice

Nancy New has just started her position as director of health information management (HIM) for a large academic medical center on the West Coast. The department includes employees who have been hired in the past few months as well as employees who have been there as long as ten years. Her most recent employee, Susan, is a newly credentialed RHIT with excellent coding skills. She is very enthusiastic about her job but sometimes fails to follow procedures that she feels are unnecessary. Some of the long-time coders are resentful of Susan's skills and new ideas and have called in sick on several occasions. Hospital management has been reluctant to send employees to continuing education programs because of the cost and time that employees lose away from work.

One of the best coders in the department, Julie, has recently returned from maternity leave. Although she enjoys her job, she has informed Nancy that she is thinking of resigning. Paying someone to care for her baby is expensive, and Julie often has difficulty concentrating on her work because she feels guilty about not being home.

Nancy has discovered that a formal training program has never been implemented for HIM department employees. Although the medical center provides a basic orientation for new employees that includes a review of basic policies and procedures, benefits, and fire safety protocols, it has no plan or budget in place for continuing education. Nancy felt that her own orientation was not comprehensive enough, and she has had to learn a great deal about her department on her own.

Concerned about these issues, Nancy has determined three major areas of focus. First, her coders are in need of updated skills. Second, she wants to upgrade the morale and interpersonal skills of both her new and long-term employees. Finally, she does not want a good employee to resign.

With her supervisor's approval, Nancy prepares an employee development plan for the department. She begins with a needs assessment on the individual as well as departmental level. She sets learning objectives for new and existing employees and prepares a departmental orientation plan to supplement the one provided by the medical center. The orientation plan includes an introduction to policies and procedures, a review of privacy regulations, and on-the-job training in the employee's specific work area. To improve cooperation within the department and to build morale, Nancy plans to involve long-term employees in revising policies and procedures and in assisting in the training efforts. Before long-term employees are permitted to train, however, they must attend a train-the-trainer session.

Nancy next requests additional funding to provide continuing education for her employees. She plans to use programs such as the AHIMA's Web-based coding programs to provide high-quality material that can be delivered to the work site, thus reducing both the cost of travel and time away from the job. All employees will be required to demonstrate competencies through annual assessments. Those with outstanding scores will be considered for promotional opportunities and merit-based salary increases.

Finally, Nancy proposes that employees be given the option to use flextime or even to work at home, provided they continue to demonstrate the ability to work independently, meet quantity and quality standards, and successfully complete periodic competency assessments.

Six months after implementing her plan, Nancy sees a marked improvement in her employees' skill levels and the elimination of unnecessary steps following a review of policies and procedures. There is a cooperative attitude among the staff, and Julie continues to work for the department as a home-based coder. Susan supported and adhered to the new processes, as did the other coders in the department.

Training Program Development

Traditional management theory differentiated between **training** for lower-level, technical employees and **development** for management staff who needed to improve skills such as decision making and interpersonal communication. However, this distinction has become outdated in the twenty-first century as organizations take a more comprehensive approach to improving employee performance. Today, the terms training and development are often used interchangeably, with the primary goal being to improve knowledge, skills, abilities, attitudes, and social behavior of workers at all levels. As employees who make up the organization grow, so does the organization.

In developing training programs, healthcare organizations must recognize that special accommodations may be required to address the needs of both a culturally diverse workforce and employees with disabilities. Employers need to understand the requirements affecting training that are included under Title VII or the 1964 Civil Rights Act, the 1991 Civil Rights Act, and the 1990 Americans with Disability Act. If completion of a training program is part of the selection process for a particular job, the organization must be able to demonstrate that the requirements are valid and do not discriminate against, or have a negative impact on, women, minorities, or disabled individuals. For example, the vocabulary in written documents used for training should match the level required for the job, and training equipment and locations should be accessible to individuals with mobility disabilities.

In addition to modifying training programs to accommodate employees with special needs, the organization should develop diversity-training programs. **Diversity training** facilitates an environment that fosters tolerance and appreciation of individual differences within the organization's workforce.

Training and development programs should be viewed as a vital part of the **strategic management** of healthcare institutions. The standards of accreditation organizations as well as healthcare plans require the demonstration of high-quality, efficient healthcare delivery. To remain financially viable, healthcare organizations must emphasize productivity, performance, and profitability. The only way to attain excellence is to challenge and encourage the workforce to work toward its highest potential.

Investment in training programs helps the organization to accomplish goals on an individual, group, and organizational level. Other important reasons for providing employee training and development include:

- To introduce new employees to the organization
- To provide a path for employee promotion and retention
- To improve employee performance and productivity
- To update skills for employees in new or restructured positions resulting from organizational or technological change
- To reduce organizational problems caused by absenteeism, turnover, poor morale, or substandard quality
- To deliver high-quality healthcare within budgetary constraints

One way to view training and development needs is as a continuum of five conceptual areas, beginning with **orientation** and extending into **career development.** Healthcare organizations are unique, and so should their development programs be. A fifty-bed long-term care facility has very different staffing and training needs than a large acute care academic medical center does. Table 24.1 presents an employee development continuum (Fottler, Hernandez, and Joiner 1998, p. 201). Each concept differs in objectives, diversity of skills, degree of emphasis on career development, training location, and frequency of delivery. There is no best way to deliver training; it must fit the context of the institution.

However, investment in employee development does not end with training. Organizations need to find ways to gain the commitment of employees so that they will remain productive. Retaining good employees and developing their potential is an area of great importance, particularly in an industry that has a shortage of qualified workers.

Table 24.1.   Employee Development Continuum

Concept	Objectives	Scope of Skill Diversity	Emphasis on Personal/Career Growth	Training Site	Frequency
Orientation training	To introduce staff to the mores, behaviors, and expectations of the organization	Narrow	Narrow	Internal	Single instance
Training	To teach staff specific skills, concepts, or attitudes			Internal	Sporadic
In-service education	To teach staff about skills, facts, attitudes, and behaviors largely through internal programs			Internal	Continuous
Continuing education	To facilitate the efforts of staff members to remain current in the knowledge base of their trade or profession through external programs designed to achieve external standards			External	Continuous
Career development	To expand the capabilities of staff beyond a narrow range of skills toward a more holistically prepared person	Broad	Broad	Internal and external	Continuous

Source: Fottler, H., S. Hernandez, and C. Joiner, editors. 1998. *Essentials of Human Resource Management in Health Service Organizations.* Albany, N.Y.: Delmar Publishers, p. 201.

Elements of Workforce Training

The goal of any institution's training program is to provide employees the skills they need to perform their jobs. Because employees are at different stages in their career development, the training program must be flexible and able to adapt to meet many needs. At any given time, some new employees will need to know basic information about the organization and long-term employees will want to improve their ability to contribute at higher levels within the organizational structure. Today's workforce needs both technical skills and so-called soft skills, such as team building and critical thinking. For example, computers have become an integral part of the work setting. Thus, whatever the primary task, most employees need to develop skills in using personal computers and related devices.

New Employee Orientation

After employees have been recruited and selected, the first step is to introduce them to the organization and their immediate work setting and functions.

Definition

New employee orientation includes a group of activities that introduce the employee to the organization's mission, policies, rules, and culture; the department or workgroup; and the specific job he or she will be performing. In addition to the basic skills needed to do the job, the employee needs to experience a period of **socialization** in which he or she learns the values, behavior patterns, and expectations of the organization.

Needs Assessment

As with all training programs, the orientation must be customized to the particular employee. New employees will require a more in-depth orientation than current employees who are starting a different position within the same institution. In a large facility, new employee orientation is usually coordinated by human resources; in a small facility, it may be performed entirely by the employee's supervisor. The orientation may consist of a brief and informal presentation, or it may be a formal program that takes place over several days on a regularly scheduled basis. Formal programs typically begin with presentations by human resources and other department heads before the new employee is introduced to his or her immediate supervisor. The supervisor then continues the orientation process within the employee's assigned department.

To develop an orientation program, it is helpful to begin with a **task analysis** to determine the specific skills required for the job. The **job description** and the **job specification** are excellent sources for this part of the process. Beyond specific tasks, all new employees need to understand matters common to the institution, such as personnel policies, benefits, and safety regulations. Federal and state governments and accreditation organizations also may require certain subjects to be included in the orientation program.

Requirements

Although the orientation program is typically done at a single point in time, a new employee may not feel completely competent for as long as a year from the date he or she was hired. The program should attempt to make employees feel that they made the right choice in accepting the position. For this to happen, they should feel welcome, comfortable in their new environment, positive about their supervisor, and confident that they are learning the skills they need to do the job. An orientation program should not just be for completing paperwork.

An effective tool used in orienting new workers is the orientation checklist. (See figure 24.1.) The orientation checklist helps the employer know that the employee is receiving the information he or she needs to begin the job and serves as an agenda for presenting the information in a logical manner. Rather than presenting everything the new employee needs to know all at once, it is helpful to spread the orientation over several days.

In addition, it is helpful to present policies and requirements that all employees must know, such as insurance programs, payroll requirements, and personnel policies, in an employee handbook given to new employees during the orientation. The handbook provides a handy reference after the immediate orientation period has ended. However, the facility must be careful not to include content that could imply conditions of an **employment contract,** either expressed or implied. If the employee views the handbook as a contract, it becomes a legally binding agreement. Employer or employee could be held liable if any conditions set out in the handbook are not strictly followed. Thus, the employee handbook must be viewed as advisory in nature and not as a legal document.

The requirements of an orientation program may be expressed on three levels: organizational, departmental, and individual.

At the *organizational level,* the orientation program provides the information that every employee who works for the company needs to know. This information typically includes:

- Background and mission of the organization
- Policies and procedures that apply to all employees, such as confidentiality agreements or infection control procedures
- Employee benefits (paid time off, insurance coverage)
- Safety regulations
- Employee/orientation handbook
- Tour of the facility

At the *departmental level,* orientation information typically includes:

- Departmental policies and procedures
- Introduction to other employees
- Tour of department

- Work hours
- Time sheet requirements
- Training in operation of equipment (for example, photocopying machines or computers)
- Safety regulations specific to the department

At the *individual level,* the new employee learns specific job tasks that, at a minimum, should include:

- Specific, measurable objectives for productivity and performance
- An explanation of each job task by the supervisor, followed by a demonstration and an opportunity for the employee to demonstrate the task

The new employee's individual orientation is usually the longest portion of the orientation program.

Components of an Orientation Program

An orientation program should be developed with input from human resources, other department heads, and the employee's supervisor. For a typical new employee in the HIM department of an acute care hospital, the orientation program might follow the schedule shown in figure 24.1. The first portion of the program introduces the employee to the institution and is typically led by the director of education or the director of human resources. The employee is given a handbook and any required forms to complete for payroll and insurance. The director of safety and security then introduces safety regulations.

To introduce the employee to the individual job setting as quickly as possible, the general portion of the orientation could be completed within the first half-day. The employee then could meet the immediate supervisor and be matched with a "buddy" to escort him or her to lunch and back to the department. Ideally, the buddy should have the same job as the new employee. On the afternoon of day one, the new worker should be introduced to coworkers, given a tour of the department, and shown his or her workstation. The first day could end with a basic overview explanation of the job's duties, including an opportunity for questions.

Figure 24.1.   Sample Orientation Checklist

Orientation Checklist

Supervisor _____   Date _____

Employee _____   Department_____

Before Worker Arrives

(Check off tasks when completed.)

___ 1. Prepare other employees.
___ 2. Have desk and supplies ready.
___ 3. Arrange for luncheon escort.

First Day

___ 1. Attend hospital orientation program.
___ 2. Receive employee handbook and (if applicable) union contract information.
___ 3. Receive benefit information.
___ 4. Review safety and security regulations, including infection control procedures.
___ 5. Introduce to immediate associates.
___ 6. Introduce to the workplace.
___ 7. Give overview of the job.
___ 8. Ask whether new employee has any questions.

Second Day

___ 1. Discuss confidentiality policy.
___ 2. Give job instructions.
___ 3. Review compensation.
___ 4. Explain hours of work.
___ 5. Discuss attendance requirements.
___ 6. Explain performance review.
___ 7. Explain quality and quantity standards.
___ 8. Encourage employee to ask questions.
___ 9. Explain where to store work overnight.

Third Day

___ 1. Explain telephone system, computer system, and fax and copier machines.
___ 2. Explain reasons for rules and policies.
___ 3. Explain insurance plans.
___ 4. Ask whether the new employee has any questions.

Fourth Day

___ 1. Give employee opportunity to describe how he or she is getting along.
___ 2. Discuss departmental policies in addition to hospital policies.
___ 3. Explain hospital continuing education program.

Fifth Day

___ 1. Describe vacation system.
___ 2. Explain bulletin board policy.

Sixth Day

___ 1. Encourage employee to talk to supervisor when necessary.
___ 2. Administer postorientation assessment.
___ 3. Give orientation evaluation form to employee to complete.

Orientation Completed _____ (Date)

Signature of Employee _____   Signature of Supervisor _____

Source: Adapted from Keeling, B., and N. Kallaus. 1996. *Administrative Office Management,* eleventh edition. Cincinnati: South-Western Publishing, p. 148.

The individual portion of the orientation then should continue as described in the suggested schedule, with some portion of each day devoted to job training and work rules so that the new employee can gradually understand the requirements of the job and become socialized to the work environment. As the new employee is trained and tested in each important aspect of the job, the supervisor should document his or her demonstrated competency. This documentation will help the organization to comply with the standards of the Joint Commission on Accreditation of Healthcare Organizations (JCAHO).

Assessment

After the orientation process, all the participants should be asked for feedback. A form should be developed and completed by the new employee. Figure 24.2 presents an example of a form for evaluating the general portion of the orientation program. Typical questions include:

- Was the program relevant to your job and needs?
- What part of the program was most useful to you?
- What part of the program was least useful to you?

Figure 24.2.   Sample Orientation Evaluation Form

Employee Orientation Program Evaluation Form

Date: _____

Job Title: _____

1. Please rate each of the following items to indicate your reaction to the session. If ranking is less than average, please comment on the back of this form.

Item	Poor	Adequate	Average	Good	Excellent
Objective 1: Applicability to your job, responsibilities, and needs					
Objective 2: Enough examples and chances to practice so you can apply your new skills at work					
Objective 3: Opportunity for discussion with other participants					
Objective 4: Length of the program relative to its objectives					

2. Which part of the program was of most value to you? Why?

3. Which part of the program was of least value to you? Why?

4a. Please use the following scale to comment on each instructor's ability to lead the program where:

1 = Needs improvement   2 = Adequate   3 = Good   4 = Excellent

Item	Instructor 1	Instructor 2
Organization/preparation of subject matter	1 2 3 4	1 2 3 4
Presentation of subject matter	1 2 3 4	1 2 3 4
Clarity of instructions	1 2 3 4	1 2 3 4
Ability to control time	1 2 3 4	1 2 3 4
Ability to link content to your job functions	1 2 3 4	1 2 3 4
Ability to stimulate productive discussions	1 2 3 4	1 2 3 4
Ability to create a productive learning environment	1 2 3 4	1 2 3 4

4b. Please comment on the instructors' abilities to lead the program:

5. How would you rate your overall reaction to the program?   1 2 3 4

6. How would you rate your level of skill/knowledge:

    a. Before the program?   1 2 3 4

    b. After the program?   1 2 3 4

7. Other comments:

Source: O'Connor, B. N., M. Bronner, and C. Delaney. 2002. *Training for Organizations,* second edition. Cincinnati: South-Western Publishing Company. Training Evaluation Form. Available online from http://workforce.com/archive.

In addition, supervisors should be asked to evaluate the effectiveness of the orientation process. For example, they should be asked for feedback on the employee's ability to apply his or her newly acquired job skills and for an assessment of the employee's comfort level with the department.

On-the-Job Training

Preparing staff to carry out the tasks and functions of their particular jobs should be an ongoing effort for both new and experienced employees. A variety of methods are available to employers. Effective training programs begin with a **needs assessment** and blend an appropriate combination of methods, media, content, and activities into a curriculum that is matched to the specific education, experience, and skill level of the audience.

Definition

On-the-job training is a method of teaching an employee to perform a task by actually performing it. Along with teaching basic skills, on-the-job training gives employees and supervisors opportunities to discuss specific problem areas and initiates socialization among the new employees and their coworkers. On-the-job training offers a number of advantages, including its relatively low cost compared to outside training programs and the fact that work is still in progress while the employee is being trained. However, employees may feel burdened if they are held responsible for work they do not accomplish during the training period and the learning process may be less than optimal if the work setting is disrupted by ongoing distractions and pressures.

Training may be performed by either a supervisor or a coworker with particular expertise. The selection of an appropriate trainer is critical to the success of this method. Even though they are very capable at performing the job being taught, some employees may not be effective teachers and may omit vital steps if not motivated to do the teaching.

Requirements of the Job

The training program should begin by reviewing the job description and the job specification. Job descriptions and job specifications should include a list of tasks performed for a job; the skills, ability, and knowledge required; and the expected quality and quantity standards of performance. Next, a performance analysis should be completed to assess the gap between expected performance and the employee's current performance level. In the case of a new employee, this may be verified through a written **competency** assessment. What the employee does not know or cannot do becomes the basis for on-the-job training. The requirements may include any of the following:

- Physical skills (for example, operation of equipment)
- Academic knowledge (for example, medical terminology or English spelling and grammar)
- Knowledge of institutional policies (for example, safety regulations)
- Technical skills, which may include both physical and mental skills (for example, use of computer programs)

Components of on-the-Job Training

On-the-job training offers a variety of delivery options, including:

- One-on-one training by a supervisor or an experienced peer
- Job rotation
- Computer-based training
- Coaching or mentoring
- Informal learning during meetings or discussions with supervisors and peers

One-on-one training is the technique used most often. In this type of training, the employee learns by first observing a demonstration and then performing the task. For this type of training to be effective, organizations may offer **train-the-trainer** workshops in which the trainer learns skills in communication and instruction. It is important to select a person to serve as a **trainer** who is not only competent in the job content, but also able to teach and interact effectively with the **trainee.** One-on-one training by the supervisor gives the supervisor an opportunity to observe how the trainee is doing and to make adjustments to meet the employee's skill level. A trainee who learns quickly can move through the steps at a faster pace; a trainee who learns slowly may need an opportunity for additional practice or a second demonstration.

In **job rotation,** the employee moves from job to job at planned intervals. This method is most useful for supervisory jobs, where the employee needs to learn a variety of tasks performed by several different employees. In **cross-training,** the employee learns to perform the jobs of many team members. This method is most useful when work teams are involved.

Computer-based training provides an opportunity to supplement job task performance with additional knowledge and/or simulation. It is effective in situations where repetition aids learning, for example, with medical terminology and tasks that cannot be duplicated entirely in the practice session, such as role-playing with different release of information scenarios.

After the trainee has demonstrated the ability to do the job, **coaching** should continue by the supervisor or an expert peer on an ongoing basis. The experienced worker observes or reviews the work of the employee in a nonthreatening manner, offering advice and suggestions for revising techniques to improve productivity and efficient work performance. In a formalized arrangement in which a specific person is assigned to follow up on a regular basis, the coach is referred to as a **mentor.** In this scenario, the mentor meets with the trainee on a regular basis and often gives advice on career growth and development within the organization.

It is estimated that approximately two-thirds of training actually results from informal interactions between the employee and his or her coworkers. Learning occurs even though it is not formally designed or monitored by the organization, for example, during hallway conversations or on lunch breaks when a work topic is discussed and other employees or supervisors offer suggestions or corrections.

On-the-job training methods can be used individually or in combination and should be adapted to each learner. Whatever technique is used, on-the-job training should follow the steps presented in figure 24.3.

Assessment

By its nature, on-the-job training provides an opportunity for immediate assessment of its effectiveness. The trainer can observe the employee's skills as part of the performance tryout and can question the employee on his or her knowledge of policies, procedures, and other academic knowledge that

Figure 24.3.   Steps in On-the-Job Training

Step 1: Preparation of the learner
   a. Put the learner at ease; relieve the tension.
   b. Explain why he or she is being taught.
   c. Create interest, encourage questions, find out what the learner already knows about his or her job or other jobs.
   d. Explain the why of the whole job and relate it to some job the worker already knows.
   e. Place the learner as close to the normal working position as possible.
   f. Familiarize the worker with the equipment, materials, tools, and trade terms.

Step 2: Presentation of the operation
   a. Explain quantity and quality requirements.
   b. Go through the job at the normal work pace.
   c. Go through the job at a slow pace several times, explaining each step. Between operations, explain the difficult parts or those in which errors are likely to be made.
   d. Again, go through the job at a slow pace several times; explain the key points.
   e. Have the learner explain the steps as you go though the job at a slow pace.

Step 3: Performance tryout
   a. Have the learner go through the job several times, slowly, explaining each step to you. Correct mistakes and, if necessary, do some of the complicated steps the first few times.
   b. You, the trainer, run the job at the normal pace.
   c. Have the learner do the job, gradually building up skill and speed.
   d. As soon as the learner demonstrates ability to do the job, let the work begin, but don't abandon him or her.

Step 4: Follow-up
   a. Designate to whom the learner should go for help if he or she needs it.
   b. Gradually decrease supervision but continue to check work against quality and quantity standards from time to time.
   c. Correct faulty work patterns that begin to creep into the work, and do it before they become a habit. Show why the learned method is superior.
   d. Compliment good work; encourage the worker until he or she is able to meet the quality/quantity standards.

Source: Dessler, G. 2000. *Human Resources Management,* eighth edition. New York City: Prentice-Hall, pp. 258–59.

may be required. If the assessment reveals areas of weakness, the training can be adjusted to reinforce knowledge or repeat steps performed incorrectly.

When the employee is working on his or her own, the supervisor should check the quantity and quality of the employee's work against performance standards from time to time. If the employee's performance is below standard, the training can be repeated before bad performance becomes a habit.

Finally, the employee should be encouraged to ask questions both during and after the training and should receive positive and negative feedback as appropriate.

Staff Development through In-Service Education

The healthcare industry grows and changes constantly. Whether it is a new law passed by the state or the federal government, new reimbursement regulations, updates to ICD-9-CM or CPT codes, new or revised accreditation standards, or upgraded software, change is a permanent factor. Preparing workers for such changes requires continuous training and retraining.

Definition

In-service education is the third step in the employee development continuum (table 24.1, p. 581). It is a continuous process that builds on the basic skills learned through new employee orientation and on-the-job training. In-service education is concerned with teaching employees specific skills and behaviors required to maintain job performance or to retrain workers whose jobs have changed. Although in-service education may include external programs, it is primarily developed and delivered at the work site.

Needs Assessment

The need for in-service education may be triggered by many events, including:

- A restructuring of the department and/or organization
- Annual updates to coding or reimbursement requirements
- Implementation of new software or hardware
- A decline in productivity or morale or an increase in absenteeism
- A new organizational policy or procedure
- An external requirement imposed by accreditation or licensing organizations, such as an annual renewal of CPR certification or retraining in infectious disease precautions or safety procedures

The amount of in-service education needed varies with the event and the education and experience of the employee. Downsizing or reorganizing organizational structure often causes changes in an individual employee's job responsibilities. Employees may need to learn other job functions within the workgroup or may even be placed in a new department. This can require a series of formal training sessions, including on-the-job training.

Renewal of training, required by external organizations, may be subject to defined content and duration, often including a test and/or demonstration of the employee's competence. On the other hand, implementation of a new policy or procedure may simply include distributing the information accompanied by a short meeting.

Decisions need to be made regarding the appropriate format of the in-service education. The following types of questions should be asked:

- Should the instruction be given as **massed training** in a highly concentrated session or as **spaced training** in several shorter sessions?
- Should the task be broken down into parts or be taught as a single unit?
- How will competence be assessed? Is the topic a skill that needs to be demonstrated by the learner, or is it a level of knowledge that should be tested with a written assessment?

As with other training categories, periodic analysis of actual-versus-desired job performance will create a list of topics that should be addressed with in-service education.

Requirements

Unlike orientation programs, which are delivered primarily at one point in time, in-service education programs need to be available on an ongoing basis. Depending on the size of the organization, some programs, such as a refresher on the response to the institution's disaster plan, may be offered on a monthly basis. The human resources department may coordinate programs on topics that affect the organization as a whole. Programs specific to health information management, such as an upgrade to a chart-tracking system, are more likely to be developed by a supervisor or manager in the HIM department.

Finally, some topics serve the needs of more than one department. For example, a program on coding updates may be given by the coding supervisor to employees from the HIM, patient accounting, and physician billing departments. This type of program probably would take place in a more formal setting and require coordination with other department managers.

Examples of in-service education topics and the individuals within the organization who are likely to have responsibility for them are shown in figure 24.4.

Steps in Conducting In-Service Education

Presenting an effective in-service program requires planning. The time frame depends on the complexity of the material and the number of participants but should include enough time to prepare materials and publicize the event. Generally, a formal in-service program should follow these steps:

- *Step 1:* Set objectives. Is the purpose of the program to teach a new job task to an individual or to improve morale within the department?

- *Step 2: Determine the audience.* Is the training intended for one employee or fifty employees? Are the participants from the same department or from several departments?
- *Step 3: Determine whether the content should be delivered as a unit or in parts (massed or spaced).* This may be determined by the availability of the employee as well as the topic.
- *Step 4: Determine the best method of instruction.* The education and experience of the audience, the time available, and the cost of preparing and delivering the instruction should all be taken into consideration. Is there a qualified expert in-house? Are videotapes or computer-based materials available for rent or purchase? Is space available to train a large group at one time? (See the discussions of adult learning strategies and delivery methods later in this chapter.)
- *Step 5: Prepare a budget.* If a specific amount has been allocated, the plan should be compared to the predetermined budget and revised, if necessary. Approval should be obtained if the proposal is a new one. In addition, the proposal should include the costs of photocopying materials, speaker fees, and training resources.
- *Step 6: Publicize the program.* Flyers and/or electronic notices should be posted to announce the program and should include the date, time, location, topic, and a summary of the content. When it is important to know the number of attendees in advance, the notice should include a method for RSVP.

Figure 24.4.   Examples of Responsibility for In-Service Education

---

Organizationwide: The human resources department typically assumes responsibility for the following topics and may include staff from other departments in the planning and presentation:
- Fire and safety awareness
- Disaster plan implementation
- Infectious disease/universal precautions
- Diversity training
- Team building
- Privacy, confidentiality, and security

Multiple Departments: The health information manager may work with managers of several departments to coordinate presentation of the following topics:
- ICD-9-CM or CPT annual updates
- Medical terminology training
- Use of office productivity software for employee productivity measurement
- Health record documentation

Health Information Management Department: The health information manager may develop in-service training within the department for the following topics:
- Release of information
- Fire, safety, and disaster preparedness
- Upgrade to DRG grouping software
- Use of new photocopier

- *Step 7: If appropriate, prepare handout materials.* Handouts would include materials to be used for instruction as well as documents to reference following the program. At a minimum, an agenda of the topics and a schedule should be developed.
- *Step 8: Practice, practice, practice!* The person presenting the program should be adequately prepared and comfortable with the content. Also, a training room should be scheduled ahead of time, and any needed equipment should be checked to ensure that it is available and in good working order. Anyone planning to use a computer or a projector should know how to operate it.
- *Step 9: Use a variety of methods, and be alert to your audience.* In addition to the lecture, the presenter should engage the audience through interactive questioning and activities. People learn by doing. Opportunities should be provided from time to time for questions and periodic breaks when the program lasts more than two hours.
- *Step 10: Obtain feedback from the audience.* It is important to give the participants an opportunity to document their reactions to the training. To that end, an evaluation form should be created and distributed. A sample in-service education evaluation form is shown in figure 24.5.

Assessment

Because some amount of cost, in terms of both time and resources, is usually involved with in-service training, it is important to determine whether its objectives have been met. Three methods for assessing the impact of in-service education are:

- *Completion of an evaluation form at the conclusion of the program:* Immediate feedback provides an assessment of the effectiveness of the delivery methods. Is the employee energized and ready to put the material to use, or was the material overwhelming?
- *Formal or informal feedback from the employee's supervisor:* Within a few days of the program, the supervisor should be contacted to determine whether the learner has applied the new skills and knowledge on the job.
- *Follow-up with the employee at a later time:* Thirty days after the in-service program, the attendees should be asked to validate the value of the program. Are they able to perform their job better? Is there something they feel they did not learn that should have been included? This may be accomplished easily via an e-mail message.

Check Your Understanding 24.1

Instructions: Answer the following questions on a separate piece of paper.

1. What are the purposes of an employee orientation program?
2. What are the three levels of an orientation program? List two items typically included at each level.
3. Who is responsible for conducting employee orientation programs?
4. What are some suggestions for making a new employee feel welcome in the new department?
5. What are the advantages and disadvantages of on-the-job training?
6. What are two examples of skills that are often included in on-the-job training programs?
7. Which is the most common technique used for on-the-job training? What key factor is essential to the success of this method?
8. When is job rotation a useful training technique?

Figure 24.5.   Sample In-Service Education Evaluation Form

In-Service Education Evaluation Form

To help us improve the quality of future programs, please complete the following evaluation of today's session.

Please use the following scale to answer questions 1–5:

1 = Needs Improvement   2 = Satisfactory   3 = Excellent

1. How satisfied were you with the content of the presentation?	1	2	3
2. How would you rate the organization of the presentation?	1	2	3
3. How would you rate the effectiveness of visual media used in the presentation?	1	2	3
4. How would you rate the delivery of the presentation?	1	2	3

5. How satisfied were you with the following aspects of the program?

a. Meeting location	1	2	3
b. Parking	1	2	3
c. Accessibility	1	2	3
d. Registration process	1	2	3
e. Meeting room setup/seating	1	2	3
f. Handout materials	1	2	3

6. What is one thing you learned that you did not know prior to attending?

7. What would you like to have learned more about?

8. Please provide any additional comments that could improve future programs.

9. What features characterize the major steps in on-the-job training?

10. What is the purpose of in-service education?

11. What events suggest a need for in-service education? List two.

12. What HIM in-service topics might be of interest to other departments? Describe at least one.

13. What printed items should always be distributed at a formal in-service program?

14. What three methods are used to assess the effectiveness of an in-service education program?

Adult Learning Strategies

Training has been defined as the process of providing individuals with the materials and activities they need to develop the knowledge, skills, abilities, attitudes, and behaviors desired in the workplace. Learning is what occurs in the individual—the changes in behavior, knowledge, attitudes, abilities, and skills that are desired. In the healthcare work environment, learning translates into achieving the goals of the institution, including improved job performance. The objective is for employees to develop effective work habits. To accomplish this objective, it is important to understand how employees learn and the factors that affect the learning environment.

Characteristics of Adult Learners

One of the most difficult tasks faced by employees is achieving balance. Ideally, people shift their time between the demands of work, the demands of home, and their own needs. Everyone wants to accomplish more with fewer and fewer hours. Although a low level of stress is positive, too much can lead to burnout. Therefore, training must be viewed as an integral part of the work environment and not as an "add-on" requirement. The individuals responsible for training need to understand that time is a very valuable resource.

Because time is scarce, employees need to see relevance in the activities that consume their time. They will be more willing to accept tasks that can be accomplished quickly, provide satisfaction or tangible benefits, and can be completed within short time frames.

Three fundamental concepts in helping adults learn are motivation, reinforcement, and knowledge of results.

Motivation

Motivation is the inner drive to accomplish a task. At different stages in life, adults are motivated by specific needs. Understanding that employees differ in the relative importance of these needs at any given time is important in designing a training program. For example, a newly credentialed health information technician in his early twenties with no dependents may be interested in working long hours. He may demonstrate an eagerness to devote extra hours to training that will advance his career. On the other hand, a young parent may value time to attend his or her children's school activities and want to limit time spent away from home.

Employees will be more motivated when they perceive a need for the training. The trainer should call attention to the important aspects of the job and help employees understand how to perform these tasks efficiently and effectively.

Moreover, employees should see a direct connection between the knowledge learned and the work goal. It is helpful when the trainer explains the reason for performing a task in a certain order and relates policies to objectives. For example, coders may be instructed to review a record in a specific order, beginning with a discharge summary and then reviewing lab reports. It is helpful when the trainer explains that the purpose of this process is to ensure appropriate evidence of diagnoses to comply with reimbursement requirements.

Reinforcement

Reinforcement is a condition following a response that results in an increase in the strength of that response. It is associated with motivation in that the strength of the response is a factor of the perceived value of the reinforcer. For example, the young parent mentioned above who values time with his or her children may be negatively reinforced by a pay increase given after a training course when the increase requires additional work hours. However, money would serve as a reinforcer for the new health information technician discussed above. Reinforcement is most effective when it occurs immediately after a correct response.

Incentive pay systems are a form of positive reinforcement. For example, transcriptionists might be compensated based on the number of lines correctly transcribed rather than on an hourly rate.

Knowledge of Results

Adults like feedback on their performance. It is important to understand the concept of the **learning curve.** When a new task is learned, productivity may decrease while a great deal of material is actually being learned. Later, there is little new learning, but productivity may increase greatly. Either situation can be frustrating, and guidance and feedback are important to help employees understand what they have accomplished. In addition, it is important to explain that the employee may reach a plateau where improvement slows or levels off and that this is normal.

Education of Adult Learners

When an organization wants its workers to improve their work habits, it must demonstrate that it values the effort behind the improvements. The organizational climate must support the continued learning and growth of its employees. Some actions the administration might take to indicate this commitment include:

- Providing training during work hours rather than outside the employees' regular work schedules
- Conducting the training off-site to avoid interruptions from day-to-day activities
- Compensating voluntary education with incentives such as bonuses and/or promotions

Adults will remember and understand material that is relevant and has value to them. Therefore, it is important to present an overall picture along with the objectives they are expected to accomplish. Performance standards should be realistic and attainable. Setting artificially high standards reduces motivation and results in feelings of frustration, anxiety, and stress. Thus, employees should feel challenged, but not overwhelmed.

Consideration should be given to the importance of motivation, reinforcement, and knowledge of results. Setting individual goals that challenge employees and satisfy their particular motivators is the ideal. Training methods that allow for the design of individualized programs, such as computer-based training or print-based programmed learning modules, should be considered. Programmed learning modules lead learners through subject material that is presented in short sections, followed immediately by a series of questions that require a written response based on the section just presented. Answers are provided in the module for immediate feedback.

Learning is accomplished best by doing; therefore, it is important to provide as many hands-on activities as possible. Correct responses should be reinforced immediately. Recognition by the trainer or feedback about achievement may be just as effective as monetary rewards in providing reinforcement.

Adults learn better in small units because their attention span is usually not long. In addition, they want to be in control of the situation and learn at their own pace. Where possible, training should be delivered in a modular fashion over a longer period of time. The employee who learns quickly can move forward whereas the slower learner can devote more time to a specific activity.

Check Your Understanding 24.2

Instructions: Answer the following questions on a separate piece of paper.

1. What role does motivation play in developing a training program?

2. Give an example of a reinforcer other than a monetary reward.

3. Performance standards should be set higher than may reasonably be accomplished. Explain why you agree or disagree with this statement.

4. What two characteristics of adult learners should be considered when training programs are developed?

Delivery Methods

There are many techniques for delivering training, just as there are many purposes of training. Factors that influence selection of a training method include:

- Purpose of the training
- Level of education and experience of the trainees
- Amount of space, equipment, and media available for training
- Number of trainees and their location
- Cost of the method in comparison to desired results
- Need for special accommodation due to disability or cultural differences among the trainees

When the purpose of training is to increase the level of knowledge or to introduce new policies, a different method is appropriate than when the goal is to teach a hands-on skill. Training that requires a lot of room and equipment located near the employees' work area will require a different method than training that needs to be delivered across a distance. Instruction in essential skills or license requirements may justify a higher expenditure than instruction that is helpful, but not mandatory.

Figure 24.6 presents the time and location requirements for various training delivery methods. Some subjects, such as demonstration of a new fire safety procedure, are best taught to a group of learners at the same time and place, for example, in a traditional classroom setting. Other subjects, such as use of online computers, may be taught to individuals at a time and place convenient for them to learn. Audioconferencing is a method used to train people located in different offices, but at one time. Each office can be equipped with a speaker and a transmitter, which enables learners to listen and respond to the same material presented by an instructor located at another site.

Self-Directed Learning

Self-directed learning allows students to progress at their own pace. It presents material, questions the learner, and provides immediate responses with either positive or negative

Figure 24.6.   Location and Time Factors of Various Training Methods

	Same Time	**Different Time**
Same Space	Traditional: Face-to-face meetings Classes	Work station: VCR Computer Interactive video disk
Different Space	Real-time distance learning: Audioconferencing Interactive television (two-way video and two-way audio) Satellite courses (one-way video and two-way audio) Synchronous computer communications	Asynchronous distance learning: Correspondence courses Video-based telecourses Online computer courses (computers and modems) Multimedia on demand (just-in-time)

© 2002 Michigan Virtual University.

Source: Levenburg, N., and H. Major. 1998. Distance learning: implications for higher education in the 21st century. Originally published in *The Technology Source.* Available online from http://ts.mivu.org/default.asp?show=article&id=66. This information is reprinted here with permission of the publisher.

reinforcement. Providing an employee with the opportunity to control the learning situation is a clear advantage. It is suitable for delivery to one or many employees and is a solution for employees who cannot attend sessions outside work hours because of home or family responsibilities.

Directed Reading

Self-directed learning was originally delivered via textbooks. Although computers have replaced them in some cases, textbooks still work very well at a relatively low cost. Learners are presented with text and diagrams and then respond to questions. Answers to the questions are provided on another page in the same book for easy checking and feedback. Other advantages to using texts are that they are easily portable and may be supported by other media, such as audiotapes. One disadvantage is that learners may not learn much more than the information in the traditional textbook, and the cost of development may not be paid back unless the book is used several times.

An example of a subject using a programmed text is medical terminology. Text and diagrams of a body system are presented, for example, and the learner is asked to label anatomical structures and to answer multiple-choice or fill-in-the-blank questions. An audiotape may be provided to give the pronunciation of the terms introduced in the text.

Computer-Based Training

Computer-based training (CBT) is another method designed to provide individual learners with training at their own pace. The students must have access to a computer on which the program is installed. The explanatory material is presented and followed by a series of questions. The text displayed is accompanied by sounds or drawings to maintain interest and present the material in a creative way. After each question is answered, there is an immediate response or reinforcement by the computer. In most systems, students can repeat sections of the material until they have mastered it. The cost of developing CBT courses is higher than classroom instruction or texts, but once developed, the cost of delivery is less because the course can be used multiple times.

Computer-based training is usually delivered via CD-ROM or DVD-ROM. Both provide an excellent way to deliver text, audio, video clips, and animation and are particularly useful for providing simulations of work situations. The advantage of DVD-ROM is a large storage capacity and high quality, with up to two hours of full-screen digital video.

Classroom Learning

When the goal is to train a large number of employees on largely factual knowledge within a short period of time, classroom learning may be the best choice. When the intention is to convey information, this method is effective and economical. However, it is not as appropriate for developing problem-solving skills or improving interpersonal competence.

Teaching a class used to mean using the **lecture** method in which the instructor delivers content and the student listens and observes—primarily one-way communication. This technique usually involves little active participation by the learner. However, because students learn more by doing, today's classroom instruction usually combines lecture with small group discussion, role-playing, student presentations, videotapes, or other means where dialogue is facilitated. Using a combination of methods has proved to be highly effective. Videotape is useful for presenting events or demonstrations not easily accomplished in lectures, such as scenarios on interpersonal communication or conflict resolution or viewing surgical procedures. The class itself may be videotaped and the videotape used to deliver the same material to other shifts or workers unable to attend the class.

Seminars and Workshops

The purpose of in-service and continuing education is to develop new skills or to retrain employees whose jobs have been affected by changes in the organization, external requirements, or new policies or procedures. This type of training is best suited for a more formal setting. Seminars or workshops are typically conducted by experts on a subject and may be held in-house or offered by professional organizations, public or private colleges, or vocational schools.

A workshop or seminar may be offered over the course of one or more days and usually consists of several sessions on specific topics related to an overall theme. Some sessions are large, general classes and others are small, "break-out" classes on topics of limited interest. The cost of workshops and seminars, especially when they are held outside the workplace, is usually high because of the costs of materials, room rental, refreshments, and speaker fees. However, the opportunity to learn from experts in the field is very worthwhile.

Distance Learning

Distance learning offers a delivery mode in which the physical classroom, the instructor, and the students are not all present at the same time and in the same location. Distance-learning systems remove barriers associated with location and timing, both individually and simultaneously. This is a particularly important issue for adult learners. In addition, distance learning supports self-directed and individual learning styles.

Methods that support different locations, but same-time delivery, include live audio- or videoconferencing or **synchronous** computer conferencing via Internet or intranet delivery. Delivery of courses at both different locations and times is accomplished via **asynchronous** Internet or intranet Web-based courses or independent study courses offered through a combination of print-based, video, and computer-based training materials.

Live Audio/Video-Based Courses

With audio- or videoconferencing, employees in several locations can learn together via telephone lines or satellite transmission. Audioconferencing enables students to listen to material delivered by a presenter while looking at handout material or books. At selected points in the presentation, the instructor pauses and students interact and share comments or ask questions about the material. The advantage of audio-conferencing is its relatively low cost compared to video or computer delivery. Moreover, it eliminates the time and expense of travel to the instruction site. It is useful for the same kind of purpose as the lecture method, which is to deliver specific content to a large group of people.

Interactive videoconferencing is delivered via satellite, television, or, most recently, computer and offers one- or two-way video together with two-way audio. With one-way video, students receive the image of the instructor and demonstrations and can both see and hear the presenter, but the instructor cannot see the students. Two-way video permits both parties to see each other and to interact. Improved technology is enhancing the quality as well as reducing the cost of this delivery method.

A teleconferencing network usually consists of video and audio recording equipment and a satellite service to broadcast the signal to televisions in a remote location. Videoconferencing permits additional flexibility in delivering courses that may be enhanced through visual as well as audio presentation, such as those that include demonstrations or simulation exercises. It is useful for training employees in organizations with multiple sites, such as integrated delivery networks with inpatient and outpatient facilities. The expense is justified for large organizations that do extensive training.

Web-Based Courses

The Internet has become a familiar entity in the lives of most people. Internet-based training permits on-demand training, removing both time and space barriers. The medium is familiar to most individuals and requires a minimum of instruction in the specific courseware used to deliver the course. This method provides instruction when, where, and at a pace suited to each learner. The instruction can be delivered in several forms. Early courses used listserv software to distribute software simultaneously to students via e-mail. Students can interact with other students and the instructor via the listserv. The most common form of delivery today is to access courses developed by training organizations or universities via a Web site. Employees are issued a log-on name and password to access the course. Material can be presented using a variety of methods, including text, audio, or video. Relevant material can be accessed through hypertext links embedded in the Web site, which students access with the click of a mouse.

After reviewing the material, students usually interact with other students and instructors either synchronously using a chat room or asynchronously in discussion boards or conferences. The discussion board format is the most frequently used, where students post comments and then review and respond at different times.

Intranets are private computer networks that use Internet technologies but are protected with security features and can only be accessed by employees of the organization. Many

hospitals use intranets to distribute policies, procedures, and education courses on a variety of topics. Material on CD-ROM can be installed and delivered via intranets for employee self-study, as well as other customized courses for specific employee needs.

The advantages of Web-based courses include the availability of the delivery medium (the Internet or intranet), which brings the course to the employee's computer at home or work, and the ability to easily update materials. Multimedia materials—including audio, video, graphics, and animation—provide an interesting way to deliver material and have been shown to result in faster learning and greater retention. They also are well suited to adult learners, meeting their needs for education on their terms of time and location. Although sometimes expensive to develop, the cost of using multimedia materials is usually less compared to the cost of classroom or seminar courses for large numbers of employees.

Intensive Study Courses

Intensive study courses allow a great deal of material to be compressed into a small time frame. A common example is the weekend college, where students attend ten to twelve hours per day on Saturday and Sunday. These courses are usually delivered on a college campus or at a hotel setting and require an overnight stay. This training method is suited for teaching special skills that can best be learned in a setting away from day-to-day operations. Examples of courses include cultural awareness, training in teamwork and empowerment, and management development.

A popular exercise is to take the organization's leadership team to an outdoor setting where they learn spirit and cooperation and the need to rely on others in order to overcome physical obstacles. The process builds trust to be transferred back to the work setting.

Check Your Understanding 24.3

Instructions: Answer the following questions on a separate piece of paper.

1. What factors should be considered in selecting a training method?

2. How is computer-based training as a learning method different from reading textbooks?

3. When is it appropriate to deliver training in a classroom setting?

4. What training obstacles are reduced with distance learning methods?

5. How would a healthcare organization use its intranet to deliver training?

6. What topics are appropriate for intensive study training?

Workforce Retention

A 1998 study by Aon Consulting identified five factors that influence employee commitment to an organization (Odgers and Keeling 2000, p. 214). They include:

- A fearless corporate culture
- Job satisfaction

- Opportunities for personal growth
- Organizational direction
- The company's recognition of employees' need for work–life balance

Many employees leave organizations because of their need for flexibility. As personal lives become more complex, managers must learn to permit their employees more control over their own time if they are to gain their loyalty.

Alternative Staffing Structures

A major resource of healthcare institutions is information. Computer-based health information can be managed in places and at times and by people other than those physically located in the institution. As security and technology advance, new staffing arrangements will present both opportunities and challenges for the health information manager. This presents an opportunity to balance work and the personal lives of employees but will require knowledge of how to manage new legal, technical, and personal issues.

Flextime

Flextime generally refers to the employee's ability to work by varying his or her starting and stopping hours around a core of midshift hours, such as 10 a.m. to 1 p.m. Depending on their position and the institution, employees may have a certain degree of freedom in determining their hours. For example, an employee may be given flexibility to start any time between 6 a.m. and 8 a.m. and leave after having worked seven hours.

Compressed workweeks permit employees to work longer days and three or four days per week rather than the usual five eight-hour days. The advantages of this arrangement include increased productivity due to fewer start-and-stop periods, a reduction in commuting time, and additional days off for personal time. The disadvantages may include fatigue and a greater impact of absenteeism and tardiness.

Another option is **flex years.** With this option, employees may choose (at six-month intervals) the number of hours they work each month for the next year. Flex hours are particularly attractive to parents of young children, who can work more hours during the school year and fewer hours during vacation periods, for example. In the HIM department, this may be a good option if an event such as an accreditation survey or the installation of a new computer system necessitates a heavier workload requiring more hours for a short period of time, but fewer hours later.

The advantages of flextime programs include a decrease in tardiness and absenteeism caused by taking time to handle personal matters, more productivity during the hours worked, the ability to adjust hours to the workload, and the opportunity to share limited resources across more employees and hours. Flextime programs also lessen the distinction between employees and supervisors and encourage the delegation of duties. However, such programs can be complex to administer and do not work well in situations where workers depend on the physical presence of others for interactive job responsibilities.

However, it is important to ensure that the flextime arrangement does not violate provisions of the Fair Labor Standards Act, the Occupational Safety and Health Act, or antidiscrimination laws. To avoid problems, the facility's policy should be clear regarding the positions that are eligible for flextime; the work schedule should not be viewed as a reward for only certain employees. In addition, it is important to understand the impact of flextime on benefit plans, which may require employees to work a certain number of hours in a given time period. For example, nonexempt employees may have different regulations than exempt employees regarding overtime pay.

Even with its minor drawbacks, flextime appears to be a viable arrangement and, in most institutions, improves morale, encourages employee responsibility, and results in an overall increase in productivity.

Successful flextime programs have the following conditions in common:

- A person appointed to oversee the program, develop policies and procedures, and resolve differences between supervisors and employees
- A written policy that clearly states the positions that are open to flextime and those that are not
- An orientation program for supervisors when the program is first introduced or as part of a new supervisor's introduction to the organization
- A job function that will benefit from flexibility, for example, one that has high and low workloads at different time periods and one that permits the employee to work independently

Job Sharing

Job sharing is a work arrangement in which two or more people share one full-time job. For example, one employee may work mornings and another afternoons, but it also can mean working different days or weeks. A distinction must be made between job sharing and part-time work. In job sharing, one full-time job is split and all employees sharing the job may perform parts of the same project. Part-time jobs involve employees who work fewer than full-time hours and perform their jobs independently of others.

The main advantage of job sharing is that it enables organizations to attract employees who otherwise may not work because of personal responsibilities. This is an attractive option for parents and employees who want to attend school. The success of job sharing depends on the individuals in the job. They must be mature and cooperative and must want to work toward achieving the objectives of the job. Frequent communication is important regarding the status of projects or unplanned events that may alter the work requirements for a given day.

The disadvantages of job sharing include lack of continuity, particularly when one employee starts a task in the morning and another is responsible for completing it later in the day, and decreased productivity when the employees are not cooperative or fail to communicate well. Job sharing also may cause confusion for other employees or the public, who have to interact with several individuals rather than one.

Home-Based Work

Computer technology has created a new option for employees who work at home—**telecommuting.** HIM departments have seen an increase in the number of coders and medical transcriptionists who choose this option. Telecommuting provides an opportunity for employees who cannot travel from home for reasons such as physical or personal limitations to become employed and helps resolve the problem of shortages of qualified employees in critical job functions. It is an excellent alternative for physically challenged individuals. Individuals who choose this option are employees of the institution and are covered by the same policies and benefits as those who work on-site. The employer usually provides a computer and any networking hardware and software, and the employee is required to submit a detailed time sheet of hours worked.

The advantages of telecommuting include freedom from the time, expense, and physical requirements of commuting; the ability to work flexible hours; increased productivity; lack of distractions from other employees; and an increase in personal time. Moreover, the institution benefits from a reduced need for physical space and improved recruitment.

The disadvantages of telecommuting include employee difficulty in separating work and personal life and feelings of isolation. The "invisible" employee also creates unique challenges for the supervisor. One way to resolve this issue is to have the employee and the manager enter into a telecommuting agreement that defines the expectations of both parties regarding location, hours, equipment, and confidentiality. (See figure 24.7 for a sample agreement.) Suggested items to include in the agreement include work schedule, communication frequency and methods, performance measures, confidentiality requirements, equipment maintenance responsibilities, and environmental safety requirements.

A particular issue for the HIM department is the confidentiality and security of personal health information transmitted over networks as records are sent for coding and dictation is sent for transcription. In addition, the information needs to be secured while in the employee's home, where it can be subject to physical damage or be viewed by the employee's family members or friends. The Health Insurance Portability and Accountability Act (HIPAA), in particular, will provide specific requirements for remote access, including secure transmission, assurance of data integrity, and authentication methods.

As with flextime, clearly stated policies should be in place regarding who is eligible for telecommuting arrangements and their impact on benefit plans. Workers' compensation issues have not been fully resolved. If an employee trips in the home, for example, is this a workers' compensation injury? The answer appears to center on whether the individual was doing work at the time of the injury.

Although many issues still need answers, it appears that telecommuting will increasingly become an important option for HIM departments as a way to recruit and retain satisfied employees.

Outsourcing

In some cases, flexible job arrangements may not be an option for employees. Another solution to the problem of a shortage of qualified staff is **outsourcing.** In this arrangement, the institution contracts with an independent company with expertise in a specific job function. The outside company then assumes full responsibility for performing the function rather than just supplying staff. Thus, the health information manager's responsibility shifts from supervising employees to managing a vendor relationship.

Common functions that are candidates for outsourcing in the HIM department include transcription, release of information, and, most recently, coding. The outsourcing company may perform the functions either at the institution or partially or completely off-site. Advances in communication and security technology have resulted in many home-based workers being employed by such independent companies.

The advantages of outsourcing to the health information manager include the ability to complete work efficiently and with high quality while avoiding the problem of staff recruitment and supervision. With the increase in companies providing these services, outsourcing also can mean a reduction in cost because of competitive bidding. The advantages to the employees of outside companies include flextime and telecommuting—the ability to work varying hours, an increase in personal time, and increased morale. The disadvantages for the health information manager include less immediate control over the quantity and quality of the work, the need to know negotiation techniques, and the reliance on the vendor. HIPAA implementation also will require special arrangements regarding security and confidentiality for outsourcing contractors.

Suggestions for successful outsourcing arrangements include:

- Seeking assistance from someone skilled in negotiation when developing the contract with the vendor
- Engaging legal counsel to review the language of the contract to ensure that it complies with the HIPAA requirements
- Requiring competitive bidding for each outsourced service at regular intervals
- Establishing expectations and performance standards for contractors
- Monitoring compliance with performance standards
- Performing periodic customer surveys to assess satisfaction with the service

Employee Development

In addition to the need to balance work and personal life, employees often look for opportunities for personal growth. By nature, they want to learn new skills and further their careers. A significant amount of training should be devoted to developing the ability of employees to help themselves—to realize that they are the ones responsible for their advancement.

Empowerment

Empowerment is the concept of providing employees with the tools and resources to solve problems themselves. In other words, employees obtain power over their work situation by assuming responsibility. Empowered employees have the freedom to contribute ideas and perform their jobs in the best possible way. The idea of empowerment actually began as part of total quality management programs, which many organizations initiated in order to improve the quality of service provided to customers and to increase their competitiveness in the marketplace. A high-quality organization strives to understand and improve work processes in order to prevent problems.

Healthcare organizations that empower their employees believe that all employees can perform—and truly want to perform—to their highest potential when given the proper resources and environment. Because they perform jobs on a regular basis, they are intimately familiar with the steps in the process. What the employees may lack are skills in analysis and problem solving. Training sessions in skills such as data analysis, use of control charts, or flowcharting will help employees to identify problems, develop alternatives, and recommend solutions.

Figure 24.7.   Sample Telecommuting Agreement

Telecommuting Agreement

I have read and understand the attached Telecommuting Policy, and agree to the duties, obligations, responsibilities, and conditions for telecommuters described in that document.

I agree that, among other things, I am responsible for establishing specific telecommuting work hours, furnishing and maintaining my remote work space in a safe manner, employing appropriate telecommuting security measures, and protecting company assets, information, trade secrets, and systems.

I understand that telecommuting is voluntary and I may stop telecommuting at any time. I also understand that the company may at any time change any or all of the conditions under which I am permitted to telecommute, or withdraw permission to telecommute.

1. Remote work location:

_____
Employee residence

_____
Company premises

_____
Description of work space at remote work location

2. Telecommuting schedule:

_____
On a weekly basis as follows

_____
On a monthly basis as follows

_____
No regular schedule (separate permission for each telecommuting day)

3. Regular telecommuting work hours:

    From _____ to _____

_____
Meal break/other breaks

4. Company assets to be used at remote work location (description and ID numbers):

5. Company information systems to be accessed from remote work location (list):

6. Noncompany equipment, software, and data used at remote work location (list):

7. Other

Source: Fletcher, D. 1999. Practice Brief: Telecommuting. *Journal of the American Health Information Management Association* 70(2):56A–D.

To perform effectively, employees also need to be given responsibility, authority, and the trust to make decisions and act independently within their area of expertise. Figure 24.8 offers suggestions on how managers can empower their employees.

Empowered employees are less likely to complain or feel helpless or frustrated when they cannot resolve a problem on their own. Moreover, they are more likely to feel a sense of accomplishment and to be more receptive to solutions that they develop themselves. In addition, they tend to demonstrate commitment and self-confidence and to produce high-quality work.

One disadvantage that is frequently mentioned by managers is that empowerment involves too much time for meetings and discussion and takes employees away from the "real work." Actually, it is much more efficient to take the time necessary to prevent problems than to solve them after they occur. In the long run, empowered employees work more efficiently and productively.

Indeed, some managers are afraid to share power. They feel that they have worked hard to gain the power they have and are reluctant to give it up. But the manager who empowers others usually increases his or her own power because a high-performing unit reflects the manager's expertise.

An example of empowerment in the HIM department would be to train employees in the release of information function to solve a slow turnaround issue. The employees are probably more aware than the supervisor of problems that prevent them from filling requests for information (missing charts, insufficient fees, incomplete records). With proper training in brainstorming and flowcharting, as well as a supportive environment, the employees may be able to develop a procedure that can be performed differently to prevent delays.

Delegation

Delegation is the process of distributing work duties and decision making to others. To be effective, delegation should be commensurate with authority and responsibility. A manager must assign responsibility, which is an expectation that another person will perform tasks. At the same time, **authority,** or the right to act in ways necessary to carry out assigned tasks, must be granted. An employee cannot be expected to perform a job for which he or she is not given authority to obtain resources. Authority should equal responsibility when work is delegated. Finally, **accountability** must be created, which is the requirement to answer to a supervisor for results. An employee must be empowered to act, given the necessary tools and skills, and held accountable for the quality of his or her work.

Successful delegation includes:

- Assigning responsibility
- Granting authority
- Creating accountability

Guidelines for delegating are presented in figure 24.9. As an employee development tool, delegation can provide employees the opportunity to try new tasks previously performed by someone in a higher position and leads to empowerment because employees are given the opportunity to contribute ideas and fully utilize their skills. At the same time, the manager should remain available to provide assistance and support.

Sometimes managers have difficulty delegating because they feel that only they can do the job correctly. In other cases, they feel threatened by the idea that another employee can do their tasks and perhaps do them better. This thinking can lead to poor morale and result in talented employees leaving the organization. In addition, it can lead to managers being overburdened with work that could be done by others and to employees being denied opportunities to learn new skills.

In some situations, employees may be unwilling to accept delegated responsibilities when they feel that they are unqualified to do the tasks or that they are being dumped on. Dumping can involve assigning an employee unpleasant or unpopular work that seems to have little value or asking an employee to take on work in addition to an already demand-

Figure 24.8.   How to Empower Employees

- Get others involved in selecting their work assignments and the methods for accomplishing tasks.
- Create an environment of cooperation, information sharing, discussion, and shared ownership of goals.
- Encourage others to take initiative, make decisions, and use their knowledge.
- When problems arise, find out what others think and let them help design the solutions.
- Stay out of the way; give others the freedom to put their ideas and solutions into practice.
- Maintain high morale and confidence by recognizing successes and encouraging high performance.

Source: Schermerhorn, J. 2002. *Management,* seventh edition. New York City: John Wiley & Sons, p. 342.

Figure 24.9.   Rules for Effective Delegation

- Create an environment of cooperation, information sharing, discussion, and shared ownership of goals.
- Carefully choose the person to whom you delegate.
- Define the responsibility; make the assignment clear.
- Agree on performance objectives and standards.
- Agree on a performance timetable.
- Give authority; allow the other person to act independently.
- Show trust in the other person.
- Provide performance support.
- Give performance feedback.
- Recognize and reinforce progress.
- Help when things go wrong.
- Don't forget your accountability for performance results.

Source: Schermerhorn, J. 2002. *Management,* seventh edition. New York City: John Wiley & Sons, p. 273.

ing workload. This results in resentment or anger. Employees may feel this way when they have a poor working relationship with their supervisor, know that others have refused the same task, or have been taken advantage of in the past.

To avoid these problems, employees should be selected who are either competent to perform the tasks or willing to undergo the necessary training. People are more willing to accept tasks that they understand, have a choice in doing, and recognize value added to the organization and their personal growth. Managers should set checkpoints, monitor how the delegate is doing, and allow the opportunity for questions and feedback.

Delegation is a skill that matches the right employee with the right task. It requires communication, support, and an environment that fosters risk taking. Effective delegation actually leads to a more efficient and productive department overall and mutually benefits the manager, the employee, and the institution.

Coaching and Mentoring

Both new employees and experienced employees who may be ready for a change can benefit from coaching or mentoring. As discussed earlier in this chapter, coaching is an ongoing process in which an experienced person offers performance advice to a less experienced person. However, coaching goes beyond teaching. A good coach is also a counselor, a resource person, a troubleshooter, and a cheerleader. Coaches deal with improving attitudes, morale, and career development in addition to giving instruction in specific tasks.

Effective coaches are dedicated leaders who display a high level of competence and are able to push or pull employees to their highest level of performance. They are role models who set a good example; show workers what is expected and how to get the job done well; provide praise or constructive feedback, where appropriate; and are ready to help with routine work alongside the employee, if necessary.

Coaching starts with orientation of the new employee and continues throughout his or her time with the organization. The more time the coach spends walking around observing and listening to employees, the more opportunities there will be to support, praise, and offer advice.

Helping employees should be done in a manner that encourages self-sufficiency. For example, when an employee comes forward with a problem, a good coach does not simply give the answer but, rather, asks the employee for suggestions. In other words, the coach's response should be "What do you think?" rather than "Here's what you should do."

Coaches defend and support their employees. They are facilitators who remove obstacles and obtain resources to enable and empower their staffs. It is important to praise performance above and beyond the expected, for example, when the employee completes a task ahead of schedule or offers to help a colleague. It is equally important to praise the worker who consistently meets objectives or improves in an area that was below standard—in other words, for doing what is

expected. To be effective, both positive and negative feedback must be timely, specific, and in the right setting (privately or publicly depending on the circumstance). Good coaches direct negative feedback at the behavior they wish to correct, not at the person.

However, coaching can be done poorly. This happens when criticism is overused or praise is undeserved. In addition, the approach needs to be adjusted to the employee. Good coaching takes time to allow flexibility and encourage the employee to perform correctly without jumping in too quickly with advice.

Mentoring is a form of coaching. A mentor is a senior employee who works with employees early in their careers, giving them advice on developing skills and career options. Several employees may be assigned as protégés to the mentor, but contact is usually one on one. Through the mentoring relationship, employees have an advisor with whom they can solve problems, analyze and learn from mistakes, and celebrate successes. Many organizations have formal mentoring programs where protégés are matched with potential mentors. Other managers voluntarily offer to work with up-and-coming employees.

Mentors share their knowledge of management styles and teach prospective supervisors specific job or interpersonal skills. They may assign challenging projects that allow employees to explore real-life learning experiences while still under the guidance of an experienced teacher. Successful mentoring depends on effective interaction between the mentor and protégé. Mentors must be chosen who enjoy passing on their experience and knowledge to others.

Promotion

Promotion may be another tool to encourage employee development and commitment. When tied to training programs, it can become a powerful incentive. Promotion usually refers to the upward progression of an employee in both job and salary. However, it also can mean a lateral move to a different position with similar job skills or to a change within the same job as a result of completing higher education or credentialing requirements. To attract, retain, and motivate employees, organizations should provide a career development system that promotes from within.

When tied to promotion, career development programs offer an incentive to ambitious employees. Goals can be incorporated into the performance review process. In the HIM department, clerical employees can be encouraged to take classes that would lead to an associate's degree in health information technology or a bachelor's degree in health information administration, making them eligible for certification exams. In addition, employees may be encouraged to enter coding certificate programs and achieve coding certification.

The higher the status of the person in the organization, the likelier it is that promotion will work as a motivator. To improve employee performance, promotion should be awarded based on competence, not on seniority. In some organizations, union contracts emphasize seniority and thus restrict the organizations' ability to use competence as a sole criterion.

Promotion based on performance is usually measured by appraising past performance against standards. However, past performance does not always predict future potential. Some organizations use testing instruments to assess this capability.

Succession planning is a specific type of promotional plan in which senior-level position openings are anticipated and candidates are identified from within the organization. The candidates are given training through formal education, job rotation, and mentoring so that they can eventually assume these positions.

To be effective, promotion criteria should be published in a formal policy and procedure, which usually includes job postings of open positions, so that all employees have the opportunity to apply for consideration. When promotions appear to be given to favored employees, or when the procedure is shrouded in secrecy, promotion ceases to be attractive.

Continuing Education

Continuing education is a requirement of most professionals, including those in health information management. It usually requires a person to complete a certain number of hours of education within a given time period to maintain a credential or license status. Accrediting organizations, such as the JCAHO, also include continuing education in their standards. The HIM field is changing rapidly, primarily in the areas of technology and legal and regulatory requirements. It is important that credentialed professionals remain current in their knowledge of the profession so that they can provide high-quality skills to the organizations for which they work.

Continuing education refers to keeping up with changes in the profession or to improving skills required to perform the same job. It is different from career development, which is geared toward preparing an individual for a new job. Sometimes this line is blurred. In health information management, management development programs may be essential for the current position, when one is already a supervisor, for example. On the other hand, preparing a technical employee to assume a new management role would be considered career development. Some organizations have tuition reimbursement policies to encourage career development.

Continuing education (CE) programs are most often provided by external organizations, such as the American Health Information Management Association (AHIMA) or local chapters. Career development, by contrast, usually includes a combination of job rotation through progressively increasing job responsibilities in-house and externally taught formal classes and workshops.

As part of the formal performance appraisal process, CE goals should be set for all employees. A record should be kept in the employee's personnel file that indicates the number of CE hours earned as well as the topic, place, and person who provided the education. Management should support

the individual's achievement by providing time off to attend workshops, flexible scheduling for formal classes offered at educational institutions, and financial reimbursement.

CE programs are delivered via many different formats to suit the individual learner. These include classroom as well as computer-based modules or Web-based courses that all employees can access, regardless of where they live or their personal or physical limitations. Continued skill development should be an important requirement for all HIM employees.

Check Your Understanding 24.4

Instructions: Answer the following questions on a separate piece of paper.

1. In what work situations would an HIM department benefit from a flextime work arrangement?
2. What is one advantage to the employee of working compressed work-weeks? To the department?
3. What potential problems with flextime should a manager be wary of? Give the possible solution to each problem.
4. What is the difference between job sharing and traditional part-time employment?
5. What items should be included in a telecommuting agreement?
6. What are two functions that the HIM department commonly outsources?
7. What factors help ensure the success of an outsourcing arrangement?
8. What are three ways managers can empower employees?
9. What two reasons might managers have for not empowering employees?
10. How are the concepts of delegation and empowerment related?
11. What three actions must be done for effective delegation?
12. When might an employee resist accepting delegated responsibilities?
13. What are the basic characteristics of effective coaches?
14. How does mentoring differ from coaching? How is it similar?
15. On what should promotion be based if it is to motivate?
16. Why do HIM professionals need continuing education?

Departmental Employee Training and Development Plan

Every healthcare organization and every HIM department have unique training needs. The level of education and experience of the employees, the tasks they perform, and the resources available will change the focus of training efforts. As table 24.1 shows, employee development is a continuum of concepts. The content, objectives, and frequency of a training program are all dependent on the specific situation that exists in an organization.

Training and Development Model

The following model can be applied on various levels and will help an organization's human resources department or a health information manager identify and fulfill the training needs of their employee group:

- *Step 1:* Perform a needs analysis.
- *Step 2:* Set training objectives.

- *Step 3:* Design the curriculum.
- *Step 4:* Determine the location and method of delivery.
- *Step 5:* Pilot the program.
- *Step 6:* Implement the program.
- *Step 7:* Evaluate the effectiveness of the program.
- *Step 8:* Make changes as needed.
- *Step 9:* Provide feedback to interested groups.

The plan should be approved and supported by upper management. Implementing a training program requires a substantial investment of time, money, and personnel. Developing a curriculum based on a systematic evaluation of needs is a much wiser investment than creating a program around the latest hot topic.

Perform a Needs Analysis

The needs analysis is critical to design of the plan. This approach typically focuses on three levels: the organization, the specific job tasks, and the individual employee. The outcome of the needs analysis is an understanding of where training is needed in the organization (entry-level, remedial, or management development). In addition, a list of the tasks to be learned at each level (based on the job description and the job specification, the specific skills and knowledge required), and an analysis of the deficiencies in knowledge and skills between the desired level and current level of employees are completed.

This information can be obtained through observation, employee and manager interviews, surveys, tests, and task analysis of the job descriptions and job specifications.

Set Training Objectives

After the needs have been established, specific, measurable training objectives should be set. Objectives specify what the employee should be able to accomplish at completion of the training program. These are based on the deficiencies that have been identified between the desired and current performance levels. It is important to set objectives before starting the program so that the results can be evaluated following completion of training.

Design the Curriculum

The curriculum is the subject content of the program that will be taught, including the sequence, activities, and materials. A budget needs to be prepared that identifies costs and available resources. Are there individuals within the organization who can develop and teach the program, or is it necessary to purchase an externally prepared program? Do materials such as videotapes or computer-based modules need to be produced? Do printed materials need to be developed and reproduced? Will the program be available over the Internet?

After these decisions are made, the curriculum must be organized into a program that supports adult learning and the stated objectives. All program elements need to be carefully prepared to ensure quality and effectiveness.

Determine the Location and Method of Delivery

Where and when the program should be delivered is an important part of the training plan. When space is available and the instructor and materials are available internally, a classroom setting might be suitable. On the other hand, when employees work over several shifts and days or in remote locations, computer-based CD-ROMs and/or Web-based delivery might permit the employee to more readily achieve the training objectives.

Pilot the Program

It is important to validate the program by introducing it to a test audience. When computer technology is part of the program delivery, all computer programs should be tested to make sure they work with a variety of hardware and/or Web browsers. Following completion of the program by a few employees, feedback should be obtained and the program revised, if necessary.

Implement the Program

The tested program now can be given to the entire audience for which it has been developed. When necessary, train-the-trainer workshops should be conducted for instructors who may not have formal training experience.

Evaluate the Effectiveness of the Program

Two issues should be addressed in evaluating training programs. The first is the method of evaluation; the second is the outcomes that will be measured.

Evaluation is most frequently assessed using a survey, such as the samples in figures 24.2 and 24.5. Opinions obtained immediately after the training, and again after a period of time, are valuable in assessing the effectiveness of the program for both trainees and managers. In addition, pretests and posttests help identify the level of knowledge or skill that has actually been learned.

When possible, an excellent method for evaluating the training program is to conduct a controlled experiment. A control group that receives no training is compared to a group that received training. Data are obtained from both groups both before and after training. It is then possible to determine the extent to which the training program caused a change in performance in the training group.

Four outcomes can be measured in evaluating effective training programs:

- *Reaction:* What is the reaction of the trainees immediately after the program? Are they excited about what they learned?
- *Learning:* What have the trainees actually learned? Can they now use a new software program?
- *Behavior:* Have supervisors noticed a change in employee behavior? Has morale improved?
- *Results:* How does the actual level of performance compare with the established objectives? Can the employees assign codes more accurately?

Make Changes as Needed

When the results of the evaluation show less-than-expected results, it is important to determine where changes may be helpful. This may include a change in the materials, the location or time of program delivery, or the subject content. In any case, it is important to adjust. A program that is not meeting the desired objectives is costly.

Provide Feedback to Interested Groups

After tallying the results of the evaluations and making any adjustments that are needed, it is important to provide feedback to the course developers, managers and supervisors of the involved departments, and the trainees. Communication is vital to maintaining interest and support for the training program. Feedback demonstrates a desire to respond to the needs of everyone involved in this important activity.

Check Your Understanding 24.5

Instructions: Answer the following questions on a separate piece of paper.

1. What are the steps in a typical training and development plan?
2. What are three outcomes of a needs analysis?
3. What is the relationship between setting objectives and evaluating a training program?
4. What are three items to consider in designing a training program?
5. What are four outcomes that should be measured in program evaluation?

Real-World Case

The employees of the HIM department in Midwest Community Hospital, a 100-bed facility located in the Chicago suburbs, have just returned from a meeting. Their director, Gary Smith, announced that the hospital was recently acquired by a large integrated delivery system, Hometown Health Systems. Gary has been with the organization for thirty years and has indicated his intention to retire when the facilities merge, which is scheduled to occur in about six months. Hometown's corporate director of health information systems, Jane Winters, will assume responsibility for managing the department, with an assistant director to be appointed at Midwest who will assume day-to-day supervisory responsibilities.

Jane knows that three employees at Midwest might be qualified to assume the position and would like to fill it through promotion. All three candidates have positive and negative factors, some of which could be remedied with training. Gary and Jane plan to discuss the best approach to selecting the new supervisor, and Gary has been asked to assist in the process by preparing the selected employee for the transition. After returning from the meeting, Gary begins to review the three employees in his mind.

Bob has worked in the release of information area of the department for three years and recently obtained his RHIT credential after attending a local community college program. He is enthusiastic about working in the department and has frequently suggested new procedures, which has led to some friction with Gary, whose motto is "If it ain't broke, don't fix it!" Now that he has the credential, Bob has mentioned that he may want to begin looking elsewhere if his ideas are not appreciated at Midwest.

Sherry is a coder who has worked at Midwest for about one year. She began her employment at the hospital in the outpatient registration area. After completing the AHIMA's online coding program, she assumed the coding position in the HIM department about six months ago. She is a single parent who is a self-proclaimed workaholic. In her spare time, she works at home as a coder for a physician's office to increase her income.

Linda currently works as the lead file clerk in the department. Of the three employees, she is the only one with supervisory experience, although she has had no formal management training. Gary had promoted her to the lead position because of her excellent attendance record and seniority. However, her employees have complained frequently to Gary that she "takes over" and corrects their work without explaining what they did wrong. Gary also knows that she does not feel comfortable disciplining employees and that she finds doing the job herself easier than working with the employee responsible for the job.

Gary will be meeting next Monday with Jane and is still unsure how to solve this dilemma.

Discussion Questions

1. What would be the advantages and disadvantages of promoting one of the employees to the assistant director position? What would be the advantages and disadvantages of selecting someone from outside the hospital?
2. What would be your approach to solving the problem?
3. Develop a training plan to prepare each employee for the supervisory position. For each employee, discuss the needs, objectives, curriculum, best delivery mode, and method to assess his or her readiness for the position.
4. Describe an appropriate succession plan for Gary after the candidate has been selected.

Summary

Employees are the healthcare institution's most valuable asset. The decreasing availability of qualified employees means that responsibility for developing staff increasingly rests with the employer. Workforce development and retention must become part of the institution's strategic plan.

Training and development needs can be viewed on a continuum of five conceptual areas: orientation, training, inservice education, continuing education, and career development. Each healthcare organization's training program must be able to adapt to the different needs of its employees.

New employees need to be introduced to the rules and culture of the organization, the department, and the specific job duties they will be performing. This function is typically performed through a formal orientation program that provides employees with information regarding organizational policies and procedures, benefits, safety regulations, and an introduction to the work area. Finally, employees begin learning the duties and responsibilities of the specific jobs they will be performing. Preparing staff to carry out their specific job tasks should be an ongoing effort. Methods used to accomplish this include on-the-job-training, job rotation, and cross-training.

In-service education builds on basic skills provided during orientation and on-the-job training. It also is used when departments are restructured or when external requirements require employees to update their competency. This training needs to be available on a continuous basis and may be conducted by department managers in formal training sessions or through self-directed learning methods.

The techniques used to deliver training should be matched with the purpose of training, the trainee's level of education and experience, location, and budget. Self-directed learning permits students to determine the pace of the learning. A number of CD-ROMs provide computer-based training for this purpose. Classroom lectures are useful for training large numbers of employees on factual knowledge in a short time period. Distance learning is an option for students who cannot be present in the classroom. Distance learning methods include audioconferencing, live teleconferencing, and synchronous or asynchronous Web-based courses.

Because training programs require a considerable investment of both time and money, the organization should encourage commitment to long-term employment. An important factor in maintaining job satisfaction is recognition by the company of employee needs for work–life balance. Alternative staffing arrangements permit employees to vary work hours and locations while still satisfying the organization's need for productivity. Options include flextime programs, job sharing, and telecommuting. For those who wish to work on a limited basis or for employers who cannot find qualified staff, outsourcing may be an option.

Another factor that enhances employee job satisfaction is the opportunity for personal growth. Employees should be empowered with the tools and resources to solve problems themselves. Successful managers delegate effectively. Effective delegation leads to a more efficient and productive department and mutually benefits the manager, the employee, and the institution.

Employees just beginning their careers may benefit from mentoring. Mentors advise and teach specific job and interpersonal skills. Coaching is a process that begins in orientation and continues throughout the employee's time with the organization. Coaches act as role models, provide praise and constructive feedback, and help with routine work when needed.

Promotion can be a powerful incentive for employees when tied to career development programs. Promotion should be awarded on competence, not seniority, and the criteria should be based on objective standards. Employees who hold professional credentials must complete continuing education requirements to remain current in their knowledge of the profession. Continued skill development should be an important requirement for all HIM employees.

Because the training needs of every department are unique, it is important to develop a formal training and development plan. The plan begins with a needs analysis and the establishment of measurable objectives. A curriculum is then designed to meet those needs.

A successful and effective plan for employee training and development requires a substantial investment of time, money, and personnel. The plan should be approved and supported by upper management and should be based on a systematic evaluation of needs.

References

Chan, S. 2000. The Invisible Factors of Telecommuting. Available online from http://www.workforce.com/archive/feature/00/06/92.

Dessler, G. 2000. *Human Resources Management,* eighth edition. New York City: Prentice-Hall.

Fletcher, D. 1999. Practice Brief: Telecommuting. *Journal of the American Health Information Management Association* 70(2):56A–D.

Flynn, Gillian. 2001. The Legalities of Flextime. Available online from http://www.workforce.com/feature/00/18.

Fottler, H., S. Hernandez, and C. Joiner, editors. 1998. *Essentials of Human Resource Management in Health Service Organizations.* Albany, N.Y.: Delmar Publishers.

Greer, C. 2001. *Strategic Human Resources Management,* second edition. New York City: Prentice-Hall.

Hutchins, Jennifer. 2000. Steps to effective orientation. *Workforce* 79(11):40. Available online from http://workforce.com/archive/feature/00/05/67/0011356.xci.

Keeling, B., and N. Kallaus. 1996. *Administrative Office Management,* eleventh edition. Cincinnati: South-Western Educational Publishing.

Levenburg, N., and H. Major. 1998. Distance learning: implications for higher education in the 21st century. Originally published in *The Technology Source.* Available online from http://ts.mivu.org/default.asp?show=article&id=66.

O'Connor, B. N., M. Bronner, and C. Delaney. 2002. *Training for Organizations,* second edition. Cincinnati: South-Western Publishing Company.

Odgers, P., and B. Keeling. 2000. *Administrative Office Management,* twelfth edition. Cincinnati: South-Western Educational Publishing.

Schermerhorn, J. 2002. *Management,* seventh edition. New York City: John Wiley & Sons.

Smith, H., and M. Fottler. 1998. Training and development. In *Essentials of Human Resources Management in Health Services Organizations,* M. D. Fottler et al., editors. Albany, N.Y.: Delmar Publishers.

Stum, D. 1998. Five ingredients for an employee retention formula. *HR Focus,* p. S10.

Training Evaluation Form. Available online from http://workforce.com/archive.

Umiker, W. 1998. *Management Skills for the New Health Care Supervisor,* third edition. Gaithersburg, Md.: Aspen Publications.

Wexley, K., and G. Latham. 2002. *Developing and Training Human Resources in Organizations,* third edition. New York City: Prentice-Hall.

Web sites for further information:

American Society for Training and Development, the association for workplace learning and performance professionals, available at www.astd.org.

Workforce, an organization that provides a variety of human resources tools, including a magazine and electronic newsletter, available at www.workforce.com/section/11/.

Application Exercises

1. You are the director of an HIM department and have just hired a recently credentialed RHIT to fill the position of transcription supervisor. She will supervise two employees who work at the hospital and five employees who are home based. Develop a checklist for her new employee orientation.

2. Your release of information section has developed a one-month backlog in responding to routine requests. The employees are complaining that they need another photocopy machine because the one they have is always being used by the transcriptionists. You are sympathetic but know there is no funding for additional equipment this year. In addition, they do not like the procedure the new supervisor has implemented for pulling charts, claiming it is much slower than the old way. The employees think they have a better idea, but the supervisor is not open to changes. What solutions would you suggest to reduce the backlog?

3. The director of human resources has asked for your expertise in developing a training program on medical terminology for clerical employees in the emergency room and outpatient registration areas. How would you perform a needs assessment to determine the amount of training needed and the best delivery mode for the current employees?

4. Use an Internet search engine or journals to locate two outsourcing companies for transcription. Contact them via their Web site, e-mail, or letter, and compare them on the following features:
   - Number of years in business
   - Number of employees
   - Services provided
   - Cost of services
   - Confidentiality agreements
   - Turnaround time
   - Another feature of your choice

   Identify which company you would select and explain your reasons.

5. Compare your experience as a student in a traditional classroom with another method described in this chapter to which you have been exposed (Web-based, online, independent study, on-the-job training, and so on. Describe what you liked or disliked about each method and suggest ways to improve them.

Review Quiz

Instructions: Complete the following sentences with the appropriate answer.

1. ___ A work schedule that requires employees to be at their job between 10:00 a.m. and 2:00 p.m. but permits them to vary their schedule during the rest of the day to fit their needs is called ___.
   a. A compressed workweek
   b. Flextime
   c. Telecommuting
   d. Job sharing

2. ___ The form of coaching in which an individual in the beginning stages of a career is matched as a protégé with a senior person is known as ___.
   a. Mentoring
   b. Cross-training
   c. Orientation
   d. Motivation

3. ___ A set of activities designed to familiarize new employees with their jobs, the organization, and the work culture is called ___.
   a. Training
   b. Job analysis
   c. Job rotation
   d. Orientation

4. ___ All of the following techniques are useful in educating adults except ___.
   a. Motivation
   b. Knowledge of results
   c. Reinforcement
   d. Setting exceptionally high standards

5. ___ A distance learning method where groups of employees in multiple classroom locations may listen to and see the material presented at the same time via satellite or telephone is called ___.
   a. Audioconferencing
   b. Computer-based training
   c. Teleconferencing
   d. DVD-ROM

6. ___ Distributing work duties to others along with the right to make decisions and take action is called ___.
   a. Delegation
   b. Coaching
   c. Accountability
   d. Communication

7. ___ On-the-job training may include all of the following delivery methods except ___.
   a. Job rotation
   b. One-on-one training by supervisor
   c. Seminars
   d. Computer-based modules

8. ___ A solution to the problem of staff recruitment for coding and transcription is ___.
   a. Outsourcing
   b. Telecommuting
   c. Job sharing
   d. All of the above

9. ___ A successful departmental training and development plan begins with ___.
   a. Designing the curriculum
   b. Performing a needs assessment
   c. Selecting the delivery methods
   d. Determining the latest hot topic

10. ___ The training method that is best used to train a large number of employees in the same location on largely factual knowledge would be ___.
    a. Classroom lecture
    b. Web-based chat rooms
    c. Teleconferencing
    d. CD-ROM

Chapter 25
Financial Management

Nadinia Davis, MBA, CIA, CPA, RHIA

Learning Objectives

- To read, understand, and use balance sheets and income statements
- To explain the difference between financial accounting and managerial accounting
- To recognize the importance of accounting to nonfinancial managers
- To calculate and identify the components of basic financial ratios
- To understand the importance of internal controls and their role in financial management
- To describe the components of operational and capital budgets
- To discuss the impact of claims processing and reimbursement on financial statements
- To describe the financial management functions of HIM professionals

Key Terms

Account	Depreciation	Income statement	Request for proposal (RFP)
Accounting	Detective control	Interim period	Reserves
Accounting rate of return	Direct method of cost allocation	Internal rate of return (IRR)	Retained earnings
Accounts payable	Discharged, no final bill (DNFB)	Inventory	Return on investment (ROI)
Accounts receivable		Journal entry	Revenue
Acid-test ratio	Disclosure	Liabilities	Securities and Exchange Commission (SEC)
Activity-based budget	Double distribution	Managerial accounting	
Assets	Entity	Matching	Simultaneous equations method
Balance sheet	Expenses	Materiality	
Bill hold	Favorable variance	Net income	Sole proprietorship
Capital budget	Financial Accounting Standards Board (FASB)	Net loss	Stable monetary unit
Chargemaster		Net present value	Statement
Claims processing	Financial data	Not-for-profit organizations	Statement of cash flow
Conceptual framework of accounting	Financial transaction	Operational budget	Statement of retained earnings
	Fiscal year	Overhead costs	
Conservatism	Fixed budget	Partnership	Statement of stockholder's equity
Consistency	Flexible budget	Payback period	
Corporation	For-profit organizations	Periodic interim payments (PIPs)	Step-down allocation
Corrective controls	Forecasting		Temporary budget variance
Cost justification	General ledger	Permanent variance	Time period
Cost report	Going concern	Preventive controls	Unfavorable variance
Credits	Government Accounting Standards Board (GASB)	Profitability index	Variance
Current ratio		Purchase order	Variance analysis
Debits		Reliability	Zero-based budget
Debt ratio			

Introduction

Every organization and every industry should have policies and procedures in place to ensure the accurate and timely collection, recording, and reporting of both inter- and intra-organizational transactions. Financial management involves the development, implementation, and oversight of such policies and procedures related to financial transactions as well as the management of funds, both long and short term.

This chapter focuses on the concepts and tools associated with planning and controlling the financial resources required to operate a department or a work unit. It presents operations, labor, and capital budgeting processes and techniques, reviews organizational and departmental financial performance measures, and explores techniques for improving financial performance at the departmental level. Finally, the chapter acquaints readers with the language of financial and managerial accounting so as to enhance their understanding of the role of the HIM professional as a manager.

Theory into Practice

Olga Paluk is director of health information services (HIS) at a 540-bed urban acute care facility and, as such, is responsible for both the HIS and the patient registration departments. She reports to the chief financial officer (CFO), who is a certified public accountant. The inpatient census has been stable for the past three years and is expected to remain so. Further, the facility is stable financially but has only limited resources for improvements and expansion.

Olga has just received her budget instruction package from the CFO's office. She will use this package to request the resources that her departments will need in the coming year. There are two open positions: a patient registrar and an inpatient coder. An inefficient incomplete-chart system and a stand-alone encoder are accommodated with an extra file clerk and a dedicated data-entry clerk. Olga knows that if she is allowed to purchase a better incomplete-chart system and interface the encoder with the main computer, she can reorganize the staffing and promote from within the departments

to fill the positions. She also knows that she will have to justify these actions to the CFO.

Olga will perform a cost analysis of the acquisition of the new equipment and the computer interface. She will compare these costs against the salaries of the eliminated positions. She will also compare the overall cost of using outsourced coding services on a regular basis with the cost of promoting from within. Olga knows that she will have to project the impact over three to five years to illustrate the long-term benefit to the organization.

Because Olga is familiar with the language of financial management and the facility's capital budget analysis process, she is able to justify the cost of the new equipment.

Healthcare Financial Management

The process of financial management involves various players within the organization's financial arena. Table 25.1 lists and describes the roles of the financial personnel who work in hospitals. However, healthcare financial management also involves a number of players outside the financial arena. For example, the process is of particular importance to health information management (HIM) professionals because they are immediately involved with the process of reimbursement.

HIM professionals are familiar with financial data as one of the components of a health record: the data related to payers and billing. To financial managers, **financial data** are the individual elements of organizational financial transactions. (The term financial refers to money and, as is discussed later, money is the measurement of financial transactions.) A **financial transaction** is the exchange of goods or services for payment or the promise of payment. Financial data are compiled into informational reports for users. The degree of detail that users require depends on their needs and is largely influenced by the relationship of the user to the origination of the transaction.

When financial transactions originate at the department level, the user may require specific detail about them. For example, the pharmacy department will review its drug transactions; the HIM department will review its purchases of

Table 25.1.   Financial Personnel and Their Roles in a Hospital

Position	Typical or Minimum Background	Financial Roles
Board of directors or trustees	Depends on the needs of the facility	Ultimate responsibility for the fiscal integrity of the organization
Chief executive officer (CEO)	Generally, master's-prepared in public administration, hospital administration, or business administration; occasionally, clinical background	Overall responsibility for administration of the organization
Chief financial officer (CFO)	Certified public accountant (CPA) or certified management accountant (CMA)	Overall responsibility for related departments, including patient accounts, internal auditing, and often HIM
Controller or accounting manager	CPA	Oversees accounting and cash disbursement, including payroll
Patient accounts manager	Bachelor's degree	Oversees claims processing

supplies and services; and so on. On the administrative level, however, such detail is not usually required. Instead, informative summaries are often more useful. For example, an organization administrator does not usually need to know the number of cases of copier paper purchased in each department. Instead, he or she would look at the total office supply purchases and evaluate whether they were at appropriate and expected levels. Additional detail or explanation would not be required unless the purchases were unusual. The accumulation and reporting of financial data within an organization is an accounting function.

Accounting

Accounting is an activity as well as a profession. Just as there are many HIM roles and functions, so are there diverse accounting roles and functions. The accounting activity involves the collection, recording, and reporting of financial data. Accountants are both the individuals who perform these activities and many of those who use the reported data. Accounting is important because it is the language that organizations use to communicate with each other to effect transactions, determine investment strategies, and evaluate performance.

The **conceptual framework of accounting** underlies all accounting activity and is based on the following ideas:

- The benefits of the financial data should exceed the costs of obtaining them.
- The data must be understandable.
- The data must be useful for decision making. In other words, the data must be relevant, reliable, and comparable.

Although some of these requirements are similar to general data quality concerns, they are discussed specifically with financial data in mind. Figure 25.1 summarizes basic accounting concepts and principles.

Accounting Concepts

Six concepts define the parameters of accounting activity:

- Entity
- Going concern
- Stable monetary unit
- Time period
- Conservatism
- Materiality

Entity

Financial data for different entities may not be mixed. An **entity** is a person or organization, such as a corporation or professional association. A business owner, for example, must not commingle business and personal data. This concept can be very difficult for small business owners, who may not understand why business receipts are not the same as personal income. It can be equally difficult for large corporations that own many different companies.

Figure 25.1.   Basic Accounting Concepts and Principles

Basic Accounting Concepts
- *Entity:* The financial data of different entities are kept separate.
- *Going concern:* Organizations are assumed to continue indefinitely, unless otherwise stated.
- *Stable monetary unit:* Money is the measurement of financial transactions.
- *Time period:* Financial data represent a specified time period.
- *Conservatism:* Resources must not be overstated, and liabilities must not be understated.
- *Materiality:* The financial data collected by an organization are relevant to its goals and objectives.

Basic Accounting Principles
- *Reliability:* Amounts represent the transactions that occurred.
- *Cost:* Transactions are recorded at historical cost.
- *Revenue:* In order to record revenue, it must be earned and measurable.
- *Matching:* Expenses are recorded in the same period as the related revenue.
- *Consistency:* When an accounting rule is followed, all subsequent periods must reflect the same rule.
- *Disclosure:* Financial reports must be accompanied by helpful explanations, when necessary.

Going Concern

For the most part, organizations are designed to continue indefinitely. Therefore, unless otherwise stated, financial data are assumed to have long-range implications. When analysis of the data shows that the organization can continue to operate for the foreseeable future, the organization is considered a **going concern.** Assuming that a business is going to continue, projections of future activities can be made based on historical trends and assumptions about future conditions. The concept of going concern also places constraints on the organization to maintain sufficient financial and other resources to ensure future stability and growth.

Stable Monetary Unit

Every financial transaction must be quantified. For quantification to be meaningful, all of an entity's transactions must be quantified using a standard measurement. Money is the generally accepted standard measurement—the **stable monetary unit.** Organizations typically use the monetary unity of the country in which they are incorporated. In the United States, financial transactions are recorded in U.S. dollars and cents.

Time Period

Financial data represent transactions during a specified period of time: hour, day, week, month, quarter, year, and so on. The specific **time period** depends on the use of the data. The **fiscal year** (also called the financial year) is defined by the tax year. Individuals generally have a tax year that coincides with the calendar year. Organizations, on the other hand, use fiscal years that correspond to their business needs, usually their business cycle, which represents the total activities of the organization. For example, the U.S. government's fiscal year ends September 30.

For financial reporting purposes, a fiscal year is divided into quarters (three-month periods) and months. Because the months generally end on the last calendar day, the quarters can be of slightly different duration. Over time, it is common to compare similar quarters from year to year, particularly when the business cycle has predictable peaks and valleys.

Conservatism

Not all financial data represent completed transactions within the period represented. Sometimes estimates are involved, or transactions are completed between periods. When this occurs, **assets** and revenue can potentially be overstated and **liabilities** and **expenses** understated. Assets are resources of the organization such as cash, land, buildings, and inventory. They also include the payments due to the organization, such as **accounts receivable.** Liabilities are amounts owed by the organization, such as **accounts payable.** When estimates of amounts are done, efforts must be made to ensure that their use does not misrepresent the actual financial transaction. Therefore, financial data must comply with **conservatism** in that they fairly represent the financial results of the period.

Materiality

Materiality refers to the thresholds below which items are not considered significant. These thresholds may be a dollar value or a percentage of a dollar value. To a $100,000 professional association with $100,000 in income, $10,000 is a significant (material) amount. To a $100 billion oil company, $10,000 is not material. This issue arises when determining the significance of errors, potential liabilities, and the necessity for disclosures (see below).

Accounting Principles

Accounting principles support the quality of financial data. Because they are data, financial data must possess the same data quality characteristics, such as timeliness and validity, as any other type of data.

Reliability

In financial data, **reliability** refers to whether the data actually represent what occurred. Are the data free of material error both in the current period and over time?

Cost

Transactions are recorded at their historical cost. In other words, the measurement of any transaction takes place at the time of the transaction. For some transactions, such as the purchase of equipment or investment in marketable securities, there may be a change in the actual or perceived value of the underlying asset or liability. In those cases, adjustments or disclosures are made when reporting the financial data. Such adjustments or disclosures reflect measurements at the time of the adjustment or disclosure.

Revenue

Revenue consists of funds, goods, or services that increase the organization's assets as a result of its activities. For a hospital, reimbursement for healthcare services, donations of equipment, and donations of volunteer time are all revenue. Revenue may only be recognized when it has been earned and can be measured.

Matching

For an organization to generate revenue, it must incur expenses. Expenses may consist of payroll, rent, travel, raw materials, and so on. Therefore, expenses are recorded in the same period as the associated revenue, thereby **matching** the expenses and revenues.

Consistency

Some accounting rules include variations, and one of the most common variations is depreciation. **Depreciation** is the systematic adjustment to the historical cost of an asset, such as equipment, in order to match the expense of the asset with the revenue that it generates and to eliminate variances in expenses that large purchases in a single period can create. Organizations may choose whatever depreciation method best suits a particular asset. However, the principle of **consistency** requires that the method not change over the life of the asset. Thus, the financial data are prepared in the same way from one period to the next. In fact, organizations sometimes change their choices. Consistency then requires that financial data be restated to show the effect of the change applied to previous periods. Interestingly, some allowed financial accounting rules differ from tax accounting rules, producing different results.

Disclosure

Sometimes the financial data alone do not provide enough information for users of the data to make informed decisions. The impact of a building fire, a potential or ongoing lawsuit, or an expiring collective bargaining agreement cannot be reflected in the financial data when no financial transaction has occurred. Therefore, notes or disclosures that help the user to make informed decisions must accompany all financial data.

Authorities

Just as clinical data are organized and reported in predetermined formats for ease of communication, financial data also are organized and reported in specific ways. Theoretically, organizations can design their own accounting systems and reporting mechanisms. Internally, this is often the case, as will be seen with budgeting. However, organizations that want to borrow funds or attract investors must follow generally accepted rules that apply to their industry. Four major sources of accounting and reporting rules apply to healthcare organizations: the Financial Accounting Standards Board, the Securities Exchange Commission, the Centers for Medicare and Medicaid Services, and the Internal Revenue Service.

Financial Accounting Standards Board

The **Financial Accounting Standards Board** (FASB) is an independent organization that sets accounting standards for businesses in the private sector. Its counterpart, the **Government Accounting Standards Board** (GASB), sets standards for accounting for government entities. The FASB promulgates the rules by which financial data are compiled and reported. These rules, which include the conceptual framework, are referred to as generally accepted accounting principles (GAAP) and generally accepted auditing standards (GAAS).

Securities and Exchange Commission

The **Securities and Exchange Commission** (SEC) is a federal agency that regulates public and some private transactions involving the ownership and debt of organizations. The SEC sets standards regarding reporting financial data, disclosures, timing, marketing, and execution of these transactions. Public transactions take place through an exchange, such as the New York Stock Exchange (NYSE) or the National Association of Securities Dealers Automated Quotation System (NASDAQ).

Centers for Medicare and Medicaid Services

The Centers for Medicare and Medicaid Services (CMS) (formerly called the Health Care Financing Administration [HCFA]) is the federal agency that administers the Medicare program and the federal portion of the Medicaid program. The federal government is the largest single payer of healthcare expenses in the United States. Although the CMS does not set accounting rules, it enforces the federal regulations regarding the reimbursement for Medicare and the federal portion of the Medicaid program and sets standards for the documentation and reporting of transactions related to such reimbursement.

Internal Revenue Service

The tax status of an organization plays a huge role in how the organization is administered. The Internal Revenue Service (IRS) regulates and collects federal taxes. Healthcare organizations fall into one of two major tax categories: for profit and not for profit. Within these categories are several legal structures, such as **sole proprietorship, partnership,** and **corporation.** A summary of legal structures is provided in table 25.2. The primary differences between for-profit and not-for-profit organizations are related to the level of accountability and the distribution of profits.

For-Profit Organizations

For-profit organizations are owned by one or more individuals or by other organizations. The owners may keep the profits (basically, the excess of revenue over expenses) or otherwise invest them as they see fit. The desire to be profitable is not the

issue, although it is certainly a common ideology. For-profit organizations may be privately or publicly owned.

Private ownership may be by an individual, a group of individuals, or an organization. Physician practices, urgent care centers, and freestanding ancillary care organizations are often privately owned. The distribution of profits from a privately owned organization is at the discretion of the owners or as defined by contract among owners.

Public ownership means that the ownership interest in the organization may be bought and sold in the financial marketplace. For example, Hospital Corporation of America (HCA) is a publicly held organization with hospitals in numerous states. Its stock is traded on the NYSE under the symbol HCA. The organization's board of directors determines the distribution of profits from publicly owned organizations. Boards are constrained in these determinations by contractual obligations, such as mortgage contracts and preferred stock obligations, stockholder expectations, and strategic organizational goals.

Not-for-Profit Organizations

Not-for-profit organizations are not owned but, instead, are held in trust for the benefit of the communities they serve. Many hospitals fall into this tax category. Other not-for-profit organizations include professional associations such as the American Health Information Management Association (AHIMA) and charitable organizations such as the American Red Cross.

There are two major categories of not-for-profit organizations: 501(c)(6) and 501(c)(3). Most professional associations are organized under 501(c)(6), which gives these organizations some tax benefits and the freedom to engage in some activities unrelated to their organizational purpose. For example, organizations under 501(c)(6) may lobby and sell goods and services, but are largely involved in activities that benefit their major interest group, which may be defined as paid membership. On the other hand, 501(c)(3) organizations are largely exempt from taxes but must confine their activities to public benefit. Donations to 501(c)(3) organizations are tax deductible to the extent that no goods or services have been received in return. For that reason, charities are generally 501(c)(3) organizations, and many 501(c)(6) organizations have charitable components that are separately incorporated. For example, the AHIMA is a 501(c)(6) organization that has a 501(c)(3) component, the Foundation on Research and Education (FORE). It is important to understand the underlying

Table 25.2.   Common Legal Structures of Organizations

Structure	Description	Healthcare Example
Sole proprietorship	One owner; all profits are owner's personal income.	Solo practitioners
Partnership	Two or more owners; all profits are owners' personal income.	Group practices
Corporation	One or many owners; profits may be either held or distributed as dividends. Dividends are income to the owners.	Hospitals
Not-for-profit organization	No owners. Profits may be held for a specific purpose or reinvested in the organization for the benefit of the community it serves.	Hospitals, professional organizations, charities

tax status of an organization because tax status affects its business decision making and long-term strategies.

For-Profit Status versus Not-for-Profit Status
Undistributed profits from a for-profit organization stay in the business as **retained earnings.** Future undistributed profits increase retained earnings and losses reduce retained earnings. There is no necessity to identify the future use for these funds, although stockholders may ultimately press for distribution when retained earnings appear excessive. Occasionally, portions of retained earnings are held in reserve for specific uses.

Unused profits from a not-for-profit organization stay in the business as **reserves.** Because all such profits must be used for the benefit of the community the organization serves, the future use of such reserves should be clearly defined.

Sources of Financial Data

Virtually every financial transaction consists of three fundamental steps:

1. The goods and/or services are provided.
2. The transaction is recorded.
3. The compensation is exchanged.

Each step may require a number of additional steps, depending on the service and the industry. In addition, the steps are not always performed in the same order. Independent contractors that perform hospital coding represent a simple example. The contractor codes the charts, submits an invoice, and receives a check from the hospital. In this case, three additional steps may be added to record the transaction: keeping a log to track the charts that have been coded, preparing an invoice to bill the hospital, and making a notation to record the activity.

In a hospital, multiple individuals and departments perform services and provide administrative support for financial transactions. Four areas are of particular concern in the context of this discussion: clinical services, patient accounts, health information management, and administration.

Clinical Services

Just as contract coders keep track of the records they have coded, so clinical, or patient care, services providers keep track of the services they perform. The documentation of original entry or source documents enables the healthcare facility to verify that the services were provided and to communicate to supporting departments that a transaction has been initiated. The source document includes two elements: the clinical documentation and the billing documentation.

The clinical documentation is the source document. In the clinical documentation is a record of who has seen the patient, why, what tests or treatments were performed: everything clinically relevant that happened to the patient during his or her interaction with the organization.

Concurrent with the recording of this source document is the capture of the associated billing information. Regardless of the reimbursement system (discussed in chapter 14 of this text), the organization must capture the billable event in such a way that the financial transaction can be completed. Otherwise, the entire health record would be sent to payers every time. Therefore, when a medication is administered to a patient, the clinical record reflects the medication, dosage, time, date and route of administration, and the clinical personnel who administered it. At the same time, the charge for the drug must be communicated to patient accounts.

Patient Accounts

The patient accounts department is responsible for collecting recorded transactions, billing the payer, and ensuring the correct receipt of reimbursement. This department depends on the reliable recording of services. This means that the capture of billing information must be timely and accurate in order to complete the financial transaction efficiently. In addition to the clinical support staff and departments, the patient accounts department relies on the HIM department for coded data.

Health Information Management

The HIM department is responsible for identifying and recording the appropriate clinical codes to describe the patient's interaction with the organization. In some cases, this coding drives the reimbursement to the facility, but in other cases, the coding is used to support the billing.

Increasingly, the reimbursement requirements mandated by the CMS and other plans and payers are commingling clinical data with coding data. For example, the minimum data set used in long-term care combines the clinical data with the codes. The HIM department should be responsible for assigning or ensuring the accuracy of the codes.

In addition to the coding activity, the HIM department is responsible for aggregating and maintaining the documentation that supports the reimbursement.

Administration

Financial transactions occur throughout the facility. Employees are paid, equipment and supplies are purchased, and departments perform services for each other. The finance department accumulates and analyzes all of the financial data. Ultimately, the entire management team participates in the review and analysis of financial data.

Uses of Financial Data

Financial data are generated virtually everywhere in a healthcare facility. Managerial and supervisory personnel use these data for four key purposes: tracking reimbursement, controlling costs, planning the future, and forecasting results.

Healthcare facilities are service organizations that derive almost all of their revenue from clinical activities. Therefore, a key use of financial data is to track reimbursement and ensure that revenues exceed expenses. In the current environment of managed care, where payers often dictate the amount of reimbursement, the provider is increasingly unable to set reimbursement levels. Therefore, expenses or costs have become the only controllable factor.

Controlling costs is best done at the departmental level. For example, the CEO of a hospital does not shop around for the best price on copier paper, and the CFO does not monitor employee productivity in the food services department. Each department is charged with responsibility for ensuring prudent management of financial resources. Departments are given this charge through the budget process, which is one of the outcomes of administrative planning.

Administrative planning reflects the organization's mission. From that mission, goals and objectives are derived that help move the organization toward meeting its mission. Financial data are used to analyze trends, develop budgets, and plan for the future. Planning cannot be accomplished by using historical data alone because the industry changes, sometimes very rapidly. Therefore, the administration must forecast future scenarios.

Forecasting is the prediction of future behavior based on historical data as well as environmental scans. It can be as simple as predicting the profits of an organization on the basis of anticipated changes in reimbursement. It also can involve complicated predictions of consumer behavior based on market research and news reports.

Check Your Understanding 25.1

Instructions: Answer the following questions on a separate piece of paper.

1. If an insurance company representative were to contact the HIM department about a claims audit, which financial personnel should he or she be directed to, and why?

2. Given that DRG payments are predetermined, why would a hospital not record revenue on the basis of the working DRG?

3. Big Medical Center earned a lot more revenue than expected this year but does not expect to earn as much next year. To make the financial reports more consistent, a junior accountant suggests that the hospital record some of next year's expenses this year. Would you agree or disagree that this is a good strategy? Why?

4. What role does the CMS play in a hospital's financial management?

5. If a hospital's HIM department has excess coding or transcription staff, can the hospital sell coding or transcription services to other hospitals? Why or why not?

Basic Financial Accounting

A basic understanding of the mechanics of financial accounting helps department managers to understand the impact of their financial transactions on the overall organization. The system of recording financial transactions is based on balancing the purpose of the transactions with their impact on the organization. For example, a facility purchases drugs with the purpose of ensuring that sufficient and appropriate drugs are on hand to treat patients. The purchase of the drugs increases the facility's pharmaceutical inventory. The impact of that purchase is the outlay of cash. After the cash is spent on drugs, it cannot be spent on something else. Recording both the increase in inventory and the outlay of cash enables the organization to understand and communicate information about its activities.

Documents of Original Entry

As previously discussed, financial transactions begin with the documents of original entry or source documents. Whether the organization's transactions are recorded on paper or via computer, there must be a way to determine the origination of the transaction.

Accounting Equation

All financial accounting is based on an equation that pictures the organization holistically, balancing what is owned against what is owed. Assets are what is owned; liabilities are what is owed. Owner's equity is the difference between the assets and liabilities. In a not-for-profit environment, owner's equity is the fund balance. Reserves and retained earnings are examples of owner's equity. These relationships can be expressed in the following equation:

$$\text{Assets} - \text{liabilities} = \text{owner's equity}$$

The purchase of a house illustrates this equation. The purchase of a house typically involves the deposit of cash and the assumption of a mortgage. The home is an asset whose value is, historically, the price that was paid at the time of the purchase. The mortgage is a liability. As mortgage payments are made, the amount of the mortgage owed declines. The deposit of cash is the owner's equity in the house. As mortgage payments are made, the amount of owner's equity in the house increases. For example, John X purchased a house for $150,000. After making a down payment (or deposit) of $30,000, he was left with a mortgage of $120,000. As the mortgage was paid over thirty years, the historical value of the house remained the same, the amount of the mortgage decreased, and the owner's equity increased. When the mortgage was completely paid, the owner's equity in the house equaled the historical value of the house, as shown in the following equations:

At purchase:
$$\text{Assets (\$150,000)} - \text{liabilities (\$120,000)} = \text{equity (\$30,000)}$$

After 10 years:
$$\text{Assets (\$150,000)} - \text{liabilities (\$100,000)} = \text{equity (\$50,000)}$$

After 20 years:
$$\text{Assets (\$150,000)} - \text{liabilities (\$50,000)} = \text{equity (\$100,000)}$$

After 30 years:
$$\text{Assets (\$150,000)} - \text{liabilities (\$0)} = \text{equity (\$150,000)}$$

Earlier, it was stated that the equation balances what is owned and what is owed. Therefore, another way to look at the accounting equation is:

$$\text{Assets} = \text{liabilities} + \text{owner's equity}$$

Using the previous mortgage example, the second version of the equation proves very useful. At every step in the following calculation, the equations balance:

At purchase:

Assets ($150,000) = liabilities ($120,000) + equity ($30,000)

After 10 years:

Assets ($150,000) = liabilities ($100,000) + equity ($50,000)

After 20 years:

Assets ($150,000) = liabilities ($50,000) + equity ($100,000)

After 30 years:

Assets ($150,000) = liabilities ($0) + equity ($150,000)

or

$150,000 = $150,000

The previous drug example mentioned cash and inventory. Although the term *cash* was used, cash refers to money in the bank as well as money in one's hands. **Inventory** is anything the organization has on hand that it plans to sell, presumably within a year (a business cycle).

Cash and *inventory* are also the terms used to express these assets in a financial transaction. Financial data are organized into **accounts.** Cash and inventory are examples of asset accounts. Each component of the accounting equation has typical accounts that are used to organize the financial data of an organization. Table 25.3 shows some common accounts and what they represent.

Double-Entry Accounting

All financial transactions are recorded with the accounting equation in mind. To simplify the recording of transactions, accountants use special terminology (debit and credit) to reflect the maintenance of a balanced equation. Visually, transactions have two sides: left and right. **Debits** are shown on the left; **credits** are shown on the right. Each account has two sides: increase and decrease. In asset accounts, the left-hand debit side represents the natural balance of the account, and debits increase the account. Conversely, credits decrease an asset account. Obviously, for the accounting equation to balance, the opposite is true of liability and equity accounts. The right-hand credit side of liability and equity accounts represents the natural balance, and credits increase the accounts.

This system of debits and credits enables us to understand immediately whether a transaction increases or decreases a particular account. Individual accounts increase and decrease in value; however, the overall equation always remains in balance. In the mortgage example, the purchase of the house involved three accounts: house, mortgage, and capital. When the equation is expanded to show the accounts, the purpose of debits and credits becomes clear:

Table 25.3.   Common Accounts

Account	Description	Example
Assets		
Cash	Money. Typically, money is represented by several accounts, depending on how the money is stored (e.g., in different banks).	Bank account
Inventory	Goods that are available for sale.	Pharmaceuticals
Accounts receivable	Amounts owed the organization for goods and services.	Claims to payers that have not yet been paid
Building	Permanent structures. The land on which they are built is often listed separately.	Office building
Equipment	Represents items that are used to generate revenue or to support the organization during more than one business cycle.	Photocopier CT scanner
Liabilities		
Accounts payable	Amounts the organization owes but has not yet paid.	Supplies purchased on credit
Loans payable	Amounts the organization has borrowed that will be paid over more than one business cycle.	Bank loan
Mortgage payable	Amounts the organization has borrowed to finance the purchase of buildings and equipment.	Building mortgage
Equity		
Capital/stock/fund balance	In a sole proprietorship or partnership, capital is the owner's equity in the organization. In a corporation, stock is the amount invested by owners in the corporation. In a not-for-profit organization, the fund balance is the amount represented by the difference between assets and liabilities.	
Retained earnings/ reserves	In a corporation, retained earnings are profits that have not been distributed. Reserves are amounts that have been designated for a specific purpose.	
Revenue	Temporary account that captures amounts earned by the organization in the current fiscal year.	The difference between revenue and expenses is net income (profits or losses). These accounts are closed at the end of every fiscal year and the net income is moved to Retained Earnings/Reserves.
Expenses	Temporary account that captures amounts disbursed by the organization in the current fiscal year to support the generation of revenue.	

Assets ($150,000) = liabilities ($120,000) + equity ($30,000)

or

Assets: House		Liabilities: Mortgage		Equity: Capital	
Debit +	Credit −	Debit +	Credit −	Debit +	Credit −
$150,000			$120,000		$30,000

Recording Transactions

Financial transactions are recorded, or posted, to the accounts described above according to a system of **journal entries.** Each journal entry will contain at least one debit and one credit, and the dollar value of all of the debits and all of the credits will be the same. Ensuring that the debits and credits equal is one aspect of ensuring the accuracy of financial data. Other aspects include posting to the correct accounts and posting in the correct time period. The following tabulation illustrates the purchase of supplies on credit. The supplies are delivered on February 24, and the supplier's invoice is paid on March 15. Note that no financial transaction is recorded until the supplies are received.

Date	Description	Debit	Credit
2/24	Supplies expense	$300	
	Accounts payable		$300
	Purchase office supplies		
3/15	Accounts payable	$300	
	Cash		$300
	Pay 2/24 office supply invoice		

The accounts payable amount is eliminated when the invoice is paid. It is common business practice to record, or accrue, liabilities as they are incurred. This accrual basis of accounting enables organizations to understand their total liabilities continuously and to match expenses with the associated revenue. Some organizations, such as small professional associations and sole proprietorships, only record transactions when the cash is paid or received. This cash basis of accounting is analogous to the way individuals handle their private transactions.

In the preceding tabulation, the supplies expense entry is a debit to increase that account. Expenses are temporary equity accounts that close annually. Revenue increases net income; expenses reduce net income. Therefore, revenue accounts have a natural credit balance and expenses have a natural debit balance.

It should be noted that all the financial accounting examples in this chapter relate to corporate and not-for-profit accounting. Government accounting activity, although a system of debits and credits, is significantly different in some respects. For example, a supply purchase would be recorded (encumbered) at the time the supplies were budgeted and then reduced at the time they were ordered.

In a paper-based accounting system, journal entries are listed chronologically in a general journal and their components are posted to the individual accounts. The list of all the individual accounts is referred to as the **general ledger.** In a computer-based environment, only the original journal entry is posted. The computer stores the entries and generates summaries of the individual accounts on request. This system is similar to a computer-based incomplete system in which the deficiencies are recorded only once but can be summarized and printed in a variety of ways, on demand.

The example in figure 25.2 is based on this chapter's original description of a financial transaction. The result of this completed transaction is an increase in cash and an increase in equity (revenue). Note that the amount in accounts receivable is eliminated when the reimbursement is received.

Nonfinancial managers are rarely required to make actual journal entries to record financial transactions. However, they do initiate the transactions themselves and receive reports that detail those transactions. Often the reports only show the department's side of the transaction. For example, a purchase of supplies would appear to the manager on a list of expenses and be added to a summary of all supplies expenses on another report. The cash and accounts payable portions of the transaction would not show because they are controlled by the accounting department. Managerial reporting activity is discussed later is this chapter.

Financial Statements

At the departmental level, individual financial transactions are reviewed for data quality and compliance with policies and procedures. On an administrative level, the overall impact of transactions is generally of more interest than the individual transactions; therefore, summary reports are prepared. These summaries also are used to communicate with lending institutions, potential investors, and regulatory agencies. A variety of summaries are useful for analyzing an organization's financial activities. The two most common reports are the balance sheet and the income statement.

Balance Sheet

The **balance sheet** is a snapshot of the accounting equation at a point in time. Because every financial transaction affects

Figure 25.2.   Example of a Financial Transaction

Service provided:	Physician sees a new patient in the office whose chief complaint is an itchy rash.
Transaction recorded:	*Clinical document:* History and physical/progress note reflects examination of rash and notation that the patient encountered poison ivy while weeding his garden. OTC topic ointment prescribed, and free sample distributed with instructions.
	Billing document: Encounter form—office visit code 99201 circled.

	Journal entry:
	    Accounts receivable—patient X 60
	    Revenue from office visits 60

Reimbursement received:	Journal entry:
	    Cash 60
	    Accounts receivable—patient X 60

the equation, theoretically, the balance sheet will look different after every transaction. To ensure a meaningful evaluation, the balance sheet is typically reviewed on a periodic basis (monthly, quarterly, semiannually, and/or annually). It is often compared to balance sheets from previous fiscal years in order to analyze changes in the organization.

The balance sheet lists the major account categories grouped under their equation headings: assets, liabilities, and equity/fund balance. Figure 25.3 shows a sample balance sheet. The dollar amount shown next to each account category is the total in each category on the date listed at the top of the report.

Income Statement

The **income statement** summarizes the revenue and expense transactions during the fiscal year. Like the balance sheet, the income statement can be reviewed at any point in time. Unlike the balance sheet, which represents all account balances at a point in time, the income statement contains only income and expense accounts and reflects only the activity for the current fiscal year.

The difference between total revenue and total expenses is **net income.** When total expenses exceed total revenue, net income is a negative number, or a **net loss.** Net income

increases owner's equity; net loss decreases owner's equity. Figure 25.4 shows the relationship between the balance sheet and the income statement.

Income statement accounts are not listed on the balance sheet because the effect of their activity is reflected in the fund balance shown on the balance sheet. At the end of the fiscal year, all income statement accounts are closed and the net results are added to, or subtracted from, the appropriate fund balance. For the purposes of periodic reporting, fund balances are adjusted in this manner every time the balance sheet is prepared. However, at the end of the fiscal year, the income and expense accounts are actually closed so that the new fiscal year begins at zero.

Analysis Statements

A number of other types of summary statements are required by users to analyze an organization's financial activity and position. Depending on the organization and their use, the additional financial statements may be required by GAAP as part of a complete financial summary report. The following statements are included for completeness of discussion and are not statements that HIM professionals will generally need to analyze:

- The **statement of cash flow** (also called the statement of changes in financial position) details the reasons that cash changed from one balance sheet period to another. It shows the analyst whether cash was used to purchase equipment or to pay down debt and whether any unusually large transactions took place.
- The **statement of retained earnings** expresses the change in retained earnings from the beginning of the balance sheet period to the end. Retained earnings are affected, for example, by net income/loss, distribution of stock dividends, and payment of long-term debt.
- The **statement of stockholders' equity** (also called the statement of fund balance) details the reasons for changes in each of the stockholders' equity accounts, including retained earnings.

Figure 25.3.   Sample Balance Sheet

Balance Sheet as of 12/31/01			
Assets		**Liabilities**	
Cash	$ 500,000	Accounts payable	$ 600,000
Accounts receivable	600,000	Mortgage	2,000,000
Inventory	400,000	Total liabilities	$2,600,000
Building	2,500,000		
		Fund Balance	
		Restricted funds	$1,000,000
		Unrestricted funds	400,000
		Total fund balance	$1,400,000
Total assets	$4,000,000	Total liabilities + Fund balance	$4,000,000

Figure 25.4.   Relationship between the Balance Sheet and the Income Statement

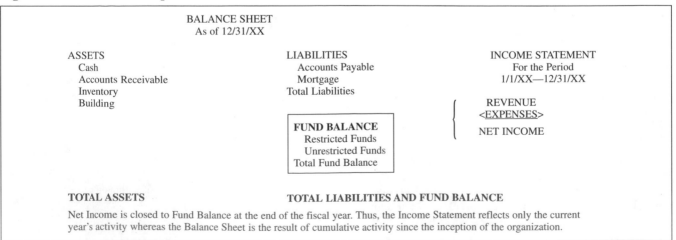

BALANCE SHEET
As of 12/31/XX

ASSETS	LIABILITIES	INCOME STATEMENT
Cash	Accounts Payable	For the Period
Accounts Receivable	Mortgage	1/1/XX—12/31/XX
Inventory	Total Liabilities	
Building		REVENUE
		<EXPENSES>
	FUND BALANCE	NET INCOME
	Restricted Funds	
	Unrestricted Funds	
	Total Fund Balance	
TOTAL ASSETS	TOTAL LIABILITIES AND FUND BALANCE	

Net Income is closed to Fund Balance at the end of the fiscal year. Thus, the Income Statement reflects only the current year's activity whereas the Balance Sheet is the result of cumulative activity since the inception of the organization.

Ratio Analysis

After the financial statements have been prepared, they are ready for analysis. Financial analysts can use financial statements, particularly the balance sheet, to determine whether an organization is using its resources similarly or differently from other organizations in that industry. In retail sales, analysts compare inventory turnover, that is, how quickly inventory is sold. In any industry, one of the most common reasons to analyze financial statements is to lend money to the organization or to invest in it. Thus, the organization's use of assets compared to its liabilities is extremely important.

Ratios are only meaningful within the context of the organization's industry. It is not useful to compare a ratio for a hospital against a ratio for an automobile manufacturer, except to state that one would expect the ratios to be different. Whether an organization's particular ratio is good or bad depends on expected ratios for similar organizations in that industry.

The Healthcare Financial Management Association publishes industry ratio medians annually as a member service. Some state hospital associations also publish ratio information. For example, the Florida Hospital Association offers *Financial and Operating Ratios for Florida Hospitals, 2001*.

Current Ratio

An organization's ability to pay current liabilities with current assets is very important to lenders. The **current ratio** compares total current assets with total current liabilities:

$$\frac{\text{Total current assets}}{\text{Total current liabilities}}$$

From the balance sheet in figure 25.3, one can take the current assets (cash plus accounts receivable plus inventory) and divide them by the current liabilities (accounts payable) to determine the current ratio:

$$\frac{1,500,000}{600,000} = \frac{15}{6} = \frac{2.5}{1.0}$$

The current ratio indicates that for every dollar of current liability, $2.50 of current assets could be used to discharge the liability, which even common sense tell us is good.

Acid-Test Ratio

Inventory is a current asset because it is presumed that inventory will be sold, or turned over, within one fiscal year. However, inventory can become obsolete very quickly, for example, in the fashion and computer industries. Pharmaceuticals can expire before they are used. For expensive items such as motor vehicles, saleable merchandise may be retained in inventory longer than expected or desirable. Therefore, a stricter measure of an organization's ability to pay current liabilities is needed. The **acid-test ratio** compares current liabilities to the current assets that are truly liquid, that is, able to be turned into cash quickly:

$$\frac{\text{Cash} + \text{short-term investments} + \text{net current receivables}}{\text{Total current liabilities}}$$

Short-term investments include money market funds, certificates of deposit, and treasury bills, for example. Using the balance sheet in figure 25.3 again, the acid-test ratio is:

$$\frac{1,100,000}{600,000} = \frac{1.1}{6.0} = \frac{1.83}{1.00}$$

In this example, the acid-test ratio reveals that for every dollar of current liabilities, there are 1.83 dollars of current assets that could be used immediately or sold quickly to discharge the liabilities.

Debt Ratio

Looking back to the mortgage example, the organization's building asset was purchased using 10 percent cash and 90 percent mortgage. Ninety percent of that asset was financed with debt. Looking at all the liabilities and all the assets together gives the analyst an overall picture of how the assets were acquired. The **debt ratio,** therefore, is total liabilities divided by total assets.

It is important to remember that all ratio analysis is industry specific and varies somewhat depending on the economic environment. Therefore, ratio analysis can be used to compare similar organizations at a specific point in time or the same organization at different points in time. However, a hospital ratio would never be compared with a professional association ratio.

Check Your Understanding 25.2

Instructions: Answer the following questions on a separate piece of paper.

1. List three assets and three liabilities.
2. Why are revenue and expense accounts part of owner's equity?
3. What inventory does a hospital have?
4. What is the difference between a debit and a credit?
5. Why is knowledge of accounting important to nonfinancial managers?
6. A lender wants to know how quickly a borrower would be able to repay a debt. What is the best ratio to use for this analysis? Why?

Basic Managerial Accounting

Managers must have some understanding of managerial accounting in order to control the financial aspects of their departments' operations. As stated earlier, managers must work within budgets that have been developed based on their organization's goals and objectives. Therefore, it is not sufficient for a manager merely to review for accuracy the financial transactions generated by the department during the period. The transactions must be compared to the expected or budgeted transactions to ensure that the goals and objectives of both the department and the organization are being met. The development, implementation, and analysis of systems that track financial transactions for managerial control purposes is called **managerial accounting.** Managerial accounting includes both budget and cost analysis systems.

Operational Budgets

The purpose of an **operational budget** is to allocate and control resources in a manner consistent with the organization's goals and objectives. These goals and objectives are tied to the organization's mission. Each department also should have its own mission, goals, and objectives that identify how the department contributes to the organization's overall mission. Every item in the operational budget should have a direct relationship to a departmental goal that supports an organizational goal.

The budget process begins with the board of directors/trustees, who approve the fiscal assumptions for the upcoming year. Those assumptions are quantified and communicated to the department managers, who develop budgets based on those assumptions. Typical assumptions include the desired growth in revenue and/or target cost reductions.

Budget Cycle

The operational budget cycle generally coincides with one fiscal year. The purpose of the operational budget is the quantification of the projected results of operations for the coming fiscal year. This process begins three to four months before the end of the current fiscal year. Projected budgets should be collected, compiled, reviewed, and approved prior to the start of the new fiscal year.

Fiscal Period

An organization's budget year coincides with its fiscal year on file with the IRS. Although the actual operational budget generally only applies to one fiscal year, financial managers often project multiple years of budgets with a variety of scenarios in order to test the financial impact of current decision making.

Interim Periods

In a computerized environment, it is relatively easy to generate financial reports as frequently as needed by management. However, monthly budget reporting is most common. Any period that represents less than an entire fiscal year is an **interim period.** Figure 25.5 provides a sample budget report for an HIM department for May. The budgeted amounts for each item are listed next to the actual amounts for the month.

As is common, the year-to-date (in this case, January through May) budget and actual amounts also are included. It is very useful for budget reports to show the differences between budgeted and actual amounts. Such differences are called **variances.** Many budget reports also show the percentage variance for each item, based on the budget. Managers may be required to explain variances that exceed a particular dollar value or a specified percentage.

In the budget report in figure 25.5, there is a large variance in May's budgeted expense for printer paper. By following that line item across to the year-to-date amount, it is evident that there is no year-to-date variance in the budget. This illustrates a timing difference between the expected expense and the actual expense. The budget may have placed that expense in April, even though the actual expense occurred in May. These types of temporary variances are the result of normal business activities, and although they may require explanation, they are usually not of concern.

Budget Components

The components of an operational budget generally follow the format of the income statement and list revenue items and expense items. Every department will be different, depending on its unique activities. However, budget reports tend to be uniform throughout the organization. Therefore, line items that do not apply to a particular department are likely to be listed with zero values rather than to be omitted.

Revenues

Revenue consists of earned, known amounts. Accounts receivable is a balance sheet account (earned revenue that has not been received) and would not be listed on the budget report. The entry to post accounts receivable includes revenue.

Clinical services are the main source of revenue for a healthcare facility. A clinical department's contribution to revenue would appear as a revenue item.

Examples of nonclinical services include employee food services, donated services, and copy fees. The materiality of these items affects how they appear on the budget. For example, copy fees that are directly related to the cost of providing copies may be considered a reimbursement of expense rather than revenue.

Figure 25.5.   HIM Department Budget Report for May

Description	May Budget	May Actual	May Variance	YTD Budget	YTD Actual	YTD Variance
Payroll	$25,000	$22,345	$2,655	$125,000	$110,321	$14,679
Fringe benefits	$8,000	$7,360	$640	$40,000	$37,870	$2,130
Contract services	$5,000	$8,000	($3,000)	$25,000	$40,000	($15,000)
Office supplies	$150	$145	$5	$750	$975	($225)
Printer paper	$100	$250	($150)	$500	$500	—
Postage	$95	$97	($2)	$475	$456	$19
Travel	$0	$0	—	$0	$0	—
Continuing education	$0	$0	—	$0	$45	($45)

Expenses

The HIM department budget consists primarily of expenses. Expenses may be incurred as a result of financial transactions outside or within the organization. Some departments, such as housekeeping and facilities maintenance, perform services for other facility departments. Therefore, charges from these departments may appear on the budget. Such charges are generally carried forward through the budget allocation process and usually are not estimated by individual managers.

Ordinarily, the single largest expense in a healthcare facility is payroll. This is typical for service organizations. Payroll can be a difficult expense to project. Employees have different anniversary dates and different salary increases.

The cost of employee benefits is part of payroll but is often listed separately. Facilities rarely expect department managers to calculate benefits budgets because this is a human resources–controlled line item. The cost of benefits tracks with payroll.

The next largest expense account is often supplies. Clinical supplies would be a substantial item on the cardiology or radiology department budget, whereas office supplies might be a large item for health information management.

Cost of goods sold is a manufacturing concept that refers to the underlying cost of making the finished goods. This concept applies to healthcare providers in the sense that there is a cost basis for providing services. For every inpatient treated, there are payroll, utility, office supplies, pharmaceutical, and equipment costs that the facility incurred. Unlike manufacturing, in which the cost of producing items is tracked very closely, healthcare facilities historically have not been good at tracking the underlying costs of providing services to individual patients. The costs of providing care are often analyzed in the aggregate.

Internal Controls

In any industry, internal controls must be in place to safeguard assets and to ensure compliance with policies and procedures. Internal controls may be designed to prevent the theft of cash or to ensure that a patient receives the correct medication. The three major categories of internal controls are preventive, detective, and corrective.

Preventive controls are implemented prior to the activity's taking place because they are designed to stop an error from happening. In financial management, pretransaction supervisory review and authorization is a preventive control.

Detective controls are designed to find errors that have already been made. Detective controls tend to be less expensive than preventive controls and can be implemented at many levels. Quantitative record reviews and computer validity edits are examples of detective controls. In accounting, the summing of debits and credits is a detective control because the two sums must always be equal. Footing and cross-footing financial reports is another detective control. (See figure 25.6.)

When an error or other problem has been detected, action must be taken to correct the error, solve the problem, or design controls to prevent future errors or problems. The error or problem must be analyzed to determine the cause. When a correction can be made, it is documented and implemented. However, some errors, such as amputation of an incorrect limb, cannot be corrected. In these cases, analysis of the root cause is important so that the error can be prevented in the future. In financial management, very few errors cannot be

Figure 25.6.   Footing and Cross-Footing Financial Reports

SUMMING OF DEBITS AND CREDITS

Cash		$1,345
	Photocopy paper	$974
	Toner	$362

In this journal entry, the debit ($1,345) does not match the credits ($1,336). This means that an error has been made. Reference back to the original documentation will reveal that the sales tax on the items was not accounted for.

FOOTING AND CROSS-FOOTING

	January	February	March	Year-to-date (Cross-foot)
Payroll	20,000	20,000	20,000	60,000
Benefits	6,000	6,000	6,000	24,000
Office supplies	1,000	1,000	1,000	3,000
Equipment service	400	500	600	500
				87,500?
Monthly Totals	27,400	27,400	27,400	82,200?
	(Foot)			

The foot is the sum of the columns; the cross-foot is the sum of the rows. Notice that in this example the sums do not match. Footing and cross-footing reports that are supposed to represent arithmetic totals is a very useful detective control, particularly with manually prepared or PC-prepared reports. A simple error in creating a formula in a spreadsheet program can cause an entire report to be wrong.

corrected. Typical errors include posting transactions to an incorrect account, posting transactions that have not been completed, and posting incorrect amounts. Even financial statement errors can be corrected and the reports redistributed. Problems that cannot always be corrected include theft of assets and failure to invest funds on a timely basis. These problems require analysis and development and implementation of controls for the future.

Corrective controls are designed to fix problems that have been discovered, frequently as a result of detective controls. Many errors and problems occur routinely, such as failing to complete forms, making computation errors, and wrongly posting transactions. Therefore, procedures must be in place to ensure the timely and accurate correction of the error or solution to the problem. In the HIM department, the incomplete-chart system is a corrective control. Incomplete charts have been detected, the source of the error identified, and the responsible individual contacted for completion of the chart. In financial management, supervisory review of transactions is typically used to detect errors and problems. The ability to correct errors in journal entries is essential.

Internal controls may be present at every level of the organization. In a service organization, such as a hospital, controls over expenditures are some of the most important responsibilities of individual managers. Two key methods of exerting such controls are through purchasing and analysis of variances.

Purchasing

Organizations handle the purchasing function differently, depending on their size and needs. Large organizations tend to maintain a central purchasing and distribution department that is responsible for the acquisition of supplies and equipment. Significant savings can be obtained by purchasing supplies in bulk and distributing them as needed to departments. Central purchasing also has the benefit of minimizing the space required for storage of items on hand. Central purchasing systems should be designed to minimize the risk of loss due to misappropriation of stored items. The periodic inventory of items on hand and the itemized distribution of stored items can assist in this process.

Maintaining a central purchasing and distribution department has direct administrative costs to the organization, for example, salary, facility maintenance, and administrative processing. Therefore, the control benefits of centralized purchasing must be weighed against the cost of such operations. Savings also can be obtained by limiting the source of supplies to one or two key vendors who offer discounts to the organization. In this scenario, managers would order items as needed, but only from approved vendors.

Finally, an organization may choose to allow individual departments to make purchases independently. Although this can result in additional supply and equipment costs, there may be overall savings in not maintaining a central purchasing department. The major disadvantages of independent, or

decentralized, purchasing are the need for use of operational areas for storage of supplies and the allocation of managerial resources to purchasing.

Regardless of the purchasing system used, controls must be in place to ensure the efficient execution of approved transactions. Purchase orders, shipping/receiving documents, and invoices are the key controls over the purchase process.

Purchase Orders

The **purchase order** system ensures that items purchased have been properly authorized prior to ordering. Authorization is often tied to dollar limits and/or the budget process. In a paper environment, a purchase order is a paper form on which all details of the intended purchase are reported. Purchase orders for routine, budgeted items often require only the authorization of a supervisor or manager. For large-dollar items, as specified in the organization's policy and procedure manual, additional authorization may be required. In a computer-based system, there may be no physical form; however, authorization levels are still required.

The purchase order shows that the appropriate individual with the appropriate authorization ordered the specific items. The order is then forwarded to the vendor. The originator of the order keeps a copy, and another copy is sent to the accounts payable department. When there is a central receiving department, that department also should receive a copy of the order.

Shipping/Receiving Documents

Items received from a vendor contain a packing slip, also known as a shipping document. This document lists the quantities and descriptions of the items sent from the vendor, but not the price. The recipient of the items must verify that the items received match the ones that were ordered. The verified shipping/receiving document is forwarded to accounts payable.

Invoices

The vendor will send an invoice (bill or request for payment) directly to accounts payable. The accounts payable department matches the invoice to the shipping/receiving document and the purchase order on file.

Statements

A **statement** is merely a list of outstanding invoices the vendor has sent, but for which no payment has been received. Some companies send statements that include all activity for the period, including payment. The statement is one way that the vendor lets the customer know that payments are late. Statements are not payable without supporting documentation. When there is no purchase order, receiving document, and invoice, accounts payable will not remit payment. Statements received for which there is no underlying documentation should be treated as suspicious. Purchases may have been made without proper authorization. On the other hand, there are unscrupulous organizations that send only statements when no transaction has taken place in the hope that the organization's controls are lax and payment will be made. This is particularly true of certain fraudulent subscriptions and advertising schemes.

Inventory Slips

In a centralized purchasing system, some mechanism must be in place to track the distribution of items to other departments. Frequently paper based, a form is completed requesting items and verifying receipt of the items. These systems are purely internal because items are on hand. The financial transaction consists of a journal entry moving the cost of the items from the purchasing department to the requesting department.

Variance Analysis

The second managerial control is **variance analysis.** A variance is the arithmetic difference between the budgeted amount and the actual amount of a line item. Variance analysis places accountability for financial transactions on the manager of the department that initiated the transaction.

Identification of Variances

Variances are often calculated on the monthly budget report. The organization's policies and procedures manual defines unacceptable variances or variances that must be explained. In identifying variances, it is important to recognize whether the variance is favorable or unfavorable and whether it is temporary or permanent.

Favorable variances occur when the actual results are better than budget projections. Actual revenue in excess of budget is a favorable variance. **Unfavorable variances** occur when the actual results are worse than what was budgeted. Actual expenditure in excess of budget is an unfavorable variance. Note that favorable and unfavorable refer to the impact on the organization rather than to the magnitude or direction of the variance. Sometimes the terms negative and positive are used instead. This can be confusing because a negative expense variance is favorable. Therefore, it is extremely important to ensure that the manager understands and correctly uses the language of the organization.

Temporary variances are not expected to continue in subsequent months. For example, a department may budget for a large purchase of file folders in May. When that purchase does not actually take place until July, there will be a temporary variance in the May and July monthly report and a temporary variance in the May and June year-to-date numbers. Figure 25.7 illustrates this point. In this example, the HIM department budgeted $250 per month for department supplies, plus an additional $9,750 in May for file folders. Because of an unexpectedly low census, the file folders were not needed until July. This created a temporary, favorable variance in expenditures in May and June.

In contrast, permanent variances do not resolve during the current fiscal year. In the preceding example, a variance still would have existed at the end of December (the close of the fiscal year) if the file folders had been budgeted in November. The department supplies variance then would be a permanent variance during the current fiscal year and would be budgeted again for the following year as an expenditure in January.

Explanation of Variances

The analysis of budget variances is a financial management control. Administration may review the monthly budget report first and ask questions of the appropriate manager. In other instances, the department managers are automatically required to respond to certain variances.

In the analysis of variance, materiality is an issue. Rarely will a manager be required to explain a $5 variance. Clearly, the cost of a manager's time to explain such an insignificant amount far exceeds the benefit of knowing why there is a $5 variance. In fact, because budgets are largely estimates, it would be quite odd if the actual amounts always matched the budgeted amounts. Therefore, dollar and/or percentage limits are set in the organization's policies and procedures manual. Variances that exceed these limits must be explained in detail.

In general, the reason for a **temporary budget variance** is the timing of the transaction. Looking back to the department supplies/file folder example in figure 25.7, there is a very simple explanation for the temporary variance. In wording the explanation to administration, the department manager should state:

- The nature of the variance (favorable or unfavorable, temporary or permanent)

Figure 25.7.   Examples of Budget Variances

May Budget Report						
	May Budget	**May Actual**	**May Variance**	**YTD Budget**	**YTD Actual**	**YTD Variance**
Department supplies	10,000	250	9,750	11,000	1,250	9,750

June Budget Report						
	June Budget	**June Actual**	**June Variance**	**YTD Budget**	**YTD Actual**	**YTD Variance**
Department supplies	250	250	0	11,250	1,500	9,750

July Budget Report						
	July Budget	**July Actual**	**July Variance**	**YTD Budget**	**YTD Actual**	**YTD Variance**
Department supplies	250	10,000	-9,750	11,500	11,500	0

- The exact amount of the variance
- The cause of the variance
- Any ameliorating circumstances or offsetting amounts

For the folder example, the explanation might be something like the following: "In department supplies, the favorable, temporary variance of $9,750 will resolve in July when the budgeted expenditure for file folders is processed." For such a temporary variance, no additional explanation is necessary; however, the administration may prefer more detail. In that case, the relationship between low census and the need for file folders could be added to the explanation.

Temporary variances are not typically of serious concern to administration. However, **permanent variances** can be a problem because management of departmental budgets is an important indicator of the competence of department managers.

Whether a variance is temporary or permanent depends on the answers to two questions:

- Are the subsequent transactions that will balance the variance likely to occur within the same fiscal year?
- Is it reasonably certain the transactions will occur as predicted?

If the balancing transactions are unlikely to take place during the current fiscal year, the result is a permanent variance in the current budget report. Sometimes the manager may not know when—or if—the transactions will actually take place. For example, the manager may have budgeted $2,000 for attendance at an unspecified continuing education conference in June. A conflict with the JCAHO survey prevented the manager from attending the conference, creating a favorable expense variance. As long as the manager believes that the amount will be spent appropriately at some time during the fiscal year, the variance is temporary. For example, the manager may be able to attend a conference later in the year. However, if the manager knows that there is no chance of attending a conference and appropriately spending the budgeted amount, the variance should be explained as permanent.

Additional explanation is probably necessary for a permanent variance. An expenditure that must be deferred until the next fiscal year is particularly important. In that case, the explanation might be something like "In department supplies, there is a favorable, permanent variance of $9,750. Because of an unexpectedly low census, the purchase of additional file folders for discharged patient records was not necessary this year. This amount is included in next year's budget."

Managers may have the opportunity to utilize favorable variances in one line item to offset unfavorable variances in another line item. For example, unused travel budget may be used for continuing education. The ability to work with the departmental budget as a whole as opposed to justifying line items is entirely dependent on the administration of the budget process. One typical example of offsetting variances occurs when an employee leaves and cannot be replaced immediately. Several things may happen. The vacancy may cause a favorable variance in payroll expense until the position is filled. The vacancy may cause an unfavorable variance in payroll expense if other employees are paid overtime to help fill the vacancy. Both of these variances may be permanent. Finally, the vacancy may cause a favorable variance in payroll expense and an unfavorable variance in consulting expenses when the vacant position is outsourced. In the latter case, the two variances at least partially offset each other, which must be explained in the monthly variance report.

Capital Budget

Unlike the operational budget, which primarily looks at projected income statement activity for the next fiscal year, the **capital budget** looks at long-term investments. Such investments are usually related to improvements in the facility infrastructure, expansion of services, or replacement of existing assets. Capital investments focus on either the appropriateness of an investment, given the facility's investment guidelines, or on choosing among different opportunities to invest. The capital budget is the facility's plan for allocating resources over and above the operating budget.

Funding for the capital budget may come from diverse sources. For example, donations or grants may fund a building project or retained earnings or unallocated reserves may fund equipment purchases. Federal and state government funds may be available to offset the cost of capital investments. Regardless of the source of the funds, capital investments are defined by facility policy and selected using financial analysis techniques.

Large-Dollar Purchases

From a departmental perspective, capital budget items are large-dollar purchases, as defined by facility budget policies and procedures. Capital budget items usually have a useful life in excess of one fiscal year, making them long-term assets, and a dollar value in excess of a predetermined amount, often $500 or $1000. The most common HIM department capital budget items include shelving, office furniture, photocopying equipment, and computer equipment. Computer software, and even some computer hardware, has a limited useful life and is often included in the operating budget. Some organizations maintain a separate capital budget and process for computer-related equipment and software. In addition, in such cases, control over the acquisition of the related long-term assets may rest with the information technology or information systems department.

Acquisitions

The acquisition of long-term assets may be controlled by the purchasing department. The purchasing department may already have a contract with a specific vendor to provide certain types of equipment or furniture. In the absence of an existing contract, it may still be the purchasing department's responsibility to ensure the appropriate acquisition of assets through the **request for proposal** (RFP) process. The RFP process is a preventive control designed to eliminate bias and to ensure competitive pricing in the acquisition of goods and services.

Cost-Benefit Analysis

An old photocopying machine breaks down at least once a week. Repair of the machine takes up to two days and is increasingly expensive. During the downtime, release of information clerks must use a machine that is located two floors below the HIM department and shared by three other departments. It seems obvious to HIM department personnel that a new machine is needed. Including a new machine in the HIM department's capital budget request is certainly warranted. However, funding for a new machine is based on specific, detailed cost justifications and is weighed in comparison to all departments' requests. Facility administration may be forced to choose between a new copier for the HIM department and several new computers for the patient accounts department. All other factors being equal, increased efficiency and productivity in claims processing is likely to be chosen over increased efficiency in release of information.

Depreciation

Certain long-term assets, such as equipment and furniture, wear out over time and must be replaced. Such assets con-tribute to revenue over multiple fiscal periods. Therefore, the cost of these assets is not booked as an expense at the time of purchase. Rather, the current asset, cash, is exchanged for a long-term asset, equipment. A portion of the historical cost of equipment then is moved from asset into expense each fiscal year. Eventually, all of the cost of equipment has been expensed and equipment is zero. This financial accounting and analysis activity is called depreciation. The purpose of depreciation is to spread the cost of an asset over its useful life. (See tables 25.4 and 25.5 [p. 620].)

Note that the depreciation of long-term assets does not have a direct relationship to the activity of actually using the asset. It is not unusual to depreciate an asset over five years, but to continue to use it for another five. For example, a facility whose equipment is fully depreciated and whose current assets are heavily financed with debt obligations may be unable to reinvest in new equipment. Thus, the capital budget is critical for the facility's continuing operations.

Capital Projects

A facility's ability to invest in capital projects is very important to the continued success of its operations. Because buildings deteriorate, equipment wears out, and new technology is

Table 25.4. Sample Depreciation Methods

Straight Line	The cost of the asset is expensed equally over the expected life of the asset. The estimated sale value of the asset at the end of its useful life is called the residual value and is subtracted from the cost prior to depreciation.	$\dfrac{\text{Cost} - \text{residual value}}{\text{\# of years (useful life)}}$
	Example: Copy machine purchased at a cost of $5,000 Useful life = 4 years Residual value = $200 Annual depreciation = $\dfrac{\$5,000 - \$200}{4}$ = $1,200 per year	
Units of Production	The cost of the asset is expensed over the expected life of the asset, measured in usage. In this case, usage would a number of copies.	$\dfrac{\text{Cost} - \text{residual value}}{\text{\# of copies (useful life)}}$
	Example: Copy machine purchased at a cost of $5,000 Useful life = 100,000 copies Residual value = $200 Depreciate rate = $\dfrac{\$5,000 - \$200}{100,000}$ = $.048 (4.8 cents) per copy Annual depreciation = $0.48 times the number of copies actually made	
Accelerated	There are several accelerated depreciation methods, all of which are designed to expense more of the asset's value early in its useful life. One such method is called double declining balance (DDB). DDB expenses the asset at double the straight-line method, based on the book value rather than on the historical cost.	Book value times twice the straight line rate Straight line rate = $\dfrac{\text{annual depreciation}}{\text{cost} - \text{residual value}}$
	Example: Copy machine purchased at a cost of $5,000 Useful life = 100,000 copies Residual value = $200 Straight line rate = $1,200/$4,800 = 25% Annual depreciation = Book value times 50%	

Note: These examples of depreciation methods are just a few of the acceptable methods in use today. The reader should be aware that there are other methods and that not all methods are acceptable for income tax purposes. Accounting for income taxes is beyond the scope of this discussion.

important to healthcare delivery, capital improvements must be implemented. Individual departments request equipment purchases and facility improvements as the needs arise. Facility administration must choose among the suggested projects to optimize the use of its resources.

In addition to capital improvements, facilities may make capital investments that improve operational efficiency. Some of these capital investments require broader analysis than the cost of the equipment. Replacing a manual incomplete tracking system, for example, with a computer-based system involves the analysis of employee time and departmental space allocations as well as the associated equipment and software costs.

Facility administration looks at capital projects differently than it reviews operational activities. Theoretically, operational activities contribute to the generation of revenue for the facility. For example, all hospital activities either provide healthcare services or in some way support departments that provide healthcare services. A hospital may elect to perform its own printing rather than outsource the printing function; however, it is unlikely that a hospital would choose to provide printing services to the general public. Printing forms supports clinical and administrative services internally; running a printing business does not. Therefore, the justification for operational budget amounts generally rests on the extent to which the underlying activities support the mission of the facility at the projected productivity levels.

Finally, budgeted capital funds generally must be expended in the time period for which they were approved. Even when allocated, capital budget items may be prioritized and timed so that purchases are made only with administrative approval. This is often the case when actual funding does not meet anticipated levels or when unforeseen circumstances change administrative priorities.

Table 25.5.   Sample Depreciation Schedule

Copy machine purchased at a cost of $5,000
Useful life = 100,000 copies
Residual value = $200

Straight Line-Depreciation (25% of Cost minus Residual Value annually)

	Book Value at Beginning of Year	Depreciation	Accumulated Depreciation	Book Value at End of Year
Year 1	$5,000	$1,200	$1,200	$3,800
Year 2	3,800	1,200	2,400	2,600
Year 3	2,600	1,200	3,600	1,400
Year 4	1,400	1,200	4,800	200
Year 5	200			

Units of Production (4.8 cents per copy annually)

	Book Value at Beginning of Year	Number of Copies Used	Depreciation	Accumulated Depreciation	Book Value at End of Year
Year 1	$5,000	20,000	$960	$960	$4,040
Year 2	4,040	20,000	960	1,920	3,080
Year 3	3,080	22,000	1,056	2,976	2,024
Year 4	2,024	25,000	1,200	4,176	824
Year 5	824	25,000	624	4,800	200

Notice that in units of production the useful life is based on the number of copies used—not on the time in service. In this example, the copier does not become fully depreciated until year 5. Also, the depreciation cannot exceed the cost less the residual value; therefore, the depreciation in year 5 is only $624.

Double Declining Balance (50% of book value annually)

	Book Value at Beginning of Year	Depreciation	Accumulated Depreciation	Book Value at End of Year
Year 1	$5,000	$2,500	$2,500	$2,500
Year 2	2,500	1,250	3,750	1,250
Year 3	1,250	625	4,375	625
Year 4	625	425	4,800	200
Year 5	200			

Notice that in DDB, the final depreciation entry in year 4 reduces the book value to the residual value (50% of $625 is really $375.50, but we added $49.50 to make the depreciation 425 so that book value drops to $200 at the end of year 4).

For capital budgets, supporting the mission of the facility is not sufficient justification. Capital projects also must satisfy predetermined levels of return on the projected investment.

Cost Justification

All departments in a facility compete for finite facility resources. Therefore, department managers must be familiar with **cost justification** techniques and with their facility's method of analyzing capital projects. Typical cost justifications are based on increased revenue, increased efficiency, improved customer service, and reduced costs. The analysis of a capital project is based on the estimated return on the investment, including the weight of costs versus the benefits to be derived from the project. The specific cost-benefit analysis method used by facility administration depends on the characteristics of the project as well as the preferences of the analyst. When no specific cash inflows are expected, return may be based on depreciation or other cost savings. Sometimes the capital budget includes the allocation of resources for assets whose acquisition will attract or retain valuable personnel or physician relationships. Even in such cases, the acquisition should be analyzed financially, not just politically.

Payback Period

The **payback period** is the time required to recoup the cost of an investment. Mortgage refinancing analysis frequently uses the concept of payback period. Mortgage refinancing is considered when interest rates have dropped. Refinancing requires up-front interest payments, called points, as well as a variety of administrative costs. The payback period is the time it takes for the savings in interest to equal the cost of the refinancing.

The advantage of using a payback period to analyze investments is that it is relatively easy to calculate and understand. For example, payback period can be used to describe the time it takes for the savings in payroll costs to equal the cost of productivity-enhancing equipment. In the previous photocopy machine example, the payroll costs would be calculated based on downtime incurred when using a copier in another area of the building.

The disadvantage of a payback period is that it ignores the time value of money. Because the funds used for one capital investment could have been invested elsewhere, there is always an inherent opportunity cost of choosing one investment over another. Hence, there is an assumed rate of return against which investments are compared and a benchmark rate of return under which a facility will not consider an investment.

Accounting Rate of Return

Another simple method of capital project analysis is the **accounting rate of return.** This method compares the projected annual cash inflows, minus any applicable annual depreciation, divided by the initial investment. Consider the purchase of a CT scanner. Reimbursement from use of the machine is the cash inflow. Depreciation is easily calculated, based on the initial investment.

Accounting rate of return is another example of a simple method of capital project analysis. However, it also ignores the time value of money. In addition, accounting rate of return is based on an estimate. If the analyst incorrectly projects annual cash inflows, the projected rate of return will be incorrect.

Return on Investment

Return on investment (ROI) is most frequently used to analyze marketable securities retrospectively. The increase in market value of the securities divided by the initial investment is the return on investment. When an income stream is associated with the investment, the income stream is added to the market value of the securities in calculating return. In comparing the ROI among different securities, the tax implications must be considered. Long-term gains are taxed differently than short-term gains. Tax-exempt investments result in different returns than taxable investments.

With respect to capital investments, the equation is similar. Divide the controllable operating profits by the controllable net investment. Operating profits are the cash inflow minus the direct costs of operation.

As with accounting rate of return and payback period, ROI is easy to calculate and understand. Similarly, it does not consider the time value of money.

Net Present Value

To take into consideration the time value of money, the analyst must establish an interest rate at which money could have otherwise been invested. From that implied interest rate and the projected future cash inflows of the investment, the present value of the cash inflows is calculated. Present value is the current dollar amount that must be invested today in order to yield the projected future cash inflows at the implied interest rate. **Net present value** is the calculated present value of the future cash inflows compared to the initial investment.

The advantage of using net present value to analyze investments is that it considers the time value of money. When choosing among like investments, net present values can be reliably compared to determine the financial advantages of the investment.

As with other analysis tools, analysts may have to estimate the projected cash flows. However, the main disadvantage of net present value is that the interest rate is subjective. Therefore, it is best used to compare multiple investment opportunities rather than to analyze one investment alone. Another disadvantage of using net present value is that it requires some knowledge of mathematics to accept its validity and understand its relevance. Fortunately, financial calculators and computer programs have made the calculation of net present value relatively simple.

Internal Rate of Return

Internal rate of return (IRR) is the interest rate that makes the net present value calculation equal zero. In other words, it is the interest rate at which the present value of the projected cash inflows equals the initial investment. IRR considers the time value of money. Individual investments can be evaluated as well as multiple investments. As with net present value, knowledge of mathematics is helpful. The main disadvantage is that a project may have multiple IRRs.

Profitability Index

Facilities cannot automatically invest in seemingly profitable projects. For example, a $500,000 radiology equipment investment may have a present value of cash inflows of $1,500,000, for a net present value of $1,000,000. At the same time, a $10,000 pharmacy computer system yields a net present value of $30,000. This seems to be a great investment; however, the facility's capital budget may be limited to $100,000. In this case, a **profitability index** helps the organization prioritize investment opportunities. For each investment, divide the present value of the cash inflows by the present value of the cash outflows. In this example, the pharmacy system has a higher profitability index, as illustrated below:

Radiology		Pharmacy
$1,500,000	Present value of cash inflows	$40,000
$500,000	Present value of cash outflows	$10,000
3	Profitability index	4

Types of Budgets

In addition to the operating and capital budgets, organizations develop and monitor other budgets, including financial budgets, cash flow budgets, and incremental budgets. These budgets are the responsibility of the finance department.

The development and monitoring of budgets is guided by the facility's policy and procedures manual and the management styles of the administrative and departmental management team. Therefore, it is extremely important for department managers to understand the facility's budgeting methods, including how administration uses budgets.

At best, a budget is a manager's best guess at the outcomes of future financial transactions. Unexpected events that influence those transactions, such as declining census, increase in interest rates, and staffing changes, create budget variances. Some budgets are specifically designed to take these fluctuations into consideration. A budget can represent virtually any projected set of circumstances. Therefore, there are many different types of budget methodologies. Common methodologies include fixed, flexible, activity-based, and zero-based budgets.

The most common type of budget is a **fixed budget.** Budget amounts are based on expected capacity. Fixed budgets do not change when expected capacity changes. For example, the HIM department would budget file folder expense on the basis of the estimated number of discharges and the historical need to replace worn folders. When the number of discharges materially increases or declines, file folder expense will increase or decrease, thus creating a budget variance.

Flexible budgets are based on projected productivity. In this case, the HIM department would budget file folder expense at several levels of discharges. As the actual dis-

charges become known, the budget reflects the estimate at that level of activity. Used primarily in manufacturing, this method of budgeting also is useful for projecting personnel budget in service areas, such as nursing units, where increased activity has a direct impact on staffing and supplies.

Activity-based budgets are based on activities or projects rather than on departments. Typically used for construction projects, an activity-based budget can be useful for any project that spans multiple budget lines or departments and for projects that span more than one fiscal year. Computer system installation and implementation should be controlled using an activity-based budget.

Different budget methodologies are developed to meet the needs of the organization. Fixed and flexible budgets are characteristic of operating budgets. Activity-based budgets are more often used for capital projects. All three types of budgets can be used by virtually any organization. **Zero-based budgets,** on the other hand, apply to organizations for which each budget cycle poses the opportunity to continue or discontinue services based on the availability of resources. Every department or activity must be justified and prioritized annually in order to effectively allocate the organization's resources. Professional associations and charitable foundations, for example, may routinely use zero-based budgeting.

Cost Reports

Prior to implementation of prospective payment systems, Medicare reimbursement to hospitals was related directly to the costs incurred by the facilities. Individual facility costs were reported to Medicare, identifying the direct and indirect costs of providing care to Medicare patients. Direct costs include nursing and radiology; indirect costs include medical records and information systems. Preparation of **cost reports** requires the definition of products or services, establishment of cost centers, and identification of service units (Dunn 1999, pp. 64-65). The expense of non-revenue-producing cost centers is allocated to revenue-producing cost centers in order to fully understand the cost of providing services.

Allocation of Overhead

The attribution of indirect or **overhead costs** to revenue-producing service units illustrates the budget concept that all activities must support the mission of the organization. There are four methods of allocation of overhead:

- The **direct method of cost allocation** distributes the cost of overhead departments solely to the revenue-producing areas. Allocation is based on each revenue-producing area's relative square footage, number of employees, or actual usage of supplies and services. (See figure 25.8.)
- **Step-down allocation** distributes overhead costs once, beginning with the area that provides the least amount of non-revenue-producing services.
- **Double distribution** allocates overhead costs twice, which takes into consideration the fact that some overhead departments provide services to each other.

Figure 25.8.   Direct Allocation versus Step Allocation

	Non-Revenue-Producing Department		Revenue-Producing Department	
	HIM Department	Business Office	Medicine	Laboratory
Direct method:				
Overhead costs before allocation	$360,000	$240,000	$400,000	$250,000
Allocation				
HIM	($360,000)		$340,000	$20,000
# discharges processed				
Business office		($240,000)	$80,000	$160,000
# labor hours used				
Total overhead after allocation	$0	$0	$820,000	$430,000
Step method:				
Overhead costs before allocation	$360,000	$240,000	$400,000	$250,000
Allocation				
HIM	($360,000)	$50,000	$300,000	$10,000
# discharges processed				
Business office		($290,000)	$90,000	$200,000
# labor hours used				
Total overhead after allocation	$0	$0	$790,000	$460,000

• The **simultaneous equations method** distributes overhead costs through multiple iterations, allowing maximum distribution of interdepartmental costs among overhead departments.

The last three methods of cost allocation above assume that overhead cost centers such as housekeeping perform services for each other as well as for revenue-producing areas. Therefore, overhead costs are distributed among overhead cost centers as well as revenue-producing areas.

Although each of these methods may produce slightly different results, the ultimate goal is to allocate overhead costs appropriately. Appropriate allocation enables the facility to express the full cost of providing services.

Impact on Reimbursement

Although cost reporting is no longer used to directly determine Medicare reimbursement, some payers still use cost reports to make reimbursement decisions. In addition, the CMS (formerly called the HCFA) uses cost reports to help determine facility-specific and regional cost adjustment factors for healthcare prospective payment systems.

Reimbursement

Chapter 14 discusses the various types of reimbursement to healthcare providers. Regardless of the reimbursement method, the facility must be able to evaluate the underlying cost of providing services and to compare its actual reimbursements to the potential reimbursements based on charges. To do this, all individual patient charges are captured in the patients' accounts. The charges themselves and the underlying costs of the services provided are maintained in a database called the chargemaster. (Several alternative terms are used for the database, for example, charge data master and charge description master.) Using the individual patient charges and the associated clinical codes, the patient accounts department is able to prepare reimbursement claims.

Chargemaster

The **chargemaster** is a database that collects information on all of the goods and services the facility provides to patients. Responsibility for maintaining the database varies among facilities, and multiple departments contribute to the data. Because many of the charges are associated with CPT/HCPCS codes, the HIM department is usually involved in the routine maintenance of this database.

The purpose of the chargemaster is to facilitate charge capture by centralizing and standardizing charge data within the facility. Grocery stores do this by linking UPC symbols to the price and description of grocery items. The customer sees the evidence of this activity on the grocery bill but does not see that the database also contains the cost of the item, the vendor, and the underlying general ledger information. Similarly, the chargemaster enables the facility to capture and record patient charges as they are incurred. For the charges to be captured accurately, the chargemaster must be updated routinely as new services emerge, costs change, and CPT code descriptions change. Use of a properly updated chargemaster also helps the facility administratively by enabling the statistical reporting of charge-related activities.

The components of the chargemaster vary, depending on the needs of the healthcare organization. At a minimum, the fields for each record include (Schraffenberger 2002, p. 119):

• Charge code
• Item description
• General ledger (GL) key
• Revenue code
• Insurance code mapping
• Charge
• Activity date/status

Figure 25.9 provides an example of a chargemaster and its components.

Maintenance of the chargemaster is a multidisciplinary activity. For example, the HIM department knows the clinical codes, the patient accounts department knows the general ledger codes, the pharmacy department knows the drugs and their costs, and the finance department knows the associated charge formulas. Pharmacy cannot realistically update radiology's data nor can finance update charges without knowledge of underlying costs.

To coordinate the update effort, a single department, usually finance, should be assigned responsibility for ensuring timely updates. That department then enlists the assistance of other disciplines. Update frequency depends on the data element to be updated, but certainly whenever underlying costs change. For example, pharmacy charges may be updated every time inventory is replenished. The entire chargemaster must be reviewed at least annually.

Claims Processing

Claims processing involves accumulating charges for services, submitting claims for reimbursement, and ensuring that claims are satisfied. As this chapter has already discussed, this is the responsibility of the patient accounts department. However, the patient accounts department can only process what the service providers have accumulated and what HIM has coded.

Claims processing is often outsourced in ambulatory care. The activity of submitting a claim is often called dropping a bill. Because reimbursement for clinical services provided is the healthcare facility's largest source of revenue, timely, accurate claims processing is necessary.

Sometimes, a facility will adopt a **bill hold** policy. This policy dictates a waiting period between the patient's discharge date and claim submission (dropping the bill). Bill hold assumes that there will be a delay in accumulating the charges incurred by a patient. By incorporating this predicted delay into normal operations, the facility creates a preventive control to avoid underbilling or having to submit late charges to the payer.

Third-party payers generally will not reimburse a claim that does not include the clinical diagnostic and procedural codes. This is true whether the reimbursement is based on a prospective payment system, actual charges, or some other method. For this reason, the patient accounts department cannot drop a bill until the patient record has been coded. Therefore, timely, accurate coding is critical to the reimbursement process and directly affects the facility's cash flow.

Accounts Receivable

During a patient's encounter with a healthcare provider, individual services are performed and associated charges are incurred. Each charge is recorded in a subledger for the specific patient account. Because each charge represents a completed transaction, the amount of the charge becomes revenue (earned and measurable) and receivable. However, from a practical standpoint, the claim to the payer is not rendered until after discharge. Therefore, after a patient is discharged, the charges incurred by the patient during the stay are finalized. For example:

Figure 25.9.   Sample Section from a Chargemaster

Charge Code	Item Description	CPT/HCPCS Code			Revenue Code	G/L Key	Activity Date
		Insurance Code A	Insurance Code B	Insurance Code C			
2110410000	ECHO ENCEPHALOGRAM	76506	76506	Y7030	320	15	12/2/1999
2110410090	F/U ECHO ENCEPHALOGRAM	76506	76506	Y7040	320	15	12/2/1999
2110413000	PORT US ECHO ENCEPHALOGRAM	76506	76506	Y7050	320	15	12/2/1999
2120411000	ULTRASOUND SPINAL CONTENTS	76800	76800	Y7060	320	15	12/2/1999
2130401000	THYROID SONOGRAM	76536	76536	Y7070	320	15	1/1/2001
2151111000	TM JOINTS BILATERAL	70330	70330	Y7080	320	15	8/12/2000
2161111000	NECK LAT ONLY	70360	70360	Y7090	320	15	10/1/1999
2162111000	LARYNX AP & LATERAL	70360	70360	Y7100	320	15	10/1/1999
2201111000	LONG BONE CHLD AP	76061	76061	Y7110	320	15	8/12/2000
2201401000	NON-VASCULAR EXTREM SONO	76880	76880	Y7120	320	15	10/1/1999
2210111000	SKULL 1 VIEW	70250	70250	Y7130	320	15	1/1/2001
2210112000	SKULL 2 VIEWS	70250	70250	Y7140	320	15	8/12/2000
2210114000	SKULL 4 VIEWS	70260	70260	Y7150	320	15	8/12/2000
2211111000	MASTOIDS	70130	70130	Y7160	320	15	1/1/2001
2212111000	MANDIBLE	70110	70110	Y7170	320	15	12/2/1999
2213111000	FACIAL BONES	70140	70140	Y7180	320	15	12/2/1999
2213114000	FACIAL BONES MIN 4	70150	70150	Y7190	320	15	12/2/1999
2214111000	NASAL BONES	70160	70160	Y7200	320	15	1/1/2001
2215111000	ORBITS	70200	70200	Y7210	320	15	1/1/2001
2217111000	PARANASAL SINUSES	70220	70220	Y7220	320	15	1/1/2001

4/15	Accounts Receivable—Patient X	$5500
	Patient Services Revenue	$5500

Total charges for account #0146589

Cumulating charges and postdischarge billing works well for ambulatory care and most acute care encounters. For long-term care, however, interim billing is necessary. When an interim bill is dropped, the reimbursement received reduces the accounts receivable for that patient.

Posting the receivable and dropping the bill are two different activities. To monitor timely claims processing, a summary report of patient receivables is generated frequently. This summary report has no standard title. It is sometimes called DNFB, which stands for **discharged, no final bill,** or merely accounts receivable, or AR.

Components of Accounts Receivable

The individual charges for a patient's account are collected in a database. The actual components of the database vary, depending on the needs of the facility. Patient identifying data and financial data collected at registration are components of the database. Individual charges incurred also are collected. Maintenance of patients' accounts in a database enables the facility to analyze these financial data in a number of ways.

Review and Analysis of Accounts Receivable

Department managers review the patient account database for different reasons. The pharmacy department may request a listing of all pharmaceutical charges in order to compare the posted charges with its records. This detective control enables the pharmacy department to ensure that all dispensed medications are charged. The chief financial officer (CFO), on the other hand, may target one number: total charges for patients who have been discharged, but for whom no final bill has been dropped. When the total charges exceed a predetermined threshold, the CFO will require an explanation from the patient accounts department.

A predetermined threshold may be a dollar amount and/or a time period, such as days in accounts receivable. For example, an acceptable level of unbilled charges may be $1,000,000. A dollar threshold would be determined taking into consideration the cash flow needs of the facility as well as the facility's historical experience in accurate billing.

An alternative or concomitant threshold would be the days in accounts receivable. This refers to the number of days that an invoice has been outstanding once it has been billed. Of course, the first step is to mail out the final bill. Because one common reason for no final bill is the lack of clinical codes, the HIM department may be involved in delivering the explanation. See the example of an accounts receivable report in figure 25.10 (p. 626).

The HIM department participates in ensuring timely claims processing by timely coding of the clinical records. Therefore, effective coding management includes the routine analysis of the DNFB. Figure 25.10 illustrates a portion of a DNFB. Notice that the report lists the outstanding charges by the patient's last name. The patient's medical record number and discharge date enable the HIM department to locate the patient's clinical record. The sample report indicates that patient number 124785 was discharged thirteen days before the report was prepared and that the accumulated charges are $18,139.45. The reason listed for failure to drop the bill is "no final diagnosis." Seeing this, the HIM department manager would have located the record, determined why it had not been coded, and taken action to solve whatever problem had prevented its coding. Typical problems include lack of a pathology report, uncertainty as to principal diagnosis, and backlog in the coding function. Table 25.6 (p. 627) lists some common coding delays and actions that can be taken to solve the underlying problem.

Another consideration in evaluating the prioritization of uncoded records is the identity of the payer. When the healthcare facility receives **periodic interim payments** (PIPs) from the CMS, unbilled records with only Medicare as a payer may not be as high a priority as unbilled records from a private insurance company that will not pay without the claim. Therefore, the HIM department personnel involved in monitoring the DNFB must be familiar with the level of priority of the payers.

Because the patients' account data are maintained in a database, theoretically, they can be retrieved in whatever format is useful to the manager. Many facilities' computer systems include sophisticated report-writing functions that enable managers to query the database for the desired data and retrieve a report in the desired format, as needed. Although this is ideal, other systems do not provide this capability. The facility's information systems (IS) department should be able to provide the manager with a customized report routinely.

The frequency with which managers review the accounts receivable data depends on the facility's policies and procedures as well as on the impact on claims processing. To proactively manage the outstanding receivables, some HIM managers review the data daily and take action on large-dollar accounts. Because the entire AR report may contain hundreds of accounts, the manager may request a report of all accounts with an amount over $10,000 that were discharged over two days ago. Even with a bill-hold policy of three or four days, a targeted report enables the HIM department to prioritize processing of high-dollar accounts quickly.

The priority of coding high-dollar accounts quickly must be balanced against the need to maintain the even distribution of workload and orderly processing of all records in the HIM department. Ten $5,000 accounts are financially equivalent to one $50,000 account. Failure to process those ten because routine was disrupted to process the one is not good financial management. Therefore, routine, timely processing of all records can obviate prioritization by dollars.

Figure 25.10. Example of an Accounts Receivable Report

Anyplace Health Systems
Accounts Not Selected for Billing—Inpatients
Patient Financial Services Version

Patient Name	Acct. #	Med Rec #	Status	Unbilled Charges	Days Since Disch.	Pt. Type	Insurance Verification			Final Dx	DRG	Open Orders	Fin. Class
							Ins. 1	Ins. 2	Ins. 3				
Axxxxxx, Rxxx	1452585	124785	Discharged	18,139.45	13	E-Inpt	Yes	Yes	Yes	No	000	No	J
Bxxxx, Vxxxx	4568972	258564	Discharged	1,173.75	26	Inpt	No	No	No	Yes	466	No	T
Cxxxx, Axxxx	7456594	256632	Discharged	10,286.70	5	E-Inpt	Yes	Yes	Yes	Yes	277	Yes	Q
Fxxxx, Txxxxx	7458961	148965	Discharged	3,425.45	15	Inpt	No	Yes	Yes	No	000	Yes	F
Plxxxxx, Gxxxxxx	8585964	745321	Discharged	15,452.25	8	Inpt	Yes	Yes	Yes	Yes	321	Yes	J
Zxxx, Mxxxxxxx	7458946	147589	Discharged	25,584.55	20	E-Inpt	Yes	Yes	Yes	No	000	No	B

Totals I/P Discharged 6   74,062.15

Reason for Rejection
- Insurance Not Verified 4
- Open Orders 4
- No Final Dx 4
- Invalid DRG 0

Anyplace Health Systems
Accounts Not Selected for Billing—Outpatients
Patient Financial Services Version

Patient Name	Acct. #	Med Rec #	Status	Unbilled Charges	Days Since Disch.	Pt. Type	Insurance Verification			Final Dx	DRG	Open Orders	Fin. Class
							Ins. 1	Ins. 2	Ins. 3				
Cxxxx, Jxxx	5869751	586462	O/P – Recur.	1,377.50	34	Recur.	No	Yes	Yes	Yes	131	No	T
Dxxx, Axxx	7469832	154783	O/P – Surg	10,850.40	16	Surgical	Yes	Yes	Yes	Yes	479	Yes	L
Gxxx, Dxxxxx	7459831	852697	O/P	12,587.75	4	Out	Yes	Yes	Yes	No	000	No	Q

Totals

		Unbilled Charges
Recurrent Outpatients	1	1,377.50
Outpatient Surgical	1	10,850.40
Outpatient General	1	12,587.75

Reason for Rejection
- Insurance Not Verified 1
- Open Orders 1
- No Final Dx. 2
- Invalid DRG 0

Table 25.6.   Remedies for Common Coding Delays

Reason for Failure to Code	Underlying Issue(s)	Possible Actions
Lack of pathology report	Pathology department may not have completed the analysis.	Ask the pathology department for an estimated completion date and a STAT dictation.
	Pathologist may not have dictated the report.	Ask the pathology department for a STAT dictation or a verbal confirmation of the pathology diagnosis.
	Pathology reports may not have been in the charts.	Search the reports for the missing one. In a computer-based environment, coders should have the ability to search for the reports on-line.
Uncertain principal or additional diagnosis	Waiting for a response to a physician query	Elevate the query to the managerial level. Meet the physician on the nursing unit during morning rounds, if necessary.
Coding backlog	Coder(s) out sick	Prioritize coding by receivable size instead of discharge date.
	Coder(s) on vacation	Consider overtime pay for staff to fill in.
	Coding function understaffed	Assign qualified supervisory personnel to assist and/or support coders.
		Plan vacation coverage in advance to avoid affecting the facility's cash flow.
		Long-term understaffing can impair coding quality. Outsourcing should be considered. Coding quality and DNFB impact are typical justifications for approving additional coding staff.

Impact of Accounts Receivable on Financial Statements

Accounts receivable represent a current asset. Delays in processing claims cause receivables to age. Aged receivables can negatively affect a facility's ability to borrow money. Failure to claim and collect receivables affects cash, which in turn negatively affects the facility's ability to discharge its current liabilities, the largest of which is payroll. Therefore, in a facility for which reimbursement is the largest revenue item and payroll is the largest expense, there is a direct relationship between getting paid and paying employees. Thus, the role of HIM becomes a critical component of maintaining the facility's fiscal integrity.

Check Your Understanding 25.3

Instructions: Answer the following questions on a separate piece of paper.

1. Compare and contrast financial accounting and managerial accounting.
2. Compare and contrast operational budgets with capital budgets.
3. A not-for-profit organization offers a variety of programs and services. Each functional department in the organization plays some role in delivering all of these programs and services. What type of operational budget would be most effective in this environment? Why?
4. Why would an organization choose a fiscal year that does not coincide with the calendar year?
5. The HIM department has a YTD budget for a payroll of $100,000. The actual YTD amount is $98,000. Is this a favorable or an unfavorable variance?

Real-World Case

Bright Hospital is a 270-bed, not-for-profit community hospital. Its largest percentage of patients consists of mothers and newborns, followed by a mix of cardiovascular-related admissions. It has an emergency department staffed by hospital employees. Bright's fiscal year follows the calendar year, ending December 31. In August, Bright began its year-end budget process by establishing its financial assumptions for the following two years. Bright assumed that revenue would remain constant, that it would continue its existing contracts with payers, that its Medicare population percentage would not change, and that no major infrastructure maintenance would be required in the upcoming fiscal year. No major capital projects were anticipated. In its operational budget, administration plans to include resources for a JCAHO steering committee and related activities to prepare for the anticipated accreditation visit in the subsequent year. Administration distributed operational and capital budget compilation packages to department managers for completion and return by September 30.

Bright Hospital does not have a large marketing department. It has one marketing professional on staff whose responsibilities include the development and publishing of brochures and coordination of patient satisfaction surveys, which are compiled and analyzed by an outside vendor. In the past two years, there has been a slight, but continuing, decline in patient satisfaction among maternity patients. Suggestions for improvement have varied, but common complaints centered on the lack of soothing ambiance in labor and delivery and the hospital policy prohibiting overnight visitors.

The maternity and newborn departments have been very concerned about declining patient satisfaction. They are worried that the current year's slight decline in maternity admissions is the result of that dissatisfaction and that patients are traveling a little further to give birth at a neighboring medical center, at which some of their physicians also have privileges. The departments would like to renovate the maternity and newborn wing, forming a women's center with increased emphasis on wellness and ancillary services. This would be a two-year capital project that would require marketing support and some minor disruption of services during construction.

The cardiology department is very excited. It has just learned that a well-respected cardiologist has retired to the area and is exploring the idea of opening a small consulting practice. The cardiologist has not yet applied for privileges at any area hospitals, but it is known that she is used to working in a facility with its own cardiac catheterization lab. Because the current chief of the medical staff at Bright is a personal friend of the cardiologist, the cardiology department believes that she could be lured on staff if the hospital had its own lab. Based on the volume of patients whom Bright currently sends out to another facility for cardiac catheterization, the cardiology department believes that patient care would be facilitated by the expansion and that the increased revenue would help justify the cost.

The HIM department has recently lost several employees to retirement and promotions within the facility. It is currently down two coders and a file clerk. The department has reduced its weekend coverage to one person, day shift only. Transcription is handled largely by the department, with a service processing any overflow. The HIM department would like to outsource all of its transcription and move to a Web-based coding system that would allow the coders to telecommute. This plan would improve productivity, decrease transcription and coding delays, and shorten billing time. In addition, the computer-based storage of documents involved in these changes would facilitate release of information. All three departments submitted capital budget requests for the projects described.

Discussion

1. If the hospital can only approve one of the proposed projects, which do you think has the best chance of being approved? Why?

2. How should Bright's finance department analyze these projects? What do you think is the best method for analyzing them under the circumstances?

3. If you were the director of the HIM department, how would you justify the project so that it is presented most favorably?

4. How should the HIM department's proposal be divided between the operational and capital budgets?

Summary

Management roles in any healthcare facility require some knowledge of accounting and financial management. The ability to read, understand, and interpret pertinent financial reports is a desirable business skill. Because of the close ties of reimbursement and HIM, this basic skill is even more important. Although the financial accounting methodologies of compiling and analyzing financial statements may not be needed routinely, the managerial accounting skills involving budget preparation and analysis are important. Also important is an awareness of the preventive, detective, and corrective controls that managers must implement to ensure the accuracy of financial data.

Operational budgets are developed annually to allocate resources for the normal functioning of the facility, according to its mission. Operational budgets focus on revenues and expenses. Capital budgets separately identify and analyze long-term asset acquisitions that are designed to maintain and improve the facility's infrastructure, improve operational efficiency, or expand business, for example. Capital budget requests are analyzed for their cost versus benefit as well as return on investment.

Efficient claims processing has a direct impact on the ability of a facility to fund its operations, including paying its bills and meeting payroll obligations. HIM plays a direct role in ensuring efficient claims processing by participating in chargemaster review, participating in the analysis and minimization of the AR totals, and ensuring efficient and accurate coding of records.

References

Dunn, Rose. 1999. *Finance Principles for the Health Information Manager.* Chicago: American Health Information Management Association.

Horngren, Charles, Walter Harrison, and Linda Bamber. 1999. *Accounting,* fourth edition. Upper Saddle River, N.J.: Prentice-Hall.

Pelfrey, Sandra. 1992. *Basic Accounting for Hospital Based Non-Financial Managers.* Albany, N.Y.: Delmar.

Schraffenberger, Lou Ann, editor. 2002. *Effective Management of Coding Services.* Chicago: American Health Information Management Association.

Shim, Jae, and Joel Siegel. 1994. *Budgeting Basics and Beyond: A Complete Step-by-Step Guide for Nonfinancial Managers.* Upper Saddle River, N.J.: Prentice-Hall.

Tinsley, Reed. 2002. *Medical Practice Management Handbook.* New York City: Harcourt Brace.

Application Exercises

1. Go to the Securities and Exchange Commission Web site (www.sec.gov) and search for healthcare organization filings. In the "Search" box, type Hospital to obtain a display of hospital organizations. Also, try HCA (Hospital Corporation of America). Look at the latest reports. Find the income statement and balance sheet. Can you calculate the ratios discussed in this chapter? The dollar amounts look as though they are hundreds or thousands of dollars. How many zeros do you think should be after each number: 000? 000,000?

2. From your library, your personal investment files, or the SEC web site, find financial statements from nonhealthcare organizations. Look at the balance sheet and income statement. How are these statements similar to or different from the healthcare statements in question 1 above? What business activities make the financial statements necessarily different?

3. Look for articles about accountants, accounting, and accounting practices in a recent *Wall Street Journal* or a large newspaper published in your area. Go to the Web site for the American Institute of Certified Public Accountants (AICPA) (www.aicpa.org) and view the home page. Is there a news release or other comment by the AICPA in response to the article? Review the news releases on the AICPA web site. Can you relate them to current events? Why do you think the AICPA puts news releases on their home page?

4. Interview a director of health information management at a local hospital. What is the operational budget process for the hospital? How long does it take? What projections and estimates does the director have to make? How are capital budgets handled?

5. Through the director of health information management at a local hospital, arrange interviews with the patient accounts manager and the chief financial officer. Find out about their career paths. Ask them how they work together to keep accounts receivable low. What are their thresholds (at what point are receivables too high)?

Review Quiz

Instructions: Select the best answers for the following questions.

1. ___ What term is used to represent the difference between the budgeted amount and the actual amount of a line item that is expected to reverse itself during a subsequent period?
   a. A permanent variance
   b. A fixed cost
   c. A temporary variance
   d. A flexible cost

2. ___ What basic accounting principle requires that helpful explanations accompany financial reports, when necessary?
   a. Disclosure
   b. Reliability
   c. Matching
   d. Consistency

3. ___ Trinity Hospital has a fiscal year end of August 31. For this hospital, the second quarter ends:
   a. November 30th
   b. February 28th or 29th
   c. May 31st
   d. August 31st

4. ___ Dr. Blake's administrative assistant purchased office supplies at an office supplies store and charged the purchase to the doctor's account. The journal entry used to record this transaction is a debit to office supplies expense and a credit to ___.
   a. Purchases
   b. Cash
   c. Accounts payable
   d. Revenue

5. ___ The following information was abstracted from Community Hospital's balance sheet:

Total assets:	$25,000,000
Current assets:	$4,000,000
Total liabilities:	$10,000,000
Current liabilities:	$5,000,000

   A vendor selling a large-dollar amount of goods to this hospital on credit would ___.
   a. Not be concerned because total assets exceed total liabilities
   b. Not be concerned because the debt ratio is less than one half
   c. Be somewhat concerned because the current ratio is less than one
   d. Not analyze the balance sheet because the vendor would care more about the income statement

6. ___ The HIM department records copy fees as revenue. Year-to-date, the budgeted fees are $25,000 and the actual fees received are $23,000. The director may be asked to explain ___.
   a. A favorable variance of $2000
   b. An unfavorable variance of $2000
   c. A favorable variance of $23,000
   d. An unfavorable variance of $23,000

7. ___ Community Hospital is purchasing a new ambulance. The ambulance will cost $100,000, which will be depreciated at $20,000 per year for five years. Related cash inflows from reimbursements are projected to be $80,000 annually. The hospital expects to replace the vehicle when it is fully depreciated. How much is the accounting rate of return on this investment?
   a. 20%
   b. 40%
   c. 60%
   d. 80%

8. ___ In 1980, Community Hospital purchased a building for its clinic for $200,000. In 2002, the hospital sold the building for $850,000. The return on this investment is ___.
   a. 24%
   b. 76%
   c. 325%
   d. 425%

9. ___ Community Hospital is evaluating three different investments. Which one has the highest profitability index?

	Radiology Investment	Cardiology Investment	Pharmacy Investment
Present value of cash inflows	$2,000,000	$1,200,000	$40,000
Present value of cash outflows	$500,000	$300,000	$10,000

   a. The radiology investment
   b. The cardiology investment
   c. The pharmacy investment
   d. All three are equally profitable

Instructions: Use the following information to answer questions 10 through 12. At the end of March, the HIM department has a YTD payroll budget of $100,000. The actual YTD amount is $95,000 because a coder resigned in February. For the past two months, the position has been filled through outsourcing. Therefore, the actual YTD amount for consulting services is $5,000, although no money was budgeted for consulting services. The reporting threshold for variances is 4 percent. The fiscal year-end is December.

10. ___ What is the best description of the payroll variance?
    a. Favorable, permanent
    b. Unfavorable, permanent
    c. Favorable, temporary
    d. Unfavorable, temporary

11. ___ What is the best description of the consulting services variance?
    a. Favorable, permanent
    b. Unfavorable, permanent
    c. Favorable, temporary
    d. Unfavorable, temporary

12. ___ Which one of the variances will the HIM director be required to explain?
    a. Only the consulting services variance
    b. Only the payroll variance
    c. Both the payroll and consulting services variances
    d. Neither because the two variances cancel each other out

Chapter 26
Project Management

Patricia B. Seidl, RHIA

Learning Objectives

- To understand how a project differs from an organization's daily operations
- To describe the components of a project
- To discuss reasons for project success versus project failure
- To describe different project team structures
- To understand the responsibilities of the project manager
- To understand the project management process and to recognize the technical and people skills involved
- To identify the components of a project proposal document
- To understand the steps in planning and organizing a project
- To estimate work, duration, and resource requirements
- To understand how to anticipate and manage project risk
- To understand how to track a project's progress and analyze variances
- To describe the types of plan revision
- To understand the concept of scope management
- To recognize the components of a communication plan

Key Terms

Assumptions
Baseline
Change control
Contingency
Critical path
Deliverables
Dependency
Duration
Issue log
Predecessor
Project charter
Project management software
Project components
Project network
Project office
Project plan
Project schedule
Project team
Resources
Risk
Roles and responsibilities
Scheduling engine
Scope
Sponsor
Stakeholders
Statement of work
Subprojects
Successor
Task
Variances
Work
Work breakdown structure
Work products

Introduction

Although health information management professionals practice in many diverse healthcare delivery systems and domains, there is a common responsibility across all lines of business: leading or participating in projects. It is important to understand the concepts and best practices of project management in order to engage fully and effectively as a project team member. Although there are many different types, all projects have similar attributes: Their objectives are of benefit to the organization, they all follow the project management process, the same characteristics of the project manager are needed, they all involve a project team, and they all result in some type of outcome.

Projects consist of organizational and behavioral components. Organizational or structural components guide the team toward its end goals. Behavioral components include the concepts of leading, motivating, politics, and interpersonal communication.

This chapter describes the different elements of a project and the different types of projects that healthcare organization might undertake. It also focuses on how projects are managed and tracked to ensure their success.

Theory into Practice

A healthcare facility is due for a Joint Commission on the Accreditation of Healthcare Organizations (JCAHO) survey later this year. The facility has strived to make compliance with JCAHO standards part of its normal operational processes and has decided to perform an assessment to ensure that any new or revised standards have been incorporated into its practices.

The facility first forms a multidisciplinary team and assigns a project manager. The project manager spearheads, and the team contributes to, preparing a plan that details the tasks that need to be accomplished. Team members are assigned tasks and decide to meet every two weeks to discuss their progress.

The team then begins the assessment. Each department conducts a review of the JCAHO standards, comparing them to the department's policies and procedures to ensure that all the standards are being met. The departments pay special attention to new standards to ensure that they are interpreting the standards correctly. When necessary, team members seeks out colleagues who have recently undergone a survey to answer questions on the standards. When a deficiency is found, it is logged and assigned to the appropriate department personnel for resolution and given a resolution due date.

After all the deficiencies have been documented, the team monitors the list and updates it regularly with the progress of the policy and procedure revisions. If the policy and proce-dure revisions are not occurring in a timely manner, the project manager needs to refer the issue to the project's sponsor.

After all the deficiencies have been addressed through updated policies and procedures, each department conducts employee educational sessions to incorporate the revisions into its daily operations.

Finally, the facility conducts a mock survey. It also prepares and executes a training program for the entire institution so that all employees know what to expect when the JCAHO surveyors arrive.

As the JCAHO survey date draws near, each team member prepares a list of items that the surveyors may request. This will help the facility to respond quickly to the requests during the actual survey.

After the JCAHO survey has been conducted and the results received by the facility, the team's final responsibility is to follow up on the survey recommendations.

The Project

An organization undertakes a project because it has determined the need for some type of change. This need may be the result of a company's strategic agenda, such as implementation of a new computer system, or may be due to the passage of a new government regulation. After the need for the project has been acknowledged, the project enters the project management life cycle or process.

Every project has an identified sponsor. The **sponsor** is the facility employee with the most vested interest in the project's success. It is a good practice to select someone who has responsibility for the organization's departments, divisions, and personnel that will be affected by the project. The project will open up many issues that, in some situations, must be resolved by an authority figure. It is much easier to obtain a decision or consensus when the sponsor already has established control over the areas involved in the project. The sponsor often approves the budget for the project and is ultimately responsible for the project expenditures.

The project also has stakeholders. A **stakeholder** is anyone in the organization who is affected by the project product. Stakeholders include personnel who are on the project team, personnel whose daily work will be changed because of the project's product, and the managers and executives for those departments involved in the project. Each stakeholder has different concerns relative to the project's objectives and goals. The **project team** wants to produce a high-quality product. Departmental personnel worry about their ability to adapt to the procedures and skills required by the new or changed product. Department managers and executives must support the functional changes that may be needed as a result of the project. Each stakeholder will evaluate the project's success based on these concerns and the expectations they hold for how the project will benefit them.

Definition of a Project

A Guide to the Project Management Body of Knowledge (PMBOK® Guide) describes a project as "a temporary endeavor undertaken to create a unique product or service" (Project Management Institute 2000, p. 4). A project has the following characteristics:

- Specific objectives or goals to be achieved
- A defined start and end date
- A defined set of resources assigned to perform the required work
- Specific deliverables or work products
- A defined budget or cost

A project differs from the day-to-day operations of an organization. Operations are concerned with the everyday jobs needed to run the business. The personnel involved in the operational aspects of the business perform the same functions on a routine basis. This work does not end. In contrast, a project has a precise, expected result produced by defined resources within a specific time frame.

Project Parameters

A well-defined project has specific objectives. After the project's objectives have been defined, all project activities should be focused toward meeting them. The project activities result in deliverables or work products. When the project activities have concluded and the project deliverables have been completed, the project ends.

The process of documenting project parameters is discussed later in this chapter.

Project Components

Lewis writes that a project's objectives include cost, performance, time, and scope. Cost is the project budget, performance relates to the quality of the project work, time is the schedule, and **scope** is the magnitude of the work to be done. He illustrates the relationship with the expression "Cost is a function of Performance, Time, and Scope." Should the cost, performance, or schedule variable change, the relationship dictates that the scope will change (Lewis 1998, pp. 61–62). The project manager and the sponsor must acknowledge this relationship and be willing to make the trade-offs that will be needed when the variables change.

When developing the **project plan**, the project manager translates the objectives into three **project components**: scope, resources, and schedule. These components have a strong dependency. Again, if one of the three changes, one of the other two parameters must change as well.

Project resources are not just people. A resource is any physical asset needed to complete a task. This includes facilities, equipment, materials and supplies. Resources can also include individuals from outside organizations, such as suppliers or vendors.

One reason why many projects fail to meet their objectives within the expected time frame and budget is that their scope begins to grow as they progress. For example, new functions or features are added to a software implementation. This is commonly known as "scope creep." The requestor presents each change as a small revision with low impact on time line or cost. However, several minor changes soon add up to a more significant modification to the original work or cost estimate. The project manager must be diligent to prevent scope creep. (This topic is discussed in detail later in this chapter.)

Project Assumptions

Assumptions are scope-limiting parameters. They provide constraints on what is and is not included in the project. For example, if the project is to implement a lab results–reporting system on the clinical units, one of the assumptions may be that the clinical personnel will look up results online, thus decreasing the number of phone calls to the laboratory.

Assumptions define answers to unknown questions. For instance, at the beginning of the project, the project manager may not know what personnel will be assigned to the project and thus will not know the skill set that will be available. One assumption might be that a project team member from a particular department on a cross-departmental project is a decision maker. In other words, when the project team meets to design the user interface for a software implementation, the decisions can be made in that meeting and will not be deferred to a person outside the team. If this assumption does not prove to be true, the project manager is faced with a potential delay because the process required for decision making was not accounted for in the project schedule.

Assumptions directly affect the project estimates for the resource and time line requirements. Therefore, it is critical that the project manager obtain agreement from the sponsor and the stakeholders on all assumptions. A lack of buy-in by all of the project participants puts the objectives at risk. Many projects immediately start down the path of failure because the assumptions were not addressed adequately at the project start.

Types of Projects

There are many different types of projects. Although they share some attributes, projects can be vastly different in several aspects. Some projects are short term and completed in the span of weeks; other projects take years to complete. One project may involve only a single department; another may require participation across the facilities in an integrated delivery system.

Following are types of projects in which health information management (HIM) professionals may be involved:

- Instituting new or revised procedures to address new regulations
- Conducting a chargemaster review
- Preparing for a Joint Commission on the Accreditation of Healthcare Organizations (JCAHO) survey

- Implementing a new dictation system
- Merging two HIM departments
- Creating a new employee orientation program
- Implementing a new business procedure or process

A complex project may comprise several **subprojects.** The subprojects share common milestones and objectives but may be managed by different project managers. Subproject information may be compiled into one report to show information across all associated projects.

Project Risk versus Project Value

Projects are undertaken to specifically incorporate some requirement or business need. Although the organization certainly expects a positive outcome, there are always some **risks** to the organization as well. One of the project manager's responsibilities is to mitigate risk. However, the organization will need to weigh the cost of potential risks against the perceived value to be gained.

Project risk can take many forms and be either of a technical or psychological nature. For example, implementing a state-of-the-art computer system may provide leading-edge technology that sets the organization apart from its competitors. However, the availability of personnel who can provide support for new technology may be limited.

Another example would be a project that introduces a significant change to a department employee's responsibilities. However, the change positions the employee out of his or her comfort zone. Before the project begins, an employee may be considered an expert in his or her job responsibilities. At the conclusion of the project, the same employee may have new duties and will not have the same proficiency in them. This could cause self-esteem problems. It is not uncommon for employee turnover to occur during a project because of this threat to job security.

Check Your Understanding 26.1

Instructions: Answer the following questions on a separate piece of paper.

1. Why does an organization start a project?
2. What are the similar responsibilities of the project's sponsor and stakeholders? What are examples of different responsibilities?
3. How do projects and organizational processes differ?
4. What is "scope creep"?

Project Management

The *PMBOK® Guide* defines **project management** as "the application of knowledge, skills, tools, and techniques to project activities to meet project requirements" (Project Management Institute 2000, p. 6). Project management is concerned with completing a project within the expected cost and time line with high-quality results. This is not easy to accomplish and, as a consequence, interest in project management best practices is very high. Many organizations are starting to stress the importance of solid project management methodologies and are establishing project offices to support the organization's project managers. A **project office** is responsible for defining project management procedures, conducting risk analyses on projects, and mentoring project managers.

Overview of Project Management

The discipline of project management has emerged as organizations have come to realize that projects cannot succeed without it. As Kleim and Ludin point out, project management has traditionally focused on project cost, schedule, and quality. They consider this to be the classical approach to project management. Their belief is that project management is now taking a more behavioral approach by viewing the project as a total system, emphasizing the project's human aspects (Kliem and Ludin 1998, p. 6).

Projects have customarily been deemed successful when they meet their objectives but do not exceed their approved cost and estimated schedule. Kliem and Ludin break down the reasons for project success and failure based on the classical or behavioral approach. These reasons are listed in table 26.1.

Lewis also proposes a different definition of project success. He challenges the commonly held belief that a project has failed when it does not meet its cost, performance, time, or scope targets by questioning how these targets were established. The targets may have been unrealistic and thus impossible to meet. By citing several studies, Lewis concludes that it is how closely the project outcomes align with the perceptions held by the key project personnel that determines project success (Lewis 1998, pp. 39–43). As an example, if a project comes in under budget but ends up solving the wrong problem, is it successful? A project may meet the schedule but have unexpected and undesirable consequences. As Thomas K. Connellan, a speaker, trainer, consultant, and senior principal of a customer relationship management consulting firm, once said, "There is no point in doing well that which you should not be doing at all."

The Project Management Life Cycle

Every project follows a project management life cycle regardless of its size or duration. Each process in the life cycle has its own importance. Any one of the processes cannot be eliminated or minimized without endangering the success of the project. The project management life cycle consists of a number of processes. (See table 26.2.) Each process is discussed in more detail later in this chapter.

The Project Team

By definition, a project results in an end product through the completion of **task** activities. The execution of these task activities is the responsibility of the project team. A project team is composed of individuals who possess the knowledge and skill set to produce the project deliverables and work products.

Table 26.1.   Reasons for Project Success and Failure

Project Success	
Classical	**Behavioral**
Well-defined goals and objectives	Agreement on goals and objectives
Detailed work breakdown structure	Commitment to achieving goals and objectives
Clear reporting relationships	High morale
Formal change management disciplines in place	Good teaming
Channels of communication exist	Cooperation among all participants
Adherence to scope	Receptivity to positive and negative feedback
Reliable estimating	Receptive culture to project management
Reliable monitoring and tracking techniques	Realistic expectations
Clear requirements	Good conflict resolution
Reasonable time frame	Executive sponsorship
Broad distribution of work	Good customer–supplier relationship
Project Failure	
Classical	**Behavioral**
Ill-defined work breakdown structure	Inappropriate leadership style
High-level schedule	No common vision
No reporting infrastructure	Unrealistic expectations
Too pessimistic or optimistic estimates	Poor informal communications and interpersonal relationships
No change management discipline	No buy-in or commitment from customer or people doing work
Inadequate formal communications	Low morale
Inefficient allocation of resources	Lack of training
No accountability and responsibility for results	Poor teaming
Poor role definition	Culture not conducive to project management
Inadequacy of tools	Lack of trust among participants
Ill-defined scope	False or unrealistic expectations
Unclear requirements	No or weak executive sponsorship
Too high, too long, or too short time frame	Mediocre knowledge transfer

Source: Reprinted from *Project Management Practitioner's Handbook.* Copyright © 1998 Ralph L. Kleim and Irwin S. Ludin. Used with permission of the publisher, AMACOM, a division of American Management Association, New York, NY. All rights reserved. *http://www.amanet.org.*

The type of project determines the size of the project team and the originating location of the resources. A project that affects only one department will typically have project team members from only that department. A project with organizationwide objectives will have a cross-departmental team, whereas a project for an integrated

Table 26.2.   Project Management Life Cycle

Project definition	This process will determine the project objectives, activities, assumptions, high-level cost estimate, and anticipated schedule.
Planning and organization	A detailed project plan is developed that delineates the tasks to be performed, the resources necessary for each task, and the estimated task duration, start, and finish. The project team is assembled.
Tracking and analysis	By tracking project progress and analyzing it against the original plan, the project manager is able to determine when the project is not moving forward as planned.
Project revisions	When the analysis reveals project deviations, the plan may need to be modified in order to still meet the project objectives.
Change control	This is the process of managing change requests to the original project definition.
Communication	This process occurs throughout the project life cycle. Project information is collected from, and disseminated to, all stakeholders.

delivery system will include representatives from all the system's facilities.

There are three types of project team structure: functional, projectized, and matrixed (Project Management Institute 2000, pp. 19–20).

Functional Team Structure

In a strictly functional organization, the project is thought to affect only one department. The functional manager may assume responsibility for managing the project. The team members are primarily from the functional department, and the functional manager confers with other functional managers on any issues affecting those departments.

Projectized Team Structure

The projectized organization has dedicated resources that are involved only in project work. Team members report to the project manager not only on project assignments, but also as their direct manager.

Matrixed Team Structure

The matrixed organization maintains the functional organization. Team members report to a functional manager and remain employees of that department. The team members receive their project assignments from the project manager.

In a matrixed organization, assigning the members of the project team can pose a dilemma for the stakeholders and the project manager. Typically, the best people to have on a project team are the ones who most intimately understand the processes and procedures affected by the project. However, these people have operational responsibilities in their respective departments that do not disappear while the project is in progress. Depending on the scope of the project, the time commitment required of the project team can be quite significant.

It is important to define the **roles and responsibilities** of the project team. In a matrixed organization, the project team members will not report to the project manager in an organizational structure. However, the project manager will hold team members accountable for their tasks.

Check Your Understanding 26.2

Instructions: Prepare a grid that lists examples of the types of projects an HIM professional may be involved in. For each project list the following:

- The project objectives
- The factors that will be used to measure project success
- The factors that may contribute to project failure
- The members of the project team

The Project Manager

The project manager is the individual with responsibility for directing the project activities from initiation through closure. Depending on the size of the project, the project manager may be a dedicated resource or may be performing these duties along with other operational assignments. For example, for a project confined to a single department, an assistant director may be asked to manage the project while the department director takes on the sponsor role. In other situations, one of the team members may be asked to be the project leader while still performing specific task assignments for the project.

In circumstances where the project manager is not fully devoted to the project, it is easy for the project management duties to fall by the wayside, especially because many of these may produce intangible results. (The functions of the project manager are discussed in a subsequent section of this chapter.) The project sponsor must ensure that an adequate percentage of the resource's time is allocated to these responsibilities.

Competencies and Skills

A project manager must possess both functional and behavioral skills. Some of his or her responsibilities are purely operational, for example, preparing a project plan. However, several skills are required that touch on the human side of projects. All projects result in a change in the organization. Facilitating an organization through the impact of these changes requires attributes that are described as "soft skills."

Project managers are very often in the position of having great responsibility, but little authority, because the project team members do not report to them from an organizational perspective. Thus, project managers must get results from the team members through leadership and influence.

Project managers should possess the following skills:

- General management skills of planning, directing, organizing, and prioritizing
- Leadership skills of influencing, motivating, providing vision, and resolving conflict
- Communication skills of being able to interact with all levels of an organization and of being able to understand different communication styles and mediums
- Facilitation skills, including negotiation, consensus building, and meeting management
- Analytical skills, including innovative thinking, problem solving, and decision making

Functions

The project manager performs several functions over the course of the project management life cycle. These functions are described in table 26.3.

Table 26.3.   Functions of the Project Manager

Set the project expectations.	As noted earlier, project success is tied to the perception that the project met the objectives. The project manager has responsibility for properly setting the project expectations and continually resetting them as the project progresses.
Create the project plan and recruit the project team.	The project manager generates a project schedule with the estimated work effort. The project team is organized, with each team member understanding his or her roles and responsibilities. The project manager leads team development efforts to form an effective, motivated team. He or she uses interpersonal skills to establish a rapport with team members.
Manage project control.	When the project is under way, the project manager must have a clear understanding of its status. Informal and formal communication methods are used to determine project progress. The project manager maintains the project plan to perform variance analysis. The project manager works with the project team to bring tasks to closure by facilitating decision-making and issue resolution. The project manager facilitates the removal of any obstacles that prevent the team from producing the project deliverables.
Recommend plan revisions.	If a plan is not progressing as scheduled, the project manager must determine what actions need to be taken to put the project back on track. He or she gains consensus on the changes from the sponsor and the stakeholders, and monitors any new risks to the plan.
Execute change control.	The project manager institutes a policy and procedure for managing change requests. He or she keeps everyone focused on the end goal.
Prepare, document, and communicate project information.	Project documentation is a key facet of project communication. The project manager creates the communication plan that will be used to determine when, how, and what information is to be gathered and distributed. He or she facilitates the dissemination of information throughout the organization. Although the project team members create much of the documentation through the project deliverables, the project manager is responsible for ensuring that documentation exists and is available.

The Project Management Process

A project follows a defined process regardless of size, type, or industry . The process is scalable, meaning that the depth to which a particular process is performed may vary according to project length, scope, or other parameters. However, to ensure the success of the project, all of these processes must be performed to some degree.

Project Definition

Project definition sets the expectation for the what, when, and how of the project. As noted under the project parameters section of this chapter, every project comprises three components: What is to be done (scope), the resources needed to accomplish the objectives, and the amount of time required to complete the project. The project definition process formally documents these variables for the project. This process is important for several reasons. First, it provides all project stakeholders, team members, and other personnel with the same information about the project—what it will accomplish, when it will be done, and what resources it will require. Second, it is then used as the basis for understanding when requested changes are out of the project's scope.

Determine Project Scope and Define Project Deliverables

The definition of the project starts with determining its goals. The project's goals or objectives should be measurable. If they are not, it would impossible for the project manager and the stakeholders to determine whether the project is successful. (Examples of objectives are shown in table 26.4.)

The next step in defining the project is to determine the tangible end results of the project. These are typically called project deliverables. The project deliverables indicate when the project activities have been completed. Typical deliverables for a software implementation, for example, include:

- System requirements
- User interface design document
- Test plans
- Training and procedure manuals
- Production software

Estimate the Project Schedule and Cost

The next step in project definition is to estimate how long the project will take and how much it will cost. At this point in the process, the project may not have been approved, so this information is needed in order for the stakeholders to make an informed decision. This also poses a dilemma for the project manager. He or she may not have enough detailed information about the project to make an estimate. (A detailed analysis occurs in the project planning phase.)

In this case, the project manager has a few options. One is to evaluate a past project that is similar in scope and to extract pertinent information from it that can be used in estimating the new project. A second option is to confer with professional colleagues who have experience in the proposed project. If a similar project is unavailable for analysis, a third alternative is for the project manager to use his or her expert judgment and intuition based on other professional experiences. Another opportunity would be available if the project manager were working with a vendor. The vendor would likely have experience in these types of projects and could assist the project manager in formulating estimates.

Prepare the Project Proposal

As stated above, one of the purposes of the project definition phase is to set project expectations. The project manager now should be ready to record the project objectives, scope, deliverables, expected time line, and anticipated cost in a written document. This document is known by various names. Typical names include **project charters, statements of work,** and project definition documents or business plans.

The project proposal contains several topics. The following information should be included:

- *Summary:* The summary provides an overview of the project and can provide any relevant background history and reasons why the project is being proposed.
- *Objectives:* The objectives state the project's goals.
- *Project activities:* This section is a high-level description of the major project tasks and maps out how the project will produce the project deliverables. These activities will be detailed during the project planning phase.
- *Assumptions:* Assumptions provide input to the estimates for the resource and time line requirements. Inclusion of the assumptions in the project definition document sets the stage for their acknowledgment and agreement. Assumptions may or may not prove to be true as the project progresses. The importance of identifying assumptions is that when one does not prove to be true, one of the project components will likely need to be altered.

Table 26.4.   Examples of Measurable and Nonmeasurable Objectives

Type of Project	Nonmeasurable Objective	Measurable Objective
Implementation of a patient accounting system	Improve communication between the HIM department and the patient accounting department	Decrease discharged, not-final-billed accounts from 10 days after discharge to 3 days
Implementation of a document imaging system	Increase availability of patient records	Decrease the number of chart requests by 50%
Institute a home coding program	Improve coder satisfaction	Decrease staff turnover by 20%

- *Roles and responsibilities:* This section defines the types of resources needed on the project and delineates who does what. Its concept is not dissimilar to defining a department's organizational structure. The purpose is to ensure that everyone is aware of everyone's duties and the lines of authority. It's a good idea to include a project organization chart. The project manager usually does not have management authority over the team so documenting the roles is crucial in order to understand how the team will function.
- *Schedule/cost:* Schedule and cost information is provided at a very high level because it will be further refined during the project planning phase. Cost estimates will include those for personnel, equipment, and supplies. If an external company will be providing some project services, this section should indicate whether the engagement is based on time and materials or fixed-fee pricing.
- *Deliverables:* The discussion of deliverables is another component of setting expectations. By documenting the tangible output from the project, everyone will understand when the project tasks are complete. This section can be specific by including the following types of information for each deliverable:
  —Type (for example, Microsoft Word)
  —Expected length or size
  —Number of copies provided
  —Mode of delivery (for example, through e-mail)

Check Your Understanding 26.3

Instructions: Prepare a project proposal document for one of the projects you listed in Check Your Understanding 26.2. Include the project objectives, deliverables, high-level project activities, assumptions, and roles and responsibilities. What needs to be considered when estimating the project cost?

Project Planning

After a project has been approved, it moves into the planning phase. The purpose of this phase is to further refine the project work effort, time line, and cost. During the project planning phase, the project manager creates a project plan that details the tasks to be performed, the resources needed to perform each task, the estimated work effort, and the estimated start and finish dates.

The project manager may use **project management software** to aid this process. Also known as a **scheduling engine,** project management software can provide the tools to automate some of the functions the project manager must perform. However, a software tool cannot perform the behavioral roles required of the project manager. Beware of software product literature promising a successful project simply by using it!

Identify Project Activities

When a project is initiated, the project manager is faced with the question, How do we complete the project objectives and produce the project deliverables? Creating a project plan that

lists each activity provides the road map to answer this question. For example, when a person decides to go on a vacation, he or she does not simply go to the airport. First, he or she has to decide where to go and how to get there and then make the appropriate reservations and so on.

A project plan starts with a **work breakdown structure** (WBS), or task list. The WBS is a hierarchical list of steps needed to complete the project. This structure provides levels that are similar to the concept of a book outline. Each level drills down to more detail. The lowest level is the task level, which is the level to which resources are assigned and work effort estimates are made.

A good place to begin in building the WBS is with the deliverables. Every deliverable should have a set of corresponding tasks to produce it. After every deliverable has been covered, the next area to address is the tasks that do not produce deliverables per se. What kind of tasks are they? One such task would be project management. Although project management tasks certainly produce plenty of documentation, the output is not a deliverable for the project itself, meaning that it does not contribute to the project objectives.

When creating the WBS, the project manager is faced with determining the level of task detail to be included. When the task level is not itemized enough, it will be difficult to assess the progress on the task. Having too much detail presents its own problems if the project manager is using project management software because he or she will spend too much time managing the project plan instead of doing the actual project. The level of detail directly correlates to the project manager's ability to control the project. He or she must determine the level of detail that provides this control.

Construct the Project Network

When all the tasks have been defined, the next step is to determine the **dependency** among tasks. The tasks in the project plan cannot all start at the same time. For example, training on a new computer system cannot begin until the training materials have been completed and the system has been thoroughly tested.

The definition of dependencies among the project tasks is the first step in scheduling the project. The purpose of the **project schedule** is to provide information on when the particular tasks can begin and when they are scheduled to end. The overall **project network** is defined through these dependencies.

Figure 26.1 shows an example of a project schedule for the JCAHO project described in the Theory into Practice section.

There are a few types of dependencies:

- *Finish-to-start:* This means that the first, or **predecessor,** task must finish before the dependent, or **successor,** task can start. Finish-to-start is the most common type of dependency.
- *Start-to-start:* This states that the successor task cannot start until the predecessor task begins. An example of

Figure 26.1.   Example of a Project Schedule

Task Name	Duration	Week 1									Week 2						
		F	S	S	M	T	W	T	F	S	S	M	T	W	T	F	S
⊟ **Readiness Assessment**	**3 days**																
Conduct assessment	1 day																
Update policies and procedures	1 day																
Conduct employee education	1 day																
⊟ **Prepare for Survey**	**3 days**																
Conduct mock survey	1 day																
Correct problem areas	1 day																
Conduct institutional training program	1 day																
Prepare list of survey requests	1 day																
⊟ **JCAHO Survey**	**2 days**																
Estimated survey date	0 days																
Review survey recommendations	1 day																
Implement plan to address recommendations	1 day																

this relationship would be in a computer system conversion. The user workstation hardware for the old system cannot be swapped out with the hardware for the new system until the old system is taken offline when the conversion process begins.

- *Finish-to-finish:* In this definition, the successor task cannot finish until the predecessor task finishes. An example of this dependency would be completing training materials when the system testing for a computer system is complete. The materials cannot be finished until the project manager is assured, via testing, that all modifications to the software have been completed.

Estimate Activity Duration and Work Effort

After the tasks have been defined, the project manager determines who will perform each task (resources), the amount of effort it will take to complete the task (work), and how long it will take to finish the task (duration). **Work** and **duration** are two different values. For example, if Emily is assigned to a task for twenty-four hours of work effort, how long will it take her to complete the task? It depends on how much of Emily's overall workday she devotes to this particular task. If she spends 100 percent of her day on this task and the assumption is that she is scheduled to work eight hours a day, she can complete the task in three days. If she can only dedicate 50 percent of her time to the task, she will complete the task in six days.

Estimating the work effort for tasks is difficult and can be time-consuming, especially if the organization does not have much experience in the type of project being performed. (Various methods for estimating work were discussed earlier in the chapter.)

It is best to get estimates from the people who will be performing the work. If the team has not been assigned, the functional manager of the area may be called on to provide this information. Either way, the project manager may still encounter unrealistic values because people tend to underestimate the effort in those instances where historical information is unavailable. Some people overcompensate in their estimate if they do have experience in projects, knowing that unforeseen circumstances can come up.

And, unfortunately, Parkinson's Law, which says that "Work expands to fill the time," complicates the estimating situation. Typically, if a resource is told that there are sixteen hours of work effort allocated for a task, he or she will expend all sixteen hours.

The assumptions for the project also play a role in defining the estimates. For example, if an assumption is that a software engineer knowledgeable in the applicable software language will be assigned to the project, the work estimates will be lower than if the assumption is that an inexperienced resource will be assigned.

After the work effort values have been determined and the task durations calculated, the project network reflects a more realistic time frame. The project finish date is calculated based on the task dependencies and task durations. Figure 26.2 (p. 640) shows how the project tasks from figure 26.1 are now scheduled.

If a project manager is using project management software, the critical path for the project can be determined. The **critical path** is the series of specific tasks that determine the overall project duration.

The critical path is important for the project manager to understand because any change in the start or finish of one of the tasks on the critical path means the expected project finish date will change. Changes to the critical path can happen in a variety of ways, including:

- The duration of a task may change because the work effort or resource availability changes.
- The expected start date for the task changes because the finish date for a predecessor task changes.

Figure 26.2.   Example of a Revised Project Schedule

Task Name	Duration	Month 1				Month 2					Month 3				Month 4	
		W1	W2	W3	W4	W5	W6	W7	W8	W9	W10	W11	W12	W13	W14	W15
⊟ **Readiness Assessment**	**21 days**															
Conduct assessment	5 days															
Update policies and procedures	15 days															
Conduct employee education	1 day															
⊟ **Prepare for Survey**	**16 days**															
Conduct mock survey	4 days															
Correct problem areas	10 days															
Conduct institutional training program	1 day															
Prepare list of survey requests	2 days															
⊟ **JCAHO Survey**	**33 days**															
Estimated survey date	0 days															
Review survey recommendations	3 days															
Implement plan to address recommendations	30 days															

- The finish date for a task changes because a resource's availability is changed. Perhaps a person schedules vacation or training for a week or his or her availability for the project changes because he or she is assigned additional duties outside the project.

The project manager also can use the critical path to determine how to shorten the overall project schedule. It is typical for the stakeholders of a project to already have a predetermined expected finish date for the project when it is proposed. It is not uncommon for this date to be earlier than the project finish date calculated by the scheduling engine software. The project manager is faced with the situation of fitting the tasks into this predetermined schedule. The way to do this is to look at the critical path tasks to determine how they could be accomplished sooner.

Conduct Risk Analysis

With the project network calculated, the project manager has a plan for the project schedule, work effort, and cost. However, it is a very ideal project; it assumes that all the tasks will occur as scheduled and estimated. For example, as soon as a predecessor task finishes, the successor task begins. It also assumes that the resources will be available on the exact day the task is scheduled to begin. At this point, the project is not accommodating delays such as illness, a delay in hardware acquisition, or the learning curve encountered when using a new technology.

If one thing can be accurately predicted about a project, it is that it will not progress as scheduled. To account for the inevitable changes, the project manager should perform a risk analysis and adjust the project schedule, work effort, or cost projections to incorporate any anticipated risk.

To conduct a risk analysis, the project manager first documents the types of risks that may occur. He or she then assigns a probability factor and an impact factor. The probability factor indicates the odds of the particular risk occur-

ring. The impact factor designates the effect the risk will have on the project if it does occur. These two factors are then multiplied together to calculate the risk factor.

A **contingency** should be put in place for any risk with a high risk factor. The contingency describes what the project team will do if the risk is realized. For example, to mitigate the risk of losing a key project team member, the project manager would ensure that the project documentation is kept up-to-date. The impact of the contingency should be reflected in the project plan. For the example cited, the project manager would make sure that a task is in the project plan for updating project documentation.

An example of a risk analysis can be illustrated by using a situation you may be familiar with—planning a vacation. (See table 26.5.) For this example, the vacation will be to a Caribbean island in November, which happens to be during hurricane season.

As with assumptions, the project manager should obtain consensus from the project team, project sponsor, and stakeholders for the contingency plans. After the initial risk assessment is documented, a synopsis can be included in the project manager's status report. This synopsis could include any changes to the risk factors, realized and unrealized risks, and changes to contingency plans. After the risk is over, it can be removed from the report.

Check Your Understanding 26.4

Instructions: Prepare a work breakdown structure for the project you initiated in Check Your Understanding 26.3. Include the following for the tasks: task name, predecessor task(s), associated deliverable(s), and a list of the team members who will work on the task. Then answer the following questions on a separate piece of paper.

1. What are methods can be used to estimate the work effort for a task?

2. What are some potential risks to the project you selected in Check Your Understanding 26.3? What contingencies can be put in place to mitigate this risk?

Table 26.5.   Example of Risk Analysis

Risk Description	Probability Factor Low = 1 Medium = 3 High = 5	Impact Factor Range is 1–10 Low = 1 High = 10	Risk Factor (Probability × Impact)	Contingency
Forget to pack an item	5	3	15	Prepare a packing list
Traffic congestion on the way to the airport	1	10	10	Check road construction hotline and radio traffic reports; allow extra travel time
Rain during the vacation	3	8	24	Plan some indoor activities
Luggage doesn't make it to the destination	1	10	10	Purchase additional baggage insurance
Hurricane strikes the resort	5	10	50	Purchase trip cancellation insurance

Project Implementation

When the project planning is complete, the organization is ready to begin the project. The project manager has prepared the project schedule, identified the work effort requirements, and anticipated potential delays. Before the project begins, he or she will capture a baseline of the project schedule and work effort. The **baseline** is a copy of the original estimates for the project. It is captured so that the progress of the project can be compared to the original plan. This comparison is discussed in further detail later in this chapter.

Hold a Project Kickoff Meeting

It is customary to hold a project kickoff meeting when the project gets under way. This meeting sets the tone for the project and helps everyone understand its importance. A typical agenda for the meeting includes the following items:

- Executive presentation, during which the key stakeholder presents the background on the project with a particular emphasis on why the organization is embarking on this endeavor
- Project objectives
- Project organization chart
- Team roles and responsibilities
- High-level WBS (approach)
- Project schedule
- Key assumptions and constraints
- Project control and communication, including project tracking, meeting schedule, project documentation, change control procedure, and issue tracking

Perform Project Tasks and Produce Deliverables

The project team now has responsibility for performing the scheduled tasks and producing the project deliverables. The project manager has responsibility for ensuring that all participants understand what is to be done and when.

At this point in the project, the team may become bogged down in indecisiveness, resistance to change, and bureaucracy. The project manager works with the team, the stakeholders, and the project sponsor to keep the project moving by getting issues resolved and decisions made. The project manager may use various problem-solving and decision-making techniques to facilitate this process. (See chapter 21 for more information on this subject.)

Track Progress and Analyze Variance

When the project is under way, the project manager needs to follow how it is progressing. He or she must be able to provide the following information to the stakeholders and the project team:

- Will the project be completed on time?
- Will the project cost more than planned?
- Will the project objectives be met?

The project manager can answer these questions only by actively tracking the project's progress and analyzing its progress against the original plan.

Project Tracking

The project is tracked through the process of collecting actual progress and remaining effort from the project team members. Each team member should provide information on a periodic basis. The frequency of progress information depends on the duration of the project. For a short project of less than two months in duration, updates may be needed more than once a week. Longer projects may require a weekly progress report. In determining tracking frequency, the project manager should consider the effort of obtaining the information and updating the project plan against the level of information needed to perform the variance analysis and, more important, should be able to adequately respond to required plan revisions when a project is in trouble.

Each project team member should report the following information for each task:

- Actual start date or new scheduled start date (when the task was not started on time)
- Percentage complete or actual work
- Remaining work or expected finish date
- Actual and remaining cost
- Actual finish date (for completed tasks)
- Issues

It is usually difficult to obtain actual progress from the project team members. There are both procedural and psychological reasons for this. With regard to procedural reasons, the project manager has to set up a mechanism for getting the information. This may be a hard-copy report, or it may be automated through project management software. Unfortunately, the process of getting the information can be tedious and project managers often neglect it to pursue other project management processes that they deem to be more important.

With regard to psychological reasons, people are inclined to overestimate their progress. They tend to tell someone what they believe that person wants to hear, rather than report true progress. People also may become defensive about their progress, especially in situations where they are behind schedule or over budget. Although some personal accountability may be involved, often the reason for the delay or overrun is not directly within the team member's control. The project manager can set the right tone for the data collection process by letting the team know how the information will be used. Honesty from team members should not result in punitive measures, unless an individual has been consistently negligent in his or her project responsibilities. When a project team member is not performing as needed, the project manager needs to address this issue. (Refer to chapter 21 for management strategies that can be used to resolve this situation.)

Variance Analysis and Project Revision

After updating the project schedule with the task progress, the project manager compares the task start date, expected finish date, estimated work effort, estimated cost, and estimated duration to what was originally planned. As stated above, all projects do not progress as originally planned. The project manager must concentrate on those **variances** that are substantially affecting the project's time line, budget, and objectives. For example, a task may start later than planned, but if it is not on the project's critical path, the delay will not affect the project finish date. However, if the task is on the critical path, the project manager must determine how to make up the delay and still complete the project on schedule. A task may have started on time but consume a higher work effort than originally estimated. Unless other tasks in the plan consume less than the original estimate, the overall project will exceed the work estimates and thus the cost estimate.

To get the project back on track, the project manager must evaluate the available options. All of these options are a variant of the variables that make up the project parameters: scope, performance, cost, and time line. The project manager needs to clearly document the options and ramifications of each and present the documentation to the project's stakeholders. The sponsor and the stakeholders will make the decision based on what is most important to the success of the project. For example, in a software implementation, it may be more important for the new system to contain all of the desired functionality than it is for the implementation to meet the budget. The sponsor may be willing to do this to obtain department satisfaction and compliance with the new system.

Table 26.6 shows the types of plan revisions the project manager may propose and the potential risk involved in using each option.

Establish Change Control

In addition to proposing project revisions to keep the project on track, the project manager is usually faced with requests for changes to the original project scope. These requests can be the result of any of the following:

- A change in a departmental procedure
- A new or revised organizational initiative
- A new or revised regulatory requirement
- A desired change in the design of a system function

Changes to project scope are inevitable and should not be automatically considered a form of project failure. It is the way project changes are handled that can have a negative impact on the success of the project. The most important factor in scope change is for the stakeholders to understand the impact of the requested change and, if approved, be willing to accept the ramifications the change will have on the project's schedule and cost. In other words, the project manager must be in control of the changes. Just as in plan revision, all changes to the plan will affect the final project outcome in terms of scope, work, time line, or cost. When the project manager, sponsor, and other stakeholders do not acknowledge the impact of the change by approving a corresponding modification to one of the other variables, the quality of the project suffers.

The procedure for **change control** should be established at the beginning of the project in order to set the proper expectations for how scope modifications will be handled. The process should be as follows:

1. The requestor completes a change request form.
2. An impact analysis is performed. Its purpose is to determine the effect the change will have on the project. For example, there may be a positive impact in relationship to the objectives of the system, but the request may increase the work effort.

Table 26.6.   Potential Risks in Revising Project Plans

Options for Plan Revision	Potential Risks
Decrease the scope of work by removing some of the project requirements. Requirements may be eliminated or deferred to a subsequent project.	Project objectives may be compromised.
Eliminate the nice-to-have features of the project to decrease the scope of work.	Project objectives may be compromised.
Add more resources to get the work done faster.	Project cost may be compromised.
Ask team members to get the work done by putting in extra time.	Project cost may be compromised.
Evaluate the project plan to determine whether some tasks can start sooner. Look for finish-to-start dependencies to determine whether the tasks can overlap.	Quality may suffer when shortcuts are taken to shorten the schedule.

3. The request is presented to the stakeholders for approval. If the change is approved, the stakeholders have indicated they are willing to accept the ramification to the project time line or cost. In other words, the benefits of the change outweighed the goal to stay within the original project budget.

Communicate Project Information

One of the success factors for a project is good project communication. All involved parties need to be kept apprised of the project's progress, understand any outstanding issues, understand the change control requests, and understand the project politics. Several forms of project communication are used during the project: project status meetings, project status reports, issue logs, and project plans.

Project Status Meetings

A project status meeting is a formal meeting attended by the project team members. Its purpose is to report accomplishments, to review the status of in-progress project tasks, and to discuss issues that are impeding the completion of any tasks.

There are a few cautions for the project manager when conducting the meeting. The first is that project team members may feel pressure to report a rosy picture of the task progress because they are among their peers. A task may be behind schedule to the point that it will most likely delay the overall project schedule, but a team member may be reluctant to report this to avoid being held accountable for the entire project missing its target finish date. Although formal status meetings are important for a project, the informal status reporting from the team members is just as important. The project manager should spend time with team members outside the meeting where the team member may feel that the environment is more conducive to an honest appraisal of the task progress.

The second problem with some status meetings is they become bogged down in discussions that cannot be resolved in the meeting. For example, team members may be discussing an issue in terms of what it is instead of actually resolving it. Although everyone must understand all project issues, it is not good use of the status meeting time to discuss the issue unless all of the decision makers are in the room. Generally, issues should be handled in separate meetings outside the project status meeting.

Project Status Reports

A project status report is the formal documentation of the project progress. Again, although formal documentation is a required component of the project, the project manager should supplement this reporting with ad hoc conversations with the team members and stakeholders. This informal reporting, sometimes referred to as "walk-around" status reporting, can elicit information on the politics, conflicts, personality disputes, and bureaucracy that tend to impede task progress.

Frequency of status reports varies depending on the overall project duration. A short project may require weekly reporting whereas a long project may require monthly reporting. Whatever frequency is selected, it should support the project manager's ability to react to changes, delays, and issues.

Topics to be included in a status report include:

- Objectives for the period
- Accomplishments during the period
- Explanation of any differences
- Objectives for next period
- Issues

When the task-tracking procedure and the formal status report follow the same frequency schedule (for example, both are completed on a weekly basis), the project manager may choose to collect this information on the same form. The feasibility of this also depends on the method selected for tracking. When task tracking is automated via project management software, the ability to also collect task status information may or may not be supported.

Issue Log

Issues are items that prevent the completion of a project task. Because all projects introduce some type of change, it is inevitable that issues will arise. The purpose of the **issue log** is to document the issues so that the project manager can ensure that they are resolved in a timely manner. The issue log should include:

- A description of each issue
- Name of the team member assigned to resolve the issue
- Priority (for example, high, medium, low)
- Date the issue was opened
- Status (open, deferred, or closed)
- The required resolution date
- A descriptive status of the issue
- Resolution date and description of the resolution

After the issue log is established, the team needs to actively be working the issues toward resolution. This is where the skills of negotiation, conflict management, and innovative thinking are critical. Consensus among the affected parties is always the best solution in any issue, but in some situations the project sponsor must be called on to end a deadlock.

The issue log also can be used to capture ideas and topics that are not either specifically pertinent to the project or within its scope. These topics are often referred to as "parking lot" items. Placing them on the issue log (with a separate priority or status) is a good time management technique that ensures that the ideas will not be forgotten.

Project Plans

Reports generated from the project plan can provide information on the status of the project tasks. These reports are usually produced for the stakeholders to provide a snapshot of the project. When the project manager is using project management software, it is able to produce a variety of reports, including:

- Gantt chart that visually displays the task start and finish dates along with the percent of progress completed
- Tasks that are behind schedule
- Task list displaying the critical path tasks
- Tasks exceeding the original work estimate
- Resource reports showing the estimated work for each resource broken down by week or month

Prepare the Final Report

When the project has been concluded, it is good practice to produce a final project report. The purpose of the report is to bring closure to the endeavor by documenting the project's final outcome. The topics to be included in the report include:

- A list of the project objectives with a description of how objective was accomplished
- A list of the project deliverables
- The final project budget, detailing the comparison of the original estimate to the actual cost
- The final project schedule, detailing the comparison of the original dates to the actual dates

Celebrate Success

Projects can be very stressful to an organization. Therefore, it is important for the stakeholders and the project manager to provide the leadership to motivate team members and departments throughout the project duration. One of the ways this can be accomplished is by emphasizing the project's importance by celebrating accomplishments. For example, several social events might be held during the project to honor key project milestones. The project stakeholder could thank project participants for the effort expended thus far and encourage the same level of commitment for the remaining project activities.

After the project is completed, a more formal celebration may take place. All project contributors should be invited and recognized for their efforts.

Check Your Understanding 26.5

Instructions: Answer the following questions on a separate piece of paper.

1. What project progress information should project team members provide to the project manager?
2. What are some of the barriers to obtaining accurate progress information from team members?
3. What is change control?
4. What are some of the problems with formal project communications methods?

Real-World Case

Reimbursement rules require that the chargemaster drive a facility's charges. To receive the optimal reimbursement for services rendered, the chargemaster must be up-to-date and all-inclusive and must meet any payer rules and regulations.

The facility has decided to undergo a review of its chargemaster to ensure that it meets the above criteria. In addition to the comprehensive evaluation, one of the other objectives of the project will be to institute the procedures to ensure that all additions, revisions, and deletions meet the chargemaster standards.

Discussion Questions

1. How will the facility measure the success of the chargemaster review project?
2. Which facility departments will be included on the project team? Describe the roles and responsibilities of each team member.
3. What company position would be most appropriate to act as the project sponsor? Who are the project stakeholders?
4. Prepare a list of tasks that need to be performed.
5. What departmental policies and procedures will need to be updated?
6. Describe the training program that should be put in place to ensure ongoing chargemaster compliance.

Summary

The art of project management encompasses a wide variety of responsibilities and skills. Project management does not just involve the creation and maintenance of a project plan. Organizations need to realize that good project management does not just happen. The concepts of project management must be understood and embraced at all levels of the organization. When the organization's executives do not support good project management methodology, the risk of project failure will outweigh any perceived benefits.

When a project is started, all parties must understand its objectives. The lack of a common vision for what the project will achieve is the first opportunity for the project to fail. All stakeholders must be willing to commit the required resources to the project and to support the procedural changes that will inevitably occur as a result of the project. All project personnel also can contribute to the success of the project by keeping proposed project changes to a minimum.

A project adheres to the project management life cycle. Depending on the size and type of project, each process is scalable. In other words, the extent to which each process is performed may vary, but all processes should be included in every project.

The project manager is in a unique position in situations where a project crosses departmental boundaries. He or she has responsibility for the project success, but generally little authority over the members of the project team. The project manager must possess technical, functional, and analytical skills as well as leadership, influential, and motivational abilities.

References

Kliem, Ralph L., and Irwin S. Ludin. 1998. *Project Management Practitioner's Handbook.* New York City: AMACOM.

Lewis, James P. 1998. *Mastering Project Management.* New York City: McGraw-Hill.

Project Management Institute. 2000. *A Guide to Project Management Body of Knowledge.*

Application Exercises

The HIM department for your facility is going to be moved to a new location within the building. The new location will be remodeled according to the department's needs. Because the new location is actually smaller than the current location, the department will be implementing a home-based coding system.

1. Prepare a project charter document that includes the project objectives, deliverables, high-level project activities, assumptions and constraints, an estimated project schedule, and estimated project costs.

2. Prepare a roles and responsibilities organizational chart for the project.

3. Prepare a project task list. For each task, indicate the task predecessor(s), the resources assigned to work on the task, and the estimated work effort for each resource.

4. Document the project risks. For each risk, indicate the probability factor, the impact factor, and the contingency plan.

5. Prepare a communication plan for the project. Include the communication mode for each type of communication.

Review Quiz

Instructions: Choose the most appropriate answer for the following questions.

1. ____ Which of the following factors is not a consideration when revising a project to keep it on track?
   a. Deferring a required feature to the next project
   b. Adding a person to help another project team member
   c. Holding a kickoff meeting
   d. Working overtime

2. ____ Which of the following circumstances could result in a change to the scope of a project?
   a. A new regulation
   b. A change in the project sponsor
   c. More copies of a deliverable
   d All of the above

3. ____ What is change control used for?
   a. Handing off deliverables from one team member to another
   b. Managing scope modifications
   c. Determining the project dependencies
   d. Documenting the project organizational chart

4. ____ What is risk?
   a. An answer to an unknown question
   b. A situation that can affect the success of the project
   c. A situation that prevents completion of a project task
   d. A change in the project scope

5. ____ What is a baseline?
   a. The documentation of the project issues
   b. The project definition document
   c. The original estimates for the work effort, cost, and project time line
   d. The tracking of project progress

6. ____ Which of the following are not attributes of both projects and daily operations?
   a. Responsible managers
   b. Roles and responsibilities
   c. Products or services
   d. Defined finish dates

7. ____ Performance, time, and scope result in which of the following?
   a. Project cost
   b. Project office
   c. Project management life cycle
   c. Project team

8. ____ Which of the following activities is not part of the project management life cycle?
   a. Preparing a project plan
   b. Conducting variance analysis
   c. Monitoring the issue log
   d. Formulating a project office

9. ____ Which of the following is not a type of project team structure according to the *PMBOK?*
   a. Tree
   b. Projectized
   c. Functional
   d. Matrixed

10. ____ What is a work breakdown structure?
    a. A list of the project deliverables
    b. A hierarchical list of the project tasks
    c. A document that defines team roles and responsibilities
    d. A list of project scope changes

Chapter 27
Strategic Management

Linda L. Kloss, RHIA, CAE

Learning Objectives

- To define and describe strategic management as an essential approach to leading health information management (HIM) services
- To explore the skills that strategic managers need to learn
- To distinguish strategic management from strategic planning
- To understand how strategic management complements other management tools and approaches
- To describe the benefits of strategic management and relate them to leadership and management principles and to the change management process
- To describe techniques for considering future HIM challenges and identifying strategic options
- To identify examples of strategic management as applied to HIM practice
- To understand how HIM strategies fit into broader information strategies and the overall strategy of the organization
- To describe the qualities and attributes of a strategic leader in health information management

Key Terms

Brainstorming
Coalition building
Environmental scanning
Forecasting
Nominal group technique
Paradigm
Scenarios
Storytelling
Strategic issue
Strategic management
Strategic planning
Strategy
Tactic
Vision

Introduction

Setting strategy is often thought of as the work of senior managers and boards of trustees. The work product is a three- to five-year strategic plan that lays out goals and key actions to meet them. As described in chapter 21, planning is important for setting direction and guiding all managers and staff to work toward a common set of goals. Simply stated, **strategy** is a course of action designed to produce a desired outcome. Management theories about the importance of strategy and how to set it are changing. This reconsideration reflects the speed of change in every facet of contemporary life, including healthcare.

This chapter explores new thinking about the importance of strategy to effective management and describes approaches to setting and implementing strategy. It illustrates how the health information management professional uses strategy to shape and effect change. Finally, it illustrates why a strategic focus is an important vehicle for organizational learning.

Theory into Practice

A large multispecialty group practice clinic has just hired its first registered health information administrator (RHIA) to manage information services. The clinic's senior management made the decision to hire an RHIA to oversee implementation of a computer-based patient record (CPR) which will allow physicians to access information from satellite clinics and from home and to communicate with patients using secure messaging technology. Senior management also wants to strengthen the clinic's overall compliance program.

Senior management has given the new director a great deal of latitude to set priorities and make decisions. The director knows that it is important to design a well-thought-out, comprehensive plan to produce tangible results early on. Further, she knows that sound planning and early tangible results will garner support and approval for the significant resources needed to achieve senior management's goals.

Early in her tenure, the RHIA discovers that most other clinical staff, physicians and nonphysicians alike, do not share senior management's understanding of the need for health information system improvements. In part, this is because there is no common understanding of the external factors, such as new regulations, that affect information management. Moreover, there is no shared vision of the benefits that can accrue to the clinic and its associates, staff, and patients if information technology is used to support patient care processes.

The director decides to approach change on two fronts at the same time. One front centers on improving the reimbursement system. A key goal is to realize early improvements in the claims rejection experience so that cash flow will improve and favorable results can be easily quantified and communicated to all. This front also involves the strategy of revamping the coding process so that data quality and timeliness can be easily monitored and tracked on an ongoing basis. Improvements in these functions will increase everyone's confidence in her abilities and garner support for the tougher second-front project.

With the reimbursement improvement initiative under way, the director convenes a series of cross-departmental visioning sessions to develop a vision for the clinic's CPR system. Given the need to expand physician and staff understanding of the CPR system, the visioning sessions are intended to educate staff about its possibilities and benefits. They also enable the director to learn more about practice management styles and the needs of various services. This information is essential in developing specifications for the technical system.

In addition, the visioning meetings will enable the director to establish a rapport with staff throughout the organization that will be essential to successful implementation of the CPR down the road. She begins to identify those who might be allies in this change agenda and those who will likely oppose it. She also learns how decisions are made, whether CPR implementation can be a top-down decision, and whether she should advise senior management that implementation must come about through consensus-building approaches. Although consensus will take longer, it might be the style that best fits with the clinic's culture. As a new employee, the director needs to assess these factors for herself because they will be essential to managing the political, cultural, and technical aspects of converting the clinic to a CPR system.

Skills of Strategic Managers

Although the definition of strategy is straightforward, the skills for setting and executing strategy are far from simple. Health information management (HIM) professionals must take advantage of opportunities to learn and develop skills for strategic management, including:

- To monitor trends in healthcare and information management
- To reflect on how trends may affect the future
- To consider how changes in one area may affect changes in other areas
- To set a course for change and help others visualize it
- To coach others to be partners in advancing a change agenda
- To implement plans effectively
- To question the status quo continually

Strategy is no longer a management domain reserved for senior managers. Today, all managers must develop a comfort level with thinking and working strategically. They can learn the skills needed to achieve their comfort level by deliberately perfecting their ability to *observe the world around them*. Strategic managers generally have a high level of curiosity and always watch for changes in the larger environment. This includes external forces and political, economic, social, and technological trends. It also includes observing the changes in thinking and action taking place within healthcare and within their own organization. For example, shifts in public policy in Washington, D.C., or in one's state capital regarding the value placed on personal privacy have implications for HIM practice at the local level.

In addition to observational skills, strategic managers learn to *continually reflect on the implications and opportunities* afforded by the forces and trends they observe in the larger environment. Whether reading a journal or discussing new ideas with others, strategic managers are always testing new ideas, identifying those that have merit, and discarding those that do not.

The best strategic managers are creative. They test various associations between ideas and new opportunities. Such relationships are not always direct, as in the example above about privacy and public policy. Many of the best strategic ideas are the result of creative thinking, effectively using information from diverse or unexpected sources to trigger innovation. For example, faced with an intractable shortage of trained coders, an HIM director instituted a program for training coders sponsored by her healthcare organization. Student tuition more than offset faculty and other costs, and the organization had the pick of the best and brightest graduates.

Strategic managers also *continually look for opportunities to improve on the status quo*. They do not accept the old adage that "If it ain't broke, don't fix it." Rather, they look for ways to make things better. They evaluate new approaches and are willing to take risks. Moreover, they learn to tolerate uncertainty. New approaches have impacts that can never be fully anticipated, and strategic managers expect that they will need to respond to the unexpected and continually make adjustments. For example, redesigning the use of physical office space to accommodate a computer-based record management system disrupts patterns of informal staff interactions, which in turn affects aspects of the department's culture.

New managers may lack the confidence to initiate change, but making change is what management is all about. Thus, while gaining experience and confidence, managers must guard against accepting or perpetuating barriers to creativity characterized by common squelchers such as "we've never done that before," "we have always done it that way," or "that's not my job." These all-too-common reasons for inaction are a trigger for the strategic manager to ask, How can we do this better?

Finally, strategic managers learn to *help others contribute to new thinking and new ideas*. They learn techniques to bring out the best thinking by all staff because they know there will be no lasting change without employee participa-

tion. As Drucker says, "the only definition of a leader is someone who has followers" (1996, p. xii). Strategic managers also need to gain the support of superiors, colleagues, and other constituents with a stake in their change agenda. For example, in pursuing a goal to shorten accounts receivable days, a health information manager realized that without record assembly, records could be coded a full day earlier. To minimize assembly, it would be necessary to transition to a universal chart order. The manager knew he would need the support of nursing to make this change. To gain that support, he involved nursing in the design of the revised system and in implementing the universal chart. Moreover, he shared the credit with nursing when the impact of this change on accounts receivable was tallied up and touted.

The skills of the strategic manager can be learned and perfected with experience. Learning begins by recognizing the importance of strategy to today's successful managers.

From Strategic Planning to Strategic Management

Strategic planning has been described in various forms in the management literature for decades. Some applications were characterized by rigorous and formal analysis of data to deduce a desired future and the steps to achieve it. In large corporations, departments of planners prepared forecasts with the aid of computer analysis. The complex reports would be delivered to senior managers who were largely uninvolved in the process. Such earlier, narrower views of strategic planning have given way to a broader concept of strategic management.

First, **forecasting** the future, particularly in such volatile times, is a near impossibility. Also, by the time a complex three- to five-year plan is finalized and delivered to senior managers, it is undoubtedly out of date. Finally, if senior managers are not involved in strategy development, the plan is unlikely to be seen as relevant and unlikely to be implemented.

Many organizations continue to use the term *strategic planning* to describe a variety of processes. It is important to go beneath the phrase and understand the characteristics of the process being followed. Strategic planning may entail a change agenda led by senior management. Rather than a three- or five-year plan, it may involve a set of three- to five-year goals with annual plans that move the organization toward those goals. Annual plans may be adjusted when new and better ideas are identified and when their effect can be evaluated. The process may involve setting goals and plans using an inclusive process of consensus, aided by, but not driven by, data analysis. Each organization's approach is a reflection of its management's philosophy and its business challenges.

Strategic management, defined as "the art and science of formulating, implementing, and evaluating cross-functional decisions that enable an organization to achieve its objectives," is an approach that keeps strategy front and center in the work of a manager (David 2001, p. 5). Rather than a periodic planning process, strategic management involves applying strategic thinking to improve organizational positioning and performance.

Again, there is no set formula for this approach. However, it does exhibit these characteristics:

- It is framed by organizational values, vision, and mission.
- It takes into account possible futures, looking to the external environment for its clues.
- It is broadly inclusive, soliciting ideas from a broad group of stakeholders.
- It integrates the work of a number of organizational functions working toward a common goal.
- It is action oriented, with a commitment to bringing about change.
- It results in organizational learning.

Strategic management is a way of advancing the organization by introducing innovation into decision making and engaging others in the change process. With the very rapid changes in HIM practice, the discussion of strategic management is central to managerial effectiveness and should be viewed as a component of each of the five functions of management discussed in chapter 21. There is a strategic management component to every aspect of management.

Elements of Strategic Management

Figure 27.1 illustrates a strategic management process that provides a framework to help health information managers apply this approach. Strategic management begins with a

vision, which is a picture of the desired future state. **Strategic issues** that need to be addressed if the vision is to be realized are identified and described. Major goals to move toward the vision are set. Strategies, the approaches that will be employed to achieve the goals and ultimately the vision, are then designed. Examples of strategies might include development of new services, phasing out existing services, joint ventures, and so on. **Tactics,** the specific plans to implement strategies, are designed and implemented. Each of these elements is discussed in detail later in this chapter.

Strategic management is not a linear process that flows neatly from step to step. Rather, it is a highly iterative process and participants are continually learning how to improve each step. As illustrated in figure 27.1, the two-directional arrows show that learning is used to improve on past and future work. For example, a manager, while establishing goals, discovers that she has failed to identify a significant strategic issue. In a bidirectional process, she would back up and evaluate the strategic issue. Also, the experience gained with a strategy may actually lead to modifying a goal. Thus, in contrast to traditional strategic planning in which all steps are neatly outlined before implementation is begun, strategic management is a process that requires continual evaluation and refinement so that new learning is applied as one goes along.

In addition, all stakeholders—employees, superiors, coworkers, and customers—are appropriately involved in strategic management activities, so there is ongoing improvement based on feedback as well as on what is being learned. In addition, there is a continual flow of new information informing and re-forming assumptions. Thus, communication is a key element of strategic management.

Check Your Understanding 27.1

Instructions: Indicate whether the following questions are true or false (T or F).

1. ___ Strategy always originates with senior management and is delegated to department(s) for implementation.
2. ___ Being a keen observer of trends and the external environment is an important skill for a strategic manager.
3. ___ In the strategic management process, vision precedes goals and tactics precede strategies.
4. ___ The bottom line goal of strategic management is to enable the organization to achieve its objectives.
5. ___ Forecasting is a reliable science, particularly in volatile times.
6. ___ Strategic management differs from strategic planning because it is a more structured process.

Establishing a Vision

According Kouzes and Posner, "A vision describes a bold and ideal image of the future" (1995, p. 94). Moreover, it is the catalyst for change. Kouzes and Posner go on to say that "if leaders are going to take us to places we've never been

Figure 27.1.   Elements of Strategic Management

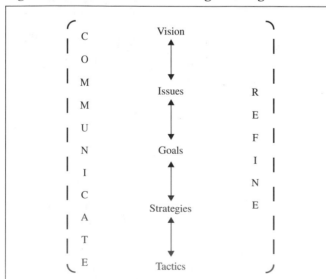

before, constituents of all types demand that they have a sense of direction" (p. 95).

A vision states the direction for change and helps motivate people to take action. Designing a compelling vision requires a solid understanding of the healthcare organization's internal and external environments. It also requires the ability to break free of the current **paradigm** and to think creatively about a new reality for the future.

Following are some examples of vision statements for health information management. A director of HIM services for a health system envisions services that would make the fullest use of technology to provide high-quality, cost-effective information to authorized users. He expressed this idealized vision as follows:

> It is our goal to utilize state-of-the-art technology and best practices grounded in applied research in every phase of the operation and to deliver accurate information in digital form to support patient care and healthcare operations. This ambitious goal will require health information services staff to become more externally focused, to gain a deeper understanding of user needs, and to work closely with others within and outside our organization. It also requires staff to work together to question all current practices and be willing to try new approaches, even if they are not all successful.

This vision lays out a very substantial challenge, yet it also provides focus. First, the overarching vision is to be able to deliver all information to all users of HIM services in digital form. It acknowledges that technology is only as good as the enabling processes; therefore, it promises use of best practices. These are not to be just what one thinks are best practices but, rather, practices substantiated by applied research that demonstrates their validity. It acknowledges that achieving this vision requires new ways of working. Success requires becoming more externally focused on those who rely on the information and on those whose collaboration is needed to achieve the vision. It also requires effective teamwork among HIM staff members who must become more comfortable with change and risk taking.

In another example, an HIM consultant for a long-term care system is having difficulty gaining support for her vision of what a CPR could contribute to the residents, staff, and the overall organizations. She developed the following description of her vision:

> All members of the care team have immediate access to complete and accurate information for each resident. This information recaps care delivered and presents the status of all health, social, ADL, and other resident-specific issues being managed. Summary reports are used as the basis for shift change briefings and for periodic care conferences. The information system prompts caregivers to actions that need to be taken and alerts them to changes in status that require special vigilance. Data entered into the system summarizing observations, care given, orders, and activities produce a record of care that meets licensing and other external requirements. The system also automatically accumulates the information needed for care and operations management and for external reporting.

This vision statement highlights the benefits of implementing a CPR from the perspective of improving management of the care process every day. It underscores that information for management and internal and external reporting is a byproduct of the system, thereby reducing redundant paperwork that currently consumes so much staff time. A careful parsing of the vision reveals the major features and functions of the system. For example, the system must be capable of producing change-in-shift summary reports recapping care processes and the status of all resident problems being managed. It also must accumulate the data needed for MDS (Minimum Data Set) and other reporting. The vision serves as a starting point for creating a more detailed set of specifications and evaluating potential system vendors.

Visions also can be more narrowly focused on a particular project. For example, a data quality manager for a multispecialty group practice clinic prepared the following vision statement to help the physicians and coding staff rally around a proposed project to improve the timeliness and accuracy of billing processes:

> During each patient visit, the physician enters problems, treatments, orders, and follow-up plans into his or her personal data assistant (PDA). PDA data are periodically uploaded to the clinical data repository throughout the day, where they are combined with other patient-specific reports and information. Codes are autoassigned by the systems, and missing data are flagged. Clinical data analysts review each visit record to check the accuracy of the autogenerated codes and determine whether the information substantiates the codes assigned. A visit record is either marked for billing or flagged as incomplete with supplementary information requested from the physician or referred service. Ninety percent of visits are billed within one business day, 95 percent within three business days, and the balance are billed within five business days.

This vision statement has three major elements. First, it sets an aggressive goal of billing 90 percent of visits on the day of service. Second, it expects physicians to initiate the process using automated tools to eliminate time-consuming handling of handwritten information. Third, it introduces the new role of clinical data analyst, which reflects the expanded role for coding specialists in data quality and compliance management.

These vision statements relate to HIM challenges. However, it is important that the HIM vision complement the organization's overall vision and mission. For example, the organization's vision is to be known for its advanced clinical services in cardiac and oncology care. To achieve this vision, the organization is pursuing a strategy of attacting clinical talent with national reputations and of expanding clinical research programs. This overall vision and strategy should be accounted for in crafting the HIM vision and strategies.

Strategic managers understand the overall organizational goals and take them into account when crafting their own plans. First, they seek ways to support and further the overall goals of the organization. For example, will the cancer registry program need to be upgraded to support the more sophisticated information needs of a world-class oncology service? As a practical matter, it is difficult to sell a plan that is out of step with priorities.

Creating a Commitment to Change

The vision sets the broad directional strategy, leaving the details to be worked out. Kotter writes that an effective vision statement has the following characteristics (1996, p. 72):

- Conveys a picture of what the future will look like
- Appeals to the long-term interests of the stakeholders
- Sets forth realistic and achievable goals
- Is clear enough to provide guidance in decision making
- Is flexible so that alternative strategies are possible as conditions change
- Is easy to describe and communicate

It is important to remember that visions are pictures of the desired future; they may never be realized in their entirety. Today's technology may not support billing 100 percent of visits within five working days, but that does not mean this bold picture should not be sketched. All health information may never be in digital form, but that does not mean this should not be the HIM department's vision. Visions must be important and worth pursuing. Otherwise, why would others become engaged?

Moreover, visions should evoke a sense of excitement and urgency from those closest to the process. If the designers are not excited about the possibilities the vision offers, it is unlikely that it will generate excitement in others. A sense of urgency is essential to overcome the forces that protect the status quo.

Understanding the Environment

Knowledge of the environment is essential to vision formulation. Sometimes called **environmental scanning,** this data-intensive process is the continuous process of gathering and analyzing intelligence about trends that are or may be affecting HIM. It is both internally focused on the healthcare organization and the HIM department and externally focused on industry and societal trends. As adapted from the work of Bryson (1995, pp. 90–92), internal environmental assessment includes analysis of:

- *Performance indicators:* Budgetary targets and results, performance and productivity measures, staff and customer feedback
- *Resources:* HIM budget and staff, information technology staff and resources, educational resources, programs, competencies, culture
- *Present strategy:* Organizationwide strategy and priorities, information management strategy, information systems plans and priorities, compliance programs, products and services, business processes

Also as adapted from Bryson (1995, pp. 87–89), external environmental assessment includes analysis of:

- *Forces and trends:* Political, economic, demographic, social, technological, and educational

- *Resource constraints:* Healthcare reimbursement systems, patient and customer trends, regulators, competitors

Current and Potential Collaborators

An HIM manager who focuses too much on his or her own department will have a difficult time succeeding as a strategic manager. Understanding the environment provides the context for the tough decisions involved in setting direction, designing strategy, and leading change. Some ways to be in touch with the environment include:

- Taking inventory of the sources of internal and external information to identify and fill information gaps
- Building performance measures to gain perspective on trends over time
- Becoming involved in projects and task forces at the organization to interact with a wide range of coworkers
- Developing a personal reading list to follow the thinking of experts in the field
- Reading what futurists are saying about how things will change
- Becoming active in the American Health Information Management Association (AHIMA) and building a network of professional colleagues
- Making full use of the information resources that the AHIMA and other organizations make available
- Contributing to the professional body of knowledge with the discovery of new HIM practice solutions

Environmental Trends

Analyzing the changing environment and envisioning the future is at the same time an analytic and a highly creative activity. Understanding trends requires analysis of:

- Relationships between trends
- The sequence of events
- Causes and effects
- Priority among items

To bring out the best thinking of a team or workgroup, it is helpful to use techniques that enable participants to consider factors from different perspectives. Group process techniques such as **brainstorming,** nominal group technique, and others may be used to help unleash each individual's creative talent.

Storytelling is one such technique. Telling stories about futures suggested by trends has a number of advantages:

- Most people are comfortable with this approach.
- Findings are presented in an understandable and real-world context.
- Stories are memorable, making it easier for others to remember essential points.
- Stories generate excitement and are fun to develop.

One storytelling technique that is used in more sophisticated strategy planning is **scenarios.** The word *scenario* literally means a script of a play or story, a projected sequence of events. Scenarios are defined as "focused descriptions of fundamentally different futures presented in coherent script-like or narrative fashion" (Schoemaker 1993, p. 195). They are plausible stories about how the future might unfold. They are not meant to predict but, rather, simply to interpret and clarify how environmental trends may play out.

Scenarios are based on analysis and interaction of environmental variables. Environmental scanning is an important preparatory step in scenario development. Based on studying the environment, three or four scenario themes reflecting alternate possible futures are developed. Stories are constructed that describe how each of these themes might be played out. The stories are refined through input and further study until they reflect the group's best thinking about what futures might be in store for the organization under various circumstances.

To understand how the clinical coding function might change in the future, an AHIMA task force studied environmental trends and developed four scenarios, each highlighting a slightly different, but plausible, future:

- The first scenario described the impact on coding of a breakthrough technology that would automate a great deal of the coding now being done manually or with the help of encoders.
- The second scenario described the impact on coding functions if healthcare organizations were strategically committed to using information to improve the quality of care information and hence the organization's strategic positioning.
- The third scenario involved the role of coding in an increasingly regulatory environment in which healthcare spending was ratcheted down and investments in technology were constrained.
- The fourth scenario involved greater consumer involvement in healthcare decision making and in maintaining personal health information.

It is easy to see that all the scenarios are plausible. The future of coding functions will be affected by all of these factors, but one or more may have a greater impact than the others. Strategic managers develop contingency plans to account for the variables that may shape the future.

The strategic manager should build a portfolio of techniques that can be used to bring out the best thinking of others. He or she might begin by perusing the business shelves of major bookstores for guidebooks containing exercises and techniques to improve group process. Another approach is to observe techniques used by facilitators.

Check Your Understanding 27.2

Instructions: Select the correct answer for the following statements.

1. ___ Which of the following is not true.
   a. A vision statement conveys a picture of a desired future state
   b. A vision statement sets out a specific course of action
   c. A vision statement is easy to describe
   d. A vision statement is flexible

2. ___ Scanning the internal environment includes:
   a. Tracking state and federal regulations
   b. Understanding the organization's strategic priorities
   c. Watching for new technology breakthroughs
   d. Following service trends in the community

3. ___ Scenarios are particularly helpful when
   a. No one can agree on the right course of action
   b. A planning group needs to think out of the box
   c. There are multiple plausible futures
   d. One wants to share a prediction about the future

4. ___ HIM professionals should incorporate the following "habits" into their professional lives to stay current:
   a. Volunteer for projects that can help to develop new skills
   b. Build and nurture a network of professional colleagues
   c. Know how to access resources
   d. All of the above

5. ___ Another word for scenario is
   a. Tale
   b. Chronicle
   c. Script
   d. Journal

From Vision to Strategy

As defined earlier, *strategy* is an action or set of actions that moves the organization toward its vision. *Strategic management* is about pursuing a new set of activities or new ways of carrying out current activities that move the organization toward its vision. For example, strategic management may:

- Take the form of new or redesigned programs or services
- Involve implementing new systems, outsourcing certain operations, or merging functions with another organizational entity
- Entail phasing out an outdated program or adopting new technologies
- Be aimed at bringing an organization into compliance with new regulations or finding new ways to reduce operating costs

The sample shown in figure 27.2 (p. 654) illustrates the thought process involved in moving from vision to strategy. This is based on the vision statement presented on page 7 regarding moving from a paper to a digital record.

The next step is to prepare a detailed tactical plan to carry out each strategy. For example, implementing the strategy to acquire and implement electronic signature software requires research into technology vendors that offer

Figure 27.2.   Vision to Strategy: Digital Information for Patient Care and Healthcare Operations

Strategic Issue #1: Physicians review, correct, and hand-sign transcribed reports on paper.	
Goals	**Strategies**
Store the output from transcription electronically.	1. Upgrade the clinical data repository to accept the output from transcribed reports. 2. Design and pilot test a plan for storing output in the data repository. 3. Design a phased plan for implementation that begins with time-sensitive dictation, such as operative reports and reports of tests and procedures (e.g., radiology, cath lab).
Physicians are able to review, modify records electronically.	1. Acquire and implement electronic signature software. 2. Design and pilot test a process whereby physicians can authenticate, make changes to, and reassign a transcribed report online. 3. Design a phased plan for implementation of online physician review that is coordinated with the availability of online access to electronic reports.

software compatible with the clinical data repository. In addition, it requires budgeting for this technology, securing support for the plan, issuing a request for proposal (RFP), checking references, and so on.

Building a strategy grounded in a vision provides a context for continually assessing whether the plan is on track and making progress.

Strategic Management versus Operations Improvement

Strategic management should not be confused with operations improvement. Operations improvement focuses on improving how existing programs and services are carried out. By definition, operations improvement is internally focused. In contrast, strategy development is a search for new programs and services that will improve the organization's fit with the external world. Techniques such as scenario development and environmental scanning are useful in formulating strategy because they shift the focus from internal to external. One cannot expect to identify new, high-impact strategies by looking at the past. Rather, in formulating strategy, one must look outside the organization and to the future.

Strategy as a Series of Trade-offs

Porter advises that the "essence of strategy is deciding what not to do" (1996, p. 70). He writes that strategy should be viewed as a series of trade-offs. This point is particularly relevant in HIM today as it transitions from managing paper to managing information using computer technology. The resources are not sufficient to maintain all paper-based processes while designing new ways of working. Major change will affect current activities and may well require their modification, or even elimination. No organization has the resources to take on major new programs without con-

sidering their impact on current programs. Making trade-offs is one of the most difficult challenges for most managers. Letting go of even a marginal program may produce a backlash. However, resources must be reallocated to those programs that will enable the organization to operate on a new plane.

To underscore the importance of making trade-offs, HIM managers should ask themselves what things they have stopped doing as a result of their new strategy. An answer of nothing is evidence of their failure to articulate a viable or significant new strategy.

Use of Tactics to Carry Out Strategy

Strategy also should not be confused with tactics. Often strategic plans are written at a tactical, rather than a strategic, level. Tactics describe how to carry out the strategy. For example, if the strategy is to redesign the coding process in order to reduce accounts receivable days, tactics may include evaluating telecommuting, hiring contract coders, and redesigning the record completion processes. When formulating strategies, the HIM manager should question whether he or she is getting too deeply into how to do something. Strategy is *what* one is going to do; tactics are *how* one plans to do it.

Check Your Understanding 27.3

Instructions: Indicate whether the following questions are true or false (T or F).

1. ____ Operations improvement and strategic management share the same goals.
2. ____ Advancing a new strategy almost always involves making tradeoffs.
3. ____ Strategic managers should hedge their bets by making few changes until it is clear the new strategy will work.
4. ____ Strategies are fundamentally oriented to the external environment and to the future.
5. ____ Once the strategy is defined, tactical plans can be prepared.

Support for Change Programs

Sound change strategies and tactics alone do not ensure success. Success depends on great execution, and this begins by securing support for the change effort. Healthcare organizations are highly complex with many competing priorities. Senior leadership must strongly support the change initiative if it is to succeed. Indeed, support must be gained from every stakeholder who may be affected by the change. For example, medical staff leadership, administration, and the staff whose work processes will change must approve of a plan to modify the requirements for record completion.

Strategic managers understand that everyone naturally resists change. Bridges identifies three phases of accepting change (1991, p. 5):

1. *The ending phase:* This phase involves the acceptance that change is necessary or, at least, the willingness to let go of the current state.

2. *The neutral zone phase:* This phase characterizes the bulk of the change process. People no longer have the safety of the familiar current state and are struggling with uncertainty, which makes then uneasy and even resistant.
3. *The beginning phase:* This phase reflects a new start as the change begins to take hold.

Individuals move through these transitional stages at their own pace. The strategic manager must be attuned to each individual's responses and transitional progress to provide appropriate support. Additional techniques are described in the following sections.

Taking a Systems Approach

According to Tichy, "the development of change strategy involves simultaneous attention to three [organizational] systems—technical, political, and cultural" (1983, p. 187). Technical systems are concerned with the business we are in and how we conduct it, for example, the processes used to manage patient information. Political systems involve the distribution of power and influence in the organization, for example, the authority of the medical staff and the approval and decision-making processes.

Cultural systems are the values and patterns of behaviors that define how the organization typically operates. Schein defines culture as a "pattern of shared basic assumptions that the group learned as it solved its problems of external adaptation and internal integration" (1992, p. 12). Culture comprises the most powerful and stable forces operating in organizations. It is like the organization's genetic code. Change agents must account for the pervasive effects of culture if they are to be successful.

Major change throws the organization into a sort of chaos as existing systems are deliberately disrupted while new ones are put in place. It is a time of great vulnerability, and strategic managers must be vigilant, watching for and reacting to unintended effects that could make it difficult to advance the effort. For example, in times of great change, employees may be more inclined to look for employment opportunities elsewhere rather than go through an unsettling period of change. Some turnover may be unavoidable in times of sustained change, but the strategic manager should be very attuned to how staff are feeling about the changes.

The technical, political, and cultural systems are highly interdependent, and any change will have an intended and unintended impact on all three systems. For example, when implementing new technology, the focus is often on features and functions of the system. Securing the right champions for the system and understanding how the new system affects the work and formal and informal interactions of staff may be as important to successful implementation as its features and functions.

This does not mean that the change should not be pursued but, rather, simply that its success will depend on how well it is managed from a systems perspective. The strategic manager must attend to all aspects of the system throughout implementation. He or she should be aware that implementation is not complete until the technical, political, and cultural systems are again in equilibrium; and this often takes time.

Managing the Politics of Change

Change leadership requires the courage to persevere even in the face of criticism. However, plowing ahead without understanding the basis for the criticicm may be folly. Criticism may signal resistance to change, but it also may indicate that there are factors the strategic manager has not considered or opinions that he or she has not taken into account. According to Bryson, managing the politics of change requires "finding ideas (visions, goals, strategies) that people can support and that further their interests . . . and making deals in which something is traded in exchange for that support" (1995, p. 225).

Political savvy entails skill in mediating conflicts and shaping compromises that are inevitable when people are offered real choices with real consequences. The strategic manager should deliberately enlist the support of opinion leaders. He or she should reach out to those who may be most threatened by the proposed change, rather than waiting for them to voice their objections. Early engagement may turn potential resisters into supporters. At the very least, it will help change leaders build their arguments and communication plan to address the concerns of the opposition.

Coalition building is one technique for managing the political dimensions of change. Change may threaten to shift the balance of power, and employees or coworkers who feel threatened may react by joining together to increase their own power so as to influence the course of events. Coalitions can be a force for thwarting change, or leaders can use coalition building as a way to build support for change. The earlier example of the health information manager who gained the support and cooperation of the nursing leadership to move ahead on a universal chart order project illustrates the power of coalition building.

The first step in building a coalition is to honestly assess subgroups in terms of how they will view the proposed change. Before embarking on a major change, the following questions should be carefully considered:

- Who will be most affected by the change?
- What benefits (for example, power) might these individuals perceive they will lose?
- Are their fears real? If so, what options are available to help overcome their fears?
- Does the change have the potential to create new benefits for these individuals?
- Can a negative reaction be avoided by engaging individuals or groups in the process?
- If the strategic manager is unsuccessful in getting the individuals opposed to change on his or her side, is their

influence likely to be strong enough to derail the change plan?

Even if the strategic manager is unsuccessful in winning over those resistant to the change, he or she will have better information about the strength of their feelings and their resolve to oppose it. At the same time the strategic manager is working to diffuse potential resistance to change, he or she should focus on building the support of the groups that are positively inclined to support it.

Implementing strategy requires broad buy-in, particularly from those whose jobs may be affected. The strategic manager reaches out to those whose support is needed through coalition building and other techniques. The strategic manager also makes certain that staff is given real roles in helping to shape change. This may involve serving on teams convened to plan and guide change. It is important to remember that no leader works alone and change happens only when systems become realigned around the new reality.

Creating a Sense of Urgency

Kotter asserts that "by far the biggest mistake people make when trying to change organizations is to plunge ahead without establishing a high enough sense of urgency" (1996, p. 4). Leaders may overestimate the extent to which they can force change on the organization.

To increase the sense of urgency, leaders must remove or minimize the sources of complacency. Examples of how this might be done include:

- Engaging employees, customers, and coworkers in a dialogue about change through a series of meetings
- Identifying opinion leaders and securing their support early on
- Presenting believable stories or scenarios that illustrate the potential futures that might occur if action is not taken
- Creating new vehicles for communication, such as a project newsletter

Taking Care to Communicate, Communicate, Communicate

Communication is key to engaging others in the vision and change process. DePree sums it up by saying that "if you're a leader and you are not sick and tired of communicating you probably aren't doing a good enough job" (1992, p. 100).

A benchmarking study of how companies successfully communicated change showed that communication is critical at three stages of the change process: as it is being planned, throughout implementation, and after it is complete (Powers 1997, p. 32). Effective communication was shown to be critical at each stage, even to the point of releasing partial information when details are incomplete.

At the planning stage, leaders should communicate the need for change and the vision. Remember, if followers do not accept the vision, the rest of the change process is likely to be very rocky. Communicating results, even when they are incomplete, is an important reinforcement. It makes the change real and maintains the necessary momentum.

Communication is most effective when the message is tailored to the recipient. It is important to identify needs and opportunities to customize the message to subgroups that have a particular set of issues. For example, the message to the medical staff will be different from the message to employees of health information services. Before implementing the use of report templates to expedite dictation, the strategic manager might design a tactical plan that details all the elements of the communication plan for each of the constituent groups affected by, or with an interest in, the project.

The communication plan must offer the opportunity for others to "talk back." As Kotter points out, the "downside of two-way communication is that feedback may suggest that you are on the wrong course and that the vision and plans need to be reformulated. But in the long run, swallowing your pride and reworking the vision and plan is far more productive than heading off in the wrong direction—or in a direction that others won't follow" (1996, p. 100).

Kotter also points out that communication comes in two forms—words and actions—and that the most effective communication is characterized by deeds. "Behavior from important people that is inconsistent with the vision overwhelms other forms of communication" (1996, p. 90). Leaders become the symbols for the change. Their motivations may be questioned and their actions scrutinized. Others will watch their actions for signs of commitment to the course of action, and they rightly insist on integrity from their leaders.

Ethics and integrity must be front and center all the time, but particularly during times of important change. At these times, the political, cultural, and technical systems are out of alignment. There is opportunity for events to take unexpected turns.

Implementation of Strategic Change

The vision and strategies are designed, the change management team is in place, and the guiding coalitions are organized. Now comes the hard work! Implementation requires all the managerial skills described in chapter 21, including planning, budgeting, monitoring, and producing results.

Creating and Communicating Short-term Wins

Major change takes time. The vision may be compelling, but if some short-term results cannot be demonstrated, the momentum for change may begin to erode. The best way to sustain the change effort is to sequence the implementation plan in such a way that visible and reinforcing short-term successes are demonstrated and celebrated. For example, in implementing a new compliance plan, the data quality manager for a group practice reported statistics to the chiefs of service showing the monthly claims rejection rate. As the rate began to decline, the data quality manager organized special events at each milestone, such as a dessert party and flowers for office managers. He also sent e-mails to physician leaders announcing major milestones and quantifying their financial impact. These actions garnered attention and maintained momentum for the project.

The implementation plan should be deliberately seeded with a number of short-term projects that have a high likelihood of success. This tactic enables the implementation team to learn to work together and assess the level of effort and resources that will be required for later phases. Moreover, it shows that the program of planned change is real and not just talk, and it strengthens the courage and commitment of the leaders and guiding coalitions.

New programs can be launched quickly by using techniques such as rapid prototyping and demonstration projects. The details do not always need to be fully worked out to create visible demonstrations. It is not necessary to secure approval for full implementation while testing an approach in order to see its value. In test mode, all operational details do not need to be worked out before "going live." There is no need to anticipate all the intricacies up front; it is most important to begin the journey and adjust as it progresses. This is the essence of the learning approach.

Pacing and Refining Plans for Change

Implementation requires managing interdependent projects at various stages of design, development, and deployment. One of the most difficult implementation challenges is deciding which phases to advance first and how quickly to move through them. Sequencing and pacing change requires a thorough knowledge of the organization and its capacity for change. Again, it is important to consider all the organizational components—cultural, political, and technical—and the available financial and managerial resources.

The timing of change is critical. Change leaders can cite examples of projects that moved too quickly and projects that moved too slowly. Lawrence sums up this challenge: "I have become convinced that the real art of leadership lies in careful pacing. Pacing means moving simultaneously in a variety of areas and keeping each area progressing so that the combined cadence does not tear the organization apart. I'm positive that nobody gets timing 100 percent right. But the winners do it less wrong" (1998, p. 298).

Implementation is a process of guiding, adjusting, and improving as one goes along. According to Walton, "Invariably, the organizational, strategic and leadership choices made during the earlier phases are only partially informed. As experience and events provide feedback to the organization, adjustments are almost always called for" (1998, p. 355).

Implementing change is a highly iterative process. The strategic manager's plans and tactics will likely need to be modified as he or she gains experience. Budgets and timetables must be created that permit frequent course corrections.

The higher the stakes, the likelier it is that a proposed change will be controversial. If the only viable approach is likely to meet with resistance, more time and effort are needed up front to gain acceptance before the approach is implemented. The importance of two-way communication throughout the process cannot be overemphasized.

Maintaining Momentum and Staying the Course

Because leading change is a process of learning and adjusting, strategic managers must learn to tolerate, and even enjoy, uncertainty. They are eager to see their well-crafted strategies take hold and inevitably feel discouraged by a lengthy process. In addition to celebrating short-term wins, strategic managers can maintain momentum and keep moving by:

- Working quickly to resolve the thorny issues.
- Reiterating what will happen when change does not occur or is watered down by compromise. If possible, focus should be placed on the consequences due to external trends.
- Keeping their eyes on the prize and putting every action in context. They should regularly revisit the vision, goals, and strategies to regenerate a sense of purpose and should help others by making the goals as tangible as possible.
- Remembering that resistance to change is natural. It should not be taken personally.
- Rethinking the tactics, sequence, and pace regularly to keep from getting bogged down. If the process does become bogged down, actions should be initiated that will produce short-term gains. It is essential to keep moving.
- Maintaining the sense of urgency. Although short-term wins should be celebrated, the celebrations should not mitigate the sense of urgency that has been created. Also, intermediate gains should not be mistaken for the bigger goals.

For maximum and sustained impact, the change that has been introduced must become part of the organization's fabric. It must become the way the organization operates, thinks, and behaves. At some point, it must become part of the culture. Even after change is implemented, there often continues to be a tug backward to the old reality. Indeed, the effect of culture can be so strong that leaders should be on the lookout for signs of slippage and for opportunities to reinforce the value of the new reality. To ensure that change is lasting and to prepare the organization for more change, leaders should:

- Quantify the impact, benefits, and value of the changes and use data to identify the direction for future change
- Continue intensive communication on issues facing HIM and the organization

- Integrate change competencies and behaviors into performance appraisal and management development programs
- Approach strategy, change, and organizational development as an ongoing process

Measuring the Results

Strategic managers are responsible for understanding the effect and effectiveness of tactics and strategy so that they can then make adjustments, manage unintended effects, and identify milestones. Depending on the strategy, this is best done by measuring performance indicators, outcomes, trends, attitudes, and levels of satisfaction. For example, a health system may determine that a central prerequisite for improving the management of patient health status is to link care across encounters and points of service so that the sum of care for each individual can be aggregated. To achieve this vision, an enterprise-wide identity management system is installed as a key element and processes for patient registration are standardized throughout the organization. Before implementation, the discrepancies in patient demographic attributes among duplicate medical records are measured to serve as a baseline for tracking improvement. Points of breakdown in the process are studied before, during, and after implementation of the enterprise system. Productivity data are also tracked throughout the change process. Information on how the linked data are used is collected to reinforce the benefits of this important change. Reporting data on the effects of change is a key way to help bolster the change initiative, and to detect negative variation in the process under scrutiny.

Environmental scanning was introduced earlier as an important prerequisite to launching major change. It also is the way to measure the impact of change and to determine what further change is needed. Whatever is done, the measures by which its success will be judged should be set forth and made part of the performance measures data set. Environmental scanning must become a core competency of the organization and part of its routine work. It need not be an elaborate system but should be systematic and ongoing, and it must include information on performance, trends, attitudes, and satisfaction.

Check Your Understanding 27.4

Instructions: Select the correct answer for the following statements

1. ___ The most difficult aspect of an organization to change is its
   a. Culture
   b. Technology systems
   c. Politics
   d. Attitudes

2. ___ According to Bridges, the neutral zone phase in accepting change is when
   a. Most don't believe there is a need to change
   b. Change begins to take hold
   c. People are struggling with uncertainty
   d. Resistance to change is overcome

3. ___ Successful strategic managers
   a. Line up support for change
   b. Learn to compromise
   c. Work at maintaining and extending support
   d. All of the above

4. ___ Which of the following is not a technique for creating a sense of urgency that helps individuals become open to change
   a. Sending out a directive
   b. Dialogue
   c. Explaining what the consequences of not acting might be
   d. Communication

5. ___ Spotlighting short term wins is critical to
   a. Getting credit for a good idea
   b. Showing the disbelievers that they were wrong
   c. Maintaining the momentum for change
   d. Laying fears to rest

6. ___ Maintaining the momentum for change is not aided by
   a. Communication
   b. Helping those who are struggling with change
   c. Avoiding problems and changing direction
   d. Regularly revisiting the vision and goals

Real-World Case

According to a recent article in the *Journal of the American Health Information Management Association,* the presence of consumer-maintained or accessible personal health records on the Web is a trend that is about to explode. As consumers become more knowledgeable about healthcare matters, they seek access to more information about their own and their family members' health and healthcare. The article points out that this trend is expected to have a profound impact on health information management as practitioners become not only patient advocates in the emerging e-world, but also knowledge and content experts. One of the experts interviewed for this article described the impact of this trend on HIM as a "sea change." This is a way of describing a profound change from which there is no turning back.

Although great change is forecast, just what forms it may take is not at all clear yet. This presents a real-life strategic challenge for HIM professionals who must consider plausible alternate futures when constructing visions and formulating strategies.

Discussion Questions

1. How might the development of personal health records on the Web change the current role of HIM professionals within the organization?

2. How might the ways in which HIM and information systems staff work together change as personal health records become more prevalent?

3. How might the working relationship between HIM professionals and physicians change as personal health records become more prevalent?

4. How might the interaction between the HIM professional and the consumer change in the future?

Summary

Health information management is a dynamic profession that offers great opportunities to advance and contribute in a variety of important roles. Among these roles are those of strategic manager and change leader. In truth, experience will be needed to perfect the skills of strategic management as will a commitment to lifelong learning.

Leading change is more than a process to be managed, it is a way of thinking and acting. Managing change is a central strategic challenge for all organizations. This challenge may be even greater in healthcare organizations because their cultures tend to be change averse and their governance structures and decision-making processes are more complicated than those of the typical business organization. Moreover, leading change requires a vision and often requires building new organizational capabilities, such as environmental scanning, creative group process, and a more external focus.

In addition, leading change must be approached as a central and fundamental role of all managers. The best way to learn how to become more strategic is just to begin. Leading change requires creativity and imagination grounded in good information, managerial competence, and effective decision making.

All change is ultimately about increasing effectiveness. To be successful, strategic managers must first understand what their "customers" want and need. This requires information and continuous two-way communication about issues, ideas, and trends. Acceptance for change strategies must be earned. Leaders must be politically savvy and know how to communicate the rationale for change, its expected results, and the consequences of nonaction. Strategic managers must be sensitive to the fact that it takes time to disseminate a change message and for the message to be assimilated at a personal level. Change projects should move at a deliberate pace, but one that takes the needs of others into account.

Successful organizations will have a bias for action because learning to lead change is a byproduct of leading change. A bias for preserving the status quo must be replaced with a bias for action. Leading change is a learning process, and success increases the sense of possibility and the excitement to tackle the next challenge. Organizations that are on the move are energized, and this energy will be felt by employees, coworkers, and superiors alike. In essence, learning to lead change is an essential skill in today's world of work.

HIM professionals who understand that leadership, change, and learning are entwined will have great opportunities ahead of them. Society talks a lot about leadership, change, and learning. What is only now becoming clear is that these concepts are highly related. As Beer states, "One cannot contemplate dramatic change occurring within an organization without the exercise of some leadership. . . . And the organization does not change fundamentally without significant reorientation and learning by its leaders and members. Without learning, the attitudes, skills, and behavior needed to formulate and implement a new strategic task will not develop" (1999, p. 127). The goal is to reorient your organization to value innovation and change. This takes time, perseverance, and courage. Nonetheless, this is what will be expected of the strategic change leader and successful HIM professional.

References

Beer, M. 1999. Leading, learning and learning to lead. In *The Leader's Change Handbook*, J. A. Conger, G. M. Spreitzer, and E. E. Lawler, editors. San Francisco: Jossey-Bass.

Bridges, W. 1991. *Managing Transitions: Making the Most of Change.* Reading, Mass.: Addison-Wesley.

Bryson, J. M. 1995. *Strategic Planning for Public and Nonprofit Organizations,* rev. ed. San Francisco: Jossey-Bass.

David, F. R. 2001. *Strategic Management Concepts and Cases,* eighth edition. Upper Saddle River, N.J.: Prentice Hall.

DePree, M. 1992. *Leadership Jazz.* New York City: Dell Publishing.

Drucker, P. 1996. Not enough generals were killed. In *The Leader of the Future,* F. Hesselbein and M. Goldsmith, editors. San Francisco: Jossey-Bass.

Kotter, J. P. 1995. Leading change: why transformation efforts fail. *Harvard Business Review* 73(2):59–67.

Kotter, J. P. 1996. *Leading Change.* Boston: Harvard Business School Press.

Kouzes, J. M., and B. Z. Posner. 1995. *The Leadership Challenge: How to Keep Getting Extraordinary Things Done in Organizations.* San Francisco: Jossey-Bass.

Lawrence, D. M. 1998. Leading discontinuous change: ten lessons from the battlefront. In *Navigating Change,* D. C. Hambrick, D. A. Nadler, and M. L. Tushman, editors. Boston: Harvard Business School Press.

Porter, M. E. 1996. What is strategy? *Harvard Business Review* 74(6): 61–78.

Powers, V. J. 1997. Benchmarking study illustrates how best-in-class achieve alignment, communicate change. *Communication World* 14(2): 30–33.

Schein, E. H. 1992. *Organizational Culture and Leadership,* second edition. San Francisco: Jossey-Bass.

Schoemaker, P. J. H. 1993. Multiple scenario development: its conceptual and behavioral foundation. *Strategic Management Journal* 14:193–213.

Tichy, N. M. 1983. *Managing Strategic Change: Technical, Political and Cultural Dynamics.* New York City: John Wiley & Sons.

Walton, E. 1998. Senior leadership and discontinuous change. In *Navigating Change,* D. C. Hambrick, D. A. Nadler, and M. L. Tushman, editors. Boston: Harvard Business School Press.

Application Exercises

1. Conduct a Web search for information on future trends affecting healthcare. Identify and describe three trends and be prepared to discuss their potential impact on HIM services in the future. Prepare a one-page summary of each trend. Include the Web address.

2. Prepare a one-page description of one group process technique or exercise that is designed to help participants think creatively about the future. You may use the library or the Internet to find an interesting technique. Your description should include instructions for facilitating

the process or exercise with a group. Provide the steps in sufficient detail so that your description could be used as a guide. Bring copies of your description to hand out to each member of the class. In this way, everyone will begin to accumulate a file of ideas for how to help groups be more creative and future oriented.

3. Identify a strategic issue that you believe will face health information managers in practice. Facilitate a discussion of the issue by a group of four to six students using one of the group process techniques distributed in the exercise above.

4. Interview a member of the senior management at an affiliation site to learn about the organization's strategic vision and plans. Prepare a paper describing the manager's assessment of the strengths and weaknesses of the process used in preparing the plan, how well the organization has embraced the vision and plan, and what impact it has had. Synthesize what you learned from the interview to identify lessons for improving the process in that organization.

5. Interview the chief information officer (CIO) at a healthcare facility to learn about the site's strategic plan for information services. Prepare a paper describing the manager's assessment of the strengths and weaknesses of the plan, how it fits with the organization's overall vision and plans, and how well it is working to guide strategy and change. Synthesize what you learned from the interview in a brief written report.

6. Based on what you learned about the information strategy through your interview with the CIO, prepare a vision statement for health information management that will complement the overall vision for information services.

Review Quiz

Instructions: Choose the best answer for the following questions.

1. ____ Which of the following descriptions does not apply when describing the characteristics of strategy?
   a. An action or set of actions
   b. A description of how one intends to achieve the goals
   c. A description of specific implementation plans
   d. Improves the organization's fit with the external world

2. ____ Which of the following best describes the role of strategic management as compared to other management tools and approaches?
   a. A component of each of the major functions of management
   b. An additional function that one learns after mastering other management functions
   c. A replacement for certain of the management functions
   d. All of the above

3. ____ Which of the following is not an element of the external environment that should be part of a manager's routine scanning?
   a. The opinions of industry experts
   b. The opinions of employees
   c. Changes in healthcare policy and regulation
   d. What is happening in similar healthcare organizations in the community

4. ____ What is the primary purpose of preparing a vision statement?
   a. To convey a picture of the future
   b. To support a request for an increased budget
   c. To set forth a specific plan of work
   d. None of the above

5. ____ Which of the following does not describe a characteristic of storytelling as a creative technique?
   a. It is comfortable and fun.
   b. It is memorable.
   c. It is familiar and understandable.
   d. It rallies a group to take action.

6. ____ Tichy describes three organizational components that must be managed in the change process. What are they?
   a. Technical, political, and social
   b. Technical, political, and cultural
   c. Political, social, and managerial
   d. Cultural, political, and human

7. ____ Which of the following is the most important consideration when securing support for a change program?
   a. Understanding that individuals accept change in their own way
   b. Clear directives from senior management
   c. Assurances that no one will loose his or her job
   d. Being clear about the rewards for those who are on board

8. ____ Bridges identifies three transitional phases in personal and organizational change. What are they?
   a. Beginning, middle, end
   b. Beginning, neutral zone, ending
   c. Ending, neutral zone, beginning
   d. Ending, neutral zone, new start

Appendices, Glossary, and Index

Appendix A
Sample Documentation Forms

Figure A.1. Example of an Admission/Discharge Record Form for a Paper-Based Health Record

Medical Record No.

ADMISSION/DISCHARGE RECORD

Last Name | First Name | Middle Name | Maiden Name | Soc. Sec. No. | Room No. | Admitting no.

Address | City | State | ZIP Code | Home Phone | Sex ☐ M ☐ F

Age-Yrs | Birth Date Mo. Day Year | Birthplace | Marital Status ☐ Married ☐ Div ☐ Single ☐ Sep ☐ Widowed ☐ Unknown | Religion

Race ☐ American Indian or Alaskan Native ☐ Asian or Pacific Islander ☐ Black ☐ White ☐ Other | Ethnicity ☐ Spanish Origin/Hispanic ☐ Non-Spanish Origin/Non-Hispanic

Occupation | Employer or Employer of Spouse | Address of Employer - Phone

Name of Spouse | Address if Other Than Above | Birthplace

Notify in Case of Emergency | Relationship | Address | Phone

Name of Father | Birthplace | Maiden Name of Mother | Birthplace

Name of Blue Cross and/or Blue Shield Plan | Group No. | Contract No. | Effective Date | Subscriber ☐ Dependent ☐ | Family Member ☐ Comprehensive Coverage ☐

Other Hospitalization Insurance | Cert. or Policy No. | Group No. | Effective Date | Medicare No.

Referring Physician's Name and Address | Attending Physician | Att. Phys. Code | Date of Last Admission

Smoker ☐ Yes ☐ No | Nature of Admission ☐ Emergency ☐ Urgent ☐ Elective ☐ Newborn | Service | Admission Date Hour AM PM | Discharge Date Hour AM PM

Admitting Diagnosis | Completed by

Principal Diagnosis: The condition established after study to be responsible for occasioning the admission of the patient to the hospital for care. | Code Name

Other Diagnoses:

Principal Procedure: The procedure performed for definitive treatment rather than for diagnostic or exploratory purposes, or to treat a complication; the procedure most related to the principal diagnosis.

Date

Other Procedures:
Date(s)

Coded By

Disposition:

Discharged
☐ To Home or Self Care
☐ Against Advice

Transferred:
☐ To Short Term Hosp.
☐ To Skilled Nurs. Fac.

Transferred (cont.)
☐ To. Int. Care/Nurs. Home
☐ To Home Health Ser.
☐ To Other Fac. (specify)

☐ Died ☐ Autopsy
☐ No Autopsy

Figure A.2.   Example of a Physician's Order

PLEASE USE BALL POINT PEN—PRESS FIRMLY

WRITE OR IMPRINT PATIENT INFORMATION BELOW

DIAGNOSIS *R10 Sepsis*	AGE 60	WEIGHT 190	SEX *M*	GENERIC EQUIVALENT MAY BE DISPENSED UNLESS CHECKED ☐
DRUG ALLERGIES —	DIET *Reg*			

DATE AND TIME	PHYSICIAN'S ORDERS	DO NOT USE THIS SHEET UNLESS RED NUMBER SHOWS.	NURSE'S INITIALS
8/10/92 15 30	Dx: Dehydration, poss sepsis, tachycardia		
	v.s. q 15' till stable		
	q 30 x 4		
	q 1° x 4		
	then, q 4°		
	NPO except for meds		
	IV = Normal saline 120/kw.		
	250 cc 5% Albumin now		
	BC x 2 for fungus		
	sputum C + S		
	urine C + S		
	Add to labs — amylase, lipase, Mg + phosphorus		
	Ca. stat		
	EKG stat		
	CT abdomen/pelvis in AM		
	Consult Dr. Smith today		
	for R/O P.E.		
	STAT PT, PTT then give		
	Heparin 4000 units IV bohist		
	start heparin drip at 800 units/hr =		
	10,000 units heparin in 250 cc NS		
	at 20 cc/hr.		
	Zantac 50 mg IV q 8°		
	Regular 10 mg IV q 8°		
	T.O. Dr. Jones / B Wilson, RN		BW/RN

PHYSICIAN'S ORDERS

TECHNIQUE SYSTEMS, INC   CHART COPY

Figure A.3. Example of a Progress Note

INTEGRATED PROGRESS NOTES

HOSPITAL STAFF
Begin Here

IDENTIFY DEPARTMENT FIRST

DATE	TIME	MEDICAL STAFF Begin Here ▼	
8/20	5P		*Nursing Admission Note*
	92		*Patient is a 63 y/o female*
			admitted per wheelchair acc.
			by friend. Oriented to room, call
			light explained and in reach, introduced
			to roommate. Scheduled for foot
			surgery in A.M. History of
			hypertension, on Aldomet, took
			med at home today. No other
			medical problems, no known
			allergies. Dr. Johnson notified,
			anes. dept. notified.
			Connie Smith, RN
8.20.92		ORTHO SVS.	
	5:30 PM		*Well developed, well (fairly) nourished F*
			admitted for resection arthroplasty ℝ foot.
			Known HBP — Aldomet. BP 160/120. Med
			consult: OR clearance requested. Pt
			will need nutritional eval & discharge
			planning help. H & P dictated. H. Johnson, MD
8-20-92	6³⁰		*Anes. PreOp – Pt seen + examined; Spinal discussed, pt.*
			agrees to same. BP 160/110. Med consult noted. No known
			reactions to anesthetic agents in the past. Last surg 10 yrs ago.
			See prlanes summary. M. Shabbeb MD

SSF-169

Figure A.3.   *(Continued)*

		INTEGRATED PROGRESS NOTES	

HOSPITAL STAFF
Begin Here

IDENTIFY DEPARTMENT FIRST

DATE	TIME	MEDICAL STAFF Begin Here ▼	HOSPITAL STAFF
8/20 92	7²⁰p		Nutrition–Dietetics
			Low sodium diet order recom. Pt wgt 115 lbs,
			ideal wgt. 130 lbs. Likes and dislikes reviewed.
			"Not a big eater" she states. Will eval. for
			nutritional risk factors.
			Mary Ryan, RD
8-21-92	7ᴬ		Pre-op holding area
			Patient received in OR #3 per cart. ID + blood
			band checked. Operative consent on chart +
			verified. Side rails up. See OR nurses notes.
			P. Gordon RN
8/21/92			Ortho Svs.
	1100		PreOp Dx degenerative joint disease
			PostOp Dx same – arith. severe hallyx
			valgus ® foot MTP joints.
			Procedure, Resection arturoplasty ® foot
			Surgeon: R. Johnson
			Asst. K. Thomas
			Anes: Spinal/Shabbeb
			EBL 100 ccs Total Time: 53 mins.
			Compl: ∅
			Send to RR in stable condition.
			R Johnson, MD

SSF-169

Figure A.4.   Example of Patient Instructions Provided at Discharge

PATIENT INSTRUCTIONS

Identification Number
_____

Medical Record Number
_____

Last Name   First Name   Middle Initial
_____

Date of Birth

WOUND CARE

1. Keep the wound clean and dry.

2. Keep covered with a clean dressing.

3. Watch for increase in redness, swelling, drainage, red streaks, and fever. Report to your physician if any of these occur.

4. The stitches must be removed in _____ days.

5. Tetanus immunization was given. Please keep a record for future reference. Tetanus shot site may become warm, swollen, red, or tender. This is normal. You may also have a low-grade fever.

6. You may wash your hair gently after suturing but then keep dry until stitches are removed.

_____   _____

Signature of individual giving instructions   Date

The above instructions have been explained to me and I understand the importance of following them.

_____   _____

Signature of individual receiving instructions   Date

Relationship to patient: _____
                                        Self/parent/guardian

Figure A.5.   Example of a Consent to Treatment

CONSENT FOR OPERATION

_____
Identification Number

_____
Medical Record Number

_____
Last Name   First Name   Middle Initial

_____
Date of Birth

I, _____ for _____ hereby consent to (nature of

operation/procedure) _____

_____

to be performed by, or under the direction of, Dr. _____)

at Community Hospital on (date of surgery/procedure) _____, _____

I further consent to the performance of any additional procedures during the course of my operation/procedure which the physician or his associates judge necessary or desirable to correct the existing conditions or any other unhealthy condition that they may discover.

I realize that an operation/procedure requires numerous assistants, technicians, nurses, and other personnel, and I give my consent to such medical procedures and care by such personnel and Community Hospital before, during, and after the operation/procedure to be performed.

I also consent to the disposal by Community Hospital of any tissue or parts that may be removed during my operation.

I have been advised by my physician about alternatives to the operation/procedure that he/she has suggested, but I believe that the treatment he/she suggests is the treatment or operation I should have.

My physician has advised me fully about the nature of the operation/procedure and the risks involved. I realize that neither the physician nor Community Hospital can guarantee any result.

I have read this authorization and understand it.

NOTE TO PATIENT: YOUR SIGNATURE BELOW INDICATES THAT YOU HAVE READ AND AGREED TO THE ABOVE, THAT THE OPERATIONS OR SPECIAL PROCEDURES HAVE BEEN ADEQUATELY EXPLAINED TO YOU BY YOUR ATTENDING PHYSICIAN OR SURGEONS, THAT YOU HAVE ALL THE INFORMATION YOU DESIRE, AND THAT YOU AUTHORIZE AND CONSENT TO THE PERFORMANCE OF THE OPERATIONS OR SPECIAL PROCEDURES MENTIONED ABOVE.

DATE: _____ SIGNATURE: _____

RELATIONSHIP (IF OTHER THAN PATIENT) _____

WITNESS' SIGNATURE: _____

Signature of physician by which he affirms that he has obtained the informed consent of the patient, or his duly authorized agent, to that which is outlined above.

DATE: _____ SIGNATURE: _____

Figure A.6.   Example of a Consent to Release Information Form

Consent to the Use and Disclosure of Health Information for Treatment, Payment, or Healthcare Operations

I understand that as part of my healthcare, this organization originates and maintains health records describing my health history, symptoms, examination and test results, diagnoses, treatment, and any plans for future care or treatment. I understand that this information serves as:

- a basis for planning my care and treatment
- a means of communication among the many health professionals who contribute to my care
- a source of information for applying my diagnosis and surgical information to my bill
- a means by which a third-party payer can verify that services billed were actually provided
- and a tool for routine healthcare operations such as assessing quality and reviewing the competence of healthcare professionals

I understand and have been provided with a *Notice of Information Practices* that provides a more complete description of information uses and disclosures. I understand that I have the right to review the notice prior to signing this consent. I understand that the organization reserves the right to change their notice and practices and prior to implementation will mail a copy of any revised notice to the address I've provided. I understand that I have the right to object to the use of my health information for directory purposes. I understand that I have the right to request restrictions as to how my health information may be used or disclosed to carry out treatment, payment, or healthcare operations and that the organization is not required to agree to the restrictions requested. I understand that I may revoke this consent in writing, except to the extent that the organization has already take action in reliance thereon.

☐   I request the following restrictions to the use or disclosure of my health information.

_____

_____

_____   _____
Signature of Patient or Legal Representative   Witness

_____   _____
Date   Notice Effective Date or Version

☐ Accepted   ☐ Denied

_____   _____   _____
Signature   Title   Date

Figure A.7.   Example of a Problem List

		PROBLEM LIST		
Identification Number				
Medical Record Number				
Last Name		First Name		Middle Initial
Date of Birth				

PROBLEM NUMBER	DATE ENTERED	LIST SIGNIFICANT ACUTE AND CHRONIC CONDITIONS INCLUDING SURGICAL PROCEDURES	PROBLEM RESOLVED	DATE RESOLVED
1				
2				
3				
4				
5				
6				
7				
8				
9				
10				
11				
12				
13				
14				
15				
16				
17				
18				
19				
20				

Appendix B
Sample Position Descriptions

Position Description: Risk Manager

Position Title: Risk Manager

Immediate Supervisor: Chief Executive Officer or Other Senior Executive

General Purpose: The Risk Manager is responsible for administering and managing the facility's risk management program.

Responsibilities:
- Develops and implements the organization's risk management program in a manner that fulfills the mission and strategic goals of the organization while complying with state and federal laws and accreditation standards related to safety and risk management.

- Develops and implements systems, policies, and procedures for the identification, collection, and analysis of risk-related information.

- Educates and trains the leadership, staff, and business associates about the risk management program and their respective responsibilities in carrying out the risk management program.

- Leads, facilitates, and advises departments in designing risk management programs within their own departments.

- Collects, evaluates, and maintains data concerning patient injuries, claims, worker's compensation, and other risk-related data.

- Investigates and analyzes root causes, patterns, or trends that could result in compensatory or sentinel events. Helps to identify and implement corrective action where appropriate.

- Provides a quarterly summary to the Board on incidents, claims, and claim payments.

- Serves as the organization's liaison to the organization's insurance carrier.

- Assists in processing summonses and claims against the facility by working with legal counsel to coordinate the investigation, processing, and defense of claims against the organization.

- Actively participates on or facilitates committees related to risk management, safety, and quality improvement.

Qualifications:
- Bachelor's degree in business administration, public health policy, or a related clinical or allied health field.

- Minimum of three years of experience in one or more of the following fields: risk management, quality improvement, health information management, healthcare administration, business administration, legal support or insurance/claims investigation and settlement, or patient care.

- Knowledge of statistics, data collection, analysis, and data presentation.

- Excellent interpersonal communication and problem solving skills.

- Knowledge of federal and state laws and regulations and accreditation standards.

Position Description: Quality Improvement Director

Position Title: Quality Improvement Director

Immediate Supervisor: Chief Operating Officer or Other Senior Executive

General Purpose: The Quality Improvement Director is responsible for administering and managing the facility's quality improvement program.

Responsibilities:

- Develops and implements the organization's quality improvement plan in accordance with the mission and strategic goals of the organization, federal and state laws and regulations, and accreditation standards.

- Develops and implements systems, policies, and procedures for the identification, collection, and analysis of performance measurement data.

- Educates and trains the leadership, staff, and business associates as to the quality improvement plan and their respective responsibilities in carrying out the quality improvement program.

- Leads, facilitates, and advises internal quality improvement teams.

- Collects and summarizes performance data, identifies opportunities for improvement, and presents findings quarterly to the Performance Improvement Committee and Board of Directors.

- Analyzes customer survey data to identify opportunities for improvement and presents findings to appropriate departments.

- Actively participates on or facilitates committees such as: Quality Improvement, Utilization Management, Patient Safety, and Risk Management.

Qualifications:

- Certification as an RHIA or RHIT or licensure as an RN and a bachelor's degree in a clinical or allied health field preferred.

- A minimum of three years of experience in health information, quality, utilization, or risk management helpful.

- Certification as a Professional in Healthcare Quality (CPHQ) preferred.

- Knowledge of statistics, data collection, analysis, and data presentation.

- Excellent interpersonal communication and problem solving skills.

- Knowledge of federal and state laws and regulations and accreditation standards.

Position Description: Utilization Management Director

Position Title:	Utilization Management Director
Immediate Supervisor:	Chief Financial Officer or Other Senior Executive
General Purpose:	The Utilization Management Director is responsible for administering and managing the facility's utilization management program.

Responsibilities:

- Develops and implements the organization's utilization management plan in accordance with the mission and strategic goals of the organization, federal and state law and regulation, and accreditation standards.

- Develops and implements systems, policies and procedures for prospective, concurrent, and retrospective case review, clinical practice guidelines, care maps, clinical protocols, and reporting quality of care issues identified during the utilization review process.

- Educates and trains the leadership, staff, and business associates as to the utilization management plan and their respective responsibilities relative to the plan.

- Collects, analyzes, and maintains data on the utilization of medical services and resources.

- Prepares and presents quarterly utilization management summaries to the Board, identifying potential areas for improvement.

- Reports quality of care issues identified during the utilization review process according to policy and procedure.

- Acts as the liaison to the Peer Review Organization (PRO), performing duties such as the preparation of replies to PRO denials.

- Obtains preapproval or precertification from third-party payers for procedures and continued stay.

- Actively participates in or facilitates selected committees such as Utilization Management and Performance Improvement.

Qualifications:

- Bachelor's degree in a clinical or allied health field, RN, RHIA, or RHIT preferred.

- Minimum of three years of experience in utilization management, health information management, nursing, quality improvement, or a related field.

- Knowledge of statistics, data collection, analysis, and data presentation.

- Excellent interpersonal communication and problem-solving skills.

- Knowledge of utilization management techniques.

- Knowledge of ICD and CPT coding

Position Description: Medical Staff Coordinator

Position Title: Medical Staff Coordinator

Immediate Supervisor: Senior Vice President

General Purpose: The Medical Staff Coordinator administers the medical staff credentialing and reappointment process and assists the medical staff in supporting the organization's mission, vision, and goals.

Responsibilities:
- Establishes and administers the credentialing, reappointment, and privileging processes.
- Coordinates procurement of DE, licensure, and malpractice insurance information. Originates or collects and maintains appropriate records.
- Assists the medical staff in the selection process for medical staff leadership.
- Orients medical staff leadership to key policies related to their roles.
- Assists medical staff leadership in the development of bylaws and related policies.
- Arranges room, food, and notices for medical staff meetings and continuing education.
- Maintains, posts, and distributes a medical staff newsletter and calendar.
- Maintains documentation of continuing medical staff education.
- Originates and maintains agendas, minutes, and postmeeting correspondence for all medical staff committees.
- Prepares credentialing reports and action items for the Board of Directors.
- Composes and disseminates correspondence from the Board to the medical staff insofar as decisions related to credentialing, privileges, and special requests.
- Develops and implements systems that allow for the flow of information to and from medical staff committees into the performance improvement structure.
- Maintains and generates performance related data for medical staff members and functions.
- Orients applicants to the medical staff bylaws, key policies, medical staff structure, and performance improvement process.
- Develops annual goals and objectives for the medical staff office in concert with the organization's strategic plan.
- Prepares and monitors the annual budget for the department.
- Stays abreast of and applies knowledge of applicable federal and state laws and regulations and accreditation standards.

Qualifications:
- Certification as a CMSC, RHIT, or RHIA.
- Proficient in computer applications (Windows, MS Office, medical staff databases, etc.).
- Knowledge of statistics, data collection, data analysis, and data presentation.
- Excellent interpersonal communication and problem-solving skills.

Position Description: Director of HIM Academic Program

Position Title: Director, HIM Academic Program

Immediate Supervisor: Chairperson, Allied Health Division or equivalent

General Purpose: The Program Director is responsible for the overall health information management education program.

Responsibilities:
- Develops and administers curriculum for students to acquire the knowledge and skills necessary for competency in accordance with the stipulations of professional and accreditation agencies.
- Develops instructional materials to include course plans, objectives, audiovisual aids, lab activities, and evaluation tools.
- Instructs students.
- Assesses course effectiveness through student evaluations.
- Works with counterparts on other campuses to establish continuity.
- Develops a student recruitment program or assists in student recruitment.
- Advises prospective students on the academic and professional aspects of the program.
- Advises current students relative to their performance and maintains appropriate documentation thereof.
- Actively participates in appropriate department, division, school, campus, or university committees.
- Engages in research/creative activities in the field of health information management, education, or related areas.
- Documents results of research/creative activities in published form.
- Develops and administers an annual program budget.
- Manages correspondence relative to the program and liaisons with all constituencies influencing health information management education.
- Establishes and monitors procedures for clinical education and evaluation.
- Administers admissions process for HIM program.
- Schedules and prepares agenda for the HIM Advisory Committee.
- Reviews faculty course evaluations.
- Schedules courses and assigns teaching loads.
- Reviews faculty performance.

Qualifications:
- Master's degree in a health-related discipline or education.
- RHIA certification by the American Health Information Management Association.
- Years of clinical experience/teaching as stipulated by university guidelines.
- Working knowledge of accreditation process desirable.

Position Description: Coder

Position Title:	Coder
Immediate Supervisor:	Director of Health Information Management, Manager of Clinical Data, or Coding Supervisor
General Purpose:	The purpose of this position is to apply the appropriate diagnostic and procedural codes to individual patient health information for data retrieval and analysis and claims processing.

Responsibilities:

- Abstracts pertinent information from patient records. Assigns ICD-9-CM or HCPCS codes, creating APC or DRG group assignments.

- Queries physicians when code assignments are not straightforward or documentation in the record is inadequate, ambiguous, or unclear for coding purposes.

- Keeps abreast of coding guidelines and reimbursement reporting requirements. Brings identified concerns to supervisor or department manager for resolution.

- Abides by the Standards of Ethical Coding as set forth by the American Health Information Management Association and adheres to official coding guidelines.

Qualifications:

- Minimum of successful completion of a coding certificate program in a program with AHIMA approval status. Certification as RHIA, RHIT, CCS, CCS-P, CPC, or CPC-H preferred.

- Coding certification from the American Health Information Management Association preferred.

- Work experience as a coder or strong training background in coding and reimbursement preferred.

Position Description: DRG Coordinator

Position Title:	DRG Coordinator
Immediate Supervisor:	Director of Health Information Management
General Purpose:	The purpose of this position is to ensure consistency and efficiency in inpatient claims processing and data collection to optimize DRG reimbursement and facilitate data quality in hospital inpatient services.

Responsibilities:

- Performs data quality reviews on inpatient records to validate the ICD-9-CM codes, DRG group appropriateness, missed secondary diagnoses, and/or procedures and ensure compliance with all DRG mandates and reporting requirements.

- Monitors Medicare and other DRG paid bulletins and manuals and reviews the current OIG work plans for DRG risk areas.

- Creates and monitors inpatient case-mix reports and the top 25 assigned DRGs in the facility to identify patterns, trends, and variations in the facility's frequently assigned DRG groups. Once identified, the DRG Coordinator evaluates the causes of the change or problems and takes appropriate steps in collaboration with the right department to effect resolution or explanation of any variances.

- Continuously evaluates the quality of clinical documentation to spot incomplete or inconsistent documentation for inpatient encounters that affect the code selection and resulting DRG groups and payment. Brings identified concerns to medical staff committee or department managers for resolution.

- Provides and/or arranges for training to facility healthcare professionals in the use of coding guidelines and practices, proper documentation techniques, medical terminology and disease processes, appropriate to the job description and function as it relates to the DRG and other clinical data quality management factors. Maintains knowledge of current professional coding certification requirements and promotes recruitment and retention of certified staff in coding positions when possible.

- Reports to the facility Compliance Committee each quarter.

- Abides by the Standards of Ethical Coding as set forth by the American Health Information Management Association and monitors coding staff for violations. Reports to the HIM Director when areas of concern are identified. Concerns involving compliance issues are forwarded to the Compliance Committee for action.

- Develops reports and collects and prepares data for studies involving inpatient stays for clinical evaluation purposes and/or financial impact and profitability.

- Serves as the facility representative for DRGs by attending coding and reimbursement workshops and bringing back information to the appropriate departments. Communicates any DRG updates published in third-party payer newsletters/bulletins and provider manuals to all facility staff that need this information.

- Keeps abreast of new technology in coding and abstracting software and other forms of automation and stays informed about transaction code sets, HIPAA requirements, and other future issues affecting the coding function.

- Demonstrates competency in the use of computer applications and DRG Grouper Software, Medicare edits, and all coding and abstracting software and hardware currently in use by the HIM department.

- Performs periodic claim form reviews to check code transfer accuracy from the abstracting system and the Chargemaster.

- Evaluates, records, and responds to the Peer Review Organization DRG change and/or denial notices. Provides appropriate documentation from required source to the PRO when appealing a PRO decision.

- Monitors unbilled accounts report for outstanding and/or uncoded discharges to reduce Accounts Receivable days for outpatients.

Qualifications:

- Minimum of associate's degree in a health services discipline. Formal HIM education with national certification (RHIA, RHIT) preferred.

- Coding certification required from the American Health Information Management Association or the American Academy of Professional Coders.

- Minimum of five years progressive coding or coding review experience in ICD-9-CM with claims processing and/or data management responsibilities a plus.

- Good oral and written communication skills and comprehensive knowledge of the DRG structure and regulatory requirements.

- Past auditing experience or strong training background in coding and reimbursement preferred.

Position Description: APC Coordinator

Position Title: APC Coordinator

Immediate Supervisor: Director of Health Information Management

General Purpose: The purpose of this position is to create consistency and efficiency in outpatient claims processing and data collection to optimize APC reimbursement and facilitate data quality in outpatient services.

Responsibilities:

- Performs data quality reviews on outpatient encounters to validate the ICD-9-CM, CPT, and HCPCS Level II code and modifier assignments, APC group appropriateness, missed secondary diagnoses and/or procedures, and compliance with all APC mandates and outpatient reporting requirements.

- Monitors medical visit code selection by departments against facility-specific criteria for appropriateness. Assists in the development of such criteria as needed.

- Monitors outpatient service mix reports and the leading medical visit, surgical service, significant procedure, and ancillary APCs assigned in the facility to identify patterns, trends, and variations in the facility's frequently assigned APC groups. Once identified, evaluates the causes of the change, and takes appropriate steps in collaboration with the right department to effect resolution or explanation of the variance.

- Continuously evaluates the quality of clinical documentation to spot incomplete or inconsistent documentation for outpatient encounters that impact the code selection and resulting APC groups and payment. Brings identified concerns to medical staff committee or department managers for resolution.

- Provides and/or arranges for training to facility healthcare professionals in the use of coding guidelines and practices, proper documentation techniques, medical terminology and disease processes, appropriate to the job description and function as it relates to the APC and other outpatient data quality management factors.

- Maintains knowledge of current professional coding certification requirements and promotes recruitment and retention of certified staff in coding positions when possible.

- Reports to the facility Compliance Committee each quarter.

- Abides by the Standards of Ethical Coding as set forth by the American Health Information Management Association and monitors coding staff for violations and reports to the HIM Director when areas of concern are identified. Concerns involving compliance issues are forwarded to the Compliance Committee for action.

- Develops reports and collects and prepares data for studies involving outpatient encounter data for clinical evaluation purposes and/or financial impact and profitability.

- Serves as the facility representative for APCs by attending outpatient coding and reimbursement workshops and bringing back information to the appropriate departments. Communicates any APC updates published in third-party payer newsletters/bulletins and provider manuals to all facility staff that need this information.

- Keeps abreast of new technology in coding and abstracting software and other forms of automation and stays informed about transaction code sets, HIPAA requirements, and other future issues impacting the coding function.

- Demonstrates competency in the use of computer applications and APC Grouper Software, OCE edits, and all coding software and hardware currently used by the HIM department.

- Performs periodic claim form reviews to check code transfer accuracy from the abstracting system and the Chargemaster.

- Evaluates, records, and responds to the Peer Review Organization APC change and/or denial notices. Provides appropriate documentation from required source to the PRO when appealing a PRO decision.

- Monitors outpatient unbilled accounts report for outstanding and/or uncoded outpatient encounters to reduce Accounts Receivable days for outpatients.

- Serves on the Chargemaster Maintenance Committee.

Qualifications:

- Minimum of associate's degree in a health services discipline. Formal HIM education with national certification, RHIA or RHIT preferred.

- Coding certification required from the American Health Information Management Association or the American Academy of Professional Coders.

- Minimum of five years progressive coding or coding review experience in ICD-9-CM, CPT, and HCPCS with claims processing and/or data management responsibilities a plus.

- Good oral and written communication skills and comprehensive knowledge of the APC structure and regulatory requirements.

- Past auditing experience or strong training background in coding and reimbursement preferred.

Position Description: Health Information Manager or Director

Position Title: Health Information Manager (or Director)

Immediate Superior: Chief Information Officer or Other Senior Executive of the Network

General Purpose: The Health Information Manager is responsible for coordinating health information management services across the multifacility integrated healthcare system.

Responsibilities:

- Working as a line manager, directs the health information management functions of all the facilities in the healthcare system.

- Develops and deploys health information management systems as part of the healthcare system's overall information system plan.

- Monitors health information management systems and sets the healthcare system's standards for data quality and ethical practice.

- Participates in the development of health information management policies and procedures on release of information, confidentiality, information security, information storage and retrieval, and record retention.

- Documents and enforces the healthcare system's health information management policies and procedures.

- Provides education and training to the healthcare system's employees in areas relevant to health information management policies and procedures.

- Supports and facilitates clinical, administrative, and external data use functions.

- Monitors local, national, and international trends in healthcare delivery.

- Monitors changes in legislation and accreditation standards that affect health information management.

- Serves as an internal consultant on health information management issues including release of information, confidentiality, information security, information storage and retrieval, and record retention as well as authorship and authentication of health record documentation, standardization of medical vocabularies, and use of classification systems.

- Performs and reports research on topics related to health information management.

- Forecasts the healthcare system's future technical and information needs.

- Coordinates specialty databases.

Qualifications:

- Master's degree in health information management or a related field.

- Certification as an RHIA.

- Experience in administrative and staff management.

- Experience in project management.

- Knowledge of information systems and healthcare applications as well as database applications and report-writing software.

Position Description: Clinical Data Specialist

Position Title: Clinical Data Specialist

Immediate Supervisor: Director of Health Information Management

General Purpose: The Clinical Data Specialist is a member of the data management team responsible for ensuring the accuracy and completeness of clinical coding; validating the information in the databases for outcomes management and specialty registries; and performing clinical research across the entire integrated healthcare system.

Responsibilities:
- Designs and uses audit tools to monitor the accuracy of clinical coding.
- Monitors compliance with policies and procedures relevant to clinical data management and makes suggestions for improvements.
- Interprets data for reimbursement applications.
- Validates data for various disease registries.
- Validates data for the outcomes management program.
- Prepares utilization analyses.
- Prepares patient demographic reports.
- Prepares provider profiles.
- Collects and analyzes data for special clinical research projects.

Qualifications:
- Bachelor's degree in health information management or a related field.
- Certification as an RHIA or RHIT.
- Certification as a CCS and CCS-P.
- Knowledge of database applications and spreadsheet design.
- Knowledge of report-writing software.

Position Description: Patient Information Coordinator

Position Title:	Patient Information Coordinator
Immediate Supervisor:	Director of Health Information Services
General Purpose:	The Patient Information Coordinator is responsible for fostering high levels of customer service in coordinating all information provided to customers and their families and caregivers and ensuring that they receive appropriate, timely, and accurate health information about the services provided by caregivers, financial services, social services, and other medical and legal entities.

Responsibilities:

- Handles all requests and inquiries for patient information; disperses the information with accountability to all regulatory entities and according to the facility's policies and procedures.

- Coordinates patient information through all caregivers, insurance companies, billing departments, and patients according to all of the facility's policies and procedures.

- Maintains information flow according to the facility's established guidelines.

- Meets one-on-one with patients to facilitate the coordination of their health information with the facility and with their insurance companies or other payers.

- Maintains the confidentiality of all patient, client, and facility information at all times, both while on and off duty.

- Performs quality reviews according to the quality improvement policies and procedures to ensure patient satisfaction; reports these results quarterly to the director of health information services.

- Demonstrates a complete understanding of the release of information process, including guidelines in training manuals, regulatory manuals, and facility policies and procedures as they relate to patient care information and billing information.

- Keeps current with ongoing or new legislative issues related to the release of information.

- Works with the IS department to incorporate new technologies.

- Plans and maintains a budget.

- Communicates effectively at all levels, internally and externally, within the organization and expresses ideas and information clearly and concisely, in verbal and written form.

- Presents educational seminars.

- Actively contributes to the morale and teamwork of the staff and facility and always presents a positive attitude and patient-minded vision, with patient satisfaction as the continuing goal.

Qualifications:

- Bachelor's degree in health information management.

- Certification as RHIA or RHIT.

- Extensive healthcare and management experience.

- Excellent communication skills, both written and verbal.

- Ability to work with a variety of customers, patients, lawyers, and other healthcare providers in a diplomatic fashion.

Position Description: Director of Data Quality Management

Position Title: Director, Data Quality Management

Immediate Superior: Vice-President, Quality

General Purpose: The Director of Data Quality Management is responsible for developing, implementing, and maintaining a data quality management (compliance) plan for coding and reimbursement, health records and documentation, and quality data in all divisions of the organization.

Responsibilities:
- Assesses current compliance activities, identifying areas of high risk and evaluating risk factors in coding and documentation practices.

- Develops, implements, and maintains a standardized, organizationwide quality data management (compliance) plan and program to ensure compliance with external regulatory and accreditation requirements, ensure consistency of quality data for the organization's internal data needs, and identify, investigate, and prevent violations.

- Reviews areas of risk, investigates identified issues, reports data analyses, and takes appropriate steps to correct violations.

- Establishes, implements, and maintains a formalized review process for compliance, including a formal review (audit) process.

- Optimizes receipt of high-quality data from parent and contract hospitals by active participation and leadership in quality-monitoring and quality improvement efforts.

- In partnership with appropriate personnel, develops and implements standardized, organizationwide coding guidelines and documentation requirements and develops and implements training and educational programs for physicians and coders.

- Provides consulting services in the area of data quality management to individuals, special projects, and executive and clinical departments throughout the organization.

Qualifications:
- Bachelor's degree in health information management or a related field and at least 10 years of professional experience, 5 of which are in data quality; or a master's degree or its equivalent and at least 7 years of experience in a clinical, operational, or data quality improvement function.

- Credentialed as an RHIA or an RHIT and a CCS.

- Experience in operational management.

- Experience in project management.

- Knowledge of health information systems and database management.

- Knowledge of applied statistics, process analysis, and outcomes analysis.

Position Description: Information Security Manager

Position Title: Information Security Manager

Immediate Superior: Director of Health Information Management, Chief Information Officer, or Other Senior Executive

General Purpose: The Information Security Manager serves as the process owner for all ongoing activities related to the availability, integrity, and confidentiality of patient, provider, employee, and business information in compliance with the healthcare organization's information security policies and procedures.

Responsibilities:

- Documents the information security policies and procedures instituted by the organization's Information Security Committee.

- Implements the organization's information security policies and procedures.

- Coordinates the activities of the Information Security Committee.

- Provides direct information security training to all employees, contractors, alliances, and other third parties.

- Monitors compliance with the organization's information security policies and procedures among employees, contractors, alliances, and other third parties and refers problems to appropriate department managers or administrators.

- Monitors internal control systems to ensure that appropriate information access levels and security clearances are maintained.

- Performs information security risk assessments and serves as the internal auditor for information security processes.

- Prepares the organization's disaster recovery and business continuity plans for information systems.

- Serves as an internal information security consultant to the organization.

- Monitors advancements in information security technologies.

- Monitors changes in legislation and accreditation standards that affect information security.

- Initiates, facilitates, and promotes activities to foster information security awareness within the organization.

- Serves as the information security liaison for users of clinical, administrative, and behavioral systems.

- Reviews all system-related information security plans throughout the organization's network and acts as a liaison to the Information Systems Department.

Qualifications:

- Bachelor's degree in health information management or a related field.

- Certification as an RHIA or an RHIT.

- Experience in project management and change management.

- Knowledge of information security and access technologies.

- Knowledge of database applications, spreadsheet design, and report-writing software.

Position Description: Data Resource Administrator

Position Title: Data Resource Administrator

Immediate Supervisor: Director of Information Services

General Purpose: The Data Resource Administrator provides overall leadership for data resource management in the organization and is responsible for developing, communicating, and monitoring data resource management policies and procedures to ensure that the organization's data are secure, accessible, accurate, and reliable for business and patient care uses.

Responsibilities:

- Works with health information management, legal services, and other departments to develop and maintain the organization's data resource management policies and procedures.

- Monitors compliance with the organization's data resource management policies and procedures.

- Works with data analysts and database managers from the information services department to develop and manage the organization's data repository and data warehouse.

- Works with data quality managers and other health information management professionals to ensure the quality of the organization's health information.

- Develops and maintains the organization's data sets, data dictionary, data standards, and data model.

- Works with health information management, legal services, information security, and information services staff to develop access and release of information policies and procedures.

- Forecasts the organization's future information system requirements.

- Participates in the planning and negotiation of acquisitions of new information system software and hardware.

- Manages the functions, staff, and budget of the data resource department.

- Performs strategic planning activities for the data resource department and participates in strategic planning for the organization.

- Assesses training needs among data users and coordinates training activities.

- Monitors advancements in information technology and health information management.

- Monitors changes in laws, regulations, and accreditation standards as they apply to data resource management.

Qualifications:

- Bachelor's degree in health information management or a related field; advanced degree or coursework in computer science desirable.

- Certification as an RHIA.

- Knowledge of health information systems, database management and design, spreadsheet design, and computer technology.

Position Description: Research Data Analyst

Position Title: Research Data Analyst

Immediate Supervisor: Department Director

Position's Purpose: The Research Data Analyst ensures the quality of data collection, coordination, and analysis for clinical research projects.

Responsibilities:

- Verifies, examines, and corrects data.

- Ensures that clinical data are quality assured, consistent, and relevant to project's and the organization's goals.

- Ensures the integrity of the data and the safe and proper management of study parameters.

- Maintains expert knowledge of relevant FDA guidelines and other regulatory procedures.

- Monitors protocol at study sites.

- Retrieves data from numerous clinical databases within the organization as well as from proprietary and nonproprietary databases available through outside sources.

- Uses structured query language and downloads data into the organization's custom databases for review and analysis.

- Manipulates and analyzes data by using statistical software, such as SPSS and SAS, and identifies and determines significant variances and trends for quality control.

- Reviews proposed research design to ensure that the data collected are adequate to meet the project's goals.

- Prepares periodic progress and monitoring reports on study recruitment, data collection, and data quality.

- Participates in team meetings.

- Prepares and provides overviews, demonstrations, and presentations to wide variety of audiences.

Qualifications:

- Master's degree in health science or related field.

- Bachelor's degree in health information management, business, or closely related area.

- Experience in health science and administration.

- Certification as RHIA preferable.

Position Description: Decision Support Specialist

Position Title: Decision Support Specialist

Immediate Supervisor: Director, Decision Support

General Purpose: The Decision Support Specialist coordinates data and research for senior managers at the corporate level of the integrated system.

Responsibilities:

- Participates and assists in the design of a comprehensive program to lend support and analysis to management.

- Performs scientific and technical planning, direction, and analysis of selected surveillance systems used by management.

- Investigates existing national data and performs descriptive and analytic studies using statistical techniques.

- Provides ongoing data analysis to entity decision makers that is relevant to the healthcare market and assists in problem solving, solution development, decision making, and strategic planning.

- Recommends focus and direction of resources toward management goals.

- Prepares and provides decision support overviews, demonstrations, and presentations to a wide variety of audiences.

- Serves as technical expert advisor and consultant to collaborating organizations in the area of management goals.

Qualifications:

- Bachelor's degree in health information management, business, healthcare, or information systems technology.

- Certification as RHIA or RHIT.

- Understanding of healthcare delivery systems and health science administration.

Position Description: HIM Compliance Specialist

Position Title: HIM Compliance Specialist

Immediate Supervisor: Corporate Compliance Officer

General Purpose: The HIM Compliance Specialist oversees and monitors implementation of the HIM compliance program.

Responsibilities:

- Develops and coordinates educational and training programs regarding elements of the HIM compliance program, such as appropriate documentation and accurate coding, to all appropriate personnel, including HIM coding staff, physicians, billing personnel, and ancillary departments.

- Maintains attendance rosters and documentation (agenda, handouts, and so on) for HIM training programs.

- Ensures that coding consultants and other contracted entities (for example, outsourced coding personnel) understand and agree to adhere to the organization's HIM compliance program.

- Conducts regular audits and coordinates ongoing monitoring of coding accuracy and documentation adequacy.

- Provides feedback and focused educational programs on the results of auditing and monitoring activities to affected staff and physicians.

- Conducts trend analyses to identify patterns and variations in coding practices and case-mix index.

- Compares coding and reimbursement profile with national and regional norms to identify variations requiring further investigation.

- Reviews claim denials and rejections pertaining to coding and medical necessity issues and, when necessary, implements corrective action plan, such as educational programs, to prevent similar denials and rejections from recurring.

- Conducts internal investigations of changes in coding practices or reports of other potential problems pertaining to coding.

- Initiates corrective action to ensure resolution of problem areas identified during an internal investigation or auditing/monitoring activity.

- Reports noncompliance issues detected through auditing and monitoring, nature of corrective action plans implemented in response to identified problems, and results of follow-up audits to the corporate compliance officer.

- Receives and investigates reports of HIM compliance violations and communicates this information to the Corporate Compliance Officer.

- Recommends disciplinary action for violation of the compliance program, the organization's standards of conduct, or coding policies and procedures to the corporate compliance officer.

- Ensures the appropriate dissemination and communication of all regulation, policy, and guideline changes to affected personnel.

- Serves as a resource for department managers, staff, physicians, and administration to obtain information or clarification on accurate and ethical coding and documentation standards, guidelines, and regulatory requirements.

- Monitors adherence to the HIM compliance program.

- Revises the HIM compliance program in response to changing organizational needs or new or revised regulations, policies, and guidelines.

- Serves on the Compliance Committee.

- Recommends revisions to the corporate compliance program to improve its effectiveness.

Qualifications:

- RHIA or RHIT, CCS preferred (for ambulatory services, CCS-P).

- Extensive knowledge of ICD-9-CM and CPT coding principles and guidelines.

- Extensive knowledge of reimbursement systems.

- Extensive knowledge of federal-, state-, and payer-specific regulations and policies pertaining to documentation, coding, and billing.

- Five years of hospital coding experience (for ambulatory services, ambulatory coding experience).

- Strong managerial, leadership, and interpersonal skills.

- Excellent written and verbal communication skills.

- Excellent analytical skills.

Position Description: Chief Privacy Officer

Position Title: Chief Privacy Officer

Immediate Supervisor: Chief Executive Officer, Senior Executive, or Health Information Management (HIM) Department Head

General Purpose: The Chief Privacy Officer oversees all ongoing activities related to the development, implementation, maintenance of, and adherence to the organization's policies and procedures covering the privacy of, and access to, patient health information in compliance with federal and state laws and the healthcare organization's information privacy practices.

Responsibilities:

- Provides development guidance and assists in the identification, implementation, and maintenance of organization information privacy policies and procedures in coordination with organization management and administration, the Privacy Oversight Committee, and legal counsel.

- Works with organization's senior management and corporate compliance officer to establish an organization-wide Privacy Oversight Committee.

- Serves in a leadership role for the Privacy Oversight Committee's activities.

- Performs initial and periodic information privacy risk assessments and conducts related ongoing compliance monitoring activities in coordination with the entity's other compliance and operational assessment functions.

- Works with legal counsel and management, key departments, and committees to ensure the organization has and maintains appropriate privacy and confidentiality consent, authorization forms, and information notices and materials reflecting current organization and legal practices and requirements.

- Oversees, directs, delivers, or ensures delivery of initial and privacy training and orientation to all employees, volunteers, medical and professional staff, contractors, alliances, business associates, and other appropriate third parties.

- Participates in the development, implementation, and ongoing compliance monitoring of all trading partner and business associate agreements, to ensure that all privacy concerns, requirements, and responsibilities are addressed.

- Establishes with management and operations a mechanism to track access to protected health information, within the purview of the organization and as required by law and to allow qualified individuals to review or receive a report on such activity.

- Works cooperatively with the HIM Director and other applicable organization units in overseeing the patient's right to inspect, amend, and restrict access to protected health information when appropriate.

- Establishes and administers a process for receiving, documenting, tracking, investigating, and taking action on all complaints concerning the organization's privacy policies and procedures in coordination and collaboration with other similar functions and, when necessary, legal counsel.

- Ensures compliance with privacy practices and consistent application of sanctions for failure to comply with privacy policies for all individuals in the organization's workforce, the extended workforce, and all business associates, in cooperation with Human Resources, the information security officer, administration, and legal counsel as applicable.

- Initiates, facilitates, and promotes activities to foster information privacy awareness within the organization and related entities.

- Serves as a member of, or liaison to, the organization's IRB or Privacy Committee, should one exist. Also serves as the information privacy liaison for users of clinical and administrative systems.

- Reviews all system-related information security plans throughout the organization's network to ensure alignment between security and privacy practices, and acts as a liaison to the information systems department.

- Works with all organization personnel involved with any aspect of release of protected health information to ensure full coordination and cooperation under the organization's policies and procedures and legal requirements.

- Maintains current knowledge of applicable federal and state privacy laws and accreditation standards and monitors advancements in information privacy technologies to ensure organizational adaptation and compliance.

- Serves as information privacy consultant to the organization for all departments and appropriate entities.

- Cooperates with the Office of Civil Rights, other legal entities, and organization officers in any compliance reviews or investigations.

- Works with organization administration, legal counsel, and other related parties to represent the organization's information privacy interests with external parties (state or local government bodies) who undertake to adopt or amend privacy legislation, regulation, or standard.

Qualifications:

- Certification as an RHIA or RHIT with education and experience relative to the size and scope of the organization.

- Knowledge and experience in information privacy laws, access, release of information, and release control technologies.

- Knowledge in and the ability to apply the principles of HIM, project management, and change management.

- Demonstrated organization, facilitation, communication, and presentation skills.

Appendix C
Standards for the Form and Content
of the Health Record

Documentation Requirements	JCAHO Standard Number	Medicare Conditions of Participation
The hospital initiates and maintains a health record for every individual assessed or treated.	IM.7.1	
A health record must be maintained for every individual evaluated or treated in the hospital.		482.24
Only authorized individuals make entries in health records.	IM.7.1.1	
Every health record entry is dated, its author identified and, when necessary, authenticated.	IM.7.8	
Hospitals establish policies and mechanisms to ensure that only an author can authenticate his or her own entry. Indications of authentication can include written signatures or initials, rubber stamps, or computer "signatures" (or sequence of keys). The medical staff rules and regulations or policies define what entries, if any, by house staff or nonphysicians must be countersigned by supervising physicians.	Intent of IM.7.8	
All entries must be legible and complete and must be authenticated and dated promptly by the person (identified by name and discipline) who is responsible for ordering, providing, or evaluating the service furnished.		482.24(c)(1)
The author of each entry must be identified and must authenticate his or her entry.		482.24(c)(1)(i)
Authentication may include signatures, written initials, or computer entries.		482.24(c)(1)(ii)
The health record contains sufficient information to identify the patient, support the diagnosis, justify the treatment, document the course and results, and promote continuity of care among healthcare providers.	IM.7.2	482.24(c)
To facilitate consistency and continuity in patient care, the health record contains very specific data and thorough information, including: • The patient's name, address, date of birth, and the name of any legally authorized representative • The legal status of patients receiving mental health services • Emergency care provided to the patient prior to arrival, if any • The record and findings of the patient's assessment • Conclusions or impressions drawn from the medical history and physical examination	Intent of IM.7 through IM.7.2	

Documentation Requirements	JCAHO Standard Number	Medicare Conditions of Participation
• The diagnosis or diagnostic impression		
• The reasons for admission or treatment		
• The goals of treatment and the treatment plan		
• Evidence of known advance directives		
• Evidence of informed consent, when required by hospital policy		
• Diagnostic and therapeutic orders, if any		
• All diagnostic and therapeutic procedures and test results		
• All operative and other invasive procedures performed, using acceptable disease and operative terminology that includes etiology, as appropriate		
• Progress notes made by the medical staff and other authorized individuals		
• All reassessments and any revisions of the treatment plan		
• Clinical observations		
• The patient's response to care		
• Consultation reports		
• Every medication ordered or prescribed for an inpatient		
• Every medication dispensed to an ambulatory patient or an inpatient on discharge		
• Every dose of medication administered and any adverse drug reaction		
• All relevant diagnoses established during the course of care		
• Any referrals and communications made to external or internal providers and to community agencies		
• Conclusions at termination of hospitalization		
• Discharge instructions to the patient and family		
• Clinical resumes and discharge summaries, or a final progress note or transfer summary. A concise clinical resume included in the health record at discharge provides important information to other caregivers and facilitates continuity of care. For patients discharged to ambulatory (outpatient) care, the clinical resume summarizes previous levels of care.		
The discharge summary contains the following information:		
• The reason for hospitalization		
• Significant findings		
• Procedures performed and treatment rendered		
• The patient's condition at discharge		
• Instructions to the patient and family		
For normal newborns with uncomplicated deliveries, or for patients hospitalized for less than 48 hours with only minor problems, a progress note may substitute for the clinical resume.		
The medical staff defines what problems and interventions may be considered minor.		
The progress note may be handwritten. It documents the patient's condition at discharge and discharge instructions.		
When a patient is transferred within the same organization from one level of care to another, and the caregivers change, a transfer summary may be substituted for the clinical resume. A transfer summary briefly describes the patient's condition at time of transfer and the reason for the transfer. When the caregivers remain the same, a progress note may suffice.		

Documentation Requirements	JCAHO Standard Number	Medicare Conditions of Participation
All records must document the following, as appropriate:		482.24(c)(2)(ii)
• Admitting diagnosis		482.24(c)(2)(iii)
• Results of all consultative evaluations of the patient and appropriate findings by clinical and other staff involved in the care of the patient		
• Documentation of complications, hospital-acquired infections, and unfavorable reactions to drugs and anesthesia		482.24(c)(2)(iv)
• Properly executed informed consent forms for procedures and treatments specified by the medical staff or by federal or state law, if applicable, to require written patient consent		482.24(c)(2)(v)
• All practitioners' orders, nursing notes, reports of treatment, medication records, radiology, and laboratory reports, vital signs, and other information necessary to monitor the patient's condition		482.24(c)(2)(iii)
All health records must document the following, as appropriate:		
• Discharge summary with outcome of hospitalization, disposition of case, and provisions for follow-up care		482.24 (c)(2)(vii)
• Final diagnosis with completion of health records within 30 days following discharge		482.24(c)(2)(viii)
A patient admitted for inpatient care has a medical history and an appropriate physical examination performed by a qualified physician. (Qualified physician: A doctor of medicine or doctor of osteopathy who, by virtue of education, training, and demonstrated competence, is granted clinical privileges by the organization to perform specific diagnostic or therapeutic procedure(s) and who is fully licensed to practice medicine.)	MS.6.2	
Qualified oral and maxillofacial surgeons may perform the medical history and physical examination, if they have such privileges, in order to assess the medical, surgical, and anesthetic risks of the proposed operative and other procedure(s).	MS.6.2.1	
Other licensed independent practitioners who are permitted to provide patient care services independently may perform all or part of the medical history and physical examination, if granted such privileges.	MS.6.2.2	
The findings, conclusions, and assessment of risk are confirmed or endorsed by a qualified physician prior to major high-risk (as defined by the medical staff) diagnostic or therapeutic interventions.	MS.6.2.2.1	
Dentists are responsible for the part of their patient's history and physical examination that relates to dentistry.	MS.6.2.2.2	
Podiatrists are responsible for the part of their patient's history and physical examination that relates to podiatry.	MS.6.2.2.3	
The medical staff determines those noninpatient services (for example, ambulatory surgery), if any, for which a patient must have a medical history taken and appropriate physical examination performed by a qualified physician who has such privileges. Except as provided in MS.6.2.1 through MS.6.2.2.3.	MS.6.3	
The patient's history and physical examination, nursing assessment, and other screening assessments are completed within 24 hours of admission as an inpatient.	PE.1.7.1	
When a history and physical examination have been performed within 30 days before admission, a durable, legible copy of this report may be used in the patient's record, provided any changes that may have occurred are recorded in the health record at the time of admission.	PE.1.7.1.1	
Before surgery, the patient's physical examination and medical history, any indicated diagnostic tests, and a preoperative diagnosis are completed and recorded in the patient's record.	PE.1.8	

Documentation Requirements	JCAHO Standard Number	Medicare Conditions of Participation
There must be a complete history and physical workup in the chart of every patient prior to surgery, except in emergencies. When this has been dictated, but not yet recorded in the patient's chart, there must be a statement to the effect and an admission note in the chart by the practitioner who admitted the patient.		482.51(b)(1)
A physical examination and medical history are to be done no more than 7 days before or 48 hours after an admission for each patient by a doctor of medicine or osteopathy or, for patients admitted only for oromaxillofacial surgery, by an oromaxillofacial surgeon who has been granted such privileges by the medical staff in accordance with state law.		482.24(c)(2)(i) 482.22(c)(5)
Plans of care are developed and documented in the patient's health record before the operative or other procedure is performed.	TX.5.3	
The hospital must ensure that the nursing staff develops and keeps current a nursing care plan for each patient.		482.23(b)(4)
All records must document all practitioners' orders.		482.24(c)(2)(vi)
All orders for drugs and biologicals must be in writing and signed by the practitioner or practitioners responsible for the care of the patient.		482.23(c)(2)
Verbal orders of authorized individuals are accepted and transcribed by qualified personnel who are identified by title or category in the medical staff rules and regulations.	IM.7.7	
When telephone or verbal orders must be used, they must be:		
• Accepted only by personnel authorized to do so by the medical staff policies and procedures, consistent with federal and state law		482.23(c)(2)(i)
• Signed or initialed by the prescribing practitioner as soon as possible		482.23(c)(2)(ii)
• Used infrequently		482.23(c)(2)(iii)
Signed X-ray reports of all examinations performed shall be made part of the patient's hospital record.		482.26(d)
The radiologist or other practitioner who performs radiology services must sign reports of his or her interpretations.		482.26(d)(1)
The health record thoroughly documents operative or other procedures and the use of sedation or anesthesia.	IM.7.3	
A preoperative diagnosis is recorded before surgery by the licensed independent practitioner responsible for the patient.	IM.7.3.1	
Operative reports dictated or written immediately after surgery record the name of the primary surgeon and assistants, findings, technical procedures used, specimens removed, and postoperative diagnosis.	IM.7.3.2	
The completed operative report is authenticated by the surgeon and filed in the health record as soon as possible after surgery.	IM.7.3.2.1	
When the operative report is not placed in the health record immediately after surgery, a progress note is entered immediately.	IM.7.3.2.2	
Postoperative documentation records the patient's vital signs and level of consciousness; medications (including intravenous fluids), blood, and blood components; any unusual events or postoperative complications; and management of such events.	IM.7.3.3	
Postoperative documentation records the patient's discharge from the postsedation or postanesthesia care area by the responsible licensed independent practitioner or according to discharge criteria.	IM.7.3.4	
Compliance with discharge criteria is fully documented in the patient's health record.	IM.7.3.4.1	

Documentation Requirements	JCAHO Standard Number	Medicare Conditions of Participation
Postoperative documentation records the name of the licensed independent practitioner responsible for discharge.	IM.7.3.5	
An informed consent for surgery shall be part of the patient's chart before surgery is performed. It must be dated, timed, and signed by the patient and the physician informant.		482.51(b)(2)
An operative report describing the reason for procedure, gross findings, operative procedure (techniques), and tissues removed or altered must be written or dictated immediately following surgery and signed by the surgeon.		482.51(b)(6)
A presedation or preanesthesia assessment is performed for each patient before beginning moderate or deep sedation and before anesthesia induction.	TX.2.1	
A preanesthesia evaluation is performed within 48 hours prior to surgery by an individual qualified to administer anesthesia.		482.52(b)(1)
An intraoperative anesthesia record is provided.		482.52(b)(2)
With respect to inpatients, a postanesthesia follow-up report is written within 48 hours after surgery by the individual who administers the anesthesia.		482.52(b)(3)
A preanesthesia evaluation is documented by an individual qualified to administer anesthesia and is performed within 48 hours prior to the anesthesia event of surgery.		482.52(b)
The hospital must maintain signed and dated reports of nuclear medicine interpretations, consultations, and procedures.		482.53(d)
The practitioner approved by the medical staff to interpret diagnostic procedures must sign and date the interpretation of these tests.		482.53(d)(2)
When emergency, urgent, or immediate care is provided, the time and means of arrival are also documented in the health record.	IM.7.5	
The health record notes when a patient receiving emergency, urgent, or immediate care left against medical advice.	IM.7.5.1	
The health record of a patient receiving emergency, urgent, or immediate care notes the conclusions at termination of treatment, including final disposition, condition at discharge, and instructions for follow-up care.	IM.7.5.2	
When authorized by the patient or a legally authorized representative, a copy of the emergency services provided is available to the practitioner or medical organization providing follow-up care.	IM.7.5.3	

Appendix D
Sample Notice of Health Information Practices

*PATIENT: This notice describes how information about you may be used
and disclosed and how you can get access to this information.
Please review it carefully.*

Understanding Your Health Record/Information

Each time you visit a hospital, physician, or another healthcare provider, a record of your visit is made. Typically, this record contains symptoms, examination and test results, diagnoses, treatment, and the plan for future care or treatment. This has the following functions:

- It serves as the basis for planning your care and treatment.

- It serves as the means of communication among the various health professionals who contribute to your care.

- It becomes the legal document that describes the care you received.

- It serves as the means by which you or a third-party payer representing you can verify that billed services were actually provided.

- It is used as a tool in the education of healthcare professionals.

- It is a source of data for medical research.

- It is a source of information for the public health officials charged with improving the health of the nation.

- It is a source of data for facility planning and marketing.

- It serves as a tool assessing and continually improving the care we render and the outcomes we achieve.

Understanding what is in your record and how your health information is used helps you to ensure its accuracy; better understand who, what, when, where, and why others may access your health information; and make more informed decisions about authorizing the disclosure of your healthcare information to other parties.

Your Health Information Rights

Although your health record is the property of the healthcare practitioner or facility that compiled it, the information in the record belongs to you. You have certain rights in connection with your health information. You have the right to:

- Request a restriction on certain uses and disclosures of your information as provided by 45 CFR 164.522.

- Obtain a paper copy of the notice of information practices upon request.

- Inspect and copy your health record as provided for in 45 CFR 164.524.

- Amend your health record as provided in 45 CFR 164.528.

- Obtain an accounting of disclosures of your health information as provided in 45 CFR 164.528.

- Request communications of your health information by alternative means or at alternative locations.

- Revoke your authorization to use or disclose health information except to the extent that action has already been taken.

Our Responsibilities

This organization has certain responsibilities in connection with your health record. We are required to:

- Maintain the privacy of your health information.

- Provide you with a notice as to our legal duties and privacy practices with respect to information we collect and maintain about you.

- Abide by the terms of this notice.

- Notify you if we are unable to agree to a requested restriction.

- Accommodate reasonable requests you may have to communicate health information by alternative means or at alternative locations.

We reserve the right to change our practices and to make the new provisions effective for all of the protected health information we maintain. Should our information practices change, we will mail a revised notice to the address you have supplied to us. We will not use or disclose your health information without your authorization, except as described in this notice.

For More Information or to Report a Problem

If you have questions and would like additional information, you may contact the director of health information management at [telephone number]. If you believe that your right to privacy has been violated, you can file a complaint with the director of health information management or with the secretary of Health and Human Services. There will be no retaliation for filing a complaint.

Examples of Disclosures for Treatment, Payment, and Health Operations

1. We will use information about you for the purposes of diagnosis and treatment.

    For example, information obtained by a nurse, physician, or other member of your healthcare team will be recorded in your record and used to determine your course of treatment. Your physician will also document his or her expectations of the members of your healthcare team in the same record. Members of your healthcare team will then record the actions they took and their observations in your health record. In that way, the physician will know how you are responding to treatment.

    We will also provide your physician or a subsequent healthcare provider with copies of various reports to assist him or her in treating you once you have been discharged from this hospital.

2. We will use your health information to request payment for the services you receive.

    For example, a bill may be sent to you or a third-party payer. The information on or accompanying the bill may include information that identifies you, as well as your diagnosis, procedures, and supply usage.

3. We will use your health information for regular health operations in our facility.

    For example, members of the medical staff, the risk or quality improvement manager, or members of the quality improvement team may use information from your health record to assess the care and clinical outcomes in your case and others like it. This information will then be used in an effort to continually improve the quality and effectiveness of the healthcare services we provide.

4. We will share your health information with our business associates only when necessary to conduct operations or provide services.

    For example, outside business associates sometimes provide physician services in the emergency department and for radiology and certain laboratory tests. In addition, we may use a copy service for making copies of your health record. When these services are contracted, we may disclose your health information to our business associates so that they can perform the job we have asked them to perform and then bill you or your third-party payer for services rendered. To protect your health information, however, we require the business associate to appropriately safeguard your information.

5. We will share limited personal information about you in our directory of patients unless you notify us that you object.

    For example, your name, location in the facility, general condition, and religious affiliation may be used for directory purposes. This information may be provided to members of the clergy and, except for religious affiliation, to other people who ask for you by name.

6. We will share limited personal information about you (your location and general condition) for the purpose of notifying your family members, personal representatives, or other people responsible for your care.

7. We will share limited personal information about you for the purpose of communication with your family or other designated individuals.

   For example, using their best judgment, healthcare professionals may disclose to a family member, relative, close personal friend, or any other person you designate health information relevant to that person's involvement in your care or payment.

8. We may disclose information to researchers when their research has been approved by an institutional review board that has reviewed the research proposal and established protocols to ensure the privacy of your health information.

9. Consistent with applicable law, we may disclose health information to funeral directors so that they can carry out their duties.

10. Consistent with applicable law, we may disclose health information to organ procurement organizations or other entities engaged in the procurement, banking, or transplantation of organs for the purpose of tissue donation and transplantation.

11. We may contact you to provide appointment reminders or information about treatment alternatives or other health-related benefits and services that may be of interest to you.

12. We may contact you as part of a fund-raising effort.

13. We may disclose to the FDA health information relative to adverse events with respect to food, supplements, product and product defects, or postmarketing surveillance information to enable product recalls, repairs, or replacement.

14. We may disclose health information to the extent authorized by, and to the extent necessary to comply with, laws relating to workers' compensation or other similar programs established by law.

15. As required by law, we may disclose your health information to public health or legal authorities charged with preventing or controlling disease, injury, or disability.

16. If you are an inmate of a correctional institution, we may disclose to the institution or agents thereof health information necessary for your health and the health and safety of other individuals.

17. We may disclose health information for law enforcement purposes as required by law or in response to a valid subpoena.

Federal law makes provision for your health information to be released to an appropriate health oversight agency, public health authority, or attorney, provided that a workforce member or business associate believes in good faith that we have engaged in unlawful conduct or have otherwise violated professional or clinical standards and are potentially endangering one or more patients, workers, or the public.

Effective Date: [DATE]

Appendix E
List of AHIMA Practice Briefs, Standards, and Position Statements

Full-text displays of the following resources may be found on the AHIMA Web site at www.ahima.org. In some cases, access is restricted to AHIMA members.

AHIMA Practice Briefs

Title	Author	Date
Accounting and Tracking Disclosures of Protected Health Information	Dougherty, Michelle	November 2001
APC Checklist	Scichilone, Rita	September 2000
Authentication of Health Record Entries (Updated)	Welch, Julie J.	March 2000
Best Practices in Medical Record Documentation and Completion	Fletcher, Donna M.	November 1999
Care and Maintenance of Charge Masters	Rhodes, Harry B.	July 1999
Checklist to Assess Data Quality Management Efforts	AHIMA Data Quality Management Task Force	March 1998
Consent for the Use/Disclosure of Individually Identifiable Health Information	Hughes, Gwen	May 2001
Correcting and Amending Entries in a Computerized Patient Record	Welch, Julie J.	September 1999
Data Quality	AHIMA Coding Policy and Strategy Committee	February 1996
Data Quality Management Model	AHIMA Data Quality Management Task Force	June 1998
Data Resource Administration: The Road Ahead	Mon, Donald, et al.	November 1998
Definition of the Health Record for Legal Purposes	Amatayakul, Margret, et al.	October 2001
Designing a Data Collection Process	Fuller, Sandra	May 1998
Destruction of Patient Health Information (Updated)	Hughes, Gwen	November 2001
Developing a Coding Compliance Policy Document	AHIMA Coding Team	July 2001
Developing a Physician Query Process	Prophet, Sue	October 2001
Developing Information Capture Tools	Rhodes, Harry B.	March 1997
Disaster Planning for Health Information	Hughes, Gwen	May 2000
Documentation Requirements for the Acute Care Inpatient Record	Smith, Cheryl M.	March 2001
E-Mail Security	Hughes, Gwen	February 2000
Electronic Signatures (Updated)	Rhodes, Harry B.	October 1998
Establishing a Telecommuting or Home-based Employee Program (Updated)	Dougherty, Michelle; Scichilone, Rita A.; Fletcher, Donna M.	July 2002

Title	Author	Date
Facsimile Transmission of Health Information	Hughes, Gwen	June 2001
Health Informatics Standards and Information Transfer: Exploring the HIM Role	Murphy, Gretchen; Brandt, Mary	January 2001
HIPAA Privacy and Security Training	Hjort, Beth	April 2002
HIPAA Privacy Checklist	Hjort, Beth	June 2001
Information Security: A Checklist for Healthcare Professionals	Carpenter, Jennifer E.	January 2000
Information Security: An Overview	Brandt, Mary D.	June 1996
Internet Resources for Health Information Professionals	Hjort, Beth	April 2001
Laws and Regulations Governing the Disclosure of Health Information	Hughes, Gwen	May 2001
Letters of Agreement/Contracts (Updated)	Hughes, Gwen	June 2001
Maintenance of Master Patient Index—Single Site or Enterprise	AHIMA MPI Task Force	October 1997
Managing Health Information in Facility Mergers and Acquisitions	Rhodes, Harry B.	November 1996
Managing Health Information Relating to Infection with HIV	Carpenter, Jennifer E.	May 1999
Managing Multimedia Medical Records: A Health Information Manager's Role	Carpenter, Jennifer E.	February 1998
Master Patient Index—Recommended Core Data Elements	AHIMA MPI Task Force	July 1997
Merging Master Patient Indexes	AHIMA MPI Task Force	September 1997
Notice of Information Practices	Hughes, Gwen	May 2001
Patient Access and Amendment to Health Records	Hughes, Gwen	May 2001
Patient Anonymity (Updated)	Rhodes, Harry B.	May 2001
Patient Photography, Videotaping, and Other Imaging (Updated)	Hjort, Beth; Brandt, Mary D.; Carpenter, Jennifer	June 2001
Portable Computer Security	Hughes, Gwen	October 2000
Preemption of the HIPAA Privacy Rule	Hughes, Gwen	February 2002
Preparing Your Organization for a New Coding System	AHIMA Coding Policy and Strategy Committee	September 1998
Protecting Patient Information After a Facility Closure	Brandt, Mary; Rhodes, Harry B.	March 1999
Recommended Regulation and Standard Acquisition for Specific Healthcare Settings	Burrington-Brown, Jill; Rhodes, Harry	June 2002
Redisclosure of Patient Health Information	Hughes, Gwen	September 2001
Release of Information for Marketing or Fund-raising Purposes	Hughes, Gwen	May 2001
Release of Information: Laws and Regulations	Rhodes, Harry B.; Larson, Joan C.	January 1999
Required Content for Authorizations to Disclose	Hughes, Gwen; Smith, Cheryl M.	November 2001
Retaining Healthcare Business Records	Tomes, Jonathan P.	March 2002
Retention of Health Information (Updated)	Fletcher, Donna M.	June 1999
Security Audits	Hjort, Beth	September 2000
Seven Steps to Corporate Compliance: The HIM Role	AHIMA Compliance Task Force	October 1999
Starting a Consulting Business	Dougherty, Michelle	May 2002
Storage Media for Health Information	Welch, Julie J.	June 2000
Telecommuting	Fletcher, Donna M.	February 1999
Telemedical Records	Fletcher, Donna M.	April 1997
Transfer of Patient Health Information Across the Continuum (Updated)	Hughes, Gwen	June 2001
Understanding the Minimum Necessary Standard	Hughes, Gwen	January 2002
Verbal/Telephone Order Authentication and Time Frames	Dougherty, Michelle	February 2001
Writing an Effective Request for Proposal	Carpenter, Jennifer E.	July 1998

Standards of Practice

Title	Author	Source	Date
AHIMA Code of Ethics	AHIMA	AHIMA Document	October 1998
Blue-ribbon Approach to Compliance	Meaney, Mark E.	*Journal of AHIMA* column	September 2001
Conduct is Their Business	Byrd, Katherine	*Journal of AHIMA* column	March 2001
Confronting Ethical Dilemmas on the Job: An HIM Professional's Guide	Harman, Laurinda B.	*Journal of AHIMA* article	May 2000
Crossing the Spectrum: Steps for Making Ethical Decisions	Navran, Frank J.	*Journal of AHIMA* article	March 2001
Drafting Policy on Business Ethics	Dingman, Barbara	*Journal of AHIMA* column	April 2001
Ethical Coding in the Physician Office	Austin, Peg; Stanfill, Mary H.	*Journal of AHIMA*—Coding Notes	March 2001
Ethics in the Age of Compliance	Kloss, Linda	AHIMA Presentation	January 1999
Health Information Management Practice Standards	AHIMA	AHIMA Book	January 1998
HIM and Ethical Decision Making: Complex Challenges	Harman, Laurinda	AHIMA Convention	October 2001
Long-term Care by the Book	Johnson, Deborah A.	*Journal of AHIMA* article	March 2001
On The Line: Professional Practice Solutions	Hjort, Beth	*Journal of AHIMA* column	July 2001
Recommended Regulation and Standard Acquisition for Specific Healthcare Settings	Burrington-Brown, Jill; Rhodes, Harry	AHIMA Practice Brief, *Journal of AHIMA*	June 2002
Recommended Regulation and Standard Acquisition for Specific Healthcare Settings	Rhodes, Harry B.	AHIMA Practice Brief	April 1998
Standards of Ethical Coding	AHIMA	*Journal of AHIMA*	March 2000
Who Should Have Access to Your Information? Privacy through the Ethics Lens	Friedman, Emily	*Journal of AHIMA* article	March 2001

AHIMA Position Statements

Title	Date
Confidential Health Information and the Internet	January 1998
Privacy Officer	February 2001
Quality Healthcare Data and Information	June 2001
Statement on Consistency of Healthcare Diagnostic and Procedural Coding	May 2002
Statement on National Healthcare Information Infrastructure	May 2002
Statement on the Health Information Management Workforce	July 2002

Appendix F
Web Resources

American Health Information Management Association (AHIMA)

www.ahima.org

AHIMA is a professional association representing more than forty thousand specially educated health information professionals who work throughout the healthcare industry. This site includes *Journal of AHIMA* indexes and articles, position statements, practice briefs, frequently asked questions, member forums, job board, hot topics, legislative issues, the fellowship program, and many other resources for HIM professionals.

AHIMA Communities of Practice

www.ahimanet.org

AHIMA Communities of Practice were launched in 2001, providing a virtual connection for AHIMA members in similar healthcare settings or with similar interests or concerns.

Accreditation Association for Ambulatory Health Care (AAAHC)

www.aaahc.org

AAAHC is committed to advocating high-quality health services in ambulatory healthcare organizations through the development of standards and survey and accreditation programs.

Accredited Standards Committee—X12N

www.x12.org

ASC X12, comprised of cross-industry representation, delivers the most widely implemented electronic data interchange (EDI) standards that interact with a multitude of e-commerce technologies and serves as the premier source for integrating electronic applications.

Agency for Healthcare Research and Quality (AHRQ)

www.ahrq.gov

Home page for the government association for research to increase quality healthcare.

American Accreditation HealthCare Commission/URAC

www.urac.org

A nonprofit organization that establishes standards for the managed care industry.

American Association for Medical Transcription (AAMT)

www.aamt.org

AAMT represents and advances the profession of medical transcription and its practitioners.

American Association of Health Plans (AAHP)

www.aahp.org

A national trade association representing health maintenance organizations, preferred provider organizations, point-of-service plans, and other health plans.

American Association of Preferred Provider Organizations (AAPPO)

www.aappo.org

A national association of network-based preferred provider organizations and affiliate organizations.

American College of Healthcare Executives (ACHE)

www.ache.org

An international society of healthcare executives, ACHE offers credentialing and educational programs.

American Hospital Association (AHA)

www.aha.org

Members of the American Hospital Association are grouped into three categories: institutional (short-term hospitals, long-term hospitals, headquarters of healthcare systems, non-hospital pre-acute and post-acute facilities, and hospital-affiliated education programs), associate, and personal.

American Hospital Association Research Data

www.ahadata.com

Detailed hospital research databank and resource for healthcare provider information.

American Health Lawyers Association

www.healthlawyers.org

Organization for lawyers associated with the health field.

American Medical Association (AMA)

www.ama-assn.org

AMA's strategic agenda remains rooted in its historic commitment to standards, ethics, excellence in medical education and practice, and advocacy on behalf of the medical profession and the patients it services.

American Medical Informatics Association (AMIA)
www.amia.org
AMIA is a nonprofit membership organization of individuals, institutions, and corporations dedicated to developing and using information technologies to improve healthcare.

American National Standards Institute (ANSI)
web.ansi.org
This web site includes a public forum for the voluntary coordination of healthcare informatics standards among all US standard developing organizations.

American Society for Testing and Materials (ASTM)
www.astm.org
An organization that sets technical standards for industries.

Association for Electronic Health Care Transactions (AFEHCT)
www.afehct.org
Supports the use of EDI to improve and reduce the cost of healthcare.

Association of State and Territorial Health Officials (ASTHO)
www.astho.org
A nonprofit organization representing the state and territorial public health agencies of the United States, U.S. territories, and the District of Columbia.

Canadian Health Record Association (CHRA)
www.chra.ca
CHRA home page.

CCH Internet Research Network (CCH)
health.cch.com/network
Links to many federal laws, regulations and programs: Balanced Budget Act, APCs, home health agency licensure, Medicare and Medicaid, OASIS, and PPS.

Centers for Disease Control and Prevention (CDC)
www.cdc.gov
CDC home page.

Centers for Medicare and Medicaid Services (CMS)
www.cms.gov
A federal agency that administers Medicare, Medicaid, and the State Children's Health Insurance Program.

Code of Federal Regulations (CFR)
www.access.gpo.gov/nara/cfr/
The CFR is a codification of the general and permanent rules published in the *Federal Register* by the executive departments and agencies of the federal government.

College of Healthcare Information Management Executives (CHIME)
www.cio-chime.org
CHIME was formed with the dual objective of serving the professional development needs of healthcare CIOs and advocating the more effective use of information management within healthcare.

Department of Health & Human Services (HHS)
www.hhs.gov
The Department of Health and Human Services is the U.S. government's principal agency for protecting the health of all Americans and providing essential human services, especially for those who are least able to help themselves.

Disease Management Association of America (DMAA)
www.dmaa.org
A nonprofit organization representing the disease management community.

Federation of American Hospitals (FAHS)
www.fahs.com
Represents owned and managed hospitals and health systems that offer traditional care, ambulatory care, psychiatric and rehabilitative care, and allied companies involved in health insurance and healthcare systems.

Health Care Compliance Association (HCCA)
www.hcca-info.org
HCCA is a forum for healthcare professionals involved in compliance serving all segments of the health care industry.

Health Information Management Listserv
shrplist.umsmed.edu/mailman/listinfo/him-l
This listserv facilitates the transition of "medical record" practitioners to "health information managers" and the discussion of current legislative, accreditation, regulatory, technological, and systems issues, as well as other issues affecting the HIM field.

Health Insurance Association of America (HIAA)
www.hiaa.org
A trade association representing the private health care system that provides health, long-term care, dental, disability, and supplemental coverage to consumers.

Health Internet Ethics
www.hiethics.org
A coalition of health sites supporting high ethical standards.

Health Level Seven (HL-7)
www.hl7.org
One of the ANSI-accredited standards-developing organizations operating in the healthcare area, producing standards for particular healthcare domains such as pharmacy, medical devices, imaging, and insurance transactions.

Health on the Net Foundation (HON)
www.hon.ch
Dedicated to realizing the benefits of the Internet and related technologies in the fields of health and medicine.

Health Privacy Project
www.healthprivacy.org
Cites, summarizes, and provides links to federal and state disclosure laws and provides articles covering privacy issues.

Health.gov

www.health.gov

This site is a portal to the Web sites of a number of multi-agency health initiatives and activities of the U.S. Department of Health and Human Services and other federal departments and agencies.

Healthcare Billing and Management Association (HBMA)

www.hbma.com

Founded in 1993, the HBMA is the only trade association representing third-party medical billers.

Healthcare Information and Management Systems Society (HIMSS)

www.himss.org

HIMSS is a trade association driving the adoption of strategic information management and technology in the health industry.

Healthcare Cost and Utilization Project (HCUP)

www.ahrq.gov/data/

National statistics, trends, and selected state statistics about hospital stays.

Healthcare Financial Management Association (HFMA)

www.hfma.org

Professional association for financial management professionals working in healthcare.

Homecare Online (NAHC)

www.nahc.org

An organization supporting the home care side of the health industry.

Human Anatomy Online

www.innerbody.com

Each anatomy topic has animations, hundreds of graphics, and thousands of descriptive links.

The Internet Public Library

www.ipl.org

An educational initiative of the University of Michigan School of Information.

International Medical Informatics Association (IMIA)

www.imia.org

IMIA home page.

Internet Healthcare Coalition (IHC)

www.ihealthcoalition.org

Healthcare resources on the Internet—affiliations include publishers of professional and consumer health information.

IPA Association of America (TIPAAA)

www.tipaaa.org

Assists independent/integrated physician associations by providing services that lead to decisions that will contribute to the implementation of appropriate operational systems, resulting in greater efficiency.

Joint Commission on the Accreditation of Healthcare Organizations

www.jcaho.org

Evaluates and accredits healthcare organizations and programs in the U.S.

Journal of the American Medical Informatics Association (JAMIA)

www.jamia.org

Articles and abstracts from *JAMIA*.

Mayo Clinic

www.mayohealth.org

The Mayo Clinic home page.

Medical Group Management Association (MGMA)

www.mgma.com

MGMA strives to improve the effectiveness of medical group practices and the knowledge and skills of those who manage and lead them.

Medical Transcription Industry Alliance (MTIA)

www.mtia.com

A nonprofit membership association serving the needs of medical transcription companies and health information management professionals.

MEDLINE

www.medlineplus.gov

A subservice of the National Library of Medicine.

***Merck Manual* Home Edition**

www.merck.com/pubs/mmanual/

Medical reference book.

National Information Center for Health Services Administration (NIC)

www.nichsa.org

The NIC is a library service available to all AHIMA members. Past *Journal of AHIMA* articles can be obtained here.

National Alliance for Health Information Technology (NAHIT)

www.nahit.org

The mission of the NAHIT is to improve quality and performance through standards-based information systems.

National Association for Healthcare Quality (NAHQ)

www.nahq.org

Web site for the organization for healthcare quality professionals.

National Association of Health Data Organizations (NAHDO)

www.nahdo.org

Membership organization dedicated to strengthening the nation's health information system by bringing together a network of state, federal, and private sector technical and policy leaders and consultants to expand health systems development and shape responsible health information policies.

National Center for Health Statistics (NCHS)

www.cdc.gov/nchs/

The federal government's principal vital and health statistics agency, part of the Centers for Disease Control and Prevention.

National Committee for Quality Assurance (NCQA)

www.ncqa.org

An independent, nonprofit organization that evaluates and reports on the quality of the nation's managed care organizations.

National Committee on Vital and Health Statistics (NCVHS)

www.ncvhs.hhs.gov

Home page for NCVHS.

National Technical Information Service (NTIS)

www.ntis.gov

NTIS acts as the central source for U.S. government scientific, technical, and business information. This growing collection, including millions of publications as well as audiovisual materials, computer datafiles, and software, originates from U.S. federal agencies, industry and university contractors with the federal government, and a worldwide compendium of research and development organizations.

National Institutes of Health (NIH)

www.nih.gov

Home page for NIH.

National Library of Medicine (NLM)

www.nlm.nih.gov/nlmhome.html

A biomedical library.

National Uniform Billing Committee (NUBC)

www.nubc.org

An organization created to meet the goals of administrative simplification as outlined in the Health Insurance Portability and Accountability Act of 1996.

National Uniform Claims Committee (NUCC)

www.nucc.org

Develops a standardized data set for use by non-institutional healthcare communities to transmit claim and encounter information to and from all third-party payers.

Physicians' Desk Reference (PDR)

www.pdr.net

Online home of the *Physicians' Desk Reference.*

Privacy Officers Association (POA)

www.privacyassociation.org

An organization for privacy officers in North America.

Professional Association of Health Care Office Managers (PAHCOM)

www.pahcom.com

Provides a support system to the managers of group and solo physician practices.

Project Management Institute (PMI)

www.pmi.org

A nonprofit professional association in the area of project management, PMI establishes project management standards, provides seminars, education programs, and professional certification.

Quality Interagency Coordination Task Force (QuIC)

www.quic.gov

Federal agencies that purchase, provide, study, or regulate health services collaborate toward the common goal of high quality and efficient healthcare systems.

Rehabilitation Accreditation Commission (CARF)

www.carf.org

A nonprofit organization offering accreditation to programs and services in rehabilitation, behavioral health, and other areas.

SNOMED

www.snomed.org

Web site for the division of College of American Pathologists that oversees the direction and scientific maintenance of the Systematized Nomenclature of Medicine, better known as SNOMED.

U.S. Government Printing Office

www.gpo.gov

Government publications.

Webopedia

www.webopedia.com

A dictionary and search engine for computer and Internet technology.

Wireless Networking Industry's Information Source (WLANA)

www.wlana.com

A nonprofit educational trade association for thought leaders and technology innovators in the local area wireless technology industry.

Workgroup for Electronic Data Interchange (WEDI)

www.wedi.org

A resource for electronic connectivity in the healthcare industry.

Glossary

Abbreviated injury scale (AIS): A set of numbers used in a trauma registry to indicate the nature and severity of injuries by body system

Ability tests: Tests used to assess the skills an individual already possesses; also called performance tests

Abstracting: The process of extracting information from a document to create a brief summary of the patient's illness, treatment, and outcome

Accept assignment: A term used to refer to a provider's or supplier's acceptance of the allowed charges (from a fee schedule) as payment in full

Acceptance theory of authority: A theory that accepts as principle the fact that employees have the freedom of will to choose whether they will follow managerial directions

Access control: The process of designing, implementing, and monitoring a system for guaranteeing that only individuals who have a legitimate need are allowed to view or amend specific data sets

Accession number: The number assigned to each case as it is entered in a cancer registry

Accession registry: A listing of cases in a cancer registry in the order in which they were entered

Account: A subdivision of assets, liabilities, and equities

Accountable: Required to answer to a supervisor for performance results

Accountable health plan: *See* Integrated provider organization (IPO)

Accounting: The collection, recording, and reporting of financial data

Accounting rate of return: The projected annual cash inflows, minus any applicable depreciation, divided by the initial investment

Accounts payable: Amounts the organization owes other entities

Accounts receivable: Records of the payments owed the organization by outside entities such as third-party payers and patients

Accreditation: A voluntary process of institutional or organizational review established by the institutions or organizations themselves in which a quasi-independent body created for this purpose periodically evaluates the quality of the entity's work against preestablished written criteria

Accreditation Association for Ambulatory Healthcare (AAAHC): A professional organization that offers accreditation programs for ambulatory and outpatient organizations such as single-specialty and multispecialty group practices, ambulatory surgery centers, college/university health services, and community health centers

Accreditation organizations: Professional organizations that set the standards against which healthcare organizations are measured to ensure the quality of their services

Accreditation standards: Preestablished statements of the criteria against which the performance of participating healthcare organizations is assessed during the voluntary accreditation process

Accredited Standards Committee, Electronic Data Interchange (ASCX X12): A subcommittee of the American National Standards Institute that develops and maintains standards for electronic data interchange

Acid-test ratio: Cash plus short-term investments plus net current receivables, divided by total current liabilities

Action steps: Specific plans the healthcare organization hopes to accomplish in the near future

Active listening: Demonstrating accurate listening skills by restating in your own words what you understand the speaker to have said

Activities of daily living (ADL): The basic activities of self-care, including grooming, bathing, ambulating, toileting, and eating

Activity-based budget: A budget based on activities or projects rather than on functions or departments

Actor: The role a user plays in a system

Acute care: Medical care of a limited duration that is provided in an inpatient hospital setting to treat an injury or a short-term illness

Acute care prospective payment system: A reimbursement system for hospital services that uses diagnosis-related groups as a classification tool

Administrative controls: Policies and procedures that address the management of computer resources

Administrative information: Information for administrative and healthcare operations purposes, such as billing and quality oversight, consent forms, and demographics

Administrative information systems: A category of healthcare information systems that supports human resources management, financial management, executive decision support, and other primarily administrative functions

Administrative law: The rules and regulations developed by various administrative bodies empowered by Congress; falls under the umbrella of public law

Administrative management: The subdivision of classical management theory that emphasizes the total organization rather than just the individual worker and delineates the major management functions

Administrative services only (ASO) contract: An agreement between an employer and an insurer to administer the employer's self-insured health plan

Admission utilization review: A review of planned services (intensity of service) and/or a patient's condition (severity of illness) to determine whether care must be delivered in an acute inpatient setting

Advance directives: The legal, written documents, such as living wills and durable powers of attorney, that specify patient preferences regarding future healthcare or the person who is authorized to make medical decisions in the event the patient is incapable of communicating his or her preferences

Affinity grouping: A technique for organizing similar ideas together in natural groupings

Age Discrimination in Employment Act: Federal legislation that prohibits employment discrimination against persons between the ages of forty and seventy and restricts mandatory retirement requirements except where age is a bona fide occupational qualification

Agency for Healthcare Research and Quality (AHRQ): The branch of the U.S. Public Health Service that supports general health research and distributes research findings and treatment guidelines with the goal of improving the quality, appropriateness, and effectiveness of healthcare services

Agenda for change: A Joint Commission on Accreditation of Healthcare Organizations initiative focused on changing the emphasis of the survey process from structure to outcomes

Aggregate data: Data extracted from individual patient records and combined to form information about groups of patients

All Patient DRGs (AP-DRGs): A case-mix system developed by 3M and used in a number of state reimbursement systems to classify non-Medicare discharges for reimbursement purposes

All Patient Refined DRGs (APR-DRGs): A system developed by 3M for assessing resource utilization in large patient populations to evaluate quality of care and cost effectiveness

Allied health professional: A healthcare worker other than a physician, nurse, psychologist, or pharmacist; for example, a physical therapist, dietitian, occupational therapist, and so on

Alphanumeric filing system: A health record filing system that uses a combination of letters and numbers to identify individual records

Alternative hypothesis: The type of hypothesis that states that there is an association between the independent and dependent variables

Ambulatory care: Preventive or corrective healthcare provided on a nonresident basis in a provider's office, clinic setting, or hospital

Ambulatory payment classification (APC) system: A hospital outpatient prospective payment system for the classification of services and procedures

Ambulatory surgery center (ASC): A freestanding or hospital-based facility for performing same-day elective surgery

American Association of Health Plans (AAHP): A trade organization for health maintenance organizations, preferred provider organizations, and other network-based health plans, created by the merger of the Group Health Association of America and the American Managed Care and Review Association

American Association of Medical Colleges (AAMC): An organization established in 1876 to standardize the curriculum for medical schools in the United States and to promote the licensure of physicians

American Association for Medical Transcription (AAMT): A professional association for medical transcriptionists

American College of Healthcare Executives (ACHE): A professional organization of healthcare administrators that provides certification services for its members and promotes excellence in the field

American College of Radiology—National Electrical Manufacturers Association (ACR-NEMA): The professional organizations (ACR) and trade associations (NEMA) that work collaboratively to develop digital-imaging standards

American College of Surgeons (ACS): A scientific and educational association of surgeons formed to improve the quality of surgical care by setting high standards for surgical education and practice

American Health Information Management Association (AHIMA): A professional membership organization for managers of health record services and healthcare information as well as coding services; provides accreditation, certification, and educational services

American Hospital Association (AHA): A national trade association for hospitals and other healthcare organizations that provides education, conducts research, and represents the hospital industry in national legislative matters

American Medical Association (AMA): A membership organization for physicians that distributes scientific information to its members and the public, informs members of legislation related to health and medicine, and represents the profession in national legislative matters

American Medical Information Association (AMIA): A membership organization composed of individuals, institutions, and corporations that develop and use information technologies in healthcare

American National Standards Institute (ANSI): An agency that coordinates the development of voluntary standards to increase global competitiveness in a variety of industries, including healthcare

American Nurses Association (ANA): A professional membership association of nurses that works for the improvement of health standards and the availability of healthcare services, fosters high professional standards for the nursing profession, and advances the economic and general welfare of nurses

American Osteopathic Association (AOA): A professional association of osteopathic physicians, surgeons, and graduates of approved colleges of osteopathic medicine that inspects and accredits osteopathic colleges and hospitals

American Society for Healthcare Risk Management (ASHRM): A professional society for healthcare risk management professionals that is affiliated with the American Hospital Association and provides educational tools and networking opportunities for its members

American Society for Quality (ASQ): A quality improvement organization whose members' interests are related to statistical process control, quality cost measurement and control, total quality management, failure analysis, and zero defects

American Society for Testing and Materials (ASTM): An organization that develops standards related to industrial material specifications, testing methods, protective equipment, and data interchange

Americans with Disabilities Act (ADA): Federal legislation that makes it illegal to discriminate against individuals with disabilities in employment, public accommodations, public services, transportation, and telecommunications

Analog: Data or information not represented in an encoded, computer-readable format

Analysis phase: The first phase of the systems development life cycle during which the scope of the project is defined, project goals are identified, current systems are evaluated, and user needs are identified

Analysis session: The process of mining a data segment

Ancillary services: Hospital diagnostic and therapeutic services provided to patients

Appellate court: In the state court system, the court that hears appeals of final judgments from state trial courts

Application controls: Security strategies, such as password management, included in application software and computer programs

Application service provider (ASP): A service company that delivers, manages, and remotely hosts standardized applications software via a network through an outsourcing contract based on fixed, monthly usage or transaction-based pricing

Applied artificial intelligence: An area of computer science dealing with algorithms and computer systems that exhibit the characteristics commonly associated with human intelligence

Applied research: A type of research that focuses on the use of scientific theories to improve actual practice as in medical research applied to the treatment of patients

Appreciative inquiry: An organizational development technique in which successful practices are identified and expanded throughout the organization

Aptitude tests: Tests that assess an individual's general ability to learn a new skill

Arbitration: The proceedings in which disputes are submitted to a third party or a panel of experts outside the judicial trial system

Architecture: The configuration, structure, and relationships of hardware in an information system

Artificial intelligence (AI): High-level information technologies used in developing machines that imitate human qualities such as learning and reasoning

Artificial neural network (ANN): A computational technique from artificial intelligence and machine learning in which the structure and operation are inspired by the properties and operation of the brain

Assembly language: Language that translates assembly-language programs into machine language

Assets: The human, financial, and physical resources of an organization

Assisted living: A freestanding long-term care facility in which residents live with varying degrees of independence

Association rule analysis: The process of extracting useful if-then rules from data based on statistical significance; also called rule induction

Assumptions: Undetermined aspects of a project that are considered to be true; for example, assuming that the project team members have the right skill set to perform their duties

ASTM Standard E1384, Standard Guide for Description of Content and Structure of an Automated Primary Record of Care: Identification of basic information to be included in electronic health records with the information organized into categories

Asynchronous: Occurring at different times

Attending Physician Statement (APS): A standardized insurance claim form created in 1958 by the Health Insurance Association of America and the American Medical Association; also called the COMB-1 form

Attributable risk (AR): The measure of the impact of a disease on a population, for example, measuring additional risk of illness as a result of exposure to a risk factor

Attributes: Data elements within an entity that become the column names or field names when the entity relationship diagram is implemented as a relational database

Attrition: *See* Mortality

Audit: A review process conducted by healthcare facilities (internally and/or externally) to identify variations from established baselines

Audit control: A method of monitoring access to a computer information system

Audit trail: A computerized record of all transactions within a computer information system

Auditing: The process of performing internal and/or external reviews to establish variations from established baselines

Audits: *See* External reviews

Authentication: Proof of authorship

Authority: The state of having the right to make decisions and take actions necessary to carry out assigned tasks

Authorization: An individual's written permission to use or disclose his or her personally identifiable health information for purposes other than treatment, payment, or healthcare operations

Authorization management: The process of protecting the security and privacy of data in a database

Autoauthentication: A procedure that allows dictated reports to be considered automatically signed unless the health information management department is notified of needed revisions within a certain time limit

Autocoding: The process of extracting and translating dictated and then transcribed free-text data (or dictated and then computer-generated discrete data) into ICD-9-CM and CPT evaluation and management codes for patient billing and medical record coding purposes

Autodialing system: A method used to automatically call and remind patients of upcoming appointments or immunizations

Autonomy: A core ethical principle centered on the individual's right to self-determination that includes respect for the individual; in clinical applications, the patient's right to determine what does or does not happen to him or her

Autopsy rate: The proportion or percentage of deaths in a healthcare organization that are followed by the performance of autopsy

Average daily census: The average number of hospital inpatients present each day for a given period of time

Average length of stay (ALOS): The average length of stay of hospital inpatients discharged during a given period of time

Balance billing: A reimbursement method that allows the provider to bill the patient for charges in excess of the amount paid by the patient's health plan or other third-party payer (not allowed under Medicare)

Balance sheet: A report containing the totals in accounts, expressed in accounting equation format, at a point in time

Balanced Budget Refinement Act (BBRA): The amended version of the Balanced Budget Act of 1997 that authorizes implementation of a per-discharge prospective payment system for care provided to Medicare beneficiaries by inpatient rehabilitation facilities

Balanced Score Card (BSC): A strategic planning tool that identifies performance measures related to strategic goals

Baldridge Award: A congressional award recognizing excellence in several areas of business

Bandwidth: The capacity of a line or network to carry information

Bar chart: A graphic technique for displaying data that fall into categories; also called bar graph

Bar coding: A labeling technique using technology that recognizes rectangular shapes and spaces to represent characters to identify forms or track the location of records

Bar coding technology: A method of encoding data that consists of parallel arrangements of dark elements, referred to as bars, and light elements, referred to as spaces, and interpreting the data for automatic identification and data collection purposes

Bar graph: *See* Bar chart

Baseline: The original estimates for the project schedule, work, and cost

Basic research: A type of research that focuses on the development of theories and their refinement

Bed count: The number of inpatient beds available on a given day; also called complement

Bed count day: A unit of measure denoting the presence of one inpatient bed, either occupied or vacant, set up and staffed for use during a twenty-four-hour period

Bed turnover rate: The number of times, on average, a bed changes occupants during a given period of time

Behavioral description interview: An interview format that requires applicants to give specific examples of how they have performed a specific procedure or handled a specific problem in the past

Benchmarking: The process of comparing the performance of an organization to a preestablished standard or to the performance of a similar group or organization

Beneficence: A legal term that means promoting good for others or providing services that benefit others, such as releasing health information that will help a patient receive care or will ensure payment for services received

Bill hold: A policy that dictates a waiting period between the date the patient is discharged and the date the claim is submitted

Bills of Mortality: Used in London during the seventeenth century to identify the most common causes of death, these documents are the first meaningful statistical study of healthcare data

Bioethics: A field of study that applies ethical principles to decisions that affect the lives of humans; bioethical decisions require decisions and actions, such as whether to approve or deny access to health information

Bit-mapped data: Data made up of pixels displayed on a horizontal and vertical grid or matrix

Bivariate: An adjective meaning the involvement of two variables

Blanket authorization: An authorization for release of confidential information from a certain point in time and any time thereafter

Blue Cross and Blue Shield (BC/BS): The first prepaid healthcare plan in the United States; Blue Cross traditionally covers hospital care, and Blue Shield covers physicians' services

Blue Cross and Blue Shield Federal Employee Program (FEP): A federal program that offers a fee-for-service plan with preferred provider organizations and a point-of-service product; also called the BCBS Service Benefit Plan

Blue Cross and Blue Shield Service Benefit Plan: *See* Blue Cross and Blue Shield Federal Employee Program (FEP)

Board of directors: The elected or appointed group of officials who bear the ultimate responsibility for the successful operation of a healthcare organization; also called board of governors or board of trustees

Board of governors: *See* Board of directors

Board of trustees: *See* Board of directors

Bounded rationality: Recognition that decision making is often based on limited time and information about a problem and that many situations are complex and rapidly changing

Brainstorming: A group problem-solving technique that involves the spontaneous contribution of a large number of creative ideas from all members of the group

Branding communications: Messages sent to increase awareness of and to enhance product image in the marketplace

Break-even analysis: A financial analysis technique for determining the level of sales at which total revenues equal the total costs; revenues beyond that are profits

Bugs: Problems in software that prevent the smooth application of a function

Bundled payments: *See* Episode-of-care (EOC) reimbursement

Bureaucracy: A formal organizational structure based on a rigid hierarchy of decision making and inflexible rules and procedures

Business associate: According to HIPAA privacy provisions, an individual (or organization) who is not a member of a covered entity's workforce, but who helps the covered entity in the performance of various functions involving the use or disclosure of individually identifiable health information

Business continuity plan: A program that incorporates policies and procedures for continuing business operations during a computer shutdown

Business intelligence: The end product or goal of knowledge management

Business process: A set of related policies and procedures that are performed step by step to accomplish a business-related function

Business process reengineering (BPR): The analysis and design of the work flow within and between organizations

Bylaws: Operating documents that describe the rules and regulations under which a healthcare organization operates; also called rules and regulations

Capital budget: The allocation of resources for long-term investments and projects

Capitated payment: A managed care term that refers to the fixed amount a physician is paid to provide services to a patient or a group of patients over a prespecified period of time

Capitation: A method of reimbursement for medical services that is based on a fixed payment for a covered group of individuals rather than fee-for-service payments

Care Map™: A proprietary care-planning tool similar to a clinical protocol; a preplanned guide outlining major aspects of treatment on the basis of diagnosis or other characteristics of the patient

Care path: A care-planning tool similar to a clinical practice guideline that has a multidisciplinary focus that emphasizes the coordination of clinical services; also called clinical or critical path or pathway, and clinical algorithm

Career development: The process of growing or progressing within one's profession or occupation

Carrier (Medicare Part B): A contract with the Centers for Medicare and Medicaid Services to serve as the financial agent that works with providers and the federal government to locally administer Medicare Part A claims

Case definition: A method of determining criteria for cases that should be included in a registry

Case fatality rate: The total number of deaths due to a specific illness during a given time period divided by the total number of cases during the same period

Case finding: A method of identifying patients who have been *seen* and/or treated in the facility for the particular disease or condition of interest to the registry

Case law: *See* Common law

Case management: An ongoing concurrent review performed by clinical professionals to ensure the necessity and effectiveness of the clinical services being provided to a patient

Case manager: The person responsible for guiding and monitoring the patient through the process of care

Case mix: A method of grouping hospital patients according to a predefined set of characteristics

Case study: A type of nonparticipant observation in which researchers investigate one person, one group, or one institution in depth

Case-control (retrospective) study: A study that investigates the development of disease by amassing volumes of data about factors in the lives of persons with the disease (cases) and persons without the disease (controls); *see also* Retrospective study

Case-mix group payment rate: The predetermined, per-discharge reimbursement amount for each case-mix group that includes all of the inpatient operating and capital costs incurred in furnishing covered rehabilitation services, but not the costs associated with bad debts, approved educational activities, and other costs not paid for under the prospective payment system

Case-mix group relative weights: Factors that account for the variance in cost per discharge and resource utilization among case-mix groups

Case-mix groups (CMGs): Ninety-seven function-related groups into which inpatient rehabilitation facility discharges are classified based on the impairment, age, comorbidities, and functional ability of the patient and other factors

Case-mix index (CMI): The sum of the weights of diagnosis-related groups for patients discharged during a given period divided by the total patients discharged

Catastrophic coverage: *See* Major medical insurance

Categorical data: A type of data that represents values or observations that can be sorted into a category

Categorically needy eligibility groups (Medicaid): Categories of individuals to whom states must provide coverage under the federal Medicaid program

Causal relationship: A type of relationship in which one factor causes a change in another factor; cause and effect

Causal-comparative research: A research design that resembles experimental research but lacks random assignment to a group and manipulation of treatment; also known as quasi-experimental design

Cause-specific death rate: The total number of deaths due to a specific illness during a given time period divided by the estimated population for the same time period

Census: The number of inpatients present in the healthcare facility at any one time

Census survey: A survey that collects data from all the members of the population

Centers for Disease Control and Prevention (CDC): A federal agency that oversees health promotion and disease control and prevention activities in the United States

Centers for Medicare and Medicaid Services (CMS): A division of the Department of Health and Human Services that is responsible for developing healthcare policy in the United States and for administering the Medicare program and the federal portion of the Medicaid program; called the Health Care Financing Administration (HCFA) prior to 2001

Certainty factor: The defined certainty percentage rate with which an occurrence must present itself to satisfy quality standards

Certification: The process by which a nongovernment agency or association recognizes the competence of individuals who have met its specific qualifications

Certified coding specialist (CCS): An AHIMA credential awarded to individuals who have demonstrated their skill in classifying medical data from patient records, generally in the hospital setting, by passing a certification examination

Certified coding specialist—Physician-based (CCS-P): An AHIMA credential awarded to individuals who have demonstrated coding expertise in physician-based settings such as group practices by passing a certification examination

Certified medical transcriptionist (CMT): A certification that is granted upon successful completion of an examination

Chain of command: A hierarchical reporting structure within an organization

Champion: A role played by an individual within an organization who believes in an innovation or change and who promotes the idea by building financial and political support

Change agent: An individual within an organization whose primary responsibility is to facilitate change

Change control: The process of performing an impact analysis and obtaining approval before modifications to the project scope are made

Change drivers: Forces in the external environment of organizations or industries that force organizations or industries to change the way they operate in order to survive

Change management: A formal process of introducing change, getting it adopted, and implementing it throughout the organization

Chargemaster: A financial management form that provides information about the organization's charges for the healthcare services it provides to patients; also called the charge description master

Charisma: The ability of a leader to inspire and motivate others to high performance and commitment

Chart tracking: A system that identifies current location of record or information

Checksheet: A tool that permits the systematic recording of observations of a particular phenomenon so that trends or patterns can be identified

Chief executive officer (CEO): The individual appointed by a governing board to direct an organization's overall management

Chief financial officer (CFO): The individual who oversees the fiscal management of the healthcare organization

Chief information officer (CIO): The senior manager responsible for the overall management of information resources in a healthcare organization

Chief nursing officer (CNO): The senior manager (usually a registered nurse with advanced education and extensive experience) responsible for the administration of patient care services

Chief security officer (CSO): The manager (usually middle level) responsible for overseeing all aspects of the healthcare organization's security plan

Children's Health Insurance Program (CHIP): *See* State Children's Health Insurance Program (SCHIP)

Circuit switching: Technology that establishes a connection between callers in a telephone network using a dedicated circuit path

Civil law: A branch of law that involves court actions between private parties, corporations, government bodies, or other organizations, typically for the recovery of private rights with compensation usually being monetary

Civil Rights Act of 1964, Title VII: Federal legislation that prohibits discrimination in employment on the basis of race, religion, color, sex, or national origin

Civil Rights Act of 1991: Federal legislation that focuses on establishing an employer's responsibility for justifying hiring practices that *seem* to adversely affect people because of their race, color, religion, sex, or national origin

Civilian Health and Medical Program—Uniformed Services (CHAMPUS): *See* TRICARE

Civilian Health and Medical Program—Veterans Administration (CHAMPVA): A healthcare benefits program for dependents of veterans rated by the Veterans Administration (VA) as having a total and permanent disability; for survivors of veterans who died from VA-rated service-connected conditions or who, at the time of death, were rated permanently and totally disabled from a VA-rated service-connected condition; and for survivors of persons who died in the line of duty

Claim: A statement submitted to a third-party payer by a healthcare provider that describes the services provided to a patient

Claims management: A function related to risk management that enables an organization to track descriptive claims information (incidents, claimants, insurance, demands, dates, and so on), along with data on investigation, litigation, settlement, defendants, and subrogation

Claims processing: The process of accumulating claims for services, submitting claims for reimbursement, and ensuring that claims are satisfied

Class: The higher level abstraction of an object that defines its properties and operations

Classification: A system that is clinically descriptive and arranges or organizes like or related entities for easy retrieval

Classification system: A system for grouping similar diseases and procedures and organizing related information for easy retrieval; a system for assigning numeric or alphanumeric code numbers to represent specific diseases and/or procedures

Client: A computer that accesses shared resources located on a server; a patient who receives behavioral and mental health services

Clinical algorithm: *See* Care path

Clinical care plans: Care guidelines created by healthcare providers for individual patients for a specified period of time

Clinical coding: The process of assigning numeric or alphanumeric classifications to diagnostic and procedural statements

Clinical data: Data captured during the process of diagnosis and treatment

Clinical data repository (CDR): A central database that focuses on clinical information

Clinical decision support system (CDSS): A special subcategory of clinical information system that is designed to help healthcare providers make knowledge-based clinical decisions

Clinical informatics: A field of information science concerned with the management of data and information used to support the practice and delivery of patient care through the application of computers and computer technologies

Clinical information systems: A category of healthcare information system that includes systems that directly support patient care

Clinical path or pathway: *See* Care path

Clinical practice guideline: A detailed, step-by-step guide used by healthcare practitioners to make knowledge-based clinical decisions related to patient care; also called clinical protocol

Clinical research: Specialized area of research that primarily investigates the efficacy of preventive, diagnostic, and therapeutic procedures; also called medical research

Clinical/medical decision support system: Data-driven decision support system that assists physicians in applying new information to patient care through the analysis of patient-specific clinical/medical variables

Clinical privileges: The authorization granted by a healthcare organization's governing board to a member of the medical staff that enables the physician to provide patient services in the organization within specific practice limits

Clinical protocol: *See* Clinical practice guideline

Clinical quality assessment: The process for determining whether the services provided to patients meet predetermined standards of care

Clinical repository: A frequently updated database that provides users with direct access to detailed patient-level data as well as the ability to drill down into historical views of administrative, clinical, and financial data; often called a data warehouse

Clinical terminology: *See* Nomenclature

Clinical Terms, Version 3 (CTV3): *See* Read Codes

Clinical trial: A controlled study involving human subjects designed to evaluate prospectively the safety and effectiveness of new drugs, tests, devices, or interventions

Clinical vocabulary: A formally recognized list of preferred medical terms; also referred to as a medical vocabulary

Clinical workstation: A single point of access that includes a common user interface to view information from disparate applications as well as to launch applications

Clinician: A healthcare provider, including physicians and others who treat the patient

Clinician/physician portals: Media for providing physician/clinician access to the provider organization's multiple sources of data from any network-connected device

Closed records: Records of patients who have been discharged from the hospital or whose treatment has been terminated

Closed-ended question: *See* Structured question

Closed-record review: A review of records after a patient has been discharged from the organization or treatment has been terminated

Closed systems: Systems that operate in a self-contained environment

Cluster sampling: The process of selecting subjects for a sample from each cluster when the population has clusters, such as families, schools, or communities

CMS-1500: A claim form used to bill third-party payers for provider services such as physician office visits

Coaching: A method of training in which an experienced person gives advice to a less-experienced worker on a formal or informal basis; also a method of discipline used as the first step for employees who are not meeting performance expectations

Coalition building: A technique used to manage the political dimensions of change within an organization by building the support of groups for change

Code of Federal Regulations (CFR): A publication that publicizes all of the final rules and regulations established by the federal government

Coded data: Data that are translated into a standard nomenclature of classification so that they may be aggregated, analyzed, and compared

Coding: The process of assigning alphabetic and/or numeric representations to clinical documentation

Coding specialist: The healthcare worker responsible for assigning numeric or alphanumeric codes to diagnostic or procedural statements

Cohort study: A study, followed over time, in which a group of subjects is identified as having one or more characteristics in common

Coinsurance: The amount an insured individual pays as a requirement of his or her insurance policy (for example, the insurer pays 80 percent and the insured pays 20 percent co-insurance)

Collaborative Stage Data Set: A new standardized neoplasm staging system developed by the American Joint Commission on Cancer

College of Healthcare Information Management Executives (CHIME): A membership association serving chief information officers through professional development and advocacy

Column/field: A basic fact within a table, such as LAST_NAME, FIRST_NAME, and date of birth

COMB-1: *See* Attending Physician Statement (APS)

Commission on Accreditation of Rehabilitation Facilities (CARF): A private, not-for-profit organization that develops customer-focused standards for behavioral healthcare and medical rehabilitation programs and accredits such programs on the basis of its standards

Common cause variation: The source of variation in a process that is inherent within the process

Common law: Unwritten law originating from court decisions where no applicable statute exists; also known as judge-made or case law

Communication standards: *See* Transmission standards

Communications: The manner in which various individual computer systems are connected (for example, telephone lines, microwave, satellite)

Communications plan: A documented approach to identifying the media and schedule for sharing information with affected parties

Community-acquired infection: An infectious disease contracted as the result of exposure before or after a patient's period of hospitalization

Comorbidity: A medical condition that coexists with the primary cause for hospitalization and affects the patient's inpatient length of stay

Compensable factor: A characteristic used to compare the worth of jobs; for example, skill, effort, responsibility, and working conditions

Competencies: Demonstrated skills that a worker should perform at a high level

Compiler: Software that looks at an entire high-level program before translating it into machine language; a third-level programming language

Complaint: A written legal statement from a plaintiff that initiates a civil lawsuit

Complement: *See* Bed count

Compliance: The process of establishing an organizational culture that promotes the prevention, detection, and resolution of instances of conduct that do not conform to federal, state, or private payer healthcare program requirements or the healthcare organization's ethical and business policies; the condition of acting in conformance with rules and regulations

Compliance program guidance: Information provided by the Office of the Inspector General of the Department of Health and Human Services to help healthcare organizations develop internal controls that promote adherence to applicable federal and state guidelines

Complication: A medical condition that arises during an inpatient hospitalization

Component alignment model (CAM): A model for strategic information systems planning that includes seven major interdependent components that should be aligned with other components in the organization

Comprehensive Drug Abuse Prevention and Control Act of 1970: *See* Controlled Substance Act

Compressed workweek: A work schedule that permits a full-time job to be completed in less than the standard five days of eight-hour shifts

Compression algorithm: The process or program for reducing a message without significantly losing information

Computer telephony: A combination of computer and telephone technologies that allows people to use a telephone handset to access information stored in a computer system or to use computer technology to place calls within the public telephone network

Computer virus: A software program that attacks computer systems and sometimes damages or destroys files

Computer-based patient record (CPR): A health record housed in an information system designed to provide users with access to complete and accurate clinical data, practitioner alerts and reminders, clinical decision support systems, and links to medical knowledge; also known as electronic health record

Computer-based Patient Record Institute (CPRI): A private organization founded in 1992 to develop a strategy to support the development and adoption of computer-based patient records

Computer-based training: Training that is delivered partially or completely using a computer

Computer–telephone integration (CTI): An integration of computer technology and public telephone services that allows people to access common computer functions such as database queries via telephone handsets or interactive voice technology

Concept: A unit of knowledge created by a unique combination of characteristics

Conceptual data model: The highest level of data model, representing the highest level of abstraction, independent of hardware and software

Conceptual framework of accounting: The concept that the benefits of financial data should exceed the cost of obtaining them and that the data must be understandable, relevant, reliable, and comparable

Conceptual skills: One of the three managerial skill categories; includes intellectual tasks and abilities such as planning, deciding, and problem solving

Concurrent analysis: A review of the health record while the patient is still hospitalized or under treatment; sometimes called concurrent review

Concurrent review: *See* Concurrent analysis

Concurrent utilization review: An evaluation of the medical necessity, quality, and cost-effectiveness of a hospital admission and ongoing patient care at or during the time that services are rendered

Conditions of Participation: The rules and regulations under which facilities are allowed to be part of the Medicare program, set forth by the Department of Health and Human Services' Centers for Medicare and Medicaid Services

Confidentiality: A legal and ethical concept that establishes the healthcare provider's responsibility for protecting health records and other personal and private information from unauthorized use or disclosure

Confounding variable: An event or a factor that is outside a study but occurs concurrently with the study; also called extraneous or secondary variable

Connectivity: The ability of one computer system to exchange meaningful data with another computer system

Consent: A voluntary permission granted by a patient to a healthcare provider allowing the provider to administer care and/or treatment or to perform surgery and/or other medical procedures

Conservatism: The concept that resources must not be overstated and liabilities not understated

Consideration: The leadership orientation of having concern for people and providing support

Consistency: The idea that all time periods must reflect the same accounting rules

Consultation: A report of an individual with expertise to provide professional advice and/or a second opinion requested by the patient's attending physician

Consultation rate: The total number of hospital inpatients receiving consultations for a given period divided by the total number of discharges and deaths for the same period

Consumer informatics: The field of information science concerned with the management of data and information used to support consumers by consumers (the general public) through the application of computers and computer technologies

Construct validity: The ability of an instrument to measure hypothetical, nonobservable traits

Content analysis: A method of research that provides a systematic and objective analysis of communication effectiveness, such as the analysis performed on tests

Content validity: The extent to which an instrument's items represent the content that the instrument is intended to measure

Context: Text that illustrates a concept or the use of a designation

Contingency: A plan of action to be taken when circumstances affect project performance

Contingency model of leadership: A leadership theory based on the idea that the success of task- or relationship-oriented leadership depends on leader–member relations, task structure, and position power

Continued-stay utilization review: A periodic review conducted during a hospital stay to determine whether the patient continues to need acute care services

Continuing education: A type of training that enables employees to remain current in the knowledge base of their profession

Continuous data: Data that represent values or observations that have an indefinite number of points along a continuum

Continuous quality improvement (CQI): A quality improvement philosophy that emphasizes the importance of knowing and meeting customer expectations, reducing variation within processes, and relying on data to build knowledge for process improvement; a continuous cycle of planning, measuring, and monitoring performance and making knowledge-based improvements

Continuous speech recognition: Computer technology that automatically translates voice patterns into written language in real time

Continuous speech technology: A method of encoding speech signals that does not require speaker pauses (but uses pauses if they are present) and of interpreting at least some of the signals' content as words or the intent of the speaker; also called voice recognition technology

Continuum of care: A term referring to the range of healthcare services provided to patients, from routine ambulatory care to intensive acute care

Contract law: A branch of law based on common law that deals with written or oral agreements that are enforceable through the legal system

Contract service: An entity that provides certain agreed-upon services for the facility, such as transcription, coding, or copying

Control: One of the four management functions in which performance is monitored in accordance with organizational policies and procedures

Control group: A comparison study group whose members do not undergo the treatment under study

Controlled Substances Act: Legislation that controls the use of narcotics, depressants, stimulants, and hallucinogens; abbreviated name for the Comprehensive Drug Abuse Prevention and Control Act of 1970

Controls: Subjects used for comparison who are not given a treatment under study or do not have the condition or risk factor that is the object of study

Convenience sample: A type of nonrandom sampling in which researchers "conveniently" use any unit that is at hand

Cooperating parties: A group of four organizations (the American Health Information Management Association, the American Hospital Association, the Centers for Medicare and Medicaid Services, and the National Center for Health Statistics) that collaborate in the development and maintenance of the *International Classification of Diseases, Ninth Revision, Clinical Modification* (ICD-9-CM)

Coordinated care plans: Organized patient care plans that meet the standards set forth in the law (for example, health maintenance organizations, provider-sponsored organizations, and preferred provider organizations)

Coordination of benefits (COB) transaction: The electronic transmission of claims and/or payment information from a healthcare provider to a health plan for the purpose of determining relative payment responsibilities

Core communications: A series of triggered, event-specific communications based on need and data such as age, sex, and health profile that give providers an appropriate time and personalized reason to communicate with the recipients

Core measure/core measure set: Standardized performance measures developed to improve the safety and quality of healthcare (for example, core measures are used in the Joint Commission on Accreditation's ORYX initiative)

Corporate negligence: A legal term referring to the failure of an organization to exercise the degree of care considered reasonable under the circumstances that resulted in an unintended injury to another party

Corporation: An organization that may have one or many owners in which profits may be held or distributed as dividends (income paid to the owners)

Correct Coding Initiative (CCI): A national initiative designed to improve the accuracy of Part B claims processed by Medicare carriers

Corrective controls: Internal controls designed to fix problems that have been discovered, frequently as a result of detective controls

Correlational research: A design of research that determines the existence and degree of relationships among factors

Cost justification: Rationale developed to support competing requests for limited resources

Cost outlier: An inpatient hospital case that is exceptionally costly when compared to other cases in the same diagnosis-related group

Cost outlier adjustment: Additional payments for certain high-cost home care cases based on the loss-sharing ratio (a percentage) of costs in excess of a threshold amount for each home health resource group

Cost report: A report that analyzes the direct and indirect costs of providing care to Medicare patients

Cost–benefit analysis: A process that uses quantitative techniques to evaluate and measure the benefit of providing products or services compared to the cost of providing them

Court of Appeals: A court that reviews decisions made by a lower court

Courts of appeal: A branch of the federal court system that is empowered to hear appeals from final judgments of the district courts

Court order: An official order issued by the judge of a court, requiring or forbidding somebody to do something

Covered entity: According to HIPAA privacy provisions, any health plan, healthcare clearinghouse, or healthcare provider that transmits specific healthcare transactions in electronic form

Credentialing: The process of reviewing and validating the qualifications (degrees, licenses, and other credentials), of healthcare practitioners, granting medical staff membership, and awarding specific clinical privileges to licensed independent practitioners to provide patient care services

Credentialing process: A screening process used by the medical staff to evaluate a physician's application for medical staff membership

Credits: The amounts on the right side of a journal entry

Criminal law: A branch of law that addresses crimes that are wrongful acts against public health, safety, and welfare, usually punishable by imprisonment and/or fine

Critic: A role in organizational innovation in which an idea is challenged, compared to stringent criteria, and tested against reality

Critical path or pathway: *See* Care path

Critical path method: A project management method for determining a logical sequence of activities, the time required to complete each, and what must be done to complete the project on time

Cross-sectional: A type of time frame that collects data at one point in time

Cross-sectional study: A biomedical research study in which both the exposure and the disease outcome are determined at the same time in each subject; also called a prevalence study

Cross-training: The training to learn a job other than the employee's primary responsibility

Crude birth rate: The number of live births divided by the population at risk

Crude death rate: The total number of deaths in a given population for a given period of time divided by the estimated population for the same period of time

Current Procedural Terminology **(CPT):** A comprehensive list of descriptive terms and codes published by the American Medical Association and used for reporting diagnostic and therapeutic procedures and other medical services performed by physicians

Current ratio: The total current assets divided by total current liabilities

Customer: An internal or external recipient of a service, product, or information

Customer relationship management (CRM): A management system whereby organizational structure and culture and customer information and technology are aligned with business strategy so that all customer interactions can be conducted to the long-term satisfaction of the customer and to the benefit and profit of the organization

Cybernetic systems: Systems that have standards, controls, and feedback mechanisms built into them

Daily inpatient census: The number of inpatients present at census-taking time each day, plus any inpatients who were admitted and discharged after the census-taking time the previous day

Data: The dates, numerals, images, symbols, letters, and words that represent basic facts about people, processes, measurements, and conditions

Data accessibility: A term referring to how obtainable healthcare data are

Data accuracy: A term referring to the correctness of healthcare data

Data administrator: An emerging role responsible for managing the less technical aspects of data, including data quality and security

Data availability: A term referring to the accessibility of healthcare data whenever and wherever they are needed

Data capture: The process of recording healthcare-related data in a health record system or database

Data comprehensiveness: A term referring to the completeness of healthcare

Data confidentiality: A term referring to the efforts made to guarantee the privacy of personal health information

Data consistency: A term referring to the reliability of healthcare data

Data currency: A term referring to how up-to-date data are; also called data timeliness

Data definition: A term referring to the meaning of healthcare data

Data definition language (DDL): A special type of software used to create the tables within a relational database, the most common of which is structured query language (SQL)

Data dictionary: A descriptive list of the data elements to be collected in an information system or database; the purpose of the list is to ensure consistency of usage

Data display: A method for presenting or viewing data

Data element: An individual fact or measurement collected in a healthcare database

Data Elements for Emergency Department Systems (DEEDS): A data set designed to support the uniform collection of data in hospital-based emergency departments

Data exchange standards: Protocols that help ensure that the transmission of data from one system to another provides comparable data

Data field: An area within a healthcare database in which the same type of information is usually recorded

Data granularity: A term referring to the level of detail at which the attributes and values of healthcare data are defined

Data input: The process of entering data into a healthcare database

Data integrity: A term referring to the completeness, accuracy, consistency, and timeliness of healthcare data

Data manipulation language (DML): A special type of software used to retrieve, update, and edit data in a relational database, of which the most common is structured query language (SQL)

Data marts: User-centered, searchable data warehouses that organize data by specific, user-defined subjects

Data miners: Individuals within the healthcare organization whose primary job function is to conduct the process and analysis of data mining

Data mining: The process of extracting information from a database and then quantifying and filtering discrete, structured data

Data modeling: The process of determining data needs and identifying the relationships among the data

Data models: Pictures or abstractions of real conditions; used extensively in database design

Data precision: A term referring to the values that data are expected to have

Data quality management: A process that ensures the integrity of an organization's data during data collection, application, warehousing, and analysis

Data relevancy: A term referring to the usefulness of healthcare data

Data repositories: Databases acting as information storage facilities for day-to-day transaction-processing capabilities and little or no analysis or querying functionality

Data resource manager: A role described by the AHIMA that ensures that the organization's information systems meet the needs of people who provide and manage patient services

Data retrieval: The process of obtaining data from a healthcare database

Data security: A term referring to the procedures followed to protect data from unauthorized alteration or destruction

Data set: A list of recommended data elements with uniform definitions

Data timeliness: *See* Data currency

Data type: A technical category of data (text, numeric, currency, date, memo, and link data) that a field in a database can contain

Data warehouse: *See* Clinical repository

Database: An organized collection of data, text, references, or pictures in a standardized format, typically stored in a computer system

Database administrator: An individual responsible for the technical aspects of designing and managing databases

Database life cycle (DBLC): Several phases representing the useful life of a database, including initial study, design, implementation, testing and evaluation, operation, and maintenance and evaluation

Database management system (DBMS): A specific set of processes used to create, modify, delete, and view the data in a database

Database model: A structure for organizing data in a healthcare database, such as in a computer-based patient record

Day outlier: An inpatient hospital stay that is exceptionally long when compared with other cases in the same diagnosis-related group

Debits: Amounts on the left side of a journal entry

Debt ratio: The total liabilities divided by total assets

Decentralization: The shift of decision-making authority and responsibility to lower levels of the organization

Decision support system (DSS): A computer-based system that gathers data from a variety of sources and assists in providing structure to the data using various analytical models and visual tools in order to facilitate and improve the ultimate outcome in decision-making tasks associated with nonroutine and nonrepetitive problems

Decision tree: A structured data-mining technique based on a set of rules useful for predicting and classifying information and making decisions

Deductive reasoning: A process of creating conclusions based on generalizations (deduction)

Default judgment: A court ruling against a defendant in a lawsuit who fails to answer a summons for a court appearance

Defendant: An individual or company against whom a civil lawsuit has been filed; in criminal cases, an individual who has been accused of a crime

Deficiency slip: A device for tracking information (for example, reports) missing from a paper-based health record

Deidentified information: Health information from which all names and other identifying descriptors have been removed to protect the privacy of patients, families, and healthcare providers

Delegation: The process by which managers distribute work to others along with the authority to make decisions and take action

Delinquent: *See* Delinquent health record

Delinquent health record: An incomplete record not finished or made complete within the time frame determined by the medical staff of the facility

Deliverables: Tangible output produced by the completion of project tasks

Delivery system: *See* Integrated provider organization (IPO)

Demographic information: Information used to identify an individual such as name, address, gender, age, and other information specifically linked to a specific person

Dental informatics: A field of information science concerned with the management of data and information used to support the practice and delivery of dental healthcare through the application of computers and computer technologies

Department of Health and Human Services (HHS): A cabinet-level federal agency that oversees all of the health- and human services–related activities of the federal government

Dependency: Relationship between two tasks in a project plan

Dependent variable: A measured variable that occurs after the manipulation; it depends upon the independent variable

Deposition: A method of gathering information for use in a litigation process

Depreciation: The allocation of the dollar cost of a capital asset over its expected life

Derived attribute: An attribute whose value is based on the value of other attributes, for example, current date minus date of birth yields the derived attribute age

Descriptive research: Research that determines and reports the current status of topics and subjects

Descriptive statistics: A set of statistical techniques used to describe data such as means, frequency distributions, and standard deviations; statistical information that describes the characteristics of a specific group or a population

Design phase: The second phase of the systems development life cycle during which all options in selecting a new information system are considered

Designated record set: A group of records maintained by or for a covered entity that may include patient medical and billing records; the enrollment, payment, claims adjudication, and cases or medical management record systems maintained by or for a health plan; or information used, in whole or in part, to make patient care-related decisions

Detective control: An internal control designed to find errors that have already been made

Development: The process of growing or progressing in one's level of skill, knowledge, or ability

Diagnostic image data: Bit-mapped images used for medical or diagnostic purposes, such as chest X rays or computed tomography (CT) scans

Diagnosis-related groups (DRGs): A case-mix system that classifies inpatient hospitalizations according to diagnosis (along with other patient data, such as age, sex, and discharge status); an element of the Medicare's acute care prospective payment system

***Diagnostic and Statistical Manual of Mental Disorders, Fourth Revision* (DSM-IV):** A nomenclature developed by the American Psychiatric Association to standardize the diagnostic process for patients with psychiatric disorders; includes codes that correspond to ICD-9-CM codes

Diagnostic codes: Numeric or alphanumeric characters used to identify diseases, conditions, and injuries

Diffusion S curve: The S-shaped curve that describes the initially gradual, then more rapid, and finally plateauing adoption of an innovation

Digital: Data or information represented in an encoded, computer-readable format

Digital dictation: A process in which vocal sounds are converted to bits and stored on computer for random access by transcriptionist and dictator

Digital Imaging and Communication in Medicine (DICOM): A standard that promotes a digital image communications format and picture archive and communications systems for use with digital images

Direct method of allocation: A budgeting concept where the cost of overhead departments is distributed solely to the revenue-producing areas

Direct relationship: *See* Positive relationship

Disaster recovery: A plan developed by an organization in anticipation of potential natural and manmade disasters that describes the actions that the organization will take to minimize damages and resume operations

Discharge abstract system: A data repository (usually electronic) for information on demographics, clinical conditions, and services rendered; data are condensed from hospital health records into coded data for the purpose of producing summary statistics about discharged patients

Discharge analysis: An analysis of the health record at or following discharge

Discharge days: *See* Total length of stay

Discharge planning: The process of coordinating the activities related to releasing a patient when inpatient hospital care is no longer needed

Discharge summary: The final conclusions at the termination of a facility stay or treatment

Discharge utilization review: A process for assessing a patient's readiness to leave the hospital

Discharged, no final bill (DNFB): A term sometimes used to refer to a summary report

Discipline: A field of study characterized by a knowledge base and perspective that is different from other fields of study

Disclosure: A helpful explanation that appears in financial reports, as needed

Discounting: The application of lower rates of payment to multiple surgical procedures performed during the same operative session under the outpatient prospective payment system; the application of adjusted rates of payment by preferred-provider organizations

Discovery: The pretrial stage in the litigation process during which both parties to a suit use various strategies to identify information about the case, the primary focus of which is to determine the strength of the opposing party's case

Discovery process: The compulsory disclosure of pertinent facts or documents to the opposing party in a civil action, usually before a trial begins

Discrete data: A type of data that represents separate and distinct values or observations

Discrete variables: A dichotomous or nominal variable whose values are placed into categories

Disease index: A listing of diseases and conditions of patients sequenced according to the code numbers of the classification system in use

Disease registry: A central collection of data used to improve the quality of care and measure the effectiveness of a particular aspect of healthcare delivery

Disposition: The place where the patient goes after discharge or at the conclusion of treatment; in regard to record retention, final destruction or final repository of record

Distance learning: A learning delivery mode in which the instructor, the classroom, and the students are not all present in the same location and at the same time

Distribution-free technique: *See* Nonparametric technique

District court: The lowest tier in the federal court system that hears cases involving felonies and misdemeanors which fall under federal statute and suits in which a citizen of one state sues a citizen of another state

Diversity training: A type of training that facilitates an environment that fosters tolerance and appreciation of individual differences within the organization's workforce

Document image data: Bit-mapped images based on data created and/or stored on analog paper or photographic film

Do not resuscitate (DNR): An order written by the treating physician stating that in the event the patient suffers cardiac or pulmonary arrest, cardiopulmonary resuscitation should not be attempted

Double distribution: A budgeting concept where overhead costs are allocated twice, taking into consideration that some overhead departments provide services to each other

Double-blind study: A type of clinical trial conducted with strict procedures for randomization in which neither the researcher nor the subject knows whether the subject is in the control group or the experimental group

Downsizing: A reengineering strategy to reduce the cost of labor and streamline the organization by laying off portions of the workforce

DRG grouper: A computer program that assigns inpatient cases to diagnosis-related groups and determines the Medicare reimbursement rate

Durable medical equipment (DME): Medical equipment designated by a doctor for patient use in the home (for example, a wheelchair)

Durable power of attorney for healthcare: A third party designated by a competent individual to make healthcare decisions for that individual should he or she become incompetent

Duration: The amount of time, usually measured in days, for a task to be completed

E codes: A supplementary ICD-9-CM classification used to identify the external causes of injuries and poisonings

E-commerce: The use of the Internet and its derived technologies to integrate all aspects of business-to-business and business-to-consumer activities, processes, and communications

E-health: The application of e-commerce to the healthcare industry

Early adopters: A category of adopters of innovations who are leaders, role models, and opinion leaders

Early majority: A category of adopters of innovations who are not leaders but are deliberate in thinking

Edit: A condition that must be satisfied before a computer system can accept data

Effectiveness: The degree to which stated outcomes are attained

Efficiency: How well a minimum of resources is used to obtain outcomes

Effort: The mental and physical exertion required to perform the job-related tasks

85/15 rule: The total quality management (TQM) assumption that 85 percent of the problems that occur are related to faults in the system rather than to worker performance

Electronic data interchange (EDI): A standard transmission format using strings of data for business information communicated among the computer systems of independent organizations

Electronic health record (EHR): Synonymous term for computer-based patient record (CPR)

Electronic medical record (EMR): A form of computer-based health record in which information is stored in whole files instead of by individual data elements; a term sometimes mistakenly used to refer to computer-based patient record or electronic health record

Electronic remittance advice (ERA): Payment information from third-party payers that is communicated electronically

Electronic signature: An exclusively assigned unique identification code entered by the author of documentation through electronic means

Emergency Maternal and Infant Care Program (EMIC): The military medical program that provides obstetrical and infant care to dependents of active-duty service personnel in the four lowest pay grades

Empiricism: The quality of being based on observed and validated evidence

Employee Retirement Income Security Act of 1974 (ERISA): Legislation designed to protect the pension rights of employees; also prohibits states from applying certain mandates to self-insured health benefit plans

Employment contract: A legal and binding agreement of terms related to an individual's work, such as hours, pay, or benefits

Employer-based self-insurance: Health plans that are funded directly by employers to provide coverage for their employees exclusively; employers establish accounts to cover their employees' medical expenses and retain control over the funds but bear the risk of paying claims greater than their estimates

Empowerment: The condition of having the environment and resources to perform a job independently

Encoder: Specialized software used as a tool in assigning diagnostic and procedural codes according the rules of the coding system

Encounter: The contact between a patient and a provider who has primary responsibility for and can use independent judgment in assessing and treating the patient

Encryption: Coding attached to data with the intent of keeping the information secure from anyone but the addressee

Ending: The first stage of Bridges's model of transition management in which people experience losses because of change

Enterprise master patient index (EMPI): Indexes that provide access to multiple repositories of information from overlapping patient populations that are maintained in separate systems and databases

Entity: An individual person or organization

Entity relationship diagram (ERD): A specific type of data modeling used in conceptual data modeling and the logical-level modeling of relational databases

Environmental assessment, internal: A collection of information about changes that have occurred within an organization during a specified time period

Environmental assessment, external: A collection of information about changes that have occurred in the healthcare industry as well as the broader U.S. economy during a specified time period

Environmental scanning: A systematic and continuous effort to search for important cues about how the world is changing outside and inside the organization

Epidemiological data: Data used to reveal disease trends within a specific population

Epidemiological studies: Studies that are concerned with finding the causes and effects of diseases and conditions

Episode-of-care (EOC) reimbursement: Payments made as lump sums to providers for all healthcare services delivered to a patient for a specific illness and/or over a specified time period; also called bundled payments because they include multiple services and may include multiple providers of care

Equal Pay Act of 1963 (EPA): Federal legislation that requires equal pay for men and women who perform substantially the same work

Ergonomics: A discipline of functional design associated with the employee in relationship to his or her work environment, including equipment, workstation, and office furniture adaptation to accommodate the employee's unique physical requirements so as to facilitate efficacy of work functions

Essential Medical Data Set (EMDS): A recommended data set designed to create a health history for an individual patient treated in an emergency service

Ethical decision making: The process of requiring everyone to consider the perspectives of others, even when they do not agree with them

Ethicist: An individual trained in the application of ethical theories and principles to problems that cannot be easily solved because of conflicting values, perspectives, and options for action

Ethics: A field of study that deals with moral principles, theories, and values; in healthcare, a formal decision-making process for dealing with the competing perspectives and obligations of the people who have an interest in a common problem

Ethnography: A method of observational research that investigates culture in naturalistic settings using both qualitative and quantitative approaches

Evaluation research: A design of research that examines the effectiveness of policies, programs, or organizations

Evidence-based management: A management system in which practices based on research evidence will be effective and produce the outcomes they claim

Evidence-based medicine: Clinical methods that have been thoroughly tested through controlled, peer-reviewed studies

Exclusive provider organization (EPO): A type of managed care organization that provides benefits to subscribers when the healthcare services are performed only by network providers

Executive dashboard: An information management system providing decision makers with regularly updated information on an organization's key strategic measures

Executive information system (EIS): An information system that provides standard, scheduled, and periodic reports that healthcare executives can use in making decisions that affect the overall organization

Executive managers: Managers who oversee broad functional areas or groups of departments or services, set the organization's future direction, and monitor the organization's operations

Exempt employees: Specific groups of employees who are identified as not being covered by some or all of the provisions of the Fair Labor Standards Act

Expectancy theory: A theory of motivation that assumes people will choose behaviors because they expect that those behaviors to lead to certain outcomes

Expenses: Amounts that are charged as costs by an organization to the current year's activities of operation

Experimental research: A design of research that establishes cause and effect

Experimental study: A controlled investigation in which subjects are assigned randomly to groups that experience carefully controlled interventions that are manipulated by the experimenter according to a strict protocol

Expert decision support system: A decision support system that uses a set of rules or encoded concepts to construct a reasoning process

Expert system: A type of information system that supports the work of professionals engaged in the design or evaluation of complex situations that require expert knowledge in a well-defined and usually limited area

Explanation of benefits: A statement sent to a healthcare provider or patient to explain services provided, amounts billed, and payments made by a health plan

Explicit knowledge: Documents, databases, and other types of recorded and documented information

Expressed consent: The spoken or written permission to provide treatment granted by a patient to a healthcare provider

Extended care facility: A healthcare facility that provides care over a long period of time

Extensible markup language (XML): A standardized language for the interchange of data as structured text

External reviews: Performance or quality reviews conducted by third-party payers or by consultants hired for the purpose; also called audits

External validity: An attribute of a study's design that allows its findings to be applied to other groups

Extraneous variable: *See* Confounding variable

Extranet: Connections of private Internet networks outside an organization's firewall that use Internet technology to enable collaborative applications among enterprises

Facilities management: Functional oversight of a healthcare organization's physical plant to ensure operational efficiency in an environment that is safe for patients, staff, and visitors

Facility-based registry: A registry that includes only cases from a particular healthcare facility, such as a hospital or a clinic

Facility-specific system: A computer information system that was developed exclusively to meet the needs of one healthcare organization

Factor comparison method: A complex quantitative method of job evaluation that combines elements of both the ranking and point methods; results indicate the degree to which different jobs vary from each other on the basis of compensable factors, which makes it possible to translate each factor value more easily into a monetary wage

Fair Labor Standards Act of 1938 (FLSA): Federal legislation that sets minimum wage and overtime payment regulations

Family and Medical Leave Act of 1993 (FMLA): Federal legislation that allows employees time off from work (up to twelve weeks) to care for themselves or their family members with the assurance of an equivalent position upon return to work

Family numbering: A numbering system, sometimes used in clinic settings, in which a number is assigned to the entire family

Favorable variance: The positive difference between the budgeted amount and the actual amount of a line item; that is, when actual revenue exceeds budget or actual expenses are less than budget

Federal Employees' Compensation Act (FECA): Legislation enacted in 1916 to mandate worker's compensation for civilian federal employees; coverage includes lost wages, medical expenses, and survivors' benefits

Federal poverty level (FPL): The income qualification threshold established by the federal government for certain government entitlement programs

Federal Register: Daily publication of the U.S. Government Printing Office that includes administrative rules and revisions to rules related to federal laws

Fee schedule: A list of healthcare services and procedures (usually CPT/HCPCS codes) and the charges associated with them developed by a third-party payer; also referred to as a table of allowances, it represents the approved payment levels for a given insurance plan

Fee-for-service basis: A method of reimbursement through which providers receive payment based on billed charges for services provided and annually updated fee schedules

Felony: A serious crime such as murder, larceny, rape, and assault for which punishment is usually severe

Fetal autopsy rate: The number of autopsies performed on intermediate and late fetal deaths for a given time period divided by the total number of intermediate and late fetal deaths for the same time period

Fetal death: A death (in a hospital facility) prior to the complete expulsion or extraction from the mother of a product of human conception (fetus and placenta), regardless of the duration of pregnancy; *early:* gestation of less than twenty weeks and weight of 500 grams or less; *intermediate:* gestation of at least twenty weeks, but less than twenty-eight and weight between 501 and 1000 grams; *late:* gestation of twenty-eight weeks or more and weight of more than 1001 grams; also called stillborn death

Fetal death rate: The number of intermediate and/or late fetal deaths for a given time period divided by the total number of live births and intermediate and late fetal deaths for the same time period

Financial Accounting Standards Board (FASB): An independent organization that sets accounting standards for businesses in the private sector

Financial data: data collected for the purpose of managing the assets of a business (for example, a healthcare organization, a product line); in healthcare, data derived from the charge generation documentation associated with the activities of care and then aggregated by specific customer grouping for financial analysis

Financial transaction: The exchange of goods or services for payment or the promise of payment

Fiscal intermediary (FI): An organization that contracts with the Centers for Medicare and Medicaid Services to serve as the financial agent between providers and the federal government in the local administration of Medicare Part B claims

Fiscal year: One business cycle or tax year, which may or may not coincide with the calendar year

Fishbone diagram: A performance improvement tool used to identify or classify the root causes of a problem or condition and to display the root causes graphically; also known as a cause-and-effect diagram

Fixed budget: A type of budget that is based on expected capacity

Flex years: A work arrangement in which employees can choose, at specific intervals, the number of hours they want to work each month over the next year

Flexible budget: A type of budget that is based on multiple levels of projected productivity (actual productivity triggers the levels to be used as the year progresses)

Flextime: A work schedule that gives employees some choice in the pattern of their work hours, usually around a core of midday hours

Flow process chart: A tool that uses standard symbols to visually present detailed information, including time and distance, of the sequential flow of work of an individual or a product as it progresses through a process

Flowchart: A graphic technique used to visually display the steps in a process in order to identify potential problems

Focused study: A study in which a researcher orally questions and conducts discussions with members of a group

Food and Drug Administration (FDA): An agency of the federal government responsible for controlling the sale and use of pharmaceuticals, including the licensing of new medications for human use

For-profit organization: A tax status that reflects ownership of an organization by one or more individuals or other organizations

Force-field analysis: A performance improvement tool used to identify specific drivers of, and barriers to, an organizational change so that positive factors can be reinforced and negative factors reduced

Forecasting: An operations management technique in which future financial outcomes are predicted on the basis of historical data as well as environmental scans

Foreign key: A key attribute used to link one entity/table to another

Fourteen principles of management: Henri Fayol's key points in the formulation of the administrative approach to management

Frame data: *See* Motion video

Fraud and abuse legislation: Federal laws that address the intentional and mistaken misrepresentation of reimbursement claims submitted to government-sponsored health programs

Free-text data: Data that are narrative in nature

Freedom of Information Act (FOIA): A federal law, applicable only to federal agencies, through which individuals can seek access to information without the authorization of the person to whom the information applies

Frequency distribution: A table or graph that displays the number of times (frequency) a particular observation occurs

Frequency polygon: A type of line graph that represents a frequency distribution

Fuzzy logic: A technique used in data mining that handles imprecise concepts

Gantt chart: A project management chart showing how sequential tasks are scheduled over time

General ledger: A master list of individual accounts maintained by an organization

Generalizability: The ability to apply research results, data, or observations to groups not originally under study

Generic screening: *See* Occurrence screening

Genetic algorithms: Optimization techniques that can be used to improve other data-mining algorithms so that they derive the best model for a given set of data

Geographic adjustment factor (GAF): Used by the Centers for Medicare and Medicaid Services to account for regional variation in the cost of ambulance service so that reimbursement amounts for this service can be determined

Geographic information system (GIS): A decision support system that is capable of assembling, storing, manipulating, and displaying geographically referenced data and information

Geographic practice cost index (GPCI): An index used for making local adjustments to the resource-based relative value scale; GPCI values include physicians' services (GPCIw), practice expenses (GPCIpe), and malpractice costs (GPCIm)

Gesture recognition technology: *See* Intelligent character recognition (ICR) technology

Global payment: A payment made for radiological and other procedures that includes professional and technical components and is paid as a lump sum to be distributed between the physician and the healthcare facility

Global surgery payment: A payment made for surgical procedures that includes the provision of all healthcare services, from the treatment decision through normal postoperative patient care

Goal: The reflection in more specific terms of what a department does or what deliverable good is provided

Going concern: An organization that is assumed to continue indefinitely unless otherwise stated

Government Accounting Standards Board (GASB): A federal agency that sets the accounting standards to be followed by government entities

Graphical user interface (GUI): An electronic interface that uses images (for example, small pictures, or icons) to represent the tasks, functions, and programs performed by the software

Graphics-based decision support system: A decision support system in which the knowledge base consists primarily of graphical data and the user interface exploits the use of graphical display

Great person theory: The belief that some people have natural leadership skills or inherit them

Grievance: A formal, written description of a complaint or disagreement

Grievance procedures: The steps employees can follow to seek resolution of disagreements with management on job-related issues

Gross autopsy rate: The number of inpatient autopsies conducted during a given time period divided by the total number of inpatient deaths for the same time period

Gross death rate: The number of inpatient deaths that occurred during a given time period divided by the total number of inpatient discharges, including deaths, for the same time period

Group health insurance: A prepaid medical plan that covers the healthcare expenses of a company's full-time employees

Group model health maintenance organization: A closed-panel health maintenance organization that provides contracted healthcare services to subscribers

Group practice without walls (GPWW): A type of managed care contract that allows physicians to maintain their own offices and share administrative services (billing, medical transcription, and so on)

Groupware: An Internet technology that consolidates documents from different information systems within the organization into a tightly integrated workflow

Habit: An activity repeated so often that it becomes automatic

Hawthorne effect: A study finding that novelty, attention, and interpersonal relations had a motivating effect on performance, giving impetus to the human relations movement

Hay method: A modification of the point method of job evaluation that numerically measures the levels of three major compensable factors: know-how, problem-solving ability, and accountability requirements; also known as the Hay Guide Chart/Profile Method of Job Evaluation

HCFA-1500: Former name of the CMS-1500 form

Health Care Financing Administration (HCFA): *See* Centers for Medicare and Medicaid Services (CMS)

Health Care Quality Improvement Program (HCQIP): A quality initiative begun in 1992 by the Health Care Financing Administration (since 2001 called the Centers for Medicare and Medicaid Services) and implemented by peer review organizations; uses patterns of care analysis and collaboration with practitioners, beneficiaries, providers, plans, and other purchasers of healthcare services to develop scientifically based quality indicators and to identify and implement opportunities for healthcare improvement

Health delivery network: *See* Integrated provider organization (IPO)

Health Industry Business Communications Council (HIBCC): A subgroup of the American Standards Committee X12 that focuses on electronic data interchange for billing transactions

Health informatics standards: A set of standards that describes accepted methods for collecting, maintaining, and/or transferring healthcare data among computer systems

Health information: According to HIPAA privacy provisions, any information (verbal or written) created or received by a healthcare provider, health plan, public health authority, employer, life insurer, school or university, or healthcare clearinghouse that relates to the physical or mental health of an individual, provision of healthcare to an individual, or payment for provision of healthcare

Health information management (HIM): A professional field that ensures that high-quality data and information are available to every type of authorized user who depends on the data or information to deliver high-quality healthcare services and to make high-quality healthcare-related decisions

Health information management professional: An allied healthcare worker who has graduated from an accredited health information technology or administration program and/or holds one or more professional credentials (RHIA, RHIT, CCS, CCS-P)

Health information services department: The department in healthcare organizations that is responsible for maintaining records of patient care in accordance with external and internal rules and regulations; formerly known as the medical records department

Health Informatics Standards Board (HISB): A subgroup of the American National Standards Institute that acts as an umbrella organization for groups interested in developing healthcare computer messaging standards

Health Insurance Portability and Accountability Act of 1996 (HIPAA): Federal legislation to specifically direct the Department of Health and Human Services to protect the confidentiality and security of electronically transmitted health information

Health Level Seven (HL7): A standards development organization accredited by the American National Standards Institute that addresses issues at the seventh, or application, level of healthcare systems interconnections

Health maintenance organization (HMO): A prepaid health plan that provides healthcare services to enrollees in return for monthly premiums; must meet the requirements of the federal HMO act

Health management information system (HMIS): A system whose purpose is to provide reports on routine operations and processing (for example, a pharmacy inventory system, radiological system, and patient-tracking system)

Health Plan Employer Information Data Set® (HEDIS®): A set of performance measures developed by the National Commission for Quality Assurance that are designed to provide purchasers and consumers of healthcare with information to compare the performance of managed care plans

Health record: A paper- or computer-based tool for collecting and storing information about the healthcare services provided to a patient; also called patient record, medical record, resident record, or client record, depending on the healthcare setting

Health record number: A unique numeric or alphanumeric identifier assigned to each patient's record upon admission to a healthcare facility

Health Resources and Services Administration (HRSA): The national organization that administers the State Children's Health Insurance Program (SCHIP) along with the Centers for Medicare and Medicaid Services

Health science librarian: A professional librarian who manages a medical library that offers local and remote access to medical information

Health services research: Research concerning healthcare delivery systems, including their organization and delivery and the effectiveness and efficiency of the care they provide

Healthcare claims (HCC) and payment/advice transaction: An electronic transmission sent by a health plan to a provider's financial representative for the purpose of providing information about payments and/or payment processing and information about the transfer of funds

Healthcare Cost and Utilization Project (HCUP): A group of healthcare databases and related software tools developed through collaboration by the federal government, state governments, and industry; this resource is sponsored by the Agency for Healthcare Research and Quality and brings together the data collection efforts of state data organizations, hospital associations, private data organizations, and the federal government to create a national information resource of patient-level health care data

Healthcare Common Procedure Coding System (HCPCS): A classification system composed of three levels (I, Current Procedural Terminology (CPT) codes; II, codes for equipment, supplies, and services not covered by CPT codes as well as modifiers that can be used with all levels of codes; and III, local codes developed by regional Medicare Part B carriers) and used to report physicians' services and supplies to Medicare for reimbursement

Healthcare Information Management and Systems Society (HIMSS): A membership association that provides leadership in healthcare for the management of technology, information, and change

Healthcare information system (HIS): A transactional system used in healthcare organizations (for example, patient admitting, accounting, receivables, and so on); also called hospital information system

Healthcare Information Systems Steering Committee: An interdisciplinary team of healthcare professionals generally responsible for developing a strategic information systems (IS) plan, prioritizing IS projects, and coordinating IS-related projects across the enterprise

Healthcare Integrity and Protection Data Bank (HIPDB): A national database that collects information on cases of healthcare fraud and abuse

Healthcare provider: An individual (such as a physician) who renders medical services (such as office visits) or a facility (such as a hospital) that provides medical services (such as outpatient surgery)

Heterogeneity: The state or fact that a thing shows variation

Hierarchy: An authoritarian organizational structure in which each member is assigned a specific rank that reflects his or her level of decision-making authority within the organization

Hierarchy of needs: Maslow's theory suggesting that needs are organized hierarchically from basic physiological to creative motives

Hill-Burton Act: Enacted in 1946 as the Hospital Survey and Construction Act, legislation that authorized grants for states to construct new hospitals and, later, to modernize old ones

Histocompatibility: The immunologic similarity between an organ donor and a recipient

Histogram: A graphic technique used to display the frequency distribution of continuous data as either numbers or percentages in a series of bars

Historical research: A design of research that investigates the past

History: The pertinent information about the patient, including chief complaint, past and present illnesses, family history, social history, and review of body systems

Home Assessment Validation and Entry (HAVEN): Data-entry software used to collect Outcome and Assessment Information Set (OASIS) data and then transmit them to state databases; imports and exports data in standard OASIS record format, maintains agency/patient/employee information, enforces data integrity through rigorous edit checks, and provides comprehensive online help

Home health agency (HHA): An organization that provides medical care in the residence of a homebound Medicare beneficiary who needs intermittent or part-time skilled nursing and/or certain other therapy or rehabilitation care

Home health care: Care provided to individuals and families in their place of residence with the goal of promoting, maintaining, or restoring health or minimizing the effects of disability and illness, including terminal illness

Home health prospective payment system (HH PPS): A reimbursement system developed by the Centers for Medicare and Medicaid Services to cover home care services provided to Medicare beneficiaries

Home health resource group (HHRG): A classification system established to support the prospective reimbursement of covered home care services provided to Medicare beneficiaries during sixty-day episodes of care

Horizontally integrated system: *See* Integrated provider organization (IPO)

Hospice: An organization that specializes in providing medical care or psychosocial support in the home or in inpatient or outpatient settings to the terminally ill, their families, or significant others

Hospice care: Medical care provided to persons with life expectancies of six months or less who elect to forgo standard Medicare benefits for treatment of their illness and to receive only palliative care

Hospital autopsy: A postmortem examination performed on the body of a person who has at some time been a hospital patient by a hospital pathologist or a physician of the medical staff who has been delegated the responsibility

Hospital autopsy rate: The total number of autopsies performed by the hospital pathologist for a given time period divided by the number of deaths of hospital patients (inpatients or outpatients) whose bodies are available for autopsy for the same time period

Hospital death rate: The number of inpatient deaths for a given period of time divided by the total number of live discharges and deaths for the same time period

Hospital discharge abstract system: A group of databases compiled from aggregate data on all patients discharged from a hospital

Hospital information system (HIS): *See* Healthcare information system (HIS)

Hospital inpatient autopsy: A postmortem examination performed on the body of a patient who died during an inpatient hospitalization by a hospital pathologist or a physician of the medical staff who has been delegated the responsibility

Hospital newborn inpatient: A patient born in the hospital at the beginning of the current inpatient hospitalization

Hospital Standardization Program: An early twentieth-century survey mechanism instituted by the American College of Surgeons aimed at identifying quality-of-care problems and improving patient care; precursor to the survey program developed by the Joint Commission on Accreditation of Healthcare Organizations (JCAHO)

Hospital-acquired infection: *See* Nosocomial infection

Hospital-based ambulatory surgery center: A hospital department that provides the surgical facilities in which same-day surgical procedures can be performed

Hospitalization insurance (HI) (Medicare Part A): A federal program that covers the costs associated with inpatient hospitalizations as well as other healthcare services provided to Medicare beneficiaries

Human relations movement: A management philosophy emphasizing the shift from a mechanistic view of workers to concern for their satisfaction at work

Human subjects: Individuals whose physiologic or behavioral characteristics and responses are the object of study in a research program

Hybrid online analytical processing (HOLAP): A data access methodology that is coupled tightly with the architecture of the database management system to allow the user to perform business analyses

Hypertext markup language (HTML): A standardized language that allows the electronic transfer of information and communications among many different information systems

Hypothesis: A statement of the research question in measurable terms

Identifier standards: Recommended methods for assigning unique identifiers to individuals (patients, clinical providers), corporate providers, and healthcare vendors and suppliers

Image processing: The ability of a computer to "take a picture" of a text block, photograph, drawing, or other image and make it available throughout an information system

Imaging technology: Health record software that is able to combine health record text files with diagnostic imaging files

Implementation phase: The third phase of the systems development life cycle during which a comprehensive plan is developed and instituted to ensure that the new information system is effectively implemented within the organization

Implied consent: The type of permission that is inferred when a patient voluntarily submits to treatment

Incentive: Something that stimulates or encourages an individual to work harder

Incentive pay: A system of bonuses and rewards based on employee productivity; often used in transcription areas of healthcare facilities

Incidence: The number of new cases of a specific disease

Incidence rate: A computation that compares the number of new cases of a specific disease for a given time period to the population at risk for the disease during the same time period

Incident: A happening that is inconsistent with the standard of care

Incident report: A quality/performance management tool used to collect data and information about potentially compensable events (events that have the potential of resulting in death or serious injuries)

Incident report review: An analysis of incident reports or an evaluation of descriptions of adverse events

Income statement: A statement that summarizes an organization's revenue and expense accounts using totals accumulated during the fiscal year

Indemnity plans: Health insurance coverage provided in the form of cash payments to patients or providers

Independent practice association (IPA): An open-panel health maintenance organization that provides contract healthcare services to subscribers through independent physicians who treat patients in their own offices; also called individual practice association or foundations model

Independent variable: An antecedent factor that researchers manipulate directly; the cause

Index: An organized (most often alphabetical) list of specific data that serves to guide, indicate, or otherwise facilitate reference to the data

Indian Health Service (IHS): The agency within the Department of Health and Human Services responsible for providing federal health services to American Indians and Alaska natives

Indicator(s): An activity, event, occurrence, or outcome that is to be monitored and evaluated, under a Joint Commission on Accreditation of Healthcare Organizations (JCAHO) standard, in order to determine whether those aspects conform to standards; commonly relates to structure, process, and/or outcome of an important aspect of care

Indicator measurement system: An indicator-based monitoring system developed by the Joint Commission on Accreditation of Healthcare Organizations (JCAHO) for accredited organizations and meant to provide hospitals with information on their performance

Individual: According to HIPAA privacy provisions, a person who is the subject of protected health information

Inductive reasoning: A process of creating conclusions based on a limited number of observations (induction)

Infant mortality rate: The number of deaths of persons under one year of age during a given time period divided by the number of live births reported for the same time period

Infection control: A system for the prevention of communicable diseases that concentrates on protecting healthcare workers and patients against exposure to disease-causing organisms and promotes compliance with applicable legal requirements through early identification of potential sources of contamination and implementation of policies and procedures that limit the spread of disease

Inference engine: The component of the decision support system that "reasons" from the available data and knowledge

Inferential statistics: A set of statistical techniques that allows researchers to make inferences about a population's characteristics (parameters) on the basis of a sample's characteristics

Informatics: The science of information management applied within an electronic (computer-based) environment for specific types of users, for example nursing informatics, dental informatics, consumer informatics, medical informatics, healthcare informatics, clinical informatics, and so on

Information: Data that have been collected, combined, analyzed, interpreted, and/or converted into a form that can be used for specific purposes

Information assets: Sources of information within an organization such as databases, documents, and employee expertise

Information kiosk: A computer station located within a healthcare facility that patients and families can use to access information

Information management: The management of the acquisition, organization, analysis, storage, retrieval, and dissemination of information to support decision-making activities

Information resource management: A concept that assumes that information is a valuable resource that must be managed, regardless of the form it takes or the medium in which it is stored

Information science: The study of the nature and principles of information

Information system (IS): An automated system that uses computer hardware and software to record, manipulate, store, recover, and disseminate data; that is, a system that receives and processes input and provides output; often used interchangeably with the term information technology (IT)

Information systems department: The department in a healthcare organization that is responsible for ensuring that the organization has the technical infrastructure and staff required to operate and manage its computer-based systems

Information technology (IT): A term used to describe the combination of computer technology (hardware and software) with telecommunications technology (data, image, and voice networks); often used interchangeably with the term information system (IS)

Information technology professional: An individual who works with computer technology in the process of managing health information

Information technology strategy: An organization's information technology (IT) goals, objectives, and strategic plans, which serve as a guide to the procurement of information systems within an organization

Informed consent: An individual's voluntary agreement to participate in research or to undergo a diagnostic, therapeutic, or preventive procedure

Initiating structure: A leadership orientation toward task, procedures, goals, and production

Injury severity score (ISS): An overall severity measurement maintained in the trauma registry and calculated from the abbreviated injury scores for the three most severe injuries of each patient

Innovators: A category of adopters of innovations who are eager to experiment with changes

Inpatient: An individual who receives healthcare services as well as room, board, and continuous nursing services in a unit or area of a hospital

Inpatient admission: A hospital's formal acceptance of a patient who is to be provided room, board, and continuous nursing services in an area of the hospital where patients generally stay at least overnight

Inpatient bed occupancy rate: The total number of inpatient service days for a given time period divided by the total number of inpatient bed count days for the same time period; also called percentage of occupancy

Inpatient coding compliance: The accurate and complete assignment of ICD-9-CM diagnosis and procedure codes, along with appropriate sequencing (for example, identification of principal diagnosis) to determine the appropriate diagnosis-related group and resultant payment

Inpatient discharge: The termination of hospitalization through the formal release of an inpatient by a hospital

Inpatient hospitalization: The period in a person's life when he or she is a patient in a single hospital without interruption except by possible intervening leaves of absence

Inpatient rehabilitation facility (IRF): A healthcare facility that specializes in providing services to patients who have suffered a disabling illness or injury in an effort to help them achieve and maintain their optimal level of functioning, self-care, and independence

Inpatient Rehabilitation Validation and Entry (IRVEN): A computerized data entry system for inpatient rehabilitation facilities

Inpatient service day: A unit of measure equivalent to the services received by one inpatient during one twenty-four-hour period

In-service education: Training that teaches employees specific skills required to maintain or improve performance, usually internal to an organization

Institute of Electrical and Electronics Engineers (IEEE): A national organization that develops standards for hospital system interface transactions, including links between critical care bedside instruments and clinical information systems

Institute of Medicine (IOM): A branch of the National Academy of Sciences whose mission is to advance and distribute scientific knowledge to improve human health

Institutional review board (IRB): An administrative body that provides oversight for the research studies conducted within an institution

Instrument: A way that is standardized and uniform to collect data

Integrated delivery system (IDS): A group of healthcare organizations that collectively provides a full range of coordinated health-related services from preventive care to complex hospital-based treatment

Integrated health record format: A system of health record organization in which all of the paper forms are arranged in strict chronological order and mixed with forms created by different departments

Integrated provider organization (IPO): An organization that manages the delivery of healthcare services provided by hospitals, physicians (employees of the IPO), and other healthcare organizations (for example, nursing facilities); also called accountable health plan, delivery system, health delivery network, horizontally integrated system, integrated service network, vertically integrated plan, or vertically integrated system

Integration: The complex task of ensuring that all elements and platforms of an information system communicate and act as a uniform entity

Integrity constraints: Limits placed on the data that can be entered into a database

Insured: A holder of a health insurance policy

Insurer: An organization that pays healthcare expenses on behalf of its enrollees; a third-party payer

Integrated service network: *See* Integrated provider organization (IPO)

Intellectual capital: The combined knowledge of an organization's employees with respect to operations, processes, history, and culture

Intelligent character recognition (ICR) technology: A method of encoding handwritten, print, or cursive characters and of interpreting the characters as words or the intent of the writer; also called gesture recognition technology

Intensity-of-service screening criteria: Preestablished standards used to determine the most efficient healthcare setting in which to safely provide needed services

Interactive voice technology (IVT): A communications technology that enables an individual to use a telephone to access information from a computer

Interface: The zone between different computer systems across which users want to pass information, for example, a computer program written to exchange information between systems or the graphic display of an application program designed to make the program easier to use

Interim payment system (IPS): A cost-based reimbursement system that was used until the home health prospective payment system was phased in

Interim period: Any period that represents less than an entire fiscal year

Intermediate care facility: A facility that provides health-related care and services to individuals who do not require the degree of care or treatment that a hospital or a skilled nursing facility provides but who still require medical care and services because of their physical or mental condition

Internal rate of return (IRR): An interest rate that makes the net present value calculation equal zero

Internal validity: An attribute of a study's design that contributes to the accuracy of its findings

***International Classification of Diseases, Ninth Revision, Clinical Modification* (ICD-9-CM):** A classification system used in the United States to report morbidity and mortality information

***International Classification of Diseases for Oncology, Second Edition* (ICD-O-2):** Classification system used for reporting incidences of malignant disease

Internet: An international network of computer servers that provides individual users with communications channels and access to software and information repositories worldwide

Internet browser: Client software that facilitates communications with World Wide Web information servers

Interpersonal skills: One of the three managerial skill categories that includes skills in communicating and relating effectively to others

Interpreter: Communications technology that converts high-level language statements into machine language one at a time

Interrater reliability: A measure of an instrument's reliability (that is, different persons using the instrument will have reasonably similar findings); consistency in data collection among different abstractors

Interrogatories: Discovery devices consisting of a set of written questions to a party, witness, or other person who has information needed in a case

Interval data: A type of data that represent observations that can be measured on an evenly distributed scale beginning at a point other than true zero

Intervention: A manipulation, treatment, or therapy; a broad term used by researchers to generically mean some act

Interview guide: A written list of all the questions to be asked during an interview

Interview survey: A type of survey in which the members of a population in question are orally questioned

Intranet: A private Internet network whose servers are located inside a firewall or security barrier so that the general public cannot gain access to information housed within the network

Intrarater reliability: A measure of an instrument's reliability meaning that the same person repeating the test will have reasonably similar findings

Intuition: Unconscious decision making based on extensive experience in similar situations

Inventor: A role in organizational innovation which requires idea generation

Inventory: The goods on hand that are available to sell, presumably within a year (a business cycle)

Inverse relationship: *See* Negative relationship

IP telephony: Communications technology that allows people to initiate real-time calls through the Internet instead of the public telephone system; also called voiceover IP, or VoIP

ISO 9000: An internationally agreed upon set of generic standards for quality management

Issue Log: Documentation describing questions, concerns, and problems that must be solved in order for a task to be completed

Job classification: A method of job evaluation that compares a written position description with the written descriptions of various classification grades; method used by the federal government to grade jobs

Job description: A list of a job's duties, reporting relationships, working conditions, and responsibilities

Job evaluation: The process of applying predefined compensable factors to jobs to determine their relative worth

Job procedure: A structured, action-oriented list of sequential steps involved in carrying out a specific job or solving a problem

Job ranking: A method of job evaluation that arranges jobs in a hierarchy on the basis of each job's importance to the organization, with jobs that are the most important at the top of the hierarchy and jobs that are the least important at the bottom

Job rotation: A job design in which workers are shifted periodically among different tasks

Job sharing: A work schedule in which a full-time job is split among two or more persons

Job description: *See* Position description

Job specification: A list of a job's required education, skills, knowledge, abilities, personal qualifications, and physical requirements

Joint Commission on Accreditation of Healthcare Organizations (JCAHO): A not-for-profit organization that offers an accreditation program for hospitals and other healthcare organizations on the basis of predefined performance standards

Journal entry: An accounting representation of a financial transaction or transfer of amounts between accounts; contains at least one debit and one credit, and the dollar value of the debits and the dollar value of the credits is the same

Judge-made law: *See* Common law

Jurisdiction: The power and authority of a court to hear and decide specific types of cases

Justice: The impartial administration of policies or laws that takes into consideration the competing interests and limited resources of the individuals or groups involved

K-nearest neighbor (K-NN): A classic technique used to discover associations and sequences when the data attributes are numeric

Key attributes: Common fields (attributes) within a relational database that are used to link tables to one another

Key field: A key or field that uniquely identifies each row in a table in a database; also called primary key

Knowledge: The information, understanding, and experience that gives individuals the power to make informed decisions

Knowledge assets: Assets that are the sources of knowledge for an organization; examples include printed documents, unwritten rules, work flows, customer knowledge, data in databases and spreadsheets, and the human expertise, know-how, and tacit knowledge within the minds of the organization's workforce

Knowledge base: A database, often a data repository, that manages not only raw data but also integrates them with information from various reference works

Knowledge management: A philosophy that promotes an integrated and collaborative approach to the process of information asset creation, capture, organization, access, and use

Knowledge worker: An employee who improves his or her performance by sharing knowledge with others

Labor organization: *See* Union

Labor relations: The human resources management activities associated with unions and collective bargaining

Laggards: A category of adopters of innovations who are very reluctant to accept proposed changes and may resist transition

Language translator: A software system that translates a program written in a particular computer language into a language that other types of computers can understand

Late majority: A category of adopters of innovation who change only in response to peer, authority, or economic pressure

Leader–member relations: A situation in contingency theory describing how well the leader is liked, respected, and followed

Leadership grid: A leadership model proposed by Blake and Mouton based on a grid measure of concern for people and production

Leading: One of the four management functions in which people are directed and motivated to achieve goals

Learning curve: The time required to acquire certain skills and to apply them so that new levels of productivity and/or performance exceed prelearning levels (productivity often is inversely related to the learning curve)

Learning organization: An organization where the emphasis is on acquiring and sharing business knowledge, along with delivering information quickly, clearly, and visually to everyone within the organization, with a strong emphasis on data integrity

Least Preferred Coworker Scale (LPC): Fiedler's use of a bipolar scale to measure task-relationship orientation in contingency theory

Lecture: A one-way method of delivering education through speaking, where the teacher delivers the speech and the student listens

Legislative law: *See* Statutory law

Length of stay (LOS): The number of calendar days an inpatient is hospitalized from admission to discharge

Lexicon: Vocabulary used in a language or a subject area, or by a particular speaker or group of speakers

Liability: Legal responsibility, often with financial repercussions, for adverse occurrences; also, an amount owed by the organization to others

Licensure: The legal authority or formal permission from authorities to carry on certain activities that by law or regulation require such permission; may be applied to institutions as well as individuals

Line authority: Authority to manage subordinates and to have them report back; based on relationships illustrated in an organizational chart

Line graph: A graphic technique that consists of a line that connects a series of points on an arithmetic scale; often used to display time trends or survival curves

Linear programming: An operational management technique using mathematical formulas to determine the optimal way to allocate resources for a project

Linkage analysis: A technique used to explore and examine relationships among a large number of variables of different types

Literature review: A systematic investigation of all the knowledge about a topic; may include books, journal articles, theses, and dissertations

Litigation: A civil lawsuit or contest in court

Local-area network (LAN): A network that connects computers in a relatively small area

Logical: A user's view of the way data or systems are organized, for example, a file that is a collection of data stored together; opposite of physical

Logical data model: The second level of data model that is drawn according to the type of database that will be developed

Long-term care: Health and/or personal care services required by the chronically ill, aged, disabled, or mentally handicapped individuals who reside in a nursing facility

Longitudinal: A type of time frame that collects data from the same participants at multiple points in time

Longitudinal record: A health record maintained across time, ideally from birth to death

Loss prevention: A risk control strategy that includes developing and revising policies and procedures that are both facilitywide and department specific

Loss reduction: A component of a risk management program that encompasses techniques used to manage events or claims that already have taken place

Low-utilization payment adjustment (LUPA): Alternative (reduced) payment made to home health agencies, instead of the home health resource group (HHRG) reimbursement rate when a patient receives fewer than four home care visits during a sixty-day episode

Machine language: A language using binary codes made up of zeroes and ones that the computer uses directly to represent precise storage locations and operations

Machine learning: An area of computer science that studies algorithms and computer programs that improve employee performance on some task by exposure to a training or learning experience

Mainframe: The second-most powerful type of computer hardware, after the supercomputer; includes small-, medium-, and large-scale computers that serve individual, hundreds, or thousands of users, respectively

Mainframe computer: A type of computer that was used for centralized computer applications in hospitals beginning in the 1960s

Maintenance and evaluation phase: The fourth and final phase of the systems development life cycle that helps to ensure that adequate technical support staff and resources are available to maintain or support the new system

Major medical insurance: A contract for prepaid healthcare benefits that includes a high limit for most types of medical expenses, usually requires a large deductible and sometimes places limits on coverage and charges, for example, room and board; also called catastrophic coverage

Managed care: A delivery system that influences or controls the utilization and reimbursement of healthcare services

Managed care organization (MCO): A healthcare organization that provides medical care under negotiated contracts between payers and providers that limit access to care or require discounted payment to providers of services

Managed fee-for-service plan: A healthcare plan that implements utilization controls (prospective and retrospective review of healthcare services) for reimbursement under traditional fee-for-service insurance plans

Management: The process of planning, organizing, and leading an organization's activities

Management by objectives (MBO): A management approach that defines target objectives for organizing work and for comparing performance against those objectives

Management functions: The functions of planning, organizing, directing, coordinating, and controlling

Management information system (MIS): A computer-based system that provides information to a healthcare organization's managers for use in making decisions that affect a variety of day-to-day activities

Management service organization (MSO): An organization, usually owned by a group of physicians or a hospital, that provides administrative and management support services to individual physicians' practices

Managerial accounting: The development, implementation, and analysis of systems that track financial transactions for management control purposes, including both budget systems and cost analysis systems

Many-to-many relationship: The concept that multiple instances of an entity may be associated with multiple instances of another entity; only occurs in a conceptual-level data model

Massed training: The condition of learning a large amount of material at one time

Master patient index: *See* Master population index

Master person index: *See* Master population index

Master population index (MPI): A list or database maintained by a healthcare facility that records the names and identifications of every patient who has ever been admitted or treated in the facility; also called master patient index or master person index

Matching expenses: Expenses that are recorded during the same period as the related revenue

Materiality: The significance of a dollar amount based on predetermined criteria

Maternal death rate (hospital-based): The total number of maternal deaths directly related to pregnancy for a given time period divided by the total number of obstetrical discharges for the same time period

Maternal mortality rate (community-based): The total number of deaths attributed to maternal conditions during a given time period divided by the total number of live births for the same time period

Mean: A measure of central tendency; arithmetic average of the observations in a frequency distribution

Measures of central tendency: Measures of location that indicate the typical value of a frequency distribution

Media controls: Policies and procedures designed to safeguard different computer media such as tapes, disks, and videos

Median: A measure of central tendency that shows the midpoint of a frequency distribution when the observations have been arranged in order from lowest to highest

Medicaid: A federal entitlement program that oversees medical assistance for individuals and families with low incomes and limited resources

Medical audits: *See* Medical care evaluation studies

Medical care evaluation studies: Audits required through the Conditions of Participation that require the use of screening criteria with evaluation by diagnosis and/or procedure; also called medical audits

Medical Data Interchange Standard (MEDIX): A set of hospital system interface transaction standards developed by the Institute of Electrical and Electronic Engineers

Medical foundation: A nonprofit organization that contracts with physician practices and acquires clinical and business assets; the foundation manages the practice's business

Medical Group Management Association (MGMA): A national organization composed of individuals actively engaged in the business management of medical groups that consist of three or more physicians in medical practice

Medical informaticians: Physicians specializing in medical information processing

Medical informatics: A field of information science concerned with the management of data and information used to diagnose, treat, cure, and prevent disease through the application of computers and computer technologies

Medical Literature, Analysis, and Retrieval System Online (MEDLINE): A computerized, online database of the bibliographic Medical Literature Analysis and Retrieval System (MEDLARS) of the National Library of Medicine

Medical malpractice: The professional liability of health-care providers in the delivery of patient care

Medical records department: *See* Health information services department

Medical research: *See* Clinical research

Medical savings account (MSA) plans: Plans that provide benefits after a single, high deductible has been met; Medicare makes an annual deposit to the MSA, and the beneficiary is expected to use the money in the MSA to pay for medical expenses below the annual deductible

Medical service bureaus: Organized groups of physicians who were paid by employers during the early 1900s to provide healthcare services to employees

Medical staff bylaws: A document adopted by a hospital's medical staff to govern its business conduct and the rights and responsibilities of its members

Medical staff classifications: Categories of clinical practice privileges assigned to individual practitioners on the basis of their qualifications

Medical transcription: The conversion of verbal medical reports dictated by healthcare providers into written form for inclusion in the health record

Medical transcriptionist: A medical language specialist who types or word processes information dictated by providers

Medically needy option (Medicaid): An option that allows states to extend Medicaid eligibility to persons who would be eligible for Medicaid under one of the mandatory or optional groups but whose income and/or resources exceed the eligibility level set by the state

Medicare: A federally funded health program established in 1965 to assist with the medical care costs of Americans sixty-five years of age and older, as well as individuals entitled to Social Security benefits

Medicare Conditions of Participation: A publication that describes the requirements that healthcare providers must meet to quality for reimbursement under the Medicare program

Medicare Economic Index (MEI): The economic index upon which Medicare reimbursement rates are based

Medicare fee schedule (MFS): Feature of the resource-based relative value system that includes a complete list of the payments Medicare makes to physicians and other providers; revised annually

Medicare prospective payment system: *See* Prospective payment system (PPS)

Medicare+Choice (Medicare Part C): A federally funded element of the Medicare program implemented as part of the Balanced Budget Act of 1997 to provide expanded options for the delivery of healthcare services

Medigap: A private insurance policy that supplements Medicare coverage

Mental ability tests: Tests that assess the reasoning capabilities of individuals

Mentoring: A form of coaching in which an individual in the beginning stages of a career is matched as a protégé with a senior person who coaches and advises

Message format standards: Another term for data exchange standards

Messaging standards: *See* Transmission standards

Metaanalysis: A method of research that involves the statistical analysis of a large collection of results from individual studies for the purpose of integrating the studies' findings

Metadata: Data about data

Method: A strategy that a researcher employs to collect, analyze, and present data

Microcomputer: A personal computer characterized by its "desktop" size and relatively fast processing speed

Microcontroller: A small, low-cost computer placed within an appliance or device to perform a specific task or program

Microfilming: A photographic process that reduces an original paper document into a small image on film; the process of miniaturizing information to save storage space

Middle managers: Managers who oversee the operations of a broad scope of functions at the departmental level or oversee defined product or service lines

Midsize computer: *See* Minicomputer

Minicomputer: A small mainframe computer; also called a midsize computer

Minimum Data Set for Long-Term Care, Version 2.0 (MDS 2.0): A federally mandated standard assessment form used to collect demographic and clinical data about nursing home residents

Minimum Data Set for Post Acute Care (MDS-PAC): A patient-centered assessment instrument completed for each Medicare patient that emphasizes a patient's care needs instead of provider characteristics

Minimum necessary: A term used to refer to the HIPAA requirement that the use, access, and disclosure of health information to healthcare providers and other covered entities must be limited to the least amount needed to accomplish an intended purpose

Misdemeanor: A crime that is less serious than a felony

Mission statement: A short description of the general purpose of an organization or group

Mode: A measure of central tendency that is the most frequently occurring observation in a frequency distribution

Model: The representation of a theory in a visual format, on a smaller scale, or with objects

Morality: Personal values about what is considered right or wrong

Morbidity: A term referring to the incidence of disease

Mortality: A term referring to the incidence of death; the loss of subjects during the course of the study; also called attrition

Motion video: The storing, manipulating, and displaying moving images in a format, such as frames, that can be presented on a computer monitor; also called frame data and streaming video

Motivation: The drive to accomplish a task

Movement diagram: A chart that depicts the location of furniture and equipment in a work area and shows the usual movement or work flow of individuals or paper as they progress through the work area

Multidimensional data structure: A structure whereby data are organized according to the dimensions associated with them

Multidimensional database management systems (MDDBMS): A database management system specifically designed to handle data organized into a multidimensional data structure

Multidimensional online analytical processing (MOLAP): A data access methodology that is coupled tightly with a multidimensional database management system to allow the user to perform business analyses

Multimedia: The combination of free-text, raster or vector graphic, sound, and/or motion video/frame data

Multivariate: An adjective meaning the involvement of many variables

Multivoting technique: A decision-making method for determining group consensus on the prioritization of issues or solutions

National Association of Healthcare Quality (NAHQ): An organization devoted to advancing the profession of healthcare quality improvement through its accreditation program

National Center for Health Statistics (NCHS): The federal agency responsible for collecting and disseminating information on health services utilization and the health status of the population in the United States

National Committee for Quality Assurance (NCQA): A private not-for-profit organization whose mission is to evaluate and report on the quality of managed care organizations; measures performance and accredits managed care organizations

National Committee on Vital and Health Statistics (NCVHS): A public policy advisory board that recommends policy to the National Center for Health Statistics and other health-related federal programs

National conversion factor (CF): A mathematical factor used to convert relative value units (RVUs) into monetary payments

National Correct Coding Initiative: A series of code edits on Medicare Part B claims

National Council on Prescription Drug Programs (NCPDP): A standards-setting organization for data interchange and processing standards for pharmacy transactions

National Guideline Clearinghouse (NGC): A partnership among the Agency for Healthcare Research and Quality, the American Medical Association, and the American Association of Health Plans that allows free online access to its clinical guidelines

National Health Care Survey: A national public health survey that contains data abstracted manually from a sample of acute care hospitals or from discharged inpatient records or that are obtained from state or other discharge databases

National Information Infrastructure—Health Information Network Program (NII-HIN): A national quasi-governmental organization that provides oversight of all healthcare information standards in the United States

National Practitioner Data Bank (NPDB): A databank established by the federal government through the 1986 Health Care Quality Improvement Act containing professional review actions on physicians and other licensed care practitioners; healthcare organizations are required to check the databank as part of the credentialing process

National provider file (NPF): A file currently being developed by the Centers for Medicare and Medicaid Services that will include all healthcare providers, including nonphysicians, and sites of care

National provider identifier (NPI): An eight-character alphanumeric identifier used to identify individual healthcare providers

National Uniform Billing Committee (NUBC): A national committee responsible for identifying data elements and designing the UB-92

National Uniform Claim Committee (NUCC): A national committee that replaced the Uniform Claim Form Task Force in 1995 and developed a standard data set to be used in the transmission of noninstitutional provider claims to and from third-party payers

National Vaccine Advisory Committee (NVAC): A national committee that acts as an advisory committee for the director of the National Vaccine Program

National Vital Statistics System (NVSS): A federal agency responsible for the collection of official vital statistics of the United States

Natural language: A fifth-generation programming language that uses human language to give people a more natural connection with computers

Natural language processing: A process by which digital text from online documents stored in the organization's information system is read directly by software and automatically coded

Natural language processing technology: The extraction of unstructured or structured medical word data, which are then translated into diagnostic or procedural codes for clinical and administrative applications

Naturalism: A philosophy of research that assumes that multiple contextual truths exist and that bias is always present; also known as qualitative approach

Naturalistic observation: A type of nonparticipant observation in which researchers observe certain behaviors and events as they occur naturally

Need-to-know principle: A principle that supports the release of information that is needed by a particular individual for a particular task, but no more than exactly what is needed

Needs assessment: A procedure performed to determine what is required, lacking, or desired by an employee or organization

Negative relationship: A relationship in which the effects move in opposite directions; also called inverse relationship

Negligence: In law, the result of an action by an individual who does not act the way a reasonably prudent person would act under the same circumstances

Neonatal mortality rate: The number of deaths of infants under twenty-eight days of age during a given time period divided by the total number of births for the same time period

Net autopsy rate: The total number of inpatient autopsies performed by the hospital pathologist for a given time period divided by the total number of inpatient deaths minus unautopsied coroner's or medical examiner's cases for the same time period

Net death rate: The total number of inpatient deaths minus the number of deaths that occurred less than forty-eight hours after admission for a given time period divided by the total number of inpatient discharges minus the number of deaths that occurred less than forty-eight hours after admission for the same time period

Net income: The difference between total revenues and total expenses

Net loss: The condition when total expenses exceed total revenue

Net present value: The current value of an investment that takes into consideration cash outlays and inflows over the life of the asset at a specified interest rate

Network: A specific technology that connects different systems so that they can share information

Network administrators: Individuals involved in installing, configuring, managing, monitoring, and maintaining network applications who are responsible for supporting the network infrastructure and controlling user access

Network controls: Methods for protecting data from unauthorized access and corruption during transmission between information systems

Network model health maintenance organization: A managed care organization that enters into contracts with two or more physician multispecialty group practices to provide healthcare services to subscribers

Network protocol: A set of conventions that governs the exchange of data between hardware and/or software components in a communications network

Network provider: A physician or another healthcare professional who is a member of a managed care network

Neural networks: Nonlinear predictive models that, using a set of data that describes what a person wants to find, detect a pattern to match a particular profile through a training process that involves interactive learning

Neutral zone: Bridges's transitional stage in organizational change in which the past has been left, but the future stage is not yet clearly established

New beginnings: Bridges's final stage of transition management in which the new organization is formed

Newborn (NB): A hospital inpatient who is born in the hospital at the beginning of the current inpatient hospitalization

Newborn autopsy rate: The number of autopsies performed on newborn deaths for a given time period divided by the total number of newborn deaths for the same time period

Newborn death rate: The number of newborns deaths divided by the total number of newborns, both alive and dead

Nomenclature: A system of terms that is structured according to preestablished naming rules; also referred to as clinical terminology

Nominal data: A type of data that represents values or observations that can be labeled or named (*nom* = name)

Nominal group technique: A group process technique in which individual group members generate ideas and then share, discuss, and rank-order their ideas into a single list

Nonexempt employees: All groups of employees covered by the provisions of the Fair Labor Standards Act

Nonmaleficence: A legal principle that means "do not harm" that is often used in conjunction with *beneficence* (for example, beneficence would require the release of health information whether or not it benefited a patient and nonmaleficence would require the denial of release of information whether or not it was known that employment or insurance discrimination would result)

Nonparametric technique: A type of statistical procedure used for variables that are not normally distributed in a population; also called distribution-free technique

Nonparticipant observation: A method of research in which researchers act as neutral observers who do not intentionally interact nor affect the actions of the population being observed

Nonparticipating provider: A healthcare provider that did not sign a participation agreement with Medicare and so is not obligated to accept assignment on Medicare claims

Nonprogrammed decision: A decision that involves careful and deliberate thought and discussion because of a unique, complex, or changing situation

Nonrandom sampling: A sample in which all members of the target population do not have an equal or independent chance of being selected; two types of nonrandom sampling are convenience sampling and purposive sampling

Normal distribution: A continuous frequency distribution characterized by a bell-shaped curve in which the mean, the median, and the mode are equal

Normalization: A formal process applied to relational database design to determine which variables should be grouped together in a table in order to reduce data redundancy across and within the tables

Normative decision model: A decision tree developed by Vroom-Yetton to determine when to make decisions independently, collaboratively, or by delegation

Nosocomial infection: An infectious disease contracted by a patient during an inpatient hospitalization; also called hospital-acquired infection

Nosocomial infection rate: The number of hospital-acquired infections for a given time period divided by the total number of inpatient discharges for the same time period

Nosology: A branch of medical science that deals with classification systems

Not-for-profit organizations: Organizations not owned by individuals, where profits may be held for a specific purpose or reinvested in the organizations for the benefit of the community they serve

Notice of privacy practice: According to HIPAA privacy provisions, a written statement provided to individual patients that describes how a covered entity will use and disclose protected health information; also describes the privacy rights of individuals and the entity's legal duties with respect to protecting such information

Notifiable disease: A disease that requires regular, frequent, and timely information on individual cases in order to prevent and control the disease

Null hypothesis: A hypothesis that states there is no association between the independent and dependent variables

Nursing informatics: A field of information science concerned with the management of data and information used to support the practice and delivery of nursing care through the application of computers and computer technologies

Nursing vocabulary: A classification system used to capture documentation on nursing care

Object: The basic component in the object-oriented database that includes both data and their relationships within a single structure

Object-oriented databases (OODB): A database that uses commands that act as small, self-contained instructional units (objects) that may be combined in various ways

Object-oriented database management system (OODBMS): A specific set of programs used to implement an object-oriented database

Object-relational database: A database that stores both objects and traditional tables; it is both object oriented and relational

Objective: A statement of the end result expected, stated in measurable terms, usually with a time limitation (deadline date) and often with a cost estimate or limitation

Observational research: A method of research in which researchers obtain data by observing rather than by asking

Observational study: An epidemiological study in which the exposure and outcome for each individual in the study is observed

Occasion of service: A specified identifiable service involved in the care of a patient that is not an encounter (for example, a lab test ordered for an encounter)

Occupational Safety and Health Act of 1970 (OSHA): Federal legislation that establishes comprehensive safety and health guidelines for employers

Occurrence screening: A risk management technique in which the risk manager reviews the health records of current and discharged hospital patients with the goal of identifying potentially compensable events; also called generic screening

Odds ratio: A relative measure of occurrence of an illness; the odds of exposure in a diseased group divided by the odds of exposure in a nondiseased group

Omnibus Budget Reconciliation Act (OBRA): Federal legislation passed in 1989 that mandated important changes in the payment rules for Medicare physicians

Online analytical processing (OLAP): A data access architecture that exploits the multidimensional data structure, allowing the user to drill down into the data by selecting and summarizing them along any combination of their dimensions and permitting the retrieval and summary of large volumes of data

Online analytical processing (OLAP) engine: An optimized query generator that can retrieve the right information from the warehouse to accommodate what-if business queries

Online/real-time analytical processing (OLAP): Online/real-time query tools, commonly found in data warehouses, data marts, and decision support systems, that allow users to analyze database information by interpreting their requests and providing data based on multiple search parameters

Online/real-time transaction processing (OLTP): Tools that allow transactions between user and database to be processed online and in real-time by accepting user requests and returning immediate answers across multiple platforms

On-the-job training: A method of training in which an individual learns a job while working at it

One-tailed hypothesis: An alternative hypothesis in which the researcher makes a prediction in one direction

One-to-many relationship: A relationship that exists when one instance of an entity is associated with multiple instances of another entity

One-to-one relationship: A relationship that exists when an instance of an entity is associated with only one instance of another entity, and vice versa

Open record: The health record of a patient who is still in the facility or an active patient of the facility

Open-ended question: *See* Unstructured question

Open-record review: A review of health records of patients currently in the hospital or under active treatment; part of the Joint Commission on Accreditation of Healthcare Organizations (JCAHO) survey process

Open systems: Systems that are affected by what is going on around them and must adjust as the environment changes

Operating system: The principal piece of software in any computer system that consists of a master set of programs that manage the basic operations of the computer

Operation index: A list of the operations and procedures performed on patients and sequenced according to the code numbers of the classification system in use

Operational budget: A type of budget that allocates and controls resources to meet an organization's goals and objectives for the fiscal year

Operational decision making: A type of decision making that involves the day-to-day operation of a business unit or the day-to-day execution of a job task

Operational goal: A short-term objective set by the organization to improve how it operates

Operational plan: A strategic plan implemented at the first-line level of daily activities

Operations management: The application of mathematical and statistical techniques to production and distribution efficiency

Operations research (OR): A scientific discipline primarily begun during World War II that seeks to apply the scientific method and mathematical models to analyze and solve a variety of management decision problems

Operations support system (OSS): An information system that facilitates the operational management of a healthcare organization

Optical character recognition (OCR) technology: A method of encoding text from analog paper into bit-mapped images and translating the images into a form, such as the American Standard Code for Information Interchange (ASCII), that is computer-readable

Optical imaging: The process by which information is scanned onto optical disks

Ordinal data: A type of data that represents values or observations that can be ranked or ordered

Organization: The planned coordination of the activities of more than one person for the achievement of a common purpose or goal

Organization development (OD): The application of behavioral science research and practices to planned organizational change

Organizational chart: A graphic representation of an organization's formal structure

Organizational pull model: A model in which the organization views information systems technology as the means to enable people in the organization to work more efficiently and effectively

Orientation: A set of activities designed to familiarize new employees with their jobs and the organization and its work culture

Orion Project: A Joint Commission on Accreditation of Healthcare Organizations (JCAHO) initiative designed to test accreditation models, develop a continuous accreditation process, and test alternative processes for reporting survey findings to hospitals

ORYX initiative: A Joint Commission on Accreditation of Healthcare Organizations (JCAHO) initiative that encourages the integration of outcomes data and other performance measurement data into the accreditation process

Outcome: A term from Donabedian's model of quality assessment that focuses on the end result of the treatment process

Outcome indicators: Measurements of the end results of a process (for example, complications, adverse effects, patient satisfaction)

Outcome measure: An assessment of the end result of care for an individual patient or for a group of patients within a specific diagnostic category

Outcomes and Assessment Information Set (OASIS): A standard core assessment data tool developed to measure the outcome of adult patients receiving home health services

Outcomes and effectiveness research (OER): Research performed to understand the end results of particular healthcare practices and interventions

Outcomes management: A systematic process in which outcomes data are collected; "ideal" care processes are identified and used, and outcomes analyzed; and care processes are further refined

Outguide: A type of tracking system used in paper-based health record systems

Out-of-pocket expenses: Healthcare costs paid by the insured (for example, deductibles, copayments, and coinsurance) after which the insurer pays a percentage (often 80 or 100 percent) of covered expenses

Outpatient: A patient who receives ambulatory care services in hospital-based clinics and departments

Outpatient and emergency department coding compliance: Accurate and complete assignment of ICD-9-CM diagnosis codes and CPT/HCPCS procedure/service codes, along with appropriate sequencing (for example, identification of the primary diagnosis)

Outpatient code editor (OCE): Software linked to the Correct Coding Initiative that applies a set of logical rules to determine whether various combinations of codes are correct and appropriately represent the services provided

Outpatient prospective payment system (OPPS): The Medicare reimbursement system for hospital outpatient services and procedures; based on ambulatory payment classification (APC) groups

Outsourcing: The hiring of an individual or company external to an organization to perform a job function either on-site or off-site

Overhead costs: In a healthcare facility, the expenses associated with supporting, but not rendering, patient care services

Packaging: Payment under the outpatient prospective payment system that includes items such as anesthesia, supplies, certain drugs, and the use of recovery and observation rooms

Packet switching: An information transmission system in which data are encoded into packets (short units) and sent through an electronic communications network

Palliative care: Medical care designed to relieve the patient's pain and suffering without attempting to cure the underlying disease

Panel interview: An interview format in which the applicant is interviewed by several interviewers at the same time

Paradigm: A mental model or way of understanding that provides a framework for perceiving, understanding, and responding to the world

Parallel work division: Concurrent handling, where one employee does several tasks and basically sees the job through from beginning to end

Parametric technique: A type of statistical procedure based on the assumption that a variable is normally distributed in a population

Pareto chart: A descending bar graph that visually displays a group's prioritization of issues, problems, or solutions

Participant observation: A research method in which researchers are also participants in the observed actions

Partnership: The venture of two or more owners for whom the profits represent the owners' personal income

Path-goal theory: A situational leadership theory that emphasizes the role of the leader in removing barriers to goals

Patient advocacy: The function performed by patient representatives (sometimes called ombudsmen) when they respond personally to complaints from patients and/or their families

Patient assessment instrument (PAI): A standardized tool used to evaluate the patient's condition after admission to, and at discharge from, a healthcare facility

Patient care system: A type of information system that has traditionally been designed for nursing documentation

Patient Self-Determination Act (PSDA): Federal legislation that requires healthcare facilities to provide written information on the patient's right to be given advance directives and to accept or refuse medical treatment

Patient-specific/identifiable data: Personal information that can be linked to an individual patient, such as age, gender, date of birth, address, and so on

Payback period: The time required to recoup the cost of an investment

Payer of last resort: A Medicaid term that means that Medicare pays for the services provided to individuals enrolled in both Medicare and Medicaid until Medicare benefits are exhausted and Medicaid benefits begin

Payment status indicator (PSI): An alphabetic code assigned to HCPCS/CPT codes to indicate whether a service or procedure is to be reimbursed under the outpatient prospective payment system

PDSA cycle: A performance improvement model designed specifically for healthcare organizations; PDSA stands for **P**lan, **D**o, **S**tudy, and **A**ct

Peer review: The process in which experts in the field evaluate the quality of a manuscript

Peer review organization (PRO): *See* Quality improvement organization (QIO)

Peer-reviewed journal: A type of journal in which content experts evaluate the articles for quality prior to publication; also called refereed journal

Percentage of occupancy: *See* Inpatient bed occupancy rate

Per-diem reimbursement: Payment for all of the services provided during one day

Per member per month (PMPM): *See* Per patient per month

Per patient per month (PPPM): A type of managed care arrangement by which providers are paid a fixed fee in exchange for supplying all of the healthcare services a patient needs for a specified period of time (usually one month); also called per member per month (PMPM)

Performance improvement (PI): A continuous process carried out by a healthcare organization to ensure that its services, processes, and outcomes are being incrementally improved on an ongoing basis

Performance indicator: A measure used by healthcare facilities to assess the quality, effectiveness, and efficiency of their services

Performance measure: A quantitative tool used to assess the clinical, financial, and utilization aspects of a healthcare provider's outcomes or processes

Performance measurement: The process of comparing the outcomes of an organization, work unit, or employee against preestablished performance plans and standards

Performance standards: The stated expectations for acceptable quality and productivity associated with a job function

Performance tests: *See* Ability tests

Peripheral: Any hardware device connected to a computer (for example, a keyboard, mouse, or printer)

Permanent variance: The difference between the budgeted amount and the actual amount of a line item that is not expected to reverse itself during a subsequent period

Personal digital assistant (PDA): A small, portable microcomputer capable of running applications such as e-mail and task managers

Personal health record (PHR): An electronic health record maintained and updated by an individual for him- or herself

Physical: The actual organization of data in a system, for example, a single file divided into many pieces scattered across a disk; opposite of logical

Physical access controls: Security safeguards that protect a healthcare organization's equipment, media, and facilities from intruders

Physical data model: The lowest level of data model with the lowest level of abstraction

Physician index: A list of patients and their physicians that is usually arranged according to the physician code numbers assigned by the facility

Physician–hospital organization (PHO): An organization that provides services to subscribers through an arrangement among physicians and hospital(s); previously known as a medical staff–hospital organization, or MeSH

Physiological signal processing systems: Systems that store vector graphic data based on the human body's signals and create output based on the lines plotted between the signals' points

Pie chart: A graphic technique in which the proportions of a category are displayed as "pieces" of a pie

Piece-rate incentive: An adjustment of the money paid a worker based on exceeding a certain level of output

Pilot study: A trial run on a smaller scale; a feasibility study

Pixel: An acronym for the term picture element, defined by many tiny bits of data or dots/points

Placebo: A medication with no active ingredients

Plaintiff: A person or group (party) initiating a civil action

Planning: One of the four managerial functions involving the examination of the future and preparation of action plans to attain goals

Point method: A method of job evaluation that places weight (points) on each of the compensable factors in a job; the total points associated with a job establish its relative worth; jobs that fall within a specific range of points fall into a pay grade with an associated wage

Point-of-care information systems: Systems that allow healthcare providers to capture and retrieve data and information at the location where the healthcare service is performed

Point-of-service (POS) plan: A type of managed care health plan in which subscribers are encouraged to select a primary care provider from within a network but may also seek care from nonnetwork providers when they are willing to pay a larger share of the cost than they would for network providers

Policy: A statement that describes how a department or an organization is supposed to handle specific situations

Policyholder: An individual who is covered by an insurance contract

Population-based registry: A type of registry that includes information from more than one facility in a specific geopolitical area, such as a state or region

Population-based statistics: Statistics based on a defined population rather than on a sample drawn from that same population

Position description: A document that outlines the work responsibilities associated with a job; also called job description

Position power: A situation in contingency theory in which the leader is perceived as having the authority to give direction

Positive relationship: A relationship in which the effect moves in the same direction; also called direct relationship

Positivism: *See* Quantitative approach

Postneonatal mortality rate: The number of deaths of persons aged twenty eight days up to, but not including, one year during a given time period divided by the number of live births for the same time period

Postoperative infection rate: The number of infections that occur in clean surgical cases for a given time period divided by the total number of operations within the same time period

Potentially compensable event (PCE): An event, injury, or accident that may result in financial liability to the organization

Practice guidelines: Protocols of care that guide the clinical care process; also known as Care Maps™, critical paths, and clinical practice guidelines

Preadmission utilization review: A type of review conducted before a patient's admission to an acute care facility to determine whether the planned service (intensity of service) or the patient's condition (severity of illness) warrants care in an inpatient setting

Precision factor: The definitive tolerable error rate to be considered when calculating productivity standards

Predecessor: A task that affects the scheduling of a successor task in a dependency relationship

Predictive modeling: A process that can be used to identify patterns that can be used to predict the odds of a particular outcome based on the observed data

Preferred provider organization (PPO): A managed care arrangement in which a group of providers contracts with an employer to provide healthcare services to employees at a discounted rate

Pregnancy Discrimination Act: Federal legislation that prohibits discrimination against women affected by pregnancy, childbirth, or related medical conditions; requires that affected women are treated the same as all other employees for employment-related purposes, including benefits

Premium: A monthly fee collected from a policyholder by an insurer

Prevalence rate: The proportion of people in a population that have a particular disease at a specific point in time or over a specified period of time

Preventive controls: Internal controls implemented prior to an activity and designed to stop an error from happening

Primary analysis: The analysis of original research data by the researchers who collected them

Primary care manager (PCM): A healthcare provider assigned to a TRICARE enrollee

Primary care physician (PCP): A physician who initially diagnoses and refers a patient and coordinates the patient's healthcare services

Primary data source: A record developed by healthcare professionals in the process of providing patient care

Primary key: *See* Key field

Primary source: An original work of the researcher who conducted the investigation

Principal diagnosis: A condition established, after study, to have resulted in an inpatient admission

Principal investigator: The individual with primary responsibility for the design and conduct of the research project

Principal procedure: A procedure performed for the definitive treatment of a condition (as opposed to a procedure performed for diagnostic or exploratory purposes) or for care of a complication

Privacy: The right of every individual to be left alone

Privacy Act of 1974: Legislation that gave individuals some control over information collected about them by the federal government

Privacy officer: The individual responsible for the development and implementation of an organization's privacy policies and procedures

Privacy rule: The standards for privacy of individually identifiable health information promulgated by the Department of Health and Human Services pursuant to the Health Insurance and Portability Act of 1996

Private branch exchange (PBX): A switching system for telephones on private extension lines that allows access to the public telephone network

Private law: The collective rules and principles that define the rights and duties of people and private businesses

Private, unrestricted fee-for-service plan: A prepaid health insurance plan that allows beneficiaries to select private healthcare providers

Privilege: The professional relationship between patients and specific groups of caregivers that affect the patient's health record and its contents as evidence

Privileging process: The process of evaluating a physician's quality of medical practice and determining the services he or she is qualified to perform

Probate court: A state court that handles wills and settles estates

Problem-oriented health record: A way of organizing information in a health record in which clinical problems are defined and documented individually

Procedural codes: The numeric or alphanumeric characters used to identify the clinical procedures performed

Procedure: A document that describes the steps involved in performing a specific function

Process: A term from Donabedian's model of quality assessment that focuses on how care is provided

Process and workflow modeling: The identification of the flow of work and information required to perform a function, including decomposition diagrams, dependency diagrams, and data flow

Process indicators: Specific measures that enable the assessment of the steps taken in rendering a service

Productivity: A unit of performance defined by management in quantitative standards

Productivity software: Computer software used for word processing, spreadsheet, and database management applications

Professional component (PC): The portion of radiological and other procedures performed by a physician

Professional standards review organization (PSRO): As mandated by the Social Security Act of 1972, an organization that reviews the medical necessity of inpatient admissions and treatment costs, along with medical records

Profitability index: An index used to prioritize investment opportunities, where the present value of the cash inflows is divided by the present value of the cash outflows for each investment, and the results are compared

Program evaluation and review technique (PERT): A project management technique developed to determine time lines and paths for project activities

Programmed decisions: An automated decision made by people or computers based on a situation being so stable and recurrent that decision rules can be applied to it

Programmers: Individuals primarily responsible for writing program codes and developing applications, typically performing the function of systems development and working closely with system analysts

Programming language: A set of words and symbols that allows programmers to tell the computer what operations to follow

Programs of All-Inclusive Care for the Elderly (PACE): State option legislated by the Balanced Budget Act of 1997 that provides an alternative to institutional care for individuals fifty-five years old or older who require the level of care provided by nursing facilities

Progress notes: The documentation provided by the healthcare provider as entries into the health record to indicate the patient's response to treatment and services provided

Progressive discipline: A four-step process for shaping employee behavior to conform with the requirements of the employee's job position; the process begins with a verbal caution and progresses to written reprimand, suspension, and dismissal upon subsequent offenses

Project charters: Documents that define projects; also known as statements of work

Project components: Related parameters of scope, resources, and scheduling with regard to a project

Project management software: Application software that provides the tools to create and track a project

Project network: The definition of the relationship between tasks in a project; determines the overall project finish date

Project office: A support function for project management best practices

Project plan: A plan that consists of a list of the tasks to be performed in a project, a defined order in which they will occur, the task start and finish dates, and the resource effort needed to complete each task

Project schedule: A portion of the project plan that deals specifically with task start and finish dates

Project team: A collection of individuals assigned to work on a project

Proportion: A type of ratio in which the numerator is always included in the denominator

Proportionate mortality ratio (PMR): The total number of deaths due to a specific cause during a given time period divided by the total number of deaths due to all causes

Prosecutor: An attorney who, on behalf of the government, prosecutes an accused for a crime

Prospective payment system (PPS): A type of reimbursement system based on preset reimbursement levels rather than on actual charges billed after the service has been provided

Prospective study: A study designed to observe outcomes or events that occur after the identification of the group of subjects to be studied

Prospective utilization review: A review of a patient's health records before admission to determine the necessity of admission to an acute care facility and to determine or satisfy benefit coverage requirements

Protected health information (PHI): According to HIPAA privacy provisions, individually identifiable information that is transmitted by electronic media, maintained in any medium (paper or electronic), or is transmitted or maintained in any other form or medium

Protocol: A rule or procedure to be followed in a clinical trial

Public assistance: A monetary subsidy provided to financially needy individuals; also called welfare

Public health: An area of healthcare that deals with the health of populations in geopolitical areas, such as states and counties

Public health services: Services concerned primarily with the health of entire communities and population groups

Public key infrastructure (PKI): A system of digital certificates and other registration authorities that verify and authenticate the validity of each party involved in a secure transaction

Public law: Legislation that involves the government and its relations with individuals and business organizations

Purchase order: A paper document or electronic screen on which all details of an intended purchase are reported, including authorizations

Purposive sampling: A strategy of qualitative research in which researchers use their expertise to select representative units and unrepresentative units to capture a wide array of perspectives

Push technology: Active computer technology that sends information directly to the end user when it becomes available

Qualified disabled and working individuals (QDWIs): Medicare beneficiaries who are eligible for assistance including disabled and working people who previously qualified for Medicare because of disability but lost entitlement because of their return to work (despite the disability)

Qualified Medicare beneficiaries (QMBs): Medicare beneficiaries who have resources at or below twice the standard allowed under the Social Security Income program and incomes at or below 100 percent of the federal poverty level

Qualifying individuals (QIs): Medicare beneficiaries whose incomes are at least 120 percent but less than 175 percent of the federal poverty level

Qualitative analysis: A review of the health record to ensure that standards are met and to determine the adequacy of entries documenting the quality of care

Qualitative approach: *See* Naturalism

Qualitative standards: Service standards in the context of setting expectations for how well or how soon work or a service will be performed

Quality: The degree or grade of excellence of goods or services, including, in healthcare, meeting expectations for outcomes of care

Quality assurance: A set of activities designed to measure the quality of a service, product, or process with remedial action, as needed, to maintain a desired standard

Quality improvement (QI): A set of activities that measures the quality of a service or product through systems or process evaluation and then implements revised processes that result in better healthcare outcomes for patients, based on standards of care

Quality improvement organization (QIO): An organization under contract with the Centers for Medicare and Medicaid Services to ensure that Medicare beneficiaries receive high-quality healthcare that is medically necessary and appropriate and meets professionally recognized standards of care; until 2002, called peer review organization

Quality indicator: A standard against which actual care can be measured to identify a level of performance for that standard

Quality review organization: A quality improvement organization or an accrediting body

Quantitative analysis: A review of the health record to determine its completeness and accuracy

Quantitative approach: A philosophy of research that assumes a single truth across time and place; assumes that researchers' are able to adopt a neutral, unbiased stance and establish causation; also known as positivism

Quantitative standards: Measures of productivity in the context of setting expectations for how efficiently or productively work will be performed

Quasi-experimental design: *See* Causal-comparative research

Questionnaire survey: A type of survey in which the members of the population are questioned with electronic or paper forms (questionnaires)

Queuing theory: An operations management technique for examining customer flow and designing ideal wait or scheduling times

Random sampling: An unbiased selection of subjects that includes methods such as simple random sampling, stratified random sampling, systematic sampling, and cluster sampling

Randomization: The assignment of subjects to groups (experimental or control) based on chance

Randomized clinical trial (RCT): A special type of clinical trial in which the researchers follow strict rules to randomly assign patients to groups

Range: A measure of variability between the smallest and largest observations in a frequency distribution

Raster image: Digital data or an image made up of pixels in a horizontal and vertical grid or a matrix instead of lines plotted between a series of points

Rate: A measure used to compare an event over time; comparison of the number of times an event did happen (numerator) with the number of times an event could have happened (denominator)

Ratio: A comparison of categories of a variable that fall into two categories, such as male to female, or of one category to the whole, such as male discharges to all discharges

Ratio data: A type of data that represents observations that can be measured on an evenly distributed scale beginning at a true zero

Read Codes: Codes developed by British physician James Read for recording and retrieving computerized primary care data; now known as Clinical Terms, Version 3 (CTV3)

Real audio data: The storing, manipulating and displaying sound in a computer-readable format; also called sound data

Record: *See* Row

Recruitment: The process of finding, soliciting, and attracting employees

Reengineering: A process of fundamental rethinking and radical redesign of business processes to achieve significant performance improvements

Refereed journal: *See* Peer-reviewed journal

Reference data: Information that interacts with the care of the individual or with the healthcare delivery system, such as a formulary, protocol, care plan, clinical alert, or reminder

Reference terminology: A set of concepts and relationships which provide a common reference (or consultation) point for comparison and aggregation of data about the entire health care process, recorded by multiple individuals, systems, or institutions

Referred outpatient: A patient referred by a physician for ambulatory or outpatient care outside the facility

Reflective learning: A cycle of reflection, interpretation, application of learning, and doing that is the basis of total quality management (TQM) and other continuous improvement practices

Refreezing: Lewin's last stage of change in which people internalize new practices following transition

Registered health information administrator (RHIA): Certification granted after completion of an AHIMA-accredited four-year program in health information management and a credentialing examination

Registered health information technician (RHIT): Certification granted after completion of an AHIMA-accredited two-year program in health information management and a credentialing examination

Rehabilitation services: Health services provided to assist patients in achieving and maintaining their level of function, self-care, and independence after some type of disability

Reimbursement: Payment for services provided

Reinforcement: The process of increasing the probability of a desired response through reward

Relational database: A type of database that stores data in predefined tables made up of rows and columns

Relational database management system (RDMS): A database management system in which data are organized and managed as a collection of tables

Relational online analytical processing (ROLAP): A data access methodology that provides users with various drill-down and business analysis capabilities similar to online analytical processing

Relationship: A type of connection between two terms

Relative risk (RR): A ratio that compares the risk of disease between two groups; also referred to as risk ratio

Relative value unit (RVU): Associated with the resource-based relative value scale (RBRVS), relative values for physician work (RVUw), practice expenses (RVUpe), and malpractice costs (RVUm)

Release of information (ROI): The process of disclosing patient information from the health record to another party

Reliability: A term that refers to the consistency with which a test measures an attribute

Remittance advice (RA): An explanation of payments (for example, claim denials) made by third-party payers

Report cards: A method used by managed care organizations (and other healthcare sectors) to report cost and quality of care provided

Request for information (RFI): A written communication often sent to a comprehensive list of vendors during the design phase of the systems development life cycle to ask for general product information

Request for production: A discovery device used to compel another party to produce documents and other items or evidence that are important to a lawsuit

Request for proposal (RFP): A type of business correspondence that asks for very specific product and contract information; often sent to a narrow list of vendors that have been preselected after a review of requests for information (RFIs) during the design phase of the systems development life cycle

Requisition: A request from a clinical or other area in a healthcare organization to charge out a medical record

Research data: Data used for the purpose of answering a proposed question or testing a hypothesis; in healthcare the data may be gathered through documentation of the activities of care in the patient's health record or may be gathered for specific research purposes in clinical trials

Research method: The particular strategy that a researcher uses to collect, analyze, and present data

Research methodology: The study and analysis of research study and theories

Reserves: Unused profits from a not-for-profit organization that stay in the business

Resident assessment instrument (RAI): A uniform assessment instrument developed by the Centers for Medicare and Medicaid Services to standardize the collection of skilled nursing facility patient data; includes the Minimum Data Set 2.0, triggers, and resident assessment protocols

Resident assessment protocol (RAP): A summary of resident problems and care needs in long-term care settings

Resident Assessment Validation and Entry (RAVEN): Data-entry software developed by the Health Care Financing Administration for long-term care facilities and used to collect Minimum Data Set 2.0 (MDS) assessments and to transmit data to state databases

Resource Utilization Groups, Version III (RUG-III): A classification system for skilled nursing facility residents that is case-mix–adjusted and based on Minimum Data Set 2.0 (MDS) assessments

Resource-based relative value scale (RBRVS) system: A payment system implemented in 1992 to reimburse physicians according to a fee schedule; based on values assigned to services

Resources: The labor, equipment, or materials needed to complete a project

Respite care: Any inpatient care provided to a hospice patient for the purpose of giving primary caregivers a break from their caregiving responsibilities

Responsibility: Accountability required as part of a job, such as supervising work performed by others

Restitution: The act of returning something to its rightful owner, of making good or giving something equivalent for any loss, damage, or injury

Resume: A document that describes a job candidate's educational background, work experience, and professional achievements

Retained earnings: Undistributed profits from a for-profit organization that stay in the business

Retention: The ability to keep valuable employees from seeking employment elsewhere

Retention schedules: Lists of how long various records are to be maintained according to rules, regulations, standards, and laws

Retrospective: A type of time frame that looks back in time

Retrospective payment system: A reimbursement system that is based on charges calculated after the delivery of healthcare services

Retrospective study: A type of research conducted by reviewing records from the past (for example, birth and death certificates and/or health records) or by obtaining information about past events through surveys or interviews; *see also* case-control (retrospective) study

Retrospective utilization review: A review of records some time after the patient's discharge to determine any of several issues, including the quality or appropriateness of the care provided

Return on investment (ROI): An increase in market value resulting from an investment divided by the initial investment

Revenue: Earned and measurable income

Revenue codes: UB-92 form locator that requires data entry to identify services provided to patients; *see also* Uniform Bill-92 (UB-92)

Risk analysis: An assessment of possible security threats to the organization's data

Risk management (RM): The process of overseeing the medical, legal, and administrative operations within a healthcare organization to minimize its exposure to liability

Risk prevention: One component of a successful risk management program

Risks: Threats to the success of a project

Roles and responsibilities: The definition of who does what on a project and the hierarchy for decision making

Root-cause analysis: A technique used in performance improvement initiatives to discover the underlying causes of a problem

Row: A set of columns or a collection of related data items in a table; also called record

Rule induction: *See* Association rule analysis

Rules and regulations: *See* Bylaws

Run chart: A type of graph that shows data points collected over time and identifies emerging trends or patterns

Safety management: A system for providing a risk-free environment for patients, visitors, and employees

Sample: A set of units selected for study that represents the population

Sample size: The number of subjects needed in the study to represent the population

Sample size calculation: The qualitative and quantitative procedures to determine the appropriate sample size

Sample survey: A type of survey that collects data from some representative members of the population

Satisficing: A decision process in which the decision maker accepts a solution to a problem that is a *satisfactory* solution rather than an optimal solution

Scalar chain: A theory in the chain of command in which everyone is included and authority and responsibility flow downward from the top of the organization

Scanning: The process by which a document is read into an optical imaging system

Scatter diagram: A graph that visually displays the linear relationships among factors

Scenarios: A storytelling technique

Scheduling engine: A specific functionality in project management software that automates the assignment of task start and finish dates and, as a result, the expected project finish date

Scientific inquiry: A process that comprises making predictions, collecting and analyzing evidence, testing alternative theories, and choosing the best theory

Scope: The amount of effort and materials needed to produce project deliverables

Scope of command: The number and type of employees who report to a specific management position in a defined organizational structure

Scope of work: The time period that an organization is under contract to perform as a quality improvement organization

Screen prototype: A sketch of the user interface of each screen that is anticipated in a project

Secondary analysis: A method of research that involves the analysis of the original work of another person or organization

Secondary data source: Data derived from the primary patient record, such as an index or a database

Secondary release of information: A type of information release in which the initial requester forwards confidential information to others without obtaining required patient authorization

Secondary source: A summary of an original work, such as an encyclopedia

Secondary storage: Permanent storage of data and programs on disks or tapes

Secondary variable: *See* Confounding variable

Securities Exchange Commission (SEC): A federal agency that regulates all public and some private transactions involving the ownership and debt of organizations

Security: The physical safety of facilities and equipment protected from theft, damage, or unauthorized access; also includes protection of data, information, and information networks from loss and damage as well as unauthorized access and alteration

Security breach: Violation of the policies or standards developed to ensure security

Security management: The oversight of facilities, equipment, and other resources, including human resources and technology, to reduce the possibility of harm or theft to these assets of an organization

Security program: A plan that outlines the policies and procedures created to protect healthcare information

Security standards: Statements that describe the processes and procedures meant to ensure that patient-identifiable health information remains confidential and protected from unauthorized disclosure, alteration, and destruction

Security threat: A situation that has the potential to damage a healthcare organization's information system

Self-directed learning: An instructional method that allows students to control their own learning and progress at their own pace

Self-monitoring: The act of observing the reactions of others to one's behavior and making the necessary behavioral adjustments to improve the reactions of others in the future

Semantics: A term that refers to comparable meaning, usually achieved through a standard vocabulary

Semistructured question: A type of question that begins with a structured question and follows with an unstructured question to clarify

Sentinel event: A term used by the Joint Commission on Accreditation of Healthcare Organizations (JCAHO) to describe an unexpected occurrence involving death or serious physical or psychological injury, or the risk thereof

Sequence diagram: A systems analysis tool for documenting the interaction between an actor and the information system

Serial filing system: A health record identification system in which a patient receives sequential unique numerical identifiers for each encounter with or admission to a healthcare facility

Serial work division: A system of work organization where each task is performed by one person who then hands the product to another person who does the next task in sequence

Serial-unit numbering system: A health record identification system in which patient numbers are assigned in a serial manner but records are brought forward and filed under the last number assigned

Server: A computer that makes it possible to share information resources across a network of client computers

Severity-of-illness screening criteria: Standards used to determine the most appropriate setting of care based on the level of clinical signs and symptoms that a patient shows upon presentation to a healthcare facility

Service: A unit of performance defined by providers and customers in qualitative standards

Seven dimensions of data quality: Characteristics used to evaluate the quality of data, including relevancy, granularity, precision, timeliness, currency, consistency, and accuracy

Severity indexing: The process of using clinical evidence to identify the level of resource consumption; a method for determining degrees of illness

Shared systems: Systems developed by data-processing companies during the 1960s and 1970s to address the computing needs of healthcare organizations that could not afford, or chose not to purchase, their own mainframe computing systems

Signal tracing data: *See* Vector graphic data

Significance level: The criterion used for rejecting the null hypothesis (alpha [α] level)

Simon's decision-making model: A model proposing that the decision-making process moves through three phases: intelligence, design, and choice

Simple random sampling: The process of selecting units from a population so that every unit has exactly the same chance of being included in the sample

Simulation and inventory modeling: Key components of a plan that are computer-simulated for testing and experimentation so that optimal operational procedures can be found

Simulation observation: A type of nonparticipant observation in which researchers stage events rather than allowing them to happen naturally

Simultaneous equations method: A budgeting concept that distributes overhead costs through multiple iterations, allowing maximum distribution of interdepartmental costs among overhead departments

Single-blinded study: A study design in which, typically, the investigator, but not the subject, knows the identity of the treatment and control groups

Skill: The ability, education, experience, and training required to perform job tasks

Skilled nursing facility (SNF): A long-term care facility that uses an organized professional staff and permanent facilities (including inpatient beds) to provide continuous nursing and other health-related, psychosocial, and personal services to residents in the nonacute phase of illness

Skilled nursing facility prospective payment system (SNF PPS): A per-diem reimbursement system implemented in July 1998 for costs (routine, ancillary, and capital) associated with covered SNF services furnished to Medicare Part A beneficiaries

Smart card: A plastic card that contains integrated circuit technology that allows information to be "written to" or "read from" the card

Snowflake schema: A modification of the star schema in which the dimension tables are further divided to reduce data redundancy

SOAP: An acronym for a component of the problem-oriented medical record that refers to how each progress note contains documentation relative to **s**ubjective observations, **o**bjective observations, **a**ssessments, and **p**lans

Social Security Act: Federal legislation providing support for state public health activities and healthcare services for mothers and children

Social Security number (SSN): A unique numerical identifier assigned to every U.S. citizen

Socialization: The process of influencing the behavior and attitudes of a new employee to adapt positively to the work environment

Software: A program that directs the hardware components of a computer system to perform the tasks required

Sole proprietorship: A venture with one owner in which all profits are considered the owner's personal income

Sound data: *See* Real audio data

Source-oriented health record format: A system of health record organization in which information is arranged according to the patient care department that provided the care

Spaced training: The process of learning a task in sections separated by time

Span of control: The number of subordinates reporting to a supervisor

Special cause variation: An unusual source of variation that occurs outside a process but affects it

Specialty software: Applications software that performs specialized, niche functions such as encoding or drawing and painting

Specified low-income Medicare beneficiaries (SLMBs): Medicare beneficiaries who have resources similar to qualified Medicare beneficiaries but who have higher incomes, although still less than 120 percent of the federal poverty level

Speech recognition: The ability of a computer application to use natural voice conversation as input

Sponsor: A person or an entity that initiates a clinical investigation of a drug (usually the drug manufacturer or research institution that developed the drug) by distributing it to investigators for clinical trials; also a role in organizational innovation that supports, protects, and promotes an idea within the organization

Stillborn death: *See* Fetal death

Structured query language (SQL): A computer programming language that gives information systems the ability to query and report on data

Stable monetary unit: Currency that is used as the measurement of financial transactions

Staff authority: The lines of reporting in the organizational chart in which the position advises or makes recommendations

Staff model health maintenance organization: A closed-panel health maintenance organization (HMO) that employs physicians to provide healthcare services to subscribers; premiums are paid directly to the HMO, and ambulatory care services are usually provided within HMO corporate facilities

Stage of the neoplasm: A classification of malignancies (cancers) according to the anatomic extent of the tumor, such as primary neoplasm, regional lymph nodes, and metastases; staging is important in determining the patient's treatment and prognosis

Stages of grief: Kubler-Ross's five-stage model describing how people progress through loss to acceptance in response to death; may be applied to similar changes employees experience in response to organizational transition

Stakeholder: An individual within the company who has an interest in, or is affected by, the results of a project

Standard: A scientifically based statement of expected behavior against which structures, processes, and outcomes can be measured; something established by authority, custom, or general consent as a model or example, or something set up and established by authority as a rule for the measure of quantity, weight, extent, value, or quality; according to HIPAA privacy provisions, a rule, condition, or requirement

Standard deviation: A measure of variability that describes the deviation from the mean of a frequency distribution in the original units of measurement; the square root of the variance

Standard of care: An established set of clinical decisions and actions taken by clinicians and other representatives of healthcare organizations in accordance with state and federal laws, regulations, and guidelines; codes of ethics published by professional associations or societies; regulations for accreditation published by accreditation agencies; usual and common practice of equivalent clinicians or organizations in a geographical regions

Standard of law: Established by professional associations, a statute or regulation, or a common practice, what an individual is expected to do or not do in a given situation unless determined otherwise by a court

Standards development organization (SDO): A private or government agency involved in the development of healthcare informatics standards at a national or international level

Standards for Privacy of Individually Identifiable Health Information (privacy rule): Standards promulgated and issued by the Department of Health and Human Services to become effective in April 2003 that refer to specific entities to which hospitals or healthcare providers will have the ability to disclose confidential health information

Star schema: A visual method of expressing a multidimensional data structure in a relational database

State Children's Health Insurance Program (SCHIP): The children's healthcare program implemented as part of the Balanced Budget Act of 1997; sometimes referred to as the Children's Health Insurance Program, or CHIP

State workers' compensation insurance funds: Funds that provide a stable source of insurance coverage for work-related illnesses and injuries and serve to protect employers from underwriting uncertainties by making it possible to have continuing availability of workers' compensation coverage

Statement: A list of unpaid invoices; sometimes a cumulative list of all transactions between purchaser and vendor during a specific time period

Statement of cash flow: A statement that details the reasons why cash amounts changed from one balance sheet period to another; also called a statement of changes in financial position

Statement of changes in financial position: *See* Statement of cash flow

Statement of fund balance: *See* Statement of stockholder's equity

Statement of retained earnings: A statement that expresses the change in retained earnings from the beginning of the balance sheet period to the end

Statement of stockholder's equity: A statement that details the reasons for changes in each stockholder's equity accounts; also called a statement of fund balance

Statements of work: *See* Project charters

Statistical process control chart: A type of run chart that includes both upper and lower control limits and indicates whether a process is stable or unstable

Statute: A law enacted by a legislative body of a unit of government (for example, the U.S. Congress, state legislatures, and city councils)

Statutory law: Written law established by federal and state legislatures; also called legislative law

Step-down allocation: A budgeting concept in which overhead costs are distributed once, beginning with the area that provides the least amount of non-revenue-producing services

Storyboard: A type of poster that includes both text and graphics to describe and illustrate the activities of a performance improvement project

Storytelling: A group process technique in which group members create stories describing the plausible future state of the business environment

Straight numeric filing system: A health record filing system in which health records are arranged in ascending numerical order

Strategic communications: Programs created to advance specific organizational goals such as promoting a new center or service, establishing a new program, or positioning the organization as a center of excellence in a specific discipline such as cardiology or oncology

Strategic decision making: Decision making that is usually limited to individuals such as boards of directors, chief executive officers, and top-level executives who make decisions about the healthcare organization's strategic direction

Strategic goals: Long-term objectives set by an organization to improve its operations

Strategic information systems (IS) planning: A process for setting information system priorities within an organization; the process of identifying and prioritizing information system (IS) needs based on the organization's strategic goals with the intent of ensuring that all IS technology initiatives are integrated and aligned with the organization's overall strategic plan

Strategic issue: A question, topic, opportunity, or concern that is addressed through strategic management

Strategic management: The art and science of formulating, implementing, and evaluating cross-functional decisions that enable an organization to achieve its objectives

Strategic plan: A broad organizationwide plan by which the facility accomplishes its strategic goals

Strategic planning: A disciplined effort to produce fundamental decisions that shape and guide what an organization is and does, and why

Strategy: A course of action designed to produce a desired (business) outcome

Stratified random sampling: The process of selecting the same percentages of subjects for a study sample as they exist in the subgroups (strata) of the population

Streaming video: *See* Motion video

Structure: A term from Donabedian's model of quality assessment that assesses an organization's ability to provide services in terms of both the physical building and equipment and the people providing the healthcare services

Structure and content standards: Common data elements and definitions of the data elements to be included in an electronic patient record

Structure indicator: A measurement that permits the assessment of an organization's capability to provide high-quality services

Structured analysis: A pattern identification analysis performed for a specific task

Structured data: Binary, computer-readable data

Structured decision: A decision made by following a formula or a step-by-step process

Structured interview: An interview format that uses a set of standardized questions that are asked of all applicants

Structured query language (SQL): A fourth-generation computer language used to create and manipulate relational databases; includes both DDL and DML components

Structured question: A type of question that limits possible responses; also called closed-ended question

Subacute care: Step-down care provided after a patient is released from an acute care hospital; includes nursing homes and other facilities that provide medical care but not surgical or emergency care

Subpoena duces tecum: A written document that directs individuals or organizations to furnish relevant documents and records

Subprojects: Smaller components of a larger project

Successor: A task in a dependency relationship between two tasks that is dependent on the predecessor task

Supercomputer: The largest, fastest, and most expensive type of computer that exists today

Supervised learning: Any learning technique that has as its purpose to classify or predict attributes of objects or individuals

Supervisory managers: Managers who oversee small (two- to ten-person) functional workgroups or teams and often perform hands-on functions in addition to supervisory functions

Supplemental medical insurance (SMI) (Medicare Part B): A voluntary medical insurance program that helps pay for physicians' services, medical services, and supplies not covered by the Medicare Part A

Supreme Court: The highest court in the U.S. legal system; hears cases from the U.S. Courts of Appeals and from the highest state courts when federal statutes, treaties, or the U.S. Constitution is involved

Survey: A method of self-report research in which the individuals themselves are the source of the data

Survey feedback: An organizational development technique in which data on practices and attitudes are gathered and participants interpret them in order to plan change

Synchronous: Occurring at the same time

Synergy: The interaction of parts to produce a greater outcome than would be obtained by the parts acting separately

Syntax: A term that refers to comparable structure or format of data, usually as they are being transmitted from one system to another

System: A set of related and highly interdependent components that are operating for a particular purpose

System catalog: An integrated data dictionary, which is a component of a database management system, that generally contains information on data tables and relationships in addition to data definitions

System design: The second phase of the systems development life cycle

System implementation: The third phase of the systems development life cycle

System maintenance and evaluation: The final phase of the systems development life cycle

System planning and analysis: The first phase of the systems development life cycle

Systematic sampling: The process of selecting a sample of subjects for a study by drawing every *n*th unit on a list

Systemized Nomenclature of Human and Veterinary Medicine (SNOMED): A comprehensive medical nomenclature designed to support the computer storage and automatic encoding of medical text

Systematized Nomenclature of Medicine Reference Terminology (SNOMED RT): Concept-based terminology consisting of more than 110,000 concepts with linkages to more than 180,000 terms with unique computer-readable codes

Systems analysis and design: A performance improvement methodology that can be applied to any type of system

Systems analyst: An individual who investigates, analyzes, designs, develops, installs, evaluates, and maintains an organization's healthcare information systems; is typically involved in all aspects of the systems development life cycle; serves as a liaison among end users and programmers, database administrators, and other technical personnel

Systems development life cycle (SDLC): A model used to represent the ongoing process of developing (or purchasing) information systems

Systems testing: Testing performed by an independent organization to identify problems in information systems

Systems theory: An approach to understanding organizations based on the organization and interconnections of their parts

Systems thinking: An objective way of looking at work-related ideas and processes with the goal of allowing people to uncover ineffective patterns of behavior and thinking and then to find ways to make lasting improvements

Table: A set of data arranged in rows and columns

Tacit knowledge: The actions, experiences, ideals, values, and emotions of an individual that tend to be highly personal and difficult to communicate (for example, corporate culture, organizational politics, and professional experience)

Tactic: A method for accomplishing an end

Tactical decision making: Decision making that usually affects departments or business units; includes short- and medium-range plans, schedules, and budgets; may also affect policies and procedures

Tactical plan: A strategic plan at the level of divisions and departments

Target population: A large group of individuals who are the focus of a study

Task: The step to be performed in order to complete a project or part of a project

Task analysis: A procedure for determining the specific duties and skills required of a job

Task structure: Leadership orientation toward goals, production, and procedures

Tax Equity and Fiscal Responsibility Act of 1982 (TEFRA): The federal legislation that modified Medicare's retrospective reimbursement system for inpatient hospital stays by requiring implementation of diagnosis-related groups and the acute care prospective payment system

Taxonomy: Principles of a classification system, such as data classification

Team building: The process of organizing and acquainting a team, and building skills for dealing with later team processes

Technical component (TC): The portion of radiological and other procedures that is facility based or nonphysician based; for example, radiology films, equipment, overhead, endoscopic suites, and so on

Technical skills: One of the three managerial skill categories; related to knowledge of the technical aspects of the business

Technology management: The planning and implementation of technological resources as needed to effectively and efficiently carry out the mission of the organization

Technology push model: The view of information technology as being able to push organizations into new business areas

Telecommunications: Voice and data communications

Telecommuting: A work arrangement in which at least a portion of an employee's work hours are spent outside the office, usually in his or her home, and the work is transmitted back to the employer by electronic means; often used by coding and transcription personnel

Telestaffing: *See* Telecommuting

Temporary Assistance for Needy Families (TANF): A federal program that provides states with grants to be spent on time-limited cash assistance for low-income families; generally limits a family's lifetime cash welfare benefits to a maximum of five years and permits states to impose other requirements

Temporary budget variance: The difference between a budgeted amount and the actual amount of a line item that is expected to reverse itself in a subsequent period; timing difference between the budget and the actual event

Temporary privileges: Privileges granted for a limited time period to a licensed, independent practitioner on the basis of recommendations made by the appropriate clinical department or the president of the medical staff

Ten-step monitoring and evaluation process: The systematic and ongoing collection, organization, and evaluation of data related to indicator development promoted by the Joint Commission on Accreditation of Healthcare Organizations (JCAHO) in the mid-1980s

Terminal-digit filing system: A health record filing system in which the last digit or group of last digits is used, followed by the middle and last groups of numbers

Terminology: A set of terms representing the system of concepts of a particular subject field

Terminology standard: A terminology adopted by the appropriate standard setting organizations for use in healthcare

Test statistics: A set of statistical techniques that examines the psychometric properties of measurement instruments

Text mining: The process of extracting and then quantifying and filtering free-text data

Text processing: The process of converting narrative text into structured data for computer processing

Theory: A systematic organization of knowledge that predicts or explains behavior or events

Theory X and Y: McGregor's management theory describing pessimistic and optimistic assumptions about people and their work potential

Third-party payer: An insurance company (for example, BC/BS) or healthcare program (for example, Medicare) that reimburses healthcare providers and/or patients for the delivery of medical services

Three-dimensional imaging: Construction of pictures generated from computer data in three dimensions

360-degree evaluation: A method of performance evaluation in which the supervisors, peers, and other staff who interact with the employee contribute information

Time and motion studies: Studies in which complex tasks are broken down into their component motions to determine inefficiencies and to develop improvements

Time ladder: A form used by employees to document the time spent on various tasks

Time period: Financial data that represent a specific time period

Toll bypass: Circumvention of the public telephone toll system to avoid the usage fees charged by public carriers

Tort: An action brought when one party believes that another party caused harm through wrongful conduct and seeks compensation for that harm

Total length of stay: The sum of the days of stay of any group of inpatients discharged during a specific period of time; also called discharge days

Total quality management (TQM): A management philosophy that includes all activities in which the needs of the customer and the organization are satisfied in the most efficient manner by using employee potentials and continuous improvement

Traditional fee-for-service (FFS) plan: A reimbursement method involving third-party payers that compensate providers after the healthcare services have been delivered; payment is based on specific services provided to subscribers

Train-the-trainer: A method of providing instruction; certain individuals are trained who then, in turn, will be responsible for training others on a task or skill

Trainee: A person who is learning a task or skill

Trainer: A person who gives instruction on a task or skill

Training: A set of activities and materials that provide the opportunity to acquire job-related skills, knowledge, and abilities

Trait approach: The belief that leaders possess a collection of traits or qualities that distinguish them from nonleaders

Transaction-processing system: A computer-based information system that keeps track of an organization's business transactions; inputs include transaction data such as admissions, discharges, and transfers in a hospital; outputs include census reports and bills

Transaction standards: *See* transmission standards

Transactional leadership: The leadership of a individual (manager) who strives to maintain high levels of efficiency in an organization by balancing task and social orientation

Transcription: The process of deciphering and typing medical dictation

Transformational leadership: The leadership of a visionary who strives to change an organization

Transmission standards: Standards that support the uniform format and sequence of data during transmission from one healthcare entity to another; also referred to as communication, messaging, and transaction standards

Traumatic injury: A wound or injury included in a trauma registry

Treatment: Manipulation, intervention, or therapy; a broad term used by researchers to generically mean some act, such as a physical conditioning program, a computer training program, a particular laboratory medium, or the timing of prophylactic medications

TRICARE: A federal healthcare program that provides coverage for the dependents of armed forces personnel and for retirees receiving care outside military treatment facilities; the federal government pays a percentage of the cost; formerly known as Civilian Health and Medical Program of the Uniformed Services (CHAMPUS)

TRICARE Extra: A cost-effective preferred provider network TRICARE option; costs for healthcare are lower than for the standard TRICARE program because a physician or medical specialist is selected from a network of civilian healthcare professionals who participate in TRICARE Extra

TRICARE Prime: A TRICARE program that provides the most comprehensive healthcare benefits at the lowest cost of the three TRICARE options; military treatment facilities serve as the principal source of healthcare, and a primary care manager is assigned to each enrollee

TRICARE Prime Remote: A program that provides active-duty service members in the United States with a specialized version of TRICARE Prime while they are assigned to duty stations in areas not served by the traditional military healthcare system

TRICARE Senior Prime: A managed care demonstration TRICARE program designed to better serve the medical needs of military retirees, dependents, and survivors who are sixty-five years old and over

Trier of fact: The judge or jury hearing a civil or criminal case

Trigger: A documented response that alerts a skilled nursing facility resident assessment instrument assessor to the fact that further research is needed to clarify an assessment

Trim point: The length of stay threshold used in determining day outliers

Turnkey system: A healthcare information system sold by various vendors to meet specific computing needs during the 1970s

Two-tailed hypothesis: A type of alternative hypothesis in which the researcher makes no prediction about the direction of the results

Type I error: A type of error in which the researcher erroneously rejects the null hypothesis when it is true

Type II error: A type of error in which the researcher erroneously fails to reject the null hypothesis when it is false

Unfavorable variance: The negative difference between the budgeted amount and the actual amount of a line item, where actual revenue is less than budget or actual expenses exceed budget

Unfreezing: Lewin's first stage of the change process in which people are presented with disconcerting information to motivate them to change

Unified Medical Language System (UMLS): A program initiated by the National Library of Medicine to build an intelligent, automated system that can understand biomedical concepts, words, and expressions and their interrelationships

Unified modeling language (UML): A common data-modeling notation used in conjunction with object-oriented database design

Uniform Ambulatory Care Data Set (UACDS): A data set developed by the National Committee on Vital and Health Statistics consisting of a minimum set of patient/client-specific data elements to be collected in ambulatory care settings

Uniform Bill-92 (UB-92): the single, standardized billing form required by Medicare for hospital inpatients and outpatients; also used for all inpatient and outpatient billing by the major third-party payers and most hospitals

Uniform Hospital Discharge Data Set (UHDDS): A data set developed by the National Center for Health Statistics consisting of a minimum set of patient-specific data elements to be collected in hospitals

Union: A collective bargaining unit that represents groups of employees and is authorized to negotiate with employers on the employees' behalf in matters related to compensation, health and safety; also called labor organization

Unique identifier: Information that refers to one and only one individual or organization

Unique physician identification number (UPIN): A unique numerical identifier created by the Health Care Financing Administration (now called the Centers for Medicare and Medicaid Services) for use by physicians who bill for services provided to Medicare patients

Unit filing system: A health record filing system in which all inpatient and outpatient visits and procedures are arranged together under a permanent unit number

Unit numbering system: A health record identification system in which the patient receives a unique medical record number at the time of the first encounter that is used for all subsequent encounters

Unit work division: A method of work organization where each task is performed by one person at the same time that another person is doing a task, but one does not have to wait for the other

United Nations International Standards Organization (ISO): An international standards organization that coordinates all international standards development

Unity of command: A human resources principle that assumes that each employee reports to only one specific management position

Univariate: A term referring to the involvement of one variable

Universal chart order: A system in which the health record is maintained in the same format while the patient is in the facility and after discharge

Universal patient identifier: A personal identifier applied to a patient, such as a number or code, that is used permanently for many and varied purposes

Universal personal identifier: A unique numerical identifier for each citizen in the United States

Universal precautions: A set of procedures designed specifically to minimize or eliminate the spread of infectious disease agents from one individual to another during the provision of healthcare services

Unstructured analysis: A pattern identification analysis performed through a database without a specific goal of discovering interesting patterns that were not conceived previously

Unstructured data: Nonbinary, human-readable data

Unstructured decision: A decision that is made without following a prescribed method, formula, or pattern

Unstructured question: A type of question that allows free-form responses; also called open-ended question

Unsupervised learning: Any learning technique that has as its purpose to group or cluster items, objects, or individuals

Upcoding: The practice of assigning diagnostic or procedural codes that represent higher payment rates than the codes that actually reflect the services provided to patients

U.S. Public Health Service: An agency of the U.S. Department of Health and Human Services that promotes the protection and advancement of physical and mental health

Use case diagram: A systems analysis technique used to document a software project from a user's perspective

User groups: Groups made up of users of a particular computer system

Usual, customary, and reasonable (UCR) charges: Charges a health plan pays a provider for a particular service or procedure, based on what is considered reasonable for that service or procedure in a community

Utility program: A software program that supports, enhances, or expands existing programs in a computer system, such as virus checking, data recovery, backup, and data compression

Utilization management (UM): The planned, systematic review of the patients in a healthcare facility against care criteria for admission, continued stay, and discharge

Utilization management organization: An organization that reviews the appropriateness of the care setting and resources used to treat a patient

Utilization review (UR): The process of determining whether the medical care provided to a specific patient is necessary according to preestablished objective screening criteria at time frames specified in the organization's utilization management plan

Utilization Review Act: Federal legislation that requires hospitals to conduct continued-stay reviews for Medicare and Medicaid patients

V codes: A set of ICD-9-CM codes used to classify occasions when circumstances other than disease or injury are recorded as the reason for the patient's encounter with healthcare providers

Validity: A term that refers to a test's ability to accurately and consistently measure what it purports to measure

Values statement: A short description that communicates an organization's social and cultural belief system

Variability: The dispersion of a set of measures around the population mean

Variable: A factor

Variance: A measure of variability that gives the average of the squared deviations from the mean; in financial management, the difference between the budgeted amount and the actual amount of a line item

Variance analysis: An assessment of a department's financial transactions to identify differences between the budget amount and the actual amount of a line item

Vector graphic data: Digital data that have been captured as points and are connected by lines (a series of point coordinates) or areas (shapes bounded by lines); also called signal tracing data

Vendor system: A computer system developed by a commercial company not affiliated with the healthcare organization

Verification service: An outside service that provides a primary source check on information that a physician makes available on an application to the medical staff

Vertical structure: The levels and relationships among positions in an organizational hierarchy

Vertically integrated plan: *See* Integrated provider organization (IPO)

Vertically integrated system: *See* Integrated provider organization (IPO)

Videoconferencing: A communications service that allows a group of people to exchange information over a network by using a combination of video and computer technology

Virtual private network (VPN): Traditionally, a dedicated set of network resources such as leased lines that provide wide-area connectivity to a large organization

Vision: A picture of the desired future that sets a direction and rationale for change

Vision statement: A short description of an organization's ideal future state

Vital statistics: Statistics related to births, deaths, marriages, and fetal deaths

Vocabulary: A collection of words or phrases with their meanings

Vocabulary standard: A common definition for medical terms to encourage consistent descriptions of an individual's condition in the health record

Voice recognition technology: *See* Continuous speech technology

Volume logs: Forms used (sometimes in conjunction with time ladders) to obtain information about the volume of work units received and processed in a day

Web appliance: A computer designed to connect to a network; does not have secondary storage capability

Web browser–based systems: Systems and applications written in one or more Web programming languages

Web content management systems: Systems in which information placed in a Web site can be labeled and tracked so that it can be easily located, modified, and reused

Web-enabled systems: Systems and applications that are launched from a Web page but are not written in one or more Web programming languages

Webmasters: Individuals who support Web applications and the healthcare organization's intranet and Internet operations

Wide-area network (WAN): A computer network that connects devices across a large geographical area

Wireless local-area network (WLAN): A data transmission network that uses an unguided medium such as radio or microwaves

Wireless technology: Technology that uses wireless networks and wireless devices to access and transmit data in real time

Wisdom: Intelligence that gives individuals the empowerment and courage to act

Word-processing services: Companies outside the healthcare facility that specialize in the deciphering and typing of medical dictation

Work: The effort, usually described in hours, needed to complete a task

Work breakdown structure: A hierarchical structure that decomposes project activities into levels of detail

Work distribution analysis: An analysis used to determine whether a department's current work assignments and job content are appropriate

Work distribution chart: A matrix that depicts the work being done in a particular workgroup in terms of specific tasks and activities, time spent on tasks, and the employees performing the tasks

Work division: A term used to describe how tasks are handled within an organization

Work flow: Any work process that must be handled by more than one person

Work measurement: The process of studying the amount of work accomplished and how long it takes to accomplish work in order to define and monitor productivity

Work products: Documents produced during the completion of a task that may be a component of, or contribute to, a project deliverable

Work sampling: A work measurement technique using random sample measurements to characterize the performance of the whole

Worker Immaturity–Maturity: Argyris's model describing how leadership should change with an employee's maturity

Workers' compensation: Medical and income insurance coverage for certain federal employees in unusually hazardous jobs

Workgroup on Electronic Data Interchange (WEDI): A subgroup of Accreditation Standards Committee X12 that has been involved in development electronic data interchange standards for billing transactions

Working conditions: The environment in which work is performed (surroundings) and the physical dangers or risks involved in the job (hazards)

Workstation: A computer designed to accept data from multiple sources to assist in managing information for daily activities and to provide a convenient means of entering data as desired by the user

World Health Organization (WHO): The international organization responsible for publishing the *International Classification of Diseases, Ninth Revision, Clinical Modification* (ICD-9-CM)

Zero-based budgets: Types of budgets in which each budget cycle poses the opportunity to continue or discontinue services based on available resources so that every department or activity must be justified and prioritized annually to effectively allocate resources

Index

(continued on next page)

RHIA Certification:
Your First Move Up the Career Ladder

Graduating from a health information administration (HIA) program gives you an excellent foundation, but it's not enough. Employers are looking for your commitment to the field and a certain competency level. The Registered Health Information Administrator (RHIA) credential helps you stand out from the crowd of resumes.

Top Five Reasons to Earn an RHIA Credential:

- Career advancement
- Proof of your HIA knowledge
- Demonstration of your dedication to quality healthcare
- Evidence of your ability to uphold industry standards and regulations
- Sets you apart from uncredentialed candidates

In recent AHIMA-sponsored research groups, healthcare executives and recruiters cited three reasons for preferring credentialed personnel:
1. Assurance of current knowledge through continued education
2. Possession of field-tested experience
3. Verification of base level competency

AHIMA is the premier organization for health information management professionals, with more than 45,000 members nationwide. Certification from AHIMA carries a strong reputation for quality—the requirements for RHIA certification are rigorous.

The RHIA exam is computer-based and available throughout the year. But most professionals who earned their RHIA certification agree: the sooner you take the exam after graduating, the better.

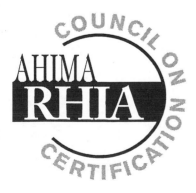

Make the right move…pair your degree with AHIMA certification and maximize your career possibilities.

For more information on the RHIA credential and how to sit for the exam, you can either visit our Web site at **www.ahima.org/certification**, send an e-mail to **certdept@ahima.org**, or call **(800) 335-5535**.

Kick Your Future into High Gear Today by Joining AHIMA!

"Becoming a member of AHIMA is an incredible deal. AHIMA has made an excellent decision to offer this membership at such an affordable cost, because it gives students an opportunity to explore AHIMA services and resources. I know I will remain a member after graduation," says Diana Spaulding of Indian River Community College in Ft. Pierce, FL.

The American Health Information Management Association (AHIMA), the name you can trust for quality healthcare education, has represented the interests of HIM professionals since 1928.

Membership Is Only $20* per Year...and It Pays for Itself!

Here are just two ways:

1. Your subscription to the *Journal of AHIMA* (worth $99), the industry's award-winning source for best practices, workplace solutions, career strategies, and more

2. A $50 savings off certification exam fees

Other benefits too good to put a price on include:

- *The Internet.* Membership provides study help, career planning, networking, and more. With Communities of Practice (CoP), AHIMA's networking tool, you can become a member of as many different professional communities as you want, or create your own.

- *Your career.* What better way to search for that perfect job than through AHIMA's network of more than 45,000 members? Use the CoP to make contacts. Put AHIMA's members-only "Job Bank" to work. Establish contacts with state and local associations.

- *Your studies.* AHIMA's searchable, members-only online library provides access to an infinite variety of HIM topics (such as legislation, reimbursement, and compliance) with professional tools, practice briefs, *Journal* articles, books, case studies, presentation materials, and more. And AHIMA's library never closes!

- *More discounts.* Savings on books and gatherings are one more way membership pays for itself.

There is no better time to join than today. Fill out an online application at **www.ahima.org/membership**, or call **(800) 335-5535** for more information.

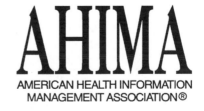

AMERICAN HEALTH INFORMATION
MANAGEMENT ASSOCIATION®

Reflects student member dues through 2003. Subject to change.

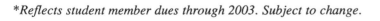

Look for These Quality AHIMA Publications at Bookstores, Libraries, and Online

Need to Know More?

Textbook details and easy ordering are available online on the AHIMA Web site at **www.ahima.org.** Click on "Professional Development." In addition to textbooks, AHIMA offers other educational products such as online training programs and audio seminars. For textbook content questions, contact **publications@ahima.org,** and for sales information contact **info@ahima.org.**

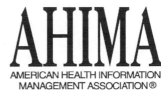

AMERICAN HEALTH INFORMATION MANAGEMENT ASSOCIATION®

Communities of Practice
What New Connections Have You Made?

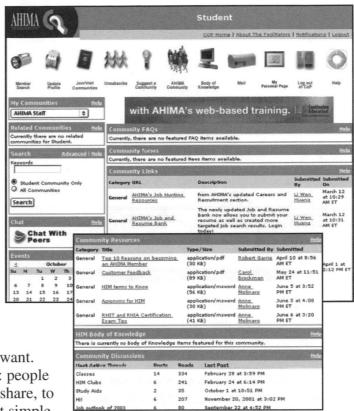

AHIMA's Communities of Practice is a vital member benefit for students. With more than 100 communities formed—focusing on everything from facilities to hot topics to job functions, including a community devoted only to students—there's a wealth of information about the health information management profession and industry.

You can join as many communities as you want. That's the whole idea behind a community: people with common interests coming together to share, to support, and to help each other out. It's that simple.

What will you find there? Each community features FAQs, News, Links, Resources, Calendar of Events, Real-Time Chats, and Discussions. The Student Community features valuable discussions on salaries and classes, and resources on sitting for certification and HIM terms to know. You can search for AHIMA members who are already in the job areas you're interested in and begin networking.

Joining a community can help you be more successful in class, read best practices, strategically plan for your future, and do fast and simple research that makes you more knowledgeable. In fact, the FORE Body of Knowledge—a great resource for class projects—provides access to:

*   All *Journal of AHIMA* articles published since January 2001
*   Most *AHIMA Advantage* articles published since January 2002
*   AHIMA practice briefs, position statements, job descriptions, and other Association information
*   Government publications such as parts of the *Federal Register* and DHHS documents
*   Links to other useful HIM documents

Communities of Practice is only open to members, so consider becoming a student member of AHIMA for only $20* a year.

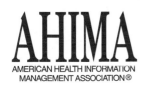

AMERICAN HEALTH INFORMATION
MANAGEMENT ASSOCIATION®

For more information about Communities of Practice, please visit **www.ahima.org** and click on "Communities of Practice."
To learn more about membership, please visit, **www.ahima.org** and click on "Membership." For technical assistance, please contact **cophelp@ahima.org.**

*Reflects student member dues through 2003. Subject to change.

AHIMA's Job Bank:
Build the career you've always dreamed of!

Members of AHIMA have a distinct advantage in the marketplace as they climb up the HIM career ladder: the AIIIMA Job Bank. The Job Bank is a Web site brimming with available positions in the HIM field. It's an exclusive way to make your talents and capabilities known to potential employers and to allow you to search for that perfect position. Very simply, the Job Bank is an exclusive arena where serious professionals can meet other serious professionals.

After logging into the Job Bank, you'll be able to:

- Post a resume, which is searchable by other AHIMA members and registered companies. Making yourself visible in this way puts you in front of hundreds of potential employers…who just might have the ability to start you up the career ladder.

- Search jobs by state, country, keyword, and job category, allowing you to customize your job search by geographical location, function, or any other parameter you want to create.

And remember: unlike other online job search engines, the AHIMA Job Bank is a TARGETED search tool, where you can customize your parameters to find exactly what you're seeking. You can search for your ideal position under more than 35 categories, including Admitting Patient Intake, Corporate Compliance, Database Management, Information Security, Patient Advocacy, Risk Management, Sales/Selling, and more!

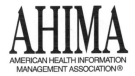

If you haven't been using the Job Bank, there's no better time than the present to check out how you can make it work for you. Simply go to **www.ahimanet.org/JobBank/Login.cfm.** For any assistance needed, please contact **info@ahima.org**

Becoming a New Voice in HIM

by Jessica Squazzo, assistant editor

Not too many recent college graduates land a position as director of quality management at a long-term care facility. Then again, not too many recent graduates are like Erin Blume, RHIA. Even before starting her position as director of quality management at the Ambassador Health System in Omaha, NE, Blume was entering the health information management (HIM) field with leaps and bounds.

A Perfect Fit

Blume, who won the 2001 Triumph Awards New Frontier Award, began her HIM career when she decided she wanted to work in healthcare but didn't want to be a healthcare provider. She earned a scholarship to the College of Saint Mary in Omaha, NE, and decided to begin the four-year accredited HIM degree program there after a family member suggested the field might suit her. Shortly after Blume began her studies, she found out that HIM was in fact a good fit. "It wasn't until I started my solid HIM classes that I knew this is what I wanted to do," she says.

Extracurricular activities also got Blume more involved with HIM and gave her a first chance at becoming an advocate for the profession. One of these activities was founding the college's HIM club, Sigma Rho Lambda. Among other club activities, Blume and other club members helped plan an annual Health Information Week, a weeklong campaign to raise awareness about the profession on campus.

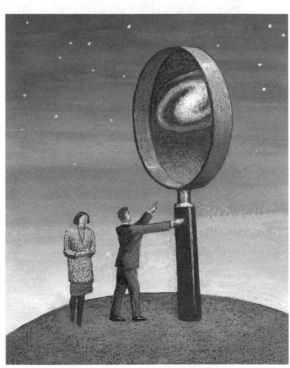

"I became a strong advocate for HIM when I was a junior [in college]," she says. "I really wanted to give HIM a voice and create awareness for it."

—Erin Blume, RHIA,
director of quality management
at The Ambassador Health System

Lifelong Learning

Besides educating others about the field, Blume is dedicated to continually educating herself, something she hasn't stopped doing since graduation. "When you're out of school, you still have to be a student," she says. One of these platforms for education is her job, where she is constantly challenged by having to learn new aspects of a changing field.

As director of quality management at the Ambassador, a three-facility system that focuses on subacute and rehabilitative care, Blume oversees three HIM departments, the corporate compliance program, and the corporate performance improvement program. Included in these responsibilities are conducting fraud and abuse investigations and implementing HIPAA.

She has been working at the Ambassador Health System since 1998, where she started as a health information associate, became a health information and improvement coordinator in 2000 (both while still a full-time student), and then came into her current role in May 2001. Blume credits her varied work experience with her understanding of HIM as a whole. "It's really liberating to work with people who see the big picture—we all affect each other," she says.

An Advocate for HIM

Being an advocate for HIM is part of Blume's current job at the Ambassador. "I use my position as a forum to demonstrate what HIM professionals do," she says. She hopes to demonstrate this to young people who are considering entering the field, a group of people she feels are sometimes neglected when it comes to spreading the word about HIM.

Blume says that if students were made more aware of the abundant opportunities available in the field, they would surely be interested. "If they knew how many different directions they could go in they would jump right in," she says. Stronger public relations campaigns to colleges and high schools and making school career counselors more aware of the field could help pique the interest of more future HIM professionals, according to Blume.

As for Blume's personal future goals, she plans on going back to school for further education ("sooner than later," she says), and hopes to eventually become more involved in education and public speaking.

A word of advice to students considering the field: be willing to work hard. As a potential future leader of HIM, Blume may be a hard act to follow.

Reprinted from an article by Jessica Squazzo, *Journal of AHIMA*, no. 4 (2002): 92.

MEDLINE Medical Literature, Analysis, and Retrieval System Online

MEI Medicare Economic Index

MFS Medicare fee schedule

MGMA Medical Group Management Association

MIS management information system

MOLAP multidimensional online analytical processing

MPI master population/patient index

MSA medical savings account plans

MSO management service organization

NAQH National Association of Healthcare Quality

NB newborn

NCHS National Center for Health Statistics

NCPDP National Council on Prescription Drug Programs

NCQA National Committee for Quality Assurance

NCVHS National Committee on Vital and Health Statistics

NII-HIN National Information Infrastructure—Health Information Network Program

NPBD National Practitioner Data Bank

NPF national provider file

NPI national provider identifier

NUBC National Uniform Billing Committee

NUCC National Uniform Claim Committee

NVAC National Vaccine Advisory Committee

NVSS National Vital Statistics System

OASIS Outcome and Assessment Information Set

OBRA Omnibus Budget Reconciliation Act

OCE outpatient code editor

OCR optical character recognition technology

OD organizational development

OER outcomes and effectiveness research

OLAP online/real-time analytical processing

OLTP online/real-time transaction processing

OODB object-oriented database

OODBMS object-oriented database management system

OPPS outpatient prospective payment system

OR operations research

OSHA Occupational Safety and Health Act of 1970

OSS operations support systems

PACE Programs of All-Inclusive Care for the Elderly

PC professional component

PCE potentially compensable events

PCM primary care manager

PCP primary care physician

PDA personal digital assistant

PERT program evaluation and review technique

PHO physician–hospital organization

PHR personal health record

PI performance improvement

PIPs periodic interim payments

PKI public key infrastructure

PMPM per member per month

PMR proportionate mortality ratio

POMR problem-oriented health record

POS point-of-service plan

PPO preferred provider organization

PPPM per patient per month

PPS prospective payment system

PRO peer review organization

PSI payment status indicator

QA quality assurance

QDWIs qualified disabled and working individuals

QI quality improvement

QIO quality improvement organization

QIs qualifying individuals

QMBs qualified Medicare beneficiaries

QRO quality review organization

RA remittance advice

RAI Resident Assessment Instrument

RAP Resident Assessment Protocol

RAVEN Resident Assessment Validation and Entry

RBRVS resource-based relative value scale

RCT randomized clinical trial

RDMS relational database management system

RFI request for information

RFP request for proposal